MEDICAL BIOCHEMISTRY

MEDICAL BIOCHEMISTRY

(For Medical, Dental, Nursing, Physiotherapy, Pharmacy, Food Science, Nutrition, and Science Students)

REVISED SECOND EDITION

N. Mallikarjuna Rao
Ph.D.
Professor and Head
Dept. of Biochemistry
Narayana Medical College
Nellore

PUBLISHING FOR ONE WORLD

NEW AGE INTERNATIONAL (P) LIMITED, PUBLISHERS
New Delhi • Bangalore • Chennai • Cochin • Guwahati • Hyderabad
Jalandhar • Kolkata • Lucknow • Mumbai • Ranchi
Visit us at **www.newagepublishers.com**

Published by New Age International (P) Ltd., Publishers
First Edition: 2000 2
Second Edition: 2006
Reprint: 2008

Branches:

- 36, Malikarjuna Temple Street, Opp. ICWA, Basavanagudi, **Bangalore**. ✆ (080) 26677815
- 26, Damodaran Street, T. Nagar, **Chennai**. ✆ (044) 24353401
- Hemsen Complex, Mohd. Shah Road, Paltan Bazar, Near Starline Hotel, **Guwahati**. ✆ (0361) 2543669
- No. 105, 1st Floor, Madhiray Kaveri Tower, 3-2-19, Azam Jahi Road, Nimboliadda, **Hyderabad**. ✆ (040) 24652456
- RDB Chambers (Formerly Lotus Cinema) 106A, Ist Floor, S.N. Banerjee Road, **Kolkata**. ✆ (033) 22275247
- 18, Madan Mohan Malviya Marg, **Lucknow**. ✆ (0522) 2209578
- 142C, Victor House, Ground Floor, N.M. Joshi Marg, Lower Parel, **Mumbai**. ✆ (022) 24927869
- 22, Golden House, Daryaganj, **New Delhi**. ✆ (011) 23262370, 23262368

ISBN (10): 81-224-1823-6

ISBN (13): 978-81-224-1823-1

Rs. 345.00

C-08-09-3104

Printed in India at Ajit Printers, Delhi.
Typeset at Monu Printers, Delhi.

PUBLISHING FOR ONE WORLD
NEW AGE INTERNATIONAL (P) LIMITED, PUBLISHERS
4835/24, Ansari Road, Daryaganj, New Delhi-110002
Visit us at **www.newagepublishers.com**

To my

Elder daughter

Late Nalluri Kiranmayi Chowdary

PREFACE TO SECOND EDITION

I attempted to provide essential information on molecular basis of health and disease that is mainly related to life of surviving cell(s) in the first edition of the book. However life cycle of cell(s) include cell(s) birth and cell(s) death apart from survival. For the last couple of years these frontier areas are advancing rapidly which is viewed by many as good sign for development of :

(*a*) new therapy or therapeutics for cancer

(*b*) immortalized cells.

The latter fuels growth of biotechnology and pharmaceutical industries also. Hence, in the second edition two chapters-1. Biochemistry of cell cycle (cell birth) 2. Biochemistry of apoptosis (cell death) are added.

As living organisms evolved from simple unicellular to highly complex multicellular mammals, several new systems and organs were developed. For example, blood which acts as vehicle or communication between various locations of body, immune system which protects body from intruders or foreign organisms.

Parkinsonism, psychosis, depression, Schizophrenia, loss of taste and olfaction are due to disturbances in nervous, taste and olfactory systems. Various organs present in body perform several organ specific functions which are essential for life. If functions of these organs are disturbed, diseases occur which may culminate in death. So, in this edition biochemistry of blood including immune response in **Chapter-32**; molecular and cellular mechanism of learning, memory, behaviour, taste and olfactory in biochemical communications in chapter tests, procedures that are done in hospital biochemistry laboratory to assess functions of liver, kidney in **Chapter-33** and thyroid in **Chapter-29** are detailed.

Depending on disease a particular constituent of blood is either elevated or lowered. Diagnosis and prognosis of disease usually involves detection and measurement of various blood constituents in hospital biochemistry laboratory. Therefore advanced techniques like high performance liquid chromatography (HPLC), affinity chromatography, and general techniques like centrifugation and dialysis, instruments from spectrophotometer to auto analyzer and methods used for detection and quantitation of blood constituents like carbohydrates, proteins, lipids, nucleic acids, enzymes, electrolytes etc., in health and disease are detailed in **Chapter-34.**

Humans and other mammals are able to remove waste products, toxins, foreign compounds from blood and organs in the form of urine. In disease, composition of urine varies from that of healthy state. So, detection, quantitation of various constituents of urine is carried out in hospital biochemistry laboratory to confirm diagnosis of diseases.

In **Chapter-34**, methods for detection and estimation of urine constituents under normal and diseases conditions are also detailed.

Most striking feature in this edition of the book is inclusion of biochemical aspects of diseases or disease causing organisms common to tropical countries like malaria, tuberculosis, peptic ulcer or gastritis, pneumonia, leishmaniasis, giardiasis, trypanosomiasis etc. Since most of the organisms are developing resistance to the existing drugs, there is need for development of new drugs which requires thorough biochemical knowledge of these diseases as well as disease causing organisms. Apart from adding new chapters, all existing chapters have been updated by adding new subject matter. References of each chapter have been updated by including reviews, books, research articles etc. Further, number of unsolved problems have been increased in most of the chapters.

I hope this edition will be well received by teachers and students of various medical, dental, pharmacy, biotechnology, physiotherapy, medical laboratory technology, biomedical engineering, life sciences under graduate and post graduate courses, Suggestions or comments from teachers and students are welcome. I am grateful to Sri R.K. Gupta, Chairman; Sri Saumya Gupta, Managing Director of New Age International, New Delhi, for publishing second edition.

N. MALLIKARJUNA RAO

PREFACE TO THE FIRST EDITION

This book explains the fundamentals of biochemical (molecular) bases of health and disease. Hence it meets medical and allied health sciences student's needs. As a teacher of medical, dental, pharmacy, biomedical engineering and science students for the last two decades, I know the problems faced by students in mastering (conceptualizing) the subject within a limited time. Most of these students need a book for their routine day-to-day study which contains only the necessary information in a simple and concise way. Therefore, this book is written in simple language in such a way that a student with very little chemistry or biology background can easily follow the various aspects of biochemistry that are presented.

This book is also useful for those who are specializing in biochemistry (M.Sc. or M.D.) because advances in frontier areas of biochemistry are presented in a systemic way. Of course advances in other areas that are relevant to medical students are also included to a limited extent. An interesting feature of this book is that the medical and biological importance of each chapter is highlighted in simple numbered statements. Further, in some chapters, diseases, drugs (treatments) or toxins of particular subject matter are described under medical importance heads. Further, each chapter's text is designed to facilitate easy flow of information in an interesting, thought provoking and logical manner. Exercises (cases) given at the end of each chapter help in mastering of the subject by student and utilization of biochemical principles by the student in solving health problems. To enthusiastic students, references given at the end of each chapter provide additional information.

There are 29 chapters in the book. First six chapters deal with the composition, structure, function and life cycle of cells and the goal of biochemistry; occurrence, chemistry, structure and functions of biomolecules like amino acids, peptides, proteins, enzymes, carbohydrates and lipids. This is then followed by chapters 7 and 8 that deal with membrane structure, various transporters that move biomolecules across membrane and disintegration of complex molecules of food and absorption of resulting products, respectively.

Chapters 9-12 deal with the production and utilization of energy in various pathways of carbohydrate, lipid and aminoacid metabolisms. Regulatory mechanisms of some of the important pathways are also outlined. Further synthesis of biologically (medically) important compounds including non-essential amino acids is detailed. In chapter 11 the ultimate way of producing energy from all energy yielding compounds in the respiratory chain is described. Changes in the flow of metabolites into various pathways of carbohydrate, lipid and protein metabolism that occur among tissues in well fed state, diabetes and starvation are described in chapter 13.

Fundamentals of molecular biology i.e., occurrence, chemistry, structure, functions, metabolism of nucleotides, nucleic acids and control of gene expression as well as applied molecular biology i.e., recombinant DNA technology are detailed in chapters 14-20. Biomedical (chemical) aspects of two major health problems of the 20th century—cancer and AIDS are briefed in chapter 21. In chapter 22 occurrence, chemistry, structure, functions and metabolism of porphyrins and hemoglobin are described.

Clinically related topics like vitamins, minerals, macro nutrients, energy, nutraceuticals of food, electrolytes, acid-base balance and detoxification are described in chapters 23-27. Chemistry, production, detection and uses of isotopes in biochemistry and medicine are detailed in chapter 28. Chapter 29 deals with mechanisms of communication between cells.

I hope both teachers and students of Biochemistry at undergraduate and postgraduate levels use this book extensively and their suggestions to improve the book further are most welcome. I express my sincere thanks to New Age International, Publishers for publishing the book.

N. MALLIKARJUNA RAO

CONTENTS

1
CHAPTER

CELL

Cell is the universal functional unit of all forms of life. On the basis of differences in cell structure, all life forms are divided into two major classes. They are prokaryotes and eukaryotes. *Prokaryotes* are simple cells and in most cases, individual cell itself is the organism. They contain cell wall and cytosol is not divided into compartments. Examples for prokaryotes are bacteria, primitive green algae and archae bacteria. All other organisms are called *eukaryotes*. They are multicellular organisms. They are plants, animals, fungi, protozoa, uni-cellular yeast and true algae.

MEDICAL AND BIOLOGICAL IMPORTANCE

1. All higher living organisms including humans are made up of cells.
2. Human body contains wide variety of cells that differ in structure and function.
3. Human cell contains subcellular structures like nucleus, mitochondria, lysosomes and peroxisomes etc.
4. Each subcellular structure the has unique shape and function.
5. Some diseases are due to a lack of subcellular structures.
6. Zellwegers syndrome is due to lack of peroxisomes.
7. Lysosomal enzymes are involved in spreading of cancer.
8. Lack of lysosomes or its enzymes results in lysosomal diseases.
9. Growth of cells requires cell divisions. Cell cycle encompasses all the events of cell division.
10. Cells are not immortal. They have finite life span. Because of this humans are not immortal.
11. Cell death is crucial for shaping of organs during development and for recovery from injuries.
12. Biochemistry explores molecular mechanisms of normal cellular processes as well as diseases.
13. Mitochondria is involved in apoptosis.

14. Endoplasic reticulum, lysosomes and golgi complex are involved in the integration of pro-apoptic signals.

MOLECULAR COMPOSITION OF CELL

Water

Water accounts for about 70-75% of the weight of the cell. Other cellular constituents are either dissolved or suspended in water.

Organic Compounds

1. Organic compounds accounts for 25-30% of the cell weight.
2. They are nucleic acids, proteins, polysaccharides (carbohydrates) and lipids. Proteins accounts 10-20% of the weight of the cell. Nucleic acids account 7-10% of the cell weight. Polysaccharides usually account for 2-5% of the cell weight. About 3% of cell weight is due to lipids. Lipids content may be higher in adipocytes or fat cells. Proteins may account more of cell weight in cells like erythrocytes.
3. Other low molecular weight organic compounds may account for 4% of cell weight. They are monosaccharides, aminoacids, fatty acids, purine and pyrimidine nucleotides, peptides, hormones, vitamins and coenzymes.

Inorganic Compounds

1. Inorganic compounds account for the rest of the cell weight.
2. They are cations like sodium, potassium, calcium, magnesium, copper, iron and anions like chloride, phosphate, bicarbonate, sulfate, iodide and fluoride.

EUKARYOTIC CELL STRUCTURE AND FUNCTION

In eukaryotes, cells aggregate to form tissues or organs and these are further organized to form whole organism. In humans, eukaryotic cells exist in large number of sizes and shapes to perform varieties of functions. For example, nerve cells differ from liver cell which differ from muscle cell and they differ in function also. Though the eukaryotic cells differ in sizes and shapes they have certain common structural features. Further, eukaryotes contain subcellular structures and well defined nucleus. Cells are surrounded by membranes. It separates the cells from surrounding and it is called as *plasma* or *cell membrane*. The other subcellular organelles are also composed in parts by membranes.

A typical eukaryotic cell is shown in Figure 1.1.

SUBCELLULAR STRUCTURES AND THEIR FUNCTIONS

Cell Membrane

Structure

1. The outermost structure of the cell that decides its contour is the cell membrane.
2. It is a lipid bi-layer. It also consist of proteins and small amounts of carbohydrates (Figure 1.1 a).

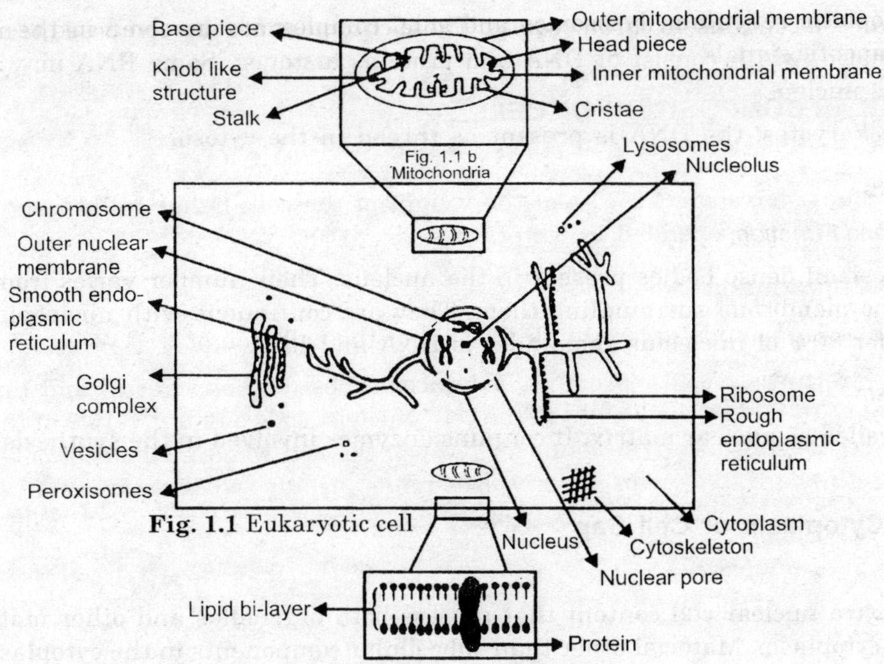

Fig. 1.1 Eukaryotic cell

Fig. 1.1 (*a*) Cell membrane

Functions

1. It is fluid and dynamic.
2. It is semi permeable, only selected compounds are allowed to pass through from outside. The selective permeability is responsible for the maintenance of internal environment of the cell and for creating potential difference across the membrane.
3. The modification of the cell membrane results in formation of specialized structures like axon of nerves, microvilli of intestinal epithelium and tail of spermatids.

Nucleus

Structure

1. Centre of the cell is nucleus.
2. It is surrounded by double-layer membrane of about 250-400 Å thick.
3. The two layers of nuclear membrane are an outer and inner membrane (layer). The two membranes fuse periodically to produce nuclear pores. Exchange of material between nucleus and rest of the cell occurs through nuclear pores.
4. The outer nuclear membrane continuous with other cytomembranes. In some eukaryotic cells, like erythrocyte nucleus is absent. In spermatozoa, nucleus accounts for 90% of cell whereas in other cells nucleus accounts for less than 10% of the cell. In prokaryotes, nucleus is not well defined.

Functions

1. Nucleus is the information centre of eukaryotic cell. More than 90% of the cellular DNA is present in the nucleus. It is mainly concentrated in the form of chromosomes.

2. Human cell contains 46 chromosomes. These chromosomes are composed of nucleoprotein chromatin, which consist of DNA and proteins histones. Some RNA may also present in the nucleus.
3. In prokaryotes, the DNA is present as thread in the cytosol.

Nucleolus

Structure and Function

These are small dense bodies present in the nucleus. Their number varies from cell to cell. There is no membrane surrounding them. They are continuous with nucleoplasm. Protein accounts for 80% of nucleolus remainder is DNA and RNA.

Nucleoplasm

It is also called as nuclear matrix. It contains enzymes involved in the synthesis of DNA and RNA.

Cytosol, Cytoplasm or Cell Sap

Structure

1. The extra nuclear cell content that possess both orgenelles and other material constitutes cytoplasm. Material other than subcellular components in the cytoplasm makes up the cytosol or cell sap.
2. Sometimes soluble portion of the cell is referred as cytosol. Cytoplasm accounts for 70-75% weight of the cytosol.

Functions

1. Numerous enzymes, proteins and many other solutes are found in cytosol.
2. Cytosol is the main site for glycolysis, HMP shunt, activation of aminoacids and fatty-acid synthesis.

Mitochondria

Structure

1. Are the second largest structures in the cell.
2. Generally mitochondria are ellipsoidal in shape and can assume variety of shapes.
3. The length of a mitochondrion is about 7 microns and has a diameter of 1 micron.
4. Mitochondria consist of outer and inner membranes. The outer membrane is composed of equal amount of protein and lipids.
5. The lipids are mainly phospholipids and cholesterol. The outer membrane functions as a limiting membrane and permeable to many compounds.
6. The inner membrane consist of 75% protein and remainder is lipid.
7. Cardiolipin is the important phospholipid of inner mitochondrial membrane.
8. The inner membrane is convoluted to form number of invaginations known as cristae extending to matrix (Figure 1.1b).
9. These cristae are covered with knob like structures, which are composed of head piece, stalk and a base piece.

Functions

1. The number of mitochondria ranges from 1-100 per cell depending on type of cell and its function. Several factors influence the size and number of mitochondria in cells. In yeast, mitochondria is present in aerobic state and absent in anaerobic state. Exposure to cold increases mitochondria by 20-30% in liver cells.
2. In highly metabolically active cells mitochondria are more and large.
3. Location of mitochondria in cell also depends on types and functions of cell. In liver cell mitochondria are scattered. In muscles they are parellely arranged. Mitochondria in liver cell may range up to 2000 whereas in kidney they may range up to 300.
4. Mitochondria is the *power house* of the cell. It is responsible for the production of energy in the form of ATP. The knob like structures function in electron transport and oxidative phosphorylation.
5. Mitochondria also contain other energy producing pathways like citric-acid cycle, fatty acid oxidation and ketone-body oxidation.
6. Some reactions of gluconeogenesis and urea cycle also occurs in mitochondria. Mitochondria is capable of synthesizing some of its proteins.
7. Mitochondria contains some DNA known as mitochondrial DNA and ribosomes.
8. Mitochondria which are essential for life because of their involvement in ATP production, also pay key role in programmed cell death of several types of cells. During apoptosis, mitochondrial membrane potential drops. This leads to permeabilization of mitochondrial membrane. Cytochrome-C or mitochondrial proteins are released into cytosol which activates death enzymes. Further alterations in mitochondrial morphology also occur during apoptosis.
9. In humans, mitochondria is derived from mother only. Hence, origin of mother of humans have been traced.
10. Outer and inner mitochondrial membranes contain translocase enzymes. They are involved in sorting of nuclear encoded proteins into mitochondrial sub-compartments as well as for their import into mitochondria. The inter mitochondrial membrane space is home for several lethal proteins like pro-death enzymes.

Lysosomes

Structure

1. They are small vesicles present in cytoplasm.
2. They are surrounded by a membrane. Lysosomes are called as 'Suicidel bags' of the cell.

Functions

1. Lysosomes are rich in hydrolytic enzymes, which are active at acidic pH. The lysosomal enzymes digest the molecules brought into the cell by phagocytosis.
2. Macrophages are rich in lysosomes.

Medical Importance

1. Lysosomal enzymes are involved in bone remodelling and intracellular digestion.

2. Disease, shock or cell death causes rupture of lysosomes and release of enzymes. In some organisms, lysosomal enzymes are responsible for cell death of larval tissues.
3. Lack of one or more of lysosomal enzymes cause accumulation of materials in the cell resulting in lysosomal diseases.
4. In some disease like arthritis and muscular dystrophy, lysosomal enzymes are released to cause uncontrolled destruction of surrounding tissues. Lysosomal proteases cathepsins are involved in spreading of cancer (metastasis).
5. As the age advances in digestible material an age pigment 'lipofuscin' occurs in some cells.
6. Lysosomol cystine transporter cystinosin is defective in cystinosis, which is a lysosomol disease. Hence, cystine transport into cytosol from lysosome is blocked.
7. Lysosomes are involved in integration of pro-apoptic signals.

Peroxisomes

Structure

1. Are also small vesicles surrounded by a membrane. They are also called as *microbodies*.

Functions

1. They contain enzymes of H_2O_2 metabolism. The concentration of protein in peroxisomes is very high and they may occur in crystallines form. The enzymes of H_2O_2 catabolism present in peroxisomes are peroxidase and catalase.
2. Peroxisomes also contain other enzymes like D, L-amino acid oxidase, uric acid oxidase and L-hydroxy fatty acid oxidation that generates H_2O_2. Glycerophospholipids are also synthesized in peroxisomes.

Medical Importance

1. Lack of peroxisomes result in Zellwegers syndrome.

Cytomembranes

There is an extensive network of membranes in the cytoplasm. These membranes are called as cytomembranes. They are divided into endoplasmic reticulum and golgi complex or apparatus. The endoplasmic reticulum is further subdivided into rough endoplasmic reticulum (RFR) and smooth endoplasmic reticulum (SER).

Rough Endoplasmic Reticulum

Structure

1. It is continuous with outer nuclear membrane.
2. The cytoplasmic surface of rough endoplasmic reticulum is coated with ribosomes. Membrane enclosed channels of endoplasmic reticulam are called *cisternae*. The ribosomes are complexes of RNA and protein.

Functions

1. Ribosomes and rough endoplasmic reticulum are involved in protein synthesis.
2. Protein synthesized, enters cisternae and later extruded.

Smooth Endoplasmic Reticulum

Structure

1. It is continuous with rough endoplasmic reticulum. It differs from RER by the absence of ribosomes. When isolated SER is called as microsomes.

Functions

1. SER of intestinal cells is involved in formation of triglycerides.
2. In the adrenal cortex, SER is the site of steroid formation.
3. Cytochrome P_{450} dependent monooxygenases are present in liver cell SER.

Golgi Apparatus

Structure

1. It consist of cluster of paired cytomembranes. The margins of these cytomembranes are flattened.
2. It also contains several small vesicles, which are pinched off from the flattened margins of membranes.

Functions

1. The golgi bodies are well developed in cells, which are involved in secretion. Material produced in the cell for export is processed by golgi body and is packaged as vesicle and is pinched off. The vesicles fuse with plasma membrane and their content is released to exterior by the process known as exocytosis. The digestive enzymes of pancreas and insulin are produced and released in this way.
2. Golgi apparatus helps in the formation of other subcellular organelles like lysosomes and peroxisomes.
3. Golgi apparatus is involved in protein targeting. It directs proteins to be incorporated into membranes of other subcellular structures. It is also involved in glycosylation and sulfation of proteins.
4. Golgi apparatus is involved in integration of proapoptic signal. It generates preapoptic mediator ganglioside GD3.

Medical Importance

Some cases of diabetes are due to defective processing of insulin in golgi complex.

Intracellular Ion Channels

Membrane of endoplasmic reticulum, golgi complex and nucleus has ion channels. They are involved in transport of ions between cytosol and these intracellular components. Calcium and chloride ion channels which are involved in their transport from these components into cytosol are known.

Vacuoles. Some animal cells contain vacuoles. They are membrane enclosed vesicles containing fluid. Mostly they contain nutrients.

Cell Coat. Some mammalian cells contain thin coat known as cell coat on the outer surface of the cell membrane. The cell coat is flexible and sticky. It is composed of mucopolysaccharides, glycolipids and glycoproteins. The adhesive properties of cell and organization of tissue is controlled by cell coat.

Cytoskeletons

These are filament like structures made up of proteins present in cytoplasm. Non-muscle cells perform mechanical work with these intracellular network of proteins.

(*a*) **Microfilaments.** They are actin like filaments. They form loose web beneath cell membrane.

(*b*) **Myosin Fibres.** Same as that of myosin of skeletal muscle.

(*c*) **Microtubules.** Tubulin is the building block of microtubules. Dendrites, axons of nerve cells and sperm cells contain microtubules. The sperm cell moves with the help of flagellum, a microtubule. These cyto skeletons are involved in the maintenance of cell shape, cell division, cell motility, phagocytosis, endocytosis and exocytosis.

(*d*) **Intermediate Filaments.** They are not involved in movement of cell. They are stable components of cytoskeleton. Neurofilament of neurons, glial filaments of glial cells and keratin of epithelial cells are some examples of intermediary filaments.

CELL CYCLE

MEDICAL IMPORTANCE

1. In all forms of life growth requires cell division.
2. However, some cells divide even after growth like erythrocytes and epithelial cells of intestine.

Sequence of events associated with cell division occur in cyclic manner. Hence, cell cycle consist of sequence of events, which occur in cyclic manner during cell division. There are four stages (phases) in cell cycle. They are

1. *S (Synthesis)-Phase*
2. *G_1 (Gap 1)-Phase*
3. *G_2 (Gap 2)-Phase*
4. *M (Mitosis)-Phase*

Sometimes, cell cycle is considered in two main events. They are mitosis and inter phase which consist of G_1, G_2 and S-phases.

1. *S (Synthesis)-Phase:* Division of a cell into two daughter cells requires duplication of DNA. During S-phase concentration of DNA precursors increases nearly 10-20 folds. In S-phase DNA synthesis occurs. Period of DNA synthesis is almost constant in all adult cells. (1 Hour)
2. *G_1 and G_2-Phases:* G_1 and G_2-phases are gaps or breaks in cell cycle. No special events occur during these phases except the size of the cell may increase. However, there may be many biochemical reactions taking place preparing the cell for division and checking that all appropriate steps are completed. The period of S_1, G_2 and M-Phases may range from 12-18 hours. But the period of G_1-phase varies, it can be few hours to months or even years.
3. *Mitosis (M)-Phase:* Many events take place in this phase of cell cycle. At the end mitosis cell divides into two daughter cells. The daughter cells are in G_1-phase.

Check Points in Cell Cycle

1. It is essential that during cell cycle, the synthesis of DNA, chromosomal segregation and cytoplasm division takes place in proper order. So, controls or check points within the cell cycle exist for all organisms.
2. During cell cycle, oscillation of cell from mitosis to interphase is controlled by many cellular proteins. Further check points exist at the G_1/S and G_2/M boundaries of cell cycle. Cell cycle with check points is illustrated in Figure 1.2.

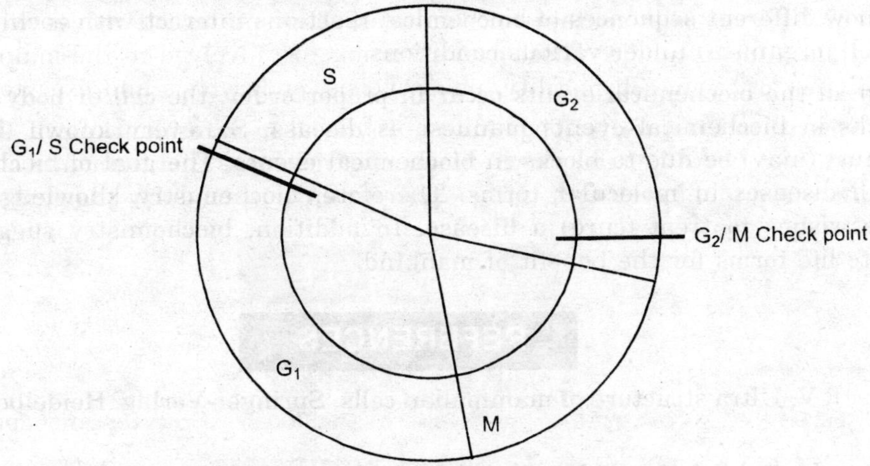

Fig. 1.2 Four phases of cell cycle with check points

CELL DEATH

MEDICAL AND BIOLOGICAL IMPORTANCE

1. Cells are not immortal i.e., they have finite life span. In the body, cells are formed and destroyed. So, cells are in dynamic state.
2. Cell division and cell death are two opposite processes required to maintain constant tissue volume (tissue homeostasis).
3. Further cell death plays an important role in shaping tissues and organs during development or during recovery from injuries.
4. Cell death may occur due to several external factors also.

There are three types of cell death.

1. *Necrosis:* It is also termed as cell murder. Cells undergo necrotic death if cell membrane is damaged or due to decreased oxygen supply and if energy (ATP) production is blocked.
2. *Apoptosis:* This type of cell death occurs in tissue turnover. Individual cells or groups of cells undergo this type of death. Aged cells in the body are removed by apoptosis. It is a genetically programmed cell death. In the initial stages of apoptosis, cell shrinks, followed by fragmentation and finally these fragments are eliminated by phagocytosis.

3. *Atrophy:* This type of cell death occurs in the absence of essential survival factors. Survival factors required by the cell are produced by other cells. Absence of nerve growth factor leads to atrophy of nerves. It is also genetically programmed cell death.

BIOCHEMISTRY, CELL AND DISEASE

Biochemistry explains all cellular or biological events in chemical terms. The chemical reactions that occur in biological systems are called *biochemical reactions*. Biochemistry also explains how different sequences of biochemical reactions interact with each other for survival of cell (organism) under various conditions.

When all the biochemical events occur in proper order, the cell or body remains normal. Blocks in biochemical events manifest as disease. So, every known (to be known) disease must (may) be due to blocks in biochemical events. The goal of biochemistry is to explain all diseases in molecular terms. Therefore, biochemistry knowledge is required when one wishes to treat (cure) a disease. In addition, biochemistry suggests ways to manipulate life forms for the benefit of mankind.

REFERENCES

1. Krstie, R.V. Ultra structure of mammalian cells, Springer-Verlag, Heidelberg, Germany, 1979.
2. Ernster, L. and Schatz, G. Mitochondria: a historical review. J. Cell Biol. **91,** 227 (S)-235 (S), 1981.
3. Rothman, J.E. The compartmental organization of golgi body. Sci. Am. **253(3),** 84-95, 1985.
4. Duive. Microbodies in livings cells. Sci. Am. **248(5),** 52-62, 1983.
5. Bainton, D.L. The discovery of lysosomes. J. Cell Biol. **91,** 665-675, 1981.
6. Zimmerman, R.A. Ins and outs of ribosome. Nature **376,** 391-392, 1995.
7. Birchmeicr, W. Cytoskeleton structure and function. Trends Biochem. Sci. **9,** 192-195, 1984.
8. Murray, A.W. and Kirschner, M.C. What controls cell cycle. Sci. Am. **264 (3),** 34-41, 1991.
9. Collins, M.K.L. and Rivas, A.L. The control of apoptosis in mammalian cells. Trends Biochem Sci. **18,** 307-309, 1993.
10. Printon, P. Puzzan, T. and Rizzuto, R. The golgi apparatus is an inositol-1, 4, 5-triphosphate Ca^{2+} store with functional properties distinct from those of endoplasmic reticulum. EMBO. J. **17,** 5298-5308, 1998.
11. Nayasawa, M. Kanzaki, M. Vinoy. Morishita, Y. and Kojima, Y. Identification of novel chloride channel expressed in the endoplasmic reticulum, golgi apparatus and nucleus. J. Biol. Chem. **276,** 20413-20418, 2001.
12. Tinacirman *et al.* Selective disruption of lysosomes in the HeLa cells triggers apoptosis mediated by cleavage of Bid by multiple papain like lysosomol cathepsins. J. Biol. Chem. **279,** 3578-3587, 2004.

13. Ferri, K.F. and Kroemer, G. Organelle specific initiation of cell death pathways. Nature Cell Biology. **3,** E255-E263, 2001.

14. Karbowski, M. and Youle, R.J. Dynamics of mitochondrial morphology in healthy cells and during apoptosis. Cell Death and Differentiation. **10,** 870-880, 2003.

15. Franklin, H.M. The way of the cell:Molecules, Organisms and order of life. Oxford University Press, 2003.

16. Cohen, R.M. and Roth, K.S. Biochemistry and disease: bridging basic science and clinical practice. Williams and Wilkins, 1996.

17. Dolman, N.J. *et al.* Stable golgi-mitochondria complexes and formation of golgi Ca^{2+} gradiants in pancreatic acinar cells. J. Biol. Chem. **280**, IS794-99, 2005.

EXERCISES

ESSAY QUESTIONS

1. Draw an animal cell diagram and label different cell organelle. Write functions of mitochondria, golgi apparatus and lysosomes.
2. Describe structure and function of each cell organelle.
3. Write about cell cycle and cell death. Mention clinical importance of each one.

SHORT QUESTIONS

1. Name organic substances present in cell.
2. Define cytoskeletons of a cell. Name them. Write their functions.
3. Define cell cycle. Name stages of cell cycle. Explain any one stage.
4. Explain apoptosis.
5. Write a note on structure and function of mitochondria.
6. Draw mitochondria. Label its various parts.
7. Name different types of cell death. Explain each one.
8. Write a note on cytomembranes.
9. Name different types of endoplasmic reticulum of cell. Write structure and function of any one.
10. Write a note on intracellular membranous network.
11. Mention functions of nucleus, nucleolus and cytosol.
12. Write a note on lysosomol role in diseases.

MULTIPLE CHOICE QUESTIONS

1. In the cell cycle check points exist

   (*a*) at G_1/S boundary
   (*b*) at G_1/G_2 boundary
   (*c*) at S/G_2 boundary
   (*d*) at G_1/M boundary

2. Lysosomes contain mainly

   (*a*) Hydrolases
   (*b*) Proteases
   (*c*) Lipases
   (*d*) Cathepsins

3. Cell death due to lack of oxygen is called as

(*a*) Necrosis (*b*) Atrophy

(*c*) Hypertrophy (*d*) Apoptosis

4. Peroxisomes are involved in

(*a*) Protein synthesis (*b*) Cell death

(*c*) Phospholipid synthesis (*d*) Triglyceride synthesis

FILL IN THE BLANKS

1. A well defined --------------- is absent in prokaryotes.
2. -------------- separates cell from its surroundings.
3. An important inner mitochondrial membrane phospholipid is -------------.
4. ---------------- are called as suicide bags of cells.
5. A cytoskeleton filament present in the axons of nerve and sperm cell ----------------.

2

CHAPTER

AMINO ACIDS AND PEPTIDES

OCCURRENCE

Amino acids and peptides are present in humans, animals, tissues, blood, microorganisms and plants.

MEDICAL AND BIOLOGICAL IMPORTANCE

1. Amino acids serve as building blocks of proteins. Some amino acids are found in free form in human blood.
2. They also serve as precursors of hormones, purines, pyrimidines, porphyrins, vitamins and biologically important amines like histamine.
3. Peptides have many important biological functions. Some of them are hormones. They are used as anti-biotics and antitumor agents.
4. Some peptides are required for detoxification reactions. Some peptides serve as neurotransmitters.
5. Amino acid proline protects living organisms against free radical induced damage.
6. Some peptides are involved in regulation of cell cycle and apoptosis.
7. Peptides of vertebrates and invertebrates act as antimicrobial agents. They are part of innate immunity. Bacterial infections at epithelial surface induce production of antimicrobial peptides, which cause lysis of microbes.
8. Peptides are enzyme inhibitors. Natural and synthetic peptide inhibitors of angiotensin converting enzyme (ACE) act as a anti hypertensives. Peptide inhibitors of ACE present in physiological foods, lowers blood pressure after they are absorbed from intestine. Lisinopril, Enalapril etc. are synthetic peptide inhibitors of ACE that are used as drugs in the treatment of hypertension.
9. Some synthetic peptides are used as enzyme substrates.

CHEMICAL NATURE OF AMINO ACIDS

Amino acids are carboxylic acids containing an amino group. In most of the amino acids, an amino group is attached to α-carbon atom next to the carboxyl group hence they are α-amino acids. The general formula is shown in Figure 2.1.

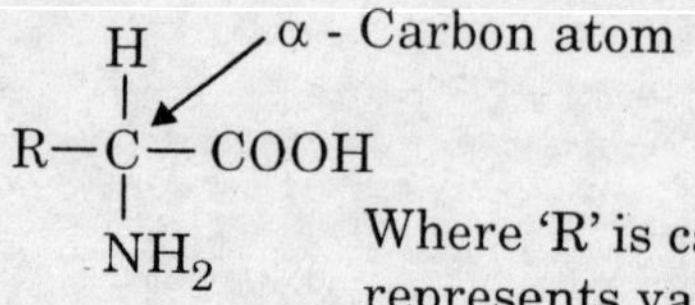

L - Amino acid

Where 'R' is called as side chain and it represents variety of structures

Fig. 2.1 Structure of an α-amino acid

COMMON AMINO ACIDS

Though more than 200 amino acids are identified in nature, only 20 amino acids serve as building blocks of body proteins. They are known as common amino acids. In addition to the common amino acids, derived amino acids are also found in proteins.

CLASSIFICATION OF AMINO ACIDS

Amino acids have been classified in various ways.

I. Based on side chain and ring structure present, amino acids are classified into 7 major classes.

1. Amino acids with aliphatic side chain. They are also called as *aliphatic amino acids*. They are glycine, alanine, valine, leucine and isoleucine (Fig. 2.2). Valine, leucine and isoleucine are called as branched chain amino acids.

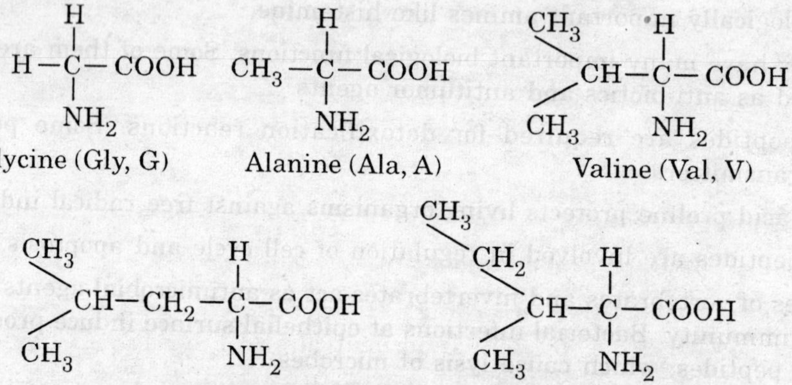

Fig. 2.2 Aliphatic amino acids

2. Amino acids with side chain containing hydroxyl groups. They are also called as hydroxy amino acids. They are serine and threonine (Fig. 2.3*a*).
3. Amino acids with side chain containing sulfur atoms. They are also called as sulfur containing amino acids. They are cysteine, methionine and cystine (Fig. 2.3*b*).
4. Amino acids with side chain containing acidic groups or their amides. They are also called as *acidic amino acids*. They are aspartic acid, aspargine, glutamic acid and glutamine (Fig. 2.4).
5. Amino acids with side chain containing basic groups. They are also called as *basic amino acids*. They are arginine, lysine, hydroxy lysine and histidine (Fig. 2.5).

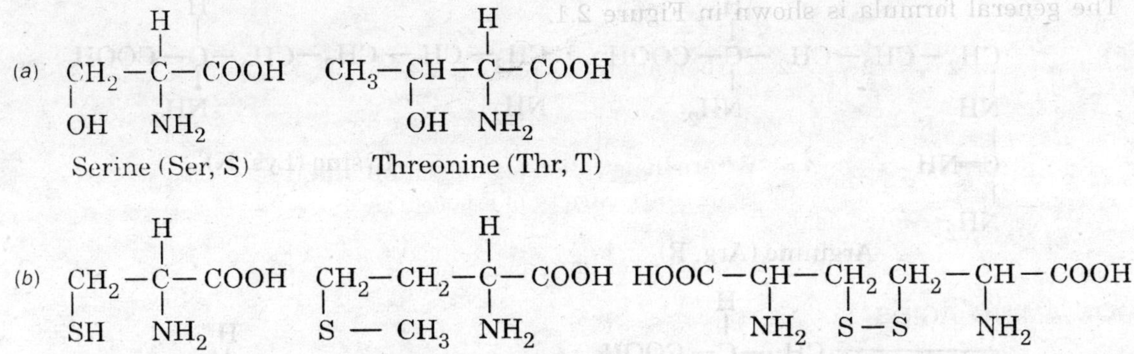

(a) Serine (Ser, S) Threonine (Thr, T)

(b) Cysteine (Cys, C) Methionine (Met, M) Cystine

Fig. 2.3 (*a*) Hydroxy amino acids (*b*) Sulfur containing amino acids

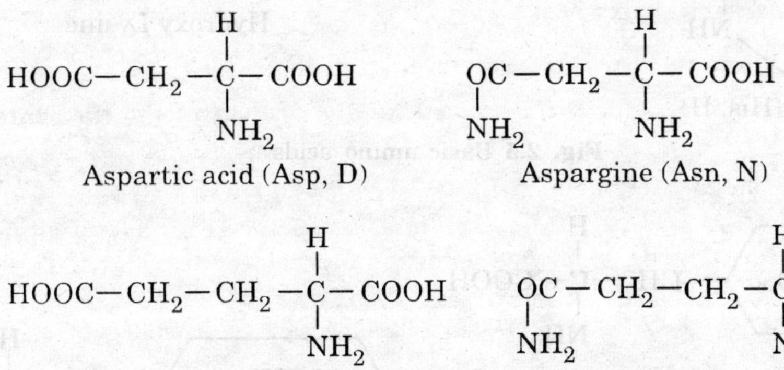

Aspartic acid (Asp, D) Aspargine (Asn, N)

Glutamic acid (Glu, E) Glutamine (Gln, Q)

Fig. 2.4 Acidic amino acids and their amides

6. Amino acids containing aromatic rings. They are also called as *aromatic amino acids*. They are phenylalanine, tyrosine and tryptophan (Fig. 2.6)
7. Imino acids. They are proline and hydroxy proline (Fig. 2.7).

II. Amino acids are also classified according to the reaction in solution or charge. They are categorized in 3 classes, acidic, basic and neutral amino acids. Acidic amino acids are aspartic acid, glutamic acid. Basic amino acids are arginine, lysine and histidine. Rest of the amino acids are neutral amino acids.

III. Another classification of amino acids is based on the number of amino and carboxyl groups present in the molecule.

Example. Mono-amino mono-carboxylic acid (Glycine), Mono-amino dicarboxylic acid (Glutamate).

IV. Amino acids are also classified according to their nutritional importance. Nutritionally amino acids are classified into

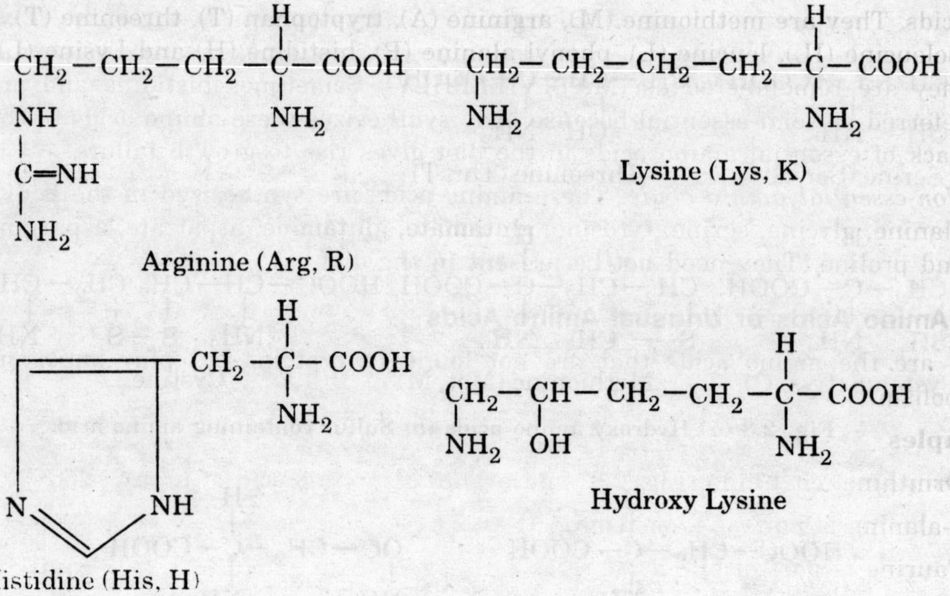

Arginine (Arg, R)

Lysine (Lys, K)

Histidine (His, H)

Hydroxy Lysine

Fig. 2.5 Basic amino acids

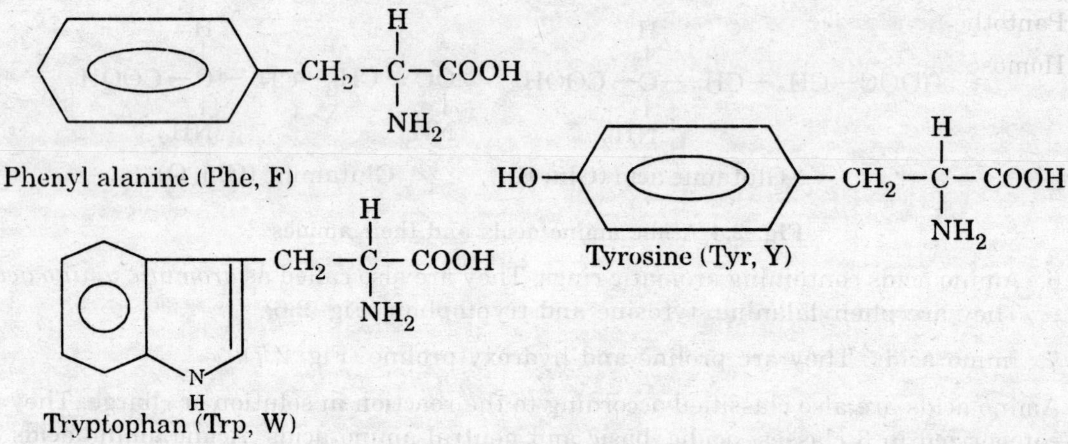

Phenyl alanine (Phe, F)

Tyrosine (Tyr, Y)

Tryptophan (Trp, W)

Fig. 2.6 Aromatic amino acids

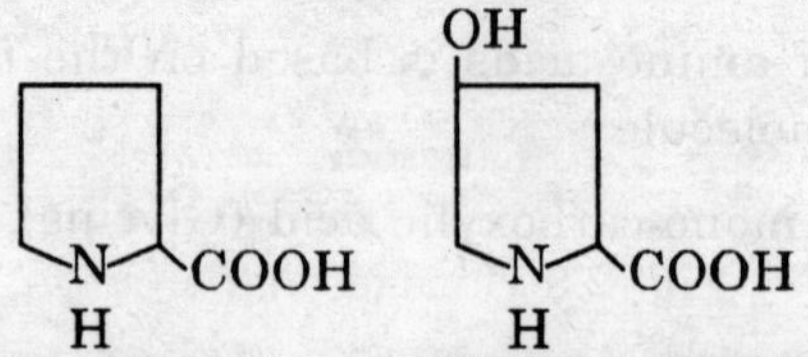

Proline (Pro, P)

Hydroxy Proline

Fig. 2.7 Imino acids

(*a*) *Essential amino acids:* These amino acids are not synthesized in the body and hence they have to be obtained from the diet. They are also referred as indispensable amino acids. They are methionine (M), arginine (A), tryptophan (T), threonine (T), valine (V), isoleucine (IL), leucine (L), phenyl alanine (P), histidine (H) and Lysine (L). Together they are remembered as (MATTVILLPHLY). Sometimes histidine and arginine are referred as semi-essential because body synthesizes these amino acids to some extent. Lack of essential amino acids in the diet gives rise to growth failure.

(b) *Non-essential amino acids*: These amino acids are synthesized in the body. They are alanine, glycine, serine, tyrosine, glutamate, glutamine, aspartate, aspargine, cysteine and proline. They need not be present in the diet.

Rare Amino Acids or Unusual Amino Acids

These are the amino acids that are not found in proteins but play important roles in metabolism.

Examples

1. Ornithine, citrulline (Fig. 2.8) and arginino succinic acid of urea cycle.
2. β-alanine is part of co-enzyme A (Fig. 2.8).
3. Taurine is part of bile acids (Fig. 2.8).
4. γ-aminobutyric acid is a neurotransmitter (Fig. 2.8).
5. Mono- and di-iodotyrosine are precursors of thyroxine.
6. Pantothenic acid is a water-soluble vitamin.
7. Homoserine is an intermediate of methionine catabolism.

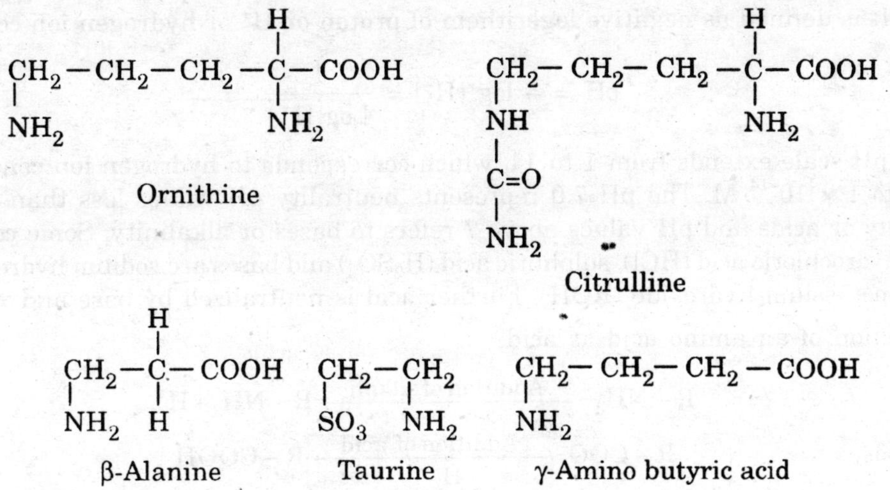

Fig. 2.8 Unusual amino acids

8. **Homocysteine.** It is also an intermediate of methionine catabolism. It is a athero-thrombogenic agent. It triggers platelet adhesion. Hence, it is considered as a risk factor for development of coronary artery disease (CAD).
9. **S-allylcysteine sulfoxide.** It is an amino acid obtained from garlic. It has many therapeutic effects. It is commonly called as alliin.

PROPERTIES OF AMINO ACIDS

1. *Optical isomerism:* All the amino acids except glycine have at least one asymmetric carbon atom because of this they exhibit optical isomerism. Presence of single asymmetric carbon atom gives rise to two optical isomers. One isomer is the mirror image of the other isomer. If a carbon atom is linked to four different groups through covalent bonds then it is called as *asymmetric carbon*. The two mirror images of amino acid serine are L-serine and D-serine (Fig. 2.9 *a* and *b*). Further, the optical isomers of amino acids are optically active. They are capable of rotating plane polarized light. Some amino acids rotate plane polarized to left and some rotate the plane polarized light to right. All the amino acids present in human proteins are L-isomers. D-isomers are usually absent but they are found in some peptide antibiotics.

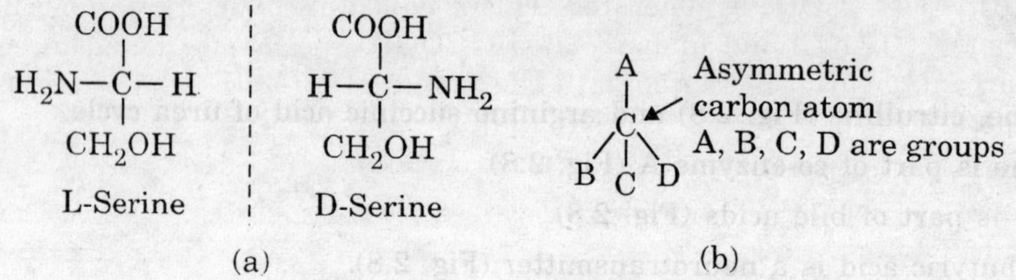

Fig. 2.9 (*a*) Optical isomers of serine (*b*) Asymmetric carbon atom

2. *Acid-base or charge properties of amino acids:* Amino acids act as acids and bases. So they are called as *ampholytes* or *amphoteric substances*. Acids are those compounds that give protons on dissociation. Bases are those compounds that combine with protons. Bases are also called as alkalies. Proton concentration is quantitatively expressed as pH. It is defined as negative logerithem of proton or H^+ or hydrogen ion concentration.

$$pH = -\log [H^+] = \frac{1}{\text{Log}[H^+]}$$

The pH scale extends from 1 to 14, which corresponds to hydrogen ion concentration of 1M to 1×10^{-14} M. The pH 7.0 represents neutrality pH values less than 7 represents acidity or acids and pH values above 7 refers to bases or alkalinity. Some common acids are hydrochloric acid (HCl), sulphuric acid (H_2SO_4) and bases are sodium hydroxide (NaOH) and potassium hydroxide (KOH). Further acid is neutralized by base and vice versa.

Function of an amino acid as acid:

$$R-NH_3^+ \xrightarrow{\text{Addition of alkali}} R-NH_2 + H^+$$

As base:

$$R-COO^- \xrightarrow[H^+]{\text{Addition of acid}} R-COOH$$

So, amino acids have two ionizable groups (–COOH, NH_3^+). The –COOH is several times more easily dissociates than $-NH_3^+$. At neutral pH both groups are ionized, i.e., the carboxyl group exist in dissociated form where as amino group exist as associated form. This doubly charged molecule of amino acid containing positive and negative charges is called as zwitter ion. It is electrically neutral so it does not move in an electrical field. The other two forms are anionic form and cationic form (Figure 2.10).

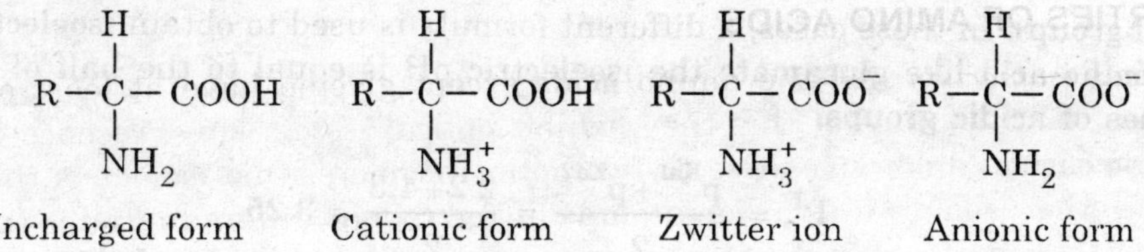

Fig. 2.10 Different forms of amino acids

The charge of an amino acid always depends on the pH of its surroundings. In other words, the charge of amino acid is altered by changing pH of its surroundings. This property is exploited for the separation of amino acids. In strong acidic conditions (pH < 2) the –COOH remains undissociated. When the pH is raised at pH of about 3 the proton from the –COOH is lost $-COO^-$ is generated. This is called pK of acid group because at this pH dissociated ($-COO^-$) and undissociated (–COOH) species are found in equal amounts. Similarly, if the pH is increased to 10, the amino group ($-NH_3^+$) dissociates to $-NH_2$ group. This pH is called the pK of amino group of amino acid because at this pH associated ($-NH_3^+$) and dissociated ($-NH_2$) species are present in equal amounts. (Fig. 2.11)

Therefore, an amino acid has two pK values corresponding to the two ionizable groups. pK values indicates strength of each group. Further an amino acid exist as zwitter ion at neutral pH and as cation at acidic pH and as anion at basic pH.

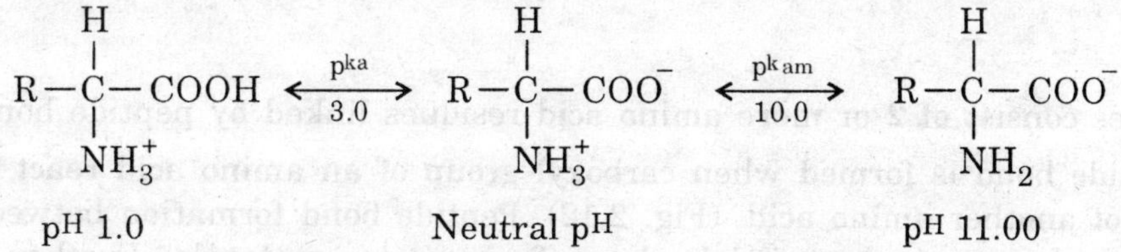

Fig. 2.11 p^H influence on amino acid charge

Example: For alanine, p^{Ka} is 2.4 and p^{Kam} is 9.7 (K is dissociation constant), the low pK value of –COOH indicates more ionizing power.

Isoelectric pH: It is the pH at which the net charge of an amino acid is zero or when the number of positive charges are equal to number of negative charges. At isoelectric pH amino acids have minimum solubility. The isoelectric pH of an amino acid having one amino group and one carboxyl group is equal to the arithamatic mean of p^{Ka} and p^{Kam} values.

$$\text{Isoelectric pH or } p^I = \frac{p^{Ka} + p^{Kam}}{2}$$

When values are substituted, isoelectric pH of alanine is

$$P^I = \frac{2.4 + 9.7}{2} = 6.05$$

For most amino acids p^I is close to 6.0. The situation differs for amino acids having more than two ionizable groups. For example, glutamate is dicarboxylic acid so it can have three pK values (two for carboxyl groups and one for amino group). Similarly, the basic amino acid lysine can have three pK values (two for amino groups and one for carboxyl group). In these cases, a different formula is used to obtain isoelectric pH. For acidic amino acid like glutamate the isoelectric pH is equal to the half of sum of two pK values of acidic groups.

$$p^I = \frac{p^{Ka1} + p^{Ka2}}{2} = \frac{2.2+4.3}{2} = 3.25$$

For basic amino acid like lysine the isoelectric pH is equal to the half of sum of two p^K values of amino groups.

$$p^I = \frac{p^{Kam1} + p^{Kam2}}{2} = \frac{9.0+10.5}{2} = 9.75$$

3. *Buffering action of amino acids:* Buffers are salts of weak acids and they resist change in pH when acid or alkali is added. Since amino acids are ampholytes they act as buffers. However, the buffering action of amino acids in the blood is insignificant because of their low concentration.
4. *Ultra violet light (UV) absorption of amino acids.* Amino acids do not absorb visible light. Aromatic amino acids absorb ultraviolet light. Tryptophan absorb ultra violet light at 280 nm. The ultra violet light absorption is also exhibited by proteins containing tryptophan. Hence, it is used for quantitative estimation of proteins and to study folding of protein molecules. Phenylalanine and tyrosine also absorb light in ultra violet region.

PEPTIDES

1. Peptides consist of 2 or more amino acid residues linked by peptide bond.
2. A peptide bond is formed when carboxyl group of an amino acid react with α-amino group of another amino acid. (Fig. 2.12). Peptide bond formation between two amino acids is always accompanied by loss of one water molecule. Further, peptide and proteins contain an amino (N–) terminus and carboxy (C–) terminus.
3. A peptide or protein is named starting with N-terminal amino acid and usually the N-terminal is located on the left hand side.

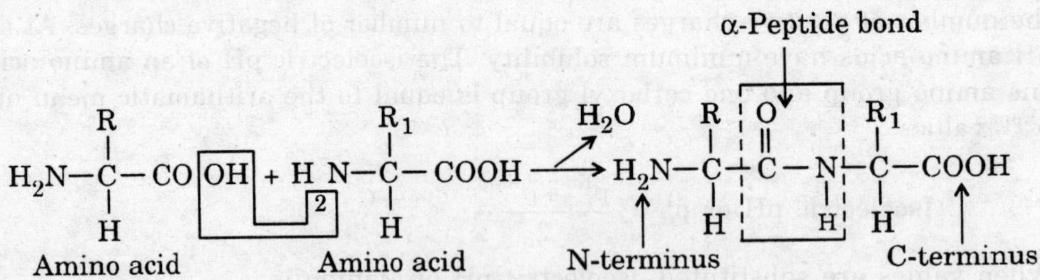

Fig. 2.12 Peptide bond formation

4. Animal, plant and bacterial cells contain wide variety of low molecular weight peptides (2-10 amino acids residues) having profound biological functions.

DIPEPTIDES

A dipeptide consist of two amino acid residues and one peptide bond.

Carnosine and Anserine

Are two peptides present in muscle and brain.

Structure

Carnosine consist of β-alanine and histidine (β-alanyl histidine). Anserine consist of β-alanine and N-methyl histidine (β-alanyl N-methyl histidine). Short hand formula for carnosine is β-ala-His.

Function

Remains unknown.

Aspartame

Structure

It consist of aspartate and phenylalanine (Aspartyl phenylalanine, Asp-Phe). It is present in African berry.

Function

It is a sweetening agent.

Tripeptides

A tripeptide consist of three amino acid residues and two peptide bonds.

Glutathione

Structure

It consist of glutamate. Cysteine and glycine. In glutathione, γ-carboxyl group of glutamate is involved in peptide linkage with cysteine hence it is named as γ-glutamyl cysteinyl glycine (Glu-Cys-Gly, G-SH, Fig. 2.13*a*).

Functions

1. It act as reducing agent in all cells. It assumes dimeric form on oxidation (Fig. 2.13*b*). It is responsible for the maintenance of –SH groups of proteins in reduced form.

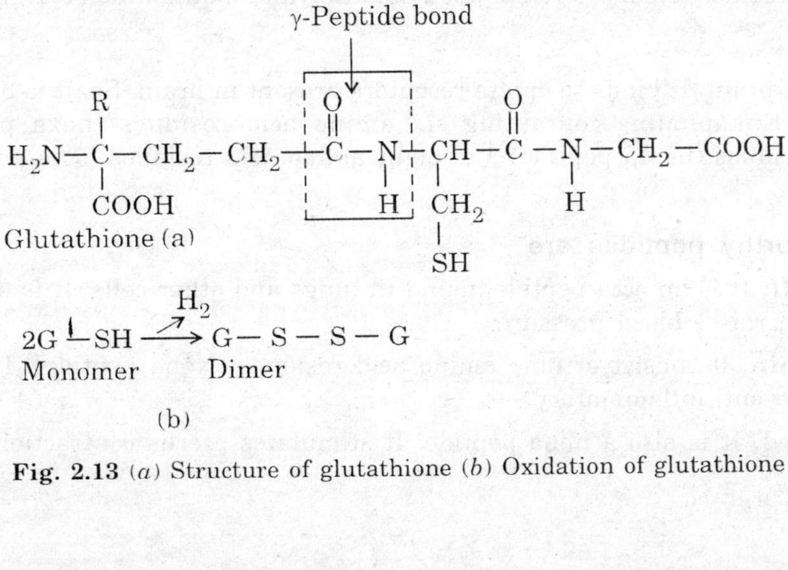

Fig. 2.13 (*a*) Structure of glutathione (*b*) Oxidation of glutathione

2. It participates in the removal of H_2O_2 in erythrocytes.
3. It is required for removal of toxins from body.
4. It is involved in release of hormones.
5. It protects body proteins from radiation effects.
6. It is involved in cellular resistance to anticancer agents.
7. Glutathione regulates telomerase activity and of the cell cycle.
8. Glutathione is involved in modulation of apoptosis.

Thyrotropin Releasing Harmone (TRH)

Structure

It consists of glutamate, histidine and proline. It is an unusual tripeptide with blocked N and C terminals.

Function

It is a hormone secreted by hypothalamus.

Chemotactic Peptide

Structure

It consists of N-Formyl methionine, leucine and phenylalanine (f met-leu-phe). Its N-terminal contains formyl (–CHO) group.

Function

It is present in leukocytes. It plays an important role in chemotaxis.

Penta Peptides

They consist of five amino acids and four peptide bonds.

Enkaphalin

Structure

It consist of tyrosine, glycine, glycine, phenylalanine and methionine (Tyr-gly-gly-phe-met).

Function

It is present in brain. It binds to opiate receptors present in brain. So, it is body own opiate or analgesic. Enkaphalins containing six amino acid residues (hexa peptide), seven amino acid residues (hepta peptide) and eight amino acid residues (octa peptide) are also found in brain.

Other noteworthy peptides are

Angiotensin II. It is an octa peptide, found in lungs and other cells. It is a powerful vaso constrictor and raises blood pressure.

Bradykinin. It consist of nine amino acid residues (Nona peptide). It is a powerful vasodilator and anti inflammatory.

Oxytocin I. It is also a nona peptide. It stimulates uterus contraction.

Vasopressin. A nona peptide produced by pituitary gland. It has a disulfide bridge. It is also known as antidiuretic harmone (ADH).

Angiotensin I and Kallidin are examples for decapeptides containing ten amino acid residues.

CYCLIC PEPTIDES

1. They differ from normal peptides.
2. In these peptides N-terminus and C-teminus are linked by peptide bond resulting in cyclization of peptide.
3. An antibiotic gramicidin-S is a cyclic peptide. It consist of ten amino acids. So gramicidin-S is a cyclic decapeptide. Further it contains D-Phenyl alanine which is usually absent in life forms.
4. Tyrocidin is another cyclic decapeptide.

TOXIC PEPTIDES

1. Some peptides act as toxins.
2. α-amanitin is a bicyclic octapeptide present in a particular variety of mushrooms. It is extremely toxic to humans.
3. It is responsible for mushroom poisoning cases around the world.
4. When the mushrooms are consumed it causes pain in the gastrointestinal tract, vomitting, diarrhoea and nausae.
5. Death occurs within a week due of impairment of liver and kidney functions.

CYCLOTIDES (CYCLIC PEPTIDES)

In some peptides disulfide bonds are more. These disulfide bonds create knot with in the molecule. Two disulfide bonds and their connecting back bone segment form ring. They are known as cyclotides. These cyclic peptides show diverse actions. Some are anti HIV, anti bacterial and insecticidal agents. Some examples are given below:

1. ***Sunflower trypsin inhibitor (SFTI).*** It is smallest circular peptide with just 14 amino acids. It is an enzyme inhibitor.
2. ***RTD-1.*** It is a circular peptide present in leucocytes. It is a defensin. It consists of only 18 amino acids.
3. ***Microsin.*** It is 21 residue cyclic peptide. It is produced by E. coli. It is an antibiotic.

REFERENCES

1. Green stein, J.P. and Winitz, M. Chemistry of amino acids. Wiley, New York, 1961.
2. Meister, A. Biochemistry of amino acids Academic Press, New York, 1965.
3. Davies, J.S. Amino acids and peptides. Chapman and Hall, 1985.
4. Weinstein, B. Ed. Chemistry and biochemistry of amino acids, peptides and proteins. Vol. 4. Mercel and Dekkar, New York, 1977.
5. Meister, A. and Anderson, M.E. Glutathione. Ann Rev. Biochem. **52**, 711-760, 1983.

6. Erdos, E.G. Johnson, A.R. and Boyden, N.J. Hydrolysis of enkaphalin by peptidyl dipeptidase. Biochem Pharmacol. **27,** 843-848, 1978.
7. Sandgreen, S. *et al.* The human antimicrobial peptide LL. 37 transfers extracellular plasmid DNA to nuclear compartment of mammalian cells via lipid raft and proteoglycan dependent endocytosis. J. Biol. Chem. **279,** 17951-17956, 2004.
8. Pierre Jolle. S.D-Amino acids in sequences of secreted peptides of multicellular organisms. Kluwer Academic Publishers, 1998.
9. Huang, L. *et al.* Novel peptide inhibitors of angiotensin converting enzyme. J. Biol. Chem. **278,** 15532-15540, 2003.
10. Borras, C. *et al.* Glutathione regulates telomerase activity in fibroblasts. J. Biol. Chem. June, 2004.
11. Korsinozky, M.L.J. *et al.* Solution structure by ^{1}H NMR of the novel cyclic trypsin inhibitor from sunflower. J. Mol. Biol. **311,** 579-591, 2001.
12. Burrett, G.C. and Elmore, D.T. Amino acids and peptides, Cambridge University Press, 1998.
13. Doonan, S. Peptides and proteins. Wiley, New York, 2003.
14. Miquel, V.P. *et al.* Structural dissection of a highly knotted peptide reveals minimal motifs with antimicrobial activity. J. Biol. Chem. **280**, 1661-1668, 2005.

EXERCISES

ESSAY QUESTIONS

1. Classify amino acids. Give examples for each class.
2. Name five biologically important peptides. Write one function for each of them.
3. Write an essay on properties of amino acids.

SHORT QUESTIONS

1. Define amino acid and isoelectric pH. Write two properties of an amino acid at isoelectric pH.
2. Write composition of glutathione. How it differs from other peptides? Write two of its functions.
3. Explain acid-base properties of amino acids.
4. Define essential amino acids. Give examples.
5. Write structures of tyrosine, methionine and valine.
6. What are unusual amino acids? Give examples.
7. Define cyclic peptide. How it differs from other peptides? Write 2 examples with functions.
8. Write a note on semi essential amino acids.
9. Calculate isoelectric point of glutamic acid. How it differs from the isoelectric point of glycine?
10. What are the functions of amino acids?
11. Draw structure of peptide. Label its various parts.

MULTIPLE CHOICE QUESTIONS

1. Most of the amino acids found in human body are
   (*a*) L-isomers (*b*) D-isomers
   (*c*) D and L-isomers (*d*) Optical isomers
2. Which of the following amino acids has more pK values.
   (*a*) Glycine (*b*) Alanine
   (*c*) Glutamate (*d*) Glutamine
3. The isoelectric pH of lysine is equal to
   (*a*) Arithamatic mean of amino groups pK values.
   (*b*) Half of sum of amino group and carboxyl group pK values.
   (*c*) Arithamatic mean of amino groups and carboxyl groups pK values.
   (*d*) None of the above.
4. An example for unusual amino acid is
   (*a*) Aspargine (*b*) Taurine
   (*c*) Cystine (*d*) Anserine
5. All of the following statements are correct regarding peptide except
   (*a*) It contains amino terminus (*b*) It contains carboxy terminus
   (*c*) It contains peptide bonds (*d*) It contains only basic amino acids

FILL IN THE BLANKS

1. -------------absorbs light in ultraviolet region.
2. --------------is a dipeptide having sweet taste.
3. In a cyclic peptide N-terminus and C-terminus are linked by --------- bond.
4. An unusual amino acid that function as neurotransmitter is -----------.

3
CHAPTER

PROTEINS

OCCURRENCE

Proteins are present in every cell of humans, animals, plant tissues, tissue fluids and in micro organisms. They account for about 50% of the dry weight of a cell. The term protein is derived from the Greek word *proteios* meaning holding first place or rank in living matter.

MEDICAL AND BIOLOGICAL IMPORTANCE

Proteins perform wide range of essential functions in mammalians.

1. Proteins are involved in the transport of substances in the body.

   Example: Haemoglobin transports oxygen.

2. Enzymes which catalyze chemical reactions in the body are proteins.
3. Proteins are involved in defence function. They act against bacterial or viral infection.

   Example: Immunoglobulins.

4. Hormones are proteins. They control many biochemical events.

   Example: Insulin.

5. Some proteins have role in contraction of muscles.

   Example: Muscle proteins.

6. Proteins are involved in the gene expression. They control gene expression and translation.

   Example: Histones.

7. Proteins serve as nutrients. Proteins are also involved in storage function.

   Examples: Casein of milk, Ferritin that stores iron.

8. Proteins act as buffers.

   Example: Plasma proteins.

9. Proteins function as anti-vitamins.

   Example: Avidin of egg.

10. Proteins are infective agents.

    Example: Prions which cause mad cow disease are proteins.

11. Some toxins are proteins.

    Example: Enterotoxin of cholera microorganism.

12. Some proteins provide structural strength and elasticity to the organs and vascular system.

    Example: Collagen and elastin of bone matrix and ligaments.

13. Some proteins are components of structures of tissues.

    Example: α-keratin is present in hair and epidermis.

In order to understand how these substances though they are all proteins play such diverse functions their structures, and composition must be explored.

CHEMICAL NATURE OF PROTEINS

All proteins are polymers of aminoacids. The aminoacids in proteins are united through "Peptide" linkage. Sometimes proteins are also called as polypeptides because they contain many peptide bonds.

PROPERTIES OF PROTEINS

1. Proteins have high molecular weight, *e.g.*, the lactalbumin of milk molecular weight is 17000 and pyruvate dehydrogenase molecular weight is 7×10^6.
2. Proteins are colloidal in nature.
3. Proteins have large particle size.
4. Different kinds of proteins are soluble in different solvents.
5. Proteins differ in their shape.
6. Some proteins yield amino acids only on hydrolysis where as others produce amino acids plus other types of molecules.
7. **Charge properties:** Charge of a protein depends on the surroundings like amino acids. So, by changing the pH of surroundings the charge of protein can be altered. This property is used for separation of proteins.

   Isoelectric point: Proteins have characteristic isoelectric points. At the isoelectric point its net charge is zero because the number of positive charges are equal to number of negative charges. So proteins are insoluble or have minimum solubility at isoelectric point. This property is used for the isolation of casein from milk. The isoelectric point for casein is 4.6. If the pH of the surrounding is raised above the isoelectric point, the protein is negatively charged *i.e.*, it exists as anion. Likewise, if the pH of the surrounding is lowered, the protein is positively charged *i.e.*, it exist as cation. Further, proteins do not move in an electrical field at isoelectric point like amino acids. However, if the pH of the medium is raised or lowered protein moves towards anode or cathode respectively. This property is exploited for the separation of proteins.
8. **Proteins act as buffers:** Since proteins are amphoteric substances, they act as buffers. Hemoglobin (Hb) of erythrocytes and plasma proteins are important buffers. Hb accounts for 60% of buffering action with in erythrocytes and plasma proteins contributes to 20% of buffering action of blood.

CLASSIFICATION OF PROTEINS

There is no single universally satisfactory system of protein classification so far.

1. One system classifies proteins according to their composition or structure.
2. One system classifies them according to solubility.
3. One system classifies them according to their shape.
4. Classification of proteins based on their function also found in literature.

Classification of proteins based on their composition

Proteins are divided into three major classes according to their structure.

1. **Simple proteins:** Simple proteins are made up of amino acids only. On hydrolysis, they yield only amino acids.

   Examples: Human plasma albumin, Trypsin, Chymotrypsin, pepsin, insulin, soyabean trypsin inhibitor and ribonuclease.

2. **Conjugated proteins:** They are proteins containing non-protein part attached to the protein part. The non-protein part is linked to protein through covalent bond, non-covalent bond and hydrophobic interaction. The non-protein part is loosely called as prosthetic group. On hydrolysis, these proteins yield non-protein compounds and amino acids.

   $$\text{Conjugated protein} \longrightarrow \text{Protein + Prosthetic group}$$

   The conjugated proteins are further classified into subclasses based on prosthetic groups.

Different classes of conjugated proteins

	Subclass	Prosthetic group	Examples	Type of linkage
1.	Lipoproteins	Lipids	Various classes of Lipoproteins. Lipovitellin of egg	Hydrophobhic Interaction
2.	Glycoproteins	Carbohydrates	Immunoglobulins of blood, Egg albumin	Covalent
3.	Phosphoproteins	Phosphorus	Casein of milk, vitellin of egg yolk	Covalent
4.	Nucleoproteins	Nucleic acids	Chromatin, Ribosomes	Non-covalent
5.	Hemoproteins/ Chromoproteins	Heme	Hemoglobin, Myoglobin, Cytochromes	Non-covalent
6.	Flavoproteins	Flavin nucleotides FMN, FAD	Succinate Dehydrogenase	Covalent
7.	Metalloproteins	Iron	Ferritin, Cytochromes	Non-covalent
8.	Visual pigments	Retinal	Rhodopsin	Covalent

3. **Derived proteins:** As the name implies this class of proteins are formed from simple and conjugated proteins. There are two classes of derived proteins.

   (*i*) *Primary derived proteins:* They are formed from natural proteins by the action of heat or alcohol etc. The peptide bonds are not hydrolysed. They are synonymous with denatured proteins.

   Example: Coagulated proteins like cooked-egg albumin.

(ii) *Secondary derived proteins:* They are formed from partial hydrolysis of proteins.

Examples: Proteoses, peptone, gelatin, and peptides.

Proteins classification according to their solubility

1. **Albumins:** Soluble in water and salt solutions.

   Examples: Albumin of plasma, egg albumin and lactalbumin of milk.

2. **Globulins:** Sparingly soluble in water but soluble in salt solutions.

   Examples: Globulins of plasma, ovoglobulins of egg, lactoglobulin of milk.

3. **Glutelins:** Soluble in dilute acids and alkalies.

   Examples: Glutenin of wheat, oryzenin of rice, zein of maize.

4. **Protamins:** Soluble in ammonia and water.

   Examples: Salmine from salmon fish, sturine of sturgeon.

5. **Histones:** Soluble in water and dilute acids.

   Example: Histones present in chromatin.

6. **Prolamines:** Soluble in dilute alcohol and insoluble in water and alcohol.

   Examples: Gliadin of wheat, zein of corn.

7. **Sclero proteins:** Insoluble in water and dilute acids and alkalies.

   Examples: Collagen, elastin and keratin.

Classification of proteins based on shape

Proteins are divided into two classes based on their shape.

1. **Globular proteins:** Polypeptide chain(s) of these proteins are folded into compact globular (Spherical) shape.

   Examples: Haemoglobin, myoglobin, albumin, lysozyme, chymotrypsin.

2. **Fibrous proteins:** Poly peptide chains are extended along one axis.

   Examples: α-keratin, β-keratin, collagen and elastin.

PROTEIN STRUCTURE

Since proteins are built from amino acids by linking them in linear fashion, it may be viewed as proteins having long chain like structures. However, such arrangement is unstable and polypeptide or protein folds to specific shape known as *conformation,* which is more stable. Various stages involved in the formation of final conformation from linear chain are divided into four levels or orders of protein structure. They are

1. Primary Structure

The linear sequence of amino acid residues in a polypeptide chain is called as primary structure. Generally disulfide bonds if any are also included in the primary structure.

Bonds responsible for the maintenance of primary structure are mainly peptide bonds and *disulfide* bonds. Both of them are covalent bonds (Fig. 3.1*a*).

Primary Structure of Insulin

This protein consist of two polypeptide chains A and B. The two chains are covalently linked by disulfide bonds. The A chain has N-terminal glycine and C-terminal aspargine. The B chain has phenylalanine and alanine as N-and C-terminal residues, respectively. Insulin is a hormone and its molecular weight is 5,700 (Fig. 3.1*b*).

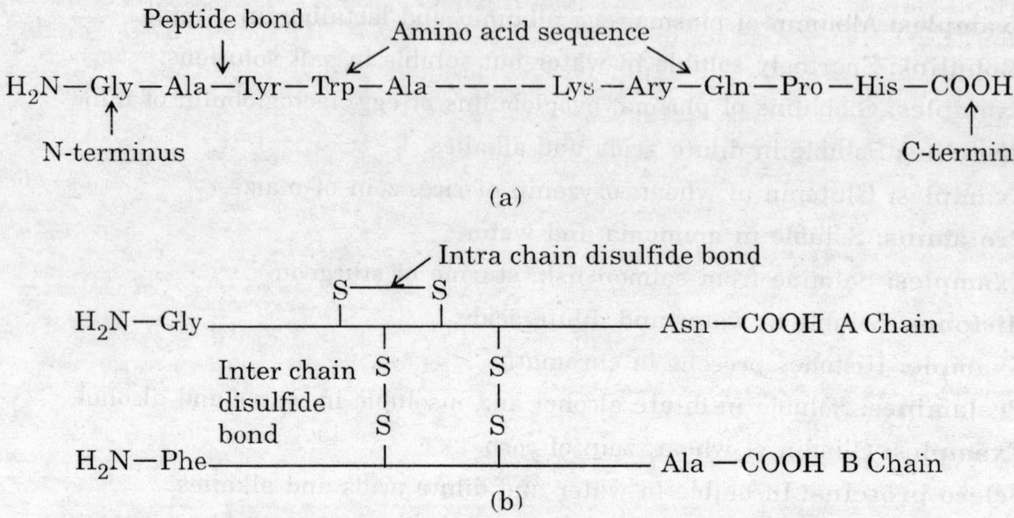

Fig. 3.1 (*a*) Primary structure of a protein (*b*) Insulin primary structure

2. Secondary Structure

Folding of polypeptide chain along its long axis is called as secondary structure of protein. Folding of polypeptide chain can be *ordered, disordered* or *random.* Secondary structure is often referred as *conformation.* So, proteins has *ordered secondary structure* or *conformation* and *random* or *disordered secondary structure* or *conformation.*

Ordered Conformation of Polypeptides

The polypeptide chain of some proteins may exist in highly ordered conformation. The conformation is maintained by *hydrogen bonds* formed between peptide residues.

Hydrogen bond

It is a weak ionic interaction between positively charged hydrogen atom and negatively charged atoms like oxygen, nitrogen, sulfur etc. It is indicated with broken lines (---).

There are two types of ordered secondary structure observed in proteins.

1. The polypeptide chain of α-keratin, which is present in hair, nails, epidermis of the skin is arranged as α-*Helix.* α-letter is given to this type of structure because it was first ordered structure noticed in proteins.
2. Polypeptide chain of β-keratin, which is present in silk fibroin and spider web is arranged in β-*pleated* sheet. The β-letter is given because it was observed later.

Main Features of α-Helix

1. In α-helix polypeptide, backbone is tightly wound round (coiled) long axis of the molecule.

2. The distance between two amino acid residues is 1.5 Å.
3. α-helix contain 3.6 amino acid residues per turn. The R-group of amino acids project outwards of the helix (Fig. 3.2*b*).
4. The pitch of the α-helix is 5.4 Å long and width is 5.0 Å (Fig. 3.2*a*).
5. The α-helix is stabilized by intra chain hydrogen bonds formed between –N–H groups and –C=O groups that are four residues back, *i.e.*, –N–H group of a 6th peptide bond is hydrogen bonded to –C=O group of 2nd peptide bond (Fig. 3.2*b*).

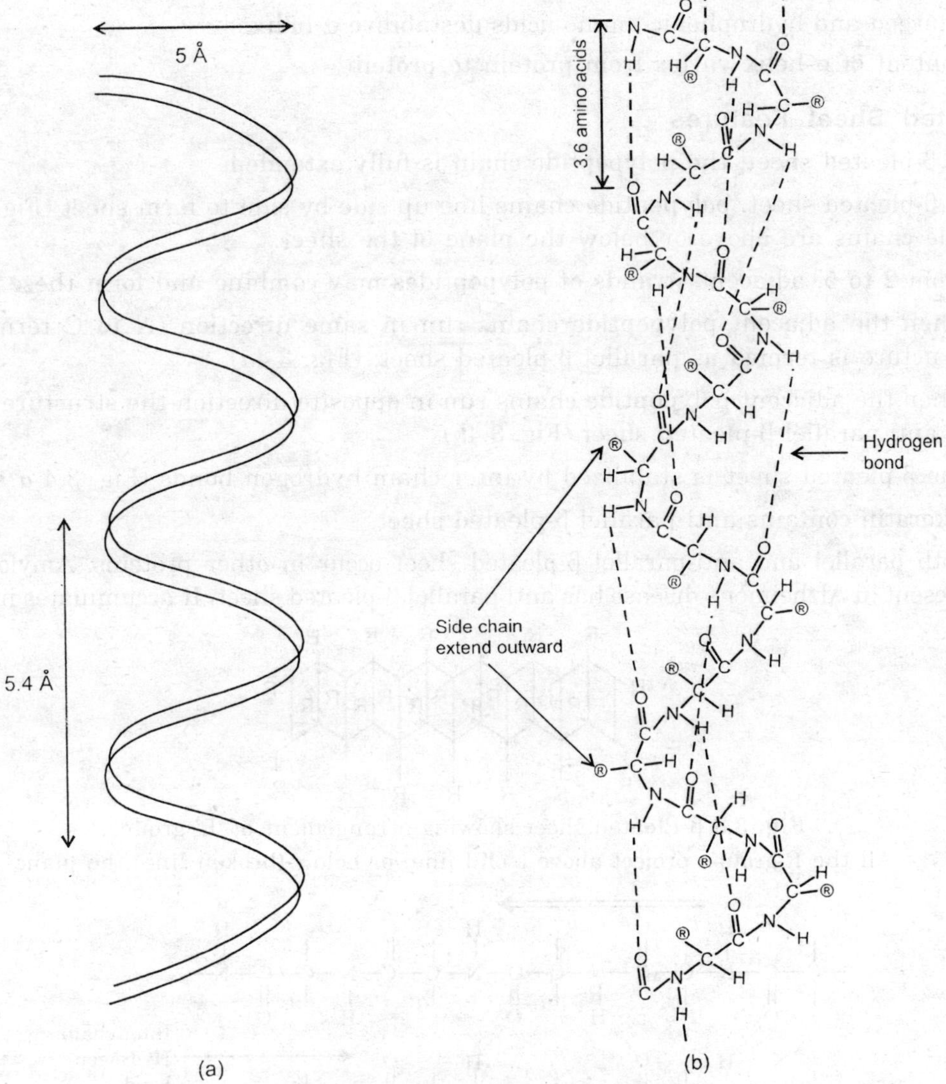

Fig. 3.2 (*a*) Right handed α-helix
(*b*) Intra chain hydrogen bonds between N–H groups and C = O groups that are four residues back

6. Each peptide bond participates in the hydrogen bonding. This gives maximum stability to α-helix.

7. α-helix present in most fibrous proteins is right handed. The right handed α-helix is more stable than the left handed helix.
8. α-helix is hydrophobic in nature because of intra chain hydrogen bonds.
9. An α-helix forms spontaneously since it is the most stable conformation of polypeptide chain.
10. Some amino acids act as terminators for α-helix.

    Example: Proline.
11. Aromatic amino acids stabilizes α-helix.
12. Charged and hydrophobic amino acids destabilize α-helix.
13. Content of α-helix varies from protein to protein.

β-Pleated Sheet Features

1. In β-pleated sheet, the polypeptide chain is fully extended.
2. In β-pleated sheet, polypeptide chains line up side by side to form sheet (Fig. 3.3). The side chains are above or below the plane of the sheet.
3. From 2 to 5, adjacent strands of polypeptides may combine and form these structure.
4. When the adjacent polypeptide chains run in same direction (N to C terminus) the structure is termed as parallel β-pleated sheet. (Fig. 3.4*a*)
5. When the adjacent polypeptide chains run in opposite direction the structure is termed as anti-parallel β-pleated sheet (Fig. 3.4*b*).
6. The β-pleated sheet is stabilized by inter chain hydrogen bonds (Fig. 3.4 *a* and *b*).
7. β-keratin contains anti parallel β-pleated sheet.
8. Both parallel and anti-parallel β-pleated sheet occur in other proteins. Amyloid protein present in Alzheimer's disease has anti parallel β-pleated sheet. It accumulates in the CNS.

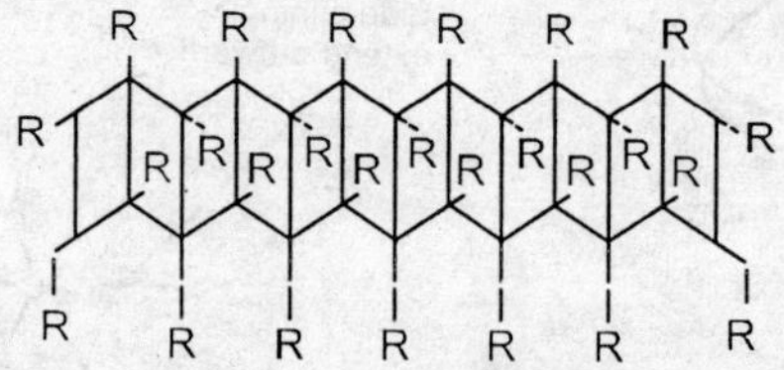

Fig. 3.3 β-Pleated sheet showing arrangement of 'R' groups. All the R-groups project above (solid line) or below (broken line) the plane

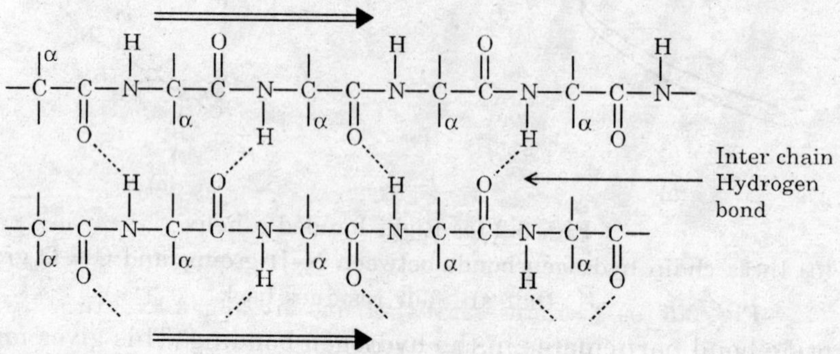

Fig. 3.4 (*a*) Parallel β-structure showing interchain hydrogen bonds

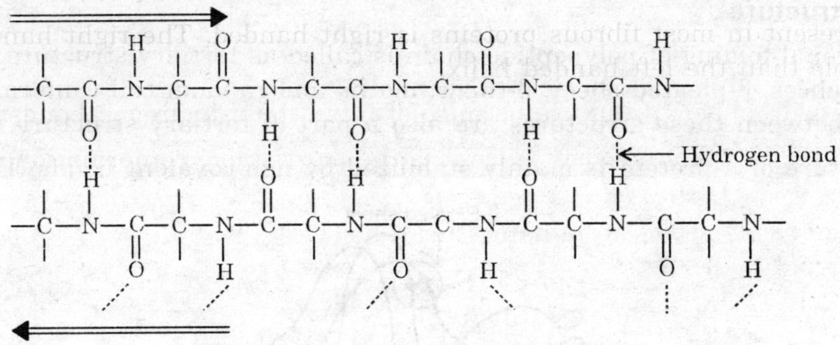

Fig. 3.4 (*b*) Anti-parallel β-structure

Random Coil (Disordered) Conformation

Regions of proteins that are not organized as helices and pleated sheet are said to be present in random coil conformation. These are also equally important for biological function of proteins as those of helices and β-pleated sheet.

β-turn or β-bends (Reverse Turn)

Hair pin turn of a polypeptide chain is called as β-turn. The change in the direction of a polypeptide chain is achieved by β-turn. β-turn connects anti parallel β-sheets. Usually four aminoacids make up β-turn. Gly, Ser, Asp, proline are involved in β-turns. (Fig. 3.5*a*)

Super Secondary Structure

In some globular proteins regions of α-helix and β-pleated sheet join to form super secondary structure or motifs. They are very important for biological function. (Fig. 3.5*b*)

Super Helix

α-keratin consist of right handed α-helix as basic unit. Three such α-helices get cross linked by disulfide bonds and form super secondary structure. (Fig. 3.5*c*)

Triple Helix

Collagen present in skin, cartilage, bone and tendons consists of left handed helix as basic unit. Three left handed helices are wrapped around each other to right handed super secondary structure triple helix.

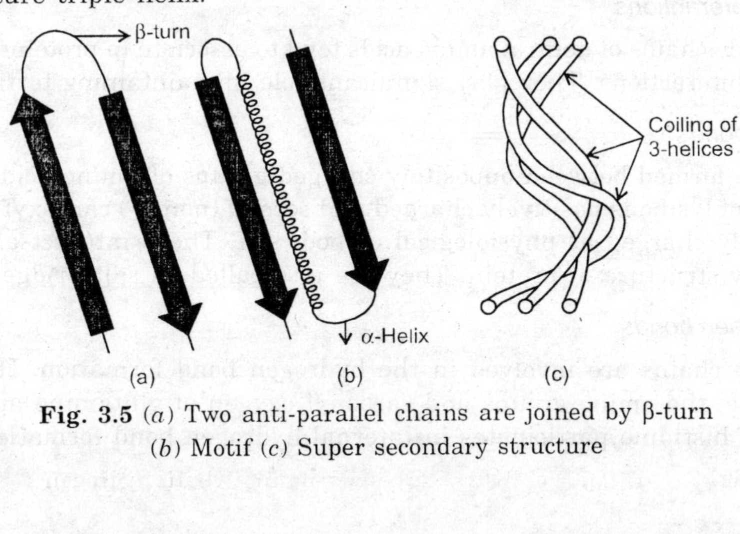

Fig. 3.5 (*a*) Two anti-parallel chains are joined by β-turn
(*b*) Motif (*c*) Super secondary structure

3. Tertiary Structure

Three-dimensional folding of polypeptide chain is called as tertiary structure. It consists of regions of α-helices, β-pleated sheet, β-turns, motifs and random coil conformations. Interrelationships between these structures are also a part of tertiary structure (Fig. 3.6).

Tertiary structure of a protein is mainly stabilized by non-covalent bonds (Fig. 3.7).

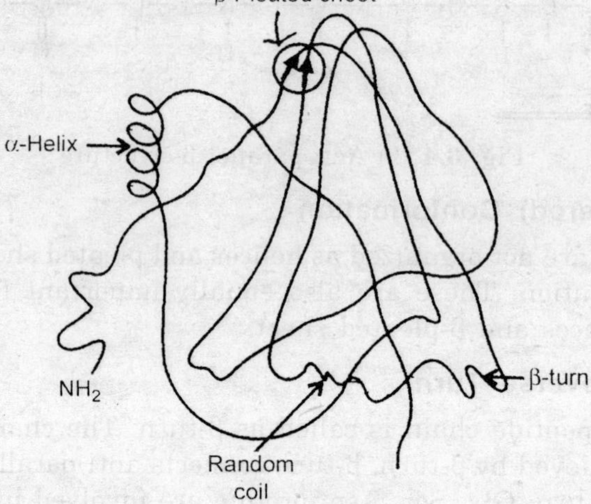

Fig. 3.6 Schematic diagram showing tertiary structure and different types of secondary structures of a protein molecule

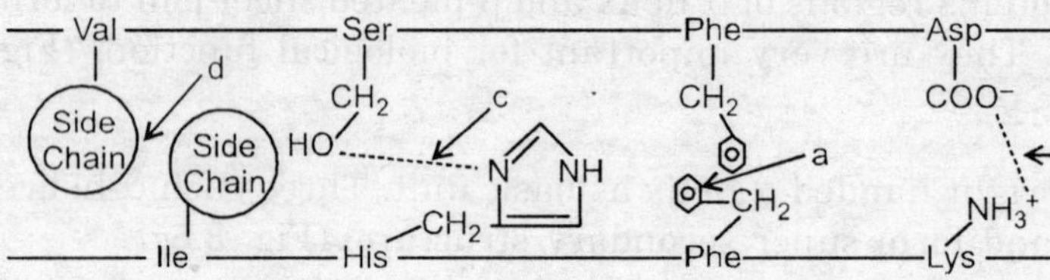

Fig. 3.7 Non-covalent bonds present in tertiary structure (*a*) Hydrophobic interaction (*b*) Electrostatic bonds (*c*) Internal hydrogen bonds (*d*) vander waal's interactions

A. Hydrophobic interactions

The non-polar side chains of neutral amino acids tend to associate in proteins. These are called as hydrophobic interactions. They play significant role in maintaining tertiary structure.

B. Electrostatic bonds

These bonds are formed between oppositely charged groups of amino acid side chains. The ε-amino groups of lysine is positively charged and second (non-α-) carboxyl group of aspartic acid is negatively charged at physiological or body pH. These interact electrostatically to stabilize tertiary structure of protein. They are also called as salt bridges.

C. Internal hydrogen bonds

Amino acid side chains are involved in the hydrogen bond formation. Hydroxyl group of serine, threonine, the amino groups and carbonyl oxygen of glutamine and aspargine, the ring nitrogen of histidine participates in internal hydrogen bond formation.

D. Vander waals interactions

These are the weak interactions between uncharged groups of protein molecule. They also contribute to the stability of proteins.

4. Quaternary Structure

Proteins containing two or more polypeptide chains possess quaternary structure. These proteins are called as *oligomers*. The individual polypeptide chains are called as protomer, *monomers* or *subunits*. The protomers are united by forces other than covalent bonds. Occasionally, they may be joined by disulfide bonds. (Fig. 3.8)

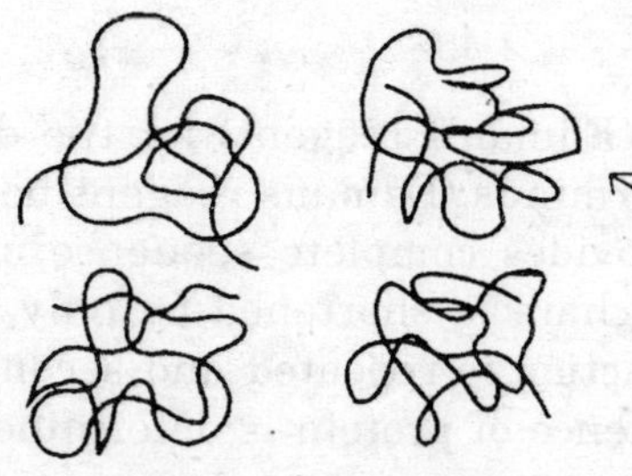

Fig. 3.8 Quaternary structure of a tetramer.

The most common oligomeric proteins contain 2 or 4 protomers and are termed dimers and tetramers.

Forces that stabilize these aggregates (assembles of monomers) are:

1. Hydrogen bonding
2. Electrostatic interactions
3. Hydrophobic interactions
4. Vander waals interactions
5. Disulfide bridges (in some proteins)

Examples: 1. Haemoglobin consist of 4 polypeptide chains.
2. Hexokinase contains 2 subunits.
3. Pryuvate dehydrogenase contains 72 subunits.

Determination of Protein Structure

The primary structure of protein directs specific folding (secondary structure) and its tertiary structure. If there is a change in one of the amino acids of protein, then conformation of polypeptide chain alters, which results change in biological function. Further, the sequence of amino acids in proteins that gives them their striking specific biological actions. Therefore knowledge of primary structure of a protein is required for the understanding of relationship of a protein's structure to its function at molecular level.

Determination of Primary Structure of Protein

1. Sanger's reagent

Sanger used FDNB (1-Fluoro-2, 4-Dinitrobenzene) to determine the amino acid sequence of a polypeptide chain from N-terminus. Sanger's reagent can be used to determine only one amino acid at a time because FDNB reacts with other amino acids. FDNB arylates free amino acid group and produces intense yellow 2, 4-dinitrophenyl residues of amino acids. These derivatives are separated by chromatography and identified (Fig. 3.9).

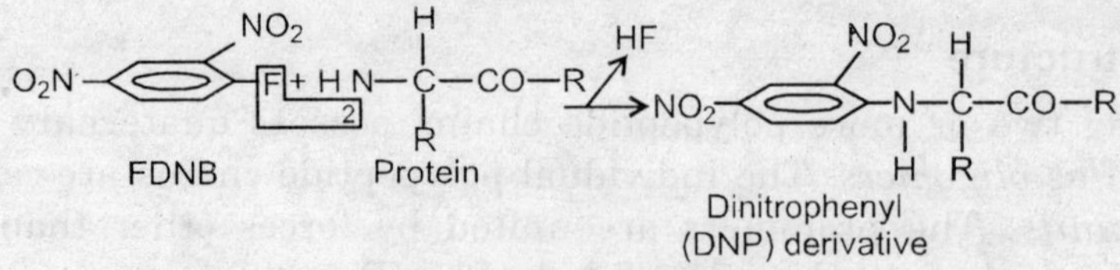

Fig. 3.9 Sanger's reaction

2. Edman's reagent

Edman used phenylisothiocyanate (Edman's reagent) for the determination of amino acid sequence of a protein from the N-terminus. Edmans reagent not only identifies N-terminus but also when used repeatedly provides complete sequence of the polypeptide chain. In Edman's reaction, the polypeptide chain is shortened by only one residue and rest of the polypeptide remains intact. The reaction is repeated and second residue is determined. By continued repetition, complete sequence of protein is determined starting from N-terminus (Fig. 3.10).

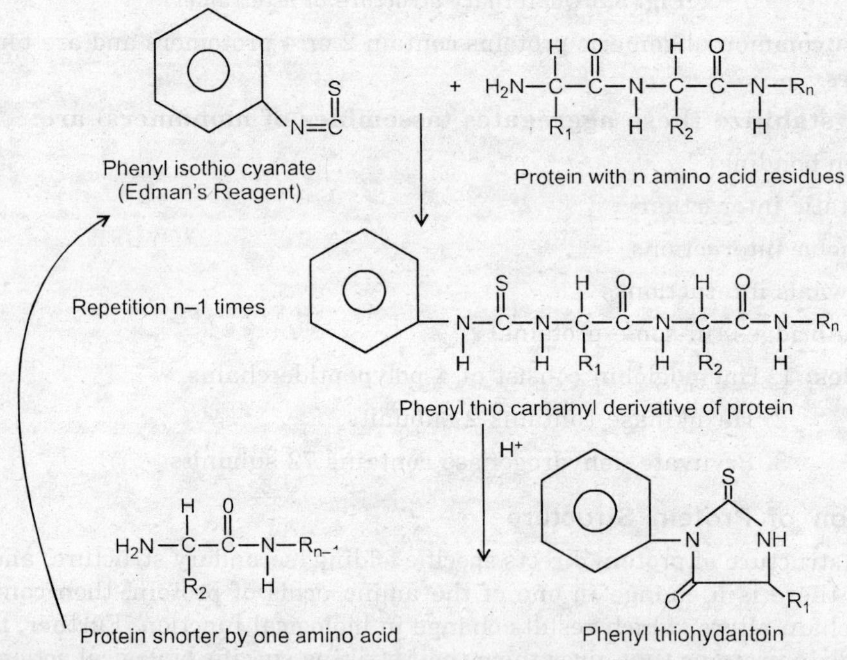

Fig. 3.10 Edman's reaction for sequence determination of protein from N-terminus

Edman's reagent react with amino group and produces phenylthiocarbamyl derivatives on treatment with acid. Phenylthiocarbamyl derivative cyclizes to phenylthiohydantoins. They are estimated using chromatography.

Protein Folding

Let us examine how polypeptide chain attains native conformation as soon as it comes out of protein synthesizing machinery. Though exact mechanisms involved in protein folding are not known due to extensive investigations carried out some information on protein folding mechanisms is available.

Stages of Protein Folding

Protein folding occurs by stages:

(a) Domains formation

α-helical, β-pleated sheet, β-bend containing domains are formed in the initial step of folding of polypeptide chain. This self assembling process mostly depends on primary structure. It involves extensive interaction among amino acids residues side chains of polypeptide chain. It is governed by thermodynamic principles like free energy etc.

(b) Molten globule

In the next step domains from molten globule state in which secondary structure predominates and tertiary structure is highly disordered.

(c) Native conformation

Finally native conformation develops from molten globule state after several minor conformational changes and rearrangements.

(d) Oligomer formation

In the case of multimeric or oligomeric proteins after attaining specific conformation protomers or sub-units may assemble into native like structure initially. After some realignments it ultimately gives rise to final conformation of oligomer.

Additional Protein Folding Factors

Though self association of polypeptide chain into ordered conformation is largely determined by amino acid sequence (primary structure) recent research has shown that in some cases folding of protein requires additional factors. Some of them are enzymes and some are protein factors.

Protein Folding Enzymes

Two protein folding enzymes are known:

(a) Disulfide isomerase

In the newly formed protein molecules –SH groups of cysteine residues may form several intra or inter disulfide linkages. However, only few disulfide linkages may be essential for proper protein folding. The disulfide isomerase favours formation of such disulfide linkages by breaking unwanted linkages formed.

(b) Cis-trans prolyl isomerase

It aids folding process by catalyzing inter conversion of *cis-trans* peptide bonds of proline residues of folding protein.

Protein Factors

Chaperons (Chaperonins)

These proteins aid protein folding process by preventing formation of aggregates. Usually aggregate formation slows down protein folding process. Chaperons accelerate protein folding by blocking protein folding pathways of unproductive nature. They bind to hydrophobic parts of protein molecules and prevent formation of aggregates. They are also involved in protein refolding that occurs when proteins cross membrane structures.

Denaturation of Proteins

Denaturation is loss of native conformation. On denaturation, physical chemical and biological properties of a protein are altered (Fig. 3.11).

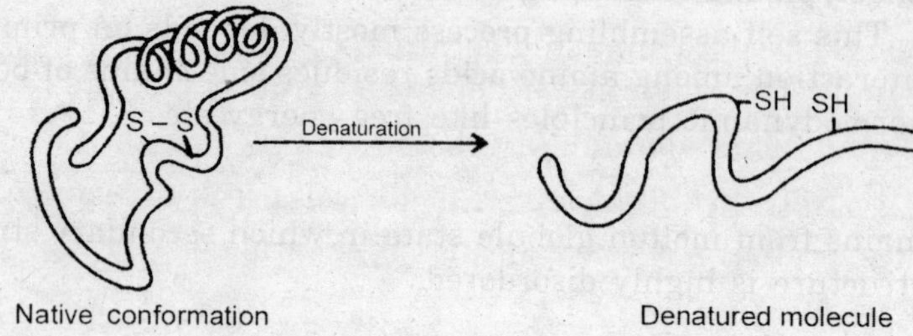

Fig. 3.11 Denaturation of protein

Some of the changes in properties are:

1. Decreased solubility
2. Unfolding of polypeptide chain
3. Loss of helical structure
4. Decreased or loss of biological activity
5. More susceptible to action of enzymes
6. Increased chemical reactivity
7. Dissociation of subunits in case of oligomeric proteins.

Causes of Denaturation

1. High temperature
2. Extreme alkaline or acidic pH
3. Use of urea and guanidine at high concentration
4. UV radiation
5. Sonication
6. Vigorous shaking
7. Detergent like sodium dodecylsulfate also denatures protein
8. Treatment with organic solvents like ethanol, acetone etc.
9. Treatment with strong acids like trichloro acetic acid, picric acid and tungstic acid
10. Exposure to heavy metals like Pb^{2+}, Ag^{2+} and Cu^{2+}

Biomedical Importance

1. These properties are exploited for the separation of serum proteins from the other compounds of clinical importance.

2. Denaturation knowledge is required when activities of enzymes in biological fluids like blood are measured for diagnosis.
3. Purification of protein from mixture of proteins also needs denaturation properties.
4. Lead poisoning cases are treated with egg white to decrease toxicity of lead in the body.

Many cases of the process of denaturation is irreversible.

Examples of Denaturation

1. When egg white is exposed to high temperature coagulum is formed because heat denatures egg albumin. The solubility of denatured protein is decreased.
2. Formation of coagulum when albumin is exposed to high temperature.
3. Heat treatment of trypsin results in loss of biological activity.
4. Monellin is a dimeric protein has sweet taste. On denaturation the sweet taste is lost.

Renaturation

Though denaturation is irreversible in majority of the cases, in few cases, renaturation is observed.

Example: Ribonuclease denatures on exposure to heat but come back to its native conformation when temperature is lowered.

PLASMA PROTEINS

Plasma is non-cellular portion of blood. The total plasma protein level ranges from 6-7 gm/dl. Plasma contains many structurally and functionally different proteins. Plasma proteins are divided into two categories.

1. **Albumin:** Not precipitated by half-saturated ammonium sulfate.
2. **Globulin:** Precipitated by half-saturated ammonium sulfate.

The albumin constitutes over half of the total protein. Albumin level ranges from 3.5-5.5 gm/dl. Globulin ranges from 2-3 gm/dl. After the age of 40, albumin gradually declines with an increase in globulins. Albumin is found to be simple protein and a single entity. But globulin has been found to contain many components. Subglobulins are detected as bands on electrophoresis. They are α_1, α_2, β and γ-globulins. Electrophoretic pattern is shown in (Fig. 3.12*a*). The different plasma protein bands are semi-quantitated using densitometer (Fig. 3.12*b*).

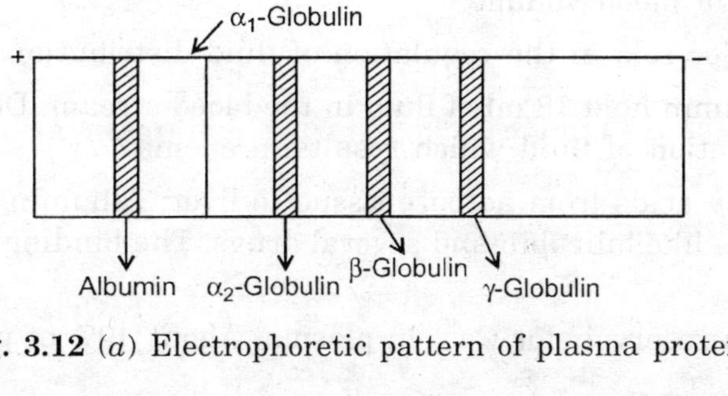

Fig. 3.12 (*a*) Electrophoretic pattern of plasma proteins

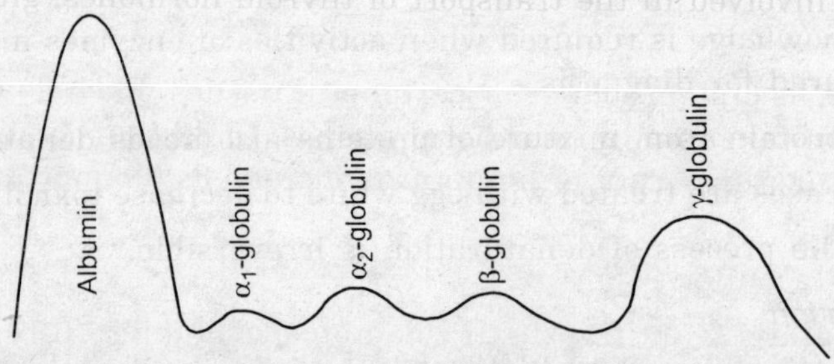

Fig. 3.12 (*b*) Densitometer scan of different plasma protein bands

Characteristics of Plasma Proteins

1. They are all glycoproteins except albumin. Sialic acid is the most important of all the sugars present in plasma proteins. Removal of sialic acid decreases the life span of plasma proteins.
2. Each plasma protein has defined life span. The half life of albumin is 20 days and haptoglobin life span is 15 days.
3. Liver is the sole source of albumin, prothrombin and fibrinogen. Most of the α and β globulins are also of hepatic origin. γ-globulins are derived from lymphocytes.

Albumin

Liver produces about 12 gms of albumin per day.

Structure

It consists of single polypeptide chain of 584 amino acid residues with a molecular weight of 66,300. Charged amino acids (glutamate, aspartate and lysine) make up a quarter of the total amino acid residues. The acidic residues out number the basic amino acids hence molecule is highly negative charged which accounts for the high mobility of albumin towards anode. Secondary structure of the protein is over half is in the α-helical conformation. 15% as β-pleated structure and remaining in random coil conformation. The tertiary structure is that of globular protein. The overall shape resembles ovoid. The hydrophobic amino acid residues are present in the hydrophobic interior and polar amino acids are arranged to face exterior of the albumin. This accounts for the high solubility of the albumin in water (aqueous solutions).

Functions

1. Albumin accounts for 75% of the osmotic pressure (25 mm Hg) in blood and responsible for maintenance of blood volume.
2. Albumin has major role in the regulation of fluid distribution.
3. One gram of albumin hold 18 ml of fluid in the blood stream. Decrease in albumin level leads to accumulation of fluid which results in edema.
4. It transports fatty acids from adipose tissue to liver. Albumin also binds many hydrophobic substances like bilirubin and several drugs. The binding of bilirubin is critical in neo-natal period.
5. Albumin act as a reservoir for Ca^{2+} in plasma. About 40% of plasma calcium is bound to albumin.

6. Albumin is also involved in the transport of thyroid hormones, glucocorticoids and sex steroids.
7. Albumin function as protein source for peripheral tissues. Each day liver replaces about 12 gm of albumin taken up by peripheral tissues. In certain conditions like stress and starvation the turn over rate of albumin is increased. Albumin is in dynamic equilibrium.
8. Albumin acts as a buffer.

α_1-Globulin: Mainly α_1-antitrypsin. It is a protease inhibitor. It is the major component of α_1-fraction and accounts more than 90%. It inhibits trypsin, chymotrypsin, elastase and neutral protease. The major function of α_1-antitrypsin is the protection of pulmonary tissue and other tissues from the destructive action of proteases.

$$\underset{(\alpha_1-\text{AT}) \text{ or AAT}}{\alpha_1-\text{antitrypsin}} \xrightarrow{\text{Elastase}} \underset{(\text{In active})}{\alpha_1-\text{AT - Elastase complex}} \longrightarrow \text{No proteolysis} \longrightarrow \text{No lung damage}$$

$$\text{Lung tissue} \xrightarrow{\text{Elastase}} \text{Proteolysis} \longrightarrow \text{Lung damage}$$

Deficiency of α_1-antitrypsin results in emphysema.

α_1-Acid glycoprotein (AAG): It is another major component of α_1-globulins. It increases in plasma in inflammatory conditions.

Other components of α_1-globulins are

α-Lipoprotein: Functions in the transport of lipids (HDL). It transports cholesterol from extra hepatic tissue to liver.

Prothrombin: Blood clotting factor.

Retinolbinding protein: Transport of Vit A.

Thyroxine binding globulin: Transport of thyroxine.

α_1-Fetoprotein: It is present only in fetal serum. Its presence in non-foetal serum indicates primary carcinoma of liver. It is referred as tumour marker.

α_2-Globulins: The α_2-fraction of globulins includes.

Haptoglobulin: It combines with haemoglobin in order to remove it from the circulation. Kidney can not filter haemoglobin-haptoglobin complex because of its larger size.

α_2-Macroglobulin: It functions as protease inhibitor. It combines with proteases and facilitates their removal from circulation. It also binds with cytokines and involved in zinc transport.

Ceruloplasmin: A copper binding plasma protein and function as ferrooxidase and converts

$$Fe^{2+} \longrightarrow Fe^{3+}$$

Erythropoietin: It is involved in erythropoiesis.

Pseudocholinesterase: It is only functional enzyme present in plasma. It hydrolyzes acetylcholine.

β-Globulins: They are

Transferrin: It accounts for about 60% of β-globulins. It is an iron transport protein.

β-Lipoproteins: Involved in the transport of cholesterol from liver to extrahepatic tissue (LDL).

Complement-3: It is one of the member of complement system present in plasma. It is involved in phagocytosis.

Other globulins present in plasma are:

Fibrinogen: It is similar to globulins because it is precipitated by half saturation with ammonium sulfate. It is a fibrous or filamentous protein. It is the precursor of fibrin, the blood clotting substances.

Prealbumin: It is a component of globulin fraction. Though it is a globulin by nature it is named as prealbumin because it migrates ahead of a albumin in electrophoresis. It is a carrier of thyroxine, Vitamin A and binds calcium.

Other blood clotting factors, plasminogen and several non-functional enzymes are also present in plasma.

Acute Phase Proteins or Reactants (APR)

1. The concentration of these proteins increases markedly during acute inflammation.
2. They are α_1-antitrypsin, haptoglobin, ceruloplasmin, complement-3, fibrinogen and c-reactive protein. Their concentration increases in conditions like surgery, myocardial infraction, infections and tumours.
3. Acute phase reaction is general to any infection. They all play part in complex defensive process of inflammation.
4. The synthesis of these proteins by liver is triggered by interleukin at the site of injury.
5. The plasma levels of these APR raises at different rates. The levels of c-reactive protein raises first followed by α_1-antitrypsin. The level of complement-3 raises at the end (Fig. 3.13).

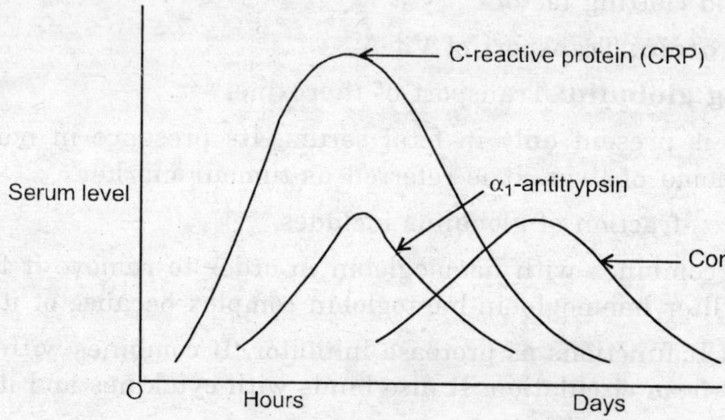

Fig. 3.13 APR levels after injury

γ-Globulins

The immunoglobulins and c-reactive protein (CRP) constitutes this fraction. C-reactive protein is so called because it forms precipitate with somatic C-polysaccharide of pneumococcus bacteria.

IMMUNOGLOBULINS

They are globulins produced as body's immune or defence against infection. Invasion of body by virus or microorganisms or foreign molecules is called *infection*. They are produced by

B-lymphocytes, bone marrow and spleen in response to infection. Entry of foreign molecule into body triggers the synthesis of specific globulin, which selectively combines with foreign molecule and lead to its inactivation. The foreign molecule is called as *antigen* where as globulin produced against it is called as antibody. Even without infection the normal plasma contains hundreds of different antibody molecules.

Classification

The immunoglobulin (Ig) proteins of plasma are divided into three major classes Ig G, Ig A, Ig M and two minor classes Ig D, Ig E based on their composition.

Structure

The composition and shape of various classes of immunoglobulins have similar pattern and are represented by the structure of major G class of molecule *i.e.,* Ig G. Each Ig G molecule consist of 4 polypeptide chains and molecular weight is 150,000. The four polypeptide chains are of two types. They are two heavy chains or H chains or about 450 amino acids (molecular weight 50,000) and two light or L chains or about 220 amino acids (molecular weight 25,000). Over all shape of the molecule represents 'Y'. Two heavy chains intertwine to form the base of the Y, a disulfide bond links the L chain to H chain to form arm of the Y. The two heavy chains are held together by disulfide bonds formed between them at the hinge region of the Y (Fig. 3.14).

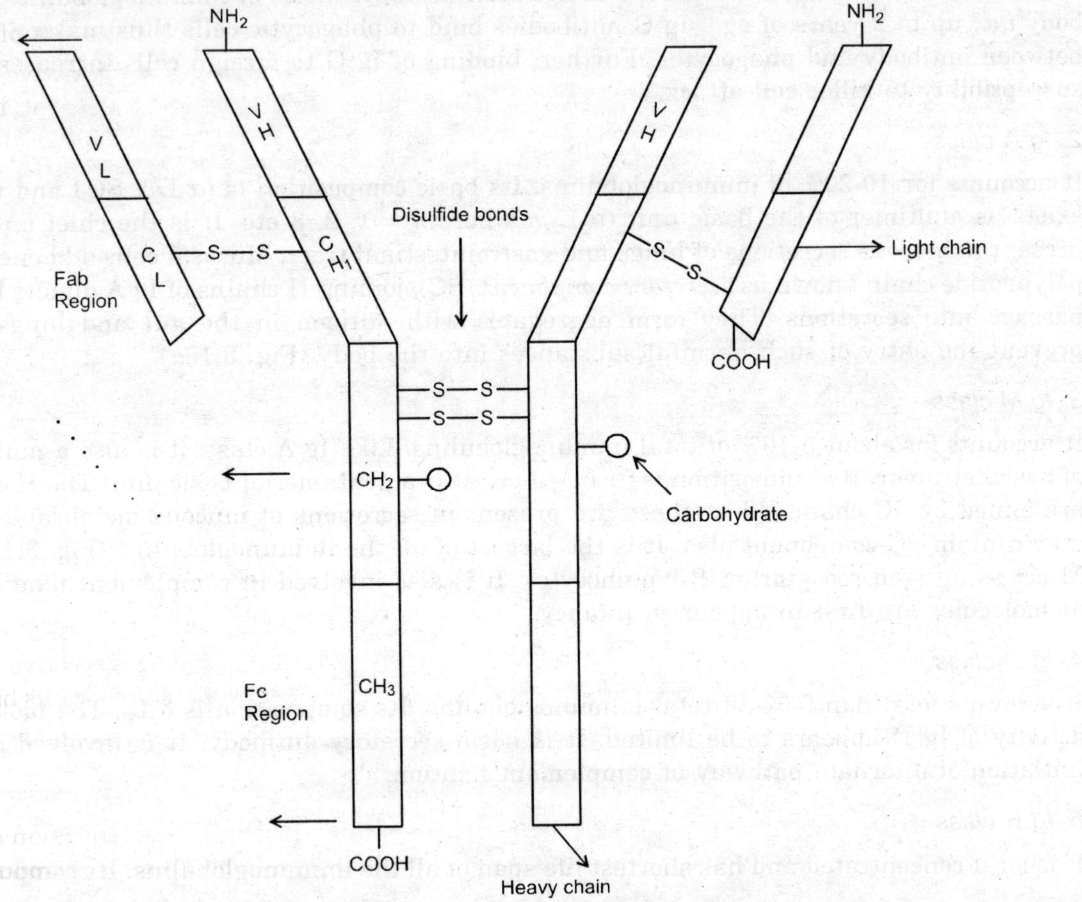

Fig. 3.14 Structure of an immunoglobulin (I_g)

The H chain contains variable region of domain (V_H) at the N-terminus and three constant domains (C_{H_1}, C_{H_2}, C_{H_3}) at the C-terminus. Like wise L chain consists of variable domain (V_L) at the N-terminus and a constant domain (C_L) at the C-terminus. The carbohydrate is attached to C_{H_2} of the heavy chain. The amino acid sequence in the variable regions of H and L chains varies and are specific to the type of antibody. In contrast amino acid sequence in constant region of H and L chains are same in each class of immunoglobulins. The antigen binding site is called as *Fab site*. It consists of light chain and N-terminal half of the heavy chain. The remaining part of the immunoglobulin is called as Fc (fragment with constant domain).

The different classes of immunoglobulins vary in their size, distribution, function and composition. The main chemical differences are found in their H chains. They are named according to the types of H chain present. There are five classes of H chains. They are γ, α, μ, δ, ε. However, there are only two classes of L chains κ or λ.

Different Classes of Immunoglobulins

1. Ig G class

It constitutes 70 to 80% serum immunoglobulins. Its composition is γ_2L_2 (γ_2k_2 or $\gamma_2\lambda_2$). It is the only class of antibody that is capable of crossing the placental barrier from the maternal to fetal circulation. It is the antibody of newborn until synthesis of immunoglobulins in the body *i.e.,* up to 2 years of age. Ig G antibodies bind to phagocytic cells thus making a link between antibody and phagocytes. Further, binding of Ig G to foreign cells increases their susceptibility to killer cell attack.

2. Ig A class

It accounts for 10-20% of immunoglobulins. Its basic composition is (α_2L_2), SCJ and it also exists as multimer of the basic unit $(\alpha_2L_2)n$ where n = 1, 2, 3 etc. It is the chief antibody present in mucous secretions of lungs and gastrointestinal tract. Mucosal cells add one more polypeptide chain known as *secretory component* (SC), joining H chains of Ig A dimers before passage into secretions. They form aggregates with antigen in the gut and lungs thus prevent the entry of such harmful substances into the body (Fig. 3.15*a*).

3. Ig M class

It accounts for about 5-10% of total immunoglobulins. Like Ig A class, it is also a multimer of basic tetramer. Its composition is $(\mu_2L_2)_5$ J *i.e.,* it is a pentamer of basic unit. The H chains are joined by JC chain. When these are present in secretions of mucous membranes they may contain SC component also. It is the largest of all the immunoglobulins (Fig. 3.15*b*) Ig M act as antigen receptor on B-lymphocytes. It is also involved in complement fixation. Ig M molecules are first to appear in infancy.

4. Ig D class

It accounts less than 0.5% of total immunoglobulins. Its composition is δ_2L_2. The biological activity of Ig D appears to be limited. It is not a secretory antibody. It is involved in the initiation of alternate pathway of complement fixation.

5. Ig E class

It is least concentrated and has shortest life span of all the immunoglobulins. Its composition is ε_2L_2. Ig E concentration increases in allergic reactions. It is a surface antibody of cells involved in anaphylactic response. The constant region of the antibody is bound to membrane receptor of leukocytes or mast cells and variable region is exposed to the outer surface. When the specific antigen reacts with antibody, it triggers the cells to release histamine and other vasoactive amines. The Ig E class also found in secretions of lungs and gut but the Ig Es lack the J chain and SC part found in Ig As and Ig Ms.

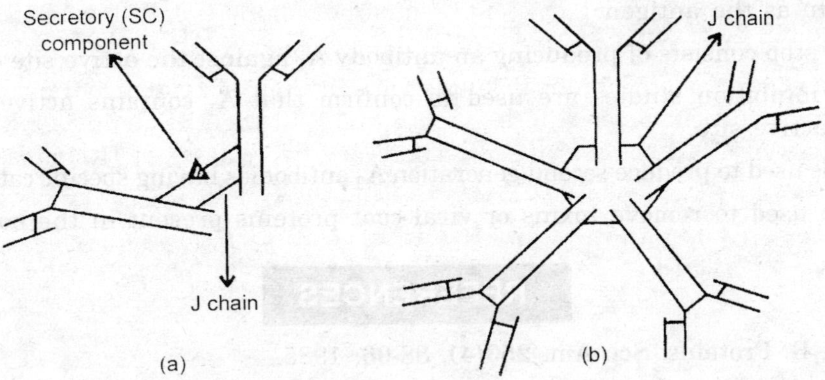

Fig. 3.15 *(a)* I_g A dimer *(b)* Structure of I_g M (pentamer)

Immunoglobulins Disorders

There are numerous disorders associated with different classes of immunoglobulins.

1. Multiplemyeloma

It is a malignant disease of single clone (cell type) of plasma cells of the bone marrow. These plasma cells proliferate throughout bone marrow. Other bone marrow cells are reduced. Tumours of the plasma cells produce myeloma proteins.

The incidence is low in individuals younger than 60 years but raises with age. Symptoms include recurrent infections, weight loss, bone lesions, anaemia and haemorrhages.

Bence-Jones proteins

They are immunoglobulins light chains present in plasma and urine of multiple myeloma patients. The molecular weight is 2500. They are found with γ-globulin fraction on electrophoresis. The characteristic property of these proteins is their behaviour on heating. The normal plasma proteins precipitates between 60-70°C. The Bence-Jones proteins precipitate at 40-60 °C completely. Redissolving of the precipitate occurs as the temperature reaches boiling point. Subsequent cooling reprecipitates the protein and boiling redissolves it. They are identified in the urine of the suspected individuals based on this property.

2. Agammaglobulinemia

It is x-chromosome linked and affects only males. γ-globulins are absent in plasma of these patients. So they are prone to infections.

3. Hypogammaglobulinemia

Production of γ-globulins is decreased in these cases.

4. Autoimmune disorders

Sometimes body rejects its own proteins which becomes antigenic. This results in auto immune disorders due to production of antibodies against its own proteins. Rheumatoid arthritis is known auto immune disorder.

Catalytic Antibodies or Abzymes

1. Immunoglobulins bearing catalytic activity of an enzyme are produced using an enzyme active site as the antigen.
2. The first step consists of producing an antibody A_1 against the active site of an enzyme.
3. Enzyme inhibition studies are used to confirm that A_1 contains active site close to enzyme active site.
4. Then A_1 is used to produce second generation A_2 antibodies having specific catalytic activity.
5. They are used to remove toxins or viral coat proteins present in the body.

REFERENCES

1. Doolittle, R. Proteins. Sci. Am. **253(4)**, 88-96, 1985.
2. Blake, C.C.F. and Johnson, L.N. Protein structure. Trends Biochem. Science **9**, 147-151, 1984.
3. Rose, G.D. Geselowitz, A.R. Lesser, G.J. Lee, R.H. and Zehfus, M.H. Hydrophobicity of amino acid residues in globular proteins. Science **229**, 834-838, 1985.
4. Brekke, O.H. Michaelson, T.E. and Sendie, I. Immunology Today **16**, 85-90, 1995.
5. Tonegawa, S. The molecules of immune system. Sci. Am. **254(4)**, 104-113, 1985.
6. Lichtenstein, L.M. Allergy and the immune system. Sci. Am. **269(6)**, 84-93, 1993.
7. Creighton, T.E. Proteins: structure and molecular properties. Freeman, Sanfrancisco, 1983.
8. Lerner, R.A. Benkovic, S.J. and Schultz, P.G. At the cross roads of chemistry and immunology: catalytic antibodies. Science **252**, 659-667, 1991.
9. Gregor. *et al.* Coordinated action of HSP 70 Chaperones. Science **303**, 98-101, 2004.
10. Chang, H-C. and Chang, G-G. Involvement of single residue tryptophan 548 in the quarternary structure stability of pigeon cytosolic malic enzyme. J. Biol. Chem. **278**, 23996-24002, 2003.
11. Frantz, S. Protein folding diseases. Raising the bar. Nature Reviews and Drug Discovery **2**, 254, 2003.
12. Fersht, A. Structure and mechanism in protein science. W.H. Freeman and Co., New York, 1999.
13. Timothy, P. Proteomics. Kluwer Academic Press, 2001.
14. Pennington, S.R. and Micheal J.D. Proteomics: from protein sequence to function. BIOS, Oxford, 2001.
15. Branden, C. and Tooze, J. Introduction to protein structure. Garland Publishing Inc., NY, USA, 1999.
16. Reichmann, D. *et al.* The modular architecture of protein-protein binding interfaces. Proc. Nats. Acad. Sci. USA **102**, 57-62, 2005.

EXERCISES

ESSAY QUESTIONS

1. Classify proteins based on composition. Give examples for each class.
2. Explain terms primary, secondary, tertiary and quaternary structure of proteins. Write various forces that stabilize protein structure.
3. Describe immunoglobulins with respect to structure, classification and functions.
4. Describe plasma proteins.
5. Write an essay on functions of proteins with examples.

SHORT QUESTIONS

1. Define denaturation. Name methods of protein denaturation and write importance of this process in medicine.
2. Write salient features of α-helix.
3. Write methods used for determination of primary structure of protein.
4. Explain primary structure of insulin.
5. Name acute phase proteins. In what conditions, they are elevated in blood ?
6. What is normal plasma protein level? Draw electrophoretic pattern of plasma proteins.
7. Write a note on super secondary structure of proteins.
8. Define abzymes. How they are produced ? Write their clinical importance.
9. Write a note on diseases associated with immunoglobulins.
10. Write briefly on Bence-Jones proteins.
11. Mention five structural features of β-pleated sheet.
12. Define primary structure. Write its importance.
13. Write about forces that stabilizes quaternary structure of protein.
14. Write normal plasma albumin level. Mention its functions.
15. Briefly write on various components of α_1-globulins.
16. Write a note on charge properties of protein.
17. Name various components of β-globulins. Mention their functions.
18. Write short note on immunoglobulin structure.
19. Define isoelectric point of protein. Give an example. Write about properties of protein at isoelectric point.
20. Write briefly about structure of albumin and collagen.
21. Name Edman's reagent. Write its importance.
22. Write about changes that occurs in protein properties on denaturation.
23. Define renaturation. Give an example.
24. Define derived proteins. Give examples.
25. Write a note on conjugated proteins.

MULTIPLE CHOICE QUESTIONS

1. All the following statements are correct regarding protein except:
   (*a*) Proteins are involved in transport of gases.
   (*b*) Proteins are involved in defence.
   (*c*) Proteins act as buffers.
   (*d*) Proteins are not found in all cells.
2. In fibrous proteins, polypeptide chains are
   (*a*) Extended (*b*) Folded
   (*c*) Twisted (*d*) Coiled
3. Hair pin turn of polypeptide chain is called as
   (*a*) β-Turn (*b*) α-Turn
   (*c*) γ-Turn (*d*) β-pleated turn
4. In the body, one gram of albumin holds
   (*a*) 10 ml of fluid (*b*) 18 ml of fluid
   (*c*) 25 ml of fluid (*d*) 20 fatty acids
5. Tumour marker present in liver cancer patient blood is
   (*a*) Haptoglobulin (*b*) Acid protein
   (*c*) α-Feto protein (*d*) Thyroxine
6. The concentration of Ig E class of immunoglobulin increases in blood in
   (*a*) Allergic reactions (*b*) Cancers
   (*c*) Cold conditions (*d*) Neonatal life

FILL IN THE BLANKS

1. --------------and -------------- are connective tissues proteins.
2. The isoelectric point of casein is --------------.
3. Gliadin of wheat is an example for --------------.
4. β-pleated sheet is stabilized by -------------- hydrogen bonds.
5. Quaternary structure of hemoglobin consists of --------------.
6. Emphysema is due to deficiency of --------------.
7. Plasma and urine of multiple myeloma patients contains --------------.
8. Immunoglobulins bearing catalytic activity are called as --------------.

4

CHAPTER

ENZYMES

OCCURRENCE

Enzymes are produced by all living organisms including humans and present only in small amounts.

MEDICAL AND BIOLOGICAL IMPORTANCE

1. Enzymes are the chemical work horses of the body. Enzymes are biological catalysts that speed up the pace of chemical reactions.
2. A chemical reaction without an enzyme is like a drive over a mountain. The enzyme bores a tunnel through it so that passage is far quicker and takes much less energy.
3. Enzymes make life on earth possible, all biology from conception to the dissolution that follows death depends on enzymes.
4. Enzymes regulates rate of physiological process. So, defects in enzyme function cause diseases.
5. When cells are injured enzymes leak into plasma. Measurement of activity of such enzymes in plasma is an integral part of modern day medical diagnosis.
6. Enzymes are used as drugs.
7. Immobilized enzymes, which are enzymes attached to solid supports are used in clinical chemistry laboratories and in industry. For example glucose in blood or urine is detected by using immobilized glucose oxidase. In pharmaceutical industry, glucose isomerase is used to produce fructose from glucose.
8. Enzymes are used as biosensors.
9. AIDS detection involves use of enzyme dependent ELISA technique.
10. Enzymes are used as cleansing agents in detergent industry.

CHEMICAL NATURE OF ENZYMES (PROPERTIES)

1. All the enzymes are proteins except ribozymes and number of enzymes are obtained in crystalline form.
2. In 1878, Kuhne, introduced term 'Enzyme' to indicate biological catalyst.
3. Enzymes cut big molecules apart and join small molecules to form big molecules.
4. Most of the chemical reactions in the body are enzyme catalysed.

5. The substance upon which an enzyme acts is called as substrate. By the action of enzyme it is converted to product. An enzyme-catalysed reaction consist of substrate, enzyme and product as shown below.

$$\text{Substrate} \xrightarrow{\text{Enzyme}} \text{Product}$$

6. The enzymes are big particles. Their molecular (size) weight ranges from few thousands to millions.
7. Enzymes have enormous power of catalysis. They increase rate of reaction to 10^5 to 10^{10} folds. For example, carbonic anhydrase can hydrate to 10^6 molecules of CO_2 per second. In the absence of enzyme hydration of CO_2 is 10^{-1} per second.
8. Enzymes are far more efficient compared to non-enzyme (man made) catalysts.
9. Enzymes are not consumed in the overall reaction.
10. Enzymes accelerate the rate of reaction but does not alter the equilibrium constant (Keq).

To know how enzymes work, physical chemistry of catalysts must be explored because enzymes are catalysts.

Catalyst

A catalyst does not change the chemical reaction but it accelerates the reaction. They are not consumed in overall reaction. But they undergo chemical or physical change during reaction and returns to original state at the end of reaction. Transition state theory was proposed to explain action of catalyst.

For a chemical reaction A $\longrightarrow$ B to occur, energy is required. When enough energy is supplied. A undergoes to transition state which is an unstable state. So, it gets converted to product B which is more stable. The amount of energy needed to convert a substance from ground state to transition state is called *activation energy*. In presence of catalyst, A undergoes to transition state very fast and requires less energy (Fig. 4.1). Hence, a catalyst accelerate the rate of reaction by decreasing the energy of activation. Likewise enzymes also speed up reaction by lowering energy of activation. Further, the activation energy is very much less for a reaction in presence of enzyme than non-enzyme catalyst (Fig. 4.1). Therefore enzymes are more efficient than non-enzyme catalyst.

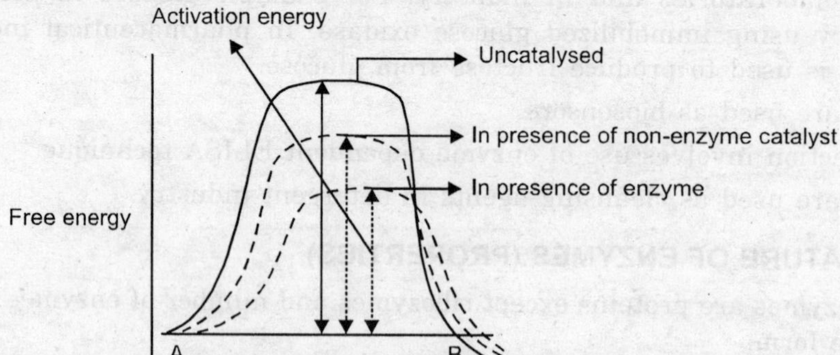

Fig. 4.1 Energy of activation for uncatalysed, non-enzyme catalysed and enzyme catalysed reactions

ENZYME SPECIFICITY

Enzymes are highly specific compared to other catalyst. An enzyme catalyzes only specific reaction. Some general types of enzyme specificity are:

1. Substrate Specificity

Enzymes are specific towards their substrates. For example, glucokinase catalyzes the transfer of phosphate from ATP to glucose. Galactokinase catalyzes transfer of phosphate from ATP to galactose. Though both enzymes catalyzes transfer of phosphate from ATP they act only on specific substrate. Similarly, transminase which catalyze transfer of amino group are specific to substrate. Aspartate transminase catalyzes the transfer of amino group from aspartate and alanine transminase catalyzes transfer of amino group from alanine only. So, they are specific towards substrate.

$$\text{Glucose} + \text{ATP} \xrightarrow{\text{Glucokinase}} \text{Glucose-6-phosphate} + \text{ADP}$$

$$\text{Galactose} + \text{ATP} \xrightarrow{\text{Galactokinase}} \text{Galactose-1-phosphate} + \text{ADP}$$

2. Reaction Specificity

A given enzyme catalyze only one specific reaction. For example, lipases only hydrolyze lipids, urease hydrolyzes urea. They do not catalyze any other type of reaction. Likewise amino acid oxidase catalyze oxidation of amino acid and decarboxylase catalyze only decarboxylation of amino acids.

$$\text{Lipids} \xrightarrow[\text{H}_2\text{O}]{\text{Lipase}} \text{Glycerol} + \text{Fatty acids}$$

$$\text{Amino acids} \xrightarrow[\text{CO}_2]{\text{Decarboxylase}} \text{Amines} \qquad \text{Urea} \xrightarrow[\text{H}_2\text{O}]{\text{Urease}} 2\text{NH}_3 + \text{H}_2\text{CO}_3$$

$$\text{Amino acids} \xrightarrow{\text{Oxidase}} \text{A-Keto acid} + \text{NH}_3$$

3. Group Specificity

Some lytic (hydrolases) enzymes act on specific groups. Proteases are specific for peptide groups, glycosidases are specific to glycosidic bonds.

$$\text{Proteins} \xrightarrow[\text{H}_2\text{O}]{\text{Protease}} \text{Amino acids} \qquad \text{Maltose} \xrightarrow[\text{H}_2\text{O}]{\text{Maltase}} \text{Glucose} + \text{Glucose}$$

$$\text{Ester} \xrightarrow[\text{H}_2\text{O}]{\text{Esterase}} \text{Acid} + \text{Alcohol}$$

4. Absolute Group Specificity

Certain lytic enzymes exhibit high order group specificity. For example, chymotrypsin is protein splitting enzyme *i.e.,* it hydrolyzes peptide bonds. But it preferentially hydrolyzes peptide bonds in which carboxyl group is contributed by aromatic amino acids phenylalanine, tyrosine and tryptophan. Likewise, trypsin another peptide bond hydrolyzing enzyme preferentially hydrolyzes peptide bonds in which carboxyl group is contributed by basic amino acids.

$$\begin{array}{c} \text{Amino peptidase} \quad \text{Chymotrypsin} \quad \text{Trypsin} \quad \text{Carboxypeptidase} \\ \downarrow \qquad\qquad \downarrow \qquad\qquad \downarrow \qquad \downarrow \\ H_2N - Ala - Gly - Val - Tyr - Glu - Ala - Ile - Arg - Ala - Gln - Asp - COOH \end{array}$$

Similarly, carboxy peptidase removes one animo acid each time from carboxy terminus and amino peptidase removes one amino acid each time from N-terminus. Thrombin of blood clotting process is highly specific for Arg-Gly-bonds.

5. Optical Specificity

Several enzymes exhibit optical specificity of substrate on which they act. It means enzymes are able to recognise optical isomers of the substrate. For example, enzymes of amino acid metabolism act only on L-isomers (L-amino acid) but not D-isomers (D-amino acids). Likewise enzymes of carbohydrate metabolism act only on D-sugars but not on L-sugars.

Enzyme Classification and Nomenclature

International Union of Biochemistry classified all enzymes into six major classes based on the type of reaction they catalyze and reaction mechanism.

Nomenclature

The name of an enzyme has two parts. The first part indicates name of its substrate and second part ending in 'ase' indicates the type of reaction it catalyzes. Further, each enzyme has code (EC) number. It is a four-digit number. The first digit indicates major class, second digit indicates sub class, third digit denotes sub sub class and final digit indicates specific enzyme.

The six major classes of enzymes with some example are:

1. Oxidoreductases

They catalyze oxidation and reduction reactions.

Examples:

(*a*) $\text{Alcohol} + NAD^+ \xrightarrow{\text{Alcohol Dehydrogenase}} \text{Aldehyde or ketone} + NADH + H^+$

(*b*) $\text{Glutamate} \xrightleftharpoons[H_2O \qquad NH_4 \\ \text{Glutamate Dehydrogenase}]{NAD^+ \qquad NADH + H^+} \alpha\text{-ketoglutarate}$

2. Tranferases

They catalyze transfer of groups

Examples:

(*a*) $\text{Hexose} + ATP \xrightarrow[Mg^{2+}]{\text{Hexokinase}} \text{Hexose-6-phosphate} + ADP$

(*b*) $\text{Acetyl-CoA} + \text{Choline} \xrightarrow[\text{Transferase}]{\text{Choline acyl}} \text{Acetyl choline} + CoA$

3. Hydrolases

They catalyze hydrolysis of peptide, ester, glycosyl etc. bonds.

Examples:

(*a*) Casein $\xrightarrow[H_2O]{\text{Trypsin}}$ Peptides

(*b*) Acetyl choline $\xrightarrow[\text{Esterase}]{\text{Choline, } H_2O}$ Choline + acetic acid

4. Lyases

They catalyze removal of groups from substrates by mechanisms other than hydrolysis forming double bonds.

Examples: (*a*)

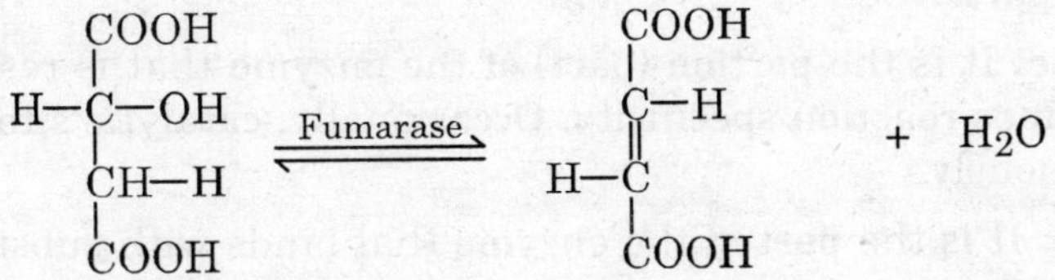

Malate Fumarate

Fig. 4.2 Fumarase catalysed reaction

(*b*) Fructose-1, 6-biphosphate $\xrightarrow{\text{Aldolase}}$ Glyceraldehyde-3-phosphate + Dihydroxyacetone Phosphate

5. Isomerases

They catalyze interconversion of optical, functional and geometrical isomers.

(*a*) Glyceraldehyde-3-Phosphate $\xrightarrow{\text{Triose phosphate isomerase}}$ Dihydroxyacetone phosphate

(*b*) L-Alanine $\xrightarrow{\text{Alanine Racemase}}$ D-Alanine

6. Ligases

They catalyze linking together of two compounds. The linking is coupled to the breaking of phosphate from ATP.

Examples:

(*a*) Glutamate + NH_4 $\xrightarrow{\text{Glutamine Synthetase}}$ Glutamine (ATP ↑, ↓ ADP + P_i)

(*b*) Acetyl-CoA + CO_2 $\xrightarrow{\text{Acetyl-CoA Carboxylase}}$ Malonyl-CoA (ATP ↑, ↓ ADP + P_i)

MECHANISM OF ENZYME ACTION

The mechanism of enzyme action deals with molecular events associated with conversion of a substrate to product in an enzymatic reaction.

Medical Importance

1. Some drugs are designed based on mechanism of enzyme action. For example, X-ray crystallographic studies on mechanism of carboxy peptidase action lead to design of specific inhibitor to angiotensin converting enzyme like captopril which is used in treatment of hypertension.
2. Enzymes with specific properties can be designed based on mechanistic studies. They may be introduced into humans to correct specific abnormalities associated with disorders.

The larger size of an enzyme molecule relative to smaller size of its substrate always puzzled biochemists. Ultimately it led to the concept that small portion of enzyme is required for enzyme action. This part of the enzyme is known as active site.

CHARACTERISTICS OF AN ENZYME ACTIVE SITE

1. It consist of two parts.
   (*a*) **Catalytic site.** It is the portion (part) of the enzyme that is responsible for catalysis. It determines reaction specificity. Occasionally, catalytic site and active site are used synonomously.
   (*b*) **Binding site.** It is the part of the enzyme that binds with substrate. It determines substrate specificity.
2. The active sites of enzyme are clefts within the enzyme molecule. For example, the active site of ribonuclease lies within cleft (Fig. 4.3).

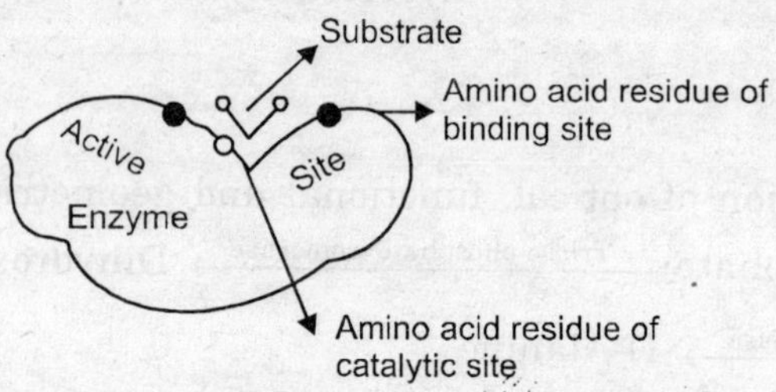

Fig. 4.3 Schematic diagram showing an enzyme active site

3. Active site consists of few amino acid residues only.
4. Active site is three dimentional.
5. The active site is contributed by amino acid residues that are far apart in the enzyme molecule. During catalysis, they are brought together.
6. The amino acids at the active site are arranged in a very precise manner so that only specific substrate can bind at the active site.
7. Usually serine, histidine, cysteine, aspartate or glutamate residues make up active site. Enzymes are named according to the active site amino acid. For example, trypsin is a serine protease and papain is cysteine protease.

MODELS OF ACTIVE SITE

Some active site models are proposed to explain enzyme specificity.

A. Lock and Key Model

1. According to this model the active site is a rigid portion of the enzyme molecule and its shape is complementary to the substrate like lock and key.
2. The complimentary shape of substrate and active site favours tightly bound enzyme. Substrate complex formation followed by catalysis (Fig. 4.4 *a*).

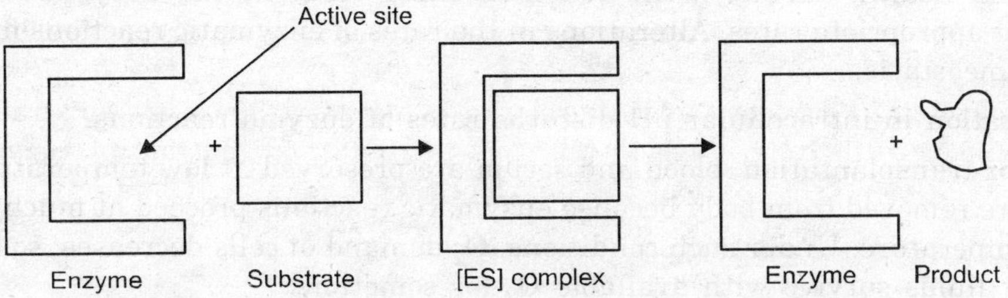

Fig. 4.4 (*a*) Lock and key model of an active site

3. This model was unable to explain the possibility of rigid active site combining with the product to form substrate in reversible reaction.

B. Induced Fit Model

1. According to this model, the active site is flexible unlike rigid type of the lock and key model.
2. In the enzyme molecule the amino acid residues that make up active site are not oriented properly in the absence of substrate.
3. When substrate combines with enzyme, it induces conformational change in the enzyme molecule in such way that amino acids that make active site are shifted into correct orientation to favour tightly bound enzyme-substrate complex formation followed by catalysis.
4. The enzyme molecule is unstable in the induced conformation and returns to its native conformation in the absence of substrate (Fig. 4.4*b*).

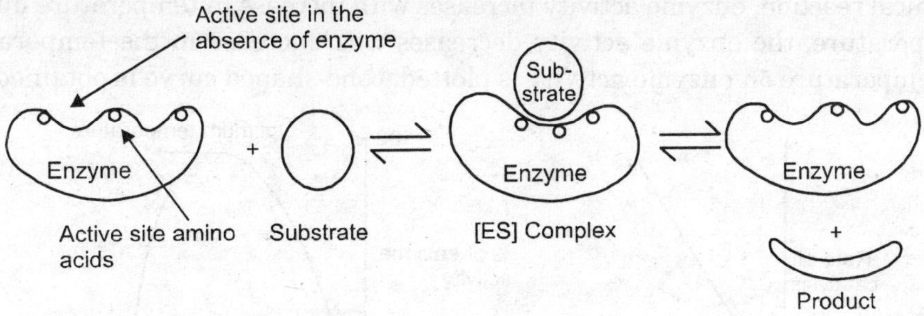

Fig. 4.4 (*b*) Induced fit model of enzyme active site

FACTORS AFFECTING ENZYME ACTION

Rates of enzyme catalyzed reactions are affected by:

1. Enzyme concentration
2. Temperature

3. Hydrogen ion concentration or pH
4. Substrate concentration
5. Inhibitors and cofactors

MEDICAL AND BIOLOGICAL IMPORTANCE

1. For normal health, all enzymatic reactions must occur in the body and they must proceed at appropriate rates. Alterations in the rates of enzymatic reactions may disturb tissue homeostasis.
2. Any alteration in intracellular pH disturbs rates of enzyme reactions.
3. Organs for transplantation, blood and serum are preserved at low temperature as soon as they are removed from body because enzymatic reactions proceed at much lower rate at low temperature. Under such conditions, O_2 demand of cells decreases, so cells of the organs or fluids survive with available O_2 for sometime.
4. Rates of enzymatic reactions are altered in fever and hypothermia because temperature influences rate of enzyme reaction.
5. An understanding of factors affecting enzyme action is required for development of drugs. Many drugs act by decreasing rate of key metabolic reaction by blocking that particular enzyme. For example, AZT used in treatment of AIDS is an inhibitor of HIV virus enzyme. Lovastatin is used in treatment of atherosclerosis is an inhibitor of HMG-CoA reductase, a cholesterol producing enzyme, captopril used in the treatment of hypertension is an inhibitor of angiotensin converting enzyme an enzyme of blood pressure regulation.
6. Some poisons work by abolishing (affecting) essential enzymatic reactions.

1. Enzyme concentration

The rate of enzyme catalyzed reaction is directly proportional to the concentration of enzyme. The plot of rate of catalysis versus enzyme concentrations a straight line (Fig. 4.5*a*).

2. Temperature

Like any chemical reaction, enzyme activity increases with increase in temperature initially. After a critical temperature, the enzyme activity decreases with increase in the temperature. When the effect of temperature on enzyme activity is plotted, cone-shaped curve is obtained (Fig. 4.5*b*).

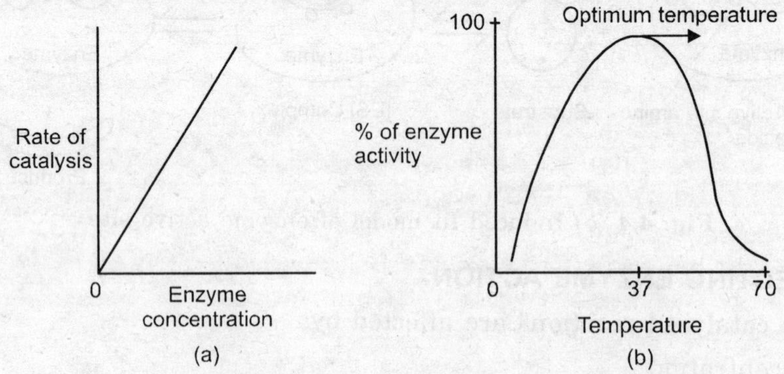

Fig. 4.5 (*a*) Effect of enzyme concentration (*b*) Effect of temperature

The figure indicates that there is an optimal temperature at which enzyme is optimally active. It is called as *optimum temperature*. For most of the enzymes, the optimum temperature is the temperature of the cell or body in which they occur. For example, human trypsin the optimum temperature in 37 °C which is the normal body temperature. The first half of the curve approaching the optimum temperature indicates that enzyme activity increased with increase in the temperature due to the increased kinetic energy of reacting molecules. The other half which corresponds to decreased catalytic activity with increased temperature is due to denaturation of enzyme.

Enzymes of plants and micro-organisms growing in hot climates or hot springs may exhibit optimal temperature close to the boiling point of water. Examples are enzymes of thermophilic bacteria, snake venom phospholipase and urease (55 °C).

3. Effect of pH or hydrogen ion concentration

Most of the enzymes are not maximally active throughout pH scale (1-14). Several enzymes has optimum activity between pH of 5 to 9. When enzyme activity measured at several pH values is plotted a bell shaped curve is obtained (Fig. 4.6 *a*).

Since enzymes are proteins pH changes affect.

1. Charged state of catalytic site.
2. Conformation of enzyme molecules.

In addition low or high pH cause denaturation of enzymes. It accounts for the less activity of enzymes at acidic or alkaline pH (Fig. 4.6*a*). For most of the enzymes, optimum pH is the pH of body or cell in which they occur. However, for some enzymes optimum pH may not be in the neutral range.

Name of the enzyme	Optimum pH
Trypsin	7.6
Pepsin	2-2.5
Acid phosphatase	5
Alkline phosphatase	9-10

In the case of oligomeric enzymes, optimum pH is required for the association of protomers. When the pH is altered, the protomers dissociate with loss of biological activity.

4. Effect of substrate concentration

If the concentration of the substrate (S) is increased while other conditions are kept constant, the initial velocity v_0 (velocity measured when little substrate is reacted) increases proportionately in the beginning. As the substrate concentration continues to increase, the increase in v_0 slows down and reaches maximum V_{max} and no further (Fig. 4.6*b*). The plot of (S) versus v_0 is rectangular hyperbola. It is called as *Michaelis plot*. To explain the reason for characteristic shape of the curve, Michaelis proposed that in an enzyme catalyzed reaction, the enzyme (E) combines with substrate (S) to form and enzyme-substrate (ES) complex which decomposes to form product (P) and free enzyme.

$$E + [S] \underset{K_2}{\overset{K_1}{\rightleftharpoons}} [ES] \xrightarrow{K_3} E + P$$

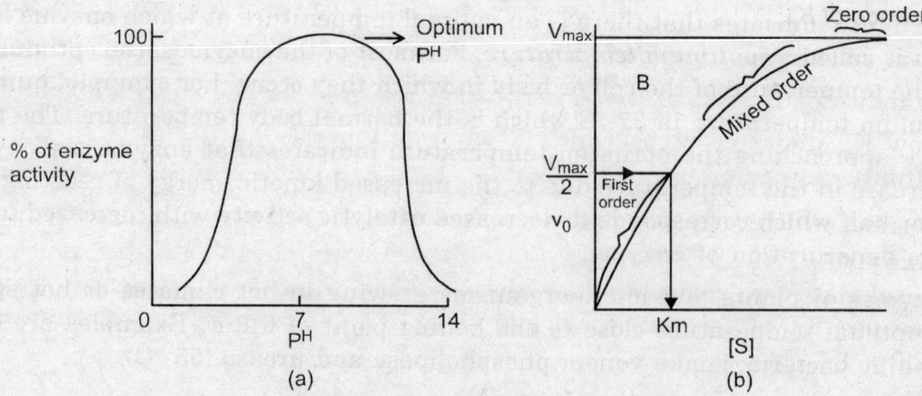

Fig. 4.6 (*a*) Effect of P^H on enzyme action
(*b*) Effect of substrate concentration

Based on this, reasons for the three phases of the curve can be interpreted.

1. In the first phase, substrate concentration is low and most of the enzyme molecules are free so they combine with the substrate molecules. Therefore, velocity is proportional to substrate concentration. At this state, enzymatic reaction shows first-order kinetics.
2. In the second phase, half of the enzyme molecules are bound to substrate, so the velocity is not proportional to substrate concentration. At this stage, enzymatic reaction shows mixed-order kinetics.
3. In the third phase, all the enzyme molecules are bound to substrate, so velocity remain unchanged because free enzyme is not available though the substrate is in excess. At this stage enzymatic reaction shows zero-order kinetics.

The Michaelis plot is used to determine Michaelis constant a characteristics of enzyme (Fig. 4.6 *b*) and type of enzyme inhibition.

Michaelis Constant or K_m

The substrate concentration that produces half the maximal velocity ($V_{max}/2$) is known as Michaelis constant. Apart from graph K_m also can be determined from Michaelis-Menten equation. It is a simple equation and describes the dependence of initial velocity (v_0) on the concentration of enzyme and substrate. It is the theoretical expression for rectangular hyperbola.

$$v_0 = \frac{V_{max}\ [S]}{K_m + [S]}$$

when $$v_0 = V_{max}/2$$

The above equation is written as

$$V_{max}/2 = V_{max}\ [S]/K_m + [S]$$

i.e., $$K_m + [S] = 2[S]$$

$$K_m = 2[S] - [S] = [S]$$

$$K_m = [S]$$

when $$v_0 = V_{max}/2\ [K_m = (K_2 + K_3)/K_1]$$

Significance of K_m

1. It is an enzyme kinetic constant.
2. It indicates the substrate concentration required for the enzyme to work efficiently.
3. Low K_m indicates high affinity of enzyme towards substrate. High K_m indicates low affinity of enzyme towards substrate. Hence, K_m and affinity are inversely related.

   ($K_m \alpha$ 1/affinity)

   Example: Hexokinase and glucokinase both phosphorylates glucose. However, hexokinase can phosphorelate glucose 2000 times more efficiently than glucokinase because K_m of hexokinase is low (1×10^{-5} M) whereas K_m of glucokinase is high (2.0×10^{-2} M).
4. K_m is required when enzymes are used as drugs.
5. Use of enzymes in immunodiagnostics (ELISA) require K_m of the enzyme.

Line Weaver–Burk Plot

1. Michaelis plot gives only approximate K_m and V_{max} values because proper V_{max} is difficult to obtain at very high substrate concentration.
2. By using Line Weaver-Burk Plot accurate K_m and V_{max} are obtained.
3. Line Weaver-Burk Plot is obtained by taking reciprocals of both sides of Michaelis-Menten equation which is given below

$$\frac{1}{v_0} = \frac{1}{\dfrac{V_{max}}{\dfrac{K_m}{S}+1}}$$

$$\frac{1}{v_0} = \frac{\dfrac{K_m}{S}+1}{V_{max}}$$

$$= \frac{K_m}{V_{max}} \cdot \frac{1}{S} + \frac{1}{V_{max}}$$

   The above equation represents Y = $ax + b$ straight line equation with slope of Km/V_{max}. Further straight line is obtained by plotting 1/S against 1/V. Since 1/S and 1/V are reciprocals of S and V, respectively. This plot is known as "double reciprocal plot".
4. The straight line intersects y-axis, which corresponds to V_{max} value. A line extended from point of intersection to x-axis of second quadrant provides K_m value (Fig. 4.6 *c*).
5. In addition to Km and V_{max} values, type of inhibition is determined using this plot.
6. Inhibition constant (K_i) of inhibitor is also determined using this plot.

Significance of K_i

1. K_i indicates affinity of inhibitor towards enzyme. Like K_m, K_i is inversely related to affinity.
2. Use of inhibitors as drugs requires knowledge of K_i. Since K_i and affinity are inversely related inhibitors of low K_i are highly potent drugs.

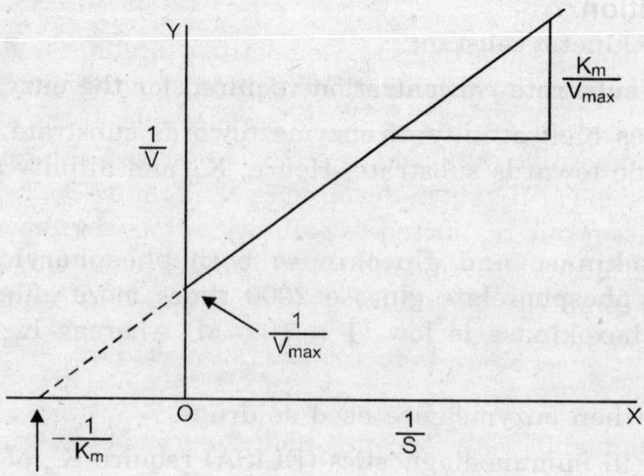

Fig. 4.6 (*c*) Line Weaver-Burk plot

Direct Linear Plot

1. Determination of K_m and V_{max} values of enzymes, which are inhibited by substrate at high concentration is not feasible with Line Weaver-Bunk plot.
2. In such cases, direct linear plot is used for K_m and V_{max} determination. They are read directly from plot without involving any calculation.
3. In this plot, each S and V are marked on X and Y axes, respectively. Then a straight line passing through two points and extending into first quadrant is drawn. When lines for all S and V values are drawn they intersect at common point which provides K_m and V_{max} (Fig. 4.6*d*).

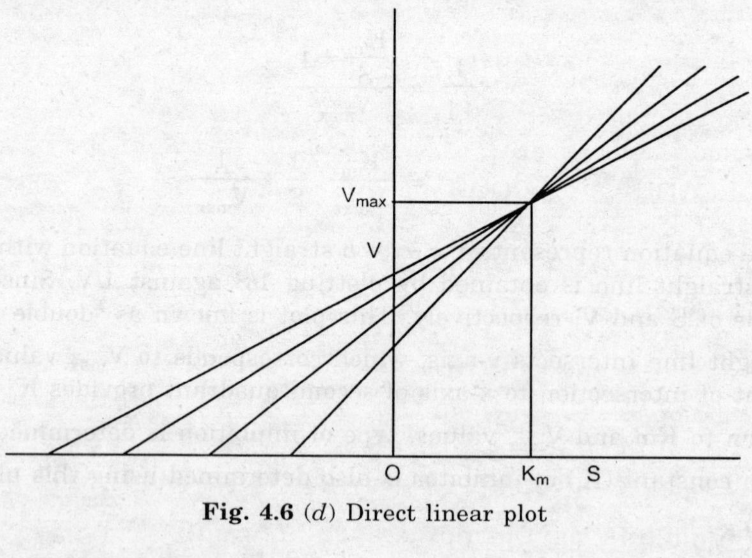

Fig. 4.6 (*d*) Direct linear plot

INHIBITORS

Substances that decrease the catalytic activity of enzymes are called as inhibitors. They may be protein or non-protein inhibitors. The decrease in enzyme activity is called as inhibition. More than two types of enzyme inhibition exist based on the mode of action of inhibitors.

Competitive Inhibition

Competitive inhibition occurs at active site. Competitive inhibitor is structurally similar to that of substrate. Hence, it competes with substrate to bind at active site. Inhibition occurs when it binds at the active site of enzyme molecule. It is reversible. If the substrate concentration is increased then the competitive inhibition is relieved. Further, the rate of formation of product from (ES) complex is same as that of in the absence of inhibitor. So, velocity (V_{max}) is not altered in competitive inhibition but K_m increases (affinity of enzyme towards substrate decreases) because of competition of substrate and inhibitor to bind at active site. The interaction of enzyme (E) substrate (S) and competitive inhibitor (I) is represented as equations below:

$$E + S \longleftrightarrow [ES] \longrightarrow E + P$$

$$E + I \longleftrightarrow [EI] \xrightarrow{\;x\;} E + P$$

In addition at high substrate concentration, the number of enzyme molecules available for the inhibitor are far less. So, the inhibition is masked. (becomes reversible.) Michaelis plot also indicates K_m alternation and unaffected V_{max} in the presence of competitive inhibitor (Fig. 4.7 *a*).

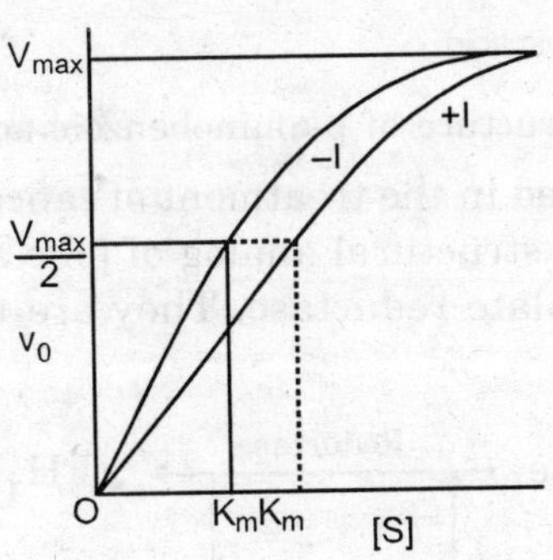

Fig. 4.7 (*a*) Michaelis plot in presence (+I) and absence (–I) of competitive inhibitor

A classical example for reversible competitive inhibition is succinate dehydrogenase enzyme. Malonate competitively inhibits the enzyme because it is structurally similar to the substrate succinate (Fig. 4.7 *b*).

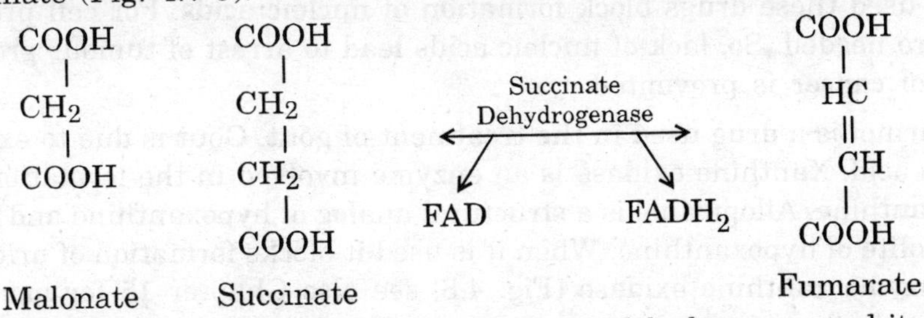

Fig. 4.7 (*b*) Reaction catalyzed by succinate dehydrogenase and its competitive inhibitor malonate

Competitive Inhibitors as Chemotherapeutic Agents

When used in clinical situations, the competitive inhibitors are called as *antagonists* or *anti metabolites* of the substrate with which they compete. The use of anti-metabolites in the treatment of diseases is called as *chemotherapy*. Therefore, competitive inhibitors are useful chemotherapeutic agents. They are used as

1. Antibiotics
2. Anti-cancer drugs
3. In the treatment of metabolic diseases like gout, atherosclerosis and hypertension.

1. Sulfonamide antibiotics are used in the treatment of bacterial infections. Bacteria synthesize folic acid from p-aminobenzoic acid (PABA). Since these sulfonamide drugs contain sulfonilamide a structural analog of PABA (Fig. 4.7 *c*), when used as chemotherapetic agent, it blocks the synthesis of folic acid in bacteria. The lack of folic acid leads to death of bacteria (see also Chapter 15). Sulfonamide act as competitive inhibitor for the enzyme involved in the formation of folic acid using PABA as substrate.

Precursor $\xrightarrow[\text{PABA blocked}]{\text{Sulfonamide}}$ Folic acid $\longrightarrow$ Bacterial growth arrest

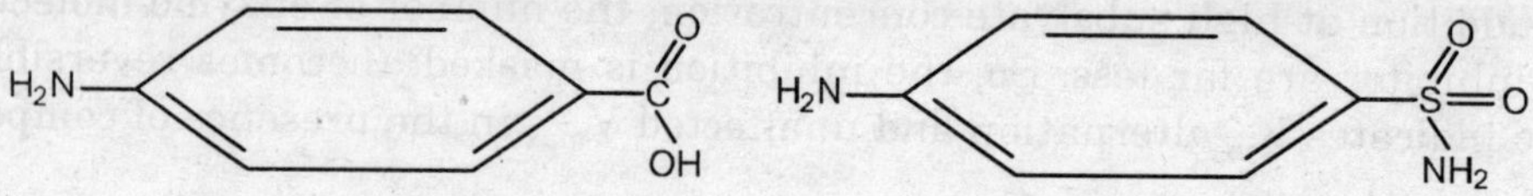

ρ-aminobenzoic acid Sulfanilamide

Fig. 4.7 (*c*) Structure of p-aminobenzoic acid and sulfanilamide.

2. Competitive inhibitors used in the treatment of cancer are aminopterin and amethopterin (methotrexate). They are structural analog of folic acid. They are competitive inhibitors for the enzyme dihydrofolate reductase. They are used in the treatment of leukaemia, a type of cancer.

(FH_2) Dihydrofolate $\xrightarrow{\text{Reductase}}$ (FH_4) Tetrahydrofolate

NADPH + H^+ $NADP^+$

Blocked in presence of aminopterin

Tumour cells growth arrest $\longleftarrow$ Nucleic acid formation

When used these drugs block formation of nucleic acids. For cell proliferation, nucleic acid are needed. So, lack of nucleic acids lead to arrest of tumour growth and advancement of cancer is prevented.

3. Allopurinol is a drug used in the treatment of gout. Gout is due to excessive production of uric acid. Xanthine oxidase is an enzyme involved in the formation of uric acid from hypoxanthine. Allopurinol is a structural analog of hypoxanthine and hence it is an antimetabolite of hypoxanthine. When it is used it blocks formation of uric acid by inhibiting the enzyme xanthine oxidase (Fig. 4.8, see also Chapter 15 for more details).

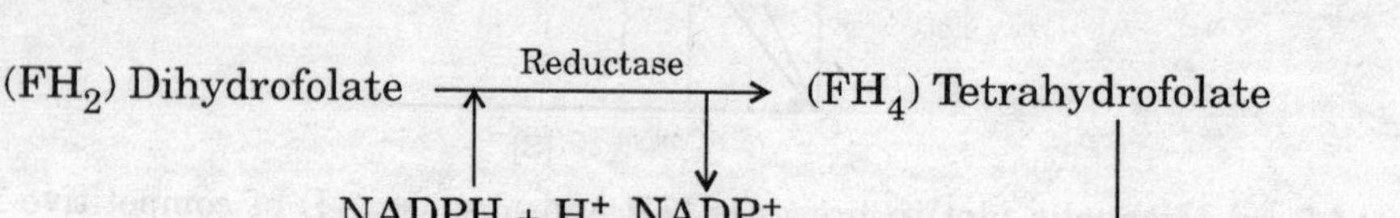

Allo purinol Hypoxanthine Xanthine Uric acid

Fig. 4.8 Reaction catalyzed by xanthine oxidase and its inhibitor

4. Lovastatin is a competitive inhibitor of enzyme HMG-CoA reductase, when used it blocks production of cholesterol. In atherosclerosis, cholesterol is more. Lovastatin reduces cholesterol formation thus arrest the advancement of atherosclerosis.
5. Competitive inhibitors used in the treatment of hypertension are captopril, lisinopril and enalapril. They competitively inhibit angiotensin converting enzyme, which is involved in regulation of blood pressure. When used they lower blood pressure by reducing activity of angiotensin converting enzyme.

Non-Competitive Inhibition

In this type of enzyme inhibition no, competition occurs between substrate and inhibitor to bind at active site of enzyme. Inhibitor is not structurally related to substrate. In addition inhibitor binds to some other site of enzyme which is far off from active site. The interaction of enzyme (E), substrate (S), and inhibitor (I) is shown below.

$$E + S \longrightarrow [ES] \xrightarrow{I} [ESI] \xrightarrow{Slow} E + P$$

$$E + I \longrightarrow [EI] \xrightarrow{S} [EIS] \xrightarrow{Slow} E + P$$

In non-competitive inhibition, the inhibitor can react with free enzyme as well as enzyme substrate complex, because its binding site is away from active site. In addition, the formation of product from enzyme substrate-inhibitor complex is not same as that of in absence of inhibitor. So, the V_{max} is decreased and K_m (affinity) remains same because no competition of substrate and inhibitor in non-competitive inhibition. Michaelis plot also indicates same in the presence of non-competitive inhibitor (Fig. 4.9).

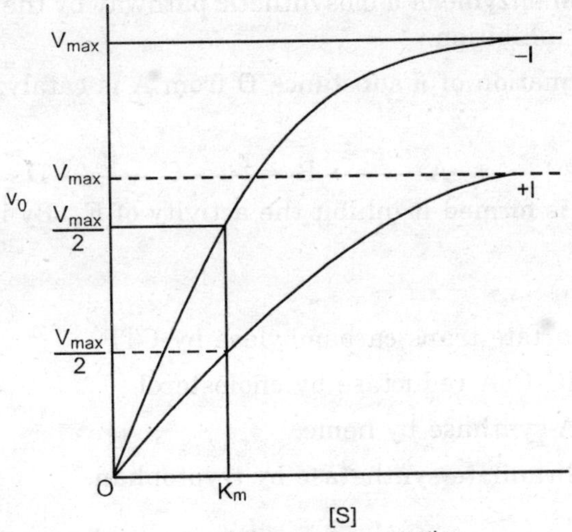

Fig. 4.9 Michaelis plot in presence (+I) and absence (–I) of non-competitive inhibitor

Examples for Non-competitive Inhibition

Reversible non-competitive inhibitors are rare. Most of the known non-competitive inhibitors are irreversible. They are referred as enzyme poisons.

1. Iodoacetate blocks the formation of 1,3-bisphosphoglycerate from glyceraldehyde-3-phosphate by inhibiting enzyme glyceraldehyde-3-phosphate dehydrogenase.

2. Fluoride blocks the action of enolase, which converts 2-phosphoglycerate to phosphoenol pyruvate.
3. Heavy metals like Hg^{2+}, Ag^{+}, Pb^{2+} and Arsenite are also enzyme poisons. They interact with –SH group of enzyme and activate it.

$$E-SH + Hg^{2+} \longrightarrow E-S-Hg + H^{+}$$

   Hg^{2+} inhibits –SH containing pyruvate dehydrogenase. Similarly, arsenite inhibits –SH containing α-ketoglutarate dehydrogenase.
4. Some non-competitive inhibitors are used as pesticides. DDT, melathion and parathion are inhibitors of enzyme choline esterase that catalyzes hydrolysis of acetylcholine.
5. Di-isopropyl fluro phosphate (DFP) is a non-competitive inhibitor used as nerve gas in World War II. It is an active site directed irreversible non-competitive inhibitor. It forms covalent linkage with –OH groups of serine residue of choline esterase. When used DFP causes constriction of larynx, pain in eyes and mental confusion.
6. CN^{-} inhibits activity of cytochrome oxidase an enzyme of respiratory chain. Bitter almonds contain some cyanide.
7. Ethylene diaminotetra acetic acid (EDTA) inhibits metalloenzymes by forming complex with metal ion.
8. Tubers, bananas and beans contain inhibitors to trypsin, chymotrypsin and elestase.

FEEDBACK INHIBITION

Inhibition of activity of enzyme of a biosynthetic pathway by the end product of that pathway is called as feedback inhibition.

For example, formation of a substance D from A is catalyzed by three enzymes E_1, E_2 and E_3.

$$A \xrightarrow{E_1} B \xrightarrow{E_2} C \xrightarrow{E_3} D$$

When enough D is formed it inhibit the activity of E_1. By inhibiting E_1, D regulates its own synthesis.

Examples:

1. Inhibition of aspartate trans carbamoylase by CTP.
2. Inhibition of HMG-CoA reductase by cholesterol.
3. Inhibition of ALA-synthase by heme.
4. Inhibition of anthranilate synthetase by tryptophan.

COFACTORS

1. Cofactors are non-protein molecules required for activity of some enzymes. They may be involved in catalysis or in structure maintenance.
2. There are two types of cofactors:
   1. Organic cofactors, and
   2. Inorganic cofactors.

   The organic cofactors are further subdivided into. 1. Prosthetic groups 2. Co-enzymes.

1. Prosthetic Groups

These organic molecules are covalently attached to the enzyme and they undergo change during catalysis but return to native state at the end of the reaction.

2. Co-enzymes

These organic molecules are loosely (non-covalent) attached to enzyme molecules. They undergo change during reaction. Since they undergo change along with substrate they are referred as co-substrates.

$$\underset{\text{(Protein)}}{\text{Apo-enzyme}} + \underset{\text{(Non-protein)}}{\text{Co-enzyme}} \longrightarrow \underset{\text{(Active)}}{\text{Holo enzyme}}$$

Examples for Organic Co-factors

The major function of water soluble vitamins is to serve as co-factors, some of them as such serve as co-factor otherwise their derivatives serve as co-factors. They are divided on the basis of their function, in enzymatic reaction.

1. Co-enzymes of oxidation reduction reactions.

   (*a*) Co-enzymes derived from niacin. They are NAD^+, $NADH + H^+$ and $NADP^+$, $NADPH + H^+$. These co-enzymes are loosely bound to apo-enzymes. Reactions where they serve as co-enzymes are given below.

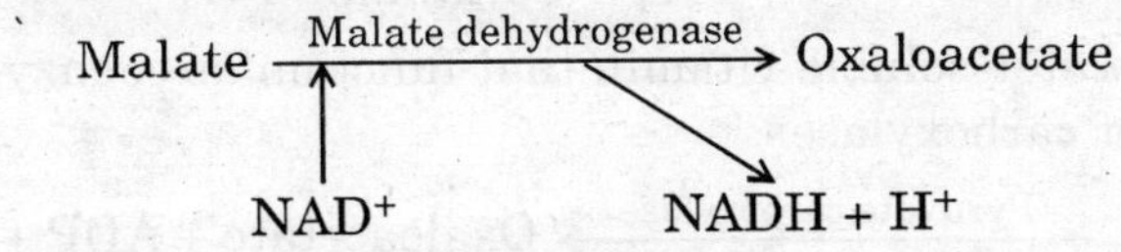

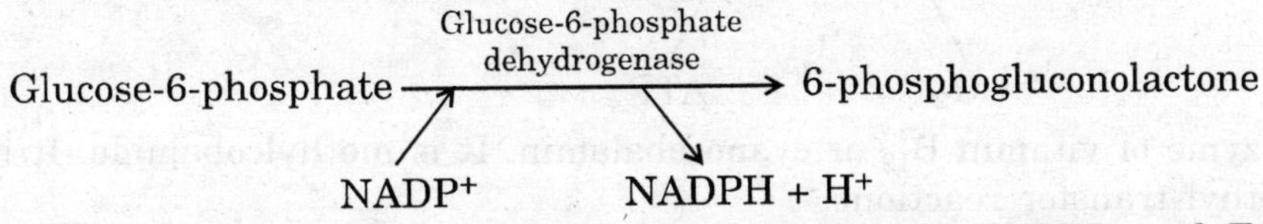

   (*b*) Co-enzymes derived from riboflavin. They are FMN, $FMNH_2$ and FAD, $FADH_2$. They are covalently linked to apo-enzymes. So, they are prosthetic groups. Enzymes to which they are prosthetic groups are given below.

(*a*)

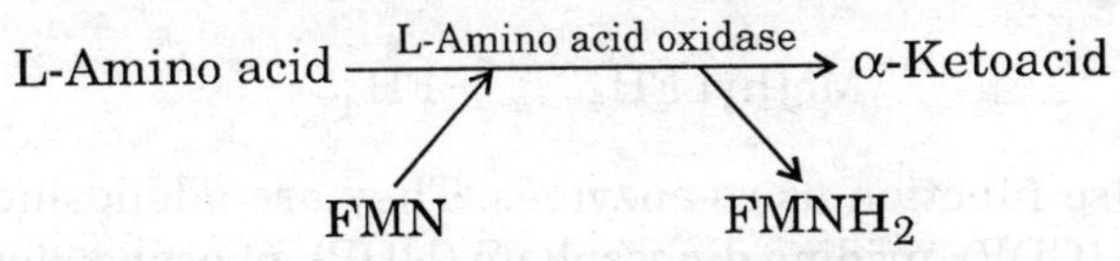

(*b*)

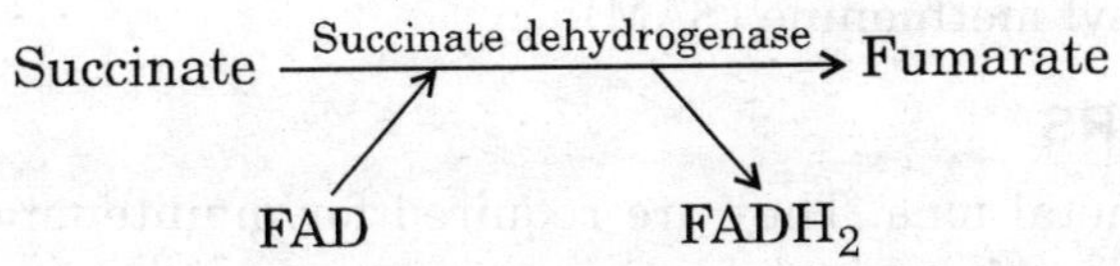

2. Coenzymes of group transfer reactions.

   (*a*) Co-enzyme of pantothenic acid. It is co-enzyme of A(CoA, CoASH). It is involved in CoA transfer reaction.

Fatty acid —(Acyl-CoA synthatase; CoA, ATP)→ Acyl-CoA + AMP + PPi

(*b*) Co-enzyme of thiamin. It is thiamnin pyro(di)phosphate (TPP, TDP). It is prosthetic group of several enzymes.

Pyruvate —(Pyruvate dehydrogenase; TPP, CoASH)→ Acetyl-CoA

(*c*) Co-enzyme of pyridoxine. It is pyridoxal phosphate (P-PO_4). It is prosthetic group of enzymes involved in amino group transfer. Other reactions where it serve as co-enzyme are decarboxylation, transulfuration etc.

Glutamate —(Decarboxylase P–PO_4)→ γ-aminobutyric acid

(*d*) Co-enzymes of folic acid. It is tetrahydrofolate (FH_4). It participates in one carbon transfer reaction.

Formiminoglutamate —(Transferase; FH_4 → Formimino-FH_4)→ Glutamate

(*e*) Biotin is the only water-soluble vitamin that function as coenzyme as such. It is the prosthetic group of carboxylases.

Pyruvate —(Pyruvate carboxylase; CO_2, ATP)→ Oxaloacetate + ADP + Pi

(*f*) Co-enzyme of vitamin B_{12} or cyanocobalamin. It is methylcobamide. It is involved in methyl transfer reactions.

Homocysteine —(Methionine Synthase, Vit. B_{12}; Methyl FH_4 → FH_4)→ Methionine

3. Many nucleotides also function as co-enzymes. They are adenosine triphosphate (ATP), cytidine diphosphate (CDP), uridine diphosphate (UDP), phosphoadenosine phosphosulfate (PAPS) and S-adenosyl methionine (SAM).

INORGANIC CO-FACTORS

Many enzymes require metal ions. They are required for maintenance of protein (enzyme) conformation and catalysis. Metal ions participate in enzymatic reactions in three ways.

1. Metallo Enzymes

Metal is tightly bound to enzyme molecule and it is an integral part of enzyme molecule. Metals are attached to enzyme through coordinate bonds. They participate in catalysis.

Examples:

(*a*) **Iron (Fe^{2+}):** It is required for cytochrome oxidase, catalase, xanthine oxidase, succinate dehydrogenase.

(*b*) **Copper (Cu^{2+}):** It is required for cytochrome oxidase, superoxidedismutase, lysyloxidase and ceruloplasmin.

(*c*) **Zinc (Zn^{2+}):** It is required for carbonic anhydrase, carboxy peptidase, alkaline phosphatase, alcohol dehydrogenase etc.

2. Metal-dependent Enzymes

Metal is loosely associated with enzyme molecule or it may be required for enzyme substrate complex formation. In the absence of metal, enzyme may not interact with substrate molecule or with co-enzyme molecule.

Examples:

(*a*) **Magnesium (Mg^{2+}):** It is needed by enzymes using ATP. Formation of Mg: ATP complex is essential. They include hexokinase, galactokinase, pyruvate kinase etc.

(*b*) **Calcium (Ca^{2+}):** It is required for the activity of calpain, a calcium-dependent protease. Others are Na^+/K^+-ATPase and Ca^{2+} ATPase.

3. Metal-activated Enzymes

In presence of metals, some enzymes get activated *i.e.,* their activity increases many folds.

Examples:

(*a*) **Chloride (Cl^-):** It activates amylase and angiotensin converting enzyme.

(*b*) **Calcium (Ca^{2+}):** It activates trypsin.

ENZYME REGULATION

Metabolic pathways are controlled by regulating enzyme activity. If enzyme activity is not regulated, it can harm cellular activities and may lead to the development of diseases. Alteration of enzyme regulation is one of the cause for cancer development. Over production of tyrosine kinase is associated with alteration of cell shape in tumour cells. Enzyme regulation can alter when drugs are used. Enzyme regulation can be altered by environmental toxins or pollutants.

Enzyme activity can be regulated by:

(*a*) changing catalytic efficiency.

(*b*) altering the amount or quantity of enzyme in cell or body.

(*a*) Catalytic efficiency of enzymes can be regulated

1. By subjecting enzyme to feedback inhibition
2. By allosteric regulation or inhibition
3. By covalent modification of enzyme molecule
4. By synthesizing enzyme in inactive form

Allosteric Inhibition

Inhibition of activity of allosteric enzymes by allosteric inhibitor is called as allosteric inhibition. Allosteric inhibition is seen in pathways that are subject to regulation. Allosteric inhibitors are not structurally similar to substrates of allosteric enzymes. They bind to enzyme at allosteric site which is different from active site. The activity of an allosteric enzyme is raised by allosteric activator. Most of the allosteric enzymes are oligomeric proteins *i.e.*, they consist of many subunits.

The most extensively studied allosteric enzyme is aspartate transcarbamolyase (Aspartate carbamolytransferase). It catalyzes first reaction unique to pyrimidine nucleotide biosynthesis.

$$\text{Carbamoylphosphate} + \text{Aspartic acid} \xrightarrow[\text{carbamoyltransferase}]{\text{Aspartate}} \text{Carbamoylaspartate} + \text{Pi}$$

The enzyme consist of catalytic and regulatory subunits. It exists in less active form and high active form. Binding of CTP to regulatory subunit converts high active form to less active form. So CTP is called as negative effector or allosteric inhibitor. In contrast, binding of ATP to regulatory subunit convert less active form to high active form. So ATP is called as positive effector or allosteric activator.

$$\underset{\text{Less active form}}{\text{Aspartate carbamoyl transferase}} \underset{\text{CTP}}{\overset{\text{ATP}}{\longleftrightarrow}} \underset{\text{High active form}}{\text{Asparatate carbamoyl transferase}}$$

Kinetics of Allosteric Enzyme

1. These enzymes does not exhibit Michaelis-Menten Kinetics. A plot of (v_S) velocity versus substrate concentration is sigmoidal or S shaped curve rather than rectangular hyperbola (Fig. 4.10).

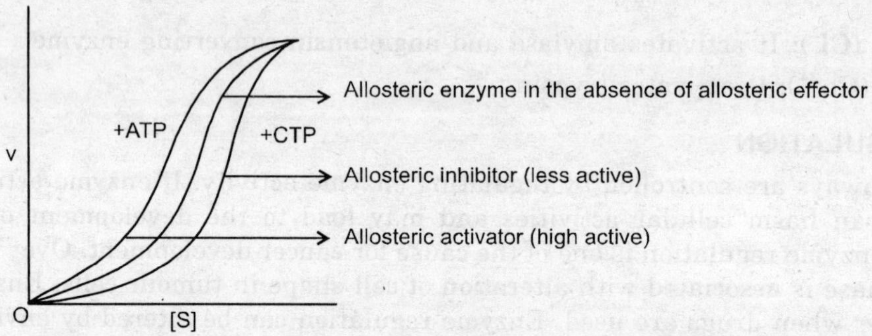

Fig. 4.10 The plot of v versus [s] for an allosteric enzyme in presence (+) of allosteric effector and in the absence of allosteric effector

2. The sigmoidel curve indicates a rapid increase in velocity after a particular substrate concentration. It is due to phenomenon of co-operativity.
3. To explain co-operativity of allosteric enzymes 'T' and 'R' model was proposed. According to this model, the oligomer (allosteric enzyme) exist in two states. A tense (T) state and relaxed (R) state. Binding of substrate (ligand) to 'T' form which is intially slow causes a conformational change (Fig. 4.11) in subunits resulting in 'R' form. Further binding of ligand (substrate) to the subunits is rapid.
4. Allosteric inhibitor stabilizes the enzyme in 'T' form, so the enzyme is less active. In contrast, allosteric activator stabilizes the enzyme in 'R' form, so the enzyme is highly active (Fig. 4.11).

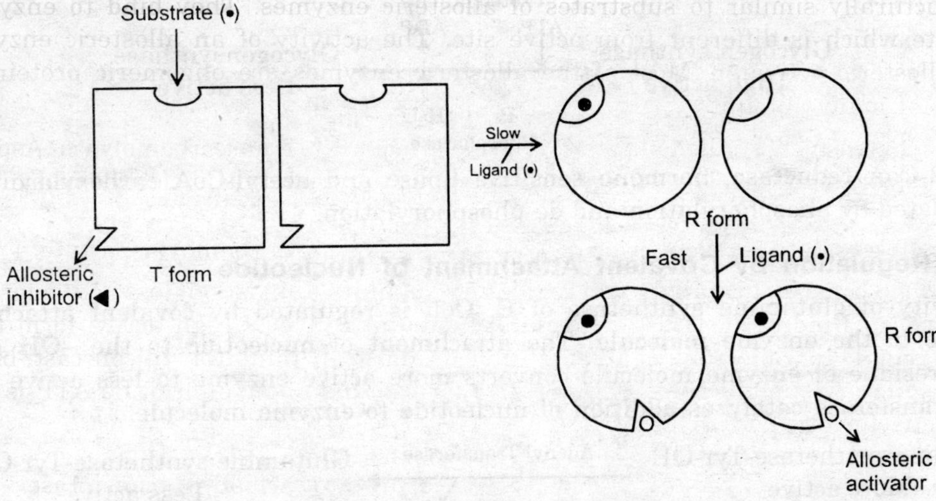

Fig. 4.11 Model for cooperativity of allosteric enzyme.

Enzyme Regulation by Covalent Modification

Enzyme activity is regulated by covalent attachment of a group to the enzyme molecule. Phosphate group is most commonly used to modify enzyme activity. Other group involved in regulation of enzyme activity by covalent modification is nucleotide. Enzymes which undergo regulation by covalent modification exist in two forms, a less active and a high active form. Depending on the enzyme, the phospho or dephospho enzyme may be less or more active, respectively. The phosphorylation (attachment of phosphate) and dephosphorylation are catalyzed by protein kinases and phosphatases, respectively. The –OH group of serine residue of the protein is the site of phosphorylation. ATP serve as donor of phosphate group.

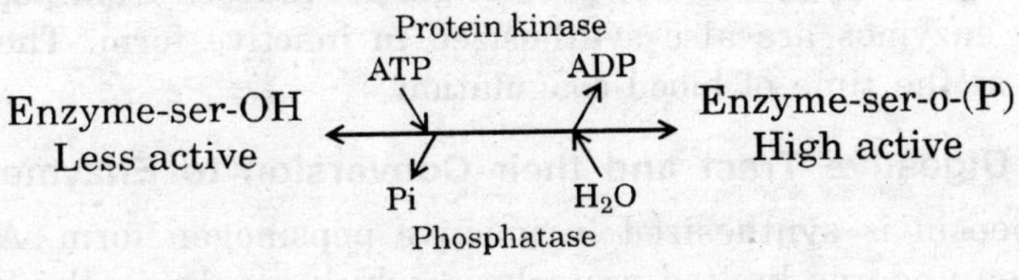

Many hormones influence the activities of proteinkinases and phosphatases.

Examples:

1. Phosphorylation of glycogen phosphorylase converts less active to high active form. Dephosphorylation converts high active to less active form.

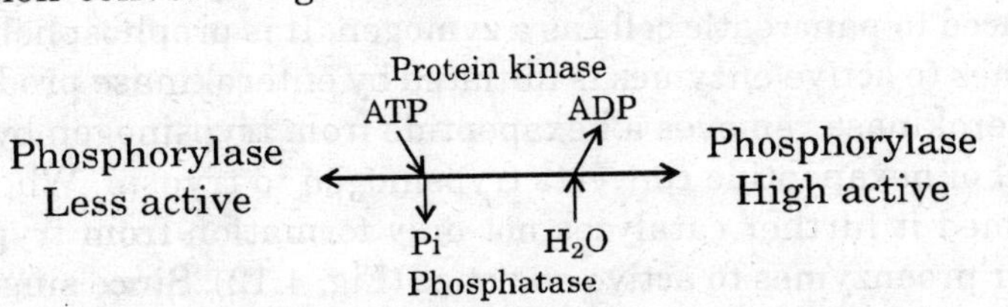

2. Phosphorylation of glycogen synthase converts high active to less active form

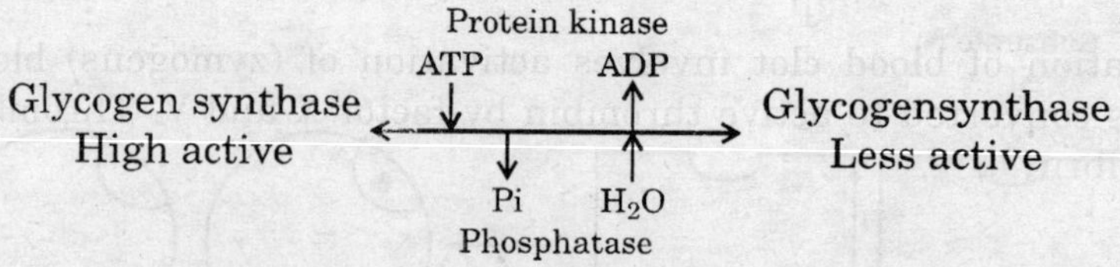

3. HMG-CoA reductase, hormone sensitive lipase and acetyl-CoA carboxylase are also regulated by phosphorylation and de-phosphorylation.

Enzyme Regulation by Covalent Attachment of Nucleotide

The activity of glutamine synthetase of E. Coli is regulated by covalent attachment of nucleotide to the enzyme molecule. The attachment of nucleotide to the –OH group of tyrosine residue of enzyme molecule converts more active enzyme to less active enzyme. Adenyl transferase catalyzes addition of nucleotide to enzyme molecule.

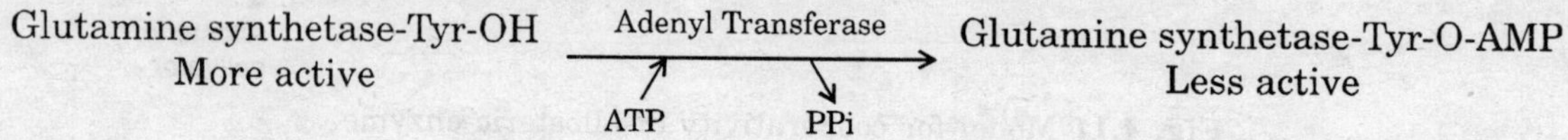

PRO-ENZYMES

One way of regulating catalytic activity of an enzyme is synthesizing enzyme in inactive (precursor) form or pro-enzyme or zymogen. They are converted to active form later when need arises. The conversion of pro-enzyme to active enzyme involves limited proteolysis. Limited proteolysis removes few aminoacids from proenzyme which results in conversion of inactive enzyme to active enzyme. So, conversion of pro-enzyme to active enzyme accompanies decrease in molecular weight of pro-enzyme due to removal of amino acids (peptides).

Most of the protein digesting enzymes of pancreas are synthesized in inactive forms to protect pancreatic cells from destructive action of proteases. Likewise, pepsin of stomach is also synthesized in pro-enzyme form to protect gastric mucosa from pepsin attack. Most of the blood clotting enzymes are also synthesized in inactive form. They are converted to active forms only at the time of blood coagulation.

Pro-enzymes of Digestive Tract and their Conversion to Enzymes

In the stomach pepsin is synthesized in inactive pepsinogen form. At the acidic pH of stomach pepsinogen undergo limited proteolysis, which results in the formation of pepsin. When once pepsin is formed it catalyzes its own formation from pepsinogen. This process is called as *autocatalysis*.

The protein splitting enzymes of pancreas are synthesized in inactive forms. They are trypsinogen, chymotrypsinogen, procarboxy peptidase and proelastase. A lipid digesting enzyme is also produced in pancreatic cells as a zymogen. It is prophospholipase. The conversion of these pro-enzymes to active enzymes is initiated by enterokinase produced by mucosal cells of duodenum. Enterokinase removes a hexapeptide from trypsinogen by hydrolysing-Lys-Ile-bond. The removal of hexapeptide converts trypsinogen to trypsin. When once few molecules of trypsin are formed it further catalyzes not only formation from trypsinogen but also the conversion of other proenzymes to active enzymes (Fig. 4.12). Since single molecule of trypsin can trigger the formation of battery of protein digesting enzymes, pancreas has another self protecting mechanism. It contains trypsin inhibitor in small amounts.

The formation of blood clot involves activation of (zymogens) blood clotting factors. Prothrombin is converted to active thrombin by factor X and V. Thrombin in turn converts fibrinogen to fibrin (Fig. 4.12).

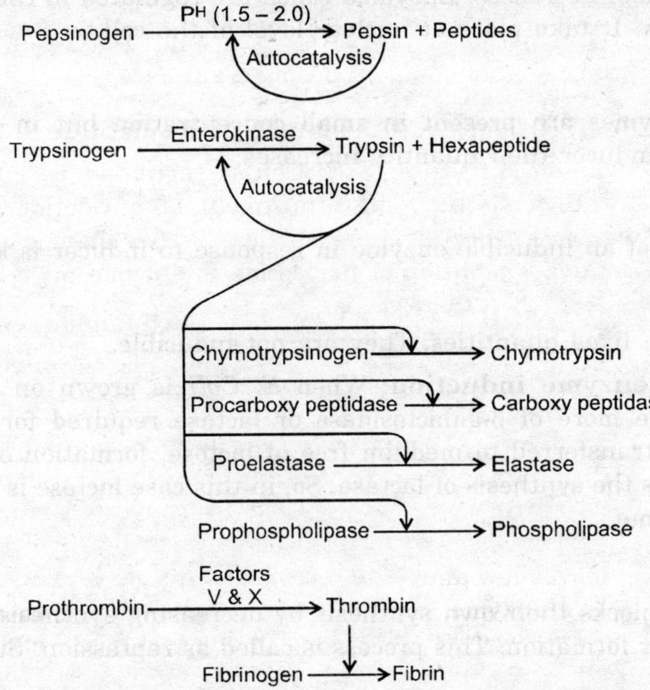

Fig. 4.12 Conversion of pro-enzymes to enzymes

Medical Importance

Though there are two in-built defensive mechanisms in the pancreas to avoid activation of pro-enzymes, in acute pancreatitis the pro-enzymes get activated and cause damage to pancreas and severe abdominal pain.

The quantity of enzyme in cell or body is regulated by

1. Enzyme degradation
2. Enzyme induction and repression

Regulation of Enzyme Activity by Degradation

Enzymes produced as a part of development or enzymes produced to overcome certain environmental conditions or enzymes produced to remove toxins are not needed any more later. Their continued presence may be harmful to the body. So, if enzymes were immortal, then it leads to creation of unwanted side effects in the body. Hence, enzymes undergo turnover. They are synthesized and degraded. Individual enzymes have life spans. Some enzymes may last few seconds or minutes in the cell. However, some enzymes may last few days in the body. There are specific mechanisms for degradation of enzymes. Enzymes that control key metabolic events are degraded very fast. Likewise if a defective enzyme is produced, it is degraded very rapidly because it is not useful any more to the body.

Enzyme Regulation by Induction and Repression

The quantity of the enzyme can be increased by increasing its synthesis and quantity of the enzyme can be decreased by decreasing its synthesis. Depending on cell needs quantity of the enzyme increases or decreases. Enzymes which are regulated in this manner are called as *inducible enzymes*. It take place at nuclear level of the cell.

Inducible Enzymes

Normally these enzymes are present in small concentration but in presence of certain substance called as inducer their quantity increases.

Induction

Increased synthesis of an inducible enzyme in response to inducer is known as induction.

Constitutive Enzymes

These are present in fixed quantities. They are not inducible.

Examples for enzyme induction: When *E. Coli* is grown on medium containing lactose, they produce more of β-galactosidase or lactase required for lactose utilization. When the cells are transferred to medium free of lactose, formation of lactase decreases. Thus, lactose induces the synthesis of lactase. So, in this case lactose is inducer and lactase is an inducible enzyme.

Repression

Certain substances blocks their own synthesis by decreasing synthesis of enzymes, which are required for their formation. This process is called as repression. Substances are called repressors.

Examples for repression: When histidine is added to the S. Typhi. containing medium synthesis of all the enzymes required for histidine formation is blocked. In this case, histidine is repressor molecule.

In humans also, induction and repression of enzymes takes place. They are called as adaptable enzymes.

Examples:

1. Arginase, an enzyme of urea-cycle formation is more in starvation and on high protein diet.
2. Pyruvate carboxylase an enzyme of gluconeogenesis is induced by glucocorticoids and repressed by insulin.
3. Phenobarbitol and anti-convulsive drug induces alkaline phosphatase.

ISO-ENZYMES OR ISOZYMES

1. They are multiple forms of enzymes.
2. The catalyze same reaction but differ in physiochemical properties. They occur in same species or in same individual.
3. They are tissue specific or species specific.
4. The are present in serum and other biological fluids and tissues.
5. Iso-enzyme for dehydrogenases, transaminases and phosphotases have been reported.

Separation of Iso-enzymes

Most commonly used technique for the separation of iso-enzymes is electrophoresis. The serum lactate dehydrogenase (LDH) iso-enzyme pattern is obtained by subjecting serum to electrophoresis at pH 8.6. On electrophoresis, iso-enzymes of lactate dehydrogenase separates into five bands. Each band exhibits same catalytic activity (Fig. 4.13). The five iso-enzymes of LDH are LDH_1, LDH_2, LDH_3, LDH_4 and LDH_5.

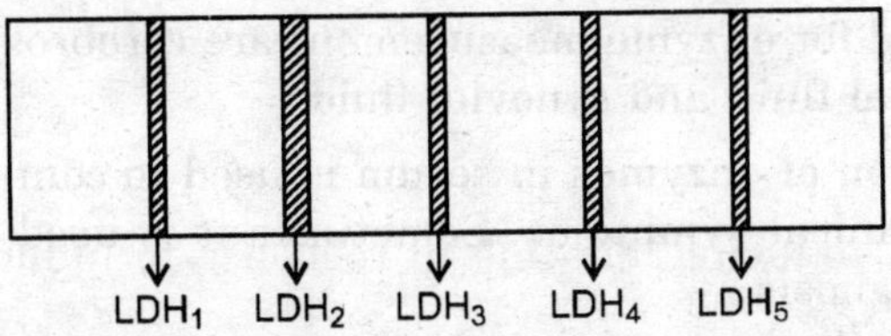

Fig. 4.13 Lactate dehydrogenase isoenzyme pattern

Structure of LDH Iso-enzymes

Lactate dehydrogenase isoenzymes differ at the level of quaternary structure. The LDH consist of 4 subunits of two types. They are H and M subunits. The subunit composition of different LDH isoenzymes are shown below:

Name of isoenzyme	Subunit composition
LDH_1	HHHH or H_4
LDH_2	HHHM or H_3M
LDH_3	HHMM or H_2M_2
LDH_4	HMMM or HM_3
LDH_5	MMMM or M_4

The synthesis of two subunits H and M is controlled by different genes. H is acidic and M is basic in nature. The molecule weight of each subunit is 35,000.

Alkaline Phosphatase Iso-enzymes

Electrophoresis is used for the separation of isoenzymes of alkaline phosphatase in serum. On electrophoresis, iso-enzymes of alkaline phosphatase separates into four bands. The four iso-enzymes of alkaline phosphatase are tissue specific. They differ in their carbohydrate content. The four isoenzymes originate from bone, liver, placenta and intestine.

Creatine Phosphokinase (CK) Iso-enzyme

CK iso-enzymes can be separated by electrophoresis. CK has three isoenzymic forms. They are CK_1, CK_2 and CK_3. They differ in subunit composition. CK is a dimer. It consist of two subunits M and B. The subunit composition of three isoenzymes of CK are BB, MB and MM for CK_1, CK_2 and CK_3 respectively.

Carbonic Anhydrase Iso-enzymes

On electrophoresis carbonic anhydrase gives three bands. The three isoenzymes differ in amino acid composition.

CLINICAL ENZYMOLOGY

1. It deals with quantitative estimation of enzymes in body fluids in normal and diseases conditions.
2. Depending on pathological conditions different body fluids are used for enzyme measurement.
3. Serum and plasma are most commonly used.
4. Other body fluids used for enzyme measurement are cerebrospinal fluid, amniotic fluid, pleural fluid, peritonial fluid and synovial fluid.
5. Quantitative estimation of enzymes in serum is used to confirm the diagnosis which is made by observing clinical symptoms. Sometimes it is used to know the effectiveness of treatment *i.e.,* prognosis.
6. Hence measurement of serum enzyme levels is of both diagnostic and prognostic importance.

Blood plasma contains several enzymes. Depending on their role they are devided into two groups.

A. Functional Enzymes

They are present in plasma at higher level than in most of tissues and they perform functions in plasma. They include lipoprotein lipase, choline esterase and enzymes of blood coagulation etc.

B. Non-functional Enzymes

The are present only at minimal concentrations in normals and have no known function in plasma. They mainly arises from normal destruction of various blood and tissues cells. So, they are mainly contributed by turnover of tissues. Increased concentration of these enzymes in plasma indicates increased tissue breakdown or damage to tissues due to disease or injury. If the plasma level cf secretory enzyme is increased it indicates block in the secretory pathway. Further distribution of enzymes among tissues varies from one organ to another organ. If an organ is rich in an enzyme, injury or damage to that organ leads to release of the enzyme into plasma in significant amounts. Some diseases or cancers of that organ also causes release of the enzyme into plasma. Quantitative measurement of the enzymes in plasma under such conditions serve as good index of disease of that organ. Further more, the amount of enzyme released is proportional to the mass of the affected tissue.

Some of the clinically important enzymes which are routinely measured in clinical chemistry laboratory are:

1. Transminases

Aspartate aminoa transferase (AST) and alanine amino transferase (ALT) are two transaminases most frequently measured. Normal levels are 3-20 U/L for AST and 4-20 U/L for ALT (Units-U). The former enzyme is also referred as GOT (Glutamate oxalo acetate transaminase) and latter is referred as GPT (Glutamate Pyruvate Transminase). These two enzymes differ in distribution. Heart is rich in AST where as liver contains both of them in equal amounts. Hence, AST estimation is most commonly done in diseases that affect heart. AST level increases in plasma following heart attack or myocardial infarction. Since liver contains more of ALT, its elevation in plasma is specific indicator of liver damage. Plasma ALT level is more in liver diseases like alcoholic cirrhosis, biliary obstruction, cancer and toxic hepatitis.

Both the enzymes are elevated in acute infective hepatitis because liver contains both of them in significant amount. After the onset of viral hepatitis, the levels of these enzymes reaches peak rapidly and come back to normal reference level within a week. Since the skeletal muscle contains appreciate amounts of ALT, its level is increased in muscle damage as in severe trauma and in muscular dystrophy. Serum transaminases are also elevated in lung disease.

2. Alkaline phosphatase

This enzyme catalyzes the hydrolysis of organic esters at alkaline pH 9.0, hence the name alkaline phosphatase. The normal level is 20-90 units/L. The level of the enzyme is elevated in rickets, obstructive jaundice, hyper para thyroidism, metastatic cancer, bone cancer and osteomalacia. In obstructive jaundice, its level is 10 times the normal level because its secretion is blocked due to obstruction. Its level also increases in some non-specific diseases like leukemia, lung and kidney damages and congestive heart failure, Hodgkin's disease and intestinal disorders.

3. Acid phosphatase

This enzyme catalyzes the hydrolysis of organic esters at acidic pH (5.0) hence the name acid phosphatase. The normal level of the enzyme is 2.5-12.0 units/L. It is increased in prostrate cancer. Small increase are seen in bone disease and breast cancer.

4. γ-glutamyl trans peptidase (GGT)

It is involved in the degradation of glutathione. Its level is increased in alcoholic cirrhosis. The normal plasma level of GGT is less than 30 units/L. Since this enzyme is secreted into bile by liver, like alkaline phosphatase γ-glutamyl trans peptidase level increases in cholestatic or obstructive jaundice. It is also elevated in brain lesions.

5. Creatine phosphokinase (CK)

The normal level of this enzyme in plasma is 12-60 U/l. Since skeletal muscle is rich in CK serum CK level raises in disease effecting skeletal muscle. Its level is elevated in muscular dystrophy, polymyositis, severe muscle exercise, muscle injury, hypothyroidism, epileptic seizures and in tetanus.

CK level is also elevated in diseases affecting cardiac muscle because of its high content in it. CK level is elevated in myocardial infarction.

6. Lactate dehydrogenase (LDH)

The LDH normal level is 70-90 units/L. LDH levels are elevated in myocardial infraction. The serum LDH level raises within 24 hours after infraction, reaches peak level around 2-3 days and returns to normal in a week. Serum LDH level is also elevated in pernicious anemia, megaloblastic anemia, acute hepatitis, blood cancer and in progressive muscular dystrophy.

7. Isocitrate dehydrogenase

The normal level of this enzyme in plasma is 1-5 Units/L. Its level is elevated in inflammatory diseases of liver like infective heptatitis, toxic hepatitis. In obstructive jaundice, its level remains normal. This enzyme is found in cerebrospinal fluid. Measurement of enzyme in C.S.F. is a valuable diagnostic aid in the cases of meningitis and brain tumors. In meningitis the level is elevated more than that of in cerebral tumors.

8. Amylase

The normal range of this enzyme in plasma is 800-1800 Units/L. This enzyme is secreted by pancreas and salivary glands. So, its level is elevated mainly in acute pancreatitis and parotitis. Its level raised in other conditions like intestinal obstruction and in mumps.

9. Lipase

It is an enzyme produced by pancreas. It is secreted into duodenum through pancreatic duct. The normal level of this enzyme is up to 150 Units/L. It is mainly elevated in acute pancreatitis and pancreas cancer. It is also elevated in patients with abdominal lesions, perforated peptic ulcer, intestinal obstruction and in acute peritonitis.

ISOENZYMES IN CLINICAL MEDICINE

1. In some cases, elevated serum enzyme level may not indicate severity and specific organ damaged, because the serum enzyme is derived from routine destruction of cells of various organs.
2. Since isoenzymes are organ specific, iso-enzyme determination gives an indication about the specific organ affected. Further, iso-enzyme distribution varies from one organ to other organ. Hence, if an organ rich in a isoenzyme is damaged or diseased, more of that iso-enzyme enters plasma.
3. By measuring that isoenzymes level in serum the specific organ diseased can be confirmed.
4. Therefore, iso-enzyme determination is useful in differential diagnosis.

(a) LDH Isoenzymes

Serum LDH is the combination of five isoenzymes. Each iso-enzyme is derived from specific organ. LDH_1 is derived from heart because heart is rich in LDH_1. Similarly, LDH_5 is derived from skeletal muscle because it is rich in LDH_5. Liver also contain LDH_2 to LDH_5 isoenzymes in different amounts. LDH isoenzymes are present in different proportions. The proportions of LDH isoenzymes in normal serum are 25%, 35%, 27%, 8% and 5% for LDH_1, LDH_2, LDH_3, LDH_4 and LDH_5, respectively.

When heart muscle is affected as in myocardial infarction, LDH_1 level increases in plasma because of release of LDH_1 from damaged heart muscle. So measurement of LDH isoenzyme in serum in myocardial infraction is more sensitive index of myocardial necrosis than the measurement of total LDH activity. Similarly, elevated levels of LDH_5 is more specific of muscle lesions and liver inflammation of hepatitis.

(b) CK Isoenzymes

The normal serum CK is composed of CK_1, CK_2 and CK_3. In normal persons, CK_2 accounts only 2% of total CK but it accounts for 20% of CK in a patient within 4 hours after heart attack.

(c) Alkaline Phosphatase Isoenzymes

The normal serum alkaline phosphatase is composed of 4 isoenzymes. They are derived from bone, liver, placenta and intestine. Measurement of isoenzymes of alkaline phosphatase is used to distinguish liver lesions from bone lesions in metastatic carcinoma.

SERUM ENZYME PROFILES

1. It involves estimations of different serum enzymes for few days following the onset of a disorder.
2. Multi enzyme determinations for a short span of time serve as good index of disorder. More over determination of more than one enzyme in a particular disease is more useful in prognosis.
3. Several serum enzymes serve as diagnostic indices of myocardial infarction. Serum AST level starts increasing by 6 hours after heart attack, reaches peak value around one to second day and returns to normal by sixth day. CK level follows a pattern similar to AST. It contrast, LDH levels raises within 24 hours of heart attack, reaches peak around 2-3 day and level remain increased even after a week (Fig. 4.14).

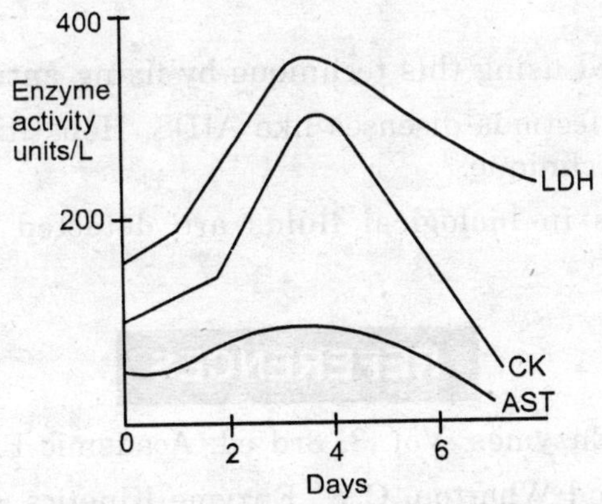

Fig. 4.14 Serum enzyme profiles in myocardial infarction

Serum enzyme levels are also determined to detect inherited disorders associated with altered enzyme levels like galactosemia, glucose-6-phosphate dehydrogenase deficiency etc.

ENZYME-LINKED IMMUNO ADSORBENT ASSAY

It is popularly known as ELISA technique. The technique combines enzymology with immunology and photometry. It is used for detection and estimation of substances which are either antigens or antibodies. It is based on immune complex formation. The immune complex consist of an antibody, antigen and second antibody with bound enzyme (antibody-antigen-antibody$_2$-enzyme). Enzyme linked to second antibody has a crucial role in detection and estimation of antigen present in sample. When it reacts with substrate color is produced. Intensity of the color is proportional to amount of antigen present in sample.

Steps of this techniques are given below:

1. Antibodies specific to an antigen of interest are produced. They are fixed to support materials using coupling agent. The support materials are cellulose, plastic, polystyrene

or glass. Plastic plates containing wells (depressions) which are coated with antibodies are commonly used.

2. Sample (serum) containing antigen is allowed to combine with antibody by placing sample in the well.
3. Unbound molecules of sample are removed by washing.
4. A second antibody linked to an enzyme is added. This also binds to antigen to form antibody-antigen-antibody$_2$-enzyme complex. Thus, second antibody linked to enzyme is fixed to support material.
5. Unbound antibody$_2$-enzyme complex is removed by washing.
6. In the final step, substrate is added. Enzyme linked to antibody$_2$ convert substrate to colored product which is measured.

Medical Importance

1. Using this technique, antigens or antibodies that are present in very small amounts (picograms) in biological fluids are detected and estimated.
2. Several hormones like insulin, TSH, hCG, Calcitonin etc. are determined world wide using this technique.
3. Antibodies are detected using this technique by fixing antigen to support material.
4. Detection of highly infectious diseases like AIDS, Hepatitis, Malaria etc. World wide involves use of this technique.
5. Some tumor markers in biological fluids are detected and estimated using this technique.

REFERENCES

1. Boyer, P.D. Ed. The Enzymes. Vol. 3, 3rd ed. Academic Press, New York, 1971.
2. Cornish-Bowden, A. and Wherton, C.W. Enzyme Kinetics. IRL Press, Oxford, 1988.
3. Kraut, J. How Do Enzymes Work ? Science **242**, 533-540, 1988.
4. Segel, I.H. Enzyme Kinetics. Wiley, New York, 1975.
5. Wei, L. Clauser, E. Alhene-Gelas, F. and Corvol, P. The Two Homologous Domains of Angiotensin Converting Enzyme Interact Differently with Competitive Inhibitors. J. Biol. Chem. **267**, 13398-13405, 1992.
6. Purich, D.L. Ed. Methods in Enzymology. Vol. 63 and 64, Academic Press, New York, 1979 and 1980.
7. Cohen, P. The Role of Protein Phosphorylation in Neural and Hormonal Control of Cellular Activity. Nature **296**, 613-620, 1982.
8. Kantowitz, E.R. and Lipscomb, W.N. E. Coli Aspartate Trans Carbamoylase, the Relation Between Structure and Function. Science **241**, 669, 1988.
9. Georgiou, G. and Dewitt, N. Enzyme Beauty. Nature Biotechnology **17**, 1161-1162, 1999.
10. Hosfield, C. *et al.* Crystal Structure of Calpain Reveals Structural Basis for Ca^{2+} Dependent Protease Activity and a Novel Mode of Enzyme Activation. The EMBO J. **18**, 6880-6889, 1999.

11. Xiao, Y. *et al.* Plugging into Enzymes: Nanowiring of Redox Enzyme by Gold Nanoparticles. Science **299**, 1877-1881, 2003.
12. Stevens, S.Y. *et al.* Delineation of the Allosteric Mechanism of Cytidylyl Transferase Exhibiting Negative Co-operativity. Nature Structural Biology **8**, 947-952, 2001.
13. Eisenmesser, E.Z. *et al.* Enzyme Dynamics During Catalysis. Science **295**, 1520-1523, 2003.
14. Eisenthal, R. Enzyme Assays: A Practical Approach. Oxford University Press, 2002.
15. A.G. Maragoni. Enzyme Kinetics. A Modern Approach. Wiley, New York, 2002.
16. Zollner, H. Hand Book of Enzyme Inhibitors. 2nd ed., VCH Publishers, New York, 1993.
17. Natesh, R. *et al.* Crystal Structure of Human Angiotensin Converting Enzyme-Lisinopril Complex, Nature **421**, 551-554, 2003.
18. Fuchs, S. *et al.* Role of N-terminal Catalytic Domain of Angiotensin Converting Enzyme Investigated by Targeted Inactivation in Mice. J. Biol. Chem. **279**, 15946-15953, 2004.
19. Dun McElheny, *et al.* Defining role of active site of fluctuations in dihydrofolate reductase catalysis. Proc. Nafd. Acad. Sci. USA. **102**, 5032-5035, 2005.

EXERCISES

ESSAY QUESTIONS

1. Classify enzymes. Give examples for each class and write reactions with cofactors they catalyze.
2. Define enzymes. Write the effect of substrate concentration, temperature and pH on enzyme activity.
3. Define active site of an enzyme. Write its characteristics and explain models of active site.
4. Define coenzyme. Name four coenzymes and write reactions with cofactors in which they act as coenzyme.
5. Define inhibition. Explain competitive and feedback inhibition with examples.
6. Describe enzyme regulation.
7. Write an essay on enzymes of diagnostic (clinical) importance.
8. Define allosteric enzymes. Describe kinetics of an allosteric enzyme with an example and model.
9. Name factors affecting enzyme catalyzed reactions. Explain each one of them with suitable examples.
10. Define cofactors. Explain their importance with suitable examples.
11. Write an essay on enzyme inhibition.

SHORT QUESTIONS

1. Define K_m. Write its significance.
2. Define proenzymes. How they are converted to enzymes ?
3. Define non-competitive inhibition. What happens to K_m and V_{max} in this type of inhibition. Give examples.
4. Explain enzyme regulation by covalent modification.

5. Competitive inhibitors are chemotherapeutic agents. Justify with examples.
6. Define isoenzymes. Write their importance in diagnosis with examples.
7. Explain clinical significance of following serum enzymes.
   (*a*) Transaminases
   (*b*) Alkaline phosphatase
8. Explain group specificity with examples.
9. Define enzyme induction and repression. Explain with examples.
10. Explain effect of substrate concentration on enzymatic reaction.
11. Explain phenomenon of cooperativity.
12. Write diagnostic importance of lactatedehydrogenase and creatine phosphokinase.
13. Define metalloenzyme. Give examples.
14. Write on coenzymes of oxidation-reduction reactions.
15. How enzymes are named? Write about E.C. number.
16. What are enzyme profiles? How they are useful in diagnosis? Explain with example.
17. Define allosteric inhibition. Explain with an example.
18. Write on enzymes of myocardial infarction.
19. Explain ELISA technique. Write its application.

MULTIPLE CHOICE QUESTIONS

1. All of the following statements are correct for enzymes. Except
   (*a*) Enzymes are proteins
   (*b*) Enzymes are catalysts
   (*c*) Enzymes speed up chemical reactions by lowering energy of activation.
   (*d*) Enzymes alters equilibrium constant of the reaction which they catalyze.
2. The pH optimum of pancreatic proteases is
   (*a*) 7.6 (*b*) 8.0
   (*c*) 6.0 (*d*) 2.5
3. A competitive inhibitor
   (*a*) Binds at active site (*b*) Does not bind at active site
   (*c*) Alters V_{max} only (*d*) Binds at allosteric site
4. A competitive inhibitor used in hypertension is
   (*a*) Malonate (*b*) Allopurinol
   (*c*) Captopril (*d*) Oxaloacetate
5. A non-competitive inhibitor that is used as nerve gas in World War II is
   (*a*) Iodo acetate (*b*) Cyanide
   (*c*) Di-isopropyl fluorophosphate (DFP) (*d*) Arsenite

6. In metalloenzymes metals are
   (a) Attached to enzyme through coordinate bonds.
   (b) Covalently attached to enzymes.
   (c) Non-covalently attached to enzymes.
   (d) Loosely attached to enzymes.
7. An allosteric enzyme
   (a) Is usually made-up of many subunits. (b) Obeys Michaelis Menten kinetics.
   (c) Undergo covalent modification. (d) Exist in pro-enzyme form.
8. γ-glutamyl transpeptidase level in blood increases in
   (a) Alcoholic cirrhosis (b) Cancer
   (c) Myocardial infarction (d) Pancreatitis

FILL IN THE BLANKS

1. In detergent industry enzymes are used as ----------------.
2. Enzymes are for more efficient than ---------------- catalysts.
3. The ability of enzymes to recognize optical isomers of a substrate is known as -------------.
4. K_m of enzymes is important when they are used as ----------------.
5. Affinity of enzyme towards substrate --------------- in competitive inhibition.
6. Heavy metals are known as enzyme ----------------.
7. Angiotensin converting enzyme is an example for --------------- enzyme and metal --------------- enzyme.
8. An allosteric enzyme exist in --------------- state --------------- state.

5
CHAPTER

CARBOHYDRATES

OCCURRENCE

Carbohydrates are present in humans, animal tissues, plants and in micro-organisms. Carbohydrates are also present in tissue fluids, blood, milk, secretions and excretions of animals.

MEDICAL AND BIOLOGICAL IMPORTANCE

1. Carbohydrates are the major source of energy for man. For example, glucose is used in the human body for energy production.
2. Some carbohydrates serve as reserve food material in humans and in plants. For example, glycogen in animal tissue and starch in plants serves as reserve food materials.
3. Carbohydrates are components of several animal structure and plant structures. In animals, carbohydrates are components of skin, connective tissue, tendons, cartilage and bone. In plants, cellulose is a component of wood and fiber.
4. Some carbohydrates are components of cell membrane and nervous tissue.
5. Carbohydrates are components of nucleic acids and blood group substances.
6. Carbohydrates are involved in cell-cell interaction.
7. Derivative of carbohydrates are drugs. For example, a glycoside ouabain is used in clinical medicine. Streptomycin an antibiotic is a glycoside.
8. Aminosugars, derivatives of carbohydrates are components of antibiotics like erythromycin and carbomycin.
9. Ascorbic acid, a derivative of carbohydrate is a water-soluble vitamin.
10. Bacterial invasion involves hydrolysis of mucopolysaccharides.
11. Survival of Antarctic fish in icy environment is due to presence of anti-freeze glycoproteins in their blood.

Chemical Nature of Carbohydrates

Carbohydrates are polyhydroxy alcohols with a functional aldehyde or keto group. They are represented with general formulae $C_n(H_2O)_n$. Usually the ratio of carbon and water is one in most of the carbohydrates hence the name carbohydrate (Carbonhydrate).

Classification of Carbohydrates

Carbohydrates are classified into three major classes based on number of carbon chains present. They are:

1. Monosaccharides
2. Oligosaccharides
3. Polysaccharides

All the three classes contain a saccharose group and hence the name saccharides.

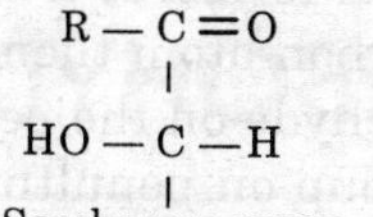

Saccharose group

MONOSACCHARIDES

Monosaccharides are those carbohydrates which can not be hydrolyzed to small compounds. Their general formula is $C_n(H_2O)_n$. They are also called as *simple sugars*. Monosaccharides containing three to nine carbon atoms occur in nature.

Nomenclature

Monosaccharides have common (trivial) names and systematic names. Systematic name indicates both the number of carbon atoms present and aldehyde or ketone group. For example, glyceraldehyde is a simple sugars containing three carbon atoms and a aldehyde group. Simple sugars containing three carbon atoms are referred as trioses. In addition, sugars containing aldehyde group or keto group are called as aldoses or ketoses, respectively. Thus, the systematic name for glyceraldehyde is aldotriose. Similarly, a simple sugar with three carbon atoms and a keto group is called as ketotriose. Some monosaccharides along with their common and systematic names are shown in Fig. 5.1.

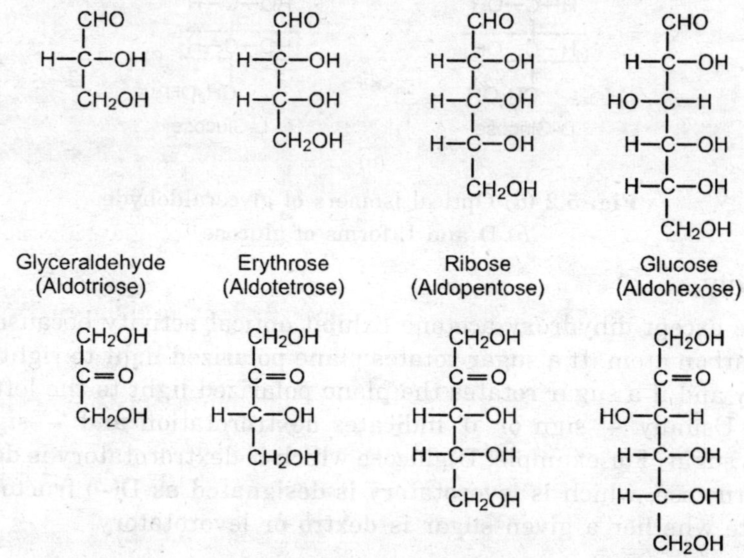

Fig. 5.1 Some important monosaccharides (systematic names are given in parenthesis)

PROPERTIES OF MONOSACCHARIDES

1. Optical Isomerism

All the monosaccharides except dihydroxyacetone contain at least one asymmetric carbon atom and hence they exhibit optical isomerism. The two optical isomers of glyceraldehyde containing one asymmetric carbon atom are D-glyceraldehyde and L-glyceraldehyde. The optical isomers are also called as *enantiomers*. The D and L forms of glyceraldehyde are shown in Fig. 5.2. Further D and L-glyceraldehyde are used as parent compounds to designate all other sugars (compounds) as D or L forms. If a sugar has the same configuration as D-glyceraldehyde on the penultimate carbon atom then it is called as 'D' sugar. If a sugar has the same configuration as L-glyceraldehyde on the penultimate carbon atom then it is called as 'L' sugar. Usually, the hydroxyl group on penultimate carbon atom points to right in 'D' glucose and D-glyceraldehyde whereas it points to left in L-glucose and L-glyceraldehyde (Fig. 5.2). Further D and L forms of glucose are mirror images like mirror images of glyceraldehyde. Though both forms of sugars are present in nature D-isomer is abundant and sugars present in the body are all D-isomers. L-fructose and L-rhamnose are two L-isomers found in animals and plants.

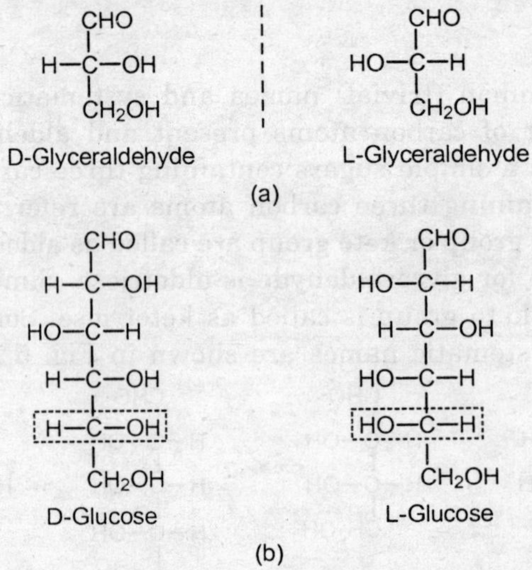

Fig. 5.2 (*a*) Optical isomers of glyceraldehyde
(*b*) D and L forms of glucose

2. Optical Activity

Monosaccharides except dihydroxy acetone exhibit optical activity because of the presence of asymmetric carbon atom. If a sugar rotates plane polarized light to right then it is called as *dextrorotatory* and if a sugar rotates the plane polarized light to the left then it is called as levorotatory. Usually '+' sign or 'd' indicates dextrorotation and '–' sign or 1 indicates levorotation of a sugar. For example, D-glucose which is dextrorotatory is designated as D(+) glucose and D-fructose, which is levorotatory is designated as D(–) fructose. The letter 'D' does not indicate whether a given sugar is dextro or levorotatory.

3. Epimers

Are those monosaccharides that differ in the configuration of –OH group on 2nd, 3rd and 4th carbon atoms. Epimers are also called as *diastereoisomers*. Glucose, galactose and mannose are examples for epimers. Galactose is an epimer of glucose because, configuration of hydroxyl group on 4th carbon atom of galactose is different from glucose. Similarly, mannose is an epimers of glucose because configuration of hydroxyl group on 2nd carbon atom of mannose is different from glucose (Fig. 5.3). Ribulose and xylulose are also epimers. They differ in the configuration of –OH group on third carbon atom (Fig. 5.3).

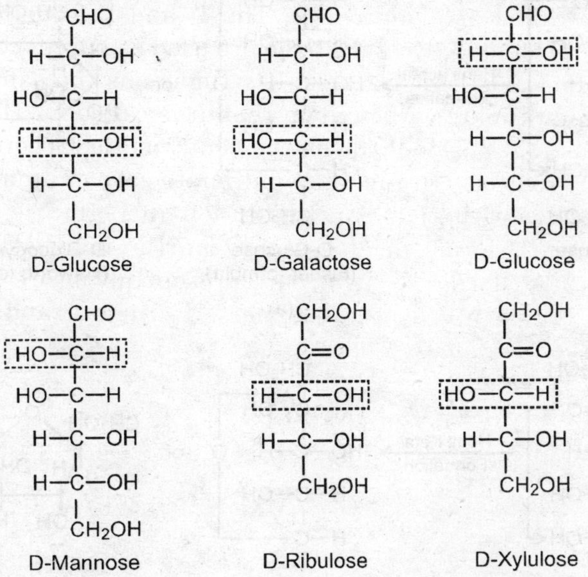

Fig. 5.3 Epimers of aldohexoses and ketopentoses

4. Functional Isomerism

Functional isomers have same molecular formulae but differ in their functional groups. For example, glucose and fructose have same molecular formulae $C_6H_{12}O_6$, but glucose contains aldehyde as functional group and fructose contains keto group (Fig. 5.4). Hence, glucose and fructose are functional isomers. This type of functional isomerism is also called as *aldose-ketose isomerism* because aldose is an isomer of ketose and vice versa.

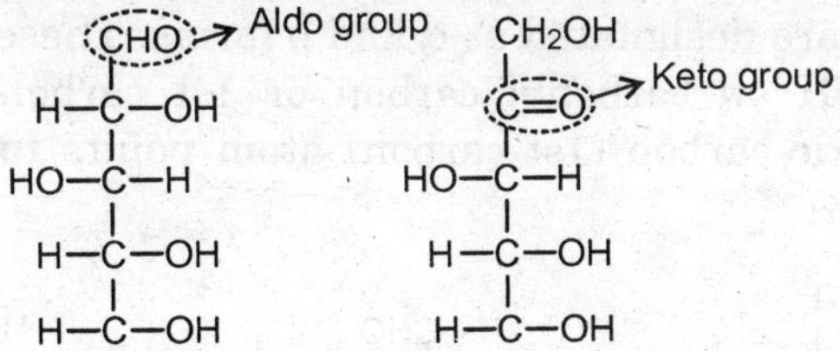

Fig. 5.4 Aldose-ketose isomerism

5. Ring Structures

In solution, the functional aldehyde group of glucose combines with hydroxyl group of 5th carbon atom. As a result a 6 numbered heterocyclic pyranose ring structure containing 5 carbons and one oxygen is formed (Fig. 5.5). The linkage between aldehyde group and alcohol is called as 'hemiacetal' linkage. Similarly, a 5 numbered furanose ring structure is formed from fructose when keto group combines with hydroxyl group on 5 carbon atom. The linkage between keto and alcohol group is called 'hemi ketal' linkage. (Fig. 5.5). Both hemi acetal and hemi ketal are internal or intra molecular linkages.

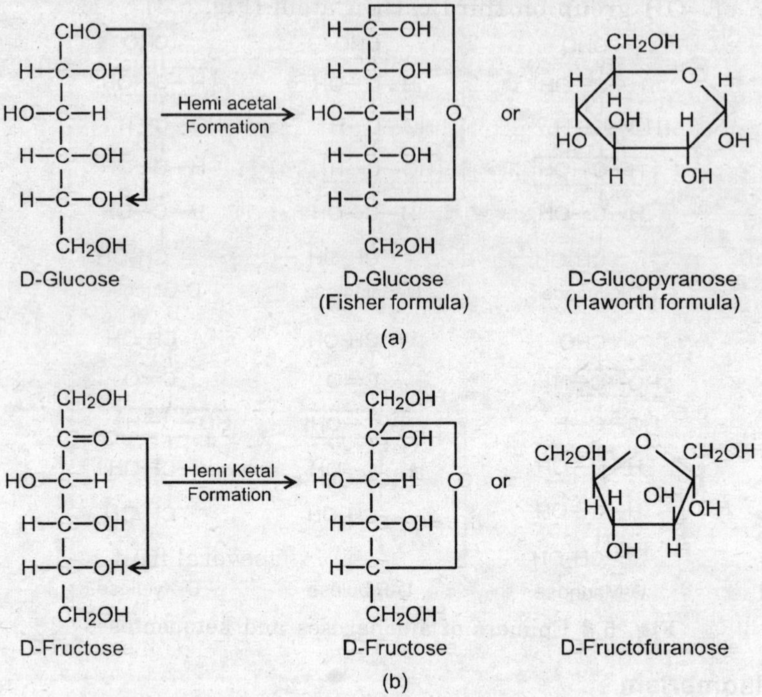

Fig. 5.5 (*a*) Glucose ring structure formation (*b*) Formation of fructose ring structure

6. Anomers

Those monosaccharides that differ in configuration of OH groups on carbonyl carbon or anomeric carbon are called as anomers. Formation of ring structure of glucose generates anomers of glucose, which are designated as α and β forms. These two forms of glucose differ in the configuration of OH on carbonyl carbon or 1st carbon atom. In the α-form the hydroxyl group on anomeric carbon (1st carbon) atom points to the right where as in the β-form to the left (Fig. 5.6).

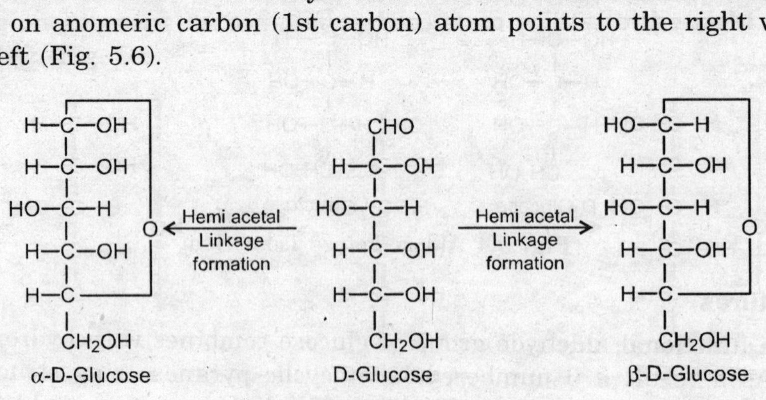

Fig. 5.6 Anomers of glucose

7. Mutarotation

Monosaccharides containing asymmetric carbon atom rotate plane polarized light. When optical rotation for α-D-glucose is measured it will be 112° and on standing the rotation decreases slowly and attains a constant value +52.5°. Likewise when optical rotation for β-D-glucose is measured the rotation changes from initial +19° to +52.5°. The changes in optical rotation for α and β forms of glucose are shown in Fig. 5.7. The change in optical rotation when either form of glucose is allowed to stand in solution is called mutarotation. It is due to conversion of cyclic form of glucose to straight chain form.

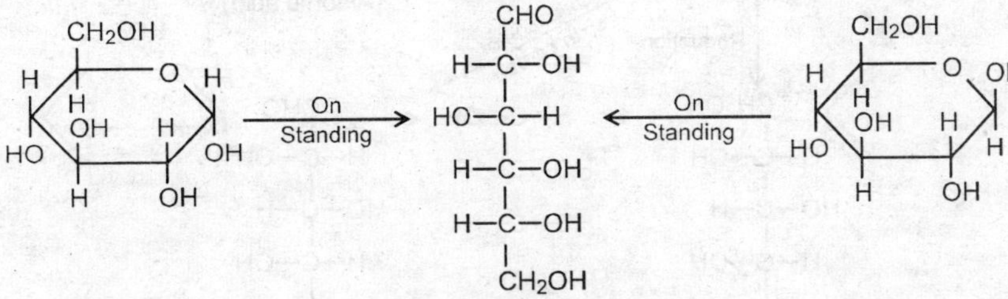

Fig. 5.7 Mutarotation of glucose

Important monosaccharides in the metabolic point of view are glucose, fructose, galactose, ribose, erythrose and glyceraldehyde. Glucose is found in several fruit juice blood of humans and in honey. Galactose is a part of lactose. Fructose is found in several fruit juices and honey. Commonly glucose is referred as dextrose. All monosaccharides containing free aldehyde or keto group reduces ions like Cu^{2+} under alkaline conditions.

Biologically Important Sugar (Glucose) Derivatives

Sugar derivatives of biological importance are sugar acids, sugar alcohols, deoxy sugars, sugar phosphates, amino sugars and glycosides.

1. Sugar acids

Oxidation of aldo group of sugars produces aldonic acids. For example, oxidation of glucose produces gluconic and (Fig. 5.8) oxidation of terminal alcohol group (–OH sixth carbon atom) of glucose produces glucuronic acid or uronic acid (Fig. 5.8). Uronic acids are components of mucopolysaccharides and required for detoxification. Ketoses are not easily oxidized. Vitamin C or ascorbic acid is also sugar acid.

2. Sugar alcohols

Reduction of aldose and keto groups of sugar produces polyhydroxy alcohols or polyols. These polyols are intermediates of metabolic reactions. Other sugar alcohols are glycerol and inositol. The alcohols formed from glucose, galactose and fructose are sorbitol, galactitol and sorbitol, respectively (Fig. 5.8).

3. Deoxy sugars

Those sugars in which oxygen of a hydroxyl group is removed leaving hydrogen. Deoxyribose is an example (Fig. 5.9). It is present in nucleic acids. Fucose is another deoxy sugar present in blood group substances.

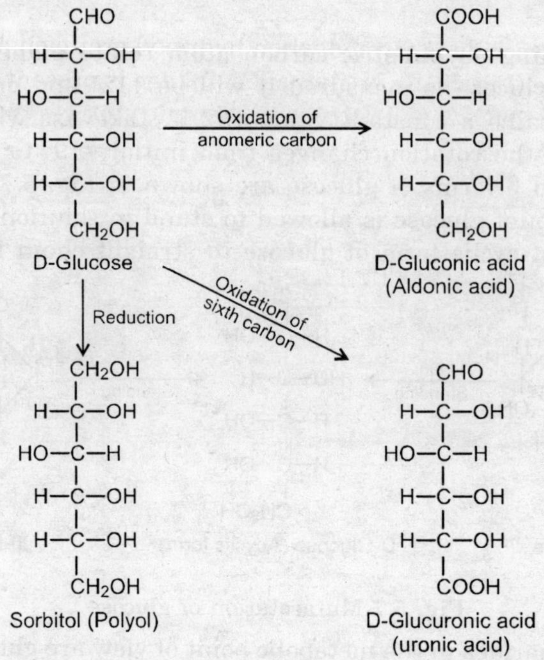

Fig. 5.8 Oxidation and reduction products of glucose

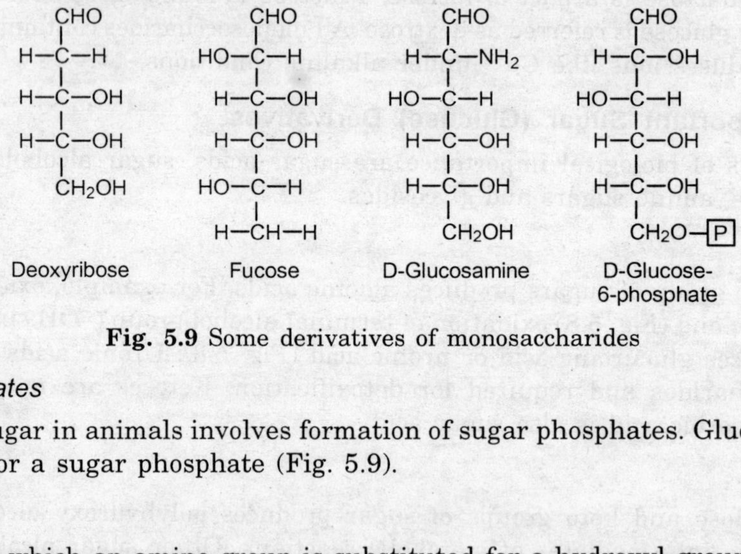

Fig. 5.9 Some derivatives of monosaccharides

4. Sugar phosphates

Breakdown of sugar in animals involves formation of sugar phosphates. Glucose-6-phosphate is an example for a sugar phosphate (Fig. 5.9).

5. Aminosugars

Those sugars in which an amino group is substituted for a hydroxyl group. D-glucosamine is an example for an amino sugar (Fig. 5.9). Amino sugars are components of mucopolysaccharides, and antibiotics.

6. Glycosides

Are of two types:

(*a*) **O-glycosides.** When hydroxyl group on anomeric carbon of a sugar reacts with an alcohol (sugar) O-glycoside is formed (Fig. 5.10). O-glycosidic linkage is present in disaccharides and polysaccharides. So, disaccharides, oligosaccharides and polysaccharides are O-glycosides.

(*b*) **N-glycosides.** N-Glycoside is formed when hydroxyl group on anomeric carbon of sugar reacts with an amine (Fig. 5.10). N-glycosidic linkage is present in nucleotides, RNA and DNA. So, nucleotides, RNA and DNA are examples for N-glycosides.

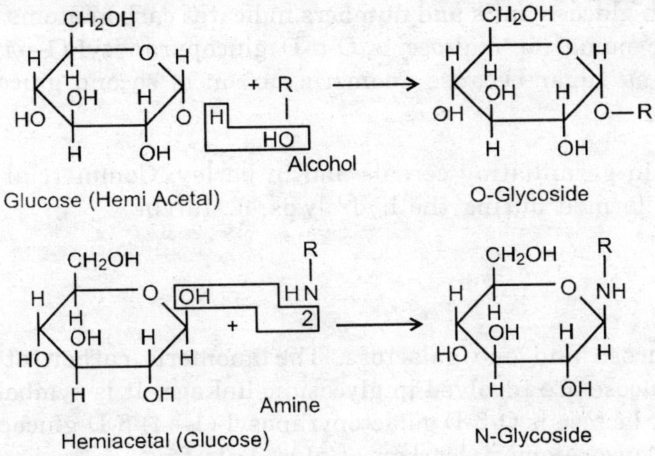

Fig. 5.10 Formation of O-Glycoside and N-Glycoside

OLIGOSACCHARIDES

They consist of 2-10 monosaccharide units. The monosaccharides are joined together by glycoside bonds. Most important oligosaccharides are disaccharides.

Disaccharides

They provide energy to human body. They consist of two monosaccharide units held together by glycosidic bond. So, they are glycosides. Most common disaccharides are maltose, lactose and sucrose (Fig. 5.11).

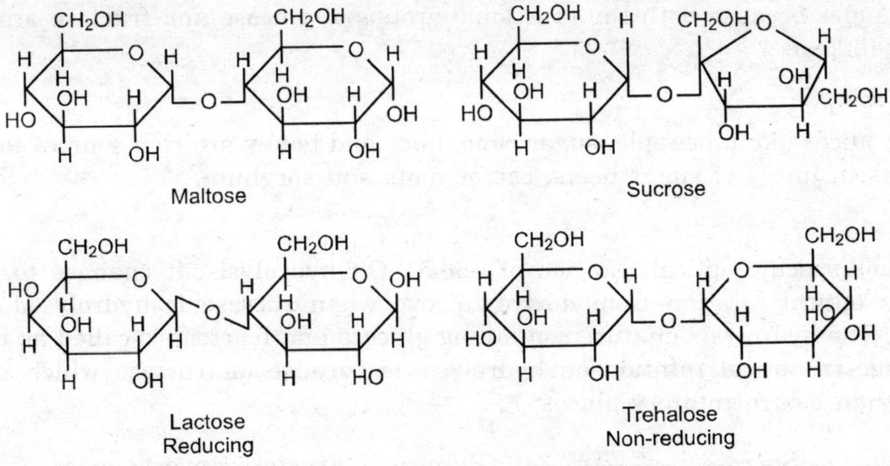

Fig. 5.11 Reducing and non-reducing disaccharides

Maltose

Structure

It contains two glucose units. The anomeric carbon atom of first glucose and carbon atom 4 of the second glucose are involved in glycosidic linkage. The glycosidic linkage of maltose is symbolized as α (1→4). In this symbol, letter α-indicates the configuration of anomeric carbon atoms of both glucose units and numbers indicates carbon atoms involved in glycosidic linkage. Systematic name for maltose is O-α-D glucopyranosyl-(1→4)-α-D glucopyranose. Maltose is a reducing sugar because anomeric carbon of second glucose is free.

Source for maltose

Maltose is present in germinating cereals and in barley. Commercial malt sugar contains maltose. It may be formed during the hydrolysis of starch.

Lactose

Structure

It contains one glucose and one galactose. The anomeric carbon atom of galactose and carbon atom 4 of glucose are involved in glycosidic linkage. It is symbolized as β (1→4). The systematic name for lactose is O-β-D galactopyranosyl-(1→4)-β-D-glucopyranose. Lactose is a reducing sugar because anomeric carbon of glucose is free.

Source for lactose

Lactose is synthesized in mammary gland and hence it occurs in milk.

Sucrose

Structure

It contains glucose and fructose. The anomeric carbon of glucose and anomeric carbon of fructose are involved in glycosidic linkage. Further, glucose is in α-form whereas fructose is in β-form in sucrose. Hence the glycosidic linkage of sucrose is designated as α, β(1→2). Its systematic name is O-α-D-glucopyranosyl-(1→2)-β-D-fructofuranose. Sucrose is a non reducing sugar because both the functional groups of glucose and fructose are involved in glycosidic linkage.

Source of sucrose

Ripe fruit juices like pineapple, sugar cane, juice and honey are rich sources for sucrose. It also occurs in juices of sugar beets, carrot roots and sorghum.

Invert sugar

Sucrose has specific optical rotation of +66.5°. On hydrolysis, it changes to –19.8°. This change in optical rotation from dextro to levo when sucrose is hydrolysed is called as *inversion*. The hydrolysis mixture containing glucose and fructose is called as invert sugar. The change in optical rotation on hydrolysis is because of fructose which is more levo rotatory than dextro rotatory glucose.

$$\underset{+66.5^\circ}{\text{Sucrose}} \xrightarrow{\text{Hydrolysis}} \underset{+52.5^\circ}{\text{Glucose}} + \underset{-92^\circ}{\text{Fructose}} \underset{-19.8^\circ}{\text{(invert sugar)}}$$

Other Disaccharides

Isomaltose

It contains two glucose units. Glycosidic linkage is $\alpha(1\rightarrow6)$. Isomaltose is the disaccharide unit present in glycogen, amylopectin and dextran.

Cellobiose

It also contains two glucose units but they are joined in $\beta(1\rightarrow4)$ linkage. It is formed from cellulose.

Trehalose

It also contains two glucose units. The glycosidic linkage is $\alpha(1\rightarrow1)$. So, it is a non-reducing disaccharide (Fig. 5.11). It is a major sugar of insect hemo lymph. In fungi it serve as reserve food material.

Other Oligosaccharides

Beans and peas contain some oligosaccharides. These oligosaccharides contain 4 to 5 monosaccharide units. Stachyose and verbascose are a few such oligosaccharides. Usually these oligosaccharides are not utilized in human body. Oligosaccharide chains are also found in glycoproteins where they have important functions. Oligosaccharides are also important constituents of glycolipids present in cell membrane.

POLYSACCHARIDES

They are polymers of monosaccharides. They contain more than ten monosaccharide units. The monosaccharides are joined together by glycosidic linkage.

Classification of Polysaccharides

Polysaccharides are classified on the basis of the type of monosaccharide present. The two classes of polysaccharides are homo-polysaccharides and hetero-polysaccharides.

(*a*) **Homopolysaccharides.** They are entirely made up of one type of monosaccharides. On hydrolysis, they yield only one kind of monosaccharide.

(*b*) **Heteropolysaccharides.** They are made up of more than one type of monosaccharides. On hydrolysis they yield more than one type of monosaccharides.

Homopolysaccharides

Important homopoly-saccharides are starch, glycogen, cellulose, dextran and inulin and chitin. All these contain glucose as repeating unit. Other name for homopolysaccharides are homoglycans.

Starch

Structure

1. It consist of two parts. A minor amylose component and a major amylopectin component.
2. Amylose is a straight-chain polymer of glucose units. $\alpha(1\rightarrow4)$ glycosidic linkage is present between glucose units.

3. In contrast amylopectin is a branched molecule (Fig. 5.12). In the linear portion of amylopectin (1→4) glycosidic linkage exist between glucose units whereas (1→6) glycosidic linkage exist at branch points between glucose residues. The branching occurs in amylopectin for every 2-30 glucose units.
4. Amylose has helical coiled secondary structure and usually 6 glucose residue make one turn (Fig. 5.12). Because of branching secondary structure of amylopectin is a random coil structure.

Function

1. It is the major polysaccharide present in our food.
2. It is also called as storage polysaccharide because it serve as reserve food material in plants.
3. It is present in food grains, tubers and roots like rice, wheat, potato and vegetables.

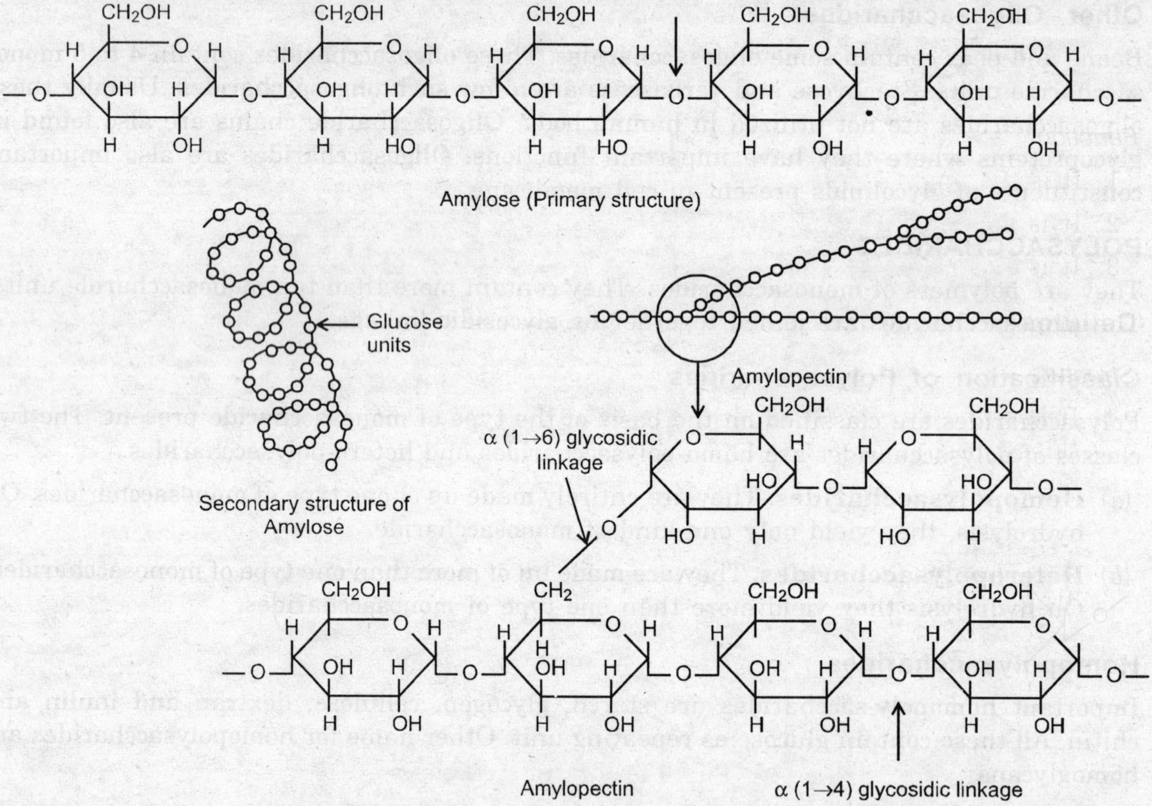

Fig. 5.12 Structures of amylose and amylopectin

Glycogen

Structure

1. The structure of glycogen is similar to that of amylopectin of starch. However, the number of branches in glycogen molecule is much more than amylopectin (Fig. 5.13).
2. There is one branch point for 6-7 glucose residues.

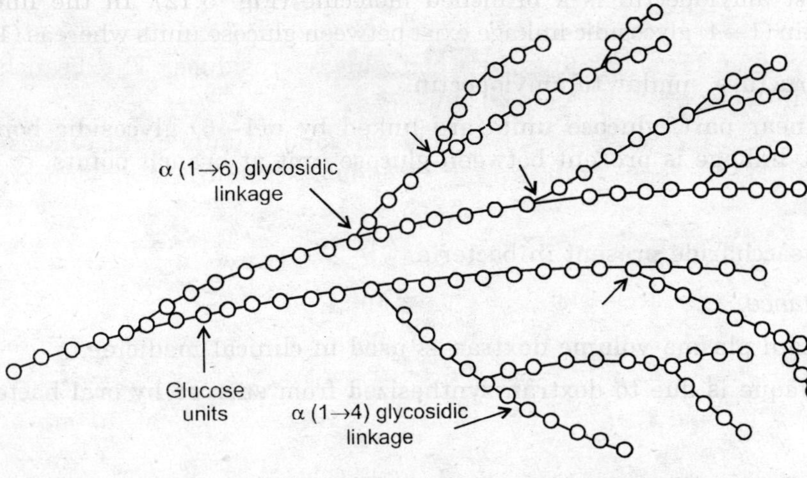

Fig. 5.13 Structure of glycogen. Each open circle represents a glucose molecule. Arrow indicates branch point

Function

1. It is the major storage polysaccharide (carbohydrate) in human body.
2. It is mainly present in liver and muscle.
3. It is also called as animal starch.

Cellulose

Structure

1. It has linear chain of glucose residues, which are linked by β(1→4) glycosidic linkage (Fig. 5.14).

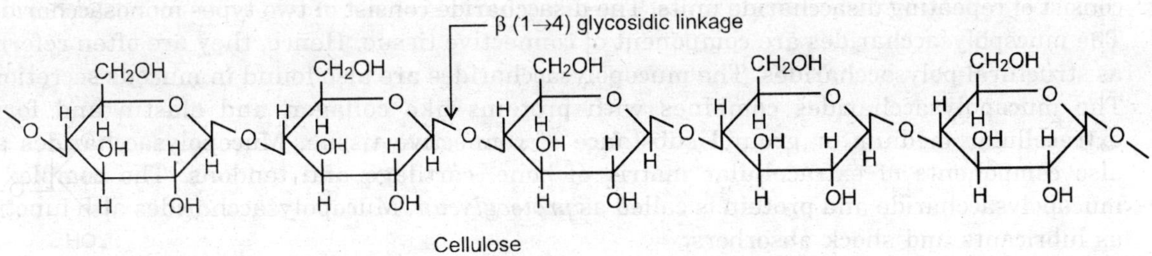

Fig. 5.14 Structure of cellulose

2. It occurs as bundle of fibres in nature.
3. The linear chains are arranged side by side and hydrogen bonding between adjacent stands stabilizes the structure.

Function

1. It is the most abundant polysaccharide in nature.
2. It is found in fibrous parts of plants like wood, cotton and straw.

Dextran

Structure

1. It has structure similar to amylopectin.
2. In the linear part, glucose units are linked by α(1→6) glycosidic bond and α(1→3) glycosidic linkage is present between glucose unit at branch points.

Function

1. It is polysaccharide present in bacteria.

Medical importance

1. To maintain plasma volume dextran is used in clinical medicine.
2. Dental plaque is due to dextran synthesized from sucrose by oral bacteria.

Inulin

(*a*) *Structure.* It is a polysaccharide composed of fructose. β(1→2) glycosidic linkage is present between fructose units.

(*b*) *Function.* It is present in tubers of chicory, dhalia and in the bulb of onion and garlic. Inulin is used to determine glomerular filteration of kidney.

Chitin

(*a*) *Structure.* A polysaccharide composed of N-acetyl glucosamine. Glycosidic linkage is β(1→4).

(*b*) *Function.* It is an important structural polysaccharide of invertebrates like crabs, lobster and insects.

HETEROPOLYSACCHARIDES

They are also called as *mucopolysaccharides* and *glycosaminoglycans*. Mucopolysaccharides consist of repeating disaccharide units. The disaccharide consist of two types monosaccharides. The mucopolysaccharides are component of connective tissue. Hence, they are often referred as structural polysaccharides. The mucopolysaccharides are also found in mucous secretions. The mucopolysaccharides combines with proteins like collagen and elastin and forms extracellular medium or ground substance of connective tissue. Mucopolysaccharides are also components of extracellular matrix of bone, cartilage and tendons. The complex of mucopolysaccharide and protein is called as *proteoglycan*. Mucopolysaccharides also function as lubricants and shock absorbers.

Few important mucopolysaccharides or glycosaminoglycans (GAGs) are:

Hyaluronic Acid (HA)

Structure

The repeating disaccharide of hyaluronic acid consist of glucuronic acid and N-acetylglucosamine.

$$—(\beta\text{-Glucuronic acid}—\text{N-acetylglucosamine})_n—$$

Hyaluronic acid

Functions

1. It is present in synovial fluid and function as lubricant.
2. It is also present in skin, loose connective tissue, umbilical cord and ovum.
3. It is present in vitreous body of eye.

Medical importance

1. As the age advances hyaluronic acid is replaced by-dermatan sulfate in synovial fluid. Dermatan sulfate is not a good lubricant, hence age related pains develop in old people.
2. In young people, vitreous is clear elastic gel in which hyaluronic acid is associated with collagen. As the age advances the elasticity of vitreous is reduced due to decreased association between collagen and hyaluronic acid. As a result, vision is affected in older people.
3. Hyaluronic acid of tumour cells has role in migration of these cells.
4. Hyaluronic acid is involved in wound healing (repair). In the initial phase of wound healing (repair), hyaluronic acid concentration increases many fold at the wound site. It allows rapid migration of the cells to the site of connective tissue development.
5. Hyaluronic acid helps in scarless repair. If suitable levels of HA are maintained during would healing scar formation is reduced or even prevented.
6. HA content of skin decreases as age advances this is the reason for increased susceptibility of aged people for scar formation.
7. Pneumonia, meningitis and bacteremia causing pathogenic bacteria contains hyaluronte lyase. Hydrolysis of HA by this enzyme facilitates invasion of host by these bacteria.

Chondroitin sulfate A and B chondroitin-4-sulfate and chondroitin-6-sulfate

Structure

1. The repeating disaccharide unit of chondroitin sulfates consist of glucuronic acid and N-acetyl galactosamine. N-acetyl galactosamine is sulfated.
2. In chondroitin-4-sulfate, 4th carbon atom of N-acetyl galactosamine is sulfated where as in chondroitin-6-sulfate the 6th carbon is sulfated.

———(β-Glucuronicacid———N-acetyl galactosamine-)$_n$———
|
sulfate

Chondrotin sulfate

Functions

1. Chondroitin sulfates are components of cartilage, bone and tendons.
2. They are also present in the cornea and retina of the eye.
3. Chondroitin sulfate content decreases in cartilage as age advances.

Heparin

Structure

1. The repeating disaccharide unit of heparin consist of glucosamine and either iduronic acid or glucuronic acid.

2. Majority of uronic acids are iduronic acids. Further amino groups of glucosamine is sulfated.

——(Iduronic acid-Glucosamine-Gluronic acid-Glucosamine)——

/ /

sulfate sulfate

Heparin

Functions

1. Heparin is a normal anti-coagulant present blood.
2. It is produced by mast cells present in the arteries, liver, lung and skin.
3. Unlike other glycosaminoglycans, heparin is an intracellular component.

Dermatan Sulfate

Structure

The repeating disaccharide consist of Iduronic acid and N-acetyl galactosamine sulfate.

——(Iduronic acid—N-acetyl galactosamine)$_n$——

|

sulfate

Dermatan sulfate

Functions

1. It is present in skin, cornea and bone.
2. It has a role in corneal transparency maintenance.

Keratan sulfates I and II

Structure

1. The repeating disaccharide consist of galactose and N-acetyl glucosamine sulfate.
2. Type I and II have different attachments to protein.

——(Galactose-N-acetyl glucosamine)$_n$——

|

sulfate

Keratan sulfate

Functions

1. They are components of cartilage, cornea and loose connective tissue.
2. Keratan sulfate l is important for corneal transparency.

GLYCOPROTEINS

They are found in mucous fluids, tissues, blood and in cell membrane. They are proteins containing short chains of carbohydrates. The carbohydrate chains are usually oligosaccharides. These oligosaccharide chains are attached to proteins by O-glycosidic and N-glycosidic bonds. Further oligosaccharide is composed of fucose, N-acetyl glucosamine, galactose and glucose. The oligosaccharide chains have important functions like:

1. Oligosaccharide present on the surface of erythrocytes are responsible for the classification of blood groups. They determine blood group and hence they are called as *blood group substances.*
2. Oligosaccharides determine the life span of proteins.
3. Cell-cell recognition depends on oligosaccharide chains of glycoproteins.
4. Glycoproteins of some invertebrates function as antifreezing agents. They are known as antifreeze glycoproteins (AFGPs). One such glycoprotein is identified in Antarctic fishes. It is very essential for their survival in such sub zero environment that exist at Antarctica. It is present in the blood of the Antarctic fishes. It prevents freezing by binding to ice, which enables these fishes to survive in the surrounding icy environment. It is surprising that this protein arose from pancreatic trypsinogen like protease.

Sialic Acids

Structure

1. Sialic acids are acyl derivatives of neuraminic acid.
2. Neuraminic acid is a 9 carbon sugar consisting of mannosamine and pyruvate. Usually amino group of mannosamine of neuraminic acid is acetylated. Hence, N-acetyl neuraminic acid (NANA) is an example for sialic acid.

Functions

1. Oligosaccharides of some membrane glycoproteins contains a terminal sialic acid.
2. Sialic acid is an important constituent of glycolipids present in cell membrane and nervous tissue.

REFERENCES

1. Pigman, W. and Horton, D. Eds. The Carbohydrates, 2nd ed. Academic Press, New York, 1972.
2. Ginsburg, V. and Robbins, P. Eds. Biology of Carbohydrates. Wiley, New York, 1984.
3. Goodwin, T.W. and Mercer, E.I. Introduction to Plant Biochemistry. Pergamon, Oxford, 1983.
4. Sharon, N. Glycoproteins, Trends Biochem. Science. **9**, 199-20, 1984.
5. Schauer, R. Sialic Acids and their Role as Biological Masks. Trends Biochem. Sci. **10**, 357-360, 1983.
6. Aspinall, G.O. Ed. The Polysaccharides. Vol. 1-3, Academic Press, New York, 1983 to 1985.
7. Cheng, C.C. and Chen, L. Evolution of Antifreeze Glycoprotein, Nature **401**, 443-444, 1999.
8. Jedrzejas. M.J. *et al*. Mechanism of Hyaluronan Degradation by *S. Pneumoniae* Hyaluronate lyase. J.Biol. Chem. **277**, 28287-28297, 2002.
9. Delpech, B. *et al.* Hyaluronan: Fundamental Principles and Applications in Cancer. J. Inter. Med. **242**, 41-48, 1997.

10. Ikan, R. Ed., Naturally Occurring Glycosides. Wiley, New York, 1999.
11. Lind horst, J.K. Essentials of Carbohydrate. Chemistry and Biochemistry, Wiley-VCH Verlag GmbH, 2003.
12. Stick, Robert, V. Carbohydrates: The Sweet Molecules of Life. Academic Press, 2001.
13. Maroclo, M.V. *et al.* Urinary glycosaminoglycan excretion during menstrual cycle in normal young women, J. Urology. **173**, 1789-1792, 2005.

EXERCISES

ESSAY QUESTIONS

1. Define carbohydrates. Classify them giving suitable examples.
2. Define polysaccharide. Classify, give examples for each class.
3. Describe properties of monosaccharides.
4. What are heteropolysaccharides? Write about structure and functions of five of them.

SHORT QUESTIONS

1. Define anomers and epimers. Give examples for each.
2. Write a note on (*a*) Mutarotation (*b*) Invert sugar
3. Name biologically important derivatives of glucose.
4. Compare starch and glycogen with respect to:
   (*a*) Source (*b*) Structure (*c*) Function
5. Write composition and functions of:
   (*a*) Hyaluronic acid (*b*) Heparin (*c*) Chondroitin sulfates
6. Define glycoproteins. Mention their functions.
7. Write four functions of carbohydrates.
8. Name non-reducing disaccharide. Write its composition, source and functions.
9. Write briefly about glycosides.
10. What are sialic acids? Write their functions.
11. Name sugar present in milk. Write its composition, linkage and function.
12. Write products of hydrolysis of sucrose, lactose and maltose.
13. Write a note on cellulose.
14. Give an account of carbohydrates functions.

MULTIPLE CHOICE QUESTIONS

1. Most of the carbohydrates found in human body are
   (*a*) D-isomers (*b*) L-isomers
   (*c*) D- and L-isomers (*d*) None of these
2. The linkage between aldehyde group of glucose and its hydroxyl group of 5th carbon atom is
   (*a*) Hemiacetal linkage (*b*) Hemiketal linkage
   (*c*) Glycosidic linkage (*d*) Ester linkage

3. Glucose and fructose are the examples for
   (*a*) Functional isomers (*b*) Optical isomers
   (*c*) Geometric isomers (*d*) Non-reducing sugars
4. Polyol is formed from
   (*a*) Oxidation of sugars (*b*) Reduction of sugars
   (*c*) Polysaccharides (*d*) Monosaccharides
5. O-glycosidic bond is formed
   (*a*) When a sugar reacts with acid.
   (*b*) When sugar reacts with alkali.
   (*c*) When an anomeric carbon of sugar reacts with an alcohol.
   (*d*) When an anomeric carbon of sugar reacts with an acid.
6. Trehalose is a disaccharide present in
   (*a*) Milk (*b*) Blood
   (*c*) Hemolymph (*d*) Tubers

FILL IN THE BLANKS

1. --------------- is reserve food material in humans.
2. A sugar acid that is water soluble vitamin is ---------------.
3. Oligosaccharide chain of erythrocyte membrane glycoproteins determines --------------- classification.
4. Non-reducing disaccharide present in cane sugar is ---------------.
5. --------------- is a nine carbon sugar present in cell membrane.

6
CHAPTER

LIPIDS

OCCURRENCE

Lipids are present in humans, animals, plants and micro-organisms to some extent. Animal fat, egg yolk, butter and cheese are lipids of animal origin, vegetable or cooking oils and vanaspati are lipids are plant origin.

MEDICAL AND BIOLOGICAL IMPORTANCE

1. Fat under skin serve as thermal insulator against cold.
2. Fat around kidney serve as padding against injury.
3. Fat serve as a source of energy for man like carbohydrates.
4. Fat is an ideal form for storing energy in the human body compared to carbohydrates and proteins because:
   (*a*) Energy content of fat is higher.
   (*b*) Only fat can be stored in a concentrated water free form which is not possible with carbohydrates and proteins
5. Lipids are structural components of cell membrane and nervous tissue.
6. Some lipids serve as precursors for the synthesis of complex molecules. For example, acetyl-CoA is used for the synthesis of cholesterol.
7. Lipoproteins, which are complexes of lipids and proteins are involved in the transport of lipids in the blood and components of cell membrane.
8. Some lipids serve as hormones and fat soluble vitamins are lipids.
9. Fats are essential for the absorption of fat soluble vitamins.
10. Fats serve as surfactants by reducing surface tension.
11. Eicosanoids which have profound biological actions are derived from the essential fatty acids.
12. Lipids present in myelinated nerves act as insulators for propagation of depolarization wave.
13. Some saturated fatty acids are anti-microbial and anti-fungal agents.
14. Lipids are an important group of antigens of parasites that cause filariasis, cysticercosis, leishmaniasis and schistosomiasis in India and other Third World countries. Anti-lipid antibodies are found in the blood of individuals affected with these diseases.

15. Some eicosanoids act as immuno modulators and mitogens.
16. Saturated free fatty acids (SFFAs) are pheromones of animals like tiger etc.

Chemical Nature of Lipids

Lipids are the group of greasy organic compounds, which are soluble in organic solvents like chloroform, ether and benzene but insoluble in water. They are fats, waxes, compound lipids, steroids, fatty acids and fat soluble vitamins. A lipid is a fat-like substance but need not be a fatty acid always.

Classification of Lipids

Based on the composition lipids are classified into 1. Simple lipids, 2. Compound lipids, 3. Derived lipids.

Simple Lipids

They are esters of fatty acids with alcohols. Fats and waxes are example for simple lipids. An ester is formed when acid reacts with alcohol (Fig. 6.1 A).

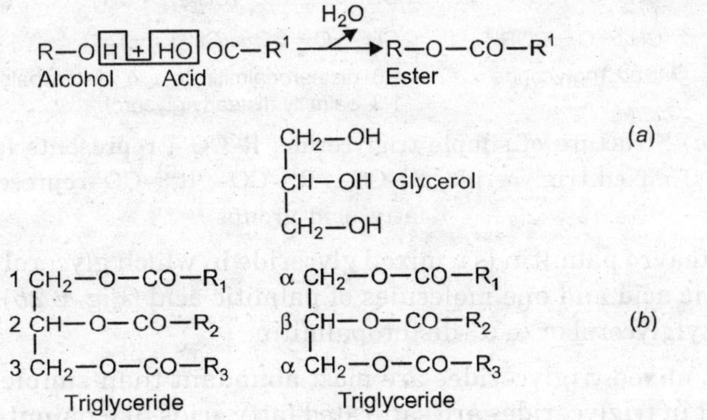

Fig. 6.1 (*a*) Ester formation; R, R^1-hydrocarbon chains.
(*b*) Triglyceride is shown with Indo-Arabic numbers and Greek alphabets.
R_1– CO–, R_2–CO–, R_3–CO– are three fatty acid groups.

Fats

They are esters of fatty acids with glycerol. They are also called as *triglycerides* or *triacylglycerols* because all the three hydroxyl groups of glycerol are esterified. Fats are also called as *neutral fats*.

Structure

The chemical structure of triglyceride or fat consist of three molecules of fatty acids esterified with one molecule of glycerol (Fig. 6.1*b*). All the three fatty acids can be same or different.

Nomenclature of Triglycerides

The carbon atoms of glycerol of triglycerides are indicated with both Indo-Arabic numbers and Greek alphabets (Fig. 6.1*b*). The former is used commonly. The triglycerides are further subdivided based on type of fatty acids esterified to glycerol. They are:

A. **Simple triglyceride.** If all the three fatty acids esterifed to glycerol are same then it is called as simple triglyceride (Fig. 6.2*a*).

Example:

(*a*) Tripalmitin in which glycerol is esterified to three molecules of palmitic acid (Fig. 6.2*a*). Other names to tripalmitin are 1,2,3-tripalmityl glycerol or α,β,α^1-tripalmitin.

(*b*) Tristearin is another simple triglyceride.

B. **Mixed triglyceride.** If the three fatty acids esterified to glycerol are different than it is called as mixed triglyceride (Fig. 6.2*b*).

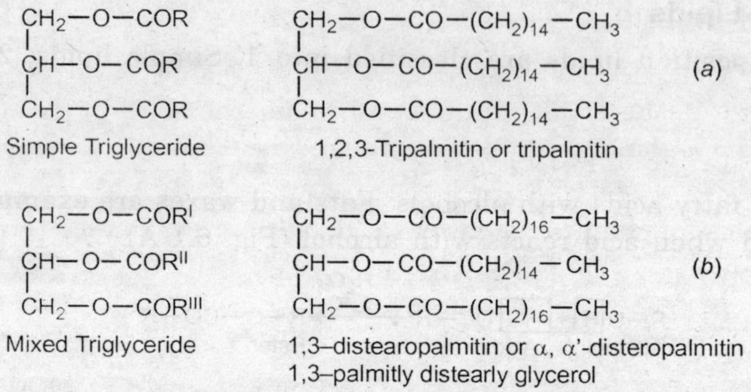

Fig. 6.2 (*a*) Structure of simple triglyceride; R–CO–, represents fatty acid group (*b*) Structure of mixed triglyceride, R^I–CO–, R^{II}–CO–, R^{III}–CO–represents three different fatty acid groups

Example: 1,3 disteavro palmitin is a mixed glyceride in which glycerol is estexdified with two molecules of steoric acid and one molecules of palmitic acid (Fig. 6.2*b*). Other names are 1,3-distearyl-2-palmitylglycerol or α, α^1-disteropalmitin.

In human, fat mixed triglycerides are most abundant than simple triglycerides. Further fatty acids present in triglycerides are saturated fatty acids like palmitic acid and stearic acid.

Shorthand Form for Fats

Writing an entire fat molecule showing structure of glycerol with attached the fatty acids is awkward, hence a shorthand form is devised. In shorthand formulae, carbon, backbone of glycerol is represented by vertical line. Horizontal lines drawn from top, middle and bottom of the vertical line represents —OH groups on 1st, 2nd and 3rd carbon atoms, respectively. (Fig. 6.3). If the hydroxyl is esterified with a fatty acid, then —OH group is replaced by 'acyl' term (Fig. 6.3).

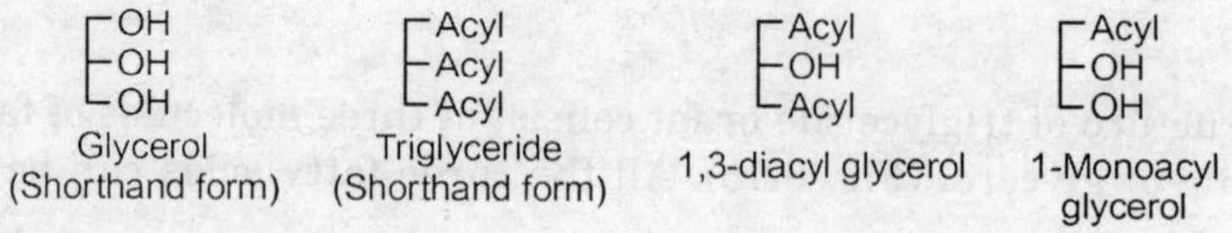

Fig. 6.3 Structures of partial acyl glycerols, Acyl represents fatty acid residue

Other Noteworthy Acyl Glycerols

1. Diacylglycerol

In which 2 fatty acids are esterified to glycerol.

Example: 1,2-diacyglycerol and 1,3-diacylglycerol. In 1,2-diacylglycerol, the 1st and 2nd–OH groups are esterified (Fig. 6.3).

2. Monoacylglycerol

In which one fatty acid is esterified with glycerol.

Example: 1-monoacylglycerol and 2-monoacylglycerol. In 1-monoacylglycerol the 1st —OH group is esterified. (Fig. 6.3). Diacylglycerol and monoacylglycerol are called as *partial acyl glycerols*.

Functions of Triglycerides

1. They function as storage lipids in animals and in plants.
2. In man adipose tissue or fat tissue found under the skin, in the abdominal cavity and in the mammary gland contain triacylglycerols. The entire cytoplasm of adipocyte is replaced by triacylglycerol.
3. In other animals and plant cells also triacylglycerols are found as tiny droplets in cytosol.
4. The fat stored under the skin serve as energy store and as insulator against cold.
5. Women have more fat than men.
6. In obese (fat) people, many kilograms of triacylglycerol is stored under the skin.
7. The antarctic and arctic animals like seals and penguins appear bloated because of high concentration of triglycerides in their bodies.

Functions of Partial Acylglycerols

They are also found in some tissues. Mainly they are formed as intermediates during the synthesis of triglycerides and during digestion of fat.

PHYSICAL PROPERTIES OF TRIGLYCERIDES

1. Pure fats have no colour, taste and odour.
2. At room temperature, fat of plant origin remains oil because it contains more unsaturated fatty acids where as animal fat remain as solid, because it contains mostly saturated fatty acids.
3. Triglycerides containing asymmetric carbon atom are optically active.

CHEMICAL PROPERTIES OF FATS

1. Saponification

When fats are boiled with bases like KOH or NaOH glycerol and salts of fatty acids are formed (Fig. 6.4*a*). This process is called as saponification. The salts of fatty acids act as soaps. Soaps are good cleansing agents, germicides and detoxicants.

2. Hydrogenation

It converts unsaturated fatty acids of triglycerides into saturated fatty acids. (Fig. 6.4*b*). Commercially hydrogenation is used to convert liquid fats of plant origin to solid cooking fats which are known as *margarines*. Since hydrogenation converts liquid fat to solid fat it is also called as *hardening*. Vanaspati (dalda) is obtained from vegetable oils through this process.

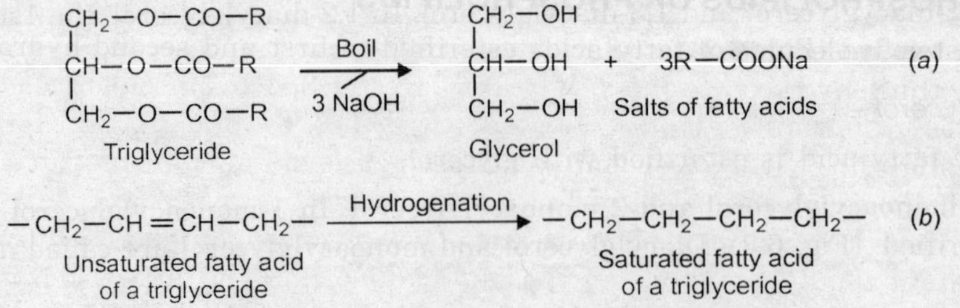

Fig. 6.4 (*a*) Saponification of triglyceride
(*b*) Hydrogenation of fat

3. Lipid Peroxidation

When natural fats are exposed to atmospheric oxygen, they develop bad smell and taste. It is called as *rancidity*. Rancidity of fat develops even on prolonged storing. It is due to formation of lipid peroxides. Atmospheric oxygen reacts with unsaturated fattly acids of triglycerides and forms lipid peroxides.

Antioxidants

Like vitamin E and ascorbic acid prevent peroxide formation. They are added to food fats to improve storage quality.

In the body also lipid peroxides are formed. Free radicals mediate lipid peroxide formation in the body. Diseases like cancer, diabetes, atherosclerosis are due to the formation of lipid peroxides in the body.

Waxes

Structure

Waxes are esters of fatty acids with long chain alcohol.

Examples:

(*a*) Lanolin or wool fat is a mixture of fatty acid esters of long chain alcohols lanosterol and agnosterol.

(*b*) Cholesterol ester is wax present in the blood (lipoprotein) and cell membranes.

(c) Bees wax is an ester of palmitic acid with myricyl alcohol.

Functions

1. Waxes serve as protective coatings on skin, fur and feathers of animals, birds and on fruit and leaves of plants. Shiny appearance of fruits and leaves is due to waxes.
2. Waxes act as water barrier for animals, birds and insects. Further wax is hard in cold climate and soft in hot climate.
3. Since wool is a wax woollen clothing provides protection against cold. Marine organisms use wax as source of energy.

COMPOUND LIPIDS

They are esters of fatty acids with alcohol containing nitrogenous bases and additional groups. Based on alcohol compounds lipids are subdivided into (*a*) Glycerophospholipids (*b*) Sphingo lipids. Compounds lipids are also divided into phospholipids and glycolipids.

GLYCEROPHOSPHOLIPIDS OR PHOSPHOLIPIDS

They contain two molecules of fatty acids esterified to first and second hydroxyl groups of glycerol. The third hydroxyl group of glycerol is esterified to phosphoric acid. Further a nitrogen base or second alcohol is also esterified to phosphoric acid (Fig. 6.5). Glycerophospholipid without second alcohol is known as *phosphatidic acid*. Some glycerophospholipids are named according to second alcohol or nitrogen base and they are considered as derivatives of phosphatidic acid. They are phosphatidyl choline, phosphatidyl serine, phosphatidyl ethanolamine and phosphatidyl inositol. The fatty acid combinations are different in each of these phospholipids.

Phosphatidylcholine

Structure

It contains two fatty acids esterified to first and second hydroxyl group of glycerol. The third hydroxyl is esterified to phosphoric acid to which second alcohol choline is also esterified. (Fig. 6.5). Phosphatidylcholine is also called as *lecithin*. Lecithin contains a saturated fattly acid at C-1 position and unsaturated fatty acid at C-2 position.

Function

It is the major phospholipid of cell membrane. It is also present in egg yolk and lipoproteins.

Phosphotidyl ethanolamine

In which second alcohol ethanolamine is esterified to phosphoric acid of phosphatidic acid (Fig. 6.5).

Phosphatidyl serine

In which aminoacid serine is esterified to phosphoric acid of phosphatidic acid (Fig. 6.5). Phosphatidyl ethanolamine and phosphatidyl serine are called as cephalins and amino-phospholipids.

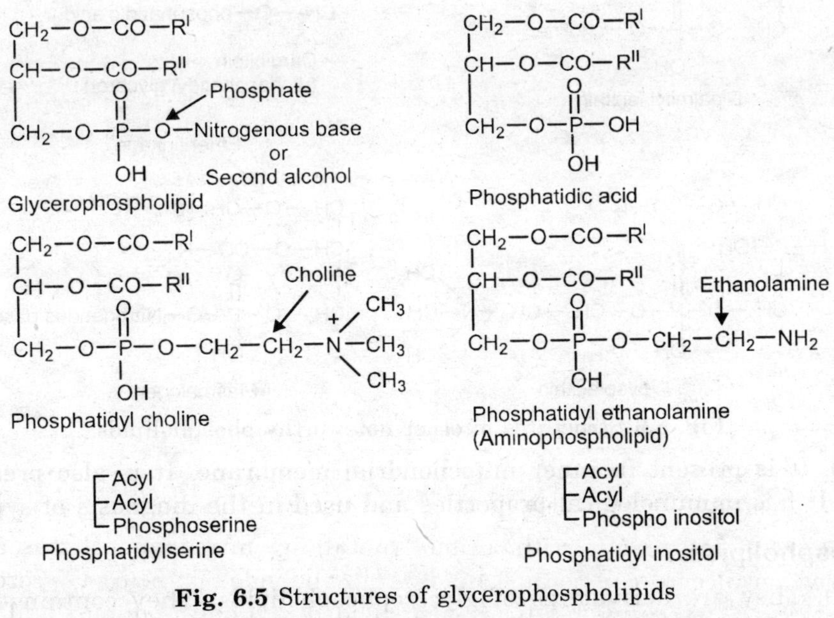

Fig. 6.5 Structures of glycerophospholipids

Phosphatidyl Inositol

In which polyol inositol is esterified to phosphoric acid of phosphatidic acid (Fig. 6.5).

Functions

1. Cephalins are major component of cell membrane, lipoproteins and nervous tissue.
2. Phosphatidyl inositol is also a component of cell membrane. Further phosphorylated phosphatidyl inositol (PIP_2) and inositol triphosphate (IP_3) are involved in signal transduction.

Other Noteworthy Phospholipids

1. Dipalmitoyl Lecithin

(*a*) *Structure.* Two molecules of palmitic acid are esterified to 1st and 2nd carbon atoms of glycerol. A phosphocoline is esterified to the third hydroxyl group (Fig. 6.6).

(*b*) *Function.* It is secreted in alveoli of lungs. It is involved in the maintenance of shape of alveoli. It acts as surfactant (surface active agent) in the lungs. It prevents the collapse of alveoli due to high surface tension of water by reducing surface tension of water. It is synthesized only after 30 weeks of gestation.

Medical importance

Its deficiency in the lungs of premature infants causes respiratory distress syndrome (RDS) which accounts for 20% mortality in premature infants.

2. Cardiolipin

(*a*) *Structure.* It is a double glycerophospholipid. It contains two phosphatidic acids esterified to C-1 and C-3 of glycerol (Fig. 6.6).

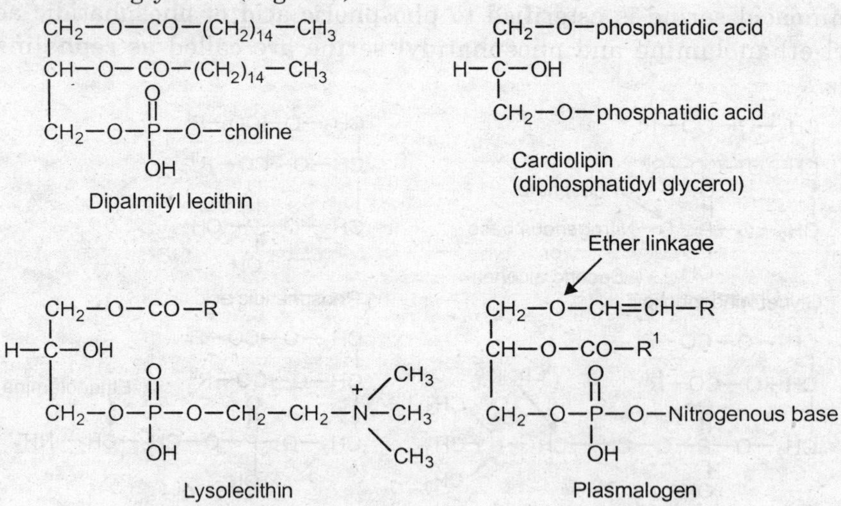

Fig. 6.6 Structures of other noteworthy phospholipids

(*b*) *Function.* It is present in inner mitochondrial membrane. It is also present in heart muscle. It has immunological properties and used in the diagnosis of syphilis.

3. Lysophospholipids

(*a*) *Structure.* They are derivatives of glycerophospholipids. They contain only one acyl group instead of two acyl groups (Fig. 6.6).

(b) *Function.* They account for 1-2% of phospholipids in living systems. They are formed from phospholipids by the action of enzymes and formed during biosynthesis of phospholipids. Lysolecithin is a component of cobra venom and a strong hemolysing agent.

4. Plasmalogens

(a) *Structure.* They are also glycero phospholipids. These compounds contain unsaturated fatty alcohol in place of fatty acid at the C-1 position. Hence, the normal ester linkage is replaced by ether linkage on the C-1 carbon of glycerol. Usually nitrogen bases are choline, serine and ethanolamine (Fig. 6.6).

(b) *Function.* They are found in brain, heart and muscle. Plasmlogen content is more in cancer cells. Platelet activating factor, which causes aggregation of platelets is a plasmalogen.

SPHINGOLIPIDS

They contain fatty acid long chain amino alcohol sphingosine (Fig. 6.7) and bases or additional groups. They are subdivided into 1. Sphingomyelins 2. Glycolipids.

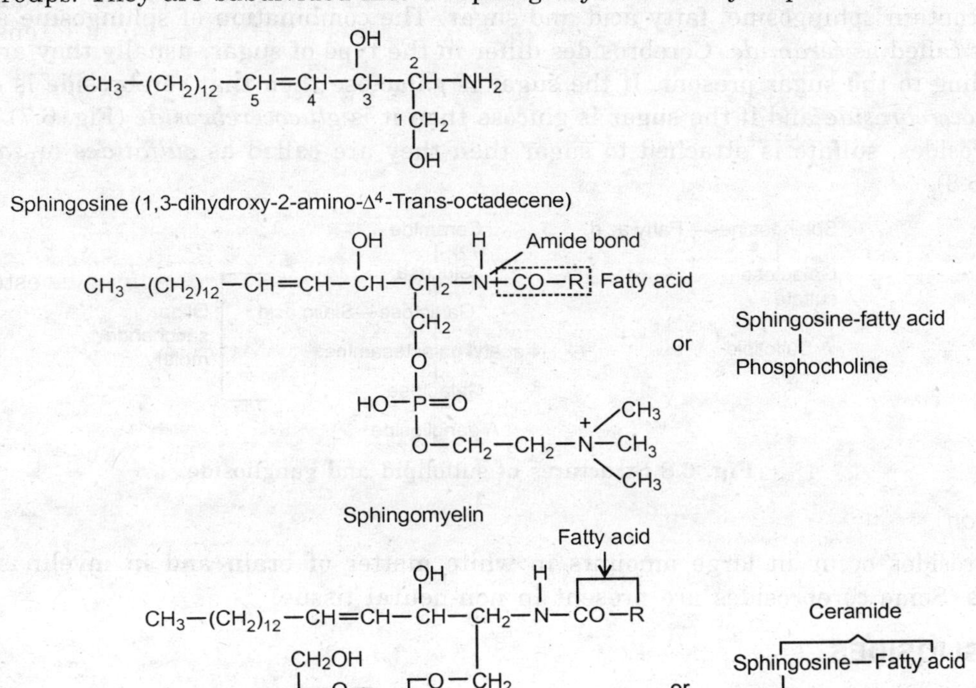

Fig. 6.7 Sphingophospholipid and glycolipid structure

SPHINGOMYELINS

Structure

In sphingomyelins, fatty acid is linked to sphingosine by an amide bond and phosphoryl choline is esterified to C-1 hydroxyl of sphingosine (Fig. 6.7). Because of the phosphorous sphingomyelins are called as sphingo phospholipids.

Functions

1. They are simple and most abundant sphingolipids.
2. They are present in most of animal membranes.
3. Myelin sheath of nerve cells is rich in sphingomyelins.
4. Grey matter also contain sphingomyelins.

GLYCOLIPIDS

They are subdivided into: 1. Cerebrosides and 2. Gangliosides.

Cerebrosides

Structure

They contain sphingosine, fatty acid and sugar. The combination of sphingosine and fatty acid is called as *ceramide*. Cerebrosides differ in the type of sugar, usually they are named according to the sugar present. If the sugar is galactose then that cerebroside is called as *galactocerebroside* and if the sugar is glucose then it is *glucocerebroside* (Fig. 6.7). In some cerebrosides, sulfate is attached to sugar then they are called as *sulfatides* or *sulfolipids* (Fig. 6.8).

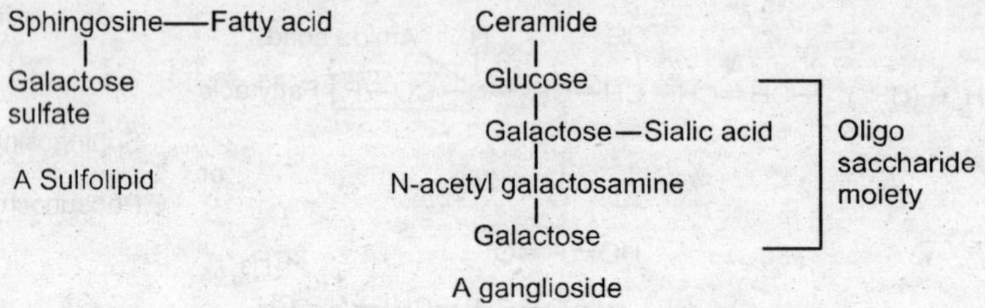

Fig. 6.8 Structures of sulfolipid and ganglioside

Function

Cerebrosides occur in large amounts in white matter of brain and in myelin sheath of nerves. Some cerebrosides are present in non-neural tissue.

GANGLIOSIDES

Structure

They are highly complex sphingolipids. They contain ceramide, oligosaccharide and sialic acid (Fig. 6.8).

Functions

1. They are abundant in grey matter of brain.
2. They are also found in non-nerval tissues.
3. They are components of hormone receptors.
4. They also function as receptors for toxins of cholera, influenza and tetanus.
5. They are also involved in cell-cell recognition, growth, differentiation and carcinogenesis.

DERIVED LIPIDS

As the name implies they are formed from simple and compound lipids by hydrolysis. They are fatty acids, steroids, glycerol and retinol.

Fatty Acids

They are acids derived from fats. They are monocarboxylic acids containing long hydro carbon side chain. Based on the nature of hydrocarbon side chain, they are divided into:

A. Saturated fatty acids

B. Unsaturated fatty acids

(a) Saturated fatty acids

In which hydrocarbon side chain is saturated (no double bonds).

(b) Unsaturated fatty acids

In which hydrocarbon side chain is unsaturated (one or more double bonds are present).

Fatty acids are also divided based on hydrocarbon chain length. They are

(*a*) **Short chain fatty acids** Fatty acids containing less than six carbon atoms.

(*b*) **Medium chain fatty acids** Fatty acids containing 6-12 carbon atoms.

(*c*) **Long chain fatty acids** In which hydrocarbon chain contains 13-20 carbon atoms.

(*d*) **Very long chain fatty acids** In which hydrocarbon chain contain 22-30 carbon atoms. Fatty acids of natural fats contain an even number of carbon atoms. Small amounts of fatty acids with odd number of carbon atoms also occurs.

Cis-trans isomerism

Because of the double bonds, unsaturated fatty acids exhibit *cis-trans* isomerism. In the *cis* isomer bulky groups are located on the same side of double bond where as in *trans* isomer they are on the opposite side of double bond (Fig. 6.9*b*). All the naturally occurring unsaturated fatty acids are *cis*-isomers.

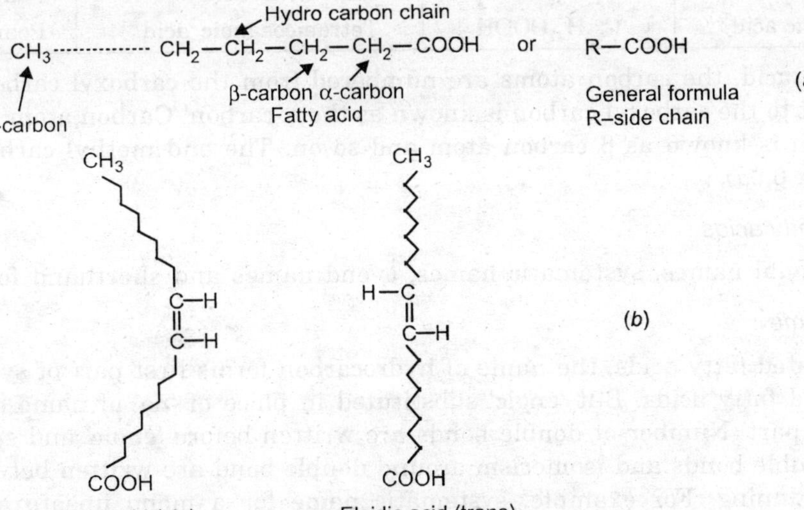

Fig. 6.9 (*a*) General structure of a fatty acid
(*b*) *Cis-trans* isomerism of unsaturated fatty acid

Function

Cis and *trans* isomers are not interchangeable in cells. Only *cis* isomers can fit into cell membrane because of bend at double bond.

Nomenclature of Fatty Acids

Saturated fatty acids

Saturated fatty acids have both trivial names and systematic names.

Systematic name

Systematic name of a saturated fatty acid consist of two parts. Name of hydrocarbon chain forms first part. 'oic' substituted in place of 'e' of hydrocarbon name forms second part. For example, systematic name for a saturated fatty acid containing 8 carbon atoms *i.e.,* (octane + oic + acid) ⟶ octanoic acid. Usually saturated fatty acids end as anoic acids. Examples of saturated fatty acids with systematic names, trivial names and with sources are given in Table 6.1. The trivial name for octanoic acid is caprylic acid.

Table 6.1 Sources, trivial and systematic names of saturated fatty acids

Fatty acid trivial name	Molecular formula	Systematic name	Sources
Butyric acid	C_3H_7COOH	Butanoic acid	Butter
Caproic acid	$C_5H_{11}COOH$	Hexanoic acid	Coconut oil
Caprylic acid	$C_7H_{15}COOH$	Octanoic acid	Coconuts
Capric acid	$C_9H_{19}COOH$	Decanoic acid	Coconuts
Lauric acid	$C_{11}H_{23}COOH$	Dodecanoic acid	Coconuts
Myristic acid	$C_{13}H_{27}COOH$	Tetradecanoic acid	Nutmegs
Palmitic acid	$C_{15}H_{31}COOH$	Hexadecanoic acid	Animal fat
Stearic acid	$C_{17}H_{35}COOH$	Octadecanoic acid	Animal fat
Arachidic acid	$C_{19}H_{39}COOH$	Eicosanoic acid	Peanuts
Lignoceric acid	$C_{23}H_{47}COOH$	Tetraeicosanoic acid	Peanuts and brain

In a fatty acid, the carbon atoms are numbered from the carboxyl carbon. The carbon atom adjacent to the carboxyl carbon is known as the α-carbon. Carbon atom adjacent to the α-carbon atom is known as β carbon atom and so on. The end methyl carbon is called as ω-carbon (Fig. 6.9*a*).

Unsaturated fatty acids

They have trivial names, systematic names, ω-end names and shorthand forms.

Systematic name

Like unsaturated fatty acids, the name of hydrocarbon forms first part of systematic name of unsaturated fatty acids. But 'enoic' substituted in place of 'ne' of name of hydrocarbon forms second part. Number of double bonds are written before 'enoic' and symbol showing position of double bonds and isomerism around double bond are written between two parts or in the beginning. For example, systematic name for a mono unsaturated fatty acid palmitoleic acid (trivial name) containing 16 carbon atoms and one double bond between 9 and 10 carbon atoms is (Hexadecane + Δ^9-*cis*-mono+enoic+acid) ⟶ Hexadeca-Δ^9-*cis*-

monoenoic acid or *cis*-9-Hexadecaenoic acid. Usually unsaturated fatty acids end as 'enoic acids'.

ω-end series

Unsaturated fatty acids are also named according to the location of double bonds(s) from ω-end. For example, palmitoleic acid containing a double bond between 9 and 10 carbon atoms is named as ω-7 fatty acid.

Shorthand forms

Number of carbon atoms, number of double bonds and location of double bonds of unsaturated fatty acid are represented with short form. For example, palmitoleic acid is written as 16:1, Δ^9 in shorthand form. First numeral indicates number of carbon atoms, later number indicates number of double bonds and Δ^9 indicates position of double bond. Example of unsaturated fatty acids with trivial names, systematic names, ω-end names, shorthand forms and along with sources are given Table 6.2.

Table 6.2 Unsaturated fatty acids with their sources.

Fatty acid trivial name	Systematic name	ω-series	Short name	Sources
Palmitoleic acid	Hexadeca - Δ^9-*cis*-mono enoic acid or *Cis*-9-hexadecaenoic acid	ω-7	16:1, Δ^9	All animal fats
Oleic acid	Octadeca-Δ^9-*cis*-enoic acid or *Cis*-9-octadecaenoic acid	ω-9	18:1, Δ^9	Many animal fats, vegetable oils
Linoleic acid	Octadeca-$\Delta^{9,12}$-dienoic acid (all *cis*) or All *cis*-9,12-octadecadienoic acid	ω-6	18:2, $\Delta^{9,12}$	Vegetable oils like peanut, coconut, sun flower etc.
Linolenic acid	Octadeca-$\Delta^{9,12,15}$-trienoic acid (all *cis*) or All *cis*-9,12,15-octadecatri-enoic acid	ω-3	18:3, $\Delta^{9,12,15}$	Lineseed oil, codliver oil, egg yolk
Arachidonic acid	Eicosa-$\Delta^{5,8,11,14}$-tetra enoic acid (all *cis*) or All *cis*-5,8,11,14-eicosatetr-aenoic acid	ω-6	20:4, $\Delta^{5,8,11,14}$	Codliver oil and egg yolk

ESSENTIAL FATTY ACIDS

They are not systhesized in the body. So they must be obtained from diet. They are also called as poly unsaturated fatty acids (PUFA). They are linoleic acid (LA), linolenic acid (LNA) and arachidonic acid (AA).

Functions

1. They are essential for the synthesis of eicosanoids.
2. They are also required for membrane lipids.

Medical Importance

1. Dietary essential fatty acids has blood cholesterol lowering effect.
2. Deficiency status of essential fatty acids are rare with normal diet. However, deficiency of these in rats causes poor growth, reproductive disorders and dermatitis.
3. Lipid transport may be impaired.
4. Infants consuming formula diets are susceptible to deficiency of essential fatty acids. They may develop skin abnormalities.

STEROIDS

Steroids are complex molecules containing four fused rings. The four fused rings make-up 'cyclopentanoperhydrophenanthrene' or 'sterane' ring (Fig. 6.10). Sterane ring is also called as *steroid nucleus*. The most abundant steroids are sterols which are steroid alcohols.

CHOLESTEROL

Structure

In animal tissue, cholesterol is the major sterol (Fig. 6.10). Cholesterol is 3-hydroxy-5, 6-cholestene. It is found in bile (chol-bile). In a normal 65 Kg adult, 200 gm of cholesterol is present. Brain is rich in cholesterol. It is also present in spinal cord and neurons. Egg yolk is also rich in cholesterol. Steroids are called as *non-saponifiable* lipids because they contain no fatty acids and they can not form soaps.

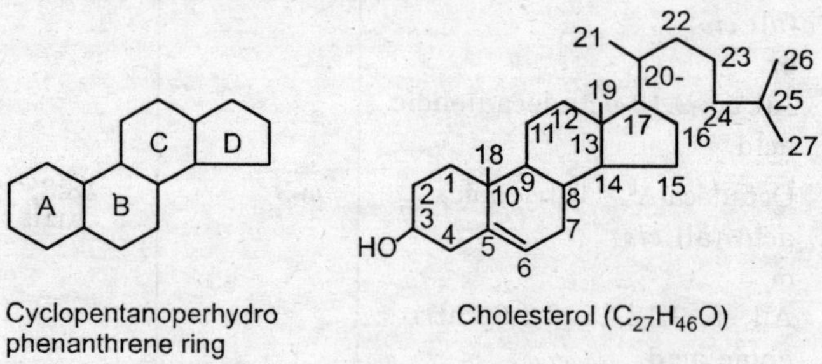

Fig. 6.10 Structures of steroid nucleus and cholesterol

Functions

1. Cholesterol and its esters are important components of cell membrane and lipoproteins.
2. Steroids with diverse physiological functions are derived from cholesterol. Some of them are given below:

   (*a*) **Vitamin D** 7-dehydrocholesterol derived from cholesterol is provitamin of vitamin D.

   (*b*) **Bile acids** They are required for the formation of bile salts.

(*c*) **Hormones of adrenal cortex** They are cortisol, corticosterone and aldosterone. They are derived form cholesterol.

(*d*) **Female sex hormones** They are progesterone and estrogen.

(*e*) **Male sex hormones** They are testosterone and androsterone.

Other Noteworthy Steroids

1. **Ergosterol** Provitamin of vitamin D found in yeast and plants.
2. **Sitosterol** Present in plants.
3. Cardiac glycosides like ouabain and streptomycin an antibiotic.
4. Coprostanol found in feces is derived from cholesterol.
5. Wool fat sterols like agnosterol and lanosterol.

CLASSIFICATION OF LIPIDS

Lipids are also classified according to their interaction with water. There are two major classes. They are 1. Polar lipids. 2. Non-polar lipids.

Polar Lipids

They are further sub-divided into 3 sub-classes.

(*a*) Class one polar lipids are non-swelling water insoluble amphipathic molecules (Amphiphiles) which forms thin lipid mono layer in water. They are tri- and di-acylglycerols, long chain free fatty acids, free cholesterol and fat soluble vitamins.

(*b*) Class two polar lipids are swelling and water insoluble amphiphiles which forms stable lipid monolayer as well as laminated lipid water structure known as *liquid crystals.* They are monoacylglycerols, ionized or dissociated free fatty acids and phospholipids.

(*c*) Class three polar lipids are water soluble amphiphiles, which contain strong polar head groups. These are water soluble only at low concentrations. They form mono-layers as well as micelles. They are salts of long chain fatty acids and bile acids.

Non-polar Lipids

They are insoluble in water. They are cholesterol esters, carotenes and hydrocarbons.

EICOSANOIDS

They are derived from eicosapolyenoic fatty acid like arachidonic acid. They are prostanoids, leukotrines (LTA) and lipoxins (LX). The prostanoids include prostaglandins (PG), prostacyclins (PGI) and thromboxanes (TXA). Often word prostaglandins is used to indicate all prostanoids.

Prostaglandins

Since they are initially found in prostate gland they are named as prostaglandins. But later they are identified in all cells and tissues except erythrocytes.

Structures

Chemically prostaglandins are derivatives of a 20 carbon prostanoic acid. Prostanoic acid is a cyclic compound with two side chains (Fig. 6.11). The cyclic ring present in prostanoic acid is a cyclopentane ring. There are some six or more types of prostaglandins. They differ in the substituents on the cyclopentane ring. They are prostaglandin A(PGA), PGB, PGC, PGD, PGE, PGF, PGG and PGH. Most widely distributed prostaglandins are PGA_1, PGA_2, PGE_1, PGE_2, PGE_3, PGF_1, PGF_2, PGF_3.

Prostacylins

Structure

They contain a second five-numbered ring in addition to the one common to all prostaglandins (Fig. 6.11).

Thromboxane

Structure

They are so named because they are identified first in thrombocytes. They contain a six numbered heterocyclic oxane ring (Fig. 6.11).

Leukotriens and Lipoxins

Structure

They are found in leukocytes. They are derivatives of arachidonic acid and contain no cyclic ring. HPETE derived from arachidonic acid serves as precursor for leukotriens (Fig. 6.11) and lipoxins.

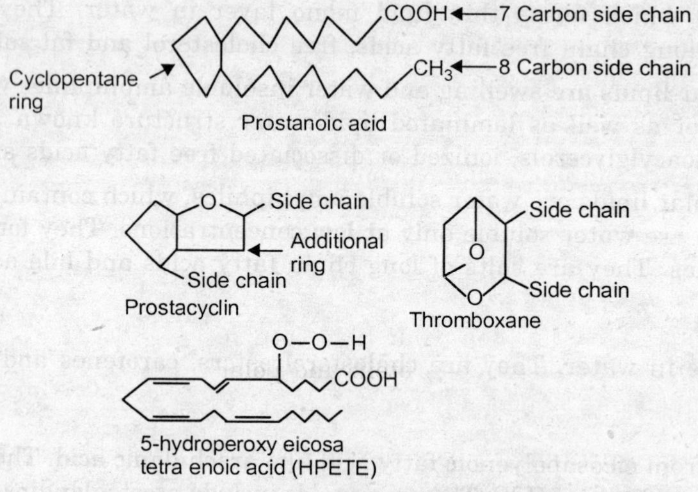

Fig. 6.11 Structures of eicosanoids

FUNCTIONS OF EICOSANOIDS

They function as local hormones. They act on several organs and produce physiological as well as pharmacological effects.

1. **Heart** PGE class prostaglandins increases cardiac output and myocardial contraction.
2. **Blood vessels** Prostaglandins (PGE) maintain blood vessel tone and arterial pressure.
3. **Blood pressure** PGA and PGE class prostaglandins lower blood pressure. So they may be useful as anti hypertensive agents.

4. **Brain** PGE class prostaglandins produce sedation and tranquilizing effect in cerebral cortex.
5. **Kidney** PGA and PGE class prostaglandins increases excretion of Na^+, K^+ and Cl^-. They may increase urine volume by increasing plasma flow.
6. **Lungs** Prostaglandins dilate bronchi, so they are useful in the treatment of asthma.
7. **Nose** Prostaglandins releive nasal congestion.
8. **Stomach** Prostaglandins decreases acid secretion in stomach. So they are useful in the treatment of peptic ulcers.
9. **Uterus.** Prostaglandins induces contraction of uterine muscle. So they are used in the termination of pregnancy. Prostaglandins also has role in fertility.
10. **Metabolism** Prostaglandins influences several metabolism by altering cAMP level. For example, they inhibit lipolysis in adipocyte by increasing cAMP level.
11. PGE class prostaglandins are involved in inflammation.
12. Prostacylins inhibit platelet aggregation.
13. Thromboxanes causes platelet aggregation and clot formation.
14. Leukotreins are involved in the regulation of neutrophil and eosinophil function. They act as mediators of immediate hyper sensitivity reaction. The slow reacting substance of anaphylaxis (SRS-A) is a leukotriene. Some leukotriens act as chemotactic agents. Lipoxins are vasoactive and immuno regulatory substances.
15. Thromboxane A_2 regulates acquired immunity. It causes construction of smooth muscle cells. It is a mitogen.

LIPOPROTEINS

They are lipid protein complexes found in plasma. They are non-covalent assemblies. The protein part of lipoprotein is called as *apolipoprotein* or *apoprotein*. The apoprotein and lipids are held together by non-covalent forces.

Structure

Lipoprotein structure consist of non-polar lipid core surrounded by apoproteins and more polar lipids (Fig. 6.12). The outer apoprotein and polar lipid coat of lipoprotein solubilizes these lipid rich particles in aqueous plasma.

Classification of Lipoproteins

1. Based on their density, the liporoteins of blood plasma are classified into 4 classes. The four classes of liporoteins can be separated by ultra centrifugation. Density of a lipoprotein is inversely related to the lipid content. The greater the lipid content, lower is the density. Different classes of lipoproteins based on the density are: 1. Chylomicrons, 2. very low density liporoteins, 3. low density liporoteins and 4. high density lipoproteins.
2. Different classes of plasma lipoproteins can be separated by electrophoresis. Based on differences in electrophoretic mobilities the plasma lipoproteins are classified into 4 classes. They are: 1. α-lipoproteins, 2. pre-β-lipoproteins, 3. β-lipoproteins and 4. chylomicrons (Fig. 6.12).

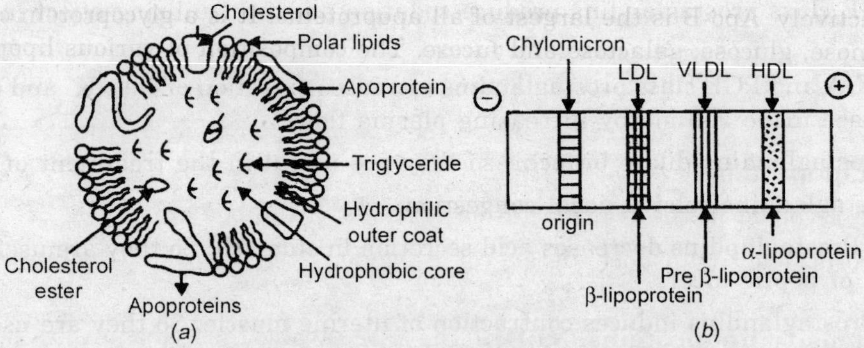

Fig. 6.12 (*a*) Lipoprotein general structure
(*b*) Electrohoresis of lipoproteins

Composition of Lipoproteins

Lipids of lipoproteins

The lipid constituents of lipoproteins are mostly triglycerides, free and esterified cholesterol and phospholipids. The non-polar triglycerides and cholesterol esters are usually present in the core of lipoproteins where as polar phospholipids along with apoproteins forms outer coat. However, the proportion of triglycerides, cholesterol and phospholipids differs in various lipoproteins (Table 6.3).

Table 6.3 Composition of various lipoproteins

Type	Density	% Lipid			% Protein	Apoproteins
		Triglycerides (TG)	Phospholipid (P)	Cholesterol (C)		
Chylomicrons	0.90-0.95	85-90	7-9	4-8	1.5-2.5	A-I, AII, B-48 C-I, II, III and E
Very low density lipoproteins (VLDL)	0.95-1.00	55-70	15-20	15-20	5-10	B-III,C-I, II, III and E
Low density lipoproteins (LDL)	1.00-1.05	7-10	15-20	40-45	20-25	B-100
High density lipoprotein (HDL)	1.05-1.20	3-50	20-35	15-18	40-55	A-I,II;C-I,II,III D and E

TG = Triglycerides, P= Phospholipid, C = Cholesterol.

Apoproteins of lipoproteins

The proportion of protein part differs in various lipoproteins (Table 6.3). Further the composition of apoprotein part also differs among various lipoproteins. There are five types of apoproteins. They are apoprotein A, apo B, apo C, apo D, and apo E. Some of the apoproteins have subtypes also. Subtypes of apo A, apo B and apo C are A-I, II; B-48, B-100 and

C-I, II, III respectively. Apo-B is the largest of all apoproteins. It is a glycoprotein contains sialic acid, mannose, glucose, galactose and fucose. The composition of various lipoproteins is shown in Table 6.3. Other little known apoproteins are apo F, apo G and apo H.

Functions of Lipoproteins

Lipoproteins are involved in the transportation of lipids in the body.

1. **Chylomicrons** They transport dietary or exogenous triglycerides from intestine to liver.
2. **Very low density lipoproteins (VLDL)** They are involved in the transport of endogenous triglycerides from liver to extra hepatic tissues.
3. **Low density lipoproteins (LDL)** LDL is the major vehicle for the transport of cholesterol from liver to extra hepatic tissues.
4. **High density lipoproteins (HDL)** HDL is the major vehicle for the transport of cholesterol from extra hepatic tissues to the liver.

Other Noteworthy Functions of Lipoproteins

In addition to their structural function, apolipoproteins have other functions also. They are:

1. Important for synthesis and degradation of lipoproteins.
2. Activators/inhibitors of some enzymes associated with lipid metabolism.

   Examples:

   1. Apo A-I activates LCAT where as Apo A-II inhibits LCAT.
   2. Apo C-II activates lipoproteinlipase.
   3. Apo E recognizes receptors on the liver cells for LDL and chylomicrons.

3. Protein components of lipoproteins has other important functions apart from solubilization of lipids in plasma.

   (*a*) Except apolipoprotein B which is the only protein component of LDL, all other apolipoproteins moves from lipoprotein particle to lipoprotein particle. Hence, they are called as *exchangeable apolipoproteins*.

   (*b*) Apolipoprotein A-I (apo A-I) and apolipoprotein E (apoE) are anti-atherogenic agents.

   (*c*) In the brain, apoE is involved in the repair of damaged nerve cells.

LIPID LAYERS, MICELLES AND LIPOSOMES

Lipids like triglycerides are insoluble in water because they contain non-polar hydrophobic hydrocarbon chain. Similarly, cholesterolester is also insoluble in water because of hydrophobic steroid nucleus.

Amphipathic Molecules

Lipids like cholesterol, phospholipids and bile salts contain both water soluble polar head group and water insoluble non-polar tail. Since they have two very different kinds of groups these molecules are called as 'amphipathic molecules' (Fig. 6.13).

Lipid monolayer

When amphipathic molecules like phospholipids are present in water, their polar head groups orient towards water phase and hydrophobic tails towards air. As a result, a unimolecular lipid layer is formed at water air interphase (Fig. 6.13).

Micelles

When amphipathic lipids are present beyond a critical concentration in aqueons medium, they aggregate into spheres. The sphere aggregates of amphipathic lipids are known as micelles (Fig. 6.13). In the sphere shaped micelles polar head groups of amphipathic lipids are on the exterior whereas non-polar tails are in the interior. Bile salts can form micelles.

Lipid Bilayer

Structure

When phospholipids are present in water oil mixture, their polar head groups orient towards water and non-polar tails towards oil. As result, a lipid bilayer is formed (Fig. 6.13). Lipid bilayer is formed even in the absence of oil phase because of hydrophobic attraction.

Function

Lipid bilayer is the basic structure of cell membrane.

Mixed Micelles

Structure

They are also micelles but they may be composed of various types of amphipathic lipids. They are formed when micelles of a particular lipid combines with other lipids. During the digestion and absorption of lipids, micelles of bile salts combines with products of lipid digestion and forms mixed micelles. (Fig. 6.13).

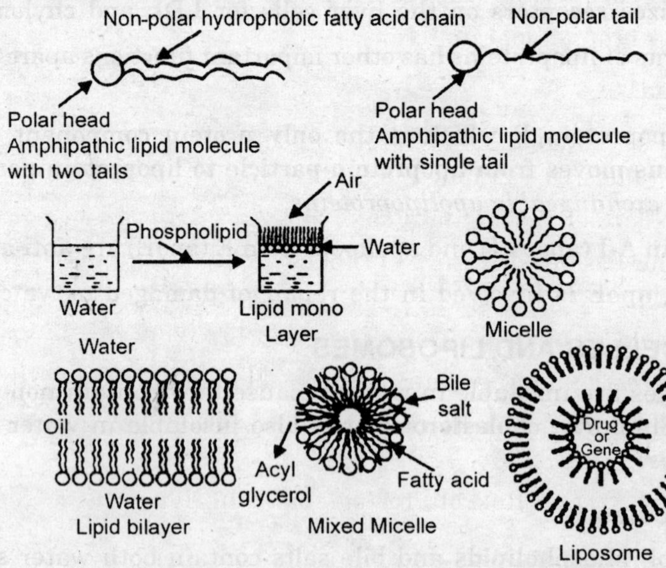

Fig. 6.13 Structures of amphipathic molecules, lipid monolayer, micelle, lipid bilayer, mixed micelle and liposomes

Function

Formation of mixed micelles is very important for digestion and absorption of lipids. Mixed micelles are also formed during cleansing action of soaps and detergents.

Liposomes

Structure

When a lipid bilayer closes on itself a spherical vesicle called as 'liposome' is formed (Fig. 6.13).

Functions

1. Liposomes are used as a carrier of certain drugs to specific site of body where they act. They can deliver drugs directly into cell because they easily fuses with cell membranes.
2. They are used in cancer therapy to deliver drugs only to cancer cells.
3. In gene therapy also they are used as vehicles for genes.

Lipoprotein X(LpX)

Structure

1. It is a variant of LDL. It contains apo C as well as albumin.
2. It is a bilammallar vesicle with an aqueous lumen. It contains equal amounts of phospholipids and cholesterol. Triglycerides and cholesterol esters are present in only small amounts (2 to 3%).

Medical Importance

1. It appears in the plasma of cholestatic patients. It may be formed in bile and enters plasma due to regurgitation that occurs in cholestatic individuals.
2. It interacts with other lipoproteins present in plasma.

REFERENCES

1. Gurr, A.I. and James, A.T. Lipid Biochemistry. 2nd ed. Halstead, New York, 1984.
2. Hanahen, D.J. Platelet Activating Factor. Ann. Rev. Biochem. **55**, 483-510, 1986.
3. Hansen, H.S. The Essential Nature of Linoleic Acid in Mammals. Trends Biochem. Res. **11**, 263-265, 1986.
4. Sabine, J.K. Cholesterol. Marcel and Dekkar, New York, 1977.
5. Hinman, J.W. Prostaglandins. Ann. Rev. Biochem. **41**, 161, 1972.
6. Scanh, A.M. and Spector, A.A. Biochemistry and Biology of Plasma Lipoproteins. Marcel and Dekkar, New York, 1986.
7. Colina-Chourio, J.A. *et al.* Role of Prostaglandins in Hypertension. J. Hum. Hypertesion. **14**, S16-S19, 2000.
8. Lucy Bird. Lymphocyte Migration: Homing in on Leukotrienes. Nat. Rev. Immunol. **3**, 777, 2003.

9. Gullaway-Stave. The Steroid Bible. Belle International, 1997.
10. Gunstone, F. Fatty Acid and Lipid Chemistry. Blackie Academic and Professional, London, 1996.
11. Yehuda, S. and Mostofsky, D.I. Eds. Handbook of essential fatty acids Biology: Biochemistry, Physiology and Behavioural Neurobiology, Humana Press, NJ, USA, 1997.
12. Lasic, D.D. Liposomes in Gene Delivery. CRC Press, Florida, USA, 1997.
13. John Betteridge. Ed. Lipoproteins in Health and Disease. Edward Arnold Publisher, 1999.
14. Mike I. Gurr. Lipid Biochemistry. Black Well, 2001.
15. Dennis E. Vance. Ed. New Comprehensive Biochemistry: Biochemistry of Lipids, Lipoproteins and Membranes. Vol. **36**, Elsevier Science, 2002.

EXERCISES

ESSAY QUESTIONS

1. Define lipids. Classify lipids giving examples.
2. What are compound lipids? Give examples along their functions.
3. Define fatty acids. Classify fatty acids giving examples.
4. Define eicosanoids. Name different eicosanoids. Explain their functions.
5. Define lipoproteins. Draw lipoprotein structure, label its various components. Classify lipoproteins. Explain their functions.
6. Define simple lipids. Classify them giving examples and mention their functions.
7. Define fatty acids. Classify them giving examples and mention their functions.
8. Define derived lipids. Give examples. Explain structure and functions of any one example.
9. Describe functions of lipids.

SHORT QUESTIONS

1. Define triglycerides. Write their functions.
2. Explain lipid peroxidation. Name diseases associated with lipid peroxidation.
3. Define waxes. Mention their functions.
4. Define essential fatty acids. Give examples. Write their functions.
5. Name the ring present in cholesterol. Write biologically important compounds derived from cholesterol.
6. Write functions of apolipo proteins.
7. Explain terms micelles, mixed micelles and liposomes. Write the importance of mixed micelles and liposomes.
8. Write briefly about physico chemical properties of fats.
9. Write a note on prostaglandins.
10. Define liposome. Mention its importance.
11. Write briefly about surfactant present in lung.
12. How lipoproteins are separated? Explain.
13. Write about ω-3 and ω-6 fatty acids.

14. Write structure, function and clinical importance of cardiolipin.
15. Write a note on lysophospolipids.
16. Name the hydrolytic products of the following:
    (*a*) Triglycerides (*b*) Lecithin (*c*) Sphingomyelin (*d*) Cerebroside

MULTIPLE CHOICE QUESTIONS

1. All of the following statements are true for lipids, except
   (*a*) Lipids are soluble in organic solvents.
   (*b*) They are present in humans, animals and plants.
   (*c*) In man they serves as energy source.
   (*d*) They are absent in cooking oil and milk.
2. An example for mixed triglyceride is
   (*a*) 1,3–distearopalmitin (*b*) Tripalmitin
   (*c*) Triolein (*d*) 1,3–diacylglycerol
3. Partial acylglycerols are formed
   (*a*) During digestion of triglycerides (*b*) From fats
   (*c*) From saponification of fats (*d*) From none of these
4. Hydrolysis of sphingomyelin yield
   (*a*) Sphingosine, 2 fatty acids, phosphate
   (*b*) Sphingosine, fatty acid, choline, phosphate
   (*c*) Sphingosine, fatty acid, glucose
   (*d*) Cerebrosides, sugars, fatty acids
5. An example for ω-3 fatty acid is
   (*a*) Palmitoleic acid (*b*) Arachidonic acid
   (*c*) Linolenic acid (*d*) Linoleic acid
6. Which of the following are susceptible to essential fatty acid deficiency
   (*a*) Adults consuming formula diet (*b*) Pregnant women
   (*c*) Infants consuming formula diet (*d*) Growing children
7. An eicosanoid acting as chemotactic agent is
   (*a*) Prostacyclin (*b*) Leukotriene
   (*c*) Lipoxin (*d*) Thromboxane

FILL IN THE BLANKS

1. Subcutaneous fat serve as --------------- against cold.
2. --------------- deficiency causes respiratory distress syndrome.
3. An example for simple triglyceride is ---------------.
4. Sialic acid is a component of ---------------.
5. Sulfolipids are cerebrosides containing ---------------.
6. Unsaturated fatty acids exhibit --------------- isomerism.
7. Amphipathic molecules contain --------------- head group and --------------- tail.
8. --------------- is basic structure of cell membrane.

7

CHAPTER

MEMBRANE AND TRANSPORT

BIOLOGICAL MEMBRANES

They are the membranes present in biological systems. They perform several functions which are essential for life.

Membrane Functions

1. Plasma membrane decides shape or individuality of cell by separating it from surroundings.
2. Membranes are permeability barriers only selected molecules can pass through the membranes.
3. Membranes are involved in the regulation of intracellular composition.
4. Membrane regulates flow of information between cell and its environment. Receptors present on the surface of membrane serve as links between cell and its surroundings.
5. Mitochondrial membrane contains energy-producing system like respiratory chain.
6. Membrane are modified to special kind of structures like axons of nerve cell, tail of sperm and villi of intestine.
7. Membranes form compartments with in the cell. Subcellular components like mitochondria, lysosomes, golgi complex and sarcoplasmic reticulum are separated by membranes.
8. Membranes are involved in the exchange of material between cell and its surroundings.
9. Exchange of material between cells is mediated by specific portions of membranes.

Medical Importance

1. Since membrane regulates intracellular composition, change in membrane structure can alter molecular, ionic and water content of cell. This may effect organ or cellular functions.
2. Some diseases are results of membrane changes. For example, hypercholesterolemia is due to lack of receptor on membrane. Similarly, congenital also goitre is due to lack of iodide transport of membrane.
3. Anaesthetics work by causing minute change in membrane structure.
4. Toxicity of snake venom is due to its action on membrane lipids.

5. Membrane proteins are altered in many diseases. A defective gene can produce altered membrane protein. For example, in cystic fibrosis due to defective gene non-functional Cl^- transporter is produced.
6. Diseases like mysthania gravis is due to change in membrane protein function. In mysthania gravis, auto antibodies to acetylcholine receptor are produced. It causes progressive muscle weakness.
7. Membrane lipids are altered in lipidoses.
8. Some forms of epilepsies are due to mutations in ion channel membrane proteins. Anti epileptic drugs work by blocking ion channels.
9. Ion channels are involved in taste signal transduction.
10. Several types of drug resistance are due to over expression of a class of membrane proteins ATP-Binding Cassette (ABC) transporters.
11. Mutations in ABC transporters cause diseases like Dubin-Johnson syndrome, Tangier disease, Adrenoleukodystropy etc. in humans.
12. Survival of parasite in host involves induction of changes in host membrane permeability and fluidity. For example, parasite *P. falciparum* that cause malaria grows and multiplies in erythrocyte. The host RBC is as such unable to meet very high nutrient requirement of rapidly multiplying parasite. So parasite increases flow of nutrients into RBC by inducing changes in membrane permeability and fluidity.

Membrane Structure

Though membranes perform diverse functions, they have some similarities with respect to their structure.

Structural Features of Membranes

1. Membranes are fluid structures.
2. Membranes are sheet like structures.
3. Membranes consist of proteins and lipids. Carbohydrates are attached to lipids and proteins.
4. Membranes lipids are amphipathic molecules. So they form bilayer which act as barrier for the movement of polar molecules.
5. Membrane proteins are embedded in lipid bilayer.
6. Membrane proteins serve as receptors, enzymes, transporters etc.
7. Proteins and lipids in membrane are held together by many non-covalent interactions. So, membranes are non-covalent assemblies.
8. Membrane and its components are in dynamic state. Membrane lipid and proteins undergo continuous degradation and resynthesis. Life span of different proteins and lipids in membrane vary widely.
9. The two sides of membrane (cytosolic side and extra-cellular side) are different.

Fluid Mosaic Model of Membrane

Singar and Nicolson proposed fluid magic model for membrane structure.

1. According to this model, membranes are two dimensional fluids of proteins and lipids.
2. Membrane lipids mostly phospholipids and glycolipids are arranged as lipid bilayer (Fig. 7.1).
3. Proteins are inserted in the lipid bilayer.
4. Some proteins float like icebergs in lipid bilayer sea and some proteins may span entire bilayer (Fig. 7.1).

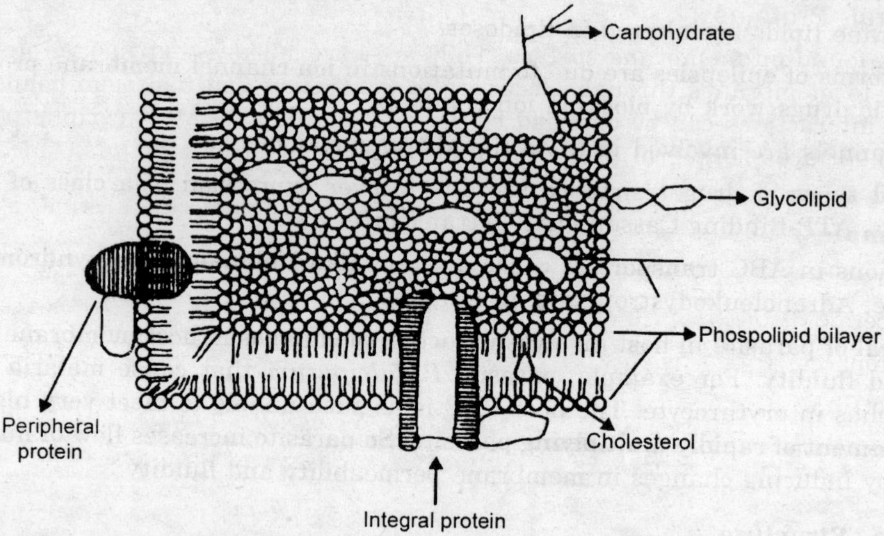

Fig. 7.1 Fluid-mosaic model of membrane

5. Usually α-helical and β-pleated sheet regions of proteins are in contact with adjacent membrane lipids.
6. The interaction of lipids with membrane proteins is essential for proper membrane function.
7. Further, the surface of membrane resembles mosaic surface. Hence, the name fluid mosaic model is given for membrane structure.

Membrane Lipids

1. Membrane consist of three types of lipids. They are phospholipids, glycolipids and cholesterol.
2. Membranes differ in their phospholipid and glycolipid content. For example, in liver and erythrocytes phospholipids accounts for 40-90% of membrane lipids where as glycolipid accounts for 5-30% of total lipid. Myelin contains phospholipids and glycolipids 43% and 30% of total lipids, respectively.
3. Cholesterol and its esters are present in eukaryotic membranes. The plasma membranes of eukaryotic cells are rich in cholesterol whereas the membranes of their organelles have lesser amount of cholesterol.

Membrane Proteins

1. Protein content differs among membranes. The protein content of plasma membrane of most cells is 50%. The protein content of inner mitochondrial membrane is highest 75%. Myelin has low protein content of about 18%.

2. The number of proteins in a membrane varies from 6 to 8 in the sarcoplasmic reticulum to more than 100 in plasma membrane.
3. The proteins can be enzymes, antigens, receptors, pumps and structural proteins.

The membrane proteins are classified into 1. Peripheral proteins and 2. integral proteins based on their association with membrane lipids.

Peripheral Proteins

They are found on membrane surface. They are also called as extrinsic proteins. They are attached to membranes through electrostatic interaction and hydrogen bonds. These non-covalent interactions can be changed by pH and adding salt. Most peripheral proteins are bound to surface of integral proteins either on cytosolic or extracellular side of membrane (Fig. 7.1).

Examples:

1. G-Protein which is involved in signal transduction
2. Glyceraldehyde-3-phosphate dehydogenase
3. Fibronectin that attaches cells to extracellular matrix
4. Spectrin of RBC
5. Cytochrome C

Integral Proteins

They are also known as intrinsic proteins. They extend all along the lipid bilayer. They interact with lipid bilayer extensively because these integral proteins possess special characteristics. They contain high proportion of hydrophobic amino acids in the protein part that is embedded in membrane (Fig. 7.1). Usually integral proteins from channel in the membranes which transport ions and molecules. Some integral membrane proteins act as enzymes also.

Examples:

1. Glycophorin of erythrocytes.
2. Anion channel in erythrocytes.
3. Adenylate cyclase.
4. Complexes of respiratory chain.

Membrane Carbohydrates

Carbohydrate content of eukaryotic membranes ranges from 2 to 10%. They may be present as glycoproteins and glycolipids (Fig. 7.1). They are located on the extracellular side of membrane. Oligo saccharides of glycophorin of RBC are responsible for antigenic specificity.

Membrane Asymmetry

The two sides of the membranes are not identical (symmetric) in many respect or ways:

1. Enzymes may be present only on one side of the membrane.
2. Cholesterol is present only on the outer side in large amounts.
3. Carbohydrates are located only on extracellular side of membrane.

4. Phospholipids are present in outer side whereas amino phospholipids are located in inner side of membrane.

Membrane Fluidity

1. Membrane fluidity depends on lipid composition.
2. The degree of fluidity of membrane depends on the degree of unsaturation and chain length of fatty acids present in the lipids.
3. Saturated fatty acids decrease membrane fluidity by increasing compactness in membrane. Saturated fatty acid chains increase compactness of membrane because hydrophobicity favours alignment of side chain (Fig. 7.2*a*).
4. In contrast unsaturated fatty acids increase membrane fluidity by decreasing compactness in membrane. Unsaturated side chains decrease compactness because of cis configuration at double bond (Fig. 7.2*b*).

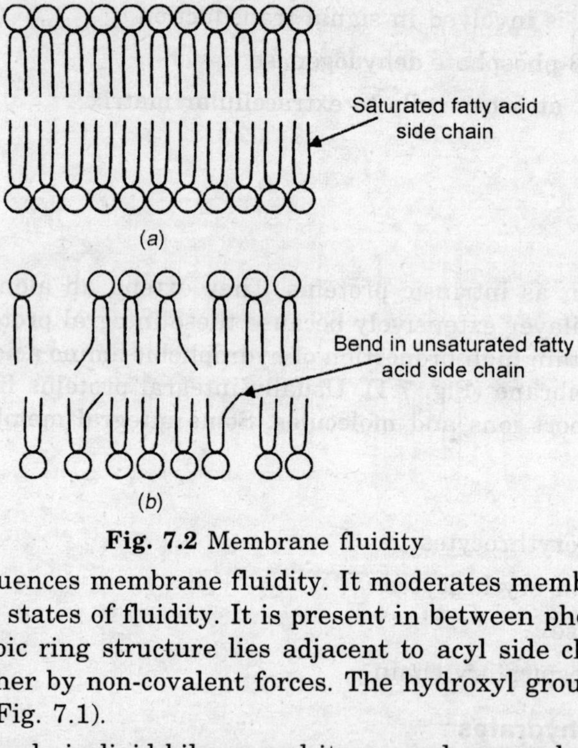

Fig. 7.2 Membrane fluidity

5. Cholesterol also influences membrane fluidity. It moderates membrane fluidity by producing intermediate states of fluidity. It is present in between phospholipid molecules. The rigid hydrophobic ring structure lies adjacent to acyl side chain of phospholipid. They are held together by non-covalent forces. The hydroxyl group of located between polar head groups (Fig. 7.1).
6. Cholesterol moves freely in lipid bilayer and it can undergo exchange with cholesterol present in the surroundings. In some organisms membrane behaviour is regulated by altering cholesterol.
7. Cholesterol present between phospholipids can decrease compactness in membrane.
8. Cholesterol has complex effect on membrane fluidity.

Changes in Membrane Fluidity

Membrane functions may be affected when membrane fluidity is altered.

1. Membrane permeability increases if fluidity is increased. So many molecules can gain entry into the cell.

2. Increased fluidity can dislocate membrane proteins like receptors. As a result membrane function is affected.
3. Many anesthetics work by increasing fluidity. So in presence of anesthetics orientation of membrane lipids and proteins is altered. Loss of sensation by anesthetics is due to the reaction at membrane level.

Motion in Membrane

1. Lipids and proteins present in cytosolic and extracellular sides of membrane are in constant motion.
2. Movement of membrane lipids parallel to membrane surface is free and rapid. It is also called as lateral movement of membrane lipids.
3. Movement of membrane lipids from one side of membrane to other side of the membrane is restricted and slow. It is called as transverse motion of lipids.
4. Usually membrane phospholipids requires few seconds to few minutes to move around the cell. Membrane proteins also move but much more slowly.
5. Transverse movement of membrane proteins is rare (Fig. 7.3).

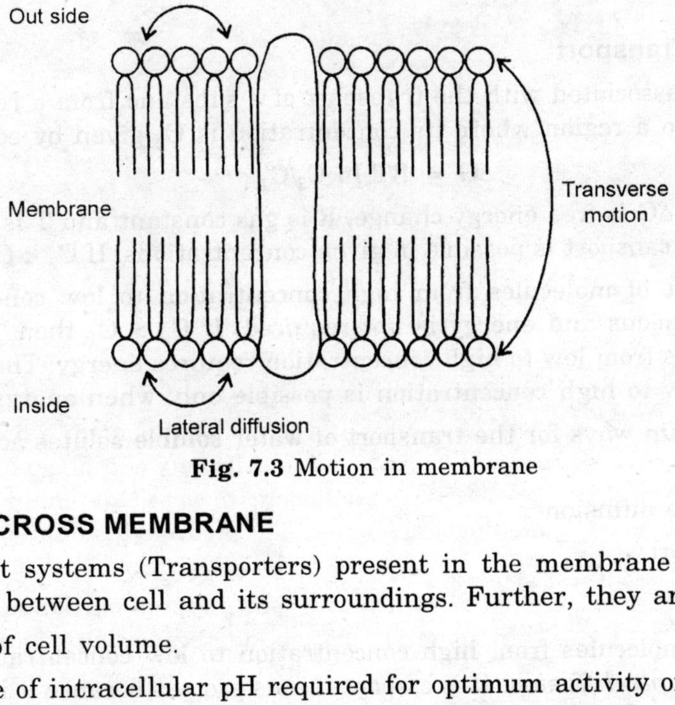

Fig. 7.3 Motion in membrane

TRANSPORT ACROSS MEMBRANE

Several transport systems (Transporters) present in the membrane regulate the flow of solute molecules between cell and its surroundings. Further, they are involved in the:

1. Regulation of cell volume.
2. Maintenance of intracellular pH required for optimum activity of cellular enzymes.
3. Uptake and concentration of nutrients from the environment.
4. Removal of toxic substances.
5. Generation of ionic gradients across membrane, which are essential for nerve impulse transmission and muscle contraction.

These transport systems (transporters) may move one solute molecule in both directions. Then the process is known as *uniport*. If the transport system moves two solute molecules in same direction then the process is symport (co transport). Sometimes, the transport system moves two solute molecules in opposite directions then the process of transport is known as *antiport* (Fig. 7.4.).

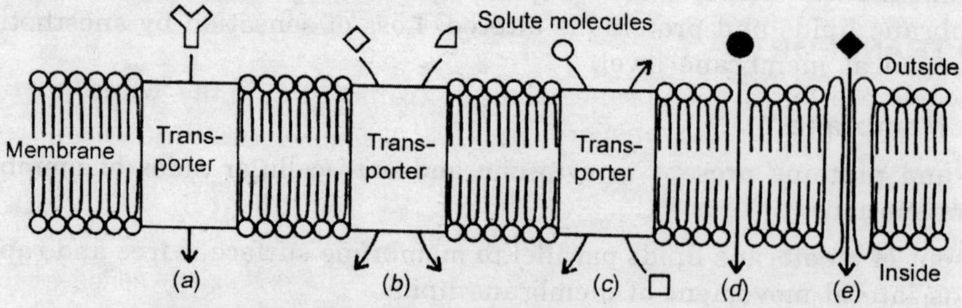

Fig. 7.4 Transport of molecules across membrane.
(*a*) Uniport (*b*) Simport (*c*) Antiport (*d*) Simple diffusion (*e*) Ion channel

The permeability of biological membrane is highly selective. The lipid or non-polar molecule can easily pass through membrane because of their solubility in membrane lipid bilayer. Even water and uncharged molecules of smaller size are freely permeable to membrane. Charged solute molecules and molecules like proteins and carbohydrates are not permeable.

Free Energy and Transport

Free energy change associated with the transport of a substane from a region in which its concentration is C_1 to a region where its concentration is C_2 given by equation.

$$\Delta G = RT \text{ In } C_2/C_1$$

In this equation, ΔG is free energy change, R is gas constant and T is temperature. ΔG determines whether transport is possible in given concentrations. If $C_2 < C_1$, then $\Delta G = -ve$.

Hence, movement of molecules from high concentration to low concentration across membrane is spontaneous and energy is not required. If $C_2 > C_1$ then $\Delta G = +ve$. Hence, transport of molecules from low to high concentration requires energy. Therefore, transport of molecules from low to high concentration is possible only when energy is supplied.

There are two main ways for the transport of water soluble solutes across membranes. They are:

1. Passive or simple diffusion
2. Mediated transport

Passive Diffusion

Transport of solute molecules from high concentration to low concentration across membrane is known as *simple diffusion*. It is a spontaneous process because it is thermodynamically favourable. It is a down hill transport and requires no energy (Fig. 7.4).

Factors influencing simple diffusion:

1. Concentration difference across membrane.
2. Permeability coefficient of the solute for the membrane.
3. Membrane potential.
4. Hydrostatic pressure across membrane.

Examples:

1. Mannose and xylose uptake by intestine.
2. Pentose uptake by intestine.

MEDIATED TRANSPORT

Carrier molecule present in membranes mediate transport of many solute molecules across membrane. Hence, mediated transport involves carrier molecules. They are known as *permeases*, *translocases*, *transporters* or *pumps*. Most of them are proteins. Mediated transport is divided into:

1. Facilitated diffusion
2. Active transport

Facilitated Diffusion or Facilitated Transport

Facilitated diffusion is faster than simple diffusion. It requires no energy. Facilitated diffusion by carrier molecule involves conformational change of carrier molecule. The carrier molecule exist in two conformations. It has binding site to solute molecule. In the native conformation the carrier is exposed to high concentration of solute. Then the solute molecules binds to the sites on carrier molecule. A conformational change in carrier molecule occurs. It exposes solute molecule to low concentration and solute molecules are released into the cell. The empty carrier returns to the native state to transport solute molecules once again (Fig. 7.5).

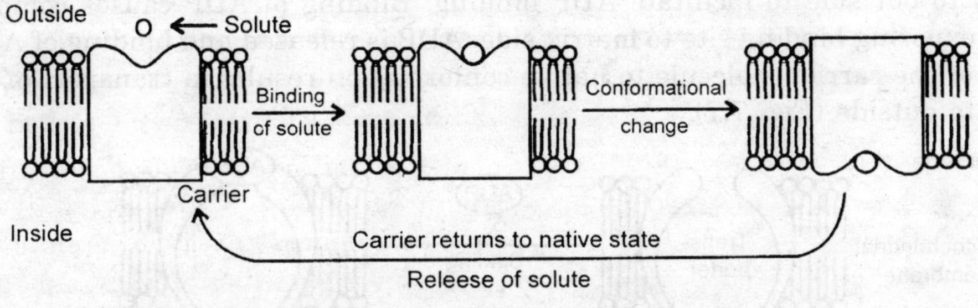

Fig. 7.5 Mechanism of facilitated diffusion by carrier

Factors Influencing Facilitated Diffusion

1. The amount of carrier available which is influenced by hormones.
2. The solute carrier interaction.
3. The rate at which conformational change occurs in carrier.

Carrier molecules which are capable of transporting one kind of solute molecule in both directions are called as uniporters, two types of solute molecules in the same direction (symporters) and two types of solute molecules in opposite directions (antiporters) are present in biological membranes. Some examples are described below:

1. Glucose uptake by erythrocytes, heart, adipose tissue, retina and brain is an example for uniport type of facilitated diffusion. The carrier molecule in erythrocyte also exhibit stereospecificity. It can bind only D-glucose, D-galactose or D-mannose but no L-type sugars. The carrier molecule in erythrocyte is known as *glucose permease*. It is an

uniporter. It is an integral membrane protein. It functions as gated pore for the transport of glucose in the erythrocyte membrane. Binding of glucose to carrier causes pore formation and transport of glucose occurs. Release of glucose causes closing of the pore. (Fig. 7.6.).

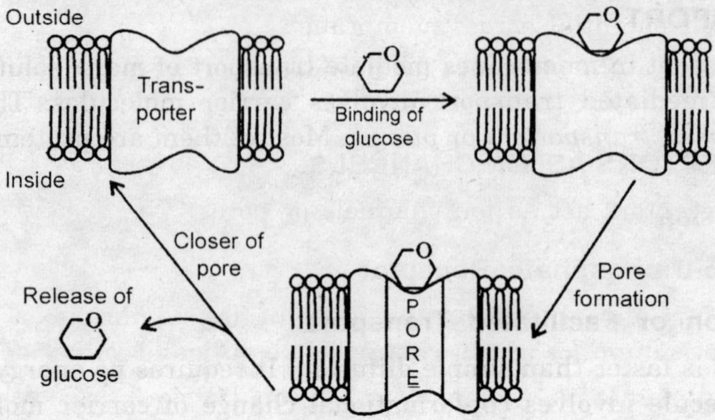

Fig. 7.6 Carrier mediated glucose transport in erythrocytes

2. **ATP.** ADP transporter present in inner mitochondrial membrane is an example for antiport type facilitated diffusion. ATP transporter is an antiporter. It transports ADP from outside to matrix of mitochondria and simultaneously moves ATP from matrix to outside. It consist of two subunits and has binding site for ATP or ADP. The mechanism of its action involves conformational change. In the native conformation, binding site is exposed to out side to facilitate ADP binding. Binding of ADP causes conformational change exposing binding site to matrix side. ADP is released and binding of ATP occurs. Return of the carrier molecule to native conformation results in transport of ATP from matrix to outside (Fig. 7.7).

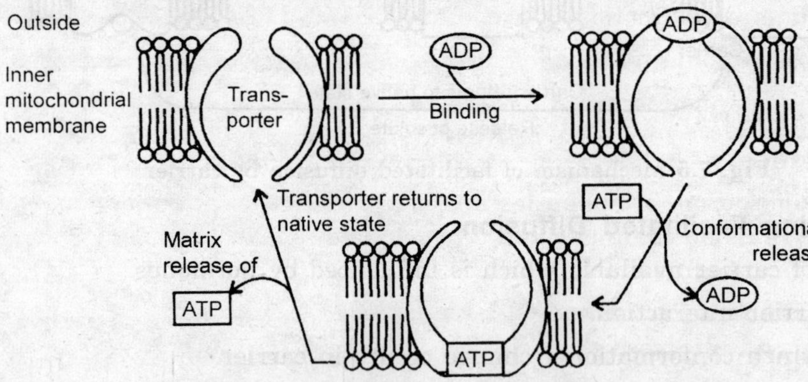

Fig. 7.7 Mechanism of ADP-ATP transporter

3. Anion channel of erythrocytes is another example for antiport type facilitated diffusion. Anion channel is an antiporter. It moves chloride from outside to inside of erythrocytes simultaneously expelling bicarbonate from inside to outside.
4. Uptake of amino acids by intestinal cells are examples for symport type facilitated transport. The carrier molecule is a symporter and moves sodium ions along with amino acids across membrane.

Ion Channels

1. In membranes, there are transmembrane channels or pore like structures. They are proteins and permit movement of ions. They are called as ion channels (Fig. 7.4).
2. The membrane of nerve cells contain ion channels. They are responsible for the generation of action potential across membrane.
3. Specific channels for Na^+, K^+ and Ca^{2+} are identified. Neurotransmitters regulate channel activity.

MEMBRANE RECEPTORS AS ION CHANNELS

Some membrane receptors act as ion channels or pores.

A. Inositol-1, 4, 5-triphosphate Receptor

1. Inositol-1, 4, 5-triphosphate receptor present in membrane of golgi complex and endoplasmic reticulum act as ion channel. It is a ligand gated ion channel.
2. It is an integral membrane protein. It is a 260 K Da glycoprotein. It has an N-terminal ligand binding cytosolic domain, a C-terminal channel domain that protrudes into cytosol and central six transmembrane domains.
3. When ligand Inositol-1, 4, 5-triphosphate binds at N-terminus, C-terminal channel domain opens for Ca^{2+}. As a result of this calcium is released into cytosol from intracellular stores.
4. Channel closes upon release of ligand from receptor.

B. Acetylcholine Receptor

1. It is also known as nicotinic-acetylcholine receptor. It is ligand gated channel. It consists of five subunits α α β γ δ.
2. When neuromuscular junction is excited release of acetylcholine takes place.
3. Binding of acetylcholine to receptor causes opening of channel to selective cations.
4. Closure of the channel occurs when acetylcholine is hydrolyzed.

Medical Importance

1. **Epilepsy.** Some forms of epilepsies are inherited diseases of ion channels. They are due to mutation in ion channel genes. They are also known as ion channelopathies. Two human epilepsy syndromes:
   (*a*) Benign familial neonatal convulsions (BFNC).
   (*b*) Generalized epilepsy with febrile seizures (GEFS) are due to mutations in potassium and sodium channel genes. Sodium valproate an antiepileptic drug work by blocking voltage dependent K^+ and Ca^{2+} channels.
2. Taste signal transduction involves ion channel interaction with tastants. The tastantion channel interaction produce depolarization of taste receptor cell by changing ion channel activity.

Active Transport

It requires energy in addition to carrier molecules. It moves solute molecules from low concentration to high concentration or against concentration gradient. Mechanisms of some active transport systems are given below:

1. Na^+/K^+–ATPase is the most extensively studied active transport system. It is integral membrane protein present in intestine, erythrocytes, kidney and brain etc. It is an antiporter. It concentrates K^+ and pump out Na^+. It is called as ATPase because it has ATP hydrolytic activity. It is responsible for the maintenance of high intracellular K^+ level which is essential for membrane potential of nerve and muscle.

   Na^+/K^+ ATPase is a glycoprotein. It has molecular weight of 300,000 and it consist of subunits of two types. They are two α subunits and β-subunits. On the cytoplasmic side it has binding sites for ATP, Na^+ and phosphate. K^+ binding site is located on the extra-cellular side of the membrane. It is closed outside and open in side (Fig. 7.8). Molecular events associated with the operation of Na^+/K^+-ATPase are:

1. Na^+ with in the cell combines with α-subunits on the cytoplasmic side.
2. ATP is hydrolysed to ADP and one of the α-subunit is phosphorylated.
3. Conformational change in α-subunits expose Na^+ to outside and Na^+ is released.
4. K^+ present outside binds to modified subunits which causes the release of phosphate.
5. The modified subunits undergo conformational change to native conformation releasing K^+ in the cell.

For every ATP molecule hydrolyzed 3 Na^+ are extruded and 2 K^+ are concentrated by the cell (Fig. 7.8).

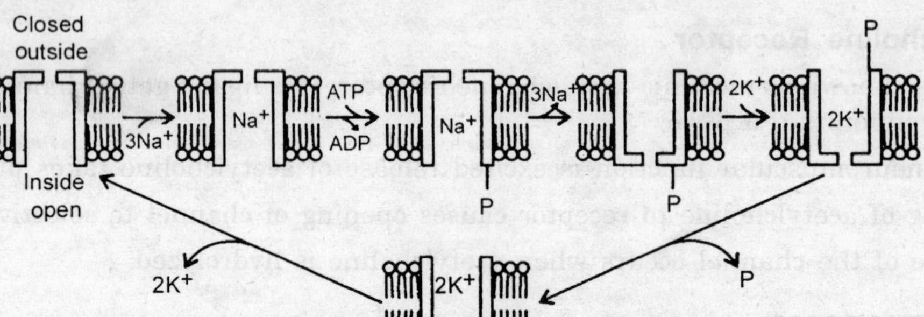

Fig. 7.8 Mechanism of Na^+/K^+–ATPase

Inhibitor of Na^+/K^+–ATPase: Ouabain a plant steroid glycoside is an inhibitor. It binds to extracellular side of α-subunits. It binds to phosphorylated form of $Na^+/K^\pm$ ATPase and prevents de phosphorylation. Because it blocks ion transport it is cardiotonic, i.e., increases cardiac muscle contraction.

2. Ca^{2+}–ATPase present in sarcoplasmic reticulum is an other example for active transport involving carrier and ATP hydrolysis. It is responsible for the concentration of Ca^{2+} in the sarcoplasmic reticulum. It is an uniporter. It transports the calcium from the cytosol to sarcoplasmic reticulum against concentration gredient. The concentration of calcium in the cytosol is 10^{-9}M whereas its concentration in sarcoplasmic reticulum is 10^{-2} M. When sarcoplasmic reticulum is excited by nerve impulse large amount of Ca^{2+} is released to facilitate muscle contraction. Ca^{2+}-ATPase transports back the calcium released from the sarcoplasmic reticulum during relaxation. Reuptake of Ca^{2+} by

sarcoplasmic reticulum involves phosphorylation and conformational change of Ca^{2+} ATPase (Fig. 7.9).

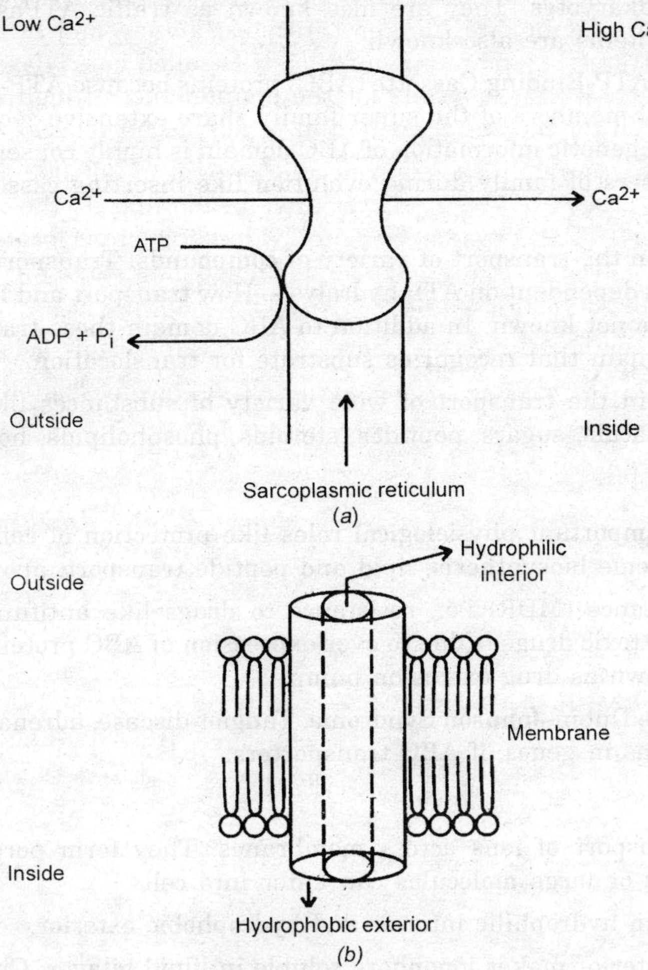

Fig. 7.9 *(a)* Ca^{2+}–ATPase of sarcoplasmic reticulum
(b) Model of an ionophore

3. $H^+/K^{\pm}$ ATPase is another active transport system present in parietal cells of stomach. It is an antiporter. It is responsible for the secretion acid (H^+ ions) into stomach. It exchanges H^+ with K^+ in opposite direction. H^+/K^+-ATPase also undergo phosphorylation and conformational change during transport of solutes.

   Sometimes active transport and facilitated diffusion are coupled. Absorption of glucose in the intestine and its reabsorption in kidney are coupled to Na^+/K^+-ATPase. Coupling of the two systems facilitates glucose uptake against concentration gradient.

Secondary Active Transport Systems

Are those active transport systems in which transport of molecules is indirectly linked to hydrolysis of ATP. One such example is glucose absorption as detailed above. ATP-Binding Cassette (ABC) proteins are also considered as secondary active transport systems.

ATP-BINDING CASSETTE (ABC) PROTEINS

1. They are rapidly growing super family of membrane transport proteins identified in prokaryotes and eukaryotes. They are also known as traffic ATPases. Several subfamilies of ABC proteins are also known.
2. They are named as ATP-Binding Cassette (ABC) proteins because ATP-Binding Cassette (ABC) domain of all members of the super family share extensive sequence homology. It indicates that the genetic information of ABC domain is highly conserved and inserted into genes of members of family during evolution like inserting cassette into cassette player.
3. They are involved in the transport of variety of compounds. Transport of molecules by ABC transporters is dependent on ATP hydrolysis. How transport and hydrolysis of ATP are exactly linked is not known. In addition to ABC domain these transporters have a transmembrane domain that recognizes substrate for translocation.
4. They are involved in the transport of wide variety of substances like heavy metals, drugs, ions, amino acids, sugars, peptides, steroids, phospholipids, hormones etc.

Medical Importance

1. ABC proteins has important physiological roles like protection of cells from cytotoxic drugs or poisons, heme biosynthesis, lipid and peptide transport, apoptosis etc.
2. Multi Drugs Resistance (MDR) i.e., resistance to drugs like antifungals, herbicides, anticancer and cyto toxic drugs is due to over expression of ABC protein P-Glycoprotein (P-gp) which is known as drug extrusion pump.
3. Human diseases like Dubin-Johnson Syndrome, Tangier disease, adrenal leukodystrophy are due to mutations in genes of ABC transporters.

Ionophores

1. They facilitate transport of ions across membranes. They form pores in membrane through which ions or large molecules can enter into cell.
2. Usually they contain hydrophilic interior and hydrophobic exterior.
3. The hydrophobic exterior makes ionophore soluble in lilpid bilayer. Charged molecules pass through the hydrophilic interior (Fig. 7.9).
4. Some antibiotics work as ionophores. They are gramicidin A and valinomycin. Diphtheria toxin also act as ionophore.

SHUTTLE SYSTEMS

For the continuation of metabolic pathways NADH of cytosol must be converted back to NAD^+. Mitochondrial membrane is impermeable to NADH. Shuttle system transfers reducing equivalent of NADH from cytosol to mitochondria and regenerates NAD^+ in the cytosol.

Malate Shuttle

1. It is active in liver, kidney and heart.
2. The shuttle begins with formation of malate from oxaloacetate using NADH as hydrogen donor. A cytosolic malate dehydrogenase catalyzes the reaction and NAD^+ is formed in the cytosol.

3. An antiport system transports malate into mitochondria. Inner mitochondrial membrane contains antiport system.
4. A mitochondrial malate dehydrogenase generates NADH by oxidizing malate to oxaloacetate. In the mitochondria NADH undergo respiratory chain oxidation to generate ATP.
5. If the oxaloacetate enters cytosol one cycle of shuttle is complete. But oxalo acetate is impermeable to mitochondrial membrane. So it enters in the form of α-ketoglutarate which is permeable to membrane.
6. Oxaloacetate is converted to α-ketoglutarate by transminase which uses glutamate and oxaloacetate as substrates.
7. The α-ketoglutarate and aspartate formed enter cytosol by facilitated diffusion.
8. In the cytosol α-ketoglutartate is converted to oxalo acetate by transaminase which uses aspartate also as substrate. Thus oxaloacetate is regenerated in the cytosol and glutamate formed is transported back to mitochondria by antiporter (Fig. 7.10).

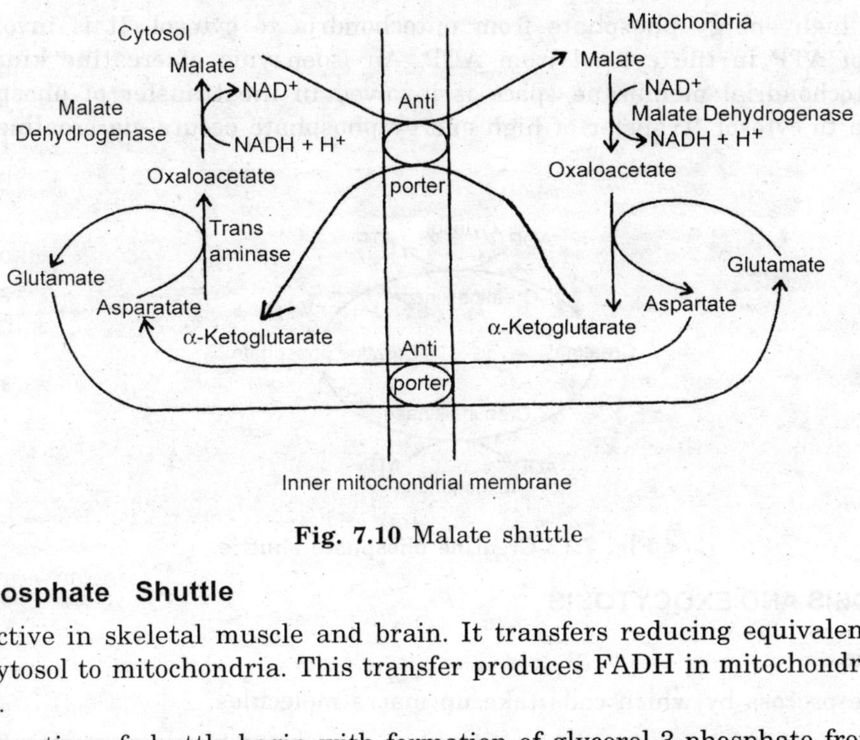

Fig. 7.10 Malate shuttle

Glycerophosphate Shuttle

1. It is active in skeletal muscle and brain. It transfers reducing equivalents of NADH from cytosol to mitochondria. This transfer produces FADH in mitochondria instead of NADH.
2. The operation of shuttle begin with formation of glycerol-3-phosphate from dihydroxy acetone phosphate catalyzed by glycerol-3-phosphate dehydrogenase in a NADH dependent reaction. As a result NAD^+ is generated in cytosol.
3. Glycerol-3-phosphate enters mitochondria where it is oxidized to dihydroxy acetone phosphate catalyzed by mitochondrial glycerol-3-phosphate dehydrogenase in a FAD dependent reaction. As a result, $FADH_2$ is generated in mitochondria which is oxidized in the respiratory chain.

4. The dihydroxy acetone phosphate enters cytosol to complete the shuttle (Fig. 7.11).

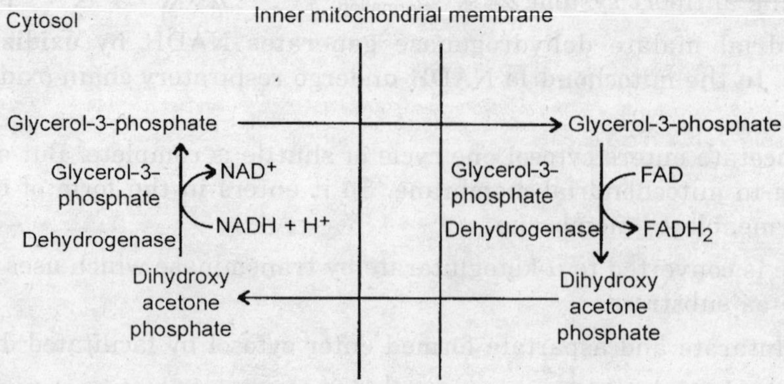

Fig. 7.11 Glycerophosphate shuttle.

Creatine Phosphate Shuttle

It transfers high energy phosphate from mitochondria to cytosol. It is involved in the generation of ATP in the cytosol from ADP. An isoenzyme of creatine kinase present between mitochondrial membrane space is involved in the transfer of phosphates from mitochondria to cytosol. Transfer of high energy phosphate occurs via creatine phosphate (Fig. 7.12).

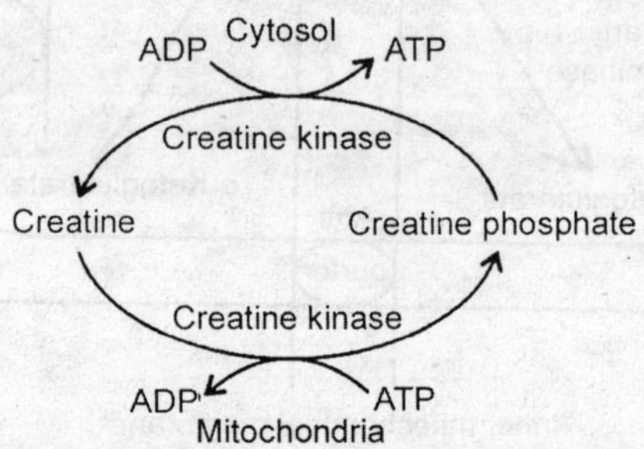

Fig. 7.12 Creatine phosphate shuttle.

ENDOCYTOSIS AND EXOCYTOSIS

Endocytosis

1. It is the process by which cells take up macro molecules.
2. The macro molecules are nutrients, hormones, viruses, bacteria, nucleic acids etc.
3. Endocytosis requires energy, extracellular Ca^{2+} and microfilaments.
4. It begins with invagination of macromolecule by cell membrane. A vesicle is formed by the fusion of plasma membrane which pinches off. The vesicle may fuse with primary lysosomes to form secondary lysosomes.
5. Lysosomal enzymes hydrolyze macromolecules to simple molecules like amino acids and sugars which diffuses into cytosol where they are used for synthesis etc. (Fig. 7.13. A).

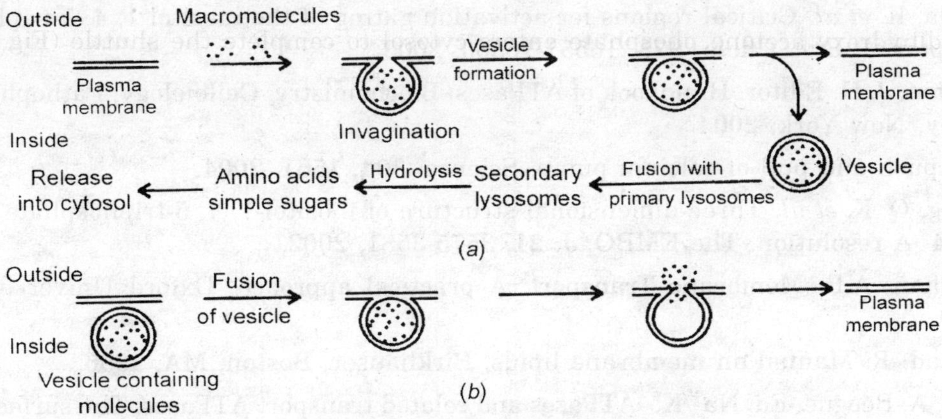

Fig. 7.13 (*a*) Process of endocytosis
(*b*) Process of exocytosis

6. Ingestion of viruses and bacteria by macrophages is similar to endocytosis and it is referred as phagocytosis.

Exocytosis

1. It is the process by which cells release macromolecules to outside.
2. In the cell molecules synthesized are stored as membrane coated vesicles. For example, digestive enzymes of pancreas are stored as vesicles in pancreatic cells. These vesicles fuses with cell membrane in response to stimulus like hormone in this case and releases digestive enzymes precursors into duct (Fig. 7.13*b*).

REFERENCES

1. Gennis, R.B. Biomembranes: Molecular structure and function. Springer-Verlag, Heidelberg, Germany, 1989.
2. Muddor, J. Origin of first cell membrane. Nature **371**, 101, 1994.
3. Singer, S.J. and Nicolson, G.I. The fluid mosaic model of the structure of cell membrane. Science **175**, 720-731, 1972.
4. Singer, S.J. The structure and insertion of integral proteins of membrane. Ann Rev. Cell Biol. **6**, 247-296, 1990.
5. Jacobson, K; Sheets, E.D. and Simson, R. Revisiting fluid mosaic model of membrane. Science. **268**, 1441-1442, 1995.
6. Lingrel, J.B. Structure-function studies of Na^+/K^+ - ATPase. Kidney Int. **44**, 32-39, 1994.
7. Jancks, W.P. How does calcium pump pump calcium. J. Biol. Chem. **264**, 18855-18858, 1989.
8. Michael, D. The human ATP-binding cassette (ABC) transporter super family, National Library of Medicine, Bethesda, MD, 2002.
9. Quick. M.W. (Editor). Transmembrane Transporters, Wiley, New York, 2002.
10. Channels and transporters, Landes Bioscience, Texas, 2004.

11. Ucida. K. *et al.* Critical regions for activation gating of the inositol-1, 4, 5-triphosphate receptor. J. Biol. Chem. **278**, 16551-16560, 2003.

12. Kaplen, J. H. Editor. Handbook of ATPases: Biochemistry, Cellbiology, Pathophysiology, Wiley, New York, 2004.

13. The push and pull of calcium pump. Science. **304**, 1561, 2004.

14. Jiang, Q. X. *et al.* Three-dimensional structure of inositol-1, 4, 5-triphosphate receptor at 24° A resolution. The EMBO. J. **21**, 3575-3581, 2002.

15. Stephan, A.B. Membrane Transport: A practical approach. Oxford University Press, 2000.

16. Prasad, R. Manual on membrane lipids. Birkhauser, Boston, MA, 1996.

17. Luis, A. Beegue, Ed. Na^+/K^+–ATPases and related transport ATPases: The surface pumps on which every living creature Relies. New York Academy of Sciences, Vol. 834, NY, 1997.

18. Richard, H. How ion channels sense membrane potential ? Proc. Natl. Acad. Sci. USA. **102**, 4929-4930, 2005.

EXERCISES

ESSAY QUESTIONS

1. Draw fluid mosaic model of cell membrane. Label its various parts. Write functions of membranes.
2. Describe various transport systems that move molecules across cell membrane.
3. Write structural components of membrane. Name salient features of fluid mosaic model of membrane.

SHORT QUESTIONS

1. Write a note on membrane proteins.
2. Write role of fatty acids and choleseterol in membrane fluidity.
3. Write functions of transport systems present in cell membrane.
4. Explain energy aspects of transport systems.
5. Write shuttle systems involved in the transport of reducing equivalents from cytosol to mitochondria.
6. Explain the following:
   (*a*) Na^+/K^+–ATPase
   (*b*) Endocytosis
   (*c*) Ionophores
7. Write a note on exocytosis.
8. Write briefly on (*a*) Ca^{2+}-ATPase (*b*) H^+/K^+-ATPase
9. Define uniport, 'symport' and antiport. Give examples.
10. Explain simple diffusion with examples.
11. Define facilitated transport. Give examples. Write mechanism of facilitated transport.

12. Write about factors influencing (*a*) Simple diffusion (*b*) Facilitated transport.
13. Define active transport. How it differs from other transport systems? Give examples.

MULTIPLE CHOICE QUESTIONS

1. The two sides of cell membrane are
   (*a*) Identical (*b*) Rich in carbohydrates
   (*c*) Not identical (*d*) Rich in cholesterol
2. Movement of membrane lipids from one side to another side of membrane is called as
   (*a*) Lateral motion (*b*) Transverse motion
   (*c*) Horizontal motion (*d*) Parallel motion
3. A symporter
   (*a*) Moves solute molecules in opposite direction.
   (*b*) Moves solute molecules in same direction.
   (*c*) Depends on energy.
   (*d*) Moves only one solute molecule.
4. Anion channel is present in
   (*a*) Erythrocytes (*b*) Leucocytes
   (*c*) Liver (*d*) Nerve

FILL IN THE BLANKS

1. ---------------in membrane serve as link between cell and its environment.
2. Congenital goitre is due to lack of --------------in membrane.
3. Anaesthetics work by causing----------------in membrane.
4. Membrane lipids and proteins are held together by --------- bonds.
5. The rate of passive transport depends on concentration --------across membrane.
6. --------------is responsible for the secretion of acid in stomach.

8
CHAPTER

DIGESTION AND ABSORPTION OF FOOD

Digestion and absorption of food occurs in gastrointestinal tract of humans, other mammals and invertebrates.

MEDICAL AND BIOLOGICAL IMPORTANCE

1. It provides substances needed for flesh formation and energy production.
2. Digestive process converts minerals and vitamins of food into easily absorbable forms.
3. Extent of digestion and absorption varies from one food stuff to another.
4. Diseases like peptic ulcer and duodenal ulcer are due to excessive production of digestive fluids. Digestion of food is also impaired in these conditions.
5. Flow of digestive fluids is obstructed in some diseases. For example, in cystic fibrosis flow of pancreatic fluid and in gallstone cases bile flow is blocked. As a result, digestion is affected in these disorders.
6. Some allergic diseases are due to absorption of partly digested products or allergins of food stuffs.
7. In some diseases like chylous fistula and filariasis products of digestion are excreted in urine.
8. Impaired digestion and absorption of food leads to increased excretion (Steatorrhea).
9. Absorption of digestive products is impaired in malabsorption syndromes.
10. Digestion and absorption of food is affected in pyloric and intestinal obstructions.
11. Parasitic infestations affect digestion and absorption in gastrointestinal tract.
12. Fat digestion and absorption impairs in cholestasis.

Chemical Nature of Digestion

Digestion is a process by which large complex organic molecules of food are disintegrated into small absorbable forms. Large molecules of diet are converted to small molecules by hydrolysis. Hydrolases of gastrointestinal tract catalyzes the hydrolysis of complex carbohydrates to monosaccharides, proteins to amino acids and lipids to glycerol, fatty acids, partial acylglycerols and cholesterol.

Chemical Nature of absorption

Transporters (carriers) present in the membrane of enterocytes are responsible for the absorption of most of the products of digestion except lipid and some monosaccharides.

Digestion and Absorption of Carbohydrates

Carbohydrates of diet

Food stuffs like rice, wheat, potato and vegetables contain polysaccharides. An adult may consume 150-300 gm of carbohydrate per day. They are mainly starch and small amounts of glycogen, dextrins and inulin. Cellulose, pentosans, inulin and oligosaccharides are not digested by non-ruminants. Milk and cane sugar of diet contributes to disaccharides lactose and sucrose. Monosaccharide content of diet is negligible under normal conditions. However, bakery products, honey and fruits may contributes some monosaccharides.

DIGESTION OF CARBOHYDRATES

Hydrolysis of dietary polysaccharides and disaccharides to monosassharides constitutes carbohydrate digestion.

In the Mouth

In the mouth, salivary amylase initiates carbohydrates digestion. Salivary amylase requires chloride ion and has optimum pH of 5.8-7.0. It catalyzes the hydrolysis of alpha-1, 4-glycosidic linkages in starch, glycogen and dextrin and convert them to maltose and oligosaccharides (Fig. 8.1). Salivary amylase acts only on cooked starch. However, the action of salivary amylase on polysaccharides is insignificant because the contact of enzyme with substrate is limited.

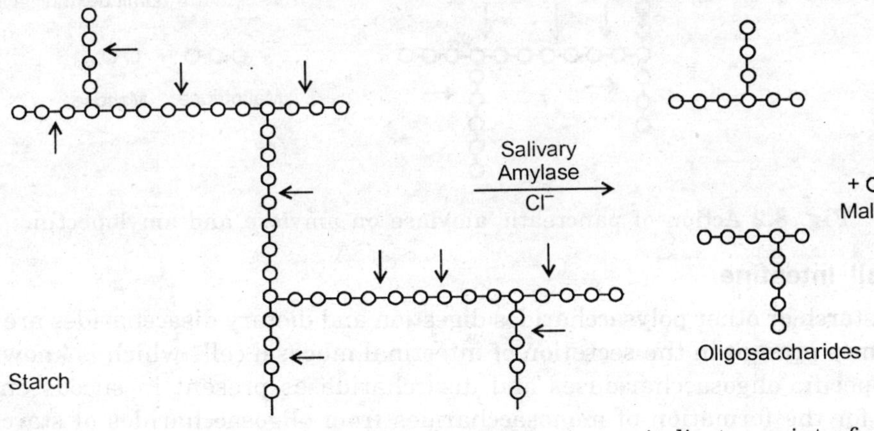

Fig. 8.1 Action of salivary amylase on starch. Arrow indicates point of attack

In the Stomach

Due to absence of enzymes in the gastric juice, no digestion of carbohydrate occurs in the stomach.

In the Duodenum

In the duodenum, pancreatic amylase acts on partly digested food. It is an endoglycosidase. It is also called as α-amylase or amylopsin. It has the optimum pH value of 7-8, which is provided by pancreatic juice bicarbonate. It catalyzes the hydrolysis of α-1, 4-glycosidic linkages and convert partially digested polysaccharide to maltose, maltotriose, oligosaccharides and α-dextrin or limit dextrin (Fig. 8.2) having 5-9 glucose residues and an α-1, 6-glycosidic bond. Generally, amylose part of starch is hydrolyzed to maltose and maltotriose but amylopectin is hydrolysed to α-dextrins and oligosaccharides in addition to maltose and maltotriose (Fig. 8.2). Further, pancreatic amylase can act on native starch. β-amylase present in plants like sweet potato releases β-anomers of maltose in stepwise manner from non-reducing ends of polysaccharides.

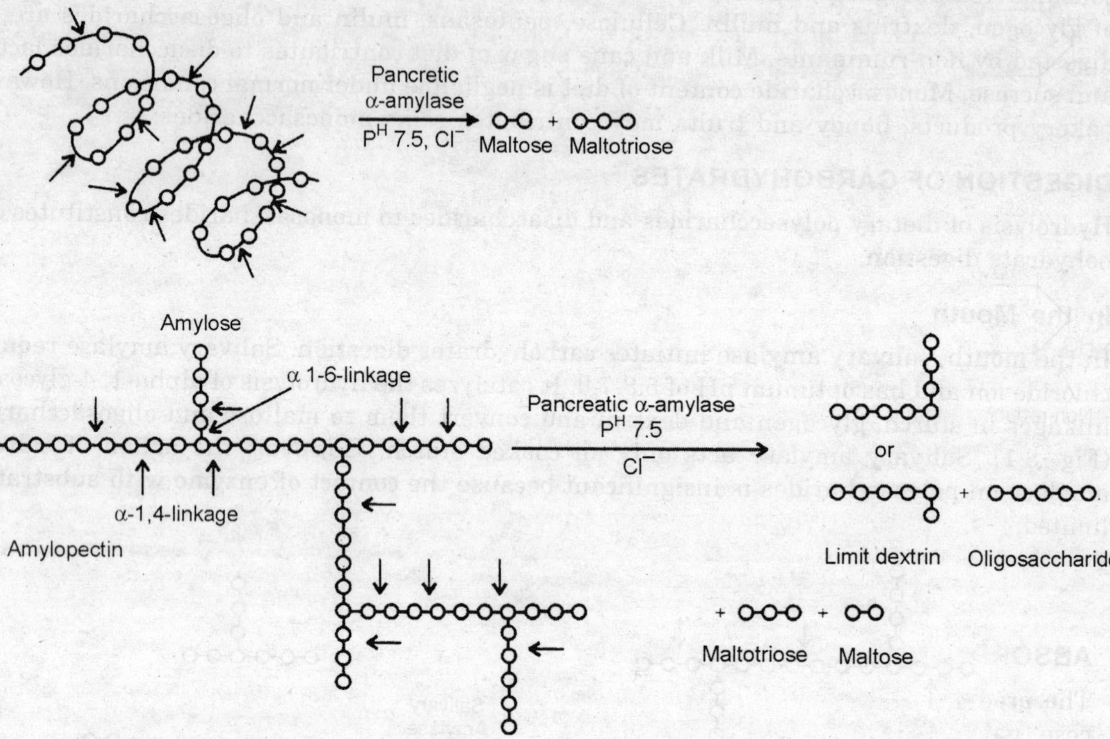

Fig. 8.2 Action of pancreatic amylase on amylose and amylopectin

In the Small Intestine

Products of starch or other polysaccharides digestion and dietary disaccharides are hydrolyzed by the enzymes present in the secretion of intestinal mucosal cells which is known as *succus entericus*. Specific oligosaccharidases and disaccharidases present in succus entericus are responsible for the formation of monosaccharides from oligosaccharides of starch digestion and disaccharides. Isomaltase or α-dextrinase an endoglycosidase catalyzes the hydrolysis of α-1, 6 bonds in the limit dextrin and converts α-limit dextrin to oligosaccharide and maltose (glucose) (Fig. 8.3). Maltase another oligosaccharidase is a exoglycosidase and catalyzes the removal of single glucose unit by hydrolyzing α-1, 4-linkages of oligosaccharides and disaccharides starting from non-reducing ends (Fig. 8.3). Sucrase also called as invertase is a disaccharidase. It catalyzes the hydrolysis of sucrose to glucose and fructose (Fig. 8.3). Lactase (β-galactosidase) another disaccharidase catalyzes the hydrolysis of lactose to glucose and galactose (Fig. 8.3). Thus by the combined action of amylases, oligosaccharidases and disaccharidases dietary polysaccharides and disaccharides are disintegrated into constituents monosaccharides.

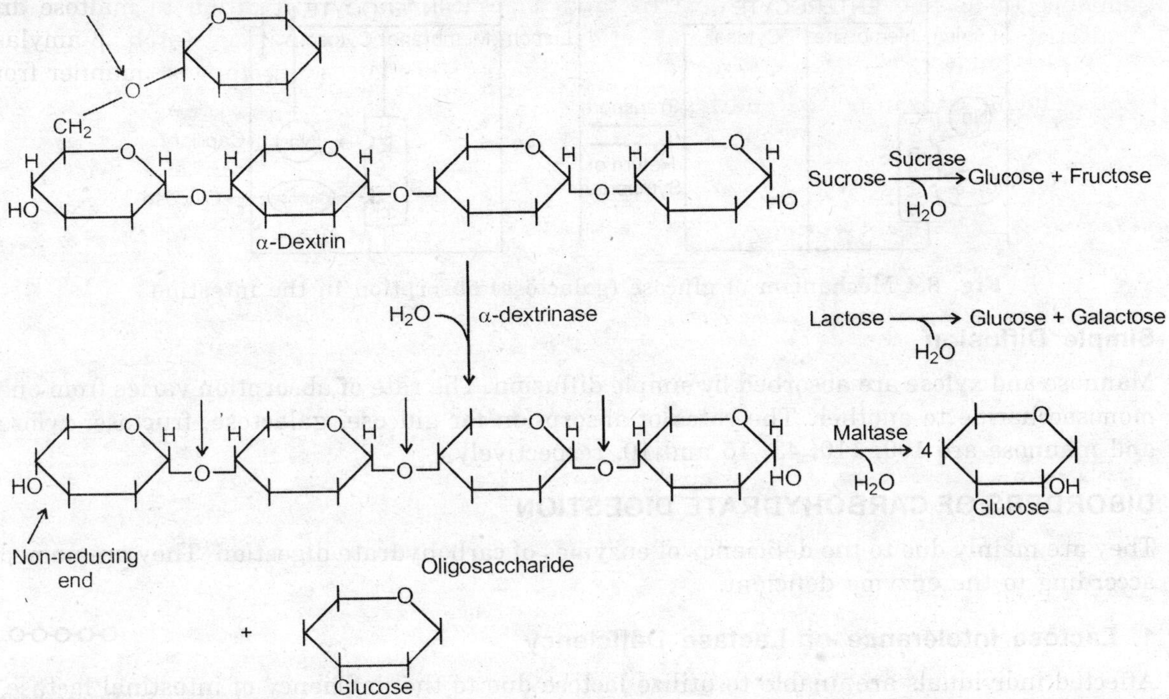

Fig. 8.3 Action of oligosaccharidases and disaccharidases

ABSORPTION OF CARBOHYDRATES

The products of dietary carbohydrate digestion are mainly monosaccharides. They are glucose, galactose, fructose, mannose and xylose. They are absorbed from the small intestine (jejunum) into blood of portal venous system. Two transport mechanisms are responsible for their absorption. They are 1. Facilitated diffusion or transport and 2. Simple diffusion. The absorbed monosaccharides reach liver through portal venous system.

Facilitated Diffusion

Glucose, galactose and fructose are absorbed by facilitated diffusion. The absorption of glucose and galactose is mediated by specific carrier molecule present in enterocyte membrane. It is a protein and often called as 'translocase'. It is a symporter. It transports Na^+ along with glucose and galactose. It is located on the external surface of membrane of intestinal cells. It has two binding sites one for monosaccharide and other for Na^+ (Fig. 8.4). The structural requirement of hexoses that are necessary for the transport by carrier molecule are 1. A pyranose ring 2. Hydroxyl on the second carbon must be same as glucose and methyl or a substitutent on C-5. When glucose and Na^+ binds to carrier protein it transports both of them through the membrane of the enterocyte and releases them into the cytosol (Fig. 8.4). From the cytoplasm glucose and galactose diffuse into blood. Na^+ is expelled out of the enterocyte through Na^+/K^+- ATPase. So the absorption of glucose and galactose by facilitated diffusion is coupled to active transport. Coupling of these two transport mechanisms facilitates absorption of glucose and galactose in the intestine.

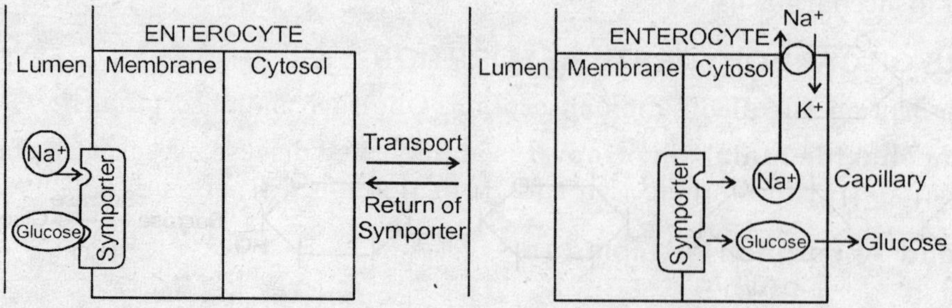

Fig. 8.4 Mechanism of glucose (galactose) absorption in the intestine

Simple Diffusion

Mannose and xylose are absorbed by simple diffusion. The rate of absorption varies from one monosaccharide to another. The rates of absorption for glucose, galactose, fructose, xylose and mannose are 100, 110, 43, 15 and 10, respectively.

DISORDERS OF CARBOHYDRATE DIGESTION

They are mainly due to the deficiency of enzymes of carbohydrate digestion. They are named according to the enzyme deficient.

1. Lactose Intolerance or Lactase Deficiency

Affected individuals are unable to utilize lactose due to the deficiency of intestinal lactase. As a result, dietary lactose accumulates in the intestine where it is acted upon by bacteria and produces fermentation products of lactose. The excess lactose and its products in the intestine causes symptoms like abdominal cramps, diarrhoea and flatulence. There are three types of lactase deficiency. They are:

A. Inherited lactase deficiency

It is a rare disorder. Feeding of lactose (milk) to the infant soon after birth produces symptoms. But these symptoms disappear on feeding lactose free diet.

B. Secondary low lactase deficiency

Intestinal diseases like colitis, gastroenteritis, tropical and non-tropical sprue and kwashiorkor can cause this disorder.

C. Primary low lactase deficiency

It is due to decreased activity of intestinal lactase in susceptible individuals. Usually it develops in the aged people.

2. Sucrase-isomaltase deficiency

It occurs in early childhood. It is an inherited deficiency of two disaccharidases namely sucrase and isomaltase. Since both these enzymes occur as single polypeptide the affected persons lacks these two enzymes.

3. Disacchariduria

It is characterized by excretion of large amounts of disaccharide in urine. It is due to deficiency of disaccharidases.

DISORDERS OF CARBOHYDRATE ABSORPTION

Defective absorption is called as malabsorption. One such malabsorption is:

1. **Monosaccharide malabsorption.** It is an inherited disease. Absorption of glucose and galactose is slow due to defective carrier in the affected persons.

Digestion and Absorption of Lipids

Dietary lipids

Foods like meat, animal fat, butter, milk, cheese, egg yolk and cooking oils and ghee contain lipids. The lipids present in them are mainly triglycerides, phospholipids, glycolipids, cholesterol and its esters, fatty acids, sterols and carotenes. An adult may consume 50-150 gms of lipid per day. However, triglycerides accounts for 90% of dietary lipids.

Digestion of Lipids

Hydrolysis of triglycerides, compound lipids and cholesterol esters to glycerol, free fatty acids, mono acylglycerols and free cholesterol constitutes the process of digestion. Since the lipids are water insoluable hydrolysis of dietary lipids by enzymes in aqueous environment of gastrointestinal tract poses a problem. The problem is solved by the emulsification of lipids by the bile salts present in bile. Sodium and potassium glycocholate, sodium and potassium taurocholate, sodium and potassium glycochenodeoxy cholate and sodium and potassium taurochenodeoxy cholate are called as bile salts. Bile salts form emulsions with lipids by reducing surface tension of water. An emulsion consist of water insoluble lipids dispersed in water. They can reduce surface tension of water because they are amphipathic molecules. The emulsification of lipids by bile salts increases surface area of lipid at water lipid interphase for the action of enzymes.

Lipid Digestion

In the mouth

Due to lack of favourable conditions like emulsification and PH, no digestion of lipid occurs in the mouth.

In the stomach

In humans, initiation of fat digestion occurs in stomach with mechanical emulsification. Gastric lipase hydrolyzes dietary triglycerides to diacylglycerol and fatty acids. About 10-30% of dietary triglycerides are hydrolyzed by gastric lipase.

In the small intestine

Small intestine is the major site of lipid digestion due to the pancreatic lipase. It requires colipase and bile salts for its activity. Colipase is a protein present in pancreatic juice along with lipase. As such lipase has no affinity towards emulsion particles of dietary lipids and bile salts. Hence, colipase forms complex with emulsion particle initially. Now the lipase attaches to emulsion particle by forming ternary complex (Fig. 8.5A). In the ternary complex lipase and colipase are bound to each other. Pancreatic lipase, is an α-lipase and an esterase. It hydrolyzes the ester linkages of triglyceride at α, α′ or (1, 3)- positions and forms 2-monoacylglycerol and free fatty acids. It can not hydrolyze the ester bond of triglyceride at 2(β) position (Fig. 8.5B). About 72% of 2-monoacylglycerol leaves emulsion particle and forms mixed micelles. The rest (about 28%) of 2-monoacylglycerol is converted to 1-monoacylglycerol by an isomerase. Now α-lipase converts 1-monoacylglycerol to glycerol and free fatty acids (22%). The rest of 1-monoacylglycerol (about 6%) is absorbed as such. Cholesterol esterase is another esterase present in pancreatic juice. It converts cholesterol esters to cholesterol and free fatty acids (Fig. 8.5B). Human cholesterol esterase also acts on triglycerides, phospholipids and lipid vitamins esters in presence of bile salts.

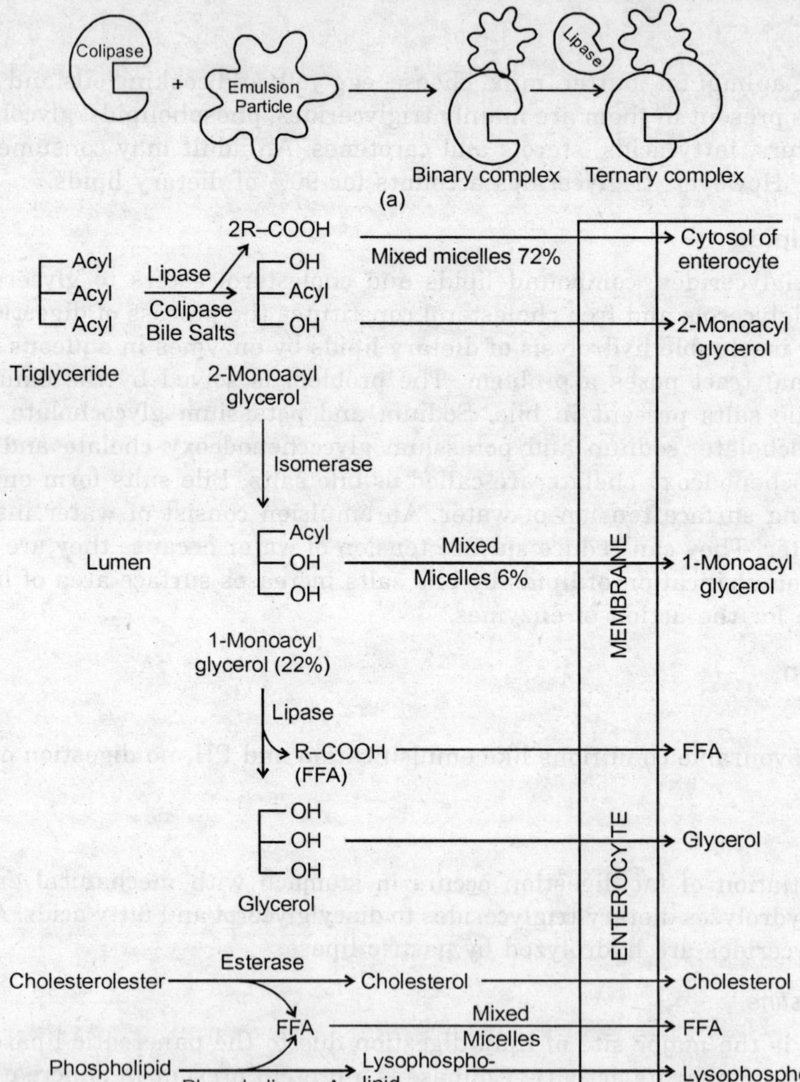

Fig. 8.5 (*a*) Formation of lipase, colipase and emulsion complex (*b*) Digestion and absorption of lipids. R–COOH indicates free fatty acids (FFA)

Pancreatic juice also contains some esterases, which acts on phospholipids. They are

1. **Phosphoplipase A_2** It is secreted in proform and activated by trypsin. It hydrolyzes ester bond at β position of phospholipid and forms lysophospholipid and fatty acid (Fig. 8.5B).
2. **Lysophospholipase** It acts on lysophospholipid and forms glycerophosphocholine and free fatty acid.

Enzymes of lipid digestion and bile secretion are hormonally regulated. In response to dietary lipids, lower part of duodenum and jejunum produces hormone cholecystokinin. It acts on pancreatic cells to release enzymes and causes contraction of gall bladder for the release of bile.

Absorption of Lipids

Proximal part of jejunum is the major site of absorption of products of lipid digestion. The monoacylglycerols, free fatty acids, cholesterol and lysophospholipids combine with bile salt micelles and form mixed micelles. These mixed micelles carry the products of lipid digestion to the brush border of mucosal cells where they are absorbed into intestinal epithelium. Under normal conditions over 98% of dietary lipid is absorbed.

Solubilization

Solubilization of products of lipid digestion is required for diffusion of these molecules from the liquid luminal contents to brush border of enterocyte. Bile salts increases the solubility of lipolytic products in the aqueous luminal phase by forming mixed micelles only. When intra luminal bile salt concentration exceeds a critical micellar concentration (CMC) mixed micelles are formed. Decreased bile salt concentration leads to formation of large sized liquid crystalline vesicles or liposomes.

Transport of Lipolytic Products into Enterocyte

Until recently it is assumed that uptake of products of lipid digestion by enterocytes involves simple diffusion. Now it is known that specific transporters are involved in the uptake of some products of lipid digestion by enterocytes.

A family of fatty acid binding proteins (FBPs) are involved in uptake of fatty acids by intestine, adipose tissue, muscle, heart, macrophages, platelets etc. Fatty acid transport protein 4 (FATP4) present in apical membrane of enterocyte is the principal intestinal transporter of very long chain fatty acids.

Sterol Transport Protein (STP) of intestinal brush border membrane is involved in the uptake of free as well as esterified cholesterol. It is an integral membrane protein anchored in the lipid bilayer through an hydrophobic domain. The active centre involved in the transport are exposed to external side of the membrane. It also mediates uptake of long chain triacylglycerols.

The absorption of monoacylglycerol (MAG) by intestinal brush border membrane involves passive diffusion down concentration gradient. MAG moves out of the mixed micelles and get incorporated into outer layer of lipid bilayer of brush border membrane of enterocyte. The mechanism of the uptake of MAG by enterocyte is a collision induced transfer.

Fate of Absorbed Lipids in Enterocyte

After translocation across membrane of enterocyte, fatty acids combine with intestinal fatty acid binding proteins (IFBP-1) which are involved in intracellular transport of fatty acids.

IFBP-1 fatty acid complex migrates to endoplasmic reticulum where it is used for triglyceride resynthesis. There are two different pathways for resynthesis of triglycerides in enterocyte. 2-monoacylglycerol (2-MAG) pathway is most important. Alpha glycerophosphate pathway is another alternative pathway for triglyceride resynthesis in enterocyte.

The absorbed cholesterol is also reesterified in enterocytes. Enzymes involved in cholesterol esterefication are acyl-COA-cholesterol acyl transferases ACAT-1 and ACAT-2. Inhibition of ACAT activity decreases absorption of dietary cholesterol. Hence, inhibitors of ACAT can act as anti-atherogenic agents.

Within the intestinal cells, monoacylglycerols and fatty acids are converted to triglycerides only. The long chain fatty acids absorbed are used for triglyceride formation (Fig. 8.6). In addition lysophospholipids absorbed are converted to phospholipids by acylation (Fig. 8.6).

Triglycerides, cholesterol esters and phospholipids so formed in intestinal cells combines with protein to form lipoproteins, which are called as *chylomicrons*. These chylomicrons are released into the lymph of intestinal lymphatics. Later these chylomicrons pass into systematic blood through the thoracic duct. Because of the absorption of dietary lipids the lymph appears milky and called as chyle (Fig. 8.6).

The absorbed short chain and medium chain fatty acids are transported into portal venous blood. Similarly, glycerol absorbed is also not utilized and enters portal venous blood (Fig. 8.6).

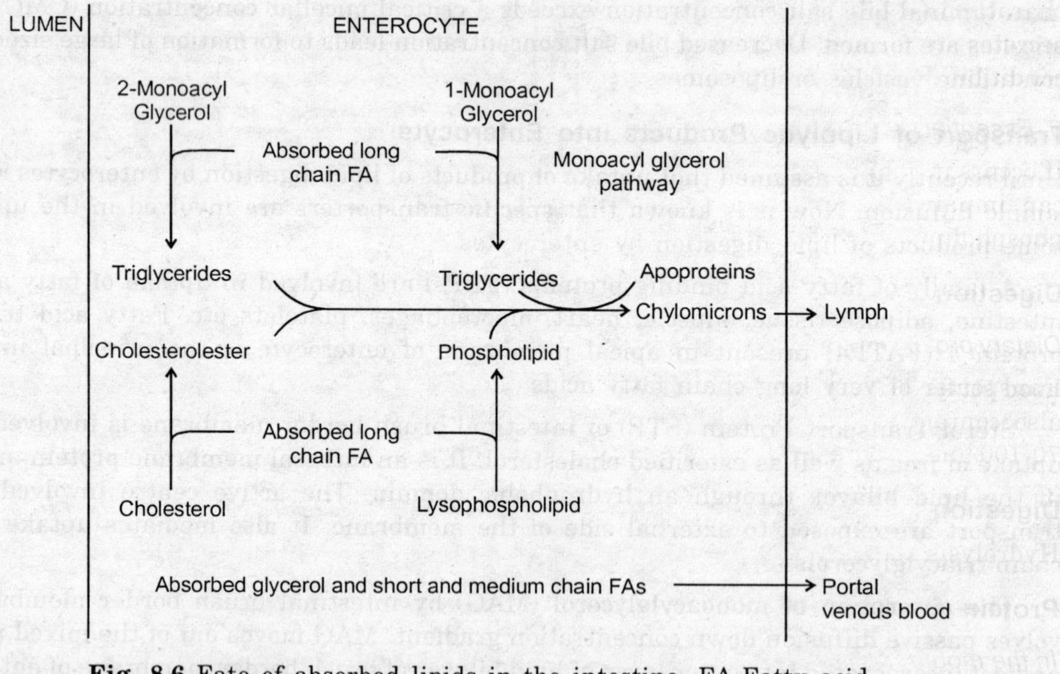

Fig. 8.6 Fate of absorbed lipids in the intestine. FA-Fatty acid

Disorders of Lipid Absorption

1. Chyluria

It is characterized by excretion of milky urine. It is due to abnormal connection between urinary tract and lymphatics of small intestine. It is also called as chylous fistula. It disappears when dietary fat is replaced with fat containing short chain and medium chain fatty acids.

2. Chylothorax

In the affected persons milky pleural fluid accumulates in pleural space due to abnormal connection between pleural space of lungs and lymphatics of small intestine. Like chyluria, chylothorax also disappears when dietary fat consist of only short and medium chain fatty acids.

3. Congenital abeta lipoproteinemia

It is of genetic origin. Triglycerides accumulates in intestinal cells due to lack of apo B-48 required for lipoprotein formation (chylomicrons).

4. Cholestasis

Lipid digestion and absorption is impaired in intra or extra hepatic cholestasis due to non availability of adequate amounts of bile salts, phospholipids and cholesterol. In cholestatic patients, liquid crystal vesicles are formed instead of mixed micelles. Proper biliary secretion of phospholipid is necessary for chylomicron formation in enterocyte and secretion of lipids into lymph.

5. Sito sterolemia

It is an autosomal recessive disorder. Elevated plasma level of plant sterol sitosterol is characteristic of this disorder. It is due to decreased activity of sterol transporter that secretes sterol into bile for elimation. Cholesterol absorption is moderately increased in this condition. Hence, atherosclerosis develops in affected individuals.

6. Essential fatty acid deficiency (EFAD)

It occurs in cholestatic patients due to malabsorption of lipids. EFAD during cholestasis itself can impair efficient lipid absorption and transport because proper biliary secretion of phospholipid is necessary for formation of mixed micelles and chylomicrons.

Digestion and Absorption of Proteins

Dietary proteins

Food stuffs like cereals, grains, milk, eggs and meat contain proteins. Vegetables and fruits also contain small amounts of proteins. Usually protein intake by an adult ranges from 70-100 gm/day.

Digestion of Proteins

Hydrolysis of dietary proteins to aminoacids constitutes the process of protein digestion.

Protein Digestion

In the mouth

Due to lack of protein splitting enzymes, no digestion of protein takes place in the mouth.

In the stomach

HCl present in gastric juice denatures proteins. The digestion of the denatured proteins is initiated by pepsin present in gastric juice. It is secreted by the chief cells of stomach in the form of inactive pro-enzyme pepsinogen. The conversion of pepsinogen to pepsin was detailed in Chapter 4.

Specificity of pepsin

Pepsin is an endo peptidase. It hydrolyzes the peptide bonds present within protein or polypeptide chain. It is optimally active at pH range of 1.5-2.5 which is provided by HCl present in gastric juice. It specifically hydrolyzes the peptide bonds of proteins in which the amino group is contributed by acidic or aromatic amino acids (Fig. 8.7). Usually pepsin transforms denaturated proteins to proteoses (large polypeptide derivatives) and peptones. Pepsin can hydrolyze only 10-15% of ingested protein.

Rennin

It is present in the infant stomach. It causes coagulation of milk. It converts casein of milk to para casein in presence of calcium ions on which pepsin acts and converts into proteoses and peptones.

In the small intestine

Pancreatic proteases and peptidases of succus entericus hydrolyzes proteoses and peptones to amino acids in the small intestine. Proteases of pancreatic juice are trypsin, chymotrypsin, elastase, carboxy peptidase and collagenease. Except collagenase all other proteases are secreted as proenzymes and their conversion to active enzymes have been described in chapter 4. All these active enzymes attack proteoses and peptones at neutral pH and produces oligopeptides and dipeptides.

1. Specificity of Pancreatic proteases

Except carboxy peptidase all others are endopeptidases. Trypsin specially catalyzes the hydrolysis of peptide bonds of proteins in which carbonyl group is contributed by basic amino acids like arginine and lysine (Fig. 8.7). Chymotrypsin is specific for the peptide bonds formed by aromatic amino acids like tyrosine and phenylalanine (Fig. 8.8). Elastase has broad specificity and catalyzes the hydrolysis of peptide bonds of proteins in which carbonyl group is contributed by glycine, alanine and serine. Collagenase attacks the collagen. All these proteases converts proteins to oligo peptides. Carboxy peptidase is an exopeptidase. It hydrolyzes polypeptides from carboxy terminal and produces one amino acid and a polypeptide shorter by one amino acid (Fig. 8.8). The action of carboxy peptidase continues on the polypeptide from carboxy terminus until the peptide is finally converted to a dipeptide. Finally the oligopeptides and dipeptides are hydrolysed to amino acids by peptidases present in succeus entericus. They are amino peptidase and dipeptidase.

2. Specificity of amino peptidase

It is an exopeptidase. It specifically hydrolyzes peptide bonds of oligopeptides from amino terminal and produces one amino acid and an oligopeptide shorter by one amino acid. It requires Mg^{2+} or Mn^{2+} for activity. The action of aminopeptidase continues from the amino terminus until the initial oligopeptide is converted to dipeptide. Dipeptidases present in succus entericus act on dipeptides and liberates amino acids (Fig. 8.9). Thus, by the combined action of these enzymes dietary proteins are hydrolyzed to amino acids. Enzymes of protein digestion are hormonally regulated. In response to partly digested proteins lower part of duodenum and jejunum produces hormone cholecystokinin. It acts on the Pancreas and causes the release of pancreatic proteases.

↓ (Glu)

H₂N — Ala — — — — — Gln — Val — Tyr — Ala — — — — — Gly — COOH

↓ Pepsin pH (1.5 – 2.5)

H₂N — Ala — — — — — Gln — Val — COOH + H₂N — Tyr — Ala — — — — — Gly — COOH

Proteoses   Peptones

↓

H₂N — Ala — — — — — Lys — Gly — — — — — Gln — Val — COOH

Proteose

↓ Trypsin pH(7.0 – 8.0)

H₂N — Ala — — — — — Lys — COOH + H₂N — Gly — — — — — Gln — Val — COOH

Oligopeptides

Fig. 8.7 Specificity of pepsin and trypsin

↓

H₂N — Tyr — Ala — — — — — Tyr — Gly — — — — — Gly — COOH

Peptone

↓ Chymotrypsin

H₂N — Tyr — Ala — — — — — Tyr — COOH + H₂N — Gly — — — — — Gly — COOH

Oligopeptides

↓

H₂N — Ala — — — — — Gln — Val — COOH

Proteose

↓ Carboxy peptidase

H₂N — Ala — — — — — Gln — COOH + Valine

Polypeptide shorter by one amino acid

↓

↓ Several steps

↓

H₂N — Ala — His — COOH + Amino acids

Dipeptide

Fig. 8.8 Action of chymotrypsin and carboxypeptidase

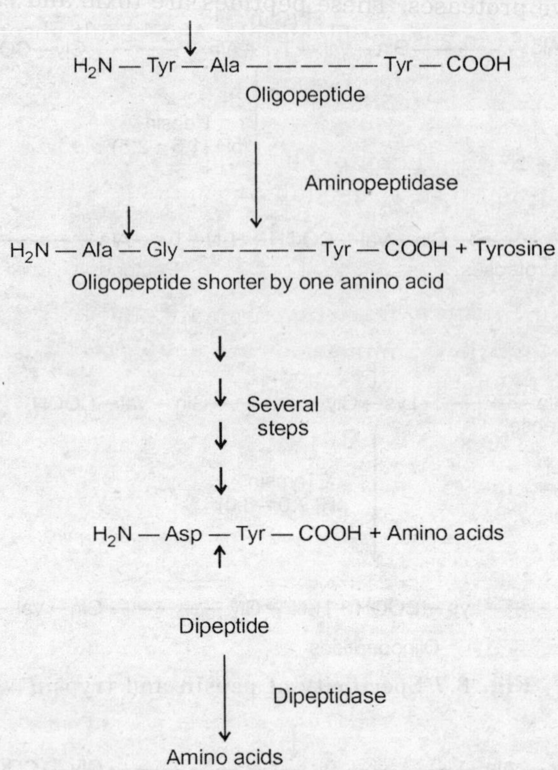

Fig. 8.9 Action of aminopeptidase and dipeptidase

ABSORPTION OF PRODUCTS OF PROTEIN DIGESTION

Amino acids formed from protein digestion are absorbed into portal venous blood. They are absorbed by mediated transport involving several carriers present in enterocyte membrane. There are different carriers for the transport of various categories of amino acids. Some of them are symporters like glucose carrier and they are called as Na^+ dependent carrier. Some carriers are Na^+ independent. There are 5 different Na^+ dependent carrier systems for the transport of amino acids. One carrier transports neutral amino acids whereas another carrier transports phenylalanine and methionine. Imino acids are transported by third carrier. Uptake of acidic amino acids is mediated by fourth carrier. Fifth carrier is involved in the transport of basic amino acids. Two different Na^+ independent carriers are involved in the transport of leucine and lysine.

DISORDERS OF AMINO ACID ABSORPTION OR PROTEIN DIGESTION

In some individuals dietary proteins are not completely hydrolysed to amino acids and these individuals absorb partly digested proteins or fragments of proteins. For example, colostrum the infant diet contains immunoglobulins which enter into blood stream of infant and act as immune system of the infant. However, in some susceptible individuals fragments act as antigens and hence individual develop immunological response. Some diseases like non-tropical sprue and celiac diseases are result of such immunological reactions.

1. Non-tropical sprue

It is due to the absorption of oligopeptide gluten derived from dietary oat, wheat and rye by the action of digestive proteases. These peptides are toxic and causes inflammation and atrophy of intestinal mucosa in susceptible people. As a result absorption is impaired in the small intestine.

2. Celiac disease

It occurs in children due to absorption of oligopeptides derived from wheat gluten. Hence, it is same as that of non-tropical sprue of adults. Symptoms of these diseases disappear when gluten is excluded from diet.

3. Hartnup disease

It is a genetic disorder. It is due to defective aromatic and hydrophobic amino acid carrier in the intestine. As a result, these amino acids are not absorbed. They are excreted in urine due to defective carrier in the kidney.

DISORDERS OF DIGESTION AND ABSORPTION

The digestion and absorption of food stuffs is impaired in some disorders.

1. Tropical sprue

It occurs due to altered intestinal flora in some individuals. The intestinal flora produces specific toxins, which cause inflammation and atrophy of mucosal cells of small intestine. As a result digestion and absorption of food is affected. Weight loss and diarrhoea are the common symptoms.

2. Cystic fibrosis

In this condition, pancreatic flow is obstructed. So digestion and absorption of fat and protein is incomplete and steatorrhea is common symptoms.

3. Gastroenteritis

The digestion and absorption of food is impaired in this condition due to inflammation of gastrointestinal tract and increased motility. Diarrhoea and abdominal cramps are the usual symptoms.

4. Gall stones

In this condition, digestion and absorption of fat is impaired due to obstruction of flow of bile which is required for the digestion and absorption of fat. Steatorrhea is common in this condition.

5. Pancreatitis

In this condition, flow of pancreatic fluid is obstructed. The proenzymes get activated and cause injury to pancreas. Inflammation and abdominal pain are common symptoms. Lack of pancreatic enzymes impairs protein and lipid digestion.

6. Parasitic infestations

In tropical countries, particularly in India, parasitic infestations occur in large population. Hook worm and round worm infestations effect digestion and absorption. Mainly the presence of these worms leads to increased motility and abdominal cramps.

REFERENCES

1. Davenport, H.W. Physiology of digestive tract. 4th ed. Year book Medical Publishers, Chicago, 1977.
2. Gray, G.M. Carbohydrate digestion and absorption. New Engl. J. Med. **292**, 1225-1230, 1975.
3. Kretchmer, M. Lactose and Lactase. Sci. Am. **227 (4)**, 74-78, 1972.
4. Rommel, K. and Bohmer (Eds.). Lipid absorption. University Park Press, Baltimore, 1976.
5. Tso, P. Gastro intestinal digestion and absorption of lipid. Adv. Lipid Res. **21**, 143, 1985.
6. Sleisener, M.H. and Kim, Y.S. Protein digestion and absorption. New Engl. J. Med. **300**, 659, 1979.
7. Michael. T. and Jansen, P.L.M. (Eds.). Fat absorption and lipid metabolism in cholestasis. Landes Bioscience, Texas, 2003.
8. Brown, J.C. Gastric inhibitory polypeptide. Springer-Verlag, 1982.
9. Donald, W.K. *et al.* (Eds.). Cancer Medicine: Alimentary tract dysfunction. BC Decker, 2003.
10. Boffelli, D. *et al.* Reconstitution and further characterization of the cholesterol transport activity of the small intestinal brush border membrane. Biochemistry. **36**, 10784-10792, 1997.
11. Berge, K.E., Tjan, Hand Graf, G. A. Accumulation of dietary cholesterol in sitosterolemia caused by mutations in adjacent ABC transporters. Science. **290**, 1771-1775, 2000.
12. Stahl, A., Hirsch, D.J. and Gimeno, R.E. Identification of the major intestinal fatty acid transport protein. Mol. Cell. **4**, 299-308, 1999.
13. Chang, C. C. *et al.* Immunological quantitation and localization of ACAT-1 and ACAT-2 in human liver and small intestine. J. Biol. Chem. **275**, 28083-28092, 2000.
14. Werner, A. *et al.* Fat malabsorption in essential fatty acid deficiency in mice is not due to impaired bile formation. Am. J. Physiol. Gastrointest. Liver Physiol. **283**, G900-G908, 2002.
15. Abumred, N. A. *et al.* Lipid transporters: Membrane transport systems for cholesterol and fatty acids. Opin. Clin. Nutr. Metab. Care. **3**, 255-262, 2000.

EXERCISES

ESSAY QUESTIONS

1. Define digestion. Explain actions of hydrolytic enzymes of digestive process.
2. Describe digestion and absorption of lipids. Explain role of bile salts in lipid digestion and absorption.
3. Name lipids present in diet. How they are digested and absorbed? Write about disease associated with digestion and absorption of lipids.
4. Name dietary carbohydrates. Write about their digestion and absorption in G.I. tract. Name diseases of this process.
5. How dietary proteins are digested and absorbed? Write disorders associated with this process.

6. Write an essay on diseases associated with digestion and absorption of food.
7. Describe about enzymes involved in digestion of food.

SHORT QUESTIONS

1. Name carbohydrates of food stuffs. Write actions of enzymes of small intestine involved in carbohydrate digestion.
2. Write a note on disorders of lipid absorption.
3. Explain absorption of products of protein digestion.
4. How products of lipid digestion are absorbed?
5. Write about diseases associated with digestion and absorption of carbohydrates.
6. Name bile salts. Write their role in digestion and absorption of lipids.
7. How glucose is absorbed in the intestine?
8. Write fate of absorbed lipids in the intestine.

MULTIPLE CHOICE QUESTIONS

1. Glucose absorption in intestine requires
   (*a*) A carrier and Na^+ (*b*) Carrier molecule
   (*c*) Na^+ only (*d*) Carrier and K^+
2. Aged people are prone to
   (*a*) Lactose intolerance (*b*) Lactase deficiency
   (*c*) Primary low lactase deficiency (*d*) Sucrase deficiency
3. All of the following statements are correct regarding congenital abeta lipoproteinemia. Except
   (*a*) It is a genetic disease
   (*b*) Triglycerides accumulates in intestine
   (*c*) Cholesterol accumulates in liver
   (*d*) It is due to lack of apo B-48
4. Peptide bonds of dietary proteins in which amino group is contributed by acidic amino acids are hydrolyzed by
   (*a*) Renin (*b*) Pepsin
   (*c*) Aminopeptidase (*d*) Exopeptidase
5. Carriers of amino acid absorption in the intestine are
   (*a*) Na^+ dependent
   (*b*) Na^+ independent
   (*c*) Na^+ dependent as well as Na^+ independent
   (*d*) None of the above.

FILL IN THE BLANKS

1. Absorption of partly digested products of proteins is responsible for ------------------ reactions.
2. Products of lipid digestion are excreted in urine of ---------patients.
3. For the absorption of hexoses by carrier molecule a ------------- ring is necessary.
4. ---------------- acts on pancreas to release enzymes.
5. Protein and lipid digestion is impaired in ------------- and ---------.

9
CHAPTER

CARBOHYDRATE METABOLISM

Metabolism can be defined as the entire chemical reactions network of the body. Other name often used is intermediary metabolism. Most of the chemical reactions in the body are enzyme catalyzed. The intermediates, substrates or products of these enzyme catalyzed reactions are called as metabolites. Sequence of enzymatic reactions that produce specific product are called as metabolic pathways. There are three types of metabolic pathways. Catabolic pathways, in which carbohydrates, lipids and proteins are degraded to small molecules by sequence of enzymatic reactions. In addition the breakdown of big molecules to small molecules is called as catabolism. Generally catabolism yields energy. Anabolic pathways: In which carbohydrates, lipids and proteins are synthesized from small molecules by sequence of enzymatic reactions. Formation of big molecules from small molecules is called as anabolism. Generally anabolism consumes energy. Amphibolic pathways have more than one function and they act as links between catabolic pathways and anabolic pathways. The three types of metabolic pathways does not occur in isolation. They interact with each other.

Usually carbohydrate metabolism consist of several pathways. Some of them are catabolic, few are anabolic and one is amphibolic pathway. Further, most of the metabolic pathways of carbohydrate metabolism either start with glucose or end with glucose. Hence, carbohydrate metabolism means it is the metabolism of glucose.

MEDICAL AND BIOLOGICAL IMPORTANCE

1. Glucose is the major fuel for all types of cells in the body. Its oxidation produces energy.
2. Glucose consumption per day varies from one organ to another.
3. Some organs like brain prefers glucose as fuel than fat and protein. Brain consumes about 100 gm of glucose per day.
4. Rate of glucose oxidation is more in cancer cells.
5. Glucose is used for the formation of glycogen, pentoses, lactose and mucopoly saccharides.
6. Since brain is totally dependent on glucose for its energy needs glucose is synthesized from glycogen or other non-carbohydrates during starvation or when food is in short supply.

7. Deficiency or absence of enzymes of glycogen metabolism causes glycogen storage diseases.
8. In erythrocytes, 2, 3-BPG is formed from glucose. 2, 3-BPG facilitates the release of oxygen from oxyhemoglobin.
9. Dietary galactose and fructose are converted to glucose.
10. Deficiency of enzymes of galactose and fructose metabolism causes galactosemia and fructosemia, respectively.
11. Most common metabolic disease diabetes mellitus is due to defective glucose metabolism.
12. Diabetes mellitus inturn causes secondary diseases like hypertension, kidney diseases and blindness.

Since most of the cells in the body extract energy from glucose, breakdown of glucose by glycolytic pathway is considered first among various pathways of carbohydrate metabolism.

GLYCOLYSIS

Degradation of glucose to two molecules of pyruvate or lactate by sequence of enzyme catalyzed reactions constitutes the process of glycolysis. It is a catabolic pathway. If glucose is degraded to pyruvate then it is called as *aerobic glycolysis*. Usually it occurs in presence of oxygen. If glucose is degraded to lactate then it is anaerobic glycolysis. Usually it occurs in the absence of oxygen. It is also called as *Embden-Meyerhof pathway,* because the reactions of glycolytic pathway were elucidated by Embden and Meyerhof.

Site of Glycolysis

Enzymes of glycolysis are present in the cytosol of most of the cells present in the body.

Source of Glucose

Dietary glucose formed from the digestion of dietary carbohydrates enter liver through portal venous system after its absorption from the intestine. Liver distributes glucose to all other organs (cells) of the body.

Entry of the Glucose in to the Cells

Glucose enters cells by facilitated transport.

1. **Liver** Glucose enters liver cells by facilitated diffusion. It is an insulin-independent transport mechanism for the transport of glucose across liver cells.
2. **Extra hepatic tissues** Glucose enters adipocytes, erythrocytes, brain and skeletal muscle by facilitated transport involving carrier molecule. The transport of glucose across the membranes of these tissues by carrier is dependent on insulin.

Reaction Sequence of Glycolysis

There are total eleven reactions in glycolysis. Extraction of energy from glucose occurs in the last six reactions of glycolysis only after some investment of energy in the first five reactions (Fig. 9.1).

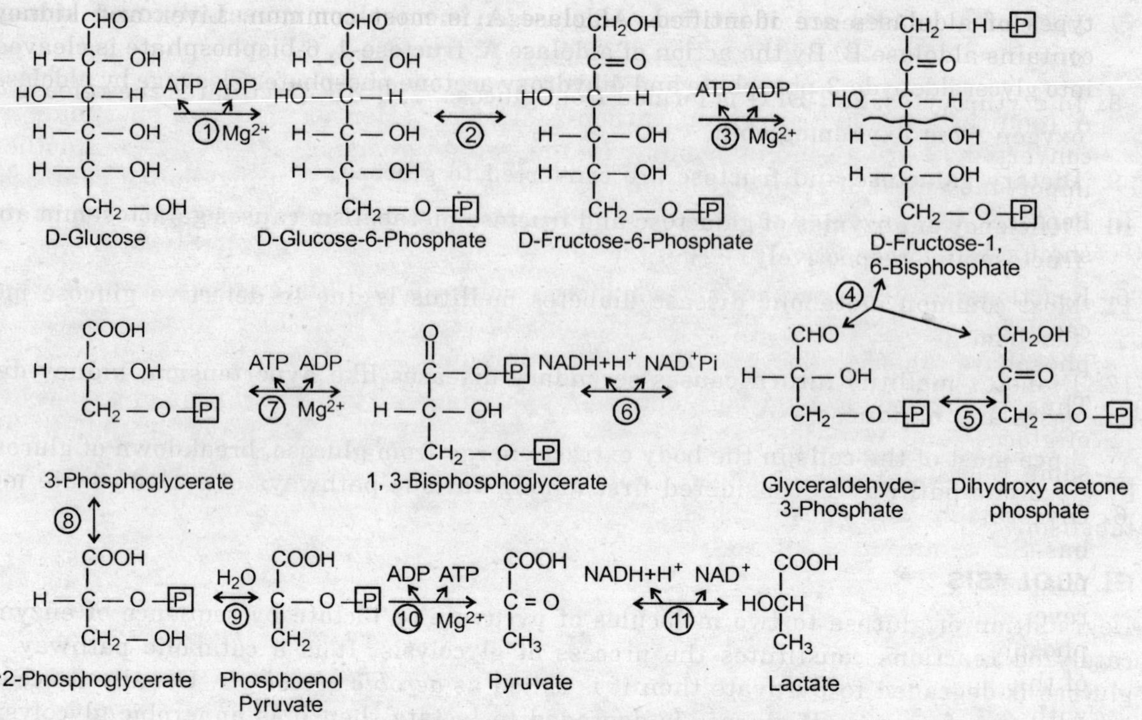

Fig. 9.1 Reaction sequence of glycolysis

1. Initial reaction of glycolysis is catalyzed by hexokinase. It is widely distributed. It phosphorylates glucose at 6 carbon in presence of Mg^{2+} and ATP. Phosphate is donated by ATP. Formation of Mg^{2+} : ATP complex is essential. Hexokinase phosphorylates other hexoses like galactose and fructose. It is an allosteric enzyme. The reaction catalyzed by this enzyme is irreversible under normal physiological conditions (Fig. 9.1). One high energy bond of ATP is used in this reaction to generate glucose-6-phosphate.

   Liver contains glucokinase, which phosporylates only glucose. It is an inducible enzyme. Its K_m for glucose is high compared to K_m of hexokinase. Hence, it phosphorylates glucose only when blood glucose concentration is high. Liver hexokinase phosphorylates glucose even blood glucose is low.
2. Second reaction of glycolysis involves aldose-ketose isomerization. The isomerization of glucose-6-phosphate (aldose) to fructose-6-phosphate (ketose) is accomplished by phospho glucose isomerase. It is a freely reversible reaction.
3. Phosphorylation once again is the third reaction of glycolysis. It is catalyzed by phosphofructokinase-1 (PFK-1) in presence of Mg^{2+} and ATP. It catalyzes the phosphorylation of fructose-6-phosphate and forms fructose-1, 6-bis phosphate. It is also irreversible like hexokinase reaction. One high energy bond of ATP is used. Phosphofructokinase is another allosteric enzyme of glycolysis and catalyzes rate limiting reaction of glycolysis.
4. Splitting of six carbon fructose-1, 6-bis phosphate to 2 triose molecules is the fourth reaction of glycolysis. It is catalyzed by aldolase. The reaction is reversible. Two

types of aldolases are identified. Aldolase A is most common. Liver and kidney contains aldolase B. By the action of aldolase A, fructose-1, 6-bisphosphate is cleaved into glyceraldehyde-3-phosphate and dihydroxy acetone phosphate. Cleavage by aldolase A requires carbonyl group on carbon-2 of sugar. Hence, glucose-6-phosphate is converted to fructose-6-phosphate in the second reaction of glycolysis. Another important aspect of second reaction of glycolysis is related to utilization of pentoses. Pentoses are converted to fructose-6-phosphate by pentose phosphate pathway as we shall see it later. The fructose-6-phosphate thus formed enter glycolysis.

5. Reaction 5 involves another aldose-ketose isomerization. Triose phosphate isomerase catalyzes conversion of dihydroxy acetone phosphate (ketose) to glyceradehyde-3-phosphate (aldose). The reaction is reversible one.

   Thus, two molecules of glyceraldehyde-3-phosphate are generated from one molecule of glucose and two high energy bonds are consumed. The two molecules follow the same reactions.

6. Glyceraldehyde-3-phosphate dehydrogenase catalyzes sixth reaction of glycolysis. It has–SH group at activesite. It catalyzes the conversion of glyceraldehyde-3-phosphate to 1, 3-bisphosphoglycerate in a NAD^+ dependent reaction. The reaction is reversible. NAD^+ is tightly bound to enzyme. The enzyme catalyzes oxidation and phosphorylation of substrate to yield high energy product. The reaction mechanism of this enzymes is shown in Fig. 9.2(*a*). The active site –SH group of enzyme reacts with aldehyde group of the substrate to form enzyme bound thiohemiacetal (*a*). NAD^+ oxidizes thiohemiacetal to high energy thiolester (*b*). As a result NAD^+ is reduced to NADH. NAD^+ replaces NADH (*c*). One molecule of orthophosphate reacts with enzyme bound thiol ester to form 1, 3-bisphosphoglycerate and free –SH at the active site of enzyme (*d*). One NADH is produced at this level of glycolysis.

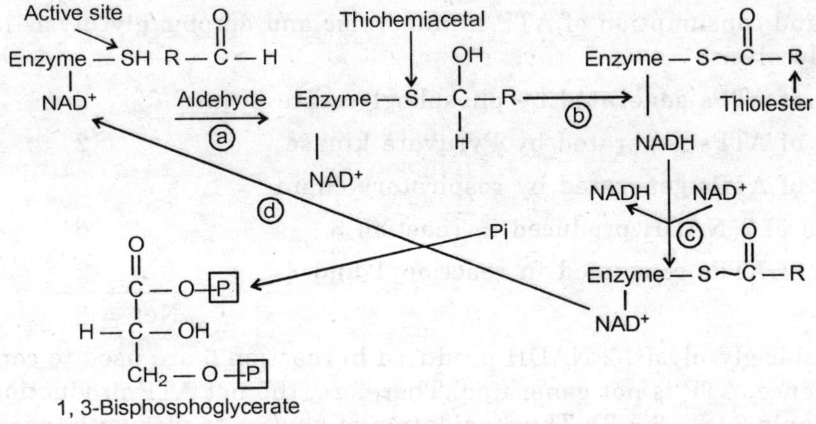

Fig. 9.2 (*a*) Mechanism of action of glyceraldehyde-3-Phosphate dehydrogenase

7. Reaction 7 involves transfer of high energy phosphate of 1, 3-bisphosphoglycerate to ADP. It is catalyzed by phosphoglycerate kinase. The reaction is reversible and requires Mg^{2+}. One ATP is formed from ADP and 1, 3-bisphosphoglycerate is converted to 3-phosphoglycerate. This reaction is an example for substrate level phosphorylation.

At this stage of glycolysis, two ATP are generated from two molecules of triose phosphates.

8. Reaction 8 involves the transfer of phosphate of 3-phosphoglycerate from carbon-3 to carbon-2 of glycerate. It is catalyzed phosphoglycerate mutase. The reaction is reversible.
9. High energy phosphate bond generation once again is the ninth reaction of glycolysis. It is catalyzed by enolase a Mn^{2+} or Mg^{2+} dependent enzyme and reaction is reversible. Removal of one molecule of water from 3-phosphoglycerate by the enzyme converts it to phosphoenolpyruvate a high energy compound.
10. Like reaction 7, reaction 10 involves transfer of high energy phosphate of phosphoenol puruvate to ADP. It is catalyzed by pyruvate kinase. The reaction is irreversible and requires Mg^{2+}. One molecule of ATP is formed and phosphoenol pyruvate is converted to pyruvate.

    At this stage of glycolysis, two ATPs and two pyruvates are generated from a molecule of glucose. Under aerobic conditions, pyruvate is the end product of glycolysis. Usually organs like liver, kidney and heart are aerobic and in these organs, NADH generated by dehydrogenation of glyceraldehyde-3-phosphate is oxidized by respiratory chain O_2. NAD^+, thus generated can be used again and glycolysis continues in the organs. Respiratory chain oxidation of one NADH generates three ATP molecules.
11. Lactate dehydrogenase catalyzes the reaction 11 of glycolysis. It reduces pyruvate to lactate using NADH generated in reaction 6 of glycolysis. This reaction occurs under anaerobic conditions. Formation of lactate using NADH as hydrogen donor is essential for the continuation of glycolysis in rapidly contracting skeletal muscle and erythrocytes because NADH can not be oxidized by respiratory chain O_2.

Energetics of Glycolysis

Generation and consumption of ATP in anaerobic and aerobic glycolysis is given below. In aerobic glycolysis:

1. Number of ATPs generated by phosphoglycerate kinase	2
2. Number of ATPs generated by Pyruvate kinase	2
3. Number of ATPs generated by respiratory chain oxidation of 2 NADH produced in reaction 6	6
4. Number of ATPs consumed in reaction 1 and 3	–2
Net =	8

In anaerobic glycolysis, 2 NADH produced in reaction 6 are used to convert pyruvate to lactate. Hence, ATP is not generated. Therefore, the net ATP production in anaerobic glycolysis is only 2 (8 – 6 = 2). Thus, oxidation of glucose to pyruvate (aerobic glycolysis) generates 8 ATP molecules whereas oxidation of glucose to lactate (anaerobic glycolysis) generates 2 ATP molecules.

Medical and Biological Importance of Glycolysis

1. Glycolysis provides energy to cells. Anaerobic glycolysis meets energy requirement of rapidly contracting skeletal muscle.

2. Since heart is mainly aerobic organ, myocardial ischemia decreases glycolytic ability of cardiac muscle. As a result energy or ATP production in heart is affected.
3. Deficiency of enzymes of erythrocyte glycolysis (pyruvate kinase) causes haemolytic anemia. This is because erythrocytes gets their energy from glycolysis.
4. Deficiency of muscle phosphofructo kinase causes decreased muscular performance and fatigue.
5. Dietary fructose and galactose are also metabolized by this pathway.
6. Glycolysis has amphibolic role also. It provides precursors for the formation of lipids and aminoacids. For example, pyruvate is converted to alanine by transamination and dihydroxy acetone phosphate serves as precursor for triglyceride formation.
7. Two glycolytic intermediates pyruvate and glyceraldehydes-3-phosphate are used for the synthesis of cholesterol, thiamine and pyridoxine in tuberculosis, malaria and gastritis causing organisms.
8. Glycolysis is the major energy source for rapidly growing malerial parasite in R.B.C. Lactate is the end product of glycolysis in malerial parasite. LDH of parasite is different from human enzyme. Unlike human LDH parasite enzyme is not subjected to inhibition by substrate pyruvate. This allows rapid formation of lactate from pyruvate and fast energy production.
9. In brain tumors lactate production is 10 times more.

Regulation of Glycolysis

Usually metabolic pathways are regulated by altering activities of few enzymes of that pathway. Glycolysis is under allosteric and hormonal control. Hexokinase phosphofructo kinase and pyruvate kinase are regulatory enzymes of glycolysis. Their activities are allosterically controlled. Further glucokinase, phosphofructokinase-1 and pyruvate kinase are under hormonal control also.

Allosteric regulation of glycolysis

Phosphofructokinase-1 is the major regulatory enzymes of glycolysis. It is an allosteric enzyme and catalyzes rate limiting reaction of glycolysis. It is inhibited by ATP and citrate. AMP and fructose-6-phosphate are activators of this enzyme. Pyruvate kinase is the second regulatory enzyme. It is inhibited by ATP and phosphoenolpyrvate. Glucose-6-phosphate inhibits activity of hexokinase. So, when ATP (energy) concentration is high glycolysis is inhibited and decrease in ATP level increases rate of glycolysis.

Hormonal regulation of glycolysis

Insulin increases rate of glycolysis by increasing concentration of glucokinase, phosphofructokinase-1 and pyruvate kinase.

Inhibitors of Glycolysis

1. Iodoacetate, arsenate and heavy metals like Hg^{2+}, Ag^{+} inhibits activity of glyceraldehyde-3-phosphate dehydrogenase. They combine with-SH of active site and makes enzyme inactive.
2. Enolase is inibited by fluoride.

Medical Importance

Inhibition of glycolysis by fluoride is exploited for accurate estimation of blood glucose level. If fluoride is not added to blood the glucose concentration in the blood decreases due to consumption of glucose by erythrocytes. Hence, inaccurate low blood glucose value is obtained on analysis.

2,3-*bis* Phosphoglycerate Cycle

It is involved in the synthesis of 2, 3-*bis* phosphoglycerate from 1, 3-*bis* phosphoglycerate in erythrocytes. Because of this energy yielding reaction catalyzed by phosphoglycerate kinase is bypassed. The formation of 2, 3-*bis* phosphoglycerate from 1, 3-bisphosphoglycerate is catalyzed by bisphosphoglycerate mutase (Fig. 9.2*b*). It is also called as Rapoport-Leubering cycle.

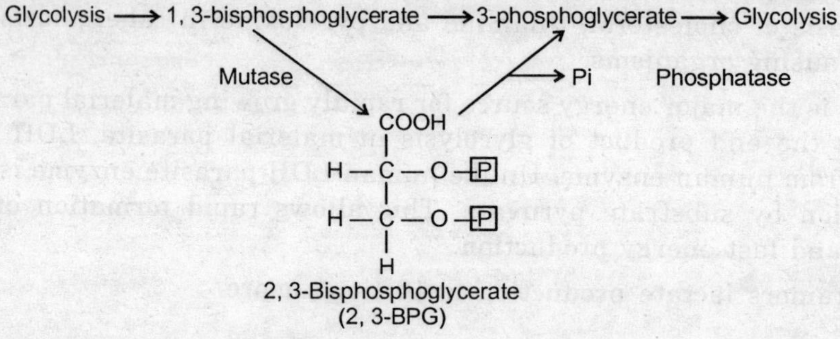

Fig. 9.2 (*b*) Formation and fate of 2, 3-bisphosphoglycerate in erythrocyte

Medical Importance

1. In the erythrocytes 2, 3-BPG aids unloading of oxygen by oxyhaemoglobin.
2. Due to the diversion of 1, 3-BPG to 2, 3-BPG production, energy yield of glycolysis is less in erythrocytes.

Fate of 2, 3-BPG

It is converted to 3-phosphoglycerate by 2, 3-bisphosphoglycerate phosphatase which enters glycolytic pathway (Fig. 9.2*b*).

Fate of Pyruvate

Under aerobic conditions, pyruvate is converted to acetyl-CoA in all tissues containing mitochondria. Both pyruvate molecules are oxidized to two acetyl-CoA molecules.

Entry of Pyruvate into Mitochondria

The mitochondrial membrane is not permeable to pyruvate, which is formed in cytosol. A specific carrier present in mitochondrial membrane transports pyruvate across mitochondrial membrane.

Fate of Pyruvate in Mitochondria

In mitochondria, pyruvate undergoes oxidative decarboxylation and remaining two carbon fragment is converted to acetyl-CoA. The reaction is irreversible and multi-step process. This reaction is catalyzed by pyruvate dehydrogenase (PDG) multi enzyme complex present in inner mitochondrial membrane. This multi enzyme complex consist of three enzymes. The first enzyme is pyruvate dehydrogenase. It contains TPP as prosthetic group and represented as E_1-TPP. The second enzyme is dihydrolipoyl transacetylase. It contains lipoic acid as prosthetic group, lipoic acid is attached to ε-amino group of lysyl residue of enzyme molecule through an amide linkage. Lipoyl lysine is called as *lipoamide*. It is represented as E_2-lipoamide. Third enzyme is dihydro lipoyl

SH SH

dehydrogenase and contains FAD as prosthetic group. It is represented as E_3-FAD. The reaction mechanisms of three enzymes are shown in Fig. 9.3.

1. In reaction-1, pyruvate dehydrogenase (E_1-TPP) reacts with substrate pyruvate to form enzyme bound anion of hydroxyethylidine-TPP. The conversion of pyruvate to enzyme bound hydroxyethylidine-TPP involves decarboxylation.
2. In reaction-2, dihydrolipoyl transacetylase first shifts hydroxyethylidine from TPP to one of -S-S-of its lipoamide to form acetyl lipoamide and E_1-TPP is released. Further shifting of acetyl moiety of acetyl lipoamide to CoA results in the formation of acetyl-CoA and reduced lipoamide.
3. In reaction-3, oxidized lipoamide is regenerated from reduced lipoamide. It is catalyzed by dihydrolipoyl dehydrogenase. This enzyme transfers electrons from reduced lipoamide to NAD^+ via FAD. Reduced NAD is produced at the end of reaction (NADH).

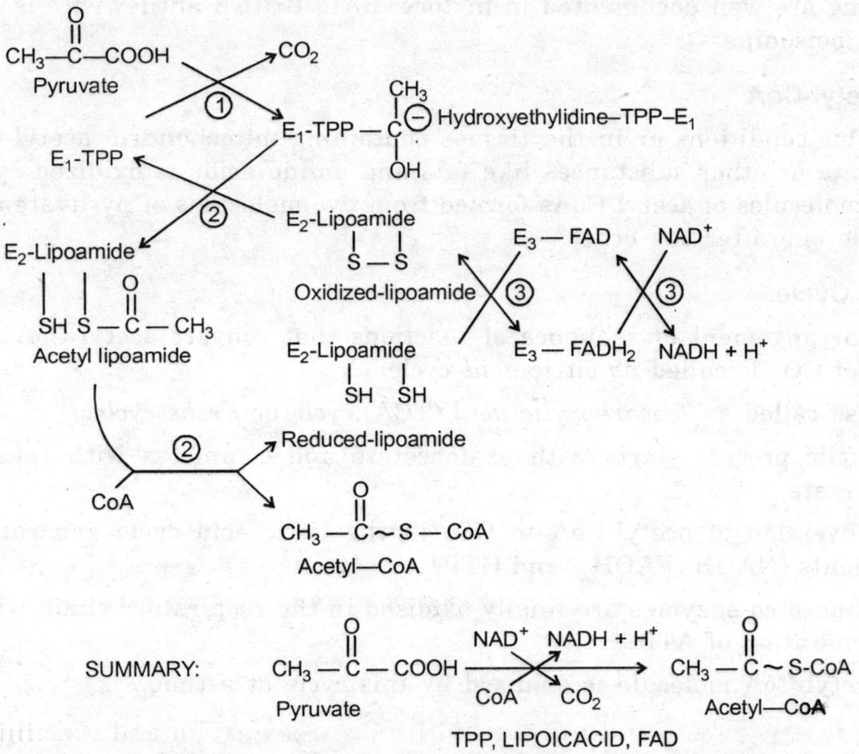

Fig. 9.3 Reaction mechanisms of enzymes of PDG complex

Energetics of Pyruvate Dehydrogenase

It indirectly produces energy. NADH oxidation generates ATP. Oxidative decarboxylation of two pyruvates yields 2 NADH. Their oxidation in respiratory chain yields 6 ATP at this level.

Regulation of Pyruvate Dehydrogenase

Pyruvate dehydrogenase activity is regulated by

1. Feedback inhibition.
2. **Covalent modification.** Acetyl-CoA and NADH inhibits activity of pyruvate dehydrogenase. Phosphorylation and dephosphorylation of this enzyme is under hormonal control Insulin increases its activity by favouring dephosphorylation.

Medical Importance

1. Pyruvate dehydrogenase serve as a link between aerobic glycolysis and citric acid cycle.
2. Since the reaction catalyzed by this enzyme is irreversible, acetyl -CoA can not be converted to pyruvate. For this reason, fat can not be converted to carbohydrate.
3. Lactic acidemia occurs in some individuals due to deficiency of pyruvate dehydrogenase.
4. Arsenic compounds inhibits this enzyme by reacting with-SH of lipoic acid. War gases and pesticides containing arsenic inhibit this enzyme. Deaths due to arsenic poisoning are well documented in history. BAL, British antilewisite is antidote for arsenic poisoning.

Fate of Acetyl-CoA

Under aerobic conditions or in the tissues containing mitochondria acetyl-CoA formed from pyruvate or other substances like fats and amino acids is oxidized by citric acid cycle. Two molecules of acetyl-CoAs formed from two molecules of pyruvate are oxidized by this cycle one after the other.

Citric Acid Cycle

1. Cyclic arrangement of sequence of reactions that convert acetyl-CoA to two molecules of CO_2 is called as citric *acid* cycle.
2. It is also called as *Tricarboxylic acid* (TCA) *cycle* or *Krebs cycle*.
3. This cyclic process starts with oxaloacetate and completes with regeneration of oxaloacetate.
4. The conversion of acetyl-CoA to CO_2 in the citric acid cycle generates reducing equivalents (NADH, $FADH_2$) and GTP.
5. The reduced co-enzymes are finally oxidized in the respiratory chain with concomitant generation of ATP.
6. One acetyl-CoA molecule is oxidized by this cycle at a time.

Site

Enzymes of citric acid cycle are present in mitochondrial matrix.

Reaction Sequence of Citric Acid Cycle

There are total eight reactions in this cycle (Fig. 9.4).

1. In the initial reaction, two carbon acetyl-CoA condenses with 4-carbon oxaloacetate to form 6 carbon citrate. A condensing enzyme citrate synthase catalyzes this reaction. Citrate formation involves carbon to carbon bond formation between methyl carbon of acetyl-CoA and carbonyl carbon of oxaloacetate. CoA is released. It is a rate limiting reaction and irreversible. One water molecule is consumed in this reaction. The remaining reactions of the cycle regenerates oxaloacetate from citrate with release of two CO_2 molecules.
2. Since citrate is tertiary alcohol it cannot be oxidized directly. Hence, in reaction-2 it is isomerized to isocitrate a secondary alcohol and can be oxidized easily. Isomerization is catalized by aconitase an iron-sulfur containing protein. Isomerization involves two steps. In the initial step, citrate is dehydrated to *cis*-aconitate. Rehydration in the next step converts *cis*-aconitate to isocitrate. The reaction is reversible.

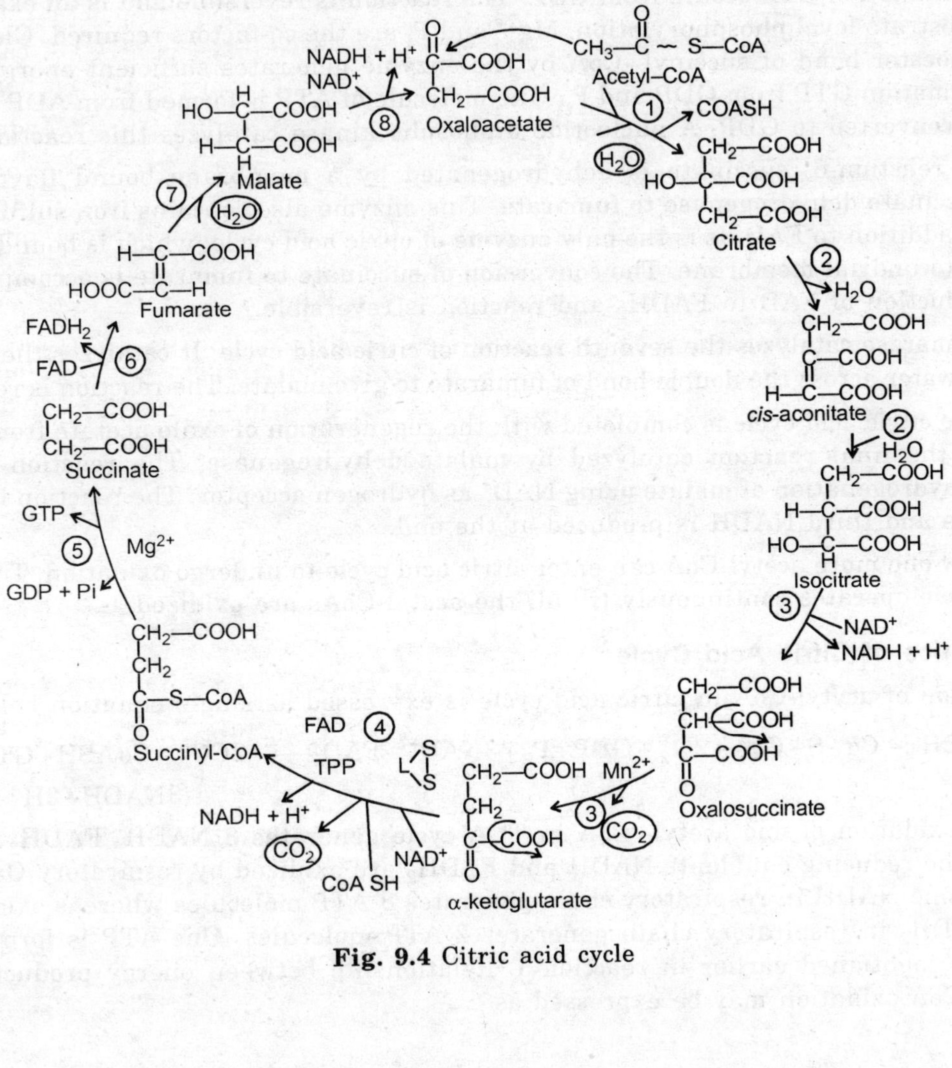

Fig. 9.4 Citric acid cycle

3. In reaction-3, isocitrate is converted to α-ketoglutarate by isocitrate dehydrogenase. The reaction is irreversible. The conversion of isocitrate to α-ketoglutarate involves two steps. In the first step, isocitrate is dehydrogenated to oxalo succinate using NAD^+ as hydrogen acceptor. Decarboxylation of oxalo succinate in the second step generates α-ketoglutarate and first CO_2 molecule. Mg^2 + or Mn^2+ are required for the decarboxylation. α-ketoglutarate is a keto acid like pyruvte. At the end of this reaction first NADH is generated.
4. In reaction-4, α-ketoglutarate undergoes oxidative decarboxylation catalyzed by α-ketoglutarate dehydrogenase multi enzyme complex to succinyl-CoA. The reaction is similar to the oxidative decarboxylation of pyruvate catalyzed by pyruvate dehydrogenase complex and requires TPP, lipoic acid, FAD, CoASH and NAD^+. The products of this reaction are succinyl-CoA, which is a thioester containing an high energy bond, second molecule of CO_2 and second NADH. The reaction is irreversible.
5. In this reaction, high energy phosphate bond is generated by the action of succinyl-CoA synthetase on succinyl-CoA. Succinate is formed from the succinyl-CoA and the formation of GTP occurs from GDP. The reaction is reversible and is an example for substrate level phosphorylation. Mg^{2+} and P_i are the co-factors required. Cleavage of thioester bond of succinyl -CoA by the enzyme generates sufficient energy for the formation GTP from GDP and P_i. One molecule of ATP is formed from ADP and GTP is converted to GDP. A nucleotide diphospho kinase catalyzes this reaction.
6. In reaction-6, succinate is dehydrogenated by a membrane bound flavo protein succinate dehydrogenase to fumarate. This enzyme also contains iron sulfur centres in addition to FAD. It is the only enzyme of citric acid cycle, which is bound to inner mitocondrial membrane. The conversion of succinate to fumarate is accompanied by reduction of FAD to $FADH_2$ and reaction is reversible.
7. Fumarase catalyzes the seventh reaction of citric acid cycle. It catalyzes the addition of water across the double bond of fumarate to give malate. The reaction is reversible.
8. The citric acid cycle is completed with the regeneration of oxalo acetate from malate in the final reaction catalyzed by malate dehydrogenase. The reaction involves dehydrogenation of malate using NAD^+ as hydrogen acceptor. The reaction is reversible and third NADH is produced at the end.

Now one more acetyl-CoA can enter citric acid cycle to undergo oxidation. Thus citric acid cycle operates continuously till all the acetyl-CoAs are oxidized.

Energetics of Citric Acid Cycle

Oxidation of acetyl-CoA in citric acid cycle is expressed as single equation below.

$$CH_3-Co-S-CoA+2O_2+GDP+P_i+3NAD^+ +FAD \longrightarrow 2CO_2+CoASH+GTP + 3NADH+3H^+ +FADH_2$$

So oxidation of one acetyl- CoA in TCA cycle generates 3 NADH, $FADH_2$ and one GTP. The reducing equalents NADH and $FADH_2$ are oxidized by respiratory O_2. Oxidation of one NADH in respiratory chain generates 3 ATP molecules whereas oxidation of one $FADH_2$ in respiratory chain generates 2 ATP molecules. One ATP is formed from GTP as mentioned earlier in reaction-5. Relationship between energy production and acetyl-CoA oxidation may be expressed as

$$\text{Acetyl–CoA} + 2O_2 + 12Pi + 12ADP \longrightarrow 2CO_2 + 12ATP + CoASH + 13H_2O$$

Generation of ATP in Citric Acid Cycle

1. Number of ATP generated by oxidation of 3 NADH	9
2. Number of ATP generated by oxidation of $FADH_2$	2
3. Number of ATP generated from GTP	1
	12

So 12 ATP are generated in citric acid cycle for every molecule of acetyl-CoA oxidized. Since glucose gives rise to two acetyl-CoA molecules aerobic oxidation of glucose yields 24 ATPs at this level.

Medical Importance

1. It is the final common metabolic pathway for oxidation of carbohydrates, fats and proteins. Some amino acids are degraded to intermediates of TCA-cycle. Acetyl-CoA arises from fat catabolism.
2. **Amphibolic role :** In the liver intermediates of TCA cycle are used for the synthesis of (*a*) Fatty acids, Cholesterol (*b*) Amino acids (*c*) Porphyrins (*d*) Glucose.
3. In some liver diseases, like hepatitis and cirrhosis amphibolic role of citric acid cycle is affected.

Regulation of Citric Acid Cycle

Enzymes of citric acid cycle are under allosteric control. Citrate synthase, isocitrate dehydrogenase and α-ketoglutarate dehydrogenase are involved in the regulation of citric acid cycle and their activities are allosterically regulated. Citrate synthase activity is inhibited by ATP and long chain acyl-CoA. Isocitrate dehydrogenase is inhibited by ATP and NADH and activated by ADP. Succinyl-CoA and NADH are allosteric inhibitors of third regulatory enzyme α-ketoglutarate dehydrogenase. So the rate of citric acid cycle incrases in the absence of ATP and decreases in the presence of ATP and NADH. The energy demand of cell determines the rate of citric acid cycle. Further Ca^{2+} seems to increase the activities of isocitrate dehydrogenase and α-ketoglutarate dehydrogenase.

Inhibitors of Citric Acid Cycle

1. Fluroacetate inhibits activity of aconitase. It is used as rodenticide. As such it is not toxic, but in the body, it is converted to fluoroacetyl-CoA, which gives rise to fluorocitrate after condensing with oxaloacetate. The aconitase is inhibited by fluoro citrate. The conversion of non-toxic compound to toxic compound inside the body is called as *lethal synthesis*.
2. α-ketoglutarate dehydrogenase is inhibited by arsenic compounds.
3. Malonate is a competitive inhibitor of succinate dehydrogenase.

Energetics of Aerobic Oxidation of Glucose

Under aerobic conditions, complete oxidation of glucose occurs in three stages. They are 1. Glycolysis 2. Pyruvate dehydrogenase complex 3. Citric acid cycle. The amount of ATP generated by each process was discussed earlier. Total yield of ATP during oxidation of glucose is obtained by adding ATP generated at each stage.

ATP Generation during Oxidation of Glucose

Process	Number of ATP/mol of glucose
1. Glycolysis	8
2. Pyruvate dehydrogenase	6
3. Citric acid cycle	24
Total	38

Thus, aerobic oxidation of glucose generates total 38 ATP molecules. However, the amount depends on shuttle used for the transfer of reducing equivalents from cytosol to mitochondria.

Efficiency of Glucose Oxidation

If all the energy released during oxidation of a compound is conserved then efficiency of that process is good (100%). Let us examine how efficient is the process of oxidation of glucose in the body. It has been estimated that oxidation of glucose in calorimeter produces 2870 KJ of energy. Aerobic oxidation of glucose in the body generates 38ATPs i.e., 38 new high energy bonds are formed. Since each high energy bond formation requires 51.6 KJ of energy about 1961 KJ (38×51.6) of energy is used for ATP synthesis. This means only 70% of energy is conserved and remainder is lost as heat. However, heat liberated keeps body temperature. Therefore, the efficiency of glucose oxidation process is 70% only.

GLYCOGENESIS

In cells, the rate of glucose oxidation largely depends on energy (ATP) demand of cell. If cell has sufficient energy (ATP) then glucose oxidation stops and excess glucose is stored as glycogen.

Glycogenesis is the Synthesis of Glycogen from Glucose

Site Though every cell can form glycogen it chiefly occurs in liver and skeletal muscle. In the muscle, about 245 gms of glycogen and in the liver about 72 gms of glycogen is stored under well fed condition. Even though-energy, rich fat is abundant in the body skeletal muscle prefers to store glucose (energy) as glycogen because

1. Fat can not be oxidized under anaerobic condition.
2. Acetyl-CoA of fat oxidation can not be converted to glucose.
3. Skeletal muscle is unable to mobilize fat rapidly.

This stored glycogen act as readily available source of glucose for glycolysis in the muscle. Glycogen granules are present in the cytoplasm. Enzymes of glycogen metabolism are also associated with these granules.

Reaction Sequence of Glycogenesis

The glucose molecules as such cannot be polymerized into glycogen. Glycogen synthesis requires activation of sugars. The active sugars transfers sugar to –OH group of an acceptor molecule. The glycogen synthesis occurs in four main reactions. Glycogenesis begins with glucose-6-phosphate an intermediate of glycolysis (Fig. 9.5).

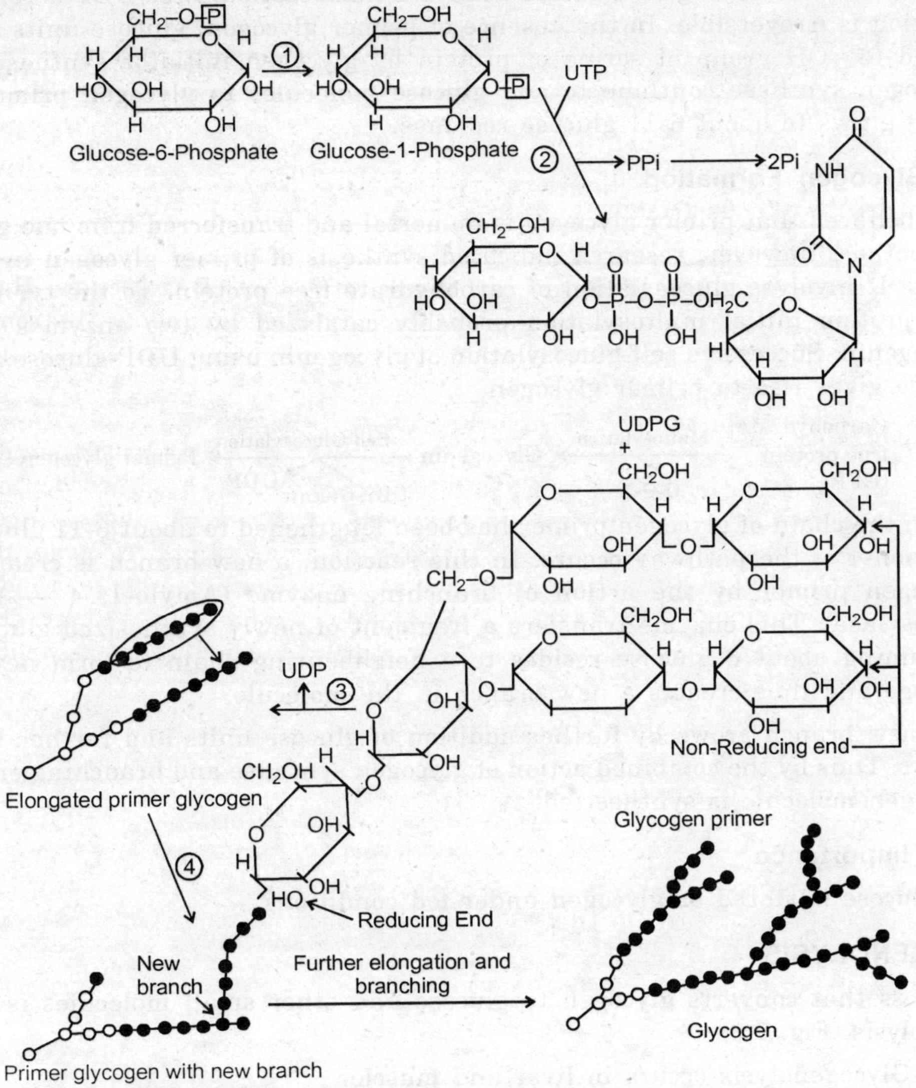

Fig. 9.5 Glycogenesis. o-Newly added glucose residues, o-Glucose units of glycogen primer

1. The first reaction leading to glycogen formation is the conversion of glucose-6-phosphate to glucose-1-phosphate. The reaction is catalyzed by phosphoglucomutase.
2. In reaction-2, glucose-1-phosphate reacts with nucleoside triphosphate UTP to form uridine diphosphate glucose (UDPG). The reaction is catalyzed by enzyme UDPG pyrophosphorylase. Even though, the reaction is reversible the immediate hydrolysis of PPi to 2 Pi by pyrophosphatase drags the reaction in the direction of UDPG formation. UDPG is active sugar. It transfers glucose residues to an acceptor.
3. Since free glucose can not accept glucose from UDP glucose to initiate chain synthesis a glycogen primer is required. A fragment of glycogen having minimum 4 glucose

residues serve as primer for glycogen synthesis. So, in reaction-3 UDP-glucose transfers glucose to non-reducing end (free-OH) of primer glycogen to form new α (1, 4) glycosidic bond. Glycogen synthase catalyzes this reaction. Free UDP is released and reaction is irreversible. In the absence of primer glycogen, glucose units are transferred to –OH group of serine of protein by glycogen initiator synthase enzyme. Glycogen synthase continue to add glucose molecules to glycogen primer till the chain grows to about 6-11 glucose residues.

Primer Glycogen Formation

4. It is believed that primer glycogen is immortal and transferred from one generation to another. However, research indicated synthesis of primer glycogen in some cell types. It involves glucosylation of carbohydrate free protein. To the tyr residue of this protein initial maltosylation probably catalyzed by two enzymes generates glycogenin. Successive self-glucosylation of glycogenin using UDP-glucose as glucose source gives rise to primer glycogen.

$$\text{Carbohydrate free protein (CFP)} \xrightarrow[\text{O-O-X}]{\text{Maltosylation}} \text{Glycogenin} \xrightarrow[\text{UDP-Glucose} \;\to\; \text{UDP}]{\text{Self Glucosylation}} \text{Primer glycogen}$$

5. When the chain of glycogen primer has been lengthened to about 6-11 glucose units reaction-4 of the pathway occurs. In this reaction, a new branch is created in the glycogen primer by the action of branching enzyme (Amylo-1, 4 → 1, 6-*trans* glycosylase). This enzyme transfers a fragment of newly synthesized glucose chain containing about 6 glucose resides to a neighbouring chain to form new α (1, 6) linkage and thus creates a new branch in the molecule.
6. The new branch grows by further addition of glucose units and further branching occurs. Thus by the combined action of glycogen synthase and branching enzyme the glycogen molecule is synthesized.

Medical Importance

Excess glucose is stored as glycogen under fed conditions.

GLYCOGENOLYSIS

The process that converts glycogen to glucose and other small molecules is called as glycogenolysis (Fig. 9.6).

Site. Glycogenolysis occurs in liver and muscle.

Degradation of glycogen is not the reversal of glycogenesis. Instead, independent enzymes are involved in glycogen break down. In the liver the end product of glycogenolysis is glucose whereas in the skeletal muscle glucose-6-phosphate or lactate is the end product.

Reaction Sequence of Glycogenolysis

There are three main reactions:

1. In reaction-1 glucose units are removed as glucose-1-phosphates from non-reducing end of glycogen by hydrolyzing α(1, 4) glycosidic bonds. The reaction is catalyzed by phosphorylase an exoglucosidase. Inorganic phosphate (Pi) is required to form glucose-1

phosphate from glucose. The enzyme is so named because of phosphorylation of glucose. Even though the reaction is reversible the *in vitro* high Pi concentration prevents backward reaction to occur. The action of phosphorylase on glycogen continues until four glucose units remain on either side of the α(1, 6) branch point. Glycogen is converted to limit dextrin by the action of phosphorylase.

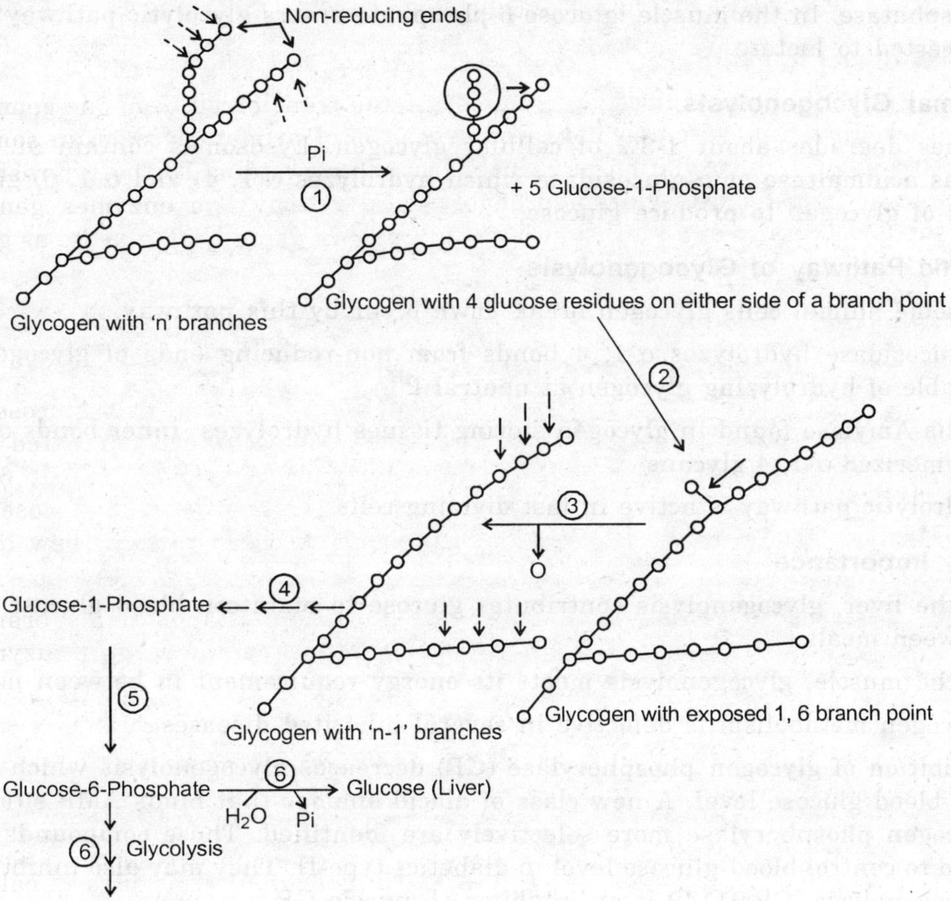

Fig. 9.6 Glycogenolysis in the liver and skeletal muscle
Broken arrows indicate cleavage sites of phosphorylase

2. In reaction-2 three glucose units from one branch are transferred to another branch to expose α(1, 6) branch point. This transfer of oligoglucan is catalyzed by oligo-α (1, 4) → α(1, 4) glucan transferase which probably involves hydrolysis and formation of α(1, 4) glycosidic bonds.
3. In reaction-3, α(1, 6) branch point is removed by hydrolyzing α(1, 6) glycosidic bond at branch point. The reaction is catalyzed by debranching enzyme. One glucose molecule is produced at this level.
4. With the removal of the branch point further action of phosphorylase occurs on the remaining glycogen molecule. Thus, by the combined action of the enzymes of

glycogenolysis the glycogen is converted to glucose-1-phosphate (90%) and glucose (10%).

5. The glucose-1-phosphate is converted to glucose-6-phosphate by the action of phosphoglucomutase.
6. In the liver, glucose-6-phosphate is converted to glucose by the action of glucose-6-phosphatase. In the muscle, glucose-6-phosphate enters glycolytic pathway and get converted to lactate.

Lysosomal Glycogenolysis

Lysosomes degrades about 1-3% of cellular glycogen. Lysosomes contain an enzyme known as acidmaltase or α-glucosidase which hydrolyzes $\alpha(1, 4)$ and $\alpha(1, 6)$ glycosidic linkages of glycogen to produce glucose.

Hydrolytic Pathway of Glycogenolysis

1. In some animal cells glycogen break down occur by this pathway.
2. α-glucosidase hydrolyzes α-1, 4 bonds from non-reducing ends of glycogen. It is capable of hydrolyzing glycogen at neutral P^H.
3. Alpha-Amylase found in glycogen storing tissues hydrolyzes inner bonds of highly polymerized α-1, 4 glycans.
4. Hydrolytic pathway is active in fast dividing cells.

Medical Importance

1. In the liver, glycogenolysis contributes glucose to maintain blood glucose level in between meals.
2. In the muscle, glycogenolysis meets its energy requirement in between meals.
3. Glycogen metabolism is defective in several inherited diseases.
4. Inhibition of glycogen phosphorylase (GP) decreases glycogenolysis which leads to low blood glucose level. A new class of diacid enalogs that binds AMP site of liver glycogen phosphorylase more selectively are identified. These compounds may be used to control blood-glucose level in diabetics type-II. They may also inhibit muscle glycogenolysis. CP-91149 is an inhibitor of muscle GP.
5. α-glucosidase activity increases in tumor cells of brain.
6. Phosphorylase activity disappears in brain tumor cells.

Glycogen Storage Diseases

These are group of inherited (genetic) diseases of glycogen metabolism. In these diseases, there is an abnormal accumulation of large amount of glycogen or its metabolites in the tissues due to deficiency or absence of enzymes of glycogen metabolism. Some of them are not serious mild disorders but few of them are fatal.

(a) Von Geirke's disease (Type-1 glycogen storage disease)

It is due to the deficiency or absence of glucose-6-phosphatase in liver, kidney and intestine. The incidence of this disease is 1 in 2,00,000. Lack of glucose-6-phosphatase cause accumulation of glycogen in liver and kidney and enlargement of liver occurs.

Hypoglycemia is common symptom other symptoms are hyperuricemia, hyperlipemia and ketosis.

(b) Pompe's disease (Type-II)

It is due to the deficiency of lysosomal α-glucosidase. Lysosomes can not utilize glycogen and accumulation of glycogen occurs in all tissues. Accumulation of glycogen in heart leads to cardiomegaly. It is a fatal disorder and death occurs before second year of life due to cardio respiratory failure.

(c) Cori's disease (Type-III)

It is due to deficiency or absence of debranching enzyme. Limit dextrin a metabolite of glycogenolysis accumulates in liver. Hence, this condition is also called as limit dextrnosis.

(d) Anderson's disease (Type-IV)

It is a fatal disease. It is due to absence of branching enzyme. Amylopectin an intermediate of glycogenesis accumulatres in liver, spleen and heart. Hence, this condition is called as amylopectinosis.

(e) Mc Ardle's syndrome (Type-V)

It is due to the absence of muscle phosphorylase. Glycogen accumulates in muscle and lactic acid production in muscle is not increased after exercise. Affected person suffer from painful muscle cramps and diminished tolerance to exercise.

(f) Her's disease (Type-VI)

It is due to the absence of liver phosphorylase. Glycogenolysis is defective and glycogen accumulates in liver.

REGULATION OF GLYCOGEN METABOLISM

1. Synthesis and degradation of glycogen are two opposite processes.
2. Simultaneous occurrence of these two processes is not desirable.
3. Hence these two processes responds to regulatory signals in opposite ways.
4. Many hormones control the synthesis and degradation of glycogen in liver and muscle.
5. The synthesis and degradation of glycogen are reciprocally regulated by hormones, In reciprocal regulation of pathways if one pathways is activated other pathway is inhibited.
6. Phosphorylase and glycogen synthase are main regulatory enzymes of glycogen metabolism.
7. Hormones indirectly control activities of regulatory enzymes of glycogen metabolism. They reciprocally regulate activities of glycogen synthase and phosphorylase.
8. They either increase or decrease cAMP which is necessary for the action of proteinkinases. The role of proteinkinases in regulating enzyme activity was discussed in chapter 4.
9. Glycogen metabolism is also under allosteric control. Regulatory enzymes are subjected to allosteric regulation.

HORMONAL REGULATION OF GLYCOGEN METABOLISM

Epinephrine and nor epinephrine increases glycogenolysis in muscle and decrease glycogenesis. Likewise glucagon increases glycogenolysis and decreases glycogenesis in liver. In contrast, insulin favours glycogenesis and suppresses glycogenolysis in liver and muscle.

We shell first examine how these hormones affect glycogenolysis in various organs. Phosphorylase, which is rate limiting enzyme of glycogenolysis has many binding sites.

1. Catalytic site where glycogen and glucose-1-phosphate binds.
2. Nucleotide binding site where AMP an allosteric effector binds.
3. Binding site for ATP and glucose-6-phosphate which are allosteric effectors.
4. Pyridoxal phosphate binding site.
5. Phosphorylation site. Ser-OH serve as site for phosphorylation.

Phosphorylase exist in two forms an active phosphorylase a form and inactive phosphorylase b form. Phosphorylation by phosphorylase b kinase converts inactive phosphorylase b to active phosphorylase a. Further dephosphorylation catalyzed by protein phosphatase converts active phosphorylase a to inactive phosphorylase b. Phosphorylase b kinase exist in two forms. Phosphorylase b kinase active and inactive phosphorylase b kinase. Phosphorylation by protein kinase converts inactive form to active form. Again here also dephosphorylation by protein phosphatase converts active phosphorylase b kinase to inactive phosphorylase b kinase. Protein kinases are dependent on cAMP for their activity. In the absence of cAMP they are inactive. A membrane bound adenylate cyclase catalyzes the formation of cAMP from ATP. Phosphodiesterese catalyzes the conversion of cAMP to AMP and hence cAMP level decreases. Protein kinases also catalyzes the phosphorylation of inactive inhibitor-1 to active inhibitor-1 phosphate which inhibits protein phosphatases activities. Epinephrine, nor-epinephrine and glucagon activates membrane bound adenylate cyclase via GTP binding protein (G-protein) thus producing more cAMP which in turn activates enzymes that favour glycogenolysis. Thus, hormones epinephrine, nor epinephrine and glucagon favours glycogenolysis by increasing cAMP level which inturn increases the activities of enzymes that favour glycogenolysis and at the same time inhibiting activities of enzymes (phosphatases) that are not favourable to glycogenolysis. In contrast insulin lowers cAMP by activating phosphodiesterase thus inhibiting enzymes that favour glycogenolysis which in turn leads to suppression of glycogenolysis. Mechanism of action of these hormones on glycogenolysis is shown in Fig. 9.7.

Now let us see mechanism by which these hormones affect glycogenesis in various organs. Like phosphorylase another regulatory enzyme of glycogen metabolism, glycogen synthase exist in two forms glycogen synthase a active form and glycogen synthase b inactive form. In contrast to phosphorylase, phosphorylation by protein kinase converts active glycogen synthase a to inactive glycogen synthese b. This explains the reason for opposite actions of hormones on glycogen metabolism. Insulin inhibits phosphorylation by lowering cAMP level. In addition, insulin promotes glycogenesis by increasing the activity of protein phosphatase that converts inactive glycogen synthase b to active glycogen synthase a. Thus, insulin favours glycogenesis by increasing glycogen synthase and lowering cAMP level. In contrast epinephrine, norepinephrine and glucagon increase cAMP level, thus suppresses glycogenesis by activating protein kinase and inhibitor-1 phosphate. Mechanism of action of these hormones on glycogenesis is shown in Fig. 9.8.

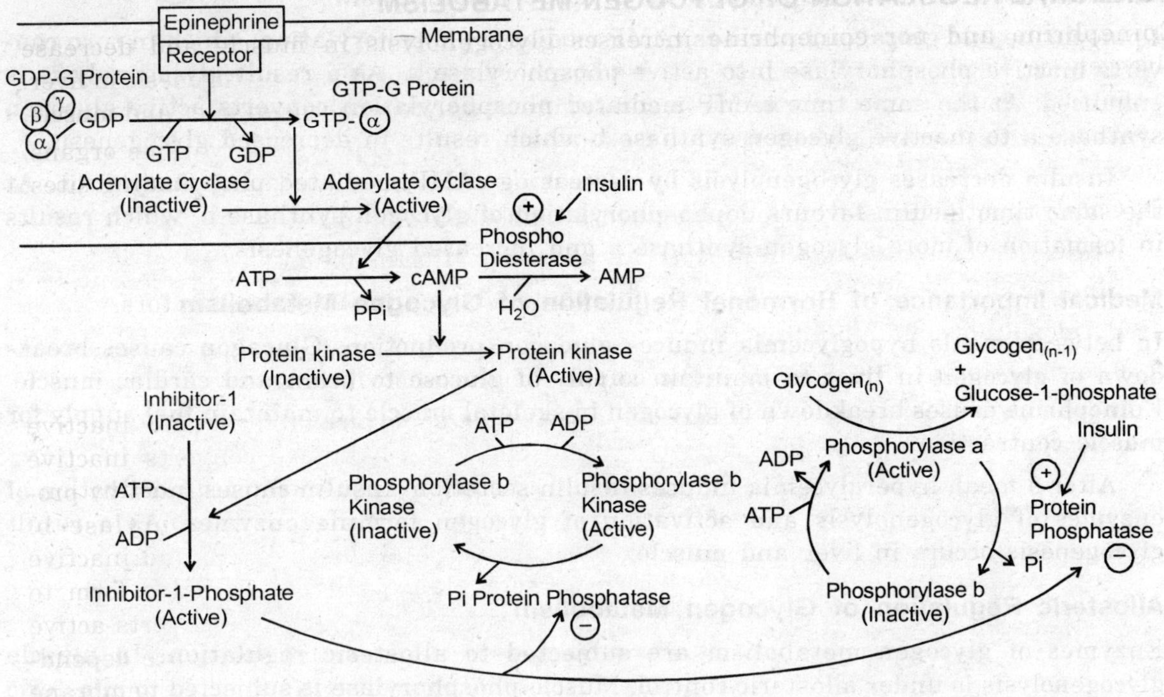

Fig. 9.7 Mechanism of action of hormones on glycogenolysis. (+) symbol indicates activation and (–) symbol indicates inhibiton. Receptor is β-adrenergic receptor

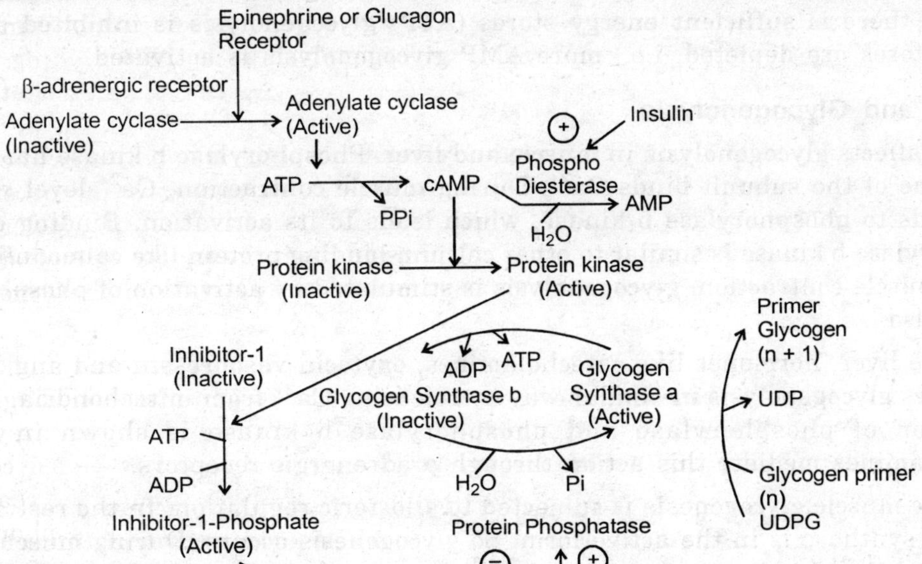

Fig. 9.8 Activation and inhibition of glycogen synthase by hormones

Summary of Hormonal Regulation of Glycogen Metabolism

Epinephrine and glucagon increases cAMP mediated phosphorylation, which in turn converts inactive phosphorylase b to active phosphorylase a. As a result glycogenolysis is enhanced. At the same time cAMP mediated phosphorylation converts active glycogen synthase a to inactive glycogen synthase b which results in decreased glycogenesis.

Insulin decreases glycogenolysis by decreasing cAMP mediated phosphorylation. At the same time insulin favours dephosphorylation of glycogen synthase b, which results in formation of more glycogen synthase a and increased glycogenesis.

Medical Importance of Hormonal Regulation of Glycogen Metabolism

In between meals hypoglycemia induces glucagon production. Glucagon causes breakdown of glycogen in liver to maintain supply of glucose to brain and cardiac muscle. Epinephrine causes breakdown of glycogen in skeletal muscle to maintain fuel supply for muscle contraction.

After a meal, hyperglycemia induces insulin secretion. Insulin causes inactivation of enzymes of glycogenolysis and activation of glycogen forming enzymes. As a result glycogenesis occurs in liver and muscle.

Allosteric Regulation of Glycogen Metabolism

Enzymes of glycogen metabolism are subjected to allosteric regulation. In muscle glycogenolysis is under allosteric control. Muscle phosphorylase is subjected to allosteric regulation. In the resting muscle it is in the inactive phosphorylase b form. Muscle contraction increases AMP which binds phosphorylase b and converts it to active phosphorylase a form. ATP and glucose-6-phosphate are allosteric inhibitors of this enzyme. So when there is sufficient energy stores (ATP) glycogenolysis is inhibited and when energy stores are depleted, i.e., more AMP glycogenolysis is activated.

Calcium and Glycogenolysis

Calcium affects glycogenolysis in muscle and liver. Phosphorylase b kinase has four subunits. One of the subunit binds Ca^{2+}. During muscle contraction, Ca^{2+} level raises and Ca^{2+} binds to phosphorylase b kinase, which leads to its activation. Binding of Ca^{2+} to phosphorylase b kinase is similar to other calcium-binding protein like calmodulin. Hence, during muscle contraction, glycogenolysis is stimulated by activation of phosphorylase b kinase also.

In the liver, hormones like catecholamines, oxytocin vasopressin and angiotensin II stimulates glycogenolysis in similar way by releasing Ca^{2+} from mitochondria. Allosteric regulation of phosphorylase and phosphorylase b kinase is shown in Fig. 9.9. Catecholamines mediate this action through α-adrenergic receptors.

In the muscle,glycogenesis is subjected to allosteric regulation. In the resting muscle glycogen synthase is in the active form. So glycogenesis occurs. During muscle contraction raised Ca^{2+} level activates calmodulin type protein kinase which converts glycogen synthase a to glycogen synthase b by phosphorylation and thus glycogenesis is prevented.

In most of the cells oxidation of glucose by glycolysis and citric acid cycle produce ATP. However, some cells are capable of oxidizing glucose to produce compound which are used for anabolic reactions or biosynthatic reactions. They are called as alternative pathways for glucose oxidation. There are two such pathways. They are pentose phosphate pathway and uronic acid pathway. Usually ATP is not generated in these pathways.

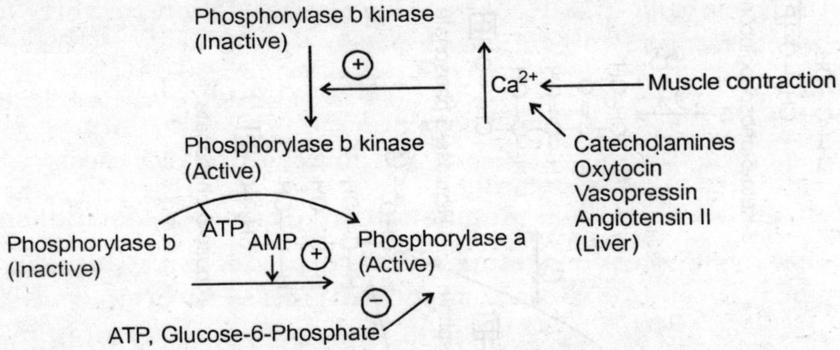

Fig. 9.9 Allosteric regulation of glycogenolysis in muscle and liver

PENTOSE PHOSPHATE PATHWAY

1. It is also called as hexose monophosphate shunt (HMP Shunt), phosphogluconate oxidative pathway and direct oxidative pathway.
2. In this pathway, oxidation of glucose generates NADPH reducing power. NADPH serves as hydrogen donor in reductive biosynthesis.
3. This pathway directly oxidizes glucose to CO_2 and hence the name direct oxidative pathway.

Site. Enzymes of this pathway are present in cytosol of liver, adipose tissue, erythrocytes, neutrophils, adrenal cortex, thyroid, testis, ovaries and lactating mammary gland. In the skeletal muscle the pathway is less active.

Reaction Sequence

The sequence of reaction of pentose phosphate pathway may be divided into three phases. The first phase converts glucose-6-phosphate into ribulose-5-phosphate. This is the oxidative phase of the pathway and consist of three irreversible reactions. In the second phase ribose-5-phosphate is generated from ribulose-5-phosphate involving inter conversion of sugars. This is accomplished by two reversible reactions.

In the third phase, ribose-5-phosphate is converted into intermediate of glycolysis. It is the non-oxidative phase of the pathway and consist of three reversible reactions (Fig. 9.10).

1. Glucose-6-phosphate an intermediate of glycolysis serves as starting compound of the pathway. Glucose-6-phosphate dehydrogenase converts glucose-6-phosphate to its internal lactone 6-phosphogluconolactone by removing –H groups of anomeric carbon in a $NADP^+$ dependent reaction. Mg^{2+} or Ca^{2+} is also necessary for the reaction. NADPH is generated by this enzyme. Internal lactone of sugar is formed when –OH and carboxyl groups interact with each other.
2. In reaction-2, lactone is hydrolysed by lactonase. It is also requires presence of metal ions like Mg^{2+} or Ca^{2+} or Mn^{2+}. 6-phosphogluconate is formed from 6-phosphogluconolactone.

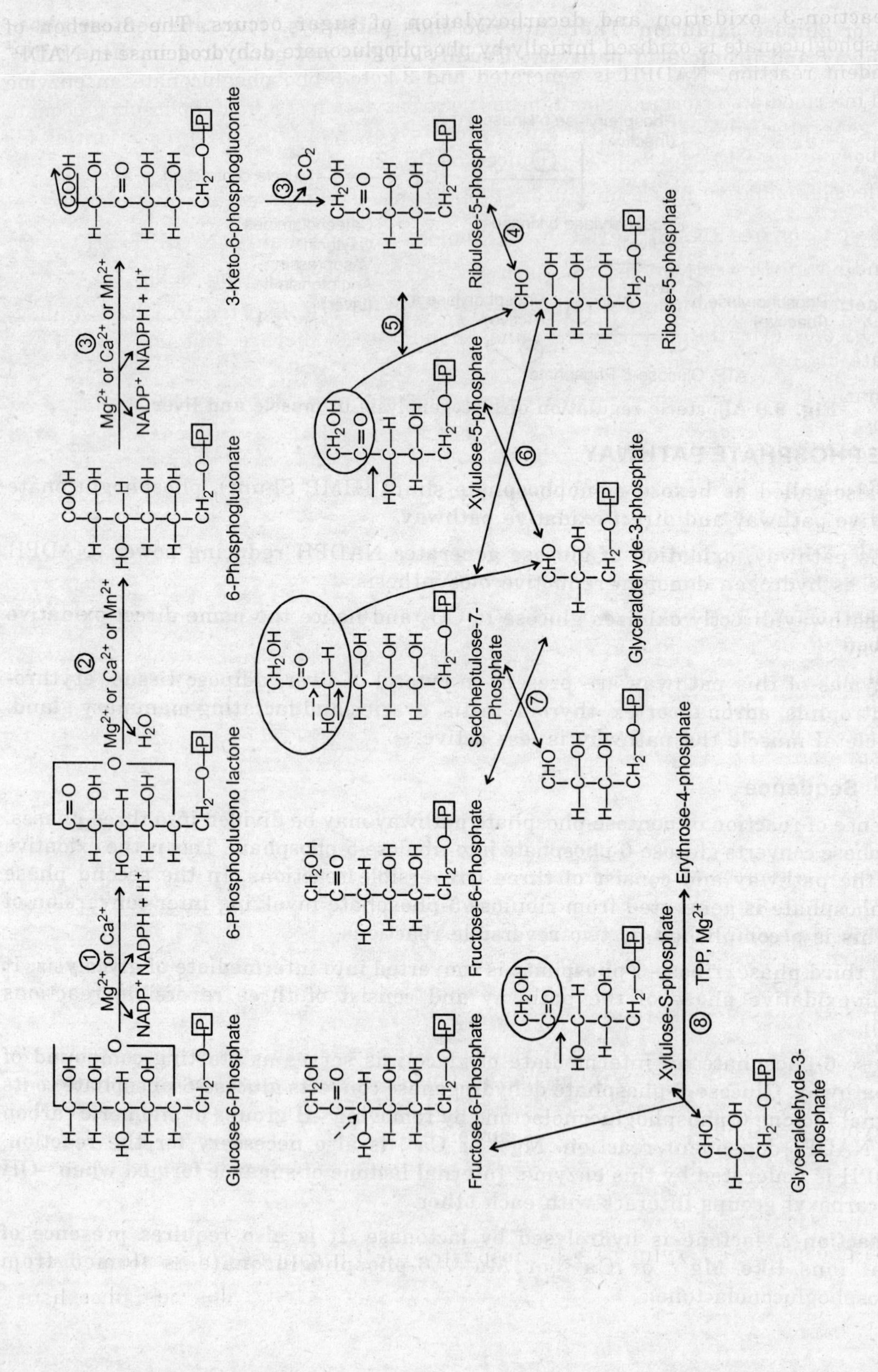

Fig. 9.10 Pentose phosphate pathway. →Indicates -C-C-Cleavage and - - →Indicates -C-C-bond formation

3. In reaction-3, oxidation and decarboxylation of sugar occurs. The 3-carbon of 6-phosphogluconate is oxidized initially by phosphogluconate dehydrogenase in $NADP^+$ dependent reaction. NADPH is generated and 3-keto-6-phosphogluconate an enzyme bound intermediate is formed. Spontaneous decarboxylation of 3-keto-6-phosphogluconate later generates ribulose-5-phosphate, which is keto pentose. Mg^{2+} is essential for decarboxylation. CO_2 molecule is produced at this stage.

Net effect of oxidative phase on glucose-6-phosphate is expressed as equation.

$$\text{Glucose}-6-\text{phosphate}+2\text{NADP}^+ + H_2O \longrightarrow \text{Ribulose}-5-\text{phosphate}+2\,\text{NADPH}+2H^+ + CO_2$$

Depending on the cell needs, the pathway can end here in some cells.

4. In reaction-4, one molecule of ribulose-5-phosphate is converted to ribose-5-phosphate by isomerization catalyzed by phosphopentose isomerase. Enediol is an intermediate of this reaction.

5. Alternatively another molecule of ribulose-5-phosphate is epimerized around 3-carbon by phosphopentose epimerase to xylulose-5-phosphate, which is also a keto pentose in reaction-5. The transformation of pentoses is given as single equation.

$$3\ \text{Ribulose-5-phosphate} \longrightarrow \text{Ribose-5-phosphate} + 2\ \text{Xylulose-5-phosphate}$$

In the third phase of the pathway conversion of ribose-5-phosphate and 2 molecules of xylulose-5-phosphate into 2 molecules of fructose-6-phosphate and glycereldehyde-3-phosphate involves carbon-carbon bond formation and cleavage among sugars.

6. Transketolase, a TPP containing enzyme catalyzes sixth reaction. It removes 1 and 2 carbon atoms of xylulose-5-phosphate which is known as glycolaldehyde or 2-carbon ketol by cleaving —C—C— bond between 2 and 3 carbons of xylulose-5-phosphate. The remaining 3-carbon atoms of xylulose-5-phosphate is released as glyceraldehyde-3-phosphate. The transfer of ketol to anomeric carbon atom of ribose-5-phosphate by the enzyme involves —C—C— bond formation. As a result ribose-5-phosphate is converted to seven carbon sedoheptulose-7-phosphate. Prosthetic group TPP participates in the transfer of ketol group. Mg^{2+} is also required for this reaction.

7. Since no pathway can utilize seven carbon sugar the 7th reaction of the pathway converts sedoheptulose-7-phosphate to 4-carbon sugar. The reaction is catalyzed by *trans* aldolase. This enzyme removes first three carbon atoms (dihydroxyacetone moiety) of sedoheptulose-7-phosphate and transfers to three carbon glyceraldehyde-3-phosphate (aldose), which is formed in sixth reaction. As a result, erythrose-4-phosphate is formed from remaining 4 carbons of sedoheptulose-7-phosphate and six carbon fructose-6-phosphate is formed from glyceraldehyde-3-phosphate.

8. Erythrose-4-phosphate so formed is converted to intermediate of glycolysis by the last reaction of the pathway involving enzyme transketolase and the reaction requires another (third) molecule of xylulose-5-phosphate. Transfer of 2 carbon moiety from xylulose-5-phosphate to the first carbon atom of erythrose-4-phosphate results in the formation of one molecule of fructose-6-phosphate and one molecule of glyceraldehyde-3-phosphate.

The transformation of pentoses is given below as equation

$$\text{Ribose-5-phosphate} + 2\ \text{xylulose} + \text{5-phosphate} \longrightarrow 2\ \text{fructose-6-phosphate} + \text{glyceraldehyde-3-phosphate}$$

Fructose-6-phosphate and glyceraldehyde-3-phosphate are intermediates of glycolysis. Their complete oxidation in glycolytic pathway generates energy. Conversely they may be transformed into glucose by the reversal of glycolysis as shown below

$$\text{Energy} \longleftarrow \text{Glycolysis} \longleftarrow \text{2 fructose-6-phosphate + glyceraldehyde-3-phosphate} \longrightarrow \text{2 glucose-6-phosphate} + \tfrac{1}{2}\,\text{glucose-6-phosphate}$$

Glucose-6-phosphate may be completely oxidized to CO_2 in this pathway. For the complete oxidation of one molecule of glucose-6-phosphate in the HMP shunt 6 molecules of glucose-6-phosphate are required. The fate of these 6 glucose-6-phosphate molecules in each of the phases discussed above is expressed as equations below.

1. $\text{6 glucose-6-phosphate} + 12NADP^+ + 6H_2O \xrightarrow{\text{Oxidative phase}} \text{6 ribulose-5-phosphate} + 12NADPH + 12H^+ + 6CO_2$

2. $\text{6 ribulose-5-phosphate} \xrightarrow[\text{of pentoses}]{\text{Inter conversion}} \text{2 ribose-5-phosphate + 4 xylulose-5-phosphate}$

3. $\text{2 ribose-5-phosphate + 4 xylulose-5-phosphate} \xrightarrow[\text{Phase}]{\text{Non-oxidative}} \text{4 fructose-6-phosphate + 2 glyceraldehyde-3-phosphate}$

4. $\text{4 fructose-6-phosphate + 2 glyceraldehyde-3-phosphate} + H_2O \xrightarrow[\text{Glycolysis}]{\text{Reversal of}} \text{5 glucose-6-phosphate + Pi}$

Now overall equation for oxidation of glucose-6-phosphate is obtained from above equations.

$$\text{6glucose-6-phosphate} + 12\,NADP^+ + 7H_2O \longrightarrow \text{5 glucose-6-phosphate} + 12\,NADPH + 12H^+ + 6CO_2 + Pi$$

This equation is further transformed by cancelling same terms on both sides as

$$\text{Glucsoe-6-phosphate} + 12NADP^+ + 7H_2O \longrightarrow 6CO_2 + 12\ NADPH + 12H^+ + Pi$$

Thus HMP shunt pathway can oxidize glucose-6-phosphate to CO_2 directly without involving citric acid cycle.

Biological Importance of HMP Shunt

1. NADPH produced in the shunt is used for biosynthesis of several important compounds in various organs.
   (*a*) In the liver, NADPH is used for fatty acid synthesis, cholesterol synthesis, bile acid synthesis, glutamate synthesis and cytochrome P_{450}-hydroxylase system.
   (*b*) In the adrenal cortex and gonads, NADPH is used for cholesterol and hormone synthesis.
   (*c*) In the adipose tissue, NADPH is used for fatty acid synthesis.
   (*d*) NADPH is used for formation of deoxy ribonucleotides and pyrimidine nucleotides.
2. In RBC, NADPH produced is used for the formation of reduced glutathione from oxidized glutathione. Glutathione reductase catalyzes this reaction. Glutathione reductase contains FAD. Electrons are transferred to FAD from NADPH. Reduced

glutathione is required for the removal of H_2O_2 by glutathione peroxidase (Fig. 9.11) for the conversion of methaemoglobin to normal hemoglobin and for maintenance of –SH groups of erythrocyte proteins. So, reduced glutathione is essential for the integrity of normal red cell structure. Usually cells with reduced glutathione level are more prone to hemolysis.

3. In neutrophils, NADPH is required for the formation of superoxide by NADPH oxidase. Respiratory burst of neutrophils during phagocytosis involves superoxide formation.
4. Pentoses produced in this pathway are used for nucleic acid synthesis and nucleotide coenzymes like NAD^+, FAD and FMN synthesis.
5. Non-oxidative phase of the pathway converts pentoses of endogenous or dietary nucleic acids into intermediates of glycolysis where they are, further oxidized to generate energy.

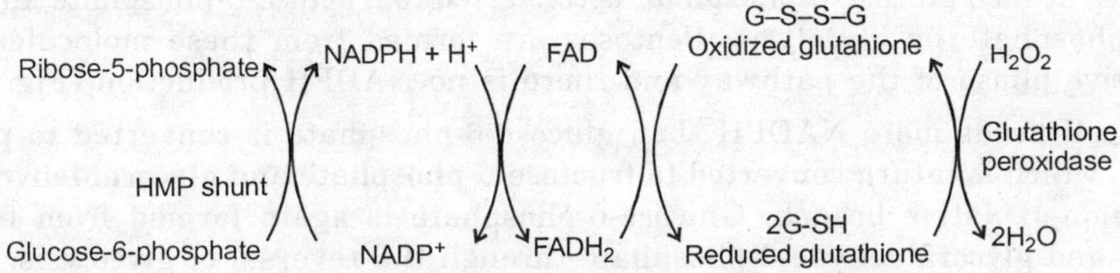

Fig. 9.11 Fate of NADPH in erythrocytes

6. Inter conversion of three, four, five, six and seven carbon sugars in the non-oxidative phase metabolically connects these sugars to glycolysis.

$$C_5 + C_5 \longleftrightarrow C_7 + C_3 \longleftrightarrow C_6 + C_4$$

$$C_5 + C_4 \longleftrightarrow C_6 + C_3$$

7. HMP shunt converts xylulose of uronic acid pathway to either glucose or intermediates of glycolysis.
8. This pathways converts glucose to CO_2 directly and hence CO_2 is the end product of the pathway.
9. In plants, a modified form of this pathway is responsible for the synthesis of glucose from CO_2.

Medical Importance of Pentose Phosphate Pathway

HMP shunt pathway is defective in some diseases.

1. **Glucose-6-phosphate dehydrogenase deficiency** In some individuals, 10-fold less active glucose-6-phosphate dehydrogenase is produced in RBC due to sex linked defective gene. About 100 million of world population carry defective gene. The rate of incidence is about 10% in American blacks. The less active glucose-6-phosphate dehydrogenase becomes inactive in presence of certain drugs. So, the affected individuals are normal until they are exposed to those drugs. Glucose-6-phosphate dehydrogenese deficiency occurs when drugs like aspirin, primaquine anti-malarial drug and sulfonamide are administered to these individuals. Since NADPH production is blocked in these individuals due to the deficiency of glucose-6-phosphate dehydrogenase the susceptibility of RBC to hemolysis is increased. Therefore, the

affected individuals develop hemolytic anemia on exposure to these drugs. Consumption of fava beans also causes glucose-6-phosphate dehydrogenase deficiency in the susceptible individuals. Favism is the name given to this type of glucose-6-phosphage dehydrogenase deficiency.

2. Transketolase deficiency can occur in thiamine deficiency cases.
3. **Wernicke-korsakoff encephalopathy** It is due to defective genes. Transketolase of affected individuals has lower affinity for TPP. The characteristic symptoms are abnormal walking and standing, memory loss and paralysis of eye movements. The disease manifests only when there is thiamine deficiency.

Regulation of HMP Shunt

According to cell needs HMP shunt produces either NADPH or pentoses. When more pentoses are needed glucose-6-phosphate is converted to fructose-6-phosphate and glyceral dehyde-3-phosphate by glycolysis. Pentoses are formed from these molecules through non-oxidative phase of the pathway and there is no NADPH production (Fig. 9.12).

When cell needs more NADPH then glucose-6-phosphate is converted to pentose-5-phosphate, which is inturn converted to fructose-6-phosphate and glyceraldehyde-3-phosphate by non-oxidative branch. Glucose-6-phosphate is again formed from fructose-6-phosphate and glyceraldehyde-3-phosphate through the reversal of glycolysis. Ribose-5-phosphats is formed from regenerated glucose-6-phosphate through the oxidative phase and thus there is no net pentose production (Fig. 9.12B).

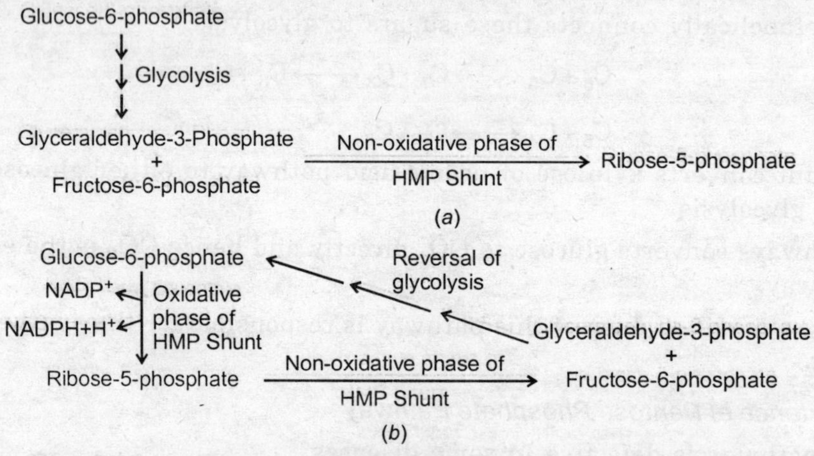

Fig. 9.12 (*a*) Formation of pentoses from glucose-6-phosphate
(*b*) Formation of NADPH from glucose-6-phosphate

Uronic Acid Pathway

In this pathway, glucose is oxidized to uronic acid. No energy is produced in this pathway like pentose phosphate pathway. Since free uronic acid can not be used for proteoglycan and other conjugation reactions it is produced as active uronic acid or UDP-glucuronic acid from UDP-Glucose. Like other activated sugars, UDP-glucuronicacid serves donor of glucuronicacid. Furhter this pathway converts free or unused glucuronicacid to D-xylulose-5-phosphate which is converted to intermediates of glycolysis by non oxidative phase of HMP shunt.

Reaction Sequence

There are eight reaction in this pathway (Fig. 9.13).

1. UDP-Glucose serves as starting-substance of the pathway. It undergoes oxidation at 6-carbon catalyzed by NAD dependent UDP-glucose dehydrogenase. The product of this reaction is UDP-glucuronicacid. The conversion of UDP-glucuronicacid involves transfer of four electrons. Two molecules of NAD^+ are reduced. UDP-glucuronate is the active form of glucuronate.
2. In reaction-2, UDP-glucuronate is converted to glucuronic acid by hydrolysis.
3. Gulonate dehydrogenase reduces glucuronate to L-gulonicacid in a NADPH dependent reduction reaction. In animals, other than man L-gulonate is converted to Vit C or ascorbic acid. In man, L-gulonate is converted to L-xylulose a pentose in two reactions involving oxidation and decarboxylation.
4. L-Gluonate is oxidized at 3-carbon by NAD^+ dependent dehydrogenase to 3-keto-L-gulonate. NADH is generated.
5. In reaction-5 of this pathway, pentose L-xylulose is generated from 3-keto-L-gulonate by removing 1-carbon of 3-keto-L-gulonate as CO_2. The reaction is catalyzed by decarboxylase. Since there is no pathway which can utilize L-xylulose it has to be converted to D-xylulose which is part of HMP shunt. The conversion of L-isomer to D-isomer involves reduction and oxidation.
6. Xylitol dehydrogenase reduces L-xylulose to xylitol in NADPH dependent reaction. NADPH is the donor of hydrogen.
7. D-xylulose dehydrogenase converts xylitol to D-xylulose by removing-H atoms from 2 carbon. NAD^+ act as hydrogen acceptor.
8. Finally phosphorylation of D-xylulose by xylulose kinase at the 5-carbon atom produces xylulose-5-phosphate and enters HMP shunt pathway. In the HMP shunt pathway, it is converted to intermediates of glycolysis and used for energy production.

Medical and Biological Importance

1. This pathway produces glucuronic acid, ascorbic acid and pentoses from glucose.
2. Glucuronic acid is used for the synthesis of proteoglycan for conjugation with bilirubin, steroid hormones and for detoxification of drugs.
3. Glucuronic acid formed from the degradation of endogenous proteoglycans by the action of lysosomal enzymes and dietary glucuronic acid are utilized for energy production by this pathway via HMP shunt after conversion to xylulose.
4. This pathways also provides means for the utilization of dietary xylitol.
5. In plants and mammals other than man Vit C is synthesized in this pathway from L-gulonate.

Formation of Vit C

(*i*) Lactonase catalyzes the formation of L-gulonolactone from L-gulonate by removing one water molecule from 1 and 4 carbons.

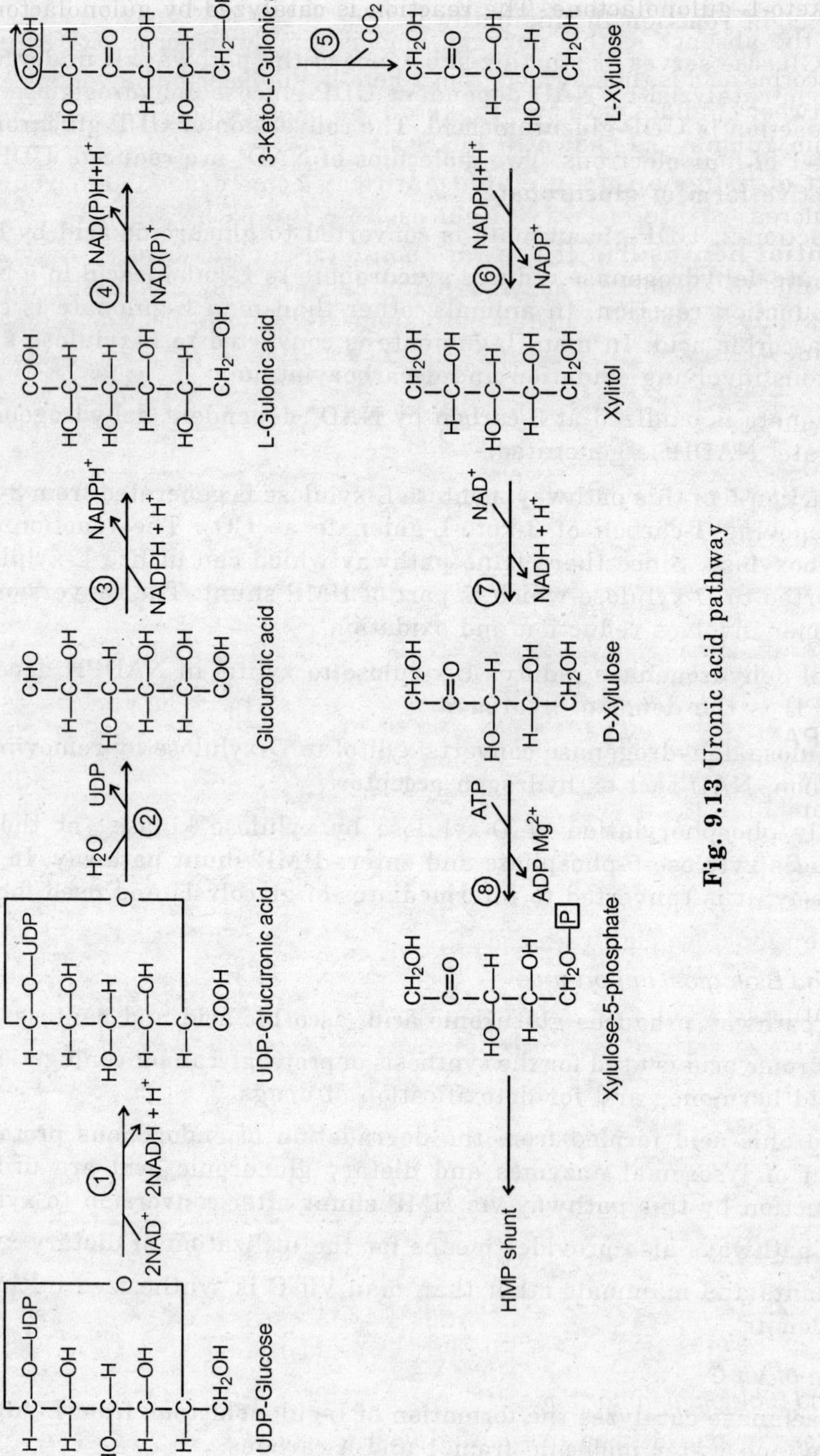

Fig. 9.13 Uronic acid pathway

(*ii*) Oxidation of L-gulonolactone at 2 carbon atom in presence of oxygen generates 2-keto-L-gulonolactone. The reaction is catalyzed by gulonolactone oxidase. Due to the absence of this enzyme, man is unable to form Vit C from L-gulonate.

(*iii*) Ascorbic acid is then formed from 2-keto-L-gulonolactone involving enediol formation between 2 and 3 carbons of 2-keto-L-gulonolactone. Reactions of Vit C formation from gulonate is shown in Fig. 9.14.

6. **Effect of drugs on uronic acid pathway** Some drugs like barbital and paracetamol increases rate of entry of glucose into the pathway.
7. **Essential pentosuria** It is a rare non-fatal genetic disease. L-xylulose appears in urine due to absence of enzyme xylitol dehydrogenase. Xylitol formation is blocked from xylulose. As a result, accumulation of xylulose in blood followed by excretion in urine occurs.

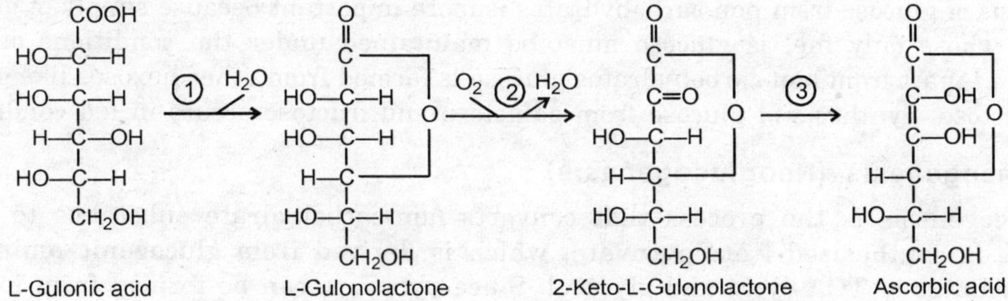

Fig. 9.14 Synthesis of ascorbic acid from gulonic acid

POLYOL PATHWAY

This pathway converts glucose to fructose. Other names of this pathway are sorbitol pathway and alditol pathway.

Reaction Sequence

The conversion of glucose to fructose occurs in two reactions (Fig. 9.15).

1. Aldose reductase catalyzes reduction of glucose of sorbitol. NADPH is the hydrogen donor.
2. Oxidation of sorbitol at 2 carbon atom by sorbitol dehydrogenase generates fructose. NAD^+ serve as hydrogen acceptor.

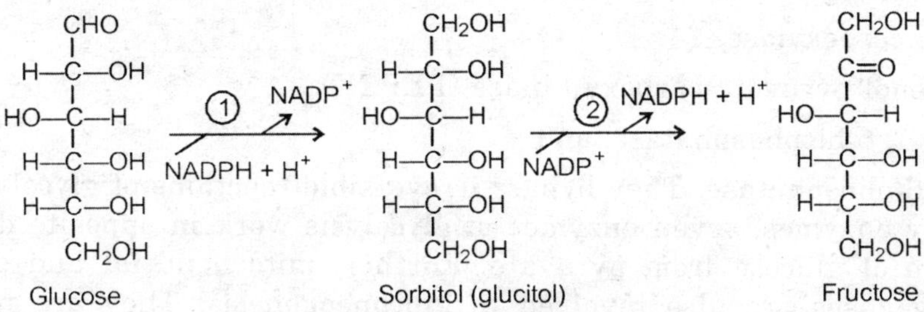

Fig. 9.15 Polyol pathway

Medical and Biological Importance

1. Fructose is synthesized in seminal vesicle where it serves as fuel for spermatozoa.
2. Placenta also produces fructose. It is source of energy for foetus.

3. In diabetics, excess glucose that enters lens is converted to sorbitol. Lens is impermeable to sorbitol, so it accumulates in the lens and cause swelling of lens. This may be ultimately responsible for cataract formation.
4. **Sorbitol intolerance.** Sorbitol is present in sugar free sweeteners used by diabetics. Sorbitol is absorbed incompletely in the intestine and liver converts it to glucose slowly. Unabsorbed sorbitol in the intestine is used by intestinal micro-organisms and thus produce abdominal pain and discomfort.

Now we shell turn our focus to pathways that produce glucose. Glucose can be produced from non-carbohydrates as well as carbohydrates (However glycogenolysis which produces glucose is not under consideration again.)

Need for Glucose Synthesis

Synthesis of glucose from non-carbohydrates is more important because supply of glucose to tissues whose only fue! is glucose must be maintained under the conditions of glucose shortage. Apart from non-carbohydrates glucose is formed from other hexoses like galactose and fructose. Synthesis of glucose from galactose and fructose occurs in fed conditions.

Gluconeogenesis (Neoglucogenesis)

Gluconeogenesis is the process that converts non-carbohydrate substance to glucose. Glucose is synthesized from pyruvate, which is derived from glucogenic amino acids, intermediates of TCA cycle and glycerol. Since pyruvate can be formed from lactate by the reversal of lactate dehydrogenase reaction synthesis of glucose occurs from lactate also. Gluconeogenesis is an energy-consuming process.

Site Gluconeogenesis occurs mainly in the liver and kidney. Enzymes of gluconeogenesis are present in mitochondria and cytosol.

Reaction Sequence

Synthesis of glucose from pyruvate is possible if the irreversible reactions of glycolysis are made reversible. The reaction catalyzed by hexokinase, phosphofructokinase and pyruvate kinase obstruct the simple reversal of glycolysis. These reactions are made reversible by specific enzymes of gluconeogenesis and they are called as key enzymes of gluconeogenesis. They are present in mitochondria and cytosol. The key enzymes of gluconeogenesis are:

1. Pyruvate carboxylase.
2. Phosphoenol pyruvate carboxy kinase (PEPCK).
3. Fructose-1, 6-bisphosphatase, and
4. Glucose-6-phosphatase. They bypass irreversible reactions of glycolysis. Apart from these key enzymes, seven enzymes of glycolysis work in opposite direction for the formation of glucose from pyruvate. Further, mitochondrial and cytosolic malate dehydrogenases are also involved in gluconeogenesis. They are required for the transfer of metabolites from mitochondria to cytosol.

Therefore, synthesis of glucose from pyruvate involves enzymes of gluconeogenesis, glycolysis, TCA cycle and cytosolic malate dehydrogenase.

Glucose formation from pyruvate is shown in Fig. 9.16.

1. In the mitochondria, gluconeogenesis starts with formation of oxaloacetate from pyruvate. The reaction is catalyzed by pyruvate carboxylase and requires biotin, CO_2 and ATP. One high energy bond is consumed in this reaction. Pyruvate carboxylase is the only key enzyme present in mitochondria.

   Oxaloacetate formed in the mitochondria is impermeable to inner mitochondrial membrane and it can not enter cytosol. So, it enters the cytosol in the form of malate which is permeable to mitochondrial membrane. Malate dehydrogenase of TCA cycle converts oxaloacetate to malate. Alternatively, Oxaloacetate is transported as aspartate. In the cytosol oxaloacetate is regenerated from malate by cytosolic malate dehydrogenase using NAD^+ as hydrogen acceptor.

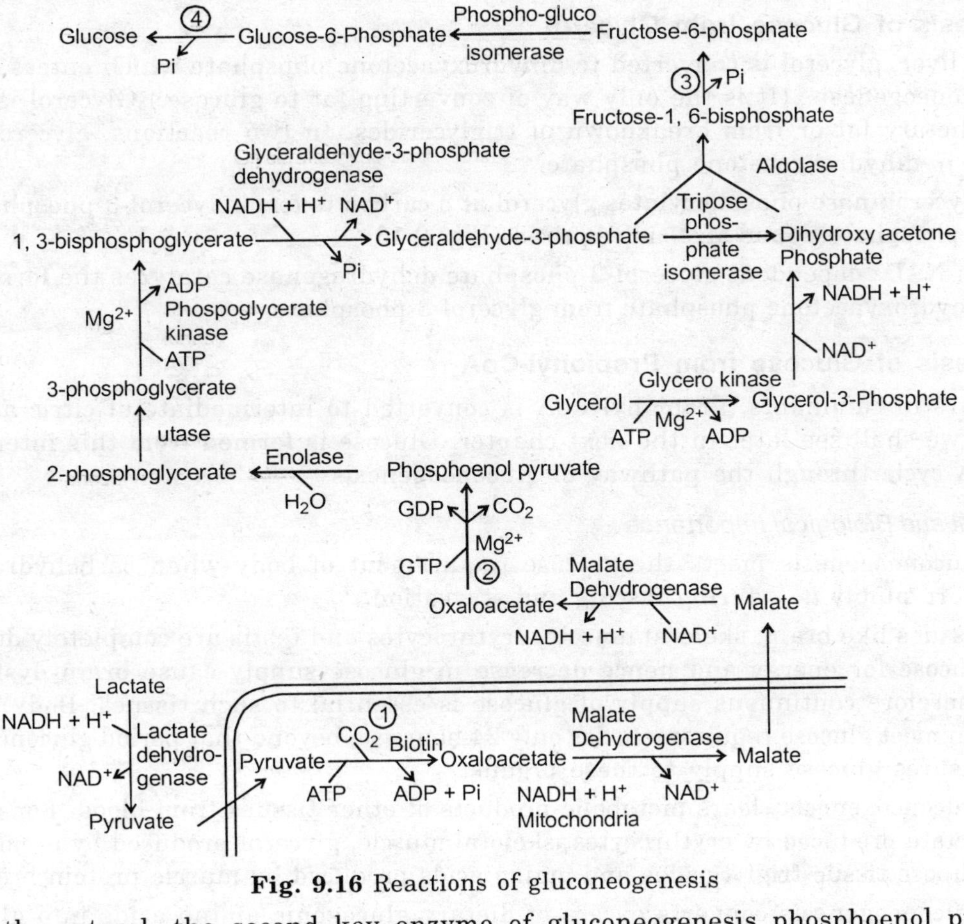

Fig. 9.16 Reactions of gluconeogenesis

2. In the cytosol, the second key enzyme of gluconeogenesis phosphoenol pyruvate carboxy kinase converts oxaloacetate to phosphoenol pyruvate using GTP as high energy phosphate donor. Mg^{2+} is essential for this kinase reaction.

   Since phosphoenol pyruvate is a metabolite of glycolysis by the six reversible reactions it is converted to fructose-1, 6-*bis*phosphate.

3. Third key enzyme of gluconeogenesis fructose-1, 6-bisphosphatase converts fructose-1, 6-*bis*phosphate to fructose-6-phosphate by removing one phosphate.

Fructose-6-phosphate is converted to glucose-6-phosphate by another enzyme of glycolysis, i.e., phosphohexose isomerase.

4. Finally glucose is formed from glucose-6-phosphate by the action of glucose-6-phosphatase.

Over all equation for the conversion of 2 molecules of pyruvate to glucose in gluconeogenesis is given below.

$$2\text{Pyruvate} + 4\text{ATP} + 2\text{GTP} + 2\text{NADH}^+ + 2\text{H}^+ + 4\text{H}_2\text{O} \longrightarrow \text{Glucose} + 4\text{ADP} + 2\text{GDP} + 2\text{NAD}^+ + 6\text{P}_i$$

The above equation indicates the energy intensive nature of gluconeogenesis. Total six high energy bonds are consumed for the synthesis of glucose from pyruvate.

Synthesis of Glucose from Glycerol

In the liver, glycerol is converted to dihydroxyacetone phosphate which enters pathway of gluconeogenesis. (It is the only way of converting fat to glucose.) Glycerol is derived from dietary fat or from breakdown of triglycerides. In two reactions, glycerol is converted to dihydroxyacetone phosphate.

1. Glycerokinase phosphorylates glycerol at 3 carbon to form glycerol-3-phosphate. ATP is phosphate donor Mg^{2+} is required (Fig. 9.16).
2. An NAD^+ dependent glycerol-3-phosphate dehydrogenase catalyzes the formation of dihydroxyacetone phosphate from glycerol-3-phosphate.

Synthesis of Glucose from Propionyl-CoA

It occurs in ruminants. Propionyl CoA is converted to intermediate of citric acid cycle which we shall see later in the next chapter. Glucose is formed from this intermediate of TCA cycle through the pathway of gluconeogenesis.

Medical and Biological Importance

1. Gluconeogenesis meets the glucose requirement of body when carbohydrate is in short supply *i.e.*, during fasting and starvation.
2. Tissues like brain, skeletal muscle, erythrocytes and testis are completely depend on glucose for energy and hence decrease in glucose supply cause brain dysfunction. Therefore continuous supply of glucose is essential to such tissues. Body glycogen can meet glucose requirement for only 24 hours so, beyond that period gluconeogenesis ensures glucose supply to these organs.
3. Gluconeogenesis clears metabolic products of other tissues from blood. For example, lactate produced by erythrocytes, skeletal muscle, glycerol produced by breakdown of adipose tissue triglycerides and amino acids produced by muscle protein breakdown.
4. Gluconeogenesis converts excess of dietary glucogenic amino acids into glucose.
5. Lactic acidosis occurs in fructose-1, 6-bis phosphatase deficiency.
6. Gluconeogenesis is impaired in alcoholics.

Regulation of Gluconeogenesis

Enzymes of gluconeogenesis are subjected to allosteric regulation and hormone regulation. Pyruvte carboxylase and fructose-1, 6-bisphosphatase regulates gluconeogenesis. They are under allosteric regulation. All the key enzymes of gluconeogenesis are under hormonal control.

Allosteric regulation

Pyruvate carboxylase is an allosteric enzyme. Acetyl-CoA is its activator. When glucose is in short supply fatty acid oxidation generates acetyl-CoA this in turn activates gluconeogenesis. Fructose-1, 6-bisphosphatase is another allosteric enzyme. AMP is its allosteric inhibitor. So when there is energy crisis gluconeogenesis is inhibited.

Hormonal regulation

Insulin decreases the synthesis of key enzymes of gluconeogenesis thus inhibit gluconeogenesis.

Reciprocal Regulation of Glycolysis and Gluconeogenesis

1. Glycolysis and gluconeogenesis are two opposite processes. Therefore, simultaneous occurrence of these pathways must be avoided.
2. Like glycogenolysis and glycogenesis, glycolysis and gluconeogenesis are subjected to reciprocal regulation.
3. Glycolysis and gluconeogenesis responds to signals in opposite ways.
4. Synthesis and degradation of glucose by different sets of enzymes allow reciprocal regulation of these two pathways.
5. Phosphofructokinese-1 (PFK-1) an enzyme of glycolysis, phosphofructokinase-2 (PFK-2) and fructose-1, 6-bisphosphatase an enzyme of gluconeogenesis are the enzymes involved in reciprocal regulation.
6. PFK-2 is under allosteric and hormonal control whereas PFK-1 and fructose-1, 6-bisphosphotase are under allosteric control.
7. PFK-2 is another form of phosphofructokinase. It is a bifunctional protein. It has kinase activity and phosphatase activity. Kinase activity phosphorylats fructose-6-phosphate to fructose-2, 6-bisphosphate whereas phosphatase activity dephosphorylates fructose-2, 6-biphosphate to fructose-6 phosphate. Both kinase and phosphatase activities are under hormonal and allosteric control. Fructose-6-phosphate stimulates kinase activity whereas cAMP mediated phosphorylation by proteinkinase activates phosphatase activity and inhibits kinase activity.
8. Fructose-2, 6-bisphosphate is an important regulator of PFK-1 and fructose-1, 6-bisphosphatase. It plays critical role in the reciprocal regulation of glycolysis and gluconeogenesis. It is a potent activator of PFK-1 compared to fructose-6-phosphate. PFK-1 is highly active in presence of small amounts of fructose-2, 6-bisphosphate. Fructose-1, 6-bisphosphatase is allosterically inhibited by fructose-2, 6-bisphosphate.

Mechanism of Reciprocal Regulation of Glycolysis and Gluconeogenesis

In the well fed state, fructose-6-phosphate concentration is more because of excess glucose. This stimulates kinase activity of PFK-2 and inhibits phosphatase activity. Thus under conditions of glucose excess fructose-2, 6-bisphosphate concentration increases which stimulates glycolysis by activating PFK-1 and at the same time gluconeogenesis is suppressed due to inhibition of fructose-1, 6-bisphosphatase (Fig. 9.17).

When the glucose is in short supply glucagon produced as response to hypoglycemia stimulates the formation of cAMP which inhibits kinase activity of PFK-2 and activates phosphatase activity through protein kinase mediated phosphorylation. Thus, under condition of glucose shortage fructose-2, 6-bisphosphate concentration decreases which favours gluconeogenesis by activating fructose-1, 6-bisphosphatase and at the same time glycolysis is inhibited due to decreased PFK-1 activity (Figure 9.17).

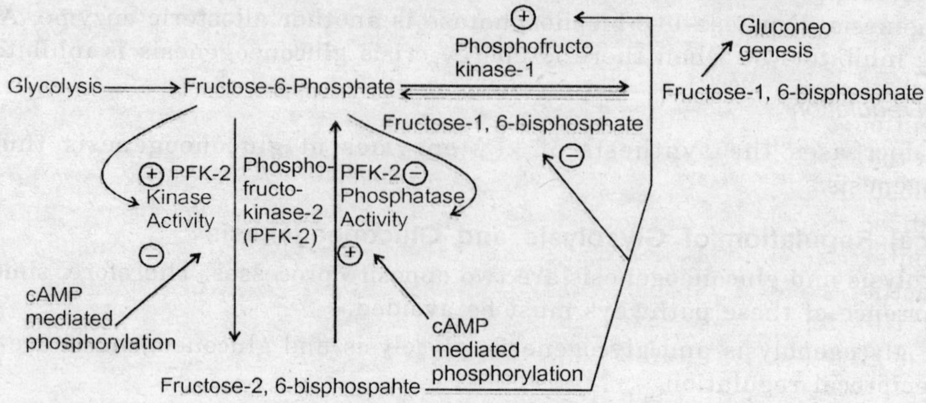

Fig. 9.17 Reciprocal regulation of glycolysis and gluconeogenesis. (+) indicates activation (–) indicates inhibition

Other note worthy reciprocal regulators of glycolysis and gluconeogenesis are acetyl-CoA and AMP.

Acetyl-CoA

As stated earlier acetyl-CoA is allosteric activator of pyruvate carboxylase and allosteric inhibitor of pyruvate dehydrogenase. Under conditions of glucose short supply fatty acid oxidation produces acetyl-CoA, which in turn stimulates gluconeogenesis by activating pyruvate carboxylase and decreases glycolysis by blocking pyruvate dehydrogenase action. Reciprocal regulation of glycolysis and gluconeogenesis by acetyl-CoA is responsible for the carbohydrate sparing action of fat (Fig. 9.18).

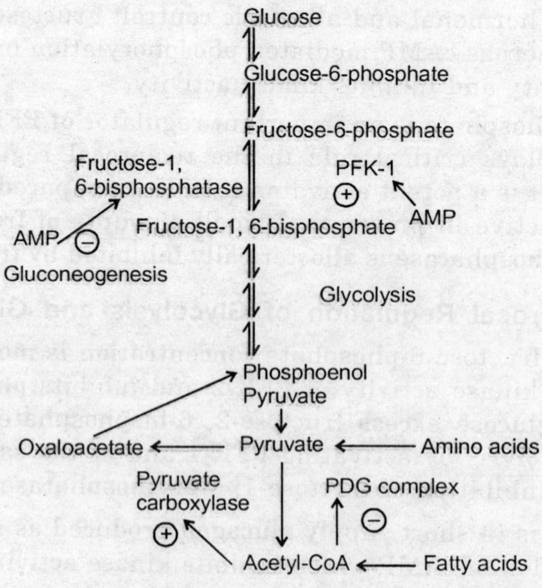

Fig. 9.18 Reciprocal regulations of glycolysis and gluconeogenesis by acetyl-CoA and AMP

AMP. As stated earlier AMP is allosteric activator of PFK-1 and allosteric inhibitor of fructose-1, 6-bisphosphatase. Under conditions of energy crisis AMP level is more and this leads to stimulation of glycolysis by activating PFK-1 and suppression of gluconeogenesis by inhibiting fructose-1, 6-bisphosphatase activity (Fig. 9.18).

Cori Cycle

As mentioned earlier the end product of glycolysis in rapidly contracting skeletal muscle and in the erythrocyte is lactate. Since the lactate is freely permeable to cells it diffuses into blood from erythrocytes and muscle. It reaches liver through circulation where it is oxidized to pyruvate. Gluconeogenic pathway converts pyruvate to glucose. Glucose then enters blood and taken up by skeletal muscle. Thus, liver furnishes glucose to the contracting skeletal muscle which produces lactate from glucose to meet its energy needs. Glucose is synthesized by liver from lactate. These reactions are called as Cori cycle or glucose-lactate cycle (Fig. 9.19).

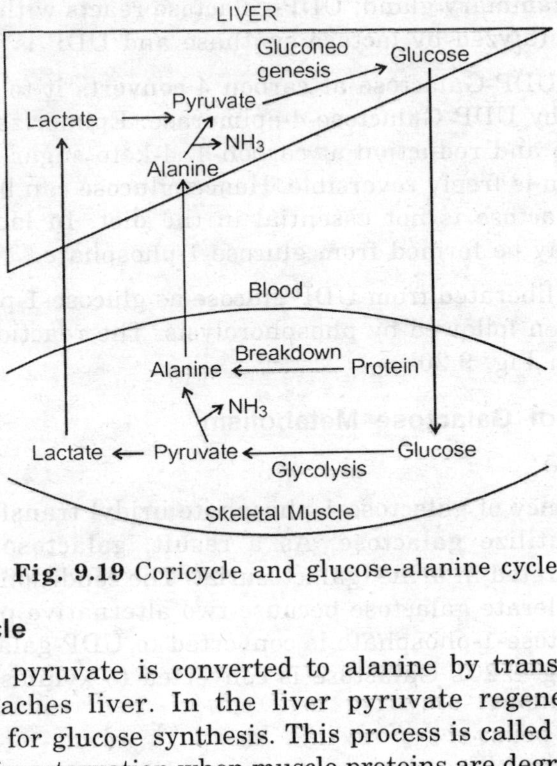

Fig. 9.19 Coricycle and glucose-alanine cycle

Glucose-alanine Cycle

In the skeletal muscle pyruvate is converted to alanine by transamination. Through the circulation alanine reaches liver. In the liver pyruvate regenerated from alanine by transamination is used for glucose synthesis. This process is called as glucose-alanine cycle. This cycle operates during starvation when muscle proteins are degraded. This cycle is meant for the transport of amino group nitrogen from muscle to liver (Fig. 9.19) also.

METABOLISM OF GALACTOSE

Source Dietary lactose is the major contributor of galactose. Lysosomal degradation of glycolipids, glyco-proteins and normal turn over of cells also contributes to galactose.

Site Galactose is converted to glucose in the liver.

Entry of galactose Entry of galactose into liver cells is not insulin dependent.

Reaction Sequence

The conversion of galactose to glucose involves active galactose formation. Active galactose serves as donor of galactose for the synthesis of galactose containing glycolipids, mucopolysaccharides, blood group substances and lactose. The reactions of active galactose formation from galactose are similar to the formation of active glucose from glucose.

1. Phosphorylation of galactose at carbon-1 is the initial reaction which is catalyzed by galactokinase. ATP is the phosphate donor and Mg^{2+} is required. Galactose-1-phosphate is the product.
2. Galactose-1-phosphate reacts with UDPG (Uridine Diphosphate Glucose) to form UDP galactose and glucose-1-phosphate. Galactose-1-phosphate uridyl transferase catalyzes this reaction. It transfers galactose to UDPG by replacing glucose. UDP-galactose is the active galactose and donates galactose to the needy reactions.

   In the lactating mammary gland, UDP-galactose reacts with glucose to form lactose. The reaction is catalyzed by lactase synthase and UDP is released.
3. Epimerization of UDP-Galactose at carbon 4 converts it to UDP-glucose. The reaction is catalyzed by UDP Galactose-4-epimerase. Epimerization involves NAD^+ dependent oxidation and reduction at carbon-4. 4-keto sugar is an intermediate. The epimerase reaction is freely reversible. Hence, glucose can be converted to galactose and therefore galactose is not essential in the diet. In lactating mammary gland UDP-galactose may be formed from glucose-1-phosphate.
4. Finally glucose is liberated from UDP glucose as glucose-1-phosphate after in corporation into glycogen followed by phosphorolysis. The reactions of galactose metabolism are shown in Fig. 9.20.

Medical Importance of Galactose Metabolism

Congenital galactosemia

It is due to the deficiency of galactose-1-phosphate uridyl transferase. The affected persons are unable to utilize galactose. As a result, galactose accumulates in blood (galactosemia) and excreted in urine (galactosuria). The condition is fatal in early life and adult galactosemics tolerate galactose because two alternative pathways develops later. In one pathway, galactose-1-phosphate is converted to UDP-galactose by UDP galactose pyrophosphorylase (Fig. 9.20). Galactose is converted to xylulose in another pathway.

Symptoms

Vomiting and diarrhoea occurs when milk is consumed. Other symptoms are mental retardation, Jaundice, liver failure and cataract due to accumulaton of galactitol a reduced product of galactose in lens. Aldose reductase catalyzes the conversion of galactose to galactitol. NADP serves as hydrogen donor. Continued intake of galactose may lead to death. So, to prevent the occurrence of death milk or milk products must be avoided.

Galactosemia due to deficiency of galactokinase and epimerase is rare.

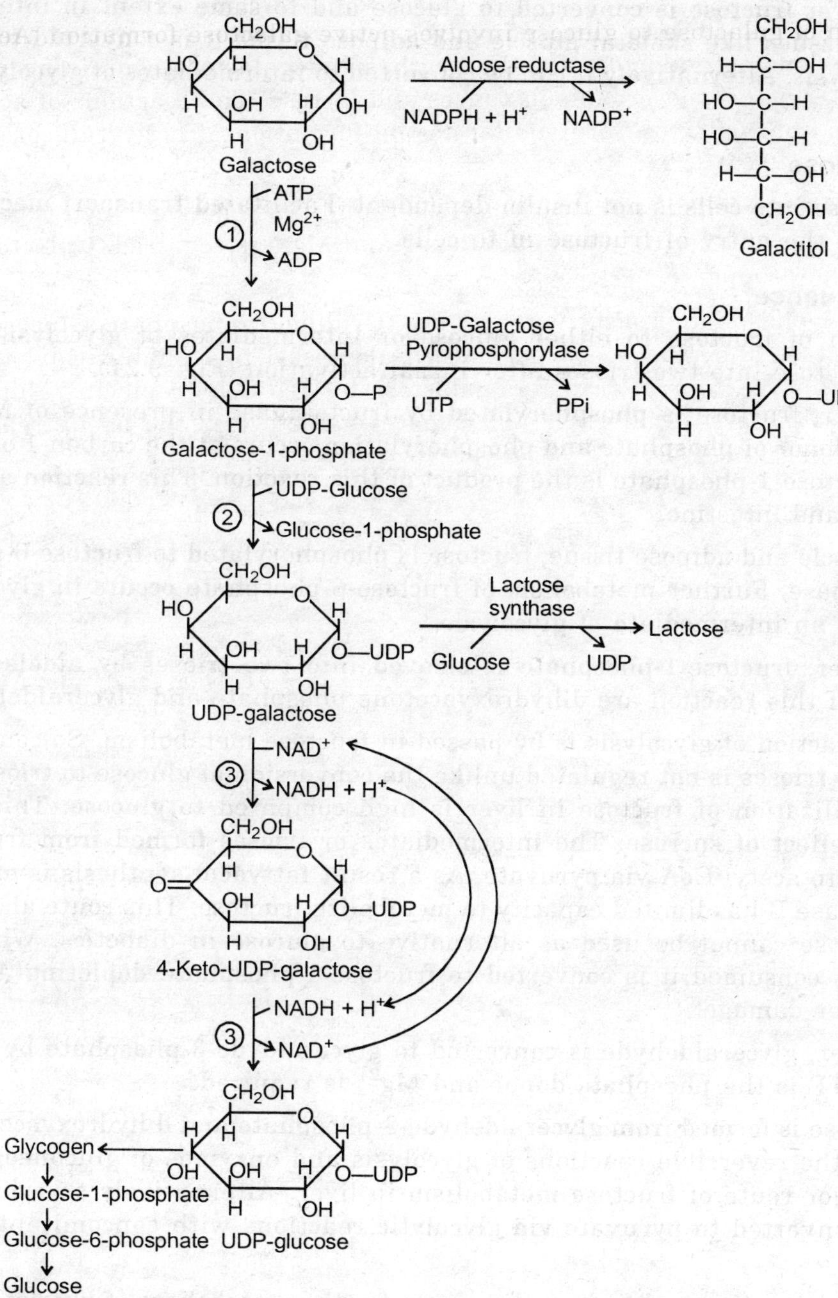

Fig. 9.20 Synthesis of glucose from galactose

FRUCTOSE METABOLISM

Source

Dietary sucrose is the main source of fructose. Honey, fruit juices, sweet potatoes and garlic bulbs also can contributes to fructose.

Site. In the liver fructose is converted to glucose and to some extent in intestine and in kidney. In tissues like skeletal muscle and adipose tissue it is converted to intermediates of glycolysis. Alternatively it can be converted to intermediates of glycolysis in the liver also.

Entry of Fructose

Entry of fructose into cells is not insulin dependent. Facilitated transport mechanism is responsible for the entry of fructose in to cells.

Reaction Sequence

The conversion of fructose to either glucose or intermediates of glycolysis involves splitting of fructose into two trioses after initial activation (Fig. 9.21).

1. In the liver, fructose is phosphorylated by fructokinase in presence of Mg^{2+}. ATP serves as donor of phosphate and phosphorylation occurs at the carbon-1 of fructose. Hence fructose-1-phosphate is the product of this reaction. This reaction also occurs in kidney and intestine.

   In the muscle and adipose tissue, fructose is phosphorylated to fructose-6-phosphate by hexokinase. Further metabolism of fructose-6-phosphate occurs in glycolysis because it is an intermediate of glycolysis.

2. In the liver, fructose-1-phosphate is cleaved into two trioses by aldolase B. The products of this reaction are dihydroxyacetone phosphate and glyceraldehyde.

   PFKase reaction of glycolysis is by passed in fructose metabolism. So conversion of fructose to trioses is not regulated unlike the conversion of glucose to trioses. Hence rate of utilization of fructose in liver is high compared to glucose. This explains lipogenic effect of sucrose. The intermediates or trioses formed from fructose are converted to acetyl-CoA via pyruvate. As a result fattyacid synthesis is more. However Aldolase B has limited capacity to metabolize fructose. This route also explains why fructose cannot be used as alternative to glucose in diabetics. When excess fructose is consumed it is converted to fructose-1-phosphate depleting ATP which causes liver damage.

3. In the liver, glyceraldehyde is converted to glyceraldyde-3-phosphate by aldehydekinase. ATP is the phosphate donor and Mg^{2+} is required.

   Now glucose is formed from glyceraldehyde-3-phosphate and dihydroxyacetone phosphate by the reversible reactions of glycolysis and enzymes of gluconeogenesis. It is the major route of fructose metabolism in liver. Alternatively triose phosphate may be converted to pyruvate via glycolytic reactions with concomitant ATP production.

   Liver and other tissues have another route for the metabolism of glyceraldehyde in which glyceraldehyde is converted to dihydroxyacetone phosphate via glycerol-3-phosphate. Both glycerol-3-phosphate and dihydroxy acetone phosphate are used for triglyceride or phospholipid synthesis.

4. Alcohol dehydrogenase converts glyceraldehyde to glycerol in a NADH dependent reduction reaction.

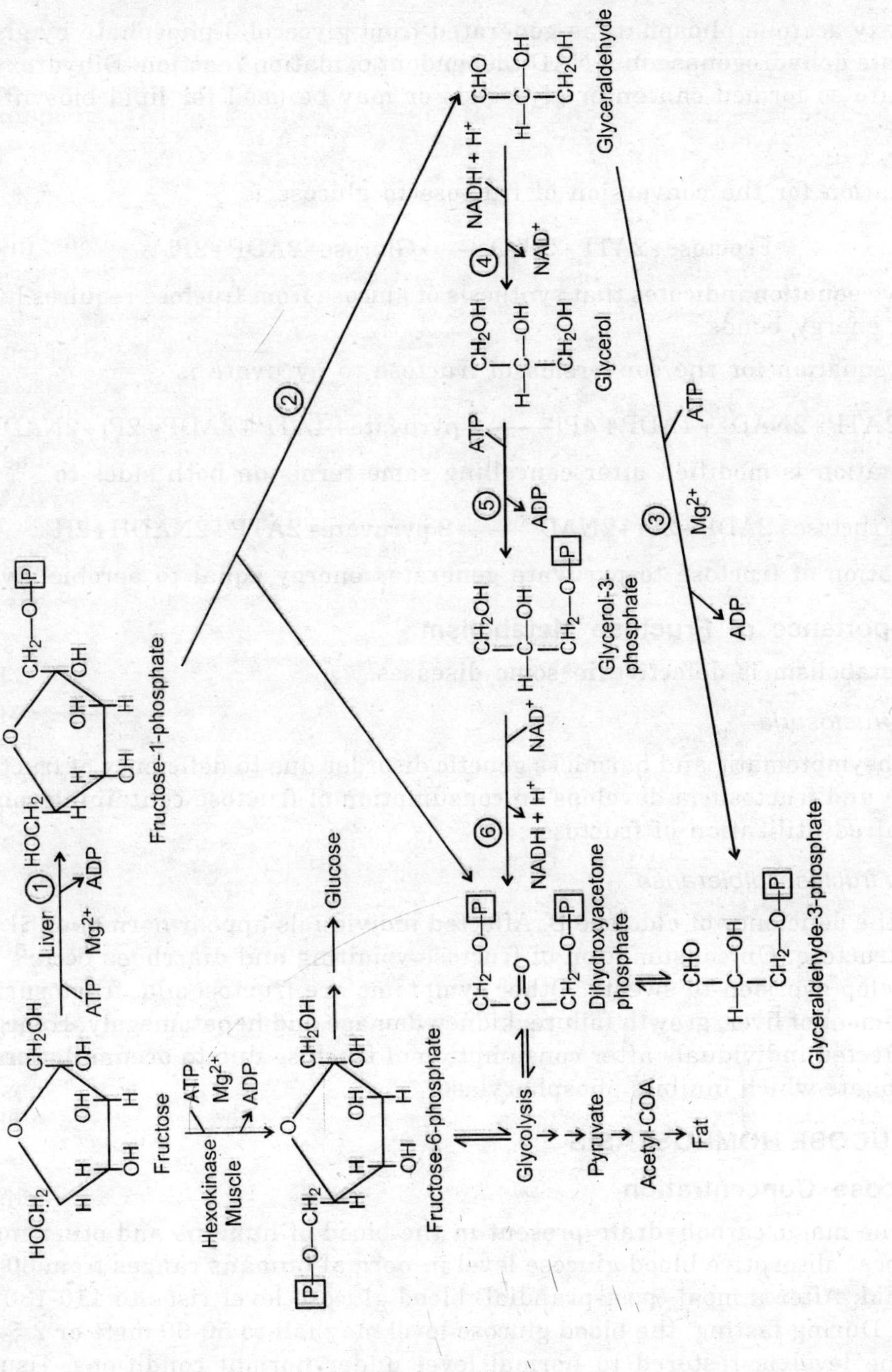

Fig. 9.21 Fructose utilization pathways.

5. Glycerokinase phosphorylates glycerol to glycerol-3-phosphate. ATP is the phosphate donor and Mg^{2+} is also required. Glycerol-3-phosphate serve as precursor for triglyceride and phospholipid synthesis.
6. Dihydroxy acetone phosphate is generated from glycerol-3-phosphate by glycerol-3-phosphate dehydrogenase in a NAD^+ dependent oxidation reaction. Dihydroxyacetone phosphate so formed can enter glycolysis or may be used for lipid biosynthesis.

Energetics

Overall equation for the conversion of fructose to glucose is

$$\text{Fructose} + 2\text{ATP} + 2\text{H}_2\text{O} \longrightarrow \text{Glucose} + 2\text{ADP} + 2\text{Pi}$$

The above equation indicates that synthesis of glucose from fructose requires hydrolysis of two high energy bonds.

Overall equation for the conversion of fructose to pyruvate is

$$\text{Fructose} + 2\text{ATP} + 2\text{NAD}^+ + 4\text{ADP} + 4\text{Pi} \longrightarrow 2\text{ pyruvate} + 4\text{ATP} + 2\text{ADP} + 2\text{Pi} + 2\text{NADH} + 2\text{H}^+$$

This equation is modified after cancelling same terms on both sides to

$$\text{Fructose} + 2\text{ADP} + 2\text{Pi} + 2\text{NAD}^+ \longrightarrow 2\text{ pyruvate} + 2\text{ATP} + 2\text{NADH} + 2\text{H}^+$$

So the oxidation of fructose to pyruvate generates energy equal to aerobic glycolysis.

Medical Importance of Fructose Metabolism

Fructose metabolism is defective in some diseases.

1. Essential fructosuria

It is a rare, asymptomatic and harmless genetic disorder due to deficiency of fructokinase. Fructosemia and fructosuria develops on consumption of fructose containing compounds due to impaired utilization of fructose.

2. Hereditary fructose intolerance

It is due to the deficiency of aldolase B. Affected individuals appear normal until they are exposed to fructose. On consumption of fructose vomiting and diarrhoea occurs. So they usually develop aversion to sweets. Other symptoms are fructosemia, fructosuria, jaundice, enlargement of liver, growth failure, kidney damage and hepatomegaly. Hypoglycemia occurs in affected individuals after consumption of fructose due to accumulation of fructose-1-phosphate which inhibits phosphorylase.

BLOOD GLUCOSE HOMEOSTASIS

Blood Glucose Concentration

Glucose is the major carbohydrate present in the blood of humans and other mammals. Fasting or post absorptive blood glucose level in normal humans ranges from 60-90 mg% or 3.5-5.0 mM. After a meal (post-prandial) blood glucose level rises to 110-130 mg% or 6.0-7.0 mM. During fasting, the blood glucose level may fall to 50-60 mg% or 2.5-3.5 mM. However, the level is restored to normal level under normal conditions. Usually the arterial blood glucose level is higher than the venous blood. In birds, the blood sugar level is higher compared to human blood glucose level. However, the blood glucose level of ruminants is lower than the human blood glucose level.

The blood glucose level is determined by two processes. They are:

1. Rate of entry of glucose into blood from different sources.
2. Rate of removal of glucose from the blood by various pathways.

Sources of Blood Glucose

1. **Dietary carbohydrates.** Mainly glucose, galactose and fructose are produced from dietary carbohydrates. They reach liver via portal vain. Galactose and fructose are also converted to glucose in liver. Dietary carbohydrate maintains blood glucose level up to 3 hours after food in take.
2. Liver glycogenolysis maintains blood sugar level up to 16 hours after food intake.
3. Gluconeogenesis maintains blood sugar level up to 36 hours after food intake. Beyond that period (If food is not taken or fasting) also gluconeogenesis is the only source of glucose.

Removal of Blood Glucose

Various pathways uses glucose for different purpose.

1. Glycolysis uses glucose for energy.
2. Glycogenesis uses glucose for glycogen formation.
3. HMP shunt and uronic acid pathways convert glucose to pentoses and mucopolysaccharides.
4. Glucose is converted to fat also as we shall see in next chapter.

Maintenance of constant level of glucose in blood is one of the finally regulated of all the homeostatic mechanisms. Liver, extra hepatic tissues and various hormones are involved in blood glucose homeostasis.

These factors regulate blood glucose level by acting at either glucose source or glucose utilization.

Liver

It plays a crucial role in the regulation of blood glucose level. Entry of glucose into liver cells is not insulin dependent. Glucose can move freely across membrane of hepatocyte. When the blood glucose level is increased liver bring down glucose level to normal by increasing glucose utilization for glycogen and fat formation. Likewise when blood glucose level falls to below normal liver raises blood sugar level to normal by forming glucose from glycogenolysis and gluconeogenesis. In starvation liver converts alanine derived from breakdown of muscle protein to glucose (glucose-alanine cycle).

Extra hepatic tissues involved in blood glucose homeostasis are skeletal muscle, kidney and erythrocytes. Entry of glucose into these tissues is dependent on insulin (not freely permeable). So entry of glucose is rate limiting in the uptake of glucose by these tissues.

Skeletal muscle

It has an indirect role in blood glucose homeostasis. It removes glucose from blood and converts it glycogen when ample glucose is present in blood. It contributes to liver gluconeogenisis by supplying lactate (Cori cycle). As mentioned above it contributes to glucose by supplying alanine during starvation.

Kidney

Kidney contributes to blood glucose by gluconeogenesis under the conditions of decreased blood glucose. Further it regulates blood glucose level when blood glucose level is above renal threshold value by eliminating glucose in urine.

Erythrocytes

They contribute lactate for gluconeogenesis. They remove glucose for NADPH, energy and 2, 3-BPG production.

Hormones

Many hormones are involved in blood glucose homeostasis. They are divided into two categories based on their action on blood glucose level.

1. **Hypoglycemic hormone** Which lowers blood glucose level. Only one hormone is known under this category. Insulin is an hypoglycemic hormone.
2. **Hyperglycemic hormones** Which raises blood glucose level. They are glucagon, epinephrine (nor-epinephrine), glucocorticoids, anterior pituitary hormones and thyroid hormone.

INSULIN

Insulin plays central role in blood glucose homeostasis. It is produced by beta (β) cells of the islets of Langerhans in the pancreas as a direct response to hyperglycemia. Insulin lowers blood glucose level by several ways.

1. Insulin increases the uptake of glucose by muscle and adipose tissue. Insulin increases transport of glucose across membrane of peripheral tissues by increasing the movement of glucose transporter from microsomes of plasma membrane. In the muscle glucose is converted to glycogen and in the adipose tissue glucose is used for fat formation. Insulin sensitive glucose transporter GLUT-4 is expressed in skeletal muscles, cardiac muscle and adipose tissue.
2. In the liver, insulin increases activities of enzymes involved in glucose utilization like glycolysis, glycogenesis, fatty acid synthesis, PDG, HMP shunt and decreases activities of enzymes of glycogenolysis and gluconeogenesis.
3. Insulin stimulates glycolysis by increasing the synthesis of glucokinase, PFK-1 and pyruvate kinase. Insulin increases activities of glucose-6-phosphate dehydrogenase and phosphogluconate dehydrogenase of HMP shunt. Insulin incrases activity of glycogen synthase. Insulin repress the synthesis of key enzymes of gluconeogenesis and decreases activity of glycogen phosphorylase.

   Oral hypoglycemic agents also causes insulin secretion.

GLUCAGON

It is the major hyperglycemic hormone produced by alpha cells of islets of Langerhans of pancreas. It is the major antagonist to insulin action. Hypoglycemia stimulates its production or secretion. It increases glucose level by enhancing gluconeogenesis in liver. It reduces the conversion of glucose to glycogen. As mentioned earlier all of these actions are mediation through cAMP.

Epinephrine

Hypoglycemia stimulates its secretion by adrenal medulla. It increases formation of glucose by enhancing glycogenolysis and gluconeogensis in liver and muscle. It prevents the use of glucose for glycogen formation.

Glucocorticoids

They are secreted by adrenal cortex. Glucocorticoids raises blood sugar level by

1. Decreasing glucose utilization by extra hepatic tissues.
2. Promoting gluconeogenesis by increasing catabolism of proteins. Glucocorticoids induces formation key enzymes of gluconeogenesis.

Anterior Pituitary Hormones

Two hormones of anterior pituitary gland elevates blood glucose level. They are growth hormone and adrenocorticotropic hormone (ACTH). Hypoglycemia stimulates growth hormone secretion. Growth hormone raises blood glucose level by

1. Decreasing the uptake of glucose by extra hepatic tissues.
2. Promoting mobilization of fat.
3. Increasing gluconeogenesis in liver.

ACTH raises blood glucose level indirectly by stimulating the production of glucocorticoids. In addition ACTH affects glycogen metabolism.

Thyroid Hormone

Thyroxine affects blood glucose through an unknown mechanism. The blood glucose level is low in hypothyroidism and high in hyper thyroidism. Further, in hyper thyroidism glycogen level found to be low in liver due to depletion of glycogen store. Thyroxine may affect glucose utilization or may be needed for glucose absorption in the intestine.

REFERENCES

1. Boyer, P.D. (Ed.) The Enzymes. Vol. 6. 3rd ed. Academic Press, New York, P. 908, 1972.
2. Frey, P.A. Advances in Enzymology and related topics in molecular biology **62**, 119, 1989.
3. Barritti, G.J. Communication with in cells. Black well, Oxford, 1992.
4. Bioteux, A. and Hess, B. Design of glycolysis. Phil. Tran. Royal Soc. London **B 293**, 5-22, 1981.

5. Wieland, O.H. The mammalian pyruvate dehydrogenase complex. Structure and regualtion. Rev. Physiol. Biochem. Pharmacol. **96**, 123, 1983.
6. Krebs, H.A. The history of TCA Cycle. Perspect. Biol. Med. **14**, 154-170, 1970.
7. Sprang, S. Structural changes in glycogen phosphorylase. Nature **336**, 215-221, 1988.
8. Linder, M.E. and Gilman, A.G. G-Proteins Sci. Am. **267 (1)**, **36-43**, 1992.
9. Wilson *et al.* (Eds.) Glycogen storage diseases. In Principles of internal Medicine. Vol. 2, 12th Ed. McGraw-Hill, New York, P. 1854, 1991.
10. Pilkus, S.J. and El-Magharbi, M.R. Hormonal regulation of hepatic glycolysis and gluconeogenesis. Ann. Rev. Biochem. **57**, 755, 1988.
11. Snell, K. Muscle alanine synthesis and hepatic gluconeogenesis. Biochem. Soc. Trans. **8,** 205, 1980.
12. Stalman, S.W. The role of liver in homeostasis of blood glucose. Curr. Top. Cell. Regul. **11**, 51, 1976.
13. Kotonski, B. Wilczek, J. Madej, J. Zurzycki, A. and Hutney, J. Activity of glycogen depolymerizing enzymes in extracts from brain tumor tissue (anaplastic astrocytoma and glial blastoma multiforme). Acta Biochimica Polonica **48(4)**, 1085-1090, 2001.
14. Lomako, J. Limako, W.M. and Whelan, W.J. The biogenesis of glycogen: Nature of the carbohydrate in protein primer. Biochem. Int. **21**, 251-260, 1990.
15. Zhou, X.Y. *et al.* Insulin regulation of hepatic gluconeogenesis through phosphorylation of CREB protein. Nature Medicine. **10**, 633-637, 2004.
16. Salway, J.W. Metabolism at a glance. Blad Well Publishers, 2003.
17. Regenold, W.T. *et al.* Postmortem evidence from human brain tissue of disturbed glucose metabolism in mood and psychotic disorders. Molecular Psychiatry, **9**, 731-733, 2004.
18. Yep, A. *et al.* Identification and characterization of a critical region in the glycogen synthase from E. Coli. J. Biol. Chem. **279**, 8359-8367, 2004.
19. Lu, Z. *et al.* A new class of glycogen phosporylase inhibitors. Bio Org. Med. Chem. Lett. **13**, 4125-4128, 2003.
20. Lerin, c. *et al.* Regulation of glycogen metabolism in cultured human muscle cells by glycogen phosphorylase inhibitor CP-91149. Biochem. J. **378**, 1073-1077, 2004.
21. Buschiazzo, A. *et al.* Crystal structure of glycogen synthase: homologous enzymes catalyzes glycogen synthesis and degradation. EMBO. J. **23**, 3196-3205, 2004.
22. Dalal, B.I. and Kollmunnsberger, C. Drug induced hemolysis and metharmoylobinemia in glucose-6-phosphate dehydrogenase deficiency. Br. J. Haematol. **29**, 291-296, 2005.

EXERCISES

ESSAY QUESTIONS

1. Describe fate of glucose in rapidly contracting skeletal muscle. Add a note on energy aspect of this process.
2. Describe citric acid cycle. Add a note on its energetics.

3. Define glycogenesis and glycogenolysis. Write reaction sequence and action of hormones for any one process.
4. Describe direct oxidative pathway of glucose. Write note on medical importance of the pathway.
5. Describe uronic acid pathway. Write its significance.
6. Trace pathway for the conversion of lactate to glucose. How it is regulated ?
7. Discuss blood glucose homeostasis.
8. Define glycolysis. Name types of glycolysis. Detail any one process along with energetics.
9. How dietary fructose and galactose are utilized in the body? Write about inherited diseases associated with their utilization.
10. Describe inherited diseases of carbohydrate metabolism.
11. Write normal blood glucose level. Name its sources. How it enters cells? Out line its fate inside cell.
12. Describe regulation of glycogen metabolism.
13. What is meant by reciprocal regulation. Explain with respect to glycolysis and gluconeogenesis.

SHORT QUESTIONS

1. Explain pyruvate dehydrogenase complex.
2. Write significance of glycolysis.
3. Write a note on 2, 3-bisphosphoglycerate cycle.
4. Give an account of glycogen storage diseases.
5. Write medical importance of hormonal regulation of glycogen metabolism.
6. Show complete oxidation of glucose in HMP shunt with appropriate equations.
7. How polyols are formed? Write importance of polyol pathway.
8. Write the role or acetyl-CoA and AMP in the reciprocal regulation of glycolysis and gluconeogenesis.
9. Write action of hypoglycemic hormones.
10. Write normal blood glucose level. In what conditions it is elevated?
11. Write a note on Cori-cycle.
12. Define gluconeogenesis. Name key enzymes of gluconeogenesis. How it is regulated?
13. Write fate of NADPH of HMP shunt in liver, RBC and WBC.
14. Write about reactions catalyzed by glucose-6-phosphate dehydrogenase and inherited diseases of this enzyme.

MULTIPLE CHOICE QUESTIONS

1. Phosphofructokinase-1 is
   (*a*) An enzyme of glycolysis
   (*b*) Inhibited by fructose-6-phosphate
   (*c*) An allosteric enzyme of glycolysis
   (*d*) Activated by ATP
2. Which one of the following statement is correct regarding pyruvate dehydrogenase?
   (*a*) It is present in cytosol
   (*b*) It is a multienzyme complex
   (*c*) It is multi enzyme complex present in mitochondria
   (*d*) Acetyl-CoA is its substrate

3. Glycogen isolated from liver of Type VI glycogen storage disease patient had normal structure. So, glycogen accumulation is due to deficiency of
   (*a*) Muscle phosphorylase (*b*) Glucose-6-phosphatase
   (*c*) Liver phosphorylase (*d*) Glycogen synthase
4. In man, uronic acid pathway is unable to produce ascorbic acid due to lack of
   (*a*) Gulonolactone oxidase (*b*) Lactonase
   (*c*) Xylulose (*d*) Xylitol
5. Synthesis of glucose from pyruvate requires
   (*a*) Six high energy bonds (*b*) Two high energy bonds
   (*c*) Reduced NADP (*d*) NADH

FILL IN THE BLANKS

1. Entire chemical reactions network of body is called as ....
2. Dietary galactose and fructose are converted to .... in liver.
3. Fluoride decreases rate of glycolysis by inhibiting ....
4. Lysosomal glycogenolysis is blocked in .... disease.
5. Congenital galactosemia is due to deficiency of ....

CASES

1. A child was brought to hospital with vomiting, dizziness and sweating. The child developed all these problems and diarrhoea only after consumption of fruits, fruit juices or sweets made from jaggery and sugar. The child mother informed on questioning that the child was normal on breast feeding. On examination his weight was found to below normal and had liver enlargement. His blood glucose level was below normal but reducing substances were found in urine. Write your diagnosis.
2. A 10-year old boy with an history of reeling sensation and sweating was brought to hospital. Physical examination showed swelling in the abdomen, liver enlargement and normal heart. Glycogen isolated from liver biopsy specimen had normal structure. Blood glucose level was below normal, uric acid and lipid levels were elevated. Write your diagnosis.

10
CHAPTER

LIPID METABOLISM

MEDICAL AND BIOLOGICAL IMPORTANCE

1. In fed condition, excess calories consumed in the form of carbohydrates are conserved in the form of lipids. Of course dietary lipids are also stored under well-fed condition.
2. Even though excess energy may be stored in the form of carbohydrate (glycogen) humans and other mammals prefers to store excess energy only in the form of lipid because
   (*a*) Energy content of lipid is 2-3 times higher.
   (*b*) Lipid can be stored without water of hydration, which is not possible with glycogen. For example 1 gm of glycogen needs 2 gm of water for storage.
   (*c*) Oxidation of lipid produces more water. For example, oxidation of glucose produces approximately 45 water molecules where as oxidation of stearic acid produces nearly 165 water molecules.
3. Usually lipid stores are greater compared to glycogen. A 70 kg individual may have lipid store of about 15 kg. However, his glycogen store is about only 0.22 kg.
4. During fasting or in between meals stored lipids are used to meet energy demands. Glycogen store get depleted within 24 hours of fasting. Later, energy requirement of the body is entirely met by stored lipid. Lipids can meet body energy requirements for weeks.
5. Desert animal camel suits well to dry conditions because it derives water and energy from large amounts of lipids stored in hump. Hibernating and migratory birds also use lipid stores to meet water and energy demands during hibernation and migration, respectively.
6. Defect or changes in the pathways of lipid metabolism are directly related to development of diseases.
7. Increased fatty acid oxidation in starvation and diabetes leads to keto acidosis. Decreased fatty acid oxidation leads to hypoglycemia.
8. Some drugs and poisons work by inhibiting pathways of lipid metabolism. Aspirin an anti inflammatory drug works by inhibiting prostaglandin formation. Hypoglycin a toxin causes hypoglycemia.

9. Transport and storage of triglycerides are affected in obesity, diabetes and hyper lipoproteinemia. Block in the movement of triglycerides cause fatty livers.
10. Abnormalities in lipoprotein metabolism cause various dyslipoproteinemias (dyslipidemias) and fatty livers.
11. Accumulation of complex lipids leads to lipidoses.
12. Cholesterol is the major player in the development of atherosclerosis. Atherosclerosis can cause coronary artery disease and other vascular diseases.
13. Excessive fat accumulation leads to obesity.
14. Cholesterol produces bile salts, which are required for digestion and absorption of dietary lipids. Inhibitors of bile acid formation are used in the treatment of atherosclerosis.

Among lipids, triglycerides serves as stored form of energy. During fasting and or in between meals they are broken down to glycerol and fatty acids. Fatty acids accounts for 95% of oxidation energy of triglycerides. The remainder is derived from glycerol. Hence oxidation of fat or lipid is nothing but oxidation of fatty acids.

FATTY ACID OXIDATION

Sources of fatty acids

(*a*) **Dietary sources** Fatty acids formed from the digestion of dietary lipids are carried to liver. From the liver, they are transported to cell in bound form with albumin.

(*b*) **Endogenous sources** As mentioned above, free fatty acids formed from body triglycerides are used for energy production.

Though the plasma free fatty acid level is lower than blood glucose level they are rapidly utilized by peripheral tissues. The plasma free fatty acid (FFA) has life of 3-4 minutes.

Site

Fatty acid oxidation occurs in the mitochondria of all types of cells like liver, heart, adipose tissue, kidney, lung, skeletal muscle and some extent in brain.

Long chain fatty acid oxidation involves

(*a*) Activation in outer mitochondrial membrane

(*b*) Transport of activated fatty acids across inner mitochondrial membrane

(*c*) Oxidation in mitochondria

The short and medium chain fatty acids are activated and oxidized in the matrix of mitochondria. Since these fatty acids are freely permeable to inner mitochondrial membrane, no transport system is required unlike long chain fatty acids.

Entry of fatty acid

At plasma membrane fatty acid dissociates from albumin and combines with membrane fatty acid binding protein, which transports fatty acid into cytosol along with Na^+.

Activation of fatty acids

Acyl-CoA synthetases present in outer mitochondrial membrane and in endoplasmic reticulum are responsible for activation of long chain fatty acids. Short and medium chain fatty acids are activated by distinct acyl-CoA synthetases present in the matrix of mitochondria. The other name of synthetase is thiokinase. ATP, Mg^{2+} and CoASH are the co-factors required.

These synthetases convert fatty acids to corresponding acyl-CoAs. ATP is hydrolyzed to AMP and PP_i. Further hydrolysis of PP_i by pyrophosphatase pulls the reaction always towards the formation of acyl-CoA (Figure 10.1).

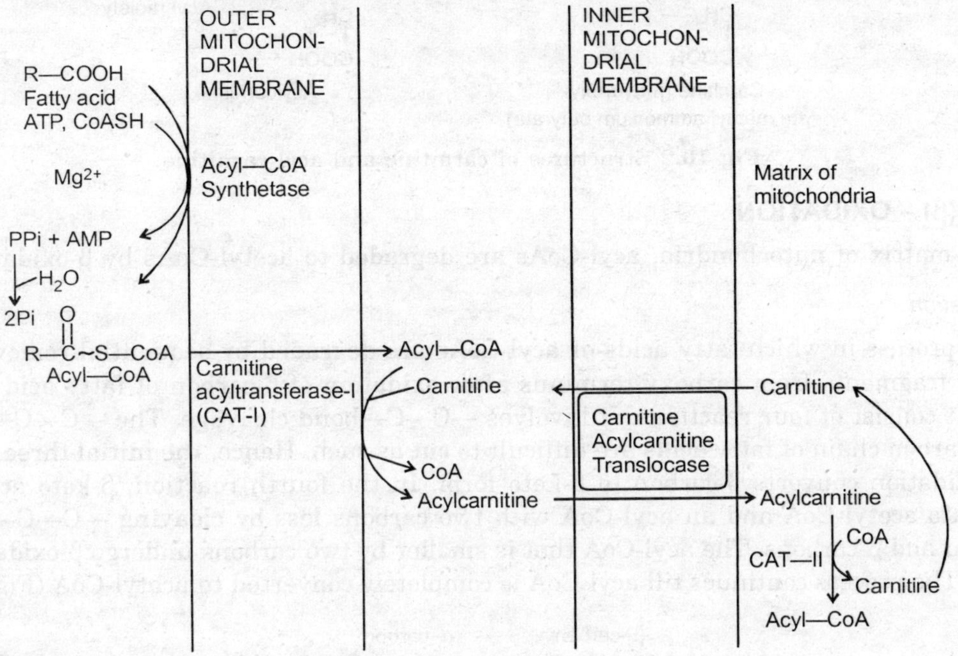

Fig. 10.1 Activation and transport of fatty acids by acyl-CoA synthetase and carnitine shuttle respectively

Transport of Fatty acyl-CoAs into mitochondria

Long chain acyl-CoAs formed are impermeable to inner mitochondrial membrane. Carnitine shuttle transfers acyl-CoAs from outer mitochondrial membrane into matrix of mitochondria. Carnitine shuttle consist of carnitine, enzymes and translocase. Carnitine is derived from amino acid lysine. Liver and kidney synthesizes carnitine from lysine.

Carnitine shuttle

1. The shuttle begins with the transfer of acyl-CoA to carnitine to form acyl carnitine. This reaction is catalyzed by carnitine acyl transferase-I (CAT-I). Acyl residue is attached to hydroxyl group of β-carbon atom of carnitine through an ester linkage (Figure 10.2). CAT-I is present in the outer mitochondrial membrane and it regulates entry of fatty acids into mitochondria (Figure 10.1).
2. Acyl carnitine is translocated into matrix of mitochondria by carnitine-acyl carnitine translocase present in inner mitochondrial membrane. Carnitine-acyl carnitine translocase is a carrier protein involved in facilitated transport.
3. Carnitine-acyl transferase-II (CAT-II) present in inside of inner mitochondrial membrane liberates acyl group from acyl carnitine as acyl-CoA.
4. To complete the shuttle, carnitine is sent back to out side of inner mitochondrial membrane by carnitine-acyl carnitine translocase. Thus, carnitine shuttle transfers acyl-CoA from outside of inner mitochondrial membrane into matrix of mitochondria.

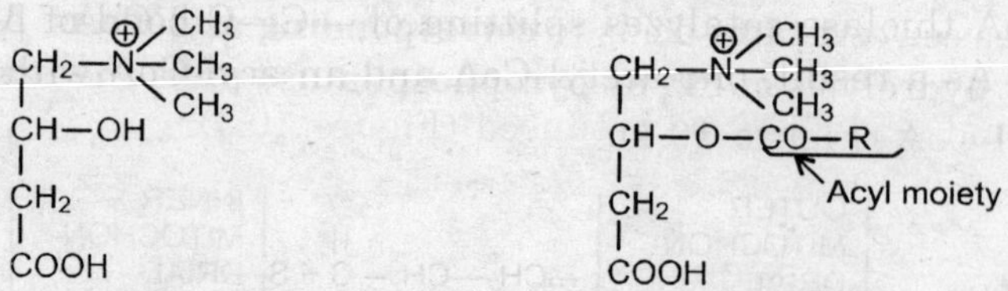

Carnitine (β-hydroxy- -γ-tri methyl ammonium butyrate) Acylcarnitine

Fig 10.2 Structures of carnitine and acyl carnitine

BETA (β) – OXIDATION

In the matrix of mitochondria, acyl-CoAs are degraded to acetyl-CoAs by β-oxidation.

β-Oxidation

It is a process in which fatty acids or acyl-CoAs are degraded by sequential removal of two carbon fragments from carboxy terminus after oxidation of β-carbon of fatty acid to β-keto form. It consist of four reactions. It involves —C—C—bond cleavage. The —C—C—bonds of hydrocarbon chain of fatty acids are difficult to cut as such. Hence, the initial three reactions of β-oxidation converts β-carbon to β-keto form. In the fourth reaction, β-keto acyl-CoA is split into acetyl-CoA and an acyl-CoA with two carbons less by cleaving —C—C—bond between α and β-carbons. The acyl-CoA that is smaller by two carbons undergo β-oxidation once again. The process continues till acyl-CoA is completely converted to acetyl-CoA (Figure 10.3)

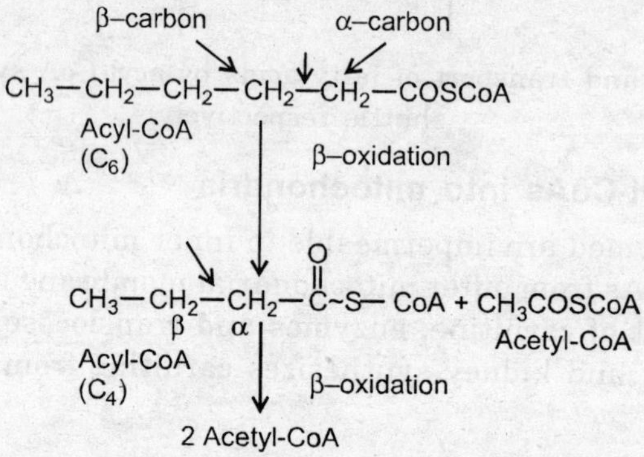

Fig. 10.3 Theory of β-oxidation of fatty acids, C—C bond cleaved is indicated by arrow

Reaction sequence of β-oxidation

1. Dehydrogenation of acyl-CoA is the first reaction of β-oxidation. It is catalyzed by FAD containing acyl-CoA dehydrogenase. Product of this reaction is Δ^2-trans-enoyl-CoA. FAD is reduced to $FADH_2$. In mitochondria, distinct acyl-CoA dehydrogenases for short, medium and long chain acyl-CoAs exist.
2. Addition of water across the double bond by Enoyl-CoA hydratase is the second reaction. Since the enzyme is stereo specific only L-isomer is formed. Thus, the product of this reaction is L-β-hydroxy acyl-CoA.
3. An NAD^+ linked β-hydroxy acyl-CoA dehydrogenase catalyzes conversion of β-hydroxy acyl-CoA to β-keto acyl-CoA. NADH is produced at the end of reaction.

4. β-keto acyl-CoA thiolase catalyzes splitting of —C—C bond of β-keto acyl-CoA at α, β-carbon atoms. As a result, one acetyl-CoA and an acyl-CoA with two carbon atoms less than the original acyl-CoA are produced (Figure 10.4).

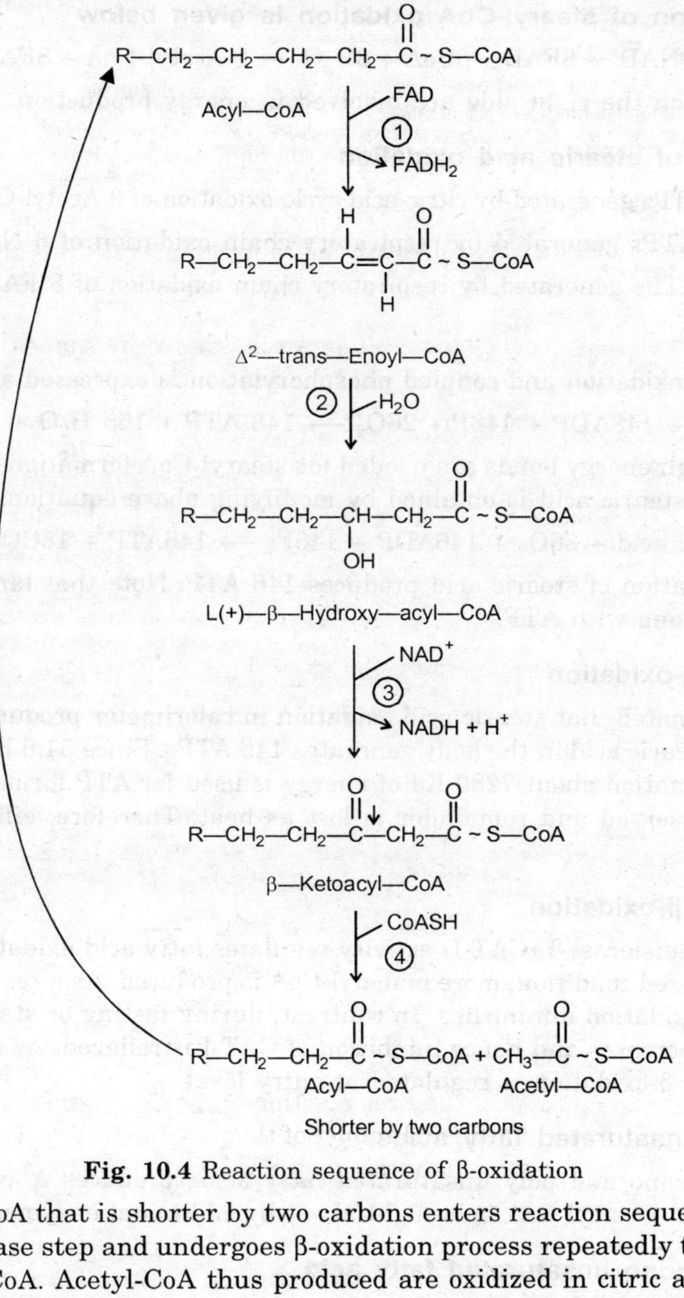

Fig. 10.4 Reaction sequence of β-oxidation

Now the acyl-CoA that is shorter by two carbons enters reaction sequence of β-oxidation at first dehydrogenase step and undergoes β-oxidation process repeatedly till it is completely oxidized to acetyl-CoA. Acetyl-CoA thus produced are oxidized in citric acid cycle.

Energetics of β-oxidation

Let us calculate the amount of energy produced when a saturated fatty acid like stearic acid is oxidized in β-oxidation. Since stearic acid is a 18-carbon fatty acid it undergoes β-oxidation

8 times producing 9 acetyl-CoA molecules (Figure 10.5). Further each β-oxidation process generates one $FADH_2$ (reaction-1) and one NADH (reaction-3). Therefore, the products of β-oxidation of stearyl-CoA are 9 acetyl-CoA, 8 $FADH_2$ and 8 NADH.

Over all equation of stearyl-CoA oxidation is given below

Stearyl–CoA + 8 NAD^+ + 8FAD + 8CoA + $8H_2O \longrightarrow$ 9 Acetyl-CoA + $8FADH_2$ + 8NADH + $8H^+$

The compounds on the right side are involved in energy production.

Energy output of stearic acid oxidation

1.	Number of ATPs generated by citric acid cycle oxidation of 9 Acetyl-CoAs	(9 × 12)	= 108
2.	Number of ATPs generated by respiratory chain oxidation of 8 NADH	(8 × 3)	= 24
3.	Number of ATPs generated by respiratory chain oxidation of 8 $FADH_2$	(8 × 2)	= 16
		Total	= 148

Stearyl-CoA oxidation and coupled phosphorylation is expressed as equation below.

Stearyl-CoA + 148ADP + 148Pi+ $26O_2 \longrightarrow$ 148 ATP + 165 H_2O + 18 CO_2 + CoASH

Since two high energy bonds are needed for stearyl-CoA formation. The net yield of ATP per molecule of stearic acid is obtained by modifying above equation.

$$\text{Stearic acid} + 26O_2 + 146\text{ADP} + 146\text{Pi} \longrightarrow 146\text{ATP} + 18CO_2 + 165H_2O$$

Thus, β-oxidation of stearic acid produces 146 ATP. Note that large amount of H_2O is also produced along with ATP.

Efficiency of β-oxidation

It has been estimated that stearic acid oxidation in calorimeter produces 1120 KJ of energy β-oxidation of stearic acid in the body generates 146 ATPs. Since 51.6 KJ of energy is needed for one ATP formation about 7280 KJ of energy is used for ATP formation. Thus, only 65% of energy is conserved and remainder is lost as heat. Therefore, efficiency of β-oxidation system is 65%.

Regulation of β-oxidation

Carnitineacyl transferase-I (CAT-I) activity regulates fatty acid oxidation. It is inhibited by malonyl-CoA. In fed condition, more malonyl-CoA is produced. As a result, CAT-I is inhibited and fatty acid oxidation diminishes. In contrast, during fasting or starvation, malonyl-CoA concentration decreases and hence inhibition of CAT-I is relieved. As a result β-oxidation is activated. Thus, β-oxidation is regulated at entry level.

Oxidation of unsaturated fatty acids

β-oxidation of mono and poly unsaturated fatty acids produces Δ^3-*cis*-acyl-CoAs. Further degradation of Δ^3-*cis*-acyl-CoA is brought about by additional enzymes.

Oxidation of mono unsaturated fatty acid

1. For example, oleyl-CoA, a mono unsaturated fatty acid undergo β-oxidation 3 times to produce 3 acetyl-CoA and Δ^3-*cis*-enoyl-CoA.

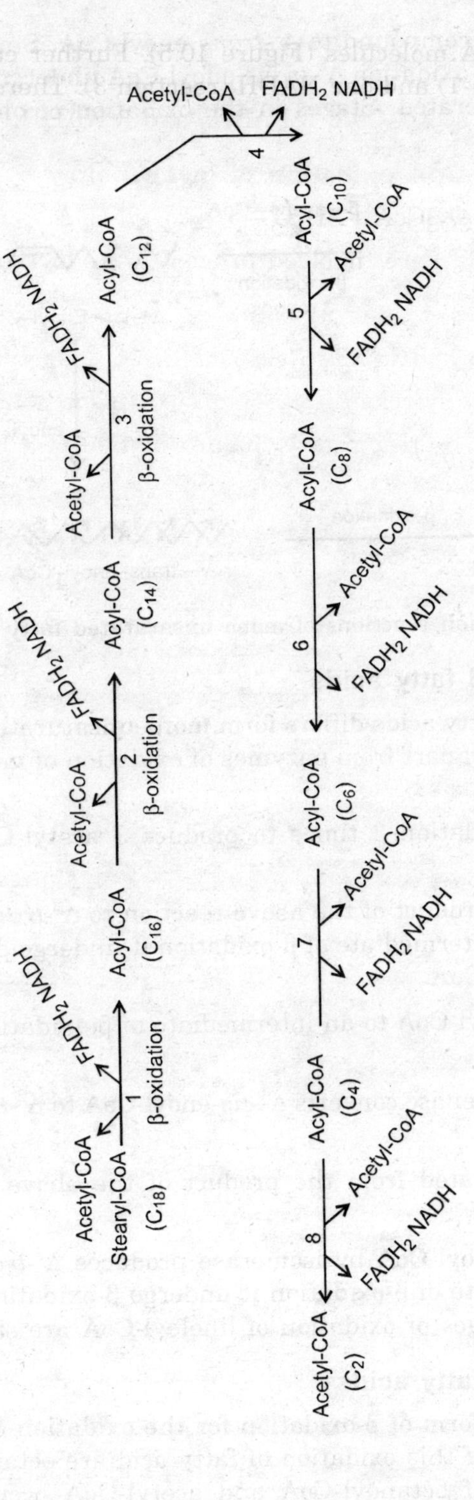

Fig. 10.5 Overall β-oxidation processes of Stearyl-CoA

2. An isomerase converts this compound to Δ^2-*trans* enoyl-CoA. Since this compound is a substrate for hydratase of β-oxidation Δ^2-*trans* enoyl-CoA undergoes β-oxidation 5 times and 6 acetyl-CoAs are generated. Stages in the oxidation of oleyl-CoA are shown in Figure 10.6.

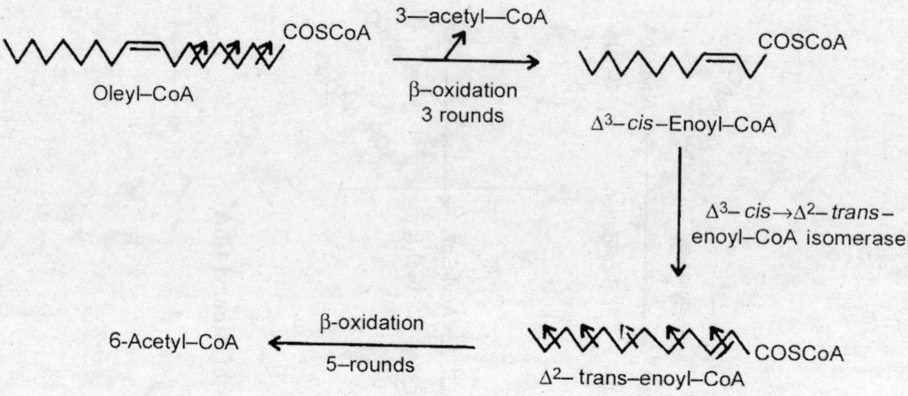

Fig. 10.6 Oxidation reactions of mono unsaturated fatty acid.

Oxidation of poly unsaturated fatty acids

Oxidation of poly unsaturated fatty acids differs form mono unsaturated fatty acid oxidation and requires additional enzymes apart from enzymes of oxidation of mono unsaturated fatty acids.

1. Linoleyl-CoA undergo β-oxidation 3 times to produce 3 acetyl-CoAs and Δ^3*cis*-Δ^6-*cis*-dienoyl-CoA.
2. An isomerase converts the product of the above reaction to Δ^2-*trans*-Δ^6-cis-dienoyl-CoA. Since this compound is an intermediate of β-oxidation it undergo β-oxidation to produce acetyl-CoA and Δ^4-*cis*-enoyl-CoA.

   The conversion of Δ^4-*cis*-enoyl-CoA to an intermediate of β-oxidation requires two additional enzymes.
3. An FAD dependent dehydrogenase converts Δ^4-*cis*-enoyl-CoA to Δ^2-*trans*-Δ^4-*cis*-enoyl-CoA by creating double bond.
4. Δ^3-*trans* enoyl-CoA is generated from the product of the above reaction by NADPH dependent reductase.
5. Isomerization of Δ^3-*trans* enoyl-CoA by isomerase produces Δ^2-*trans* enoyl-CoA. Since this compound is intermediate of β-oxidation it undergo β-oxidation 4 times to produce 5 acetyl-CoAs. Different stages of oxidation of linoleyl-CoA are shown in Figure 10.7.

Oxidation of very long chain fatty acids

Peroxisomes contain a modified form of β-oxidation for the oxidation of long and very long chain fatty acids. The products of this oxidation of fatty acid are octanoyl-CoA, acetyl-CoA and H_2O_2. Further, oxidation of octanoyl-CoA and acetyl-CoA occurs in mitochondria. Peroxisomal fatty acid oxidation may boost mitochondrial β-oxidation by partially oxidizing long chain fatty acids.

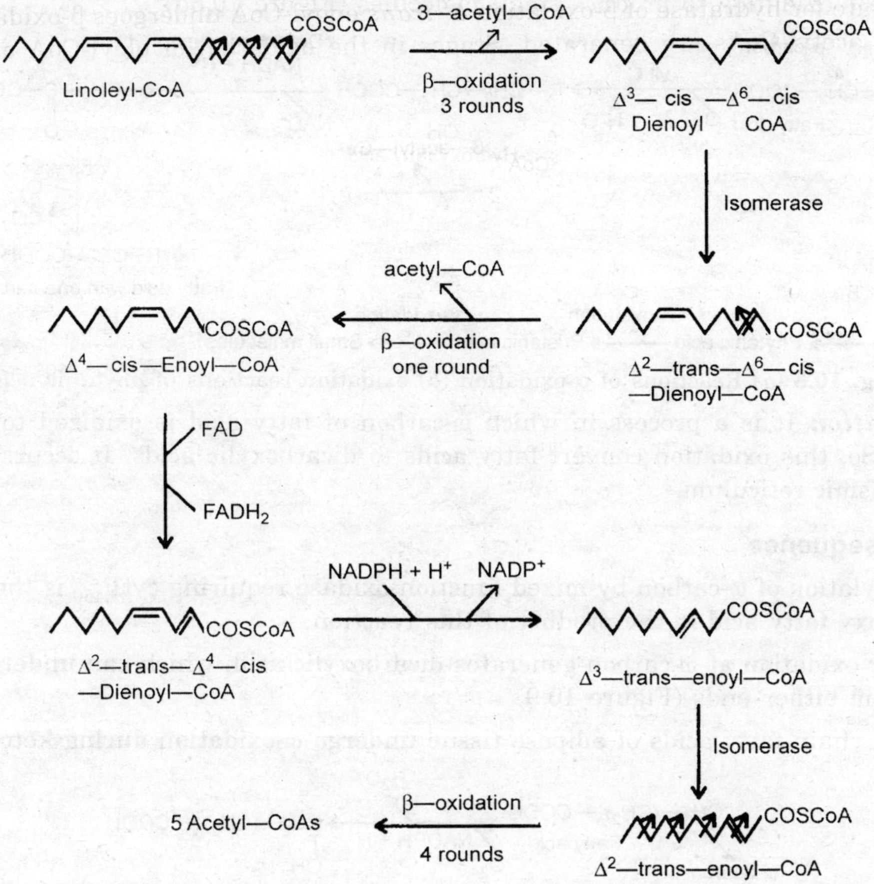

Fig. 10.7 Oxidation reactions of poly unsaturated fatty acid

Other types of fatty acid oxidation

1. **α-oxidation** It is a process in which fatty acid is degraded by sequential removal of one carbon from the carboxyl end after the oxidation of α-carbon to α-keto form. It occurs in peroxisomes and mitochondria and in plants. Unlike β-oxidation, it does not generate energy and requires no CoA intermediates.

Reaction sequence

1. Hydroxylation of α-carbon of fatty acid is the first reaction of this oxidative pathway. Mono-oxygenase catalyzes this reaction. Vit. C, O_2 and Fe^{2+} are other co-factors of this reaction. α-Hydroxy fatty acid is the product of this reaction. In the brain, hydroxy fatty acids are formed by this route.
2. Dehydrogenation and oxidative decarboxylation converts hydroxy fatty acid to a fatty acid shorter by one carbon (Figure 10.8*a*)

   Phytanic acid is the only fatty acid oxidized by α-oxidation. It is derived from plant alcohol phytol, which is present in dairy products. It can not undergo β-oxidation due to methyl group at β-carbon. α-Oxidation converts phytanic acid to pristanic acid, which undergo β-oxidation to produce small molecules (Figure 10.8*b*).

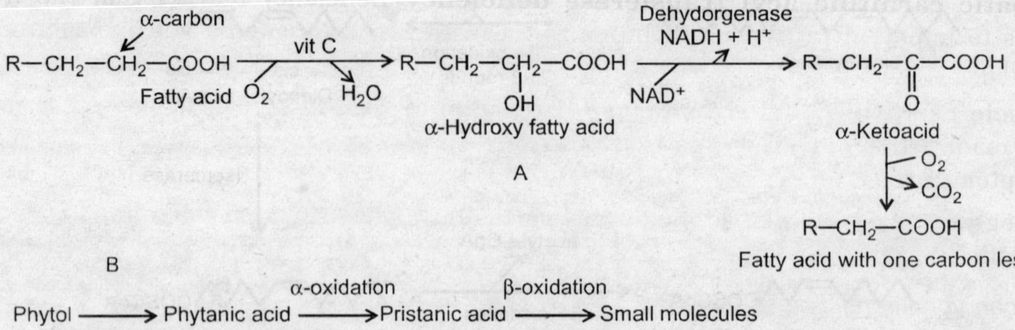

Fig. 10.8 (*a*) Reactions of α-oxidation (*b*) oxidation reactions of phytanic acid

2. ***ω-oxidation*** It is a process in which ω-carbon of fatty acid is oxidized to carboxylic group. So, this oxidation convert fatty acids to dicarboxylic acids. It occurs in smooth endoplasmic reticulum.

Reaction sequence

1. Hydroxylation of ω-carbon by mixed function oxidase requiring cytP_{450} is the first step. ω-hydroxy fatty acid is the product of this reaction.
2. Further oxidation at ω-carbon generates dicarboxylic acid, which can undergo β-oxidation from either ends (Figure 10.9).

Medium chain fatty acids of adipose tissue undergo ω-oxidation during ketosis.

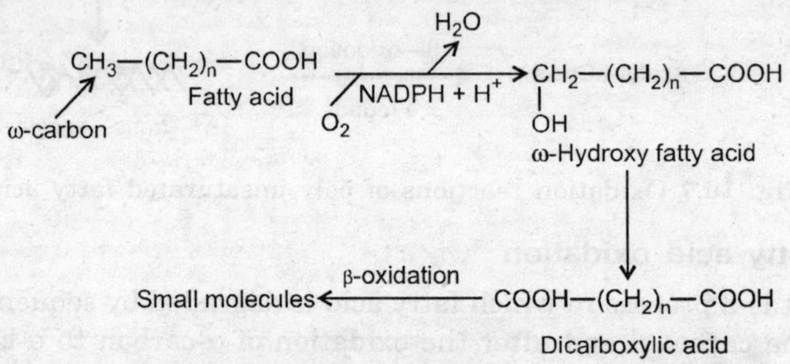

Fig. 10.9 ω-oxidation reaction sequence

Disorders of Fatty acids oxidation or Medical importance

Fatty acid oxidation is impaired in many diseases.

1. Carnitine deficiency

It occurs in premature infants and in new-borns. It is due to inadequate formation or loss in urine due to renal leakage. Lack of carnitine results in impaired transport of acyl-CoAs into mitochondria. The plasma-free fatty acid level raises due to decreased β-oxidation. Main symptom is hypoglycemia, because all tissues use glucose for energy production, other symptoms are lipid accumulation, muscle weakness and hypoketonemia. Oral supplementation of carnitine results in disappearance of symptoms.

2. Carnitine acyl transferase deficiencies

(*a*) **Hepatic carnitine acyl transferase deficiency** Deficiency of CAT-I in the liver leads to impaired fatty acid oxidation. As a result, hypoketonemia and hypoglycemia develops.

(*b*) **Muscle carnitine acyl transferase-II deficiency** Due to deficiency of CAT-II fatty acid oxidation is impaired in muscle. Muscle weakness and myoglobinuria are the main symptoms.

(*c*) Hypoglycemic agents like sulfonylureas particularly glyburide and tolbutamide used in diabetics inhibit transferases.

3. *Jamaican vomiting sickness*

It occurs when unripe fruit of akee tree is consumed. An unusual amino acid hypoglycin present in the fruit is the causating agent. It inhibits or inactivates short and medium chain acyl-CoA dehydrogenases. As a result, these fatty acid's oxidation is blocked and hypoglycemia develops. However, the short and medium chain fatty acids undergo ω-oxidation to produce corresponding dicarboxylic acids, which may be excreted in urine.

4. Dicarboxylic acid uria

It occurs due to lack of mitochondrial medium chain acyl-CoA dehydrogenase. As a result β-oxidation of these fatty acids is impaired. However, they undergo ω-oxidation to produce dicarboxylic acids, which are excreted in urine.

5. Refsum's disease

It is an inherited disease. α-Oxidation of phytanic acid is blocked in this disease. As a result phytanic acid accumulates in the blood and liver. In corporation of phytanic acid in the cell membrane affects membrane fluidity. Main symptoms are abnormalities in the skin, bone and peripheral neuropathy. Consumption of phytanic acid free diet relieves symptoms.

6. Zell weger's syndrome

It is a rare disorder associated with absence of peroxisomes in most of the tissues. Affected individuals are unable to utilize very long chain fatty acids. So, accumulation of these fatty acids particularly occurs.

Propionate Metabolism

Medical and biological importance

1. Propionate is mainly produced in the rumen of reminants by bacteria. In ruminants propionate meets 25% of energy needs.
2. In humans, propionyl-CoA arises from β-oxidation of fatty acids with odd number carbons, α-oxidation of phytanic acid, methionine and isoleucine catabolism and cholesterol catabolism.
3. However, human colon contains some propionate.
4. Propionyl-CoA may be used for the synthesis of odd number fatty acids in adipose tissue.
5. Propionate and propionyl-CoA are converted to glucose. Alternatively, they are oxidized via citric acid cycle to produce energy.
6. Propionate metabolism is defective in some diseases.

Reaction sequence

1. In ruminants, propionate reaches liver from rumen through circulation. In the liver propionate is activated by thiokinase in presence of ATP and Mg^{2+}. The activation is similar to fatty acid activation. Propionyl-CoA is the product of this reaction.
2. Biotin dependent carboxylation of propionyl-CoA is the next reaction of propionate metabolism. The reaction is catalyzed by propionyl-CoA carboxylase. ATP and CO_2 are the co-factors required. D-methyl malonyl-CoA is the product of this reaction.
3. Methyl malonyl-CoA racemase isomerizes the product of above reaction to L-isomer, i.e., L-methyl malonyl-CoA.
4. Finally succinyl-CoA is generated from L-Methyl malonyl-CoA by shifting-COSCoA to methyl carbon. The reaction is catalyzed by vit B_{12} (deoxy adenosyl cobalamin) containing mutase.

Succinyl-CoA can be used for energy production or may be converted to glucose. Reaction sequence of propionate metabolism is shown in Figure 10.10

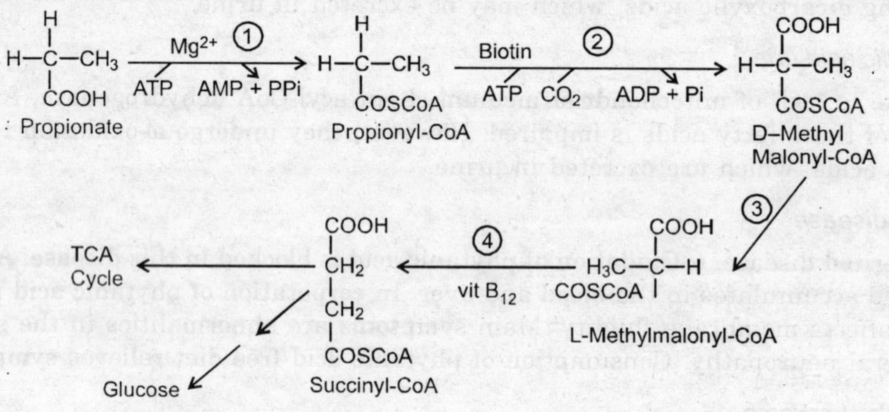

Fig. 10.10 Reaction sequence of propionate metabolism

Disorders of Propionate Metabolism

Utilization of propionate and propionyl-CoA is impaired in some diseases.

1. Congenital propionyl-CoA carboxylase deficiency

Symptoms of this condition are vomiting and ketosis. Since propionyl-CoA conversion to D-methyl malony-CoA is impaired due to lack of propionyl-CoA carboxylase propionyl-CoA combines with oxaloacetate to form methyl citrate in presence of citrate synthase. This causes depletion of oxaloacetate and impaired acetyl-CoA utilization by citric acid cycle. Accumulated acetyl-CoA is converted to ketone bodies, which leads to ketosis.

2. Mutase deficiency

It is characterized by excretion of more methyl-malonic acid in urine. In the absence of mutase, methyl malonic acid can not be coverted to succinyl-CoA. So, methyl malonic acid accumulates and methylmalonic aciduria occurs. Since vit. B_{12} is the prosthetic group of mutase methyl malonic aciduria occurs in vit B_{12} deficiency also. However, this methyl malonic acid uria disappears on administration of vit B_{12}.

Metabolism of Ketone bodies

Ketone bodies are, 1. Acetoacetic acid 2. β-Hydroxy butyric acid 3. Acetone. Acetoacetic acid is the primary ketone body. The other two ketone bodies are derived from acetoacetic acid.

Ketone body metabolism consist of two phases.

1. Ketogenesis
2. Ketolysis

Ketogenesis

1. Synthesis of ketone bodies is called as ketogenesis.
2. Under certain conditions, production of acetyl-CoA either from β-oxidation or pyruvate oxidation is more rapid than it can be utilized for other metabolic processes.
3. Liver converts the excess acetyl-CoA to ketone bodies. Hence, liver can be considered as net producer of ketone bodies.

Biological importance

1. The major purpose of ketone body formation in liver is to distribute excess fuel (acetyl-CoA) to other tissues.
2. Even number fatty acids are more ketogenic than odd number fatty acids.
3. Fat is more ketogenic than carbohydrate because fat generates more acetyl-CoA.

Reaction sequence

Enzymes responsible for ketone body formation are present in liver mitochondria. Acetyl-CoA is the starting material for ketogenesis.

1. Condensation of two acetyl-CoA molecules to form acetoacetyl-CoA is the first reaction of ketogenesis. The reaction is catalyzed by thiolase. It is reversal of final reaction of β-oxidation. Condensation involves —C—C— bond formation. Alternatively, aceto acetyl-CoA may be directly formed from fatty acid β-oxidation.

   There are two pathways for the formation of aceto acetate from acetoacetyl-CoA.
2. In one pathway, aceto acetyl-CoA further condenses with one more acetyl-CoA to form 3-hydroxy-3-methylglutaryl-CoA (HMG-CoA). The reaction is catalyzed by HMG-CoA synthase. This pathway is the major route of ketone body formation. This condensation also involes $-\overset{|}{\underset{|}{C}}-\overset{|}{\underset{|}{C}}-$ bond formation.
3. HMG-CoA lyase splits HMG-CoA to acetoacetate and acetyl-CoA. The reaction involves —C—C— bond cleavage.
4. In another pathway, acetoacetate is formed from aceto acetyl-CoA by deacylation. The reaction is catalyzed by thiol esterase.
5. β-hydroxy butyrate is formed from acetoacetate on reduction. The reaction is catalyzed by NADH-dependent dehydrogenase.
6. Non-enzymatic decarboxylation of aceto acetate produces acetone.

   Ketogenic amino acids contributes ketone bodies. Reactions of ketogenesis are shown in Figure 10.11.

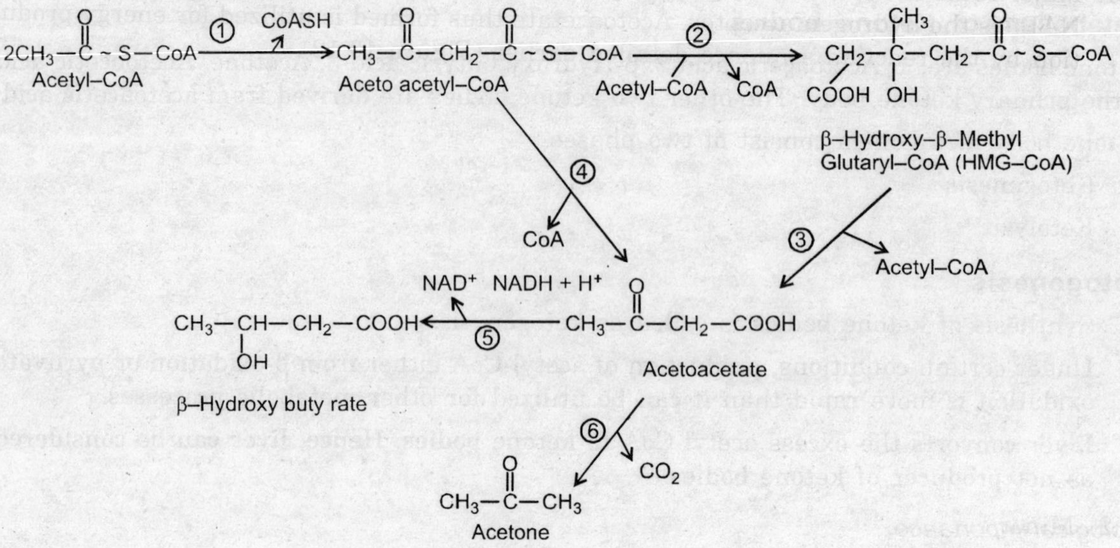

Fig. 10.11 Ketogenesis reactions sequence

Ketolysis

1. Degradation of ketone bodies is called as ketolysis.
2. Ketone bodies produced in liver reaches peripheral tissues through circulation.
3. Heart, kidney cortex, brain and to some extent skeletal muscle uses ketone bodies for energy production.

Biological importance

1. Heart and kidney cortex prefers to use ketone bodies rather than glucose. During prolonged starvation, brain derives most of energy from ketone bodies.
2. Liver is unable to use ketone bodies due to lack of enzymes.

Reaction sequence of acetoacetate utilization

Activation of acetoacetate is the first step for its utilization. There are two ways for the acetoacetate activation.

1. Acetoacetate is activated by acetoacetyl-CoA synthetase in presence of ATP, Mg^{2+} and CoA to acetoacetyl-CoA. This reaction is similar to fatty acid activation. AMP and PP_i are produced.
2. Acetoacetate activation in another route involves transfer of CoA-SH from succinyl-CoA in presence of enzyme succinyl-CoA: acetoacetate CoA transferase or thiophorase to aceto acetate. Product of this reaction is aceto acetyl-CoA.
3. Thiolase cleaves aceto acetyl-CoA to two molecules of acetyl-CoA. The acetyl-CoAs are subsequently oxidized by citric acid cycle. Steps involved in utilization of acetoacetate are shown in Figure-10.12.

β-Hydroxy butyrate utilization

There are two ways for the utilization of β-Hydroxy butyrate.

1. Major route is the conversion of β-Hydroxy butyrate to acetoacetate by dehydrogenase. NAD^+ is the hydrogen acceptor. Acetoacetate thus formed is utilized for energy production by the reaction sequence detailed earlier (Figure 10.12).

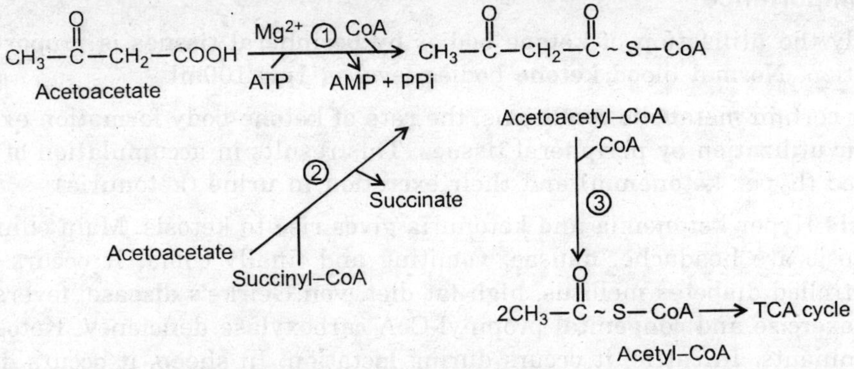

Fig. 10.12 Reactions of acetoacetate utilization

2. Minor route is the direct activation of β-hydroxy butyrate by synthetase to β-hydroxy butyryl-CoA followed by dehydrogenation to acetoacetyl-CoA, which is catalyzed by dehydrogenase (Figure 10.13).

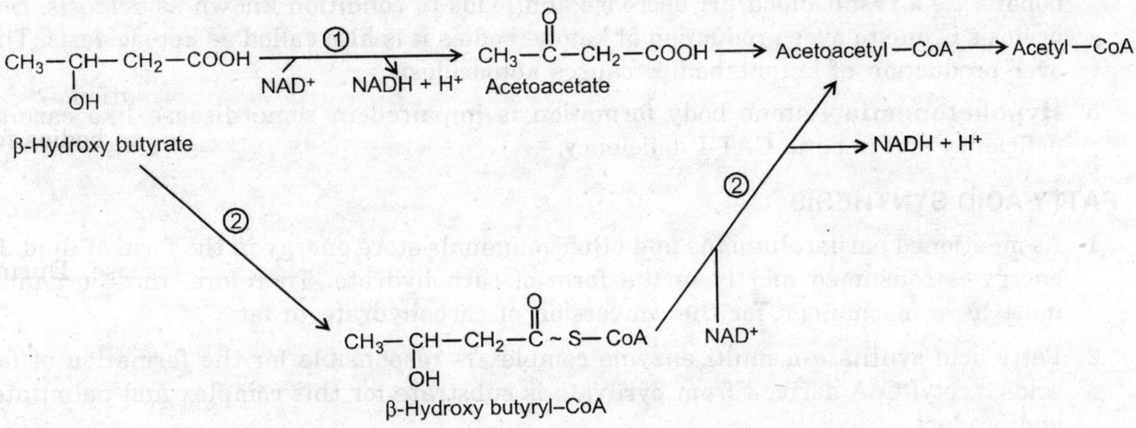

Fig. 10.13 Reactions of β-hydroxybutyrate utilization

Utilization of Acetone

Utilization of acetone by extra hepatic tissue is slow. It is removed by excretion in urine and as CO_2 through lungs.

Regulation of ketogenesis

There are several ways for regulation of Ketogenesis

1. Mobilization of free fatty acids from adipose tissue controls ketogenesis. Any condition that increases mobilization of fat increase ketone body formation.
2. Liver carnitine-acyl transferase-I activity determines rate of ketone body formation. Under fed conditions, CAT activity is inhibited by malonyl-CoA. Hence, ketogenesis is decreased due to less acetyl-CoA. During starvation, CAT-I activity is high due to low malonyl-CoA. Hence, ketogenesis is more due to plenty of acetyl-CoA.

3. ATP level in the cell controls ketogenesis. More ATP level favours ketogenesis whereas low ATP level prevents ketogenesis.

Medical Importance

1. Usually the utilization of ketone bodies by peripheral tissues is proportional to their formation. Normal blood ketone bodies level is 1mg/100ml.
2. Under certain metabolic conditions, the rate of ketone body formation exceeds the rate of their utilization by peripheral tissues. This results in accumulation of ketone bodies in blood (hyper ketonemia) and their excretion in urine (ketonuria).
3. **Ketosis** Hyper ketonemia and ketonuria gives rise to ketosis. Main clinical symptoms of ketosis are headache, nausae, vomiting and finally coma. It occurs in starvation, uncontrolled diabetes mellitus, high fat diet, von Geirke's disease, fevers, severe muscular exercise and congenital propinyl-CoA carboxylase deficiency. Ketosis also occurs in ruminants. In cattle, it occurs during lactation. In sheep, it occurs due to toxemia of pregnancy.
4. **Ketoacidosis** Under normal conditions, ketone bodies acetoacetate and β-hydroxy butyrate are neutralized by blood bicarbonate to maintain constant blood pH. Their formation in large quantities in starvation and diabetes causes depletion of blood bicarbonate. As a result blood pH decrease and leads to condition known as *acidosis*. Since acidosis is due to over production of ketone bodies it is also called as ketoacidosis. Thus, over production of ketone bodies causes ketoacidosis.
5. **Hypoketonemia** Ketone body formation is impaired in some disease like carnitine deficiency and hepatic CAT-I deficiency.

FATTY ACID SYNTHESIS

1. As mentioned earlier, humans and other mammals store energy in the form of lipid. But energy is consumed mostly in the form of carbohydrate. Therefore, these organisms must have mechanism for the conversion of carbohydrate to fat.
2. Fatty acid synthase a multi enzyme complex is responsible for the formation of fatty acids, acetyl-CoA derived from pyruvate is substrate for this complex and palmitate is end product.
3. Fatty acids are formed by the condensation of two carbon units. This condensation involves $-\overset{|}{\underset{|}{C}}-\overset{|}{\underset{|}{C}}-$ bond formation. So, fatty acid formation is the reversal of β-oxidation. However, enzymes are different for two processes.
4. Existence of two separate sets of enzymes for synthesis and degradation of fatty acids allows reciprocal regulation and prevents simultaneous operation of these pathways.
5. NADPH required for the formation of fatty acids is provided by HMP shunt, malic enzyme and isocitrate dehydrogenase.
6. **Site** Fatty acid synthesis occurs in the cytosol of liver, kidneys, brain, lung, adipose tissue and mammary gland.
7. Cytosolic synthesis of fatty is called as *de novo (total) synthesis* of fatty acids.

Transport of acetyl-CoA

1. Acetyl-CoA, which is the building block of fatty acids, is produced in the mitochondria from pyruvate. But acetyl-CoA is not permeable to mitochondrial membrane and hence it can not enter cytosol, which is the site of fatty acid synthesis.
2. The transport of acetyl-CoA into cytosol is achieved in a circuitous manner. The acetyl-CoA enters cytosol in the form of citrate, which is freely permeable.
3. Acetyl-CoA is converted to citrate by citrate synthase of citric acid cycle.
4. Tricarboxylate transporter present in mitochondrial membrane transports citrate into cytosol.
5. Acetyl-CoA is regenerated from citrate in the cytosol by ATP: citrate lyase cofactors are ATP and CoA.
6. Oxaloacetate formed in the above reaction is reduced to malate by NADH-dependent cytosolic malate dehydrogenase.
7. Cytosolic malic enzyme converts malate to pyruvate in $NADP^+$, dependent reaction. NADPH produced in this reaction is used for fatty acid synthesis. Therefore, acetyl-CoA transport from mitochondria to cytosol indirectly provides NADPH required for fatty acid synthesis.
8. To complete the circuit, pyruvate generated in the above reaction re-enters mitochondria. Acetyl-CoA transport is shown in Figure 10.14.

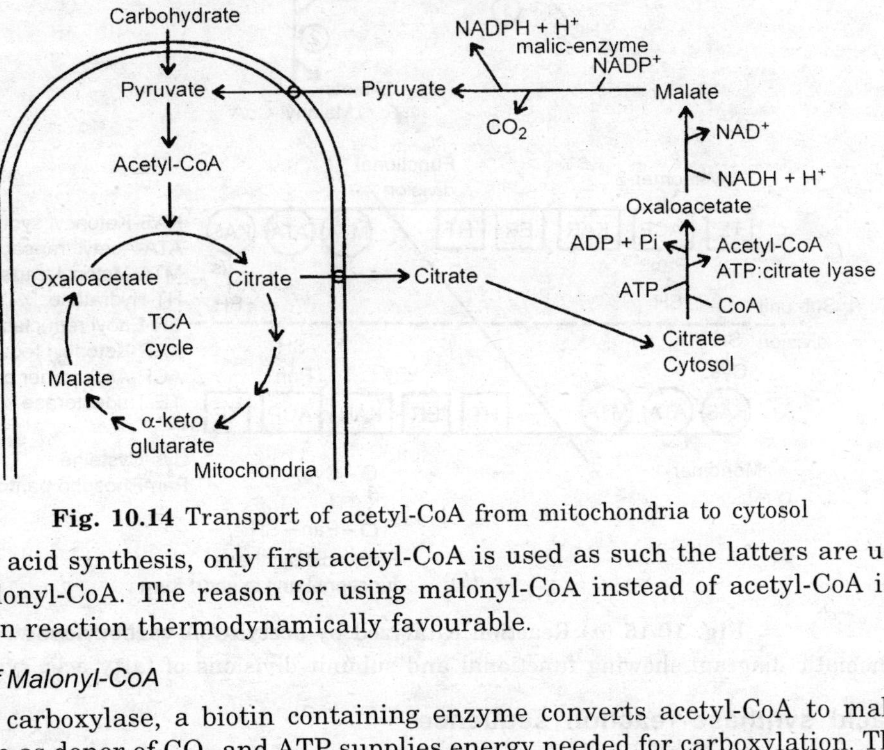

Fig. 10.14 Transport of acetyl-CoA from mitochondria to cytosol

In the fatty acid synthesis, only first acetyl-CoA is used as such the latters are used in the form of malonyl-CoA. The reason for using malonyl-CoA instead of acetyl-CoA is to make condensation reaction thermodynamically favourable.

Formation of Malonyl-CoA

Acetyl-CoA carboxylase, a biotin containing enzyme converts acetyl-CoA to malonyl-CoA. HCO_3^- serve as donor of CO_2 and ATP supplies energy needed for carboxylation. The enzyme is a multimeric protein. It contains biotin, biotin carboxyl carrier protein, transcarboxylase and regulatory site. The reaction occurs in two steps.

1. In presence of ATP, first biotin of biotinyl enzyme is carboxylated.
2. Transfer of carboxyl to acetyl-CoA to form malonyl-CoA occurs in second step and biotinyl enzyme is formed (Figure 10.15*a*). Acetyl-CoA carboxylase is regulatory enzyme of fatty acid synthesis.

Fatty acid synthase complex

1. Mammalian fatty acid synthase complex is a dimer consisting of two monomers.
2. Each monomer contain an acyl carrier protein (ACP), 7 different enzymes and two free-SH groups.
3. Two-SH groups are contributed by cysteine residue of a monomer at one end phospho pantotheine of ACP at the other end.
4. Further cysteine-SH of one monomer is in close proximity to phosphopantotheine-SH of other monomer indicating head to tail arrangement of monomers.
5. Individual monomers are not active only dimer is active.
6. Functional unit consist of one half a monomer interacting with complementary half of the other monomer. Hence, only dimer is active and two fatty acids are produced simultaneously. Organization of fatty acid synthase complex is shown in Figure 10.15*b*.

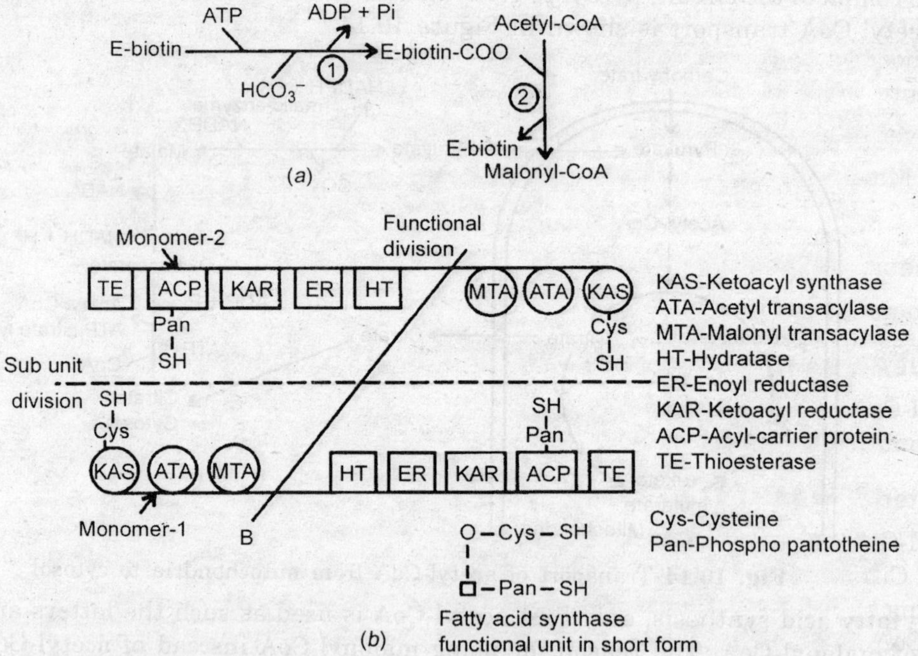

Fig. 10.15 (*a*) Reaction catalyzed by acetyl-CoA carboxylase
(*b*) Schematic diagram showing functional and subunit divisions of fatty acid synthase complex

Fatty acid synthase reaction sequence

1. Transfer of a molecule of acetyl-CoA to -cys-SH group of one of the monomer by acetyl trans acylase is the initial reaction of fatty acid synthesis.

2. Likewise malonyl transacylase catalyzes the transfer of a malonyl-CoA to-pan-SH group of the other monomer in this reaction.
3. A condensing enzyme β-keto acyl synthase catalyzes first —C—C— bond formation between carbonyl of acetyl residue and α-carbon of malonyl residue in the third reaction. In this special condensation reaction, acetyl group attacks methyl group of malonyl residue to form β-keto acyl residue on-pan-S-. As a result-cys-SH group occupied by acetyl residue becomes free. Further, the condensation is accompanied by release of CO_2, which drags the reaction towards C—C bond synthesis.
4. Reduction of β-keto acyl residue by β-keto acyl reductase to β-hydroxy acyl residue is the fourth reaction. NADPH is the hydrogen donor.
5. In the next step, hydratase (dehydratase) removes one water molecule from β-hydroxy acyl residue to form α, β-unsaturated acyl enzyme.
6. Another NADPH-dependent reduction reaction converts α,β-unsaturated acyl enzyme to butyryl enzyme. The reaction is catalyzed by enoyl reductase.

For the synthesis of 16-carbon palmityl residue reactions from 2 to 6 are repeated six times. One malonyl-CoA and 2 NADPH are utilized in each reaction sequence (Figure 10.16).

7. Release of palmityl residue from multi enzyme complex by the last enzyme thioesterase of the enzyme complex is the final reaction of fatty acid biosynthesis.

   Fatty acid synthase complex can not generate fatty acid other than palmitic acid because thioesterase is less active on other fatty acids and-cys-SH of the complex can not hold more than 14 carbon atoms.

   Overall equation for palmitic acid synthesis is

$$7\text{ Malonyl-CoA} + \text{Acetyl-CoA} + 14\text{NADPH} + 14\text{H}^+ \longrightarrow \text{Palmitic acid} + 7\text{CO}_2 + 14\text{NADP}^+ + 6\text{H}_2\text{O} + 8\text{CoA}$$

Synthesis of fatty acids with odd number carbons

Ruminants contain C_{15}-C_{17} fatty acids. They are synthesized from propionyl-CoA.

REGULATION OF FATTY ACID SYNTHESIS

Acetyl-CoA carboxylase activity regulates fatty acid biosynthesis. It is under allosteric and hormonal control.

Allosteric regulation

Acetyl-CoA carboxylase exist in two forms. An inactive protomer form and active polymer form. Citrate is the allosteric activator and long chain acyl-CoA is the allosteric inhibitor. Binding of citrate to monomer converts inactive form to active form. In contrast, long chain acyl-CoA and malonyl-CoA prevents polymerization of monomer to active form. Usually, the activity of acetyl-CoA carboxylase is inversely related to plasma-free fatty acid level. Any condition that increases free fatty acid (Acyl-CoA) level inhibits fatty acid biosynthesis. Thus, in starvation, high fat diet and diabetes fatty acid synthesis is diminished.

Hormonal regulation

Glucagon inhibits fatty acid synthesis by inhibiting acetyl-CoA carboxylase. It increases cAMP mediated phosphorylation that converts active acetyl-CoA carboxylase to inactive

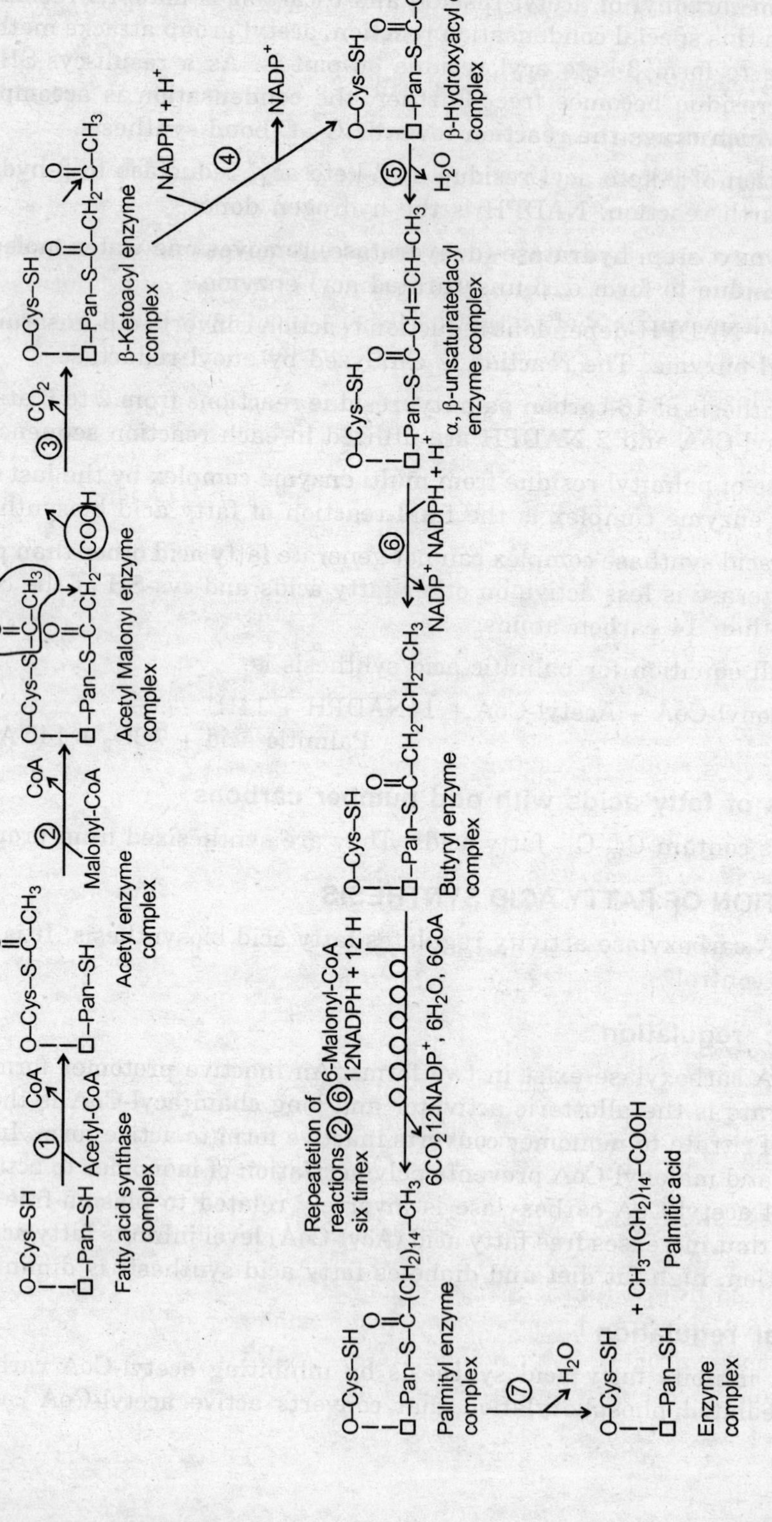

Fig. 10.16 Reaction sequence of fatty acid synthase complex ↓ indicates —C—C— bond formation.

acetyl-CoA carboxylase. In contrast, insulin favours fatty acid synthesis by activating acetyl-CoA carboxylase. It promotes fatty acid synthesis by

1. Decreasing cAMP.
2. Increasing phosphatase activity that converts inactive acetyl-CoA carboxylase to active form.
3. By increasing the availability of glucose.

Medical Importance

1. Few of the drugs used in the treatment of obesity work by inhibiting fatty acid synthesis.
2. **Hydroxy citrate is one such drug** ATP citrate lyase is the target of its action. In presence of hydroxy citrate, the enzyme can not act on its natural substrate citrate. As a result, availability of acetyl-CoA for fatty acid synthesis is impaired. Garcinia cambogia (malabar tamarind) contains hydroxy citrate.
3. In malarial parasite, fatty acid synthesis is brought about fatty acid synthesis system type-II in which reactions of the pathway are catalyzed by independent enzymes. This is different from that of host in which multi-enzyme complex of fatty acid synthase system type-I is involved in fatty acid synthesis. It is of great pharmacological importance. It allows development of new drugs for treatment of malaria, which act by blocking action of each of independent enzyme of parasite fatty acid synthesis. Triclosan and cerulenin are inhibitors of enoyl reductase and ketoacyl synthase, respectively. They are effective in killing malarial parasite in *in vitro and in vivo.*

Reciprocal regulation of fatty acid oxidation and synthesis

1. Fatty acid oxidation and synthesis are two opposite processes. Their simultaneous occurrence results in wasting of cellular resources.
2. In fed conditions, malonyl-CoA formation is increased due to activation of acetyl-CoA carboxylase by citrate. Malonyl-CoA inhibits CAT-I activity. As a result, fatty acid oxidation is decreased. Therefore, under fed conditions fatty acid synthesis is promoted and fatty acid oxidation is inhibited.
3. In starvation, diabetes and high fat diet consumption raised plasma acyl-CoA inhibit fatty acid synthesis by inactivating acetyl-CoA carboxylase. Less of malonyl-CoA formation due to inactivation of acetyl-CoA carboxylase stimulates CAT-I activity. This results in more fatty acid oxidation. Therefore, under above mentioned conditions, fatty acid synthesis is inhibited and at the same time fatty acid oxidation is favoured.
4. Thus, malonyl-CoA is the reciprocal regulator of fatty acid oxidation and fatty acid synthesis.

Fatty acid chain elongation

Since fatty acid synthase produces only palmitic acid, stearic and other long-chain fatty acids are produced from palmitic acid in endoplasmic reticulum by addition of two carbon atoms. Malonyl-CoA serves as donor of two-carbon fragment. Elongation process also requires NADPH as donor of hydrogen. Intermediates of the elongation process are CoA thioesters, which makes this process different from fatty acid synthesis. The reactions involved in elongation are shown in Figure 10.17. In most of the tissues, this process stops with formation of stearyl-CoA. However, in the brain, stearyl-CoA can be elongated to C_{24} fatty acids.

Mitochondria has another chain elongation system. Though it is not a major route for the synthesis of long chain fatty acids from palmitic acid, it is effective in converting short and medium chain fatty acids to long chain fatty acids. It requires acetyl-CoA and NAD (P) H.

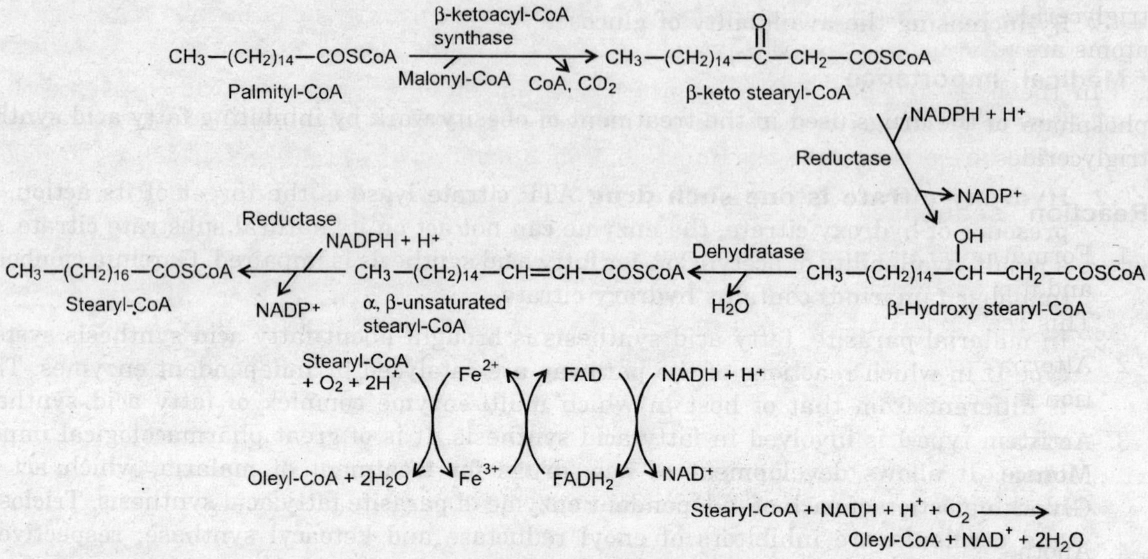

Fig. 10.17 (*a*) Fatty acid elongation
(*b*) Δ^9-desaturase system

UNSATURATED FATTY ACID BIOSYNTHESIS

In animals Δ^9-desaturase system of liver microsomes is responsible for the formation of oleyl-CoA from stearyl-CoA. It consist of $cyth_5$ and two enzymes. They are NADH-$cytb_5$ reductase and desaturase (Figure 10.17*b*). However, animals lack enzyme system that can introduce double bonds beyond C-9 of fatty acid. Hence, they can not synthesize linoleic, linolenic and arachidonic acid. But animals have an endoplasmic reticular system, which can create double bonds between existing double bond and carboxyl end. Thus, animals can synthesize only arachidonic acid from linoleic acid and are unable to synthesize linoleic acid from oleic acid (Figure 10.18).

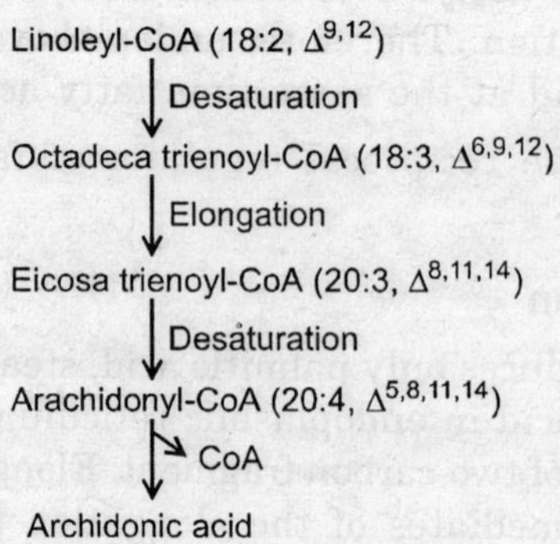

Fig. 10.18 Biosynthesis of arachidonic acid

TRIGLYCERIDE METABOLISM

Triglyceride biosynthesis

It occurs in the liver, adipose tissue and intestine of non-ruminants. Triglycerides synthesized in liver and intestine are transported to other tissues where as in adipose tissue triglycerides are stored. Both saturated and unsaturated fatty acids having 16-18 carbon atoms are used for triglycerides formation after activation. They are used in the CoA form.

In the liver, triglyceride are synthesized from either free glycerol, dihydroxyacetone phosphate of glycolysis or both. In the adipose tissue from dihydroxyacetone, phosphate triglycerides are produced. In the intestine, from 2-monoacylglycerol triglycerides are formed.

Reaction sequence

1. Formation of glycerol-3-phosphate from dihydroxy acetone phosphate is the first step and it is catalyzed by glycerol-3-phosphate dehydrogenase. NADH is the hydrogen donor. This reaction occurs in liver and adipose tissue.
2. Alternatively, in the liver glycerol-3-phosphate is formed from free glycerol. The reaction is catalyzed by glycerokinase. ATP and Mg^{2+} are required.
3. Activated fatty acid is incorporated into glycerol-3-phosphate in this reaction. Monoacylglycerol-3-phosphate or lysophosphatidate is the product of the reaction. Glycerophosphate acyl transferase catalyzes this reaction.
4. Another molecule of fatty acid is transferred to 2-carbon of lyso phosphatidate by monoacyl glycerol-3-phosphate acyl transferase to form phosphatidate. Phosphatidate is required for compound lipid synthesis also.
5. 1, 2-diacyl glycerol is generated from phosphatidate by removing phosphate. The reaction is catalyzed by phosphatase an hydrolase.
6. In the intestine 1, 2-diacyl glycerol is formed from monoacyl glycerol by the transfer of fatty acid. The reaction is catalyzed by monoacyl glycerol acyl transferase.
7. Further esterification of 1, 2-diacyl glycerol with another molecule of fatty acid at 3-carbon hydroxyl group result in the formation of trigyceride. The reaction is catalyzed by 1,2- diacyl glycerol acyl transferase. Reaction sequence of triglyceride biosynthesis is shown in Figure 10.19. Reactions 1,2 occurs in cytosol and remaining reactions occur in endoplasmic reticulum.

Medical importance

1. Diet influences the type of fat produced in adipose tissue. Carbohydrate or starchy diets produce hard fat where as diets rich is peanut oil or corn oil produce soft fat.
2. Triglyceride formation is marked in well fed state and decreased in starvation, diabetes. High fat diet also decreases fat formation.
3. Usually triglyceride biosynthesis is directly related to fatty acid biosynthesis.

FAT MOBILIZATION OR TRIGLYCERIDE DEGRADATION OR LIPOLYSIS

Medical importance

1. Triglycerides stored in adipose tissue are degraded when there is stress or in energy deficient conditions like starvation or diabetes.

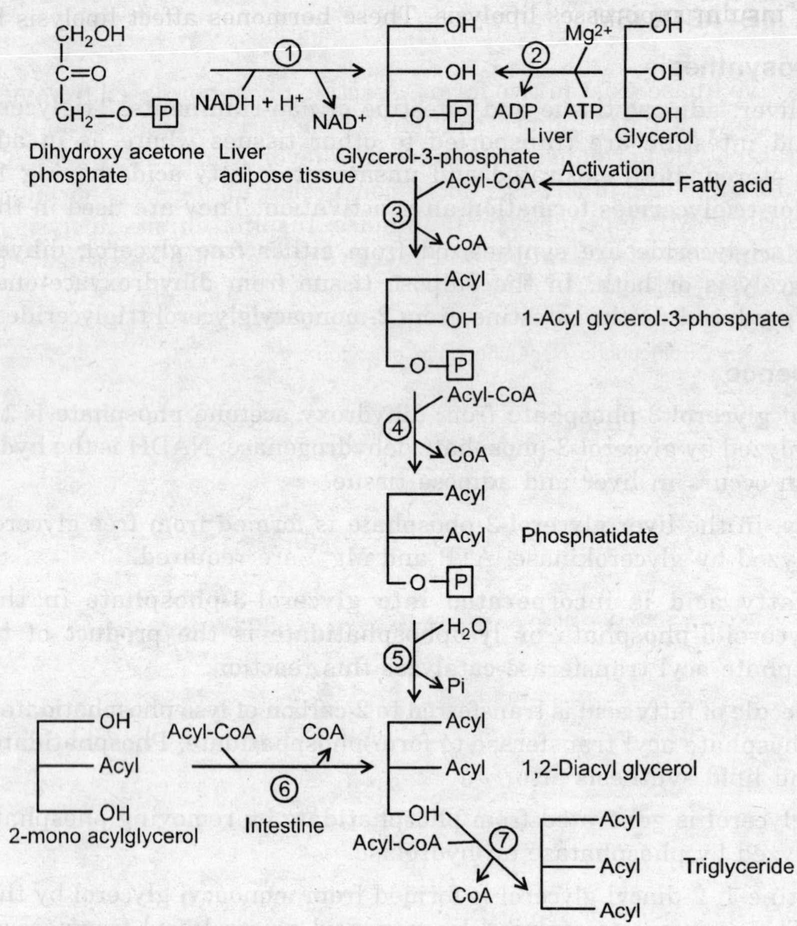

Fig. 10.19 Reaction sequence of triglyceride biosynthesis

Reaction sequence

1. Hormone sensitive lipase present in adipose tissue converts triglycerids to di or monoglycerides and fatty acids.
2. Additional di or monoglyceride lipase converts mono or diglyceride to free fatty acids and glycerol (Figure 10.20).

Fate of free fatty acids and glycerol

1. The free fatty acids are released into circulation. They reach other tissues after combining with plasma albumin. Most of them are used for energy production in peripheral tissues. Liver converts them into ketone bodies($^1/_3$).
2. The glycerol is also released into circulation because adipose tissue cannot utilize glycerol. Glucose is formed from glycerol in liver.

Action of hormones on lipolysis

Triglyceride breakdown in adipose tissue is under hormonal control. Hormones like epinephrine, nor epinephrine, glucagon, ACTH, MSH, TSH and growth hormone favours lipolysis where as insulin suppresses lipolysis. These hormones affect lipolysis by altering cAMP level.

Hormones sensitive lipase exist in two forms. A active phosphorylated from and in active dephosphorylated form. cAMP depend proteinkinase-A converts in active form to active form by phosphorylation. Lipolytic hormones increases cAMP level by activating adenylate cyclase. This inturn leads to increased lipolysis due to conversion of inactive hormone sensitive lipase to active form by cAMP dependent proteinkinase. Insulin inhibits lipolysis by decreasing cAMP level. Mechanism of activation and inactivation of hormone sensitive lipase by hormones is shown in Fig. 10.20.

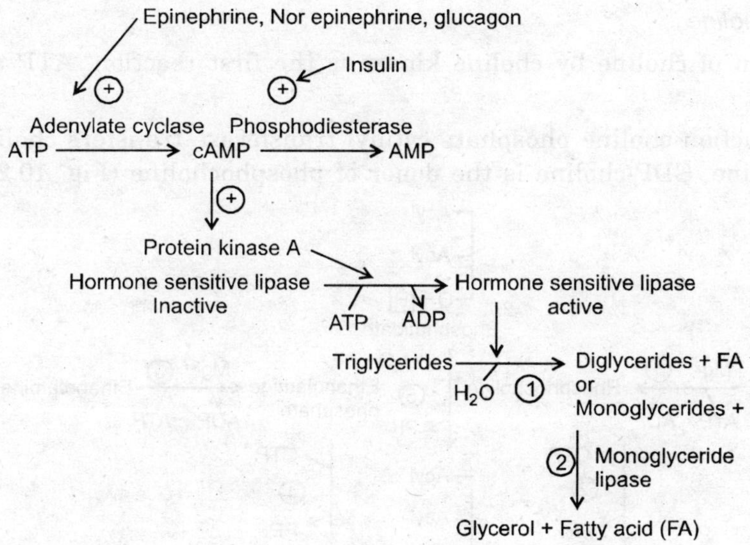

Fig. 10.20 Action of hormone sensitive lipase and lipolysis reaction sequence

Medical importance

1. Under stressful conditions or starvation, hormones like epinephrine and glucagon are released. They stimulate lipolysis to meet energy requirement of the tissues.
2. In diabetes lack of insulin causes increased lipolysis.
3. In pheochromocytoma plasma free fatty acid level is increased due to increased lipolysis.

BIOSYNTHESIS OF COMPOUND LIPIDS

Major compound lipids present in mammalian membranes are phospholipids and glycolipids.

Phospholipid Biosynthesis

Phosphatidyl choline or lecithin, phosphatidyl ethanolamine or cephalin and sphingo myelins are major components of human cell membrane. Cardiolipin is another important phospholipid of mitochondrial membrane. Phosphatidyl inositol is one of the phospholipid whose importance in signal transduction has been established recently.

Biosynthesis of lecithin and cephalin

1. It occurs in liver and adipose tissue.

2. Phosphatidic acid serves as precursor for the synthesis of lecithin and cephalin. It is the major route for the synthesis of these lipids.
3. Nitrogenous bases are activated prior to their incorporation into phospholipids. Activation occurs in the cytosol.

Formation of activated nitrogenous bases

Activated nitrogenous bases required for lecithin and cephalin formation are CDP-choline and CDP-ethanolamine.

REACTIONS OF LECITHIN AND CEPHALIN BIOSYNTHESIS

Synthesis of CDP-Choline

1. Phosphorylation of choline by choline kinase is the first reaction. ATP and Mg^{2+} are other cofactors.
2. In the next reaction choline phosphate cytidyl transferase transfers choline to CTP to form CDP-choline. CDP-choline is the donor of phosphocholine (Fig. 10.21).

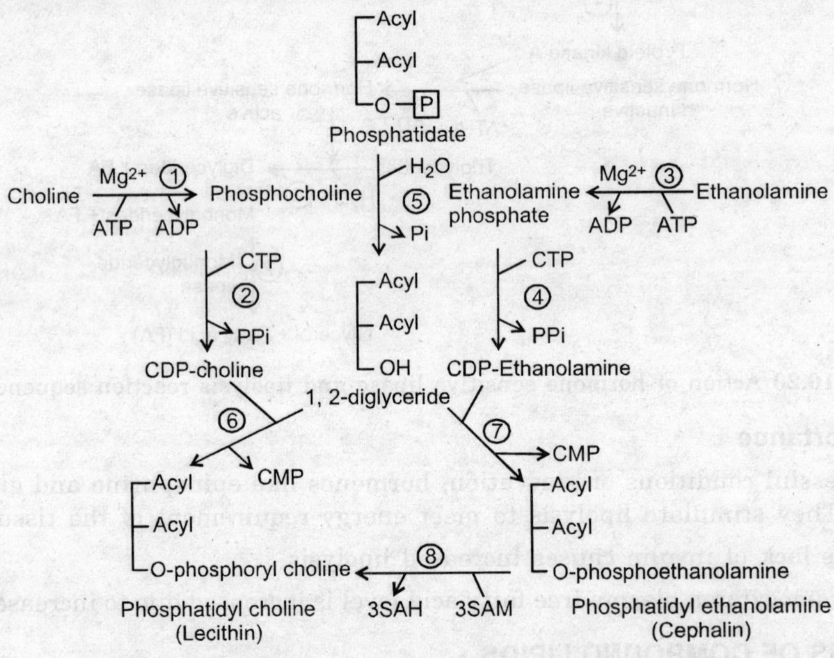

Fig. 10.21 Reactions of lecithin and cephalin biosynthesis

Synthesis of CDP-Ethanolamine

Formation of CDP-ethanolamine also involves initial phosphorylation followed by transfer of ethanolamine phosphate to CTP. Reactions 3 and 4 in Fig. 10.21. Ethanolamine kinase catalyzes reaction 3 and phosphoethanolamine cytidyltransferase catalyzes reaction 4.

Synthesis of lecithin

5. 1, 2- diglyceride formed from phosphatidic acid by the action of phosphatase is used for the formation of lecithin. The reaction occurs in endophasmic reticulum.

6. Transfer of phosphocholine from CDP choline results in the formation of phosphatidyl choline or lecithin. The reaction is catalyzed by phosphocholine transferase and CMP is released. The enzyme is localized in endoplasmic reticulum.

Synthesis of cephalin

7. Transfer of phosphoethanolamine from CDP-ethanolamine to 1,2-diglyceride results in the formation of phosphatidyl ethanolamine or cephalin. The reaction is catalyzed by phosphoryl ethanolamine transferase and CMP is released.

Synthesis of lecithin from cephalin

8. Lecithin may be formed from cephalin by using S-adenosyl methionine as methyl source. The reaction is catalyzed by methyl transferase. Biosynthetic reactions of lecithin and cephalin are shown in Fig. 10.21.

Biosynthesis of cardiolipin and phosphatidyl inositol

Phosphatidic acid serves as starting material for the synthesis of cardiolipin and phosphatidyl inositol. CDP-diglyceride is an important intermediate in this synthesis (Fig. 10.22).

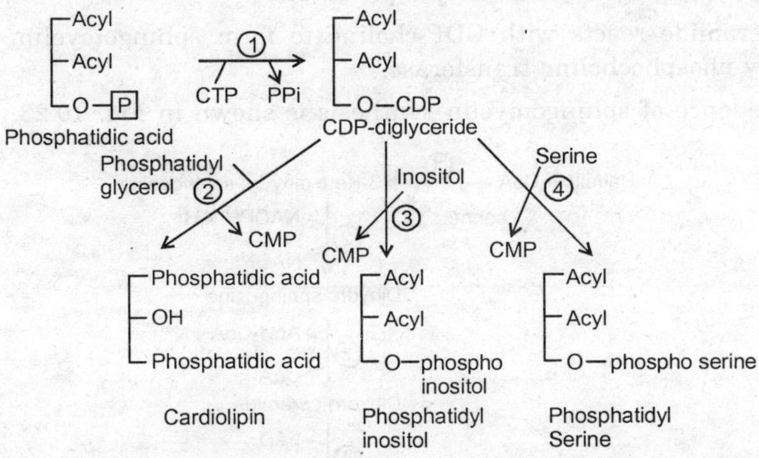

Fig. 10.22 Reactions of cardiolipin, phosphatidyl inositol and phosphatidyl serine biosynthesis

Reactions of this biosynthetic Pathway

1. Formation of CDP-diglyceride from phosphatidic acid is the first reaction of the pathway. It is catalyzed by CTP phosphatidate cytidyl transferase.
2. CDP-diglyceride reacts with phoshatidyl glycerol to form cardiolipin. CMP is released. Reaction is catalyzed by a transferase.
3. Transfer of inositol to 1,2-diglyceride generates phosphatidyl inositol. The reaction is catalyzed by inositol transferase.
4. Phosphatidyl serine is also formed from 1, 2-diglycearide by the transfer of serine (Fig. 10.22).

Biosynthesis of sphingomyelin

1. Enzymes involved in sphingomyelin synthesis are present in endoplasmic reticulum and golgi complex.

2. Sphingosine required for sphingomyelin (other sphingolipid) biosynthesis is formed from palmitoyl-CoA and serine in the form dihydrosphingosine.
3. Ceramide is an important intermediate of sphingolipid formation.

Reaction sequence of sphingomyelin formation

First four reactions occur in endoplasmic reticuluim and final reaction occurs in golgi complex.

1. In the first step palmitoyl-CoA condenses with serine. The reaction is catalyzed by 3-keto dihydrosphingosine synthase enzyme. 3-keto dihydro sphingosine is the product of this reaction and CO_2 is released.
2. Reduction of 3-keto dihydrosphingosine by NADPH dependent reductase produces dihydrosphingosine in the second reaction. $NADP^+$ is formed.
3. Acyl transferase catalyzes the transfer of acyl group from acyl-CoA to N-atom of dihydrosphingosine in the next reaction. Dihydroceramide is the product of this reaction.
4. FAD dependent dehydrogenation of dihydroceramide produces ceramide. The reaction is catalyzed by dehydrogenase. $FADH_2$ is produced.
5. Now the ceramide reacts with CDP-choline to form sphingomyelin. The reaction is catalyzed by phosphocholine transferase.

Reaction sequence of sphingomyelin synthesis is shown in Fig. 10.23.

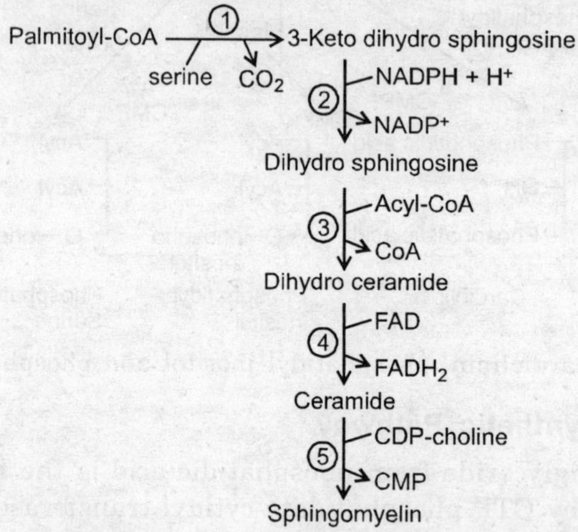

Fig. 10.23 Reaction sequence of sphingomyelin biosynthesis

Biosynthesis of glycolipids

1. Caramide is the starting material for the formation of cerebrosides, sulfolipids and gangliosides.
2. Enzymes of glycolipid synthesis are present in golgi complex.
3. They are formed by the stepwise addition of sugars or sulfate to the ceramide. Activated sugars or sugar derivatives act as donors of sugar. Active sulfate serves as donor of sulfate.

Synthesis of cerebrosides and sulfatides

UDP-galactose serves as donor of galactose. PAPS serve as donor of sulfate.

1. Galactosyl transferase catalyzes the transfer of galactose to ceramide to form galactocerebroside.
2. A galacto sulfatide is formed from galactocerebroside by reacting with PAPS which donates sulfate. The reaction is catalyzed by sulfokinase and PAP is released (Figure 10.24*a*).

Synthesis of gangliosides

1. Gangliosides are formed ceramide by stepwise addition of activated sugars like UDP-glucose, UDP-galactose, CMP-NANA and UDP- N-acetyl galactosamine. Pathway for the formation of gangliosides is shown schematically in Figure 10.24*b*.
2. Glycosyltransferases present in golgi complex are involved in the transfer of sugars from nucleotides.

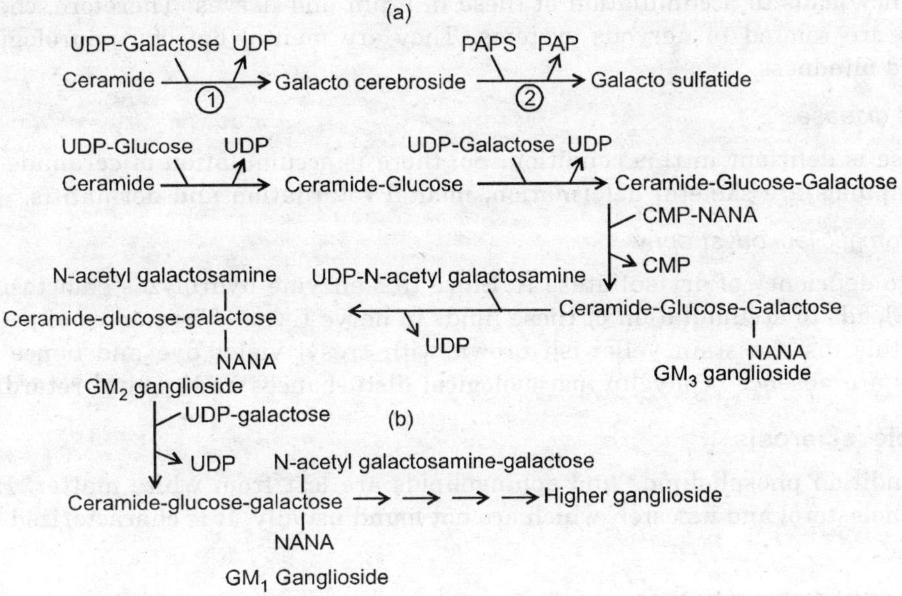

Fig. 10.24 (*a*) Reactions of cerebrosides and sulfatides biosynthesis
(*b*) Biosynthetic pathway of gangliosides

Medical Importance

Several diseases are due to impaired metabolism of compound lipids.

A. Lipid storage diseases or lipidoses

Under normal conditions, synthesis and degradation of compound lipids is well balanced. Deficiency or lack of enzymes of their degradation causes accumulation of these lipids in tissues. Abnormal accumulation of compound lipids in various tissues lead to lipidoses or lipid storage diseases. They are all inherited. Some of them are mentioned below.

1. Gaucher's disease

It is due to deficiency of β-glucosidase. Since this enzyme is involved in the breakdown of glucocerebroside. Its deficiency leads to accumulation of glucocerebrosides in liver and spleen. Therefore, the characteristic symptoms are enlarged liver and spleen.

2. Krabbe's disease

Galactocerebrosidase is deficient in this condition. Accumulation of galactocerebrosides, mental retardation and absence of myelin are the symptoms.

3. Neimann-Pick disease

It is due to defective sphingomyelinase. So, sphingomyelin accumulates in liver and spleen. As a result, spleen and liver are enlarged. It is a serious condition and usually occurs in infancy and causes death in few months.

4. Tay-Sachs disease

Hexosaminidase A is deficient in this disease. Since this enzyme degrades GM_2 gangliosides. Its deficiency leads to accumulation of these in brain and nerves. Therefore, characteristic symptoms are related to nervous systems. They are mental defects, neurological disturbances and blindness.

5. Farber's disease

Ceramidase is deficient in this condition. So, there is accumulation of ceramide in tissues. Other symptoms are skeletal deformation, mental retardation and dermatitis.

6. Metachromatic leukodystrophy

It is due to deficiency of arylsulfatase A. Since this enzyme hydrolyzes galactosulftides, its deficiency leads to accumulation of these lipids in nerve tissue. The nerves of people suffering form this disease stain yellowish brown with cresyl violet dye and hence the name. Symptoms are absence of myelin, psychological disturbances and mental retardation.

B. Multiple sclerosis

In this condition phospholipids and sphingolipids are lost from white matter. However, it contains cholesterol and its ester, which are not found usually. It is characterized by absence of myelin.

LIPOPROTEIN METABOLISM

Metabolism of chylomicrons

Synthesis

1. In the smooth endoplasmic reticulum of intestinal mucosal cells trigly cerides (TG) and cholesterol (C) formed from dietary fat are coated with phospholipids (PL) and apoA-I, A-II and apo B-48 to generate chylomicrons.
2. These chylomicrons then emerge from enterocyte into lymphatics.
3. Chylomicron that enters lymphatics from intestine is called as *nascent chylomicron*.
4. Through the thoracic duct nascent chylomicrons enters blood.
5. In the circulation nascent chylomicrons combines with apo C and apo E to form mature chylomicrons.

Degradation

1. Mature chylomicrons are rapidly removed from circulation by extra-hepatic tissues.
2. Half-life of plasma chylomicron is less than an hour in humans.
3. Lipoprotein lipase present in the walls of blood capillaries attacks triglycerides of mature chylomicrons.
4. The enzyme is anchored to capillary wall through heparin sulfate.
5. Apo C-II and phosphlipids are required for its activity.
6. Hydrolysis occurs when chylomicron binds to the enzyme on the endothelium. Apo C-II promotes binding of chylomicron to the enzyme.
7. Triglycerides are hydrolyzed to glycerol (G) and free fatty acids (FFA). Most of the fatty acids released are taken up by peripheral tissues.
8. Action of lipoprotein lipase on chylomicrons results in the loss of 90% of triglycerides, apo A, apo C and small amounts of phospholipids.
9. The size of the mature chylomicron is reduced to half and it is called as *chylomicron remnant*.
10. The chylomicron remnants are taken up by liver through apo E receptors.
11. In the liver, remaining triglycerides and cholesterol ester (if any) are hydrolyzed and metabolized.
12. Lipoprotein lipase is also found in heart, adipose tissue, spleen, lung, renal medulla, aorta, diaphram and lactating mammary gland. However, it is absent in liver. Further, the affinity of the enzyme depends on its origin. For example, heart enzyme is ten times more active than adipose tissue enzyme. Lactating mammary gland lipoprotein lipase plays an important role in the secretion of triglycerides into milk. In Fig. 10.25, steps involved in the synthesis and degradation of chylomicrons are shown.

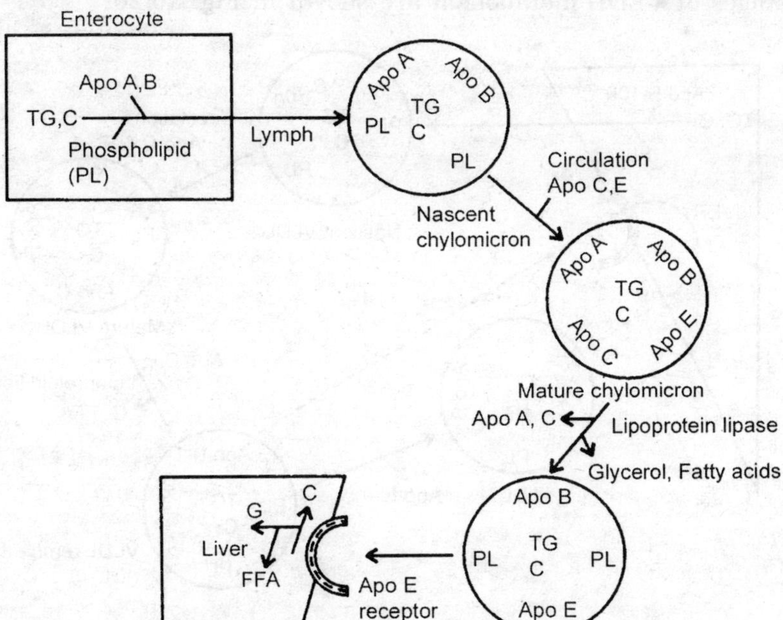

Fig. 10.25 Synthesis and degradation of chylomicrons

Metabolism of VLDL

Synthesis

1. Liver mainly synthesizes VLDL.
2. In hepatocytes, synthesized triglycerides combines with phospholipids, cholesterol and apo B-100 to generate VLDL.
3. This VLDL is called as *nascent* VLDL.
4. Nascent VLDL are secreted into hepatic sinusoids and from there they enters circulation.
5. Addition of apo C and apo E in the circulation generates mature VLDL from nascent VLDL.

Degradation

1. VLDL are rapidly removed from circulation by extra hepatic tissues.
2. Half life of plasma VLDL is about 1-3 hours.
3. Action of lipoprotein lipase on VLDL results in the loss of triglycerides and apo C. Free fatty acids and glycerol are metabolized.
4. Loss of triglycerides and apo C results in the formation of intermediate density lipoproteins (IDL) or VLDL remnants.
5. Only one IDL particle is formed from each of VLDL particle.
6. In humans, most of the VLDL remnants are taken up by the liver and converted to LDL. Uptake is through the apo E receptor mechanism.
7. However, LDL may be generated in the circulation from IDL by removing apo E Various stages of VLDL metabolism are shown in Fig. 10.26.

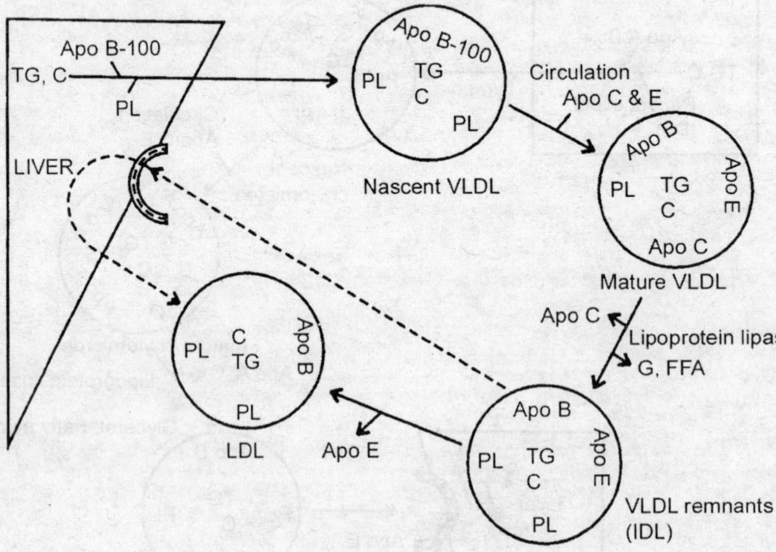

Fig. 10.26 Formation and fate of VLDL

Metabolism of LDL

Synthesis

1. Liver directly produces LDL. It is also formed from IDL in the circulation.
2. In the liver, synthesized cholesterol combines with triglycerides, phospholipids and apoproteins to generates LDL. Apo B is the only apoprotein used for LDL formation.

Degradation

1. Each day, 50% of LDL is removed from circulation. Extra hepatic tissues removes half of this and remainder is removed by liver.
2. The uptake of LDL by extra hepatic tissues is mediated by cell surface receptor. The receptors are present in clathrin coated pits. Apo B-100 of LDL is recognized by the receptor and LDL binds to the receptor. Then the LDL particles are taken up by endocytosis.
3. With in the cells LDL are broken down by lysosomal enzymes in 5-6 minutes.
4. Cholesterolesters and apo proteins are hydrolyzed by lysosomal hydrolases. Free cholesterol released may be reesterified. It regulates intra cellular cholesterol synthesis.
5. Uptake of LDL by liver is mediated through a specific LDL receptor. In the liver, free cholesterol released may be esterified and apoprotein is hydrolyzed to amino acids. Steps of LDL synthesis and degradation are shown in Fig. 10.27.

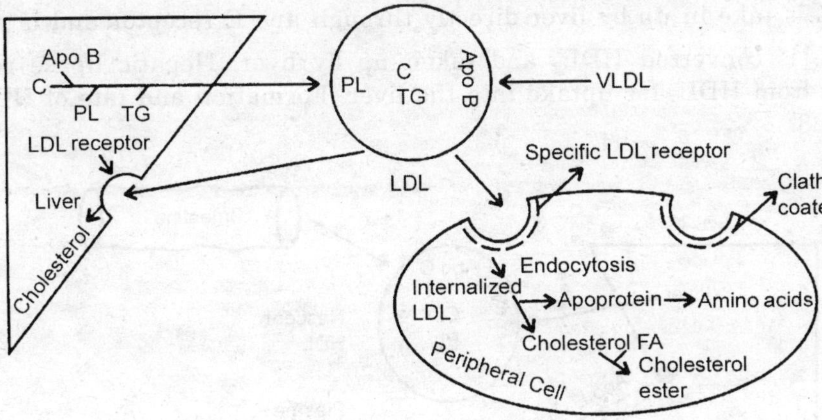

Fig. 10.27 Synthesis and degradation of LDL

Regulation of LDL up take by extra hepatic tissues

1. Free cholesterol in cells regulates uptake of LDL by extra hepatic tissue.
2. Uptake of LDL by receptors depends on number of receptors on membrane surface which are in turn regulated by cellular need for cholesterol.
3. If the cell has enough cholesterol then LDL receptors are not synthesized. So this blocks entry of LDL or excess cholesterol into cells.

METABOLISM OF HDL

Synthesis

1. Liver mainly synthesizes HDL and intestine synthesizes to some extent.

2. HDL secreted by liver (intestine) is called as nascent HDL and is composed of cholesterol, phospholipid and apo A, apo C and apo E. Nascent HDL has flat discoid shape.
3. In plasma cholesterol of HDL is esterified by LCAT. Apo A-I activates LCAT.
4. LCAT system is also involved in the removal of free cholesterol from extra herpatic tissues.
5. Cholesterolester (CE) formed by the action of LCAT moves from periphery to the center of disc and HDL assumes spherical shape.

Degradation

1. Though the half life of HDL in blood has been established as 5 days, the exact fate of HDL remains uncertain. It is a subject of intensive research.
2. However, three fates for HDL have been identified.
3. HDL may transfer cholesterolesters to other lipoproteins like VLDL, LDL. Apo D component of HDL promotes transfer of cholesterolester from HDL to LDL or VLDL. It is called as cholesterolester transfer protein. The cholesterolester of LDL or VLDL is taken up by liver. Thus HDL mainly function as tissue cholesterol scavenging agent. Since HDL removes free cholesterol from extra hepatic cells the incidence of atherosclerosis or coronary artery disease (CAD) is inversely related to plasma HDL concentration.
4. Some HDL is take in up by liver directly through apo E receptor and is metabolized.
5. Some HDL is converted HDL_2 and taken up by liver. Hepatic lipase releases free cholesterol from HDL_2 for uptake into the liver. Formation and fate of HDL is shown is Fig. 10.28.

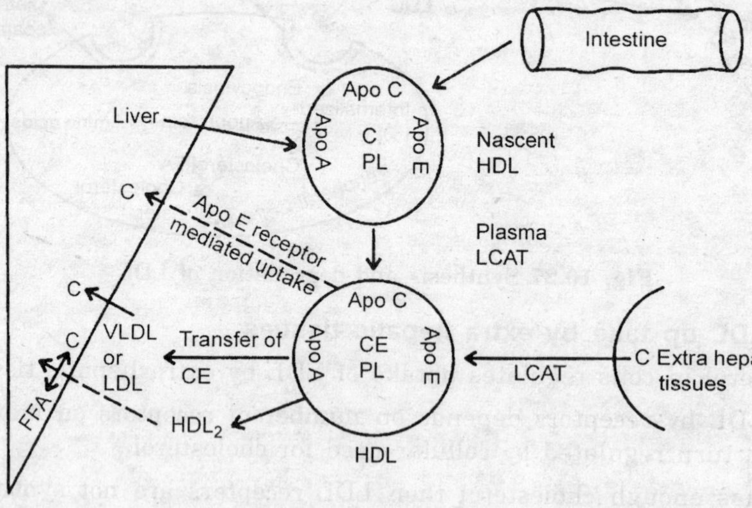

Fig. 10.28 Formation and fate of HDL

Medical Importance

Plasma lipoproteins are altered in several diseases.

Lipoproteinemias (Dyslipoproteinemias)

They are groups of genetic disorders associated with increased or decreased lipoproteins in plasma. They are mainly due to defects in either production, transport or catabolism of lipoproteins. Most of them are harmless.

They are of two types.

1. Hypolipoproteinemias: in which plasma lipoprotein is decreased.
2. Hyperlipoproteinemias: in which plasma lipoprotein is increased.

HYPOLIPOPROTEINEMIAS

A beta lipoproteinemia

1. This condition is due to block in apo B production.
2. Since apo B is required for VLDL and chylomicron their formation is affected. Further LDL formation is also affected. Hence, LDL, chylomicrons and VLDL are absent in plasma.
3. Plasma triglyceride and cholesterol levels are low.
4. Triglycerides accumulates in liver and intestine due lack of chylomicrons and VLDL.

Bassen-Kornzweig syndrome

1. It resembles abeta lipoproteinemia.
2. Plasma triglyceride and cholesterol levels are low and they accumulates in tissues.
3. Characteristic symptoms are acanthocytosis (spike like projections on erythrocytes), atypical retinitis and extensive demyelination.

Familial hypo beta lipoproteinemia

1. The condition is characterized by low LDL and normal chylomicron levels in plasma.
2. It is not a serious condition affected individuals are normal and healthy.
3. Plasma cholesterol level is low.

Familial alpha-lipoprotein deficiency (Tangier disease)

1. It was first identified in Tangier island. The condition is characterized by the absence of HDL in plasma. HDL formation is impaired due to lack of apo C-II.
2. Cholesterolesters accumulate in the tissues and plasma, cholesterol level is low.
3. Symptoms are hepato splenomegaly due to accumulation of cholesterol and orange yellow tonsils.

HYPER LIPOPROTEINEMIAS (LIPIDEMIAS)

Type-I hyper lipoproteinemia

1. Lipoprotein lipase is deficient in this condition.
2. It is a rare condition and deficiency of lipoprotein lipase is due to decreased formation of apo C-II, which is required for its activity.
3. Lipoprotein lipase deficiency impairs chylomicron clearance from plasma. As a result, chylomicron accumulates in plasma (hyper chylomicronemia).

4. Plasma triglycerides and cholesterol levels are elevated.
5. Xanthomas (collection of lipids in skin or tendon sheaths), abdominal pain are common symptoms in this condition.

Type-II hyper lipoproteinemia or Familial hyper cholesterolemia

1. It is most common among others.
2. It is due to slow clearance of LDL from circulation owing to defective LDL receptors.
3. Plasma LDL, triglycerides and cholesterol level are elevated.
4. Severe xanthomas and deposition of lipid in tissues are major features. Hence, this condition is associated with atherosclerosis and coronary artery disease.
5. Feeding of diet containing PUFA is beneficial to these individuals.

Wolman disease

1. It is a rare genetic disorder.
2. Lysosomal acid lipase, which hydrolyzes cholesterolester and triglyceride is absent in this condition.
3. Plasma LDL level is elevated, cholesterolester accumulates in tissues.
4. It is fatal condition and death can occur in the first six months of life.

Familial hyper lipoproteinemia (Broad beta disease)

1. It is a rare condition, in which chylomicron catabolism is impaired.
2. In this condition production of apo E is defective and conversion of VLDL remnants to LDL is also impaired.
3. Hence, both chylomicrons and VLDL remnants are more in plasma and condition is referred as *remnant disease*. Plasma cholesterol and triglceride levels are elevated.
4. Symptoms are xanthomas and atherosclerosis.

Familial hyper triacylglycerolemia

1. The condition is characterized by increased triglycerides and cholesterol in blood (Endogenous hyperlipidemia).
2. The biochemical defect in this disorder is not clear.
3. The condition may progress to atherosclerosis.

Familial hyper lipoproteinemia

1. In this condition, both chylomicrons and VLDL are elevated in plasma.
2. Apo B is over produced and plasma cholesterol and triglyceride levels are elevated.
3. Xanthoma is the main symptom.

LCAT deficiency

1. A familial deficiency of this enzyme has been reported.
2. Lecithin and cholesterol levels are high in plasma of the affected individuals.

3. Symptoms are accumulation of free cholesterol in erythrocytes, corneal infiltration, hemolytic anemia and kidney damage.

In addition to the above, hyper lipoproteinemias also manifest as secondary complication of diseases like diabetes, atherosclerosis, excessive use of oral contraceptives, hypothyroidism and nephrotic syndrome.

Fatty livers

1. Liver contains about 5% lipid. Of this, about 1/4 is triglyceride.
2. Extensive accumulation of lipid in the liver leads to condition known as *fatty liver*. In the fatty livers, the lipid content increases to 25-30%. Further, triglycerides and fatty acid may occupy entire cytoplasm of hepatocyte.

Several factors causes accumulation of lipid in liver

1. Raised plasma free fatty acid level

When there is a mobilization of fat from adipose and extrahepatic tissues plasma free fatty acid level increases. Liver takes up increasing amounts of fatty acids and esterifies them. Hence rate of triglyceride synthesis is more. However, the synthesis of VLDL occurs only at normal rate. As a result triglycerides accumulate and cause fatty liver. The plasma free fatty acid level is elevated in (*a*) starvation (*b*) diabetes (*c*) high fat diet (*d*) carnitine deficiency. Hence, in these conditions fatty liver occurs.

2. Metabolic block in the production of lipoproteins

Block in VLDL formation causes fatty liver even though the rate of triglyceride synthesis is normal because VLDL transports triglyceride from liver to extra hepatic tissues. VLDL formation may be blocked if substance (s) required for its formation are deficient. However, when deficient substances are supplied fat accumulation cease.

Lipotropic factors Are compounds that relieve or prevent excess accumulation of lipids in the liver. They are choline, methionine and betaine. These lipotropic factors cure fatty liver due to choline or methionine deficiency. Choline deficiency may result from impaired transmethylation reactions associated with methionine catabolism.

Choline deficiency leads to block in choline dependent phospholipid biosynthesis. This in turn impairs formation of membranes needed for lipoprotein synthesis. Thus choline deficiency results in block in VLDL formation and causes accumulation of fat in liver. Choline deficiency may impairs carnitine biosynthesis also.

Other noteworthy lipotropic factors are PUFA, vit E, pyridoxine and pantothenic acid. The deficiency of any one of these substances causes fatty liver. However, they can not prevent occurrence of fatty liver due to choline deficiency.

3. Toxic substances

Several hepato toxic agents like carbon tetrachloride, chloroform, phosphorus, lead, arsenic, alcohol and orotic acid causes fatty liver. Substances, which inhibit protein synthesis like puromycin and ethionine, a methionine analog also cause fatty liver.

Medical Importance

Effect of fatty liver When accumulation of lipid in liver becomes chronic fibrotic changes takes place in hepatocytes, which progress to cirrhosis and finally impaired liver function.

ALCOHOL METABOLISM

Sources

(*a*) **Endogenous** Small amounts of alcohol in the blood may be produced by intestinal flora.

(*b*) **Exogenous** Alcohol consumed by pleasure seekers is absorbed easily all along gastro intestinal tract and reaches liver.

Site Liver is the major site of alcohol metabolism.

There are two pathways for alcohol degradation.

1. Major pathway

In this pathway alcohol is converted to acetate by the action of cytosolic alcohol dehydrogenase and mitochondrial aldehyde dehydrogenase (Fig. 10.29). Acetyl-CoA may be formed from acetate which enters TCA cycle or fatty acid biosynthetic pathway.

2. Minor pathway

In this pathway alcohol is converted to acetaldehyde by microsomal cytP_{450}-dependent ethanol oxidizing system (Fig. 10.29). It is an inducible pathway and become prominent in chronic alcoholics.

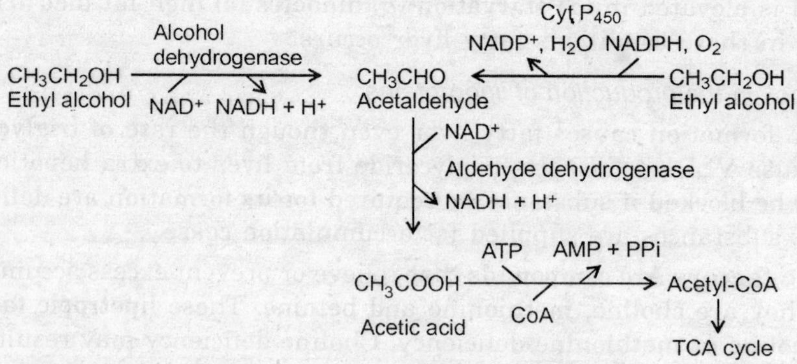

Fig. 10.29 Reactions of alcohol utilization

Medical Importance

1. It serves as energy source like carbohydrate. However, if consumed excess (chronic alcoholism) leads to fatty liver development.
2. Some individuals (chronic alcoholics) develop vit A and thiamin deficiency.
3. Lactic acidemia occurs due to excess NADH in the cytosol.
4. Women are more susceptible to alcohol effects than men.
5. Moderate consumption of alcohol was found to be beneficial to stroke patients. HDL level is higher in people consuming small amount of alcohol daily.
6. Clearance of toxins from circulation by liver becomes slow and some compounds get converted to carcinogens in chronic alcoholics.
7. Alcohol consumption aggravates gout and porphyrias.

Lipid peroxidation

1. As stated in chapter-6 action of atmospheric oxygen on fats results in formation of peroxides.
2. In the body (*in vivo*) also, lipid peroxidation occurs.
3. Lipid peroxidation is a chain reaction.
4. Free radicals initiate lipid peroxidation chain reaction. Free radicals can be defined as molecules having unpaired electrons in outer orbitals. They are highly reactive. They all contain oxygen hence they often called as reactive oxygen species (ROS).

In biological systems, free radicals are generated by

1. Oxygen radicals

Oxygen radical are involved in lipid peroxidation. Hydrogen of methylene (—CH_2—) group of PUFA is susceptible to extraction due to adjacent double bonds. Hence, in presence of oxygen free radical of PUFA is generated by extracting a methylene hydrogen from membrane PUFA. Reaction of PUFA free radical with O_2 forms peroxy PUFA radical, which in turn reacts with another molecule of PUFA to form PUFA free radical and endoperoxide (Fig. 10.30) Ultimately malondialdehyde (MDA) and other small molecules are formed. Usually MDA estimation used to assess extent of lipid peroxidation.

2. Superoxide

As such super oxide (O_2^-) can not initiate lipid peroxidation. It generates reactive oxygen species (ROS) or free radicals like singlet oxygen ($\dot{O}_2$) and hydroxyl radical ($\dot{OH}$). These may initiate lipid peroxidation.

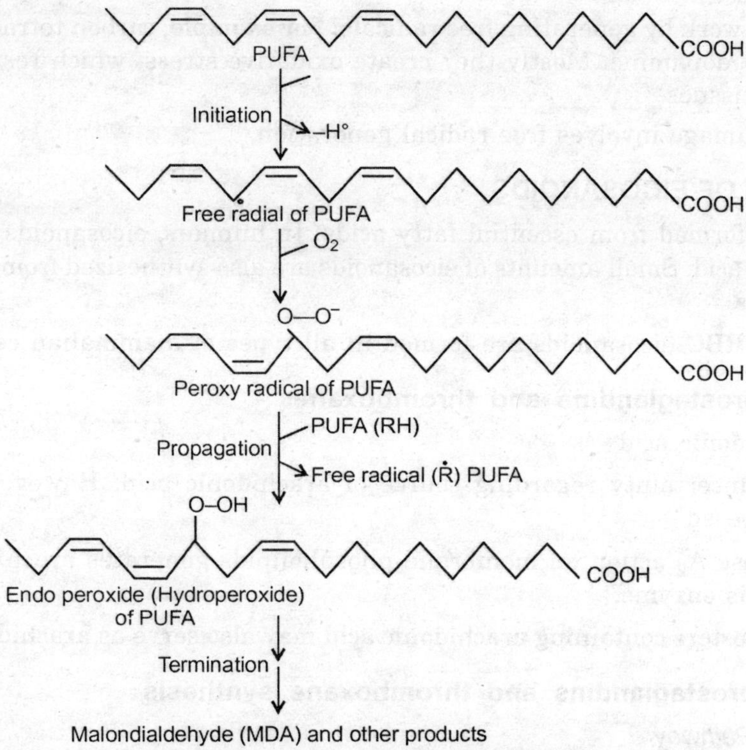

Fig. 10.30 Lipid peroxidation mechanism

Apart from the above two systems, light or metals also can generate free radical, which in turn can initiate lipid peroxidation.

Medical Importance

1. Membrane lipids particularly PUFA are in contact with O_2 and metal rich environment. So, they are susceptible to lipid peroxidation which in turn can cause membrance dysfunction.
2. Lipid peroxidation is associated with several diseases or conditions like ageing, diabetes, cancer, necrosis, epilepsy, inflammatory or autoimmune disorders and cardiovascular diseases like atherosclerosis.
3. **Free radical scavenger systems (FRSS)** Since free radicals initiate lipid peroxidation body devised ways to remove free radicals.
   (*a*) **Enzymatic free radical scavenger system (EFRSS)** It consist of antioxidant enzymes like superoxide dismutase, glutathione-s-transferase, catalase, peroxidase and glutathione peroxidase.
   (*b*) **Non-enzymatic free redical scavenger system (NEFRSS)** It consist of several compounds, which act as antioxidants. Most of them are naturally occurring. They are glutathione, melatonin, tocopherol (vit E), ascorbic acid (vit C), lipoic acid, uric acid, carotenes, caffeine and bilirubin.

Some artificial or synthetic antioxidants are widely used in preservation of processed fat foods. They are butylated hydroxy toluene (BHT), butylated hydroxy anisole (BHA) and propyl gallate (PG).

4. Some toxins work by generating free radicals. For example, carbon tetrachloride, alloxan and hydroxy dopamine. Mostly they create oxidative stress, which results in impaired function of tissues.
5. Radiation damage involves free radical generation.

BIOSYNTHESIS OF EICOSANOIDS

Eicosanoids are formed from essential fatty acids. In humans, eicosanoids are synthesized from arachidonic acid. Small amounts of eicosanoids are also synthesized from dietary linolenic and linoleic acids.

Site Except RBC eicosanoids are formed in all types of mammalian cells.

Synthesis of prostaglandins and thromboxanes

Source of arachidonic acid

There is some uncertainty regarding source of arachidonic acid. However, two alternate sources are proposed.

1. Phospholipase A_2 action on membrane phospholipids generates arachidonic acid. Ca^{2+} activates this enzyme.
2. Cholesterol esters containing arachidonic acid may also serve as arachidonic acid source.

Reactions of prostaglandins and thromboxane synthesis

Cyclooxygenase Pathway

1. First reaction is catalyzed by cyclooxygenase component of prostaglandin cyclooxygenase

complex. It converts arachidonicacid to PGG_2 using 2 oxygen molecules. It is a hemeprotein and located in microsomes. The enzyme complex has two components (*a*) Cyclo oxygenase and (*b*) endoperoxidase components. Cyclooxygenase gets in activated after operating 15-30 times by hydroperoxy group generated.

2. The PGG_2 is converted to PGH_2 by reduced glutathione dependent endoperoxidase component of prostaglandin cyclooxygenase complex.

   Specific enzymes present in different tissues catalyzes the formation of PGD, E, F series, prostacyclins and thromboxanes from PGH_2.

3. In the kidney and spleen PGE_2 and PGF_2, are produced from PGH_2 by the action of isomerase and reductas, respectively.
4. In the platelets, lung thromboxane A_2 is formed from PGH_2 by the action of thromboxane A_2 synthase.
5. In the blood vessels, PGI is produced from PGH_2 by the action of synthase. Formation of some prostaglandins and thromboxanes are shown in Fig. 10.31.

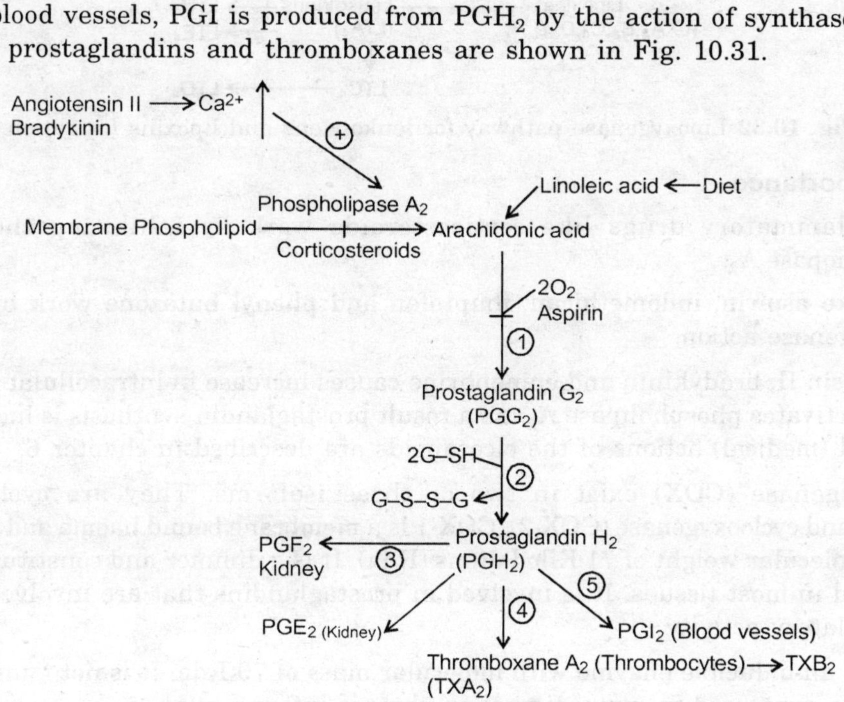

Fig. 10.31 Cyclooxygenase pathway for prostaglandins and thromboxane biosynthesis

Synthesis of leukotriens and lipoxins

Lipoxygenase pathway

Lipoxygenases are enzymes present in various tissues. They exhibit positional specificity and oxygenate arachidonic acid at different positions. Addition of O_2 by these enzymes to arachidonic acid generates hydroperoxides. Lipoxygenases are named according to position they oxygenate.

Leucocytes and neutrophils have 5-lipoxygenase. Likewise kidney, platelets have 12-lipoxygenase and lymphocytes, neutrophils and reticulocytes have 15-lipoxygenase.

Reactions of leukotriene and lipoxin formation

1. In leucocytes 5-lipooxygenase adds O_2 to 5-position of arachidonic acid. This results in the formation of 5-hydroxy eicosa tetraenoate (5-HPETE).
2. Leukotriene LTA_4 is generated from 5-HPETE by dehydration catalyzed by dehydrase.
3. By the action of 15-lipoxygenase on LTA_4 lipoxins are produced.

   Formation of leukotriens and lipoxins is shown in Fig. 10.32.
4. LTA_4 also serve as precursor for the formation of LTB_4, LTC_4 LTD_4 and LTE_4.

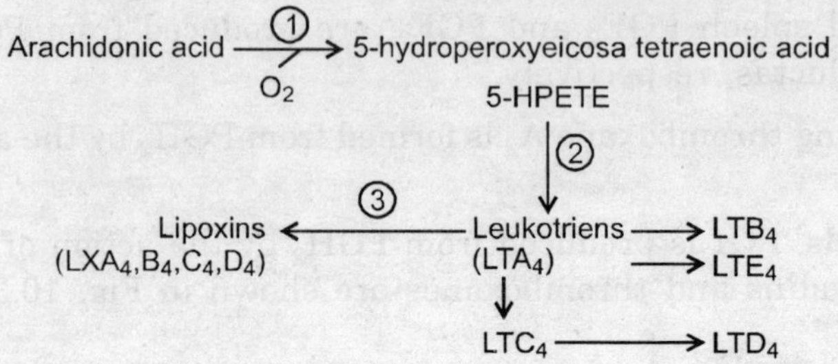

Fig. 10.32 Lipoxygenase pathway for leukotriens and lipoxins formation

Medical importance

1. Anti inflammatory drugs like corticosteroids work by inhibiting the action of phospholiopase A_2.
2. Drugs like aspirin, indomethican, ibuprofen and phenyl butazone work by inhibiting cyclooxygenase action.
3. Angiotensin II, bradykinin and epinephrine causes increase in intracellular Ca^{2+}, which in turn activates phospholipase A_2. As a result prostaglandin synthesis is increased. The biological (medical) actions of the eicosanoids are described in chapter 6.
4. Cyclooxygenase (COX) exist in two or three isoforms. They are cyclooxygenase (COX-1) and cyclooxygenase (COX-2). COX-1 is a membrane bound haemo and glycoprotein with a molecular weight of 71 Kilodaltons (Kda). It is a dimmer and constitutive enzyme expressed in most tissues. It is involved in prostaglandins that are involved in normal cell regulatory activity.

   COX-2 is an inducible enzyme with molecular mass of 70 Kda. It is not found in resting cells. It is expressed in many tissues in chronic inflammation.
5. Side effects associated with use of nonsteroidal anti inflammatory drugs (NSAIDS) like aspirin, indometacin or ibuprofen are gastrointestinal ulcers and renal disturbances. They are due to inhibition of both the isoforms of COX by these drugs. Aspirin inhibits by irreversible acetylation where as indomethican or ibuprofen inhibit reversibly by competing with substrate. Since COX-2 is expressed in inflammatory conditions selective NSAIDS that inhibits only COX-2 are free from side effects. At least two selective COX-2 inhibitors are introduced into market at present Nimesulide and Celecoxib are two such selective NSAID that work by inhibiting COX-2.
6. COX-2 over expression occurs in Alzheimer's disease and colorectal cancer.

CHOLESTEROL METABOLISM

Biosynthesis of cholesterol

1. About 1 gm of cholesterol is synthesized in the body per day.
2. **Site.** Cholesterol synthesis takes place in all nucleated cells particularly liver, adrenal cortex, testis, ovaries, brain, placenta, aorta and skin. The enzymes of cholesterol biosynthesis are present in micro somes and cytosol of the cells.
3. **Precursors.** Acetyl-CoAs generated from the break down of carbohydrates, fats and aminoacids act as precursors of cholesterol. Acetyl-CoAs are transported from mitochondria to cytosol by similar mechanism described for fatty acid biosynthesis. HMP shunt generates NADPH required for cholesterol synthesis.
4. Synthesis of cholesterol takes place in several stages and involves condensation of two and five carbon fragments. Further each condensation reaction involves –C–C– bond formation. First 3 acetyl-CoA molecules condense to form 6 carbon mevalonate. In the next stage 5 carbon isoprenoid unit is generated from mevalonate by loss of CO_2. Then six isoprenoid units condense in a specific stepwise manner to form 30 carbon polyisoprenoid squalene. The squalene undergo cyclization to generate first sterol lanosterol. Formation of cholesterol from lanosterol occurs after several steps.

$$\underset{(C_2)}{\text{3 Acetyl-CoA}} \longrightarrow \underset{(C_6)}{\text{Mevalonate}} \longrightarrow \underset{(C_5)}{\text{Isoprenoid}}$$

$$\underset{(C_{27})}{\text{Cholesterol}} \twoheadleftarrow\!\!\twoheadleftarrow \underset{(C_{30})}{\text{Lanosterol}} \longleftarrow \underset{(C_{30})}{\text{Squalene}}$$

REACTIONS OF CHOLESTEROL SYNTHESIS

Formation of cholesterol from acetyl-CoA involves participation of numerous enzymes, which catalyzes complex reactions. For the elucidation of this most complex and extra ordinary pathway Bloch, Lynen and Corn forth were awarded Nobel Prize in 1964.

1. Synthesis of cholesterol begins with condensation of two acetyl-CoAs. The reaction is catalyzed by β-ketothiolase or thiolase and acetoacetyl-CoA is the product. In this reaction –C–C– bond is formed between methyl carbon of one acetyl-CoA and carbonyl carbon of another acetyl-CoA. Alternatively aceto acetyl-CoA may be obtained from acetoacetate by activation.
2. The acetoacetyl-CoA condenses with another molecule of acetyl-CoA in this reaction. HMG-CoA synthase catalyzes the condensation and –C–C– bond is formed between β-carbon of aceto acetyl-CoA and methyl carbon of acetyl-CoA. HMG-CoA is the product of this reaction. HMG-CoA is key cholesterol precursor.

   HMG-CoA is also an intermediate in ketogenesis which was described earlier. However, the enzymes forming HMG-CoA from acetyl-CoA leading to formation of Cholesterol are present in cytosol where as enzymes of HMG-CoA synthesis which needed for ketogenesis are located in mitochondria.

   HMG-CoA is the precursor of two isoprenoid intermediates of cholesterol synthesis. They are isopentenyl pyrophosphate and dimethylallyl pyrophosphate. The formation of isopentenyl pyrophosphate occurs in the next four reactions.

3. The carbonyl of thioestergroup HMG-CoA is reduced to an alcohol in an NADPH dependent four electron reduction reaction catalyzed by HMG-CoA reductase. Mevalonate is the product of this reaction.
4. Mevalonate-5-phosphotransferase phosphorylates new-OH group of mevalonate in a ATP dependent reaction. Mevalonate-5-phosphate is the product of this reaction.
5. Phosphomevalonate kinase converts product of the above reaction to mevalonate-5-pyrophosphate in another ATP dependent reaction.
6. Pyrophosphomevalonate is converted to 5-carbon isopentenyl pyrophosphate by pyrophosphomevalonate decarboxylase in a ATP-dependent decarboxylation reaction.

   The reaction involves formation of 3-phospho-5-pyrophosphomevalonate as a transient intermediate. It is formed by phosphorylation on 3 carbon atom of pyrophosphomevalonate (*a*) Decarboxylation of this intermediate results in dehydration and loss of P_i (*b*) All these phosphorylation, dehydration and loss of CO_2 and P_i occur in a concerted reaction.
7. In this reaction, dimethylallyl pyrophosphate is formed from the isopentenyl pyrophosphate by the action of isopentenyl pyrophosphate isomerase. It is a reversible reaction.

   The two isomers isopentenyl pyrophosphate and dimethyl allylpyrophosphate are responsible for remaining carbon to carbon bond forming condensation reaction in cholesterol synthesis. Since isopentenyl pyrophosphate acts as nucleophils (x^-) and dimethyl allyl pyrophosphate acts as electrophile (y^+) they undergo head-to-tail condensation.
8. In this reaction, prenyl transferase (Farnesyl pyrophosphate synthase) catalyzes head to tail condensation of dimethylallyl pyrophosphate and isopentenyl pyrophosphate. As a result carbon-carbon bond is formed between 1 carbon of dimethylallylpyrophosphate and 4 carbon of isopentenyl pyrophosphate. Product of this reaction is geranyl pyrophosphate.
9. Prenyl transferase catalyzes another head to tail condensation ($1 \rightarrow 4$) of geranyl pyrophosphate and isopentenyl pyrophosphate. A carbon-carbon bond is formed between 1 carbon of geranyl pyrophosphate and 4 carbon of isopentenyl pyrophosphate in this reaction.
10. Squalene synthase now catalyzes head-to-head condensation of two farnesyl pyrophosphate molecules. Formation of product squalene occurs in complex two-step reactions.

    (*a*) In the first step, 1 carbon of one of farnesyl pyrophosphate is inserted into–C_2=C_3– bond of second farnesyl pyrophosphate. This leads to formation of presqualene pyrophosphate by eliminating pyrophosphate. In this reaction two –C–C– bonds are formed between 1 carbon of one farnesyl pyrophosphate and 2,3 carbons of second farnesyl pyrophosphate molecule.

    (*b*) In the second step, presqualene pyrophosphate undergoes reduction and rearrangement in presence of NADPH, which leads to formation of squalene with loss of another pyrophosphate.

    Intermediates of squalene to cholesterol are bound to squalene sterol carrier protein which allows them to react in the aqueous phase of cell. In the next two reactions squalene an open chain 30 carbon compound is cyclized to form tetracyclic steroid skeleton lanosterol.

11. Microsomal an NADPH-dependent squalene mono-oxygenase or squalene epoxidase catalyzes oxidation of squalene to form squalene-2, 3-epoxide or 2, 3-oxidosqualene.
12. Squalene oxidocyclase converts squalene-2, 3-epoxide to lanosterol involving complex cyclization process. In Fig. 10.33 reactions of lanosterol formation from acetyl-CoA are shown.

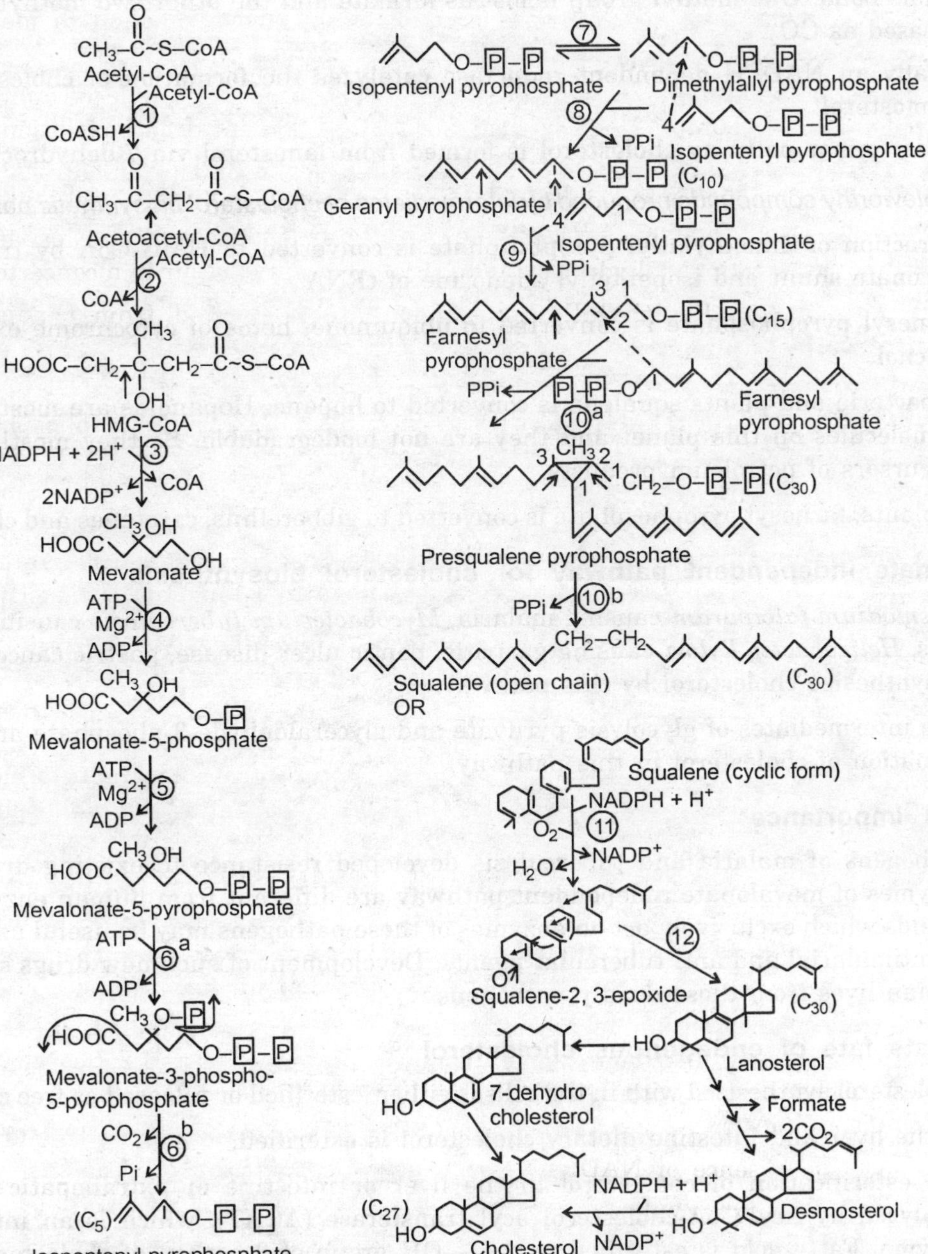

Fig. 10.33 Cholesterol biosynthetic pathway. ↑ Indicates —C—C— bond formation. ↑ Indicates head to tail condensation

Formation of cholesterol form lanosterol

Conversion of lanosterol to cholesterol involves several steps and they are shown in Figure-10.33. Briefly they are

1. Lanosterol gives rises to desmosterol after the loss of three methyl groups and shift of double bond. One methyl group is lost as formate and the other two methyl group are released as CO_2.
2. Finally an NADPH dependent reductase catalyzes the formation of cholesterol from desmosterol.

In another minor pathway cholesterol is formed from lanosterol via 7-dehydrocholesterol.

Other noteworthy compounds produced by intermediates of cholesterol biosynthetic pathway are

1. A fraction of dimethylallyl pyrophosphate is converted to HMG-CoA by transmethyl gluconate shunt and isopentenyl adenosine of tRNA.
2. Farnesyl pyrophosphate is converted to ubiquinone, heme of cytochrome oxidase and dolichol.
3. In bacteria and plants squalene is converted to hopane. Hopanoids are most abundant biomolecules on this planet and they are not biodegradable. So they mostly serve as precursors of petroleum products.
4. In plants, farnesyl pyrophosphate is converted to gibberellins, carotenes and chlorophyll.

Mevalonate independent pathway for cholesterol biosynthesis

1. *Plasmodium falciparam* causing malaria, *Mycobacterium tuberculosis* causing tuberculosis, *Helicobacter Pylori* causing gastritis, peptic ulcer disease, gastric cancer are able to synthesize cholesterol by this pathway.
2. Two intermediates of glycolysis pyruvate and glyceraldehyde-3-phosphate are used for formation of cholesterol in this pathway.

Medical importance

1. Pathogens of malaria and tuberculosis developed resistance to existing drugs. Since enzymes of mevalonate independent pathway are different from human enzymes compounds which exclusively act on enzymes of these pathogens may be useful as new class of antimalarial and anti tubercular agents. Development of such new drugs saves more human lives from these deadly pathogens.

Immediate fate of endogenous cholesterol

1. Cholesterol synthesized with in the cells is either esterified or released as free cholesterol.
2. In the liver and intestine dietary cholesterol is esterified.
3. The esterification of cholesterol in the liver or intestine or extrahepatic tissues is catalyzed by Acyl-CoA-cholesterol acyl transferase (ACAT), which is an intracellular enzyme. Fatty acid is esterified to the —OH group of 3 carbon of cholesterol.

$$\text{Acyl-CoA+Cholesterol} \xrightarrow[\text{CoA}]{\text{ACAT}} \text{cholesterolester}$$

Transport of cholesterol

(a) Transport of dietary and hepatic cholesterol

1. In the intestine dietary cholesterol and cholesterol synthesized is incorporated into chylomicrons and transported to liver.
2. In the liver, cholesterol is released from chylomicrons and incorporated into VLDL and LDL.
3. VLDL and LDL secreted by liver contains cholesterol of dietary origin and also cholesterol synthesized in the liver. So they transport cholesterol from liver to plasma.
4. In plasma highest proportion of cholesterol is found in LDL and most of it is in the esterified form. The free form undergoes exchange between different lipoprotein fractions and cell membrane.
5. Extra hepatic tissues take up LDL through receptor mediated endocytosis.

   In extrahepatic tissues, LDL are broken down and lysosomal lipase hydrolyzes cholesterolesters. The liberated free cholesterol may undergo either storage or for cell membrane formation (Fig. 10.34)

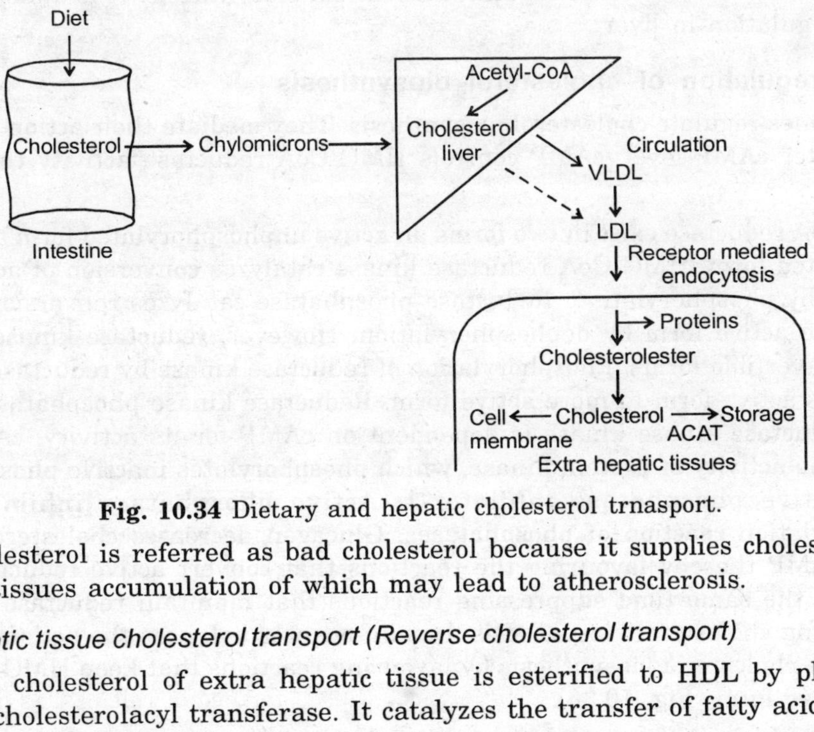

Fig. 10.34 Dietary and hepatic cholesterol trnasport.

6. LDL-cholesterol is referred as bad cholesterol because it supplies cholesterol to extra hepatic tissues accumulation of which may lead to atherosclerosis.

(b) Extra hepatic tissue cholesterol transport (Reverse cholesterol transport)

1. The free cholesterol of extra hepatic tissue is esterified to HDL by plasma (LCAT) lecithin-cholesterolacyl transferase. It catalyzes the transfer of fatty acid in position 2 of lecithin to cholesterol.

$$\text{Lecithin of HDL + cholesterol} \rightleftharpoons \text{lysolecithin + cholesterolester}$$

2. The cholesterol ester so generated diffuses into the core of HDL and transported to liver. Lysolecithin combines with plasma albumin.
3. Thus, HDL-LCAT reaction plays important role in the transfer of extrahepatic tissue cholesterol to liver.

4. However, in plasma some cholesterol ester of HDL may be transferred to other lipoproteins by cholesterolester transfer protein.
5. In liver cholesterol is eliminated as bile acids or as free cholesterol in bile (Fig. 10.35). This process is called as *reverse cholesterol transport.*

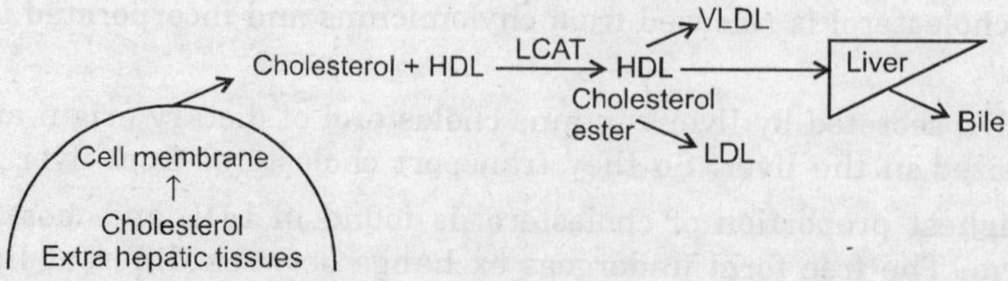

Fig. 10.35 Extra hepatic tissue cholesterol transport. (Reverse cholesterol transport)

6. HDL-cholesterol is referred as good cholesterol because it transports extrahepatic tissue cholesterol to liver for elimination.

Regulation of cholesterol biosynthesis

Activity of HMG-CoA reductase regulate cholesterol biosynthesis. It is under hormonal and feed back regulation in liver.

Hormonal regulation of cholesterol biosynthesis

Many hormones regulate cholesterol biosynthesis. They mediate their action through cAMP. They can alter cAMP level. cAMP controls HMG-CoA reductase activity through covalent modification.

HMG-CoA reductase exist in two forms an active unphosphorylated form and an in active phosphorylated form. HMG-CoA reductase kinase catalyzes conversion of active form to in active form by phosphorylation. Reductase phosphatase catalyzes conversion of less active form to more active form by dephosphorylation. However, reductase kinase itself exist in two inter convertible forms. Phosphorylation of reductase kinase by reductase kinase kinase converts less active form to more active form. Reductase kinase phosphatase reverses this process. Reductase kinase kinase is dependent on cAMP for its activity. cAMP is also required for the activity of protein kinase, which phosphorylates inactive phosphatase inhibitor-1 to active phosphatase inhibitor-1. Active phosphatase inhibitor-1 inhibits dephosphorylation reaction of phosphatases. Glucagon decreases cholesterol synthesis. It increases cAMP thereby favouring the reactions that convert active reductase to inactive form and at the same time suppressing reactions that maintain reductase in active form thus inhibiting cholesterol biosynthesis. Insulin counter balances the action of glucagon. It increases the cholesterol biosynthesis by favouring reactions that keep HMG-CoA reductase in more active form (Fig. 10.36).

Other hormones that influence cholesterol biosynthesis are thyroxine and cortisol. Thyroxine increases cholesterol synthesis where as cortisol decreases cholesterol synthesis.

Feed back regulation of cholesterol biosynthesis

HMG-CoA reductase is subjected to feed back regulation by cholesterol. Cholesterol inhibits HMG-CoA reductase by allosteric mechanism. Hence cholesterol diets reduces HMG-CoA reductase activity.

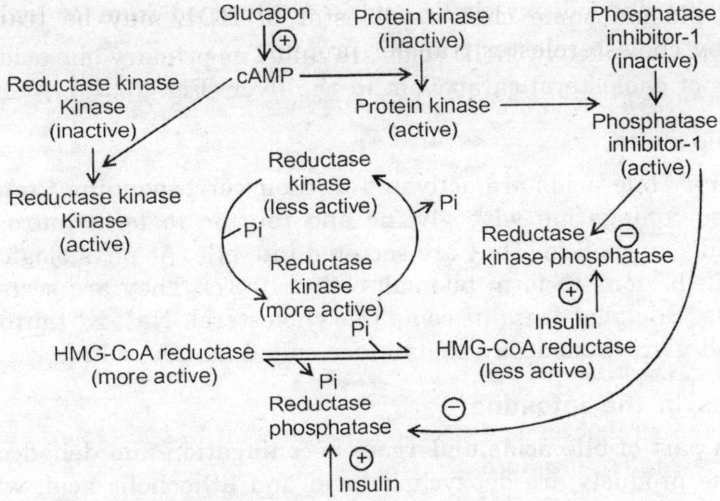

Fig. 10.36 Regulation of HMG-CoA reductase activity by hormones
⊖ indicates inhibition ⊕ indicates activation

Other noteworthy regulatory mechanisms are

1. **LDL receptor synthesis** Cholesterol synthesis is regulated in directly in extra hepatic tissues by regulating rate of LDL receptor synthesis. High intracellular cholesterol concentration inhibits LDL receptor synthesis whereas low intracellular cholesterol concentration stimulates LDL receptor synthesis. Thus, in extra hepatic tissues cholesterol synthesis is regulated at entry level.
2. **Esterification** In extra hepatic tissues cholesterol synthesis is influenced by the rate of its esterification by ACAT.

Catabolism of cholesterol

Humans lack enzyme system which can break steroid nucleus of cholesterol. So cholesterol is not degraded to small compounds in the body. However, it is converted to bile acids in the liver and eliminated through the bile.

Formation of bile acids

1. It is the major pathway of cholesterol catabolism. About 80% cholesterol is converted to primary and secondary bile acids in liver and intestine. However, only small portions of bile acids are excreted through feces.
2. About 0.5 gm of bile acids are formed per day in the body.
3. 7α-hydroxylase a cytP$_{450}$ - NADPH-dependent microsomal monooxygenase catalyzes first reaction of bile acid formation. Vit. C is required for this reaction. 7α-hydroxylase is the regulatory enzyme of bile acid biosynthesis and subjected to feed back inhibition.
4. In one pathway, 7α-hydroxy cholesterol undergoes further hydroxylations and oxidation of side chain to give trihydroxy coprostanoic acid. Loss of propionate results in the formation of cholic acid from trihydroxy coprostanoic acid. In humans, cholic acid is the major bile acid.

5. In another route chenodeoxy cholic acid is synthesized from 7α-hydroxy cholesterol.
6. Cholic acid and chenodeoxy cholic acids are called as primary bile acids and they are the end products of cholesterol catabolism in the liver (Fig. 10.37).

Formation of bile salts

In the liver, primary bile acids are activated to their corresponding CoAs. These activated bile acids undergo conjugation with glycine and taurine to form tauro, glycocholate and tauro, glycochenodeoxy cholate. They are secreted into bile. At physiological pH of bile, they combine with Na^+, K^+ ions to form bile salts (Fig. 10-37). They are secreted into intestine as bile salts of bile. Bile also contains come free cholesterol. Na^+, K^+ tauro and glycocholate, Na^+, K^+ tauro and glycochenodeoxy cholate are called as bile salts.

Fate of bile salts in the intestine

In the intestine a part of bile acids undergoes deconjugation and dehydroxylation by intestinal bacteria. The products are deoxycholic acid and lithocholic acid, which are called as secondary bile acids (Fig. 10.37).

Enterohepatic circulation

Most of primary and secondary bile acids are absorbed in ileum. About 99% of bile acids secreted into intestine returns to liver through portal circulation. This is known as enterohepatic circulation (from intestine to liver and back).

Only a small part of bile acids (400 mg/day) escaps reabsorption in the ileum. Lithocholic acid is not reabsorbed because of its less solubility. So, it is eliminated through the feces along with other bile that escaped reabsorption.

Other catabolic fates of cholesterol

1. Another important catabolic fate of cholesterol relates to steroid hormones.
2. Steroid hormones are synthesized in various tissues using cholesterol as starting material. Finally, they are excreted in urine after conjugation.

Formation of Steroid Hormones

1. Five classes of steroid hormones are synthesized from cholesterol. They are progesterone, testosterone, cortisol, aldosterone and estradiol.
2. Corpus luteum and placenta synthesizes progesterone. Testis and ovaries produce testosterone and estradiol, respectively. Adrenal cortex produces aldosterone and cortisol.
3. NADPH is another important substance needed for steroid hormone formation.
4. **Site** Most of the reactions of steroid hormone formation occurs in mitochondria and smooth endoplasmic reticulum.
5. Pregnenolone is the common intermediate of all the five classes of steroid hormone biosynthetic pathways.
6. Enzymes involved in steroid hormone formation are dehydrogenases, hydroxylases and lyases.
7. **Formation of pregnenolone** A mitochondrial cyt P_{450} dependent cholesterol desmolase converts cholesterol to pregnenolone by cleavage of side chain.

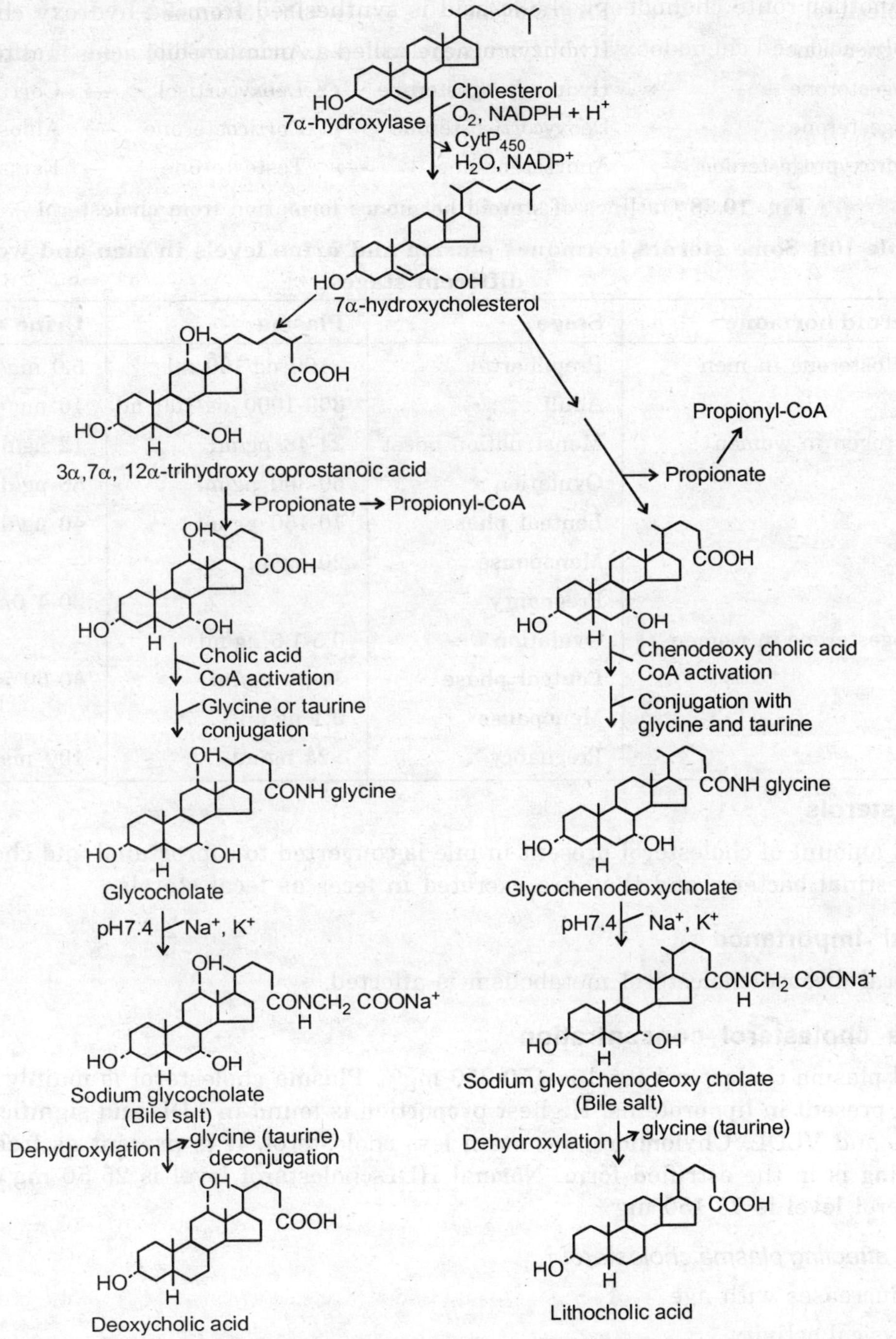

Fig. 10.37 Reactions of cholesterol catabolism

8. Formation of steroid hormones from pregnenolone is out lined in Fig. 10.38.
9. Plasma and urinary levels of testosterone, estradiol and progesterone in men and women at different stages are presented in Table 10.1.

Cholesterol	⟶	Pregnenolone	⟶	Progesterone		
Prognenolone	⟶	Hydroxypregnenolone	⟶	Andostenediol	⟶	Testosterone
Progesterone	⟶	Hydroxyprogesterone	⟶	Deoxycortisol	⟶	Cortisol
Progesterone	⟶	Deoxycorticosterone	⟶	Corticosterone	⟶	Aldosterone
Hydroxyprogesterone	⟶	Androstendione	⟶	Testosterone	⟶	Estradiol

Fig. 10.38 Outlines of steroid hormones formation from cholesterol

Table 10.1 Some steroid hormones plasma and urine levels in men and women of different stages.

Steroid hormone	Stage	Plasma	Urine
Testosterone in men	Prepubertal	<100 ng/100 ml	5.0 mg/day
	Adult	300-1000 ng/100 ml	10 mg/day
Estrogen in women	Menstruation onset	24-48 pg/ml	12 μg/day
	Ovulation	50-300 pg/ml	56 μg/day
	Leuteal phase	70-150 pg/ml	40 μg/day
	Menopause	20 pg/ml	–
	Pregnancy	–	20-4 0mg/day
Progesterone in women	Ovulation	0.5-1.5 ng/ml	–
	Leuteal phase	10-20 ng/ml	40-50 mg/day
	Menopause	0.1 ng/ml	
	Pregnancy	>24 ng/ml	100 mg/day

Fecal sterols

A small amount of cholesterol present in bile is converted to coprostanol and cholestanol by the intestinal bacteria and they are excreted in feces as fecal sterols.

Medical Importance

In several disease cholesterol metabolism is affected.

Plasma cholesterol concentration

Normal plasma cholesterol level is 150-250 mg%. Plasma cholesterol is mainly due to cholesterol present in lipoproteins. Highest proportion is found in LDL and significant amount in HDL and VLDL. Chylomicrons contain less cholesterol. It is present as free (30%) and remaining is in the estrified form. Normal HDL-cholesterol level is 25-50 mg% and LDC-cholesterol level is 75-150 mg%.

Factors affecting plasma cholesterol

1. It increases with age
2. Physical activity
3. Life style
4. Dietary fat
5. Smoking
6. Genetic factors

Hyper cholesterolemia

Plasma cholesterol level is high in atherosclerosis, coronary artery disease, diabetes, xanthomatosis, nephrotic syndrome, hypothyroidism and obstructive jaundice.

Hyper cholesterolemia and incidence of coronary artery disease

Though there are many lipids in plasma relative risk of developing Coronary Artery Disease (CAD) is related to raised plasma cholesterol level. However, the most useful index of coronary artery disease incidence is LDL:HDL cholesterol ratio. This ratio is used to predict incidence of coronary disease.

Effect of PUFA of diet on plasma cholesterol

The polyunsaturated fatty acids (PUFA) in diet decreases plasma cholesterol where as saturated fatty acids increase plasma cholesterol level. The mechanism is not clear. Hence, consumption of diets rich in PUFA reduces incidence of coronary artery disease. Wheat germ oil, safflower oil, sunflower oil, rice bran oil and peanut oil are rich sources of PUFA.

Cholesterol lowering drugs (Hypocholesterolemic drugs)

Since raised cholesterol level is associated with development of coronary artery disease, several drugs are used to lower blood cholesterol level. Lowering of plasma cholesterol level decreases incidence of coronary artery disease. For example, at the age of 40, a decrease in blood cholesterol level from 250 to 200mg% lowers incidence of coronary artery disease by 50%.

Hypocholesterolemic drugs lower plasma cholesterol level by affecting cholesterol metabolism at several stages.

1. **Lovastatin (Mevinolinate)** It is a competitive inhibitor of HMG-CoA reductase. It reduces plasma cholesterol level with minimal side affects. Compactin or mevastatin is another competitive inhibitor.
2. **Nicotinic acid** It decreases plasma cholesterol by interfering with the mobilization of free fatty acids.
3. **Neomycin** It interferes with bile acid re-absorption and absorption of dietary cholesterol. As a result, elimination of cholesterol is more from the body. This leads to decrease in plasma cholesterol level.
4. **Probucol** It also decreases blood cholesterol level by increasing excretion of cholesterol and bile acids.
5. **Cholesteramine (Questran)** It lowers blood cholesterol level by decreasing re-absorption of bile acids.
6. **Clofibrate (Astromid-S)** It blocks cholesterol formation in liver and increases excretion of cholesterol and bile acids. As a result, blood cholesterol level is decreased.
7. **Dextro thyroxine (D-thyroxine)** It lowers blood cholesterol level by accelerating cholesterol catabolism thereby increasing fecal cholesterol excretion.
8. **β-Sitosterol** It is a plant sterol. It decreases blood cholesterol by blocking absorption of dietary cholesterol.
9. **Plant lectins and gums** They lower blood cholesterol level by interfering with absorption of cholesterol and bile acids.

10. **Guava** Consumption of this tropical fruit for three months bring down plasma cholesterol from 250 mg% to 200 mg%.

Hypocholesterolemia

Plasma cholesterol level is decreased in hyper thyroidism, liver disease malabsorption syndrome and hemolytic anaemia.

Gall stones

Since cholesterol solubility is less in bile, an increase in cholesterol amount in bile favours gall stone formation. However, genetic factors are mainly involved in gall stone formation. Cholesterol content of gallstone is very high about 80%. Normally cholesterol is precipitated around nucleus of protein and bilirubin. Bacterial infections also promote gall stone formation. Further, woman are three times more susceptible to this condition. Cholelithiasis affected individuals have gallstones in biliary tract.

Atherosclerosis

1. It is an abnormality associated with cholesterol metabolism. Blood cholesterol level is always high in atherosclerosis.
2. However, genetic factors are also involved in the development of this disease.
3. In this condition, initially cholesterol esters particularly cholesterol oleates of arterial smooth muscle cells deposits in arterial intima. This leads to fatty streaks formation and condition is reversible. If condition is not controlled continued extracellular deposition of cholesterol esters along with apo B-100 of lipoproteins results in the formation of plaque in the arterial wall.
4. Plaque formation in the arterial wall causes narrowing of arterial lumen.
5. Blood vessel narrowing due to deposition of cholesterolester and apo B-100 is called as atherosclerosis.
6. Plaque in arteries promotes clot formation.
7. If clot formation occurs in coronary artery, the blood and O_2 supply to cardiac muscle diminishes. This manifest as myocardial infarction or stroke because anoxia causes necrosis of cardiac tissue.
8. Thus atherosclerosis cause coronary artery, disease (CAD)
9. Atherosclerosis may develop as secondary complication of diseases like diabetes, hypothyroidism, lipid nephrosis and other type of dyslipoproteinemias.
10. Some atherosclerotic lesions occurs even with normal blood cholesterol level. Inflammatory factors, low HDL levels are involved in this type of atherosclerosis development. Decreased HDL level leads to monocyte in filtration into arterial wall, macrophage, foam cell formation and lesion.

Antiatherogenic action of apoA-I of HDL

Let us examine how decreased HDL triggers atherosclerotic lesion despite normal cholesterol level.

1. ApoA-I major apolipoprotein component of HDL inhibits atherosclerosis without altering plasma cholesterol level by its antioxidant effect on LDL.

2. It inhibits formation of minimally modified LDL (MM LDL) or oxidized LDL.
3. MM LDL is formed from LDL when hydroperoxide formation from LDL surface fatty acids like arachidonic acid or linolenic acid reached a critical level by lipoxygenase pathway.
4. In the arterial endothelium MM LDL produces monocyte chemotactic protein (MCP) which causes monocyte in filtration.
5. Once monocyte enters into arterial wall they undergo MM LDL mediated transformation into macrophages that takes up more cholesterol form LDL. This leads to formation of foam cells and atherosclerotic lesion.
6. ApoA-I removes hydroperoxides formed on surface of LDL. Hence formation of MM LDL is prevented.
7. Thus apoA-I inhibits atherosclerosis through its antioxidant effect.
8. Since apoA-I is component of HDL, decreases HDL leads to atherosclerotic lesion.

Cancer

Regulation of HMG-CoA reductase activity is lost in cancer cells particularly in hepatomas. As a result, excess cholesterol is produced which in turn is used by growing cells for membrane formation.

Obesity

Hydroxycitrate is used in treatment of obesity. It works by blocking cholesterol synthesis.

Lipoprotein (a) and coronary artery disease

It is a LDL variant present in plasma, which contains apo-A. It is cholesterolester rich lipoprotein. Asian Indians have higher levels of this lipoprotein in plasma than most of the other ethnic groups. High levels of lipoprotein (a) increases the risk of premature coronary artery disease. Its level is also elevated in diabetes, nephrotic syndrome and renal failure. High levels of this lipoprotein in plasma promotes fat deposition and clot formation in blood vessel walls.

Brown Fat

1. It is a special type of adipose tissue. It is present in humans, hibernating animals like grizzly bear, dormouse and mammals that live in cold environment.
2. Large number of mitochondria present are responsible for characteristic colour.
3. Brown adipose tissue mitochondrial respiratory chain does not produce ATP. It generates heat.
4. Thermogenin, an inner mitochondrial protein act as proton channel. Hence, protons pumped out by respiratory chain flows back into mitochondria. As a result, respiratory chain energy is released as heat instead of ATP.

Medical importance

1. In humans, it is present in front and back side of upper chest and neck.
2. In cold environment, epinephrine stimulates fat mobilization oxidation of fatty acids produce heat rather than ATP. Thus, in cold environment, brown fat act as warming oven.

3. Brown fat is less or absent in obese people.
4. Brown fat may be more in people who can eat but not get fat.

REFERENCES

1. Wakil, S.J. (Ed.) Lipid Metabolism. Academic Press, New York, 1970.
2. Mcgarry, J.D. and Foster, D.W. Regulation of hepatic fatty acid oxidation and ketone body production. Ann. Rev. Biochem. **49**, 395, 1980.
3. Jelliffe, D.B. and Stuart, K.L. Acute toxic hypoglycemia in the vomiting sickness of Jamaica, Brit, Med. J.**1**, 75-77, 1954.
4. Wakil, S.J. and Stoops, J.K. Structure and mechanism of fatty acid synthase in the Enzymes. Vol. 16. P.D. Boyer (Ed.) 3rd ed. Academic Press, New York.
5. Wakil, S.J. Stoops, J.K. and Joshi, V.R. Fatty acid synthesis and its regulation. Ann. Rev. Biochem. **52**, 537-579, 1983.
6. Reed, L.J. Multi enzyme complexes. Acco. Chem. Res. **7,** 43, 1974.
7. Needle, P.J. Turk, B.A. and Leftkowith, J.B. Arachidonic acid metabolism. Ann. Rev. Biochem. **55**, 69-102, 1986.
8. Eisenberg, S, and Levy, R.I. Lipoprotein metabolism. Adv. Lipid. Res. **13,** 1, 1975.
9. Brown, M.S. and Goldstein, J.L. A receptor mediated Pathway for cholesterol homeostasis. Science **232**, 34-47, 1986.
10. Goldstein, J.L. and Brown, M.S. Familial hypercholesterolemia. In Scriver, C.R. et al. (Eds.). The Methabolic Basis of Inherited Disease 6th ed. McGraw-Hill, New York 1989.
11. Norum, K.R. Gjone, E. and Glomset, J.A. Familial lecithin cholesterol acyl transferase deficiency. In Scriver, C.R. et al. (Eds.). The metabolic Basis of Inherited Disease. 6th ed. McGraw-Hill, New York, 1989.
12. Morrisett, J.D. *et al.* In Lipoprotein (a). Scanu. A.M. (Ed.). Academic Press, San Diego, pp. 53-74, 1990.
13. Doren, M.V. *et al.* HMG-CoA reductase guides migrating primordial germ cells. Nature. **401**, 443-444, 1999.
14. Vanden Berg, B. *etal.* Crystal structure of long chain fatty acid transporter Fad L. Science. **304**, 1506-1509, 2004.
15. Starai, V.J. *et al.* Sir-2 dependent activation of acetyl-CoA synthetase by deacylation of active lysine Science. **298**, 2390-2392, 2002.
16. Shartt, A.R. *et al.* Coronary heart disease prediction from lipoprotein cholesterol level, triglycerides, lipoproteins (a), apolipoproteins A-1 and B and HDL density sub fractions, Circulation. **104,** 1108-1113, 2001.
17. Halliwell Barry and Gutteridge John, M.L. Free radicals in biology and medicine, Oxford Press, 2003.
18. Gotto, Mannual of lipid disorders: reducing the risk of coronary heart disease. Lippincot Williams and Wilkins, 2003.

19. Kim, E.K. *et al.* C 75 a fatty acid synthase inhibitor reduces food in take via hypothalamic AMP activated protein Kinase. J. Biol. Chem. **279**, 19970-19976, 2004.

20. Jamie Llorda *et al.* Emigration of monocyte derived cells from atherosclerotic lesion characterize regressive but not progressive plaques. Proc. Natl. Acad. Sci. USA **101**, 11779-11784, 2004.

21. Fransisco J. Asturias *et al.* structural and molecular organization of mammalian fatty acid Synthase. Structural and Molecular Biology Nature. **12**, 225-232, 2005.

EXERCISES

ESSAY QUESTIONS

1. Define β-oxidation. Describe β-oxidation of myristic acid. Add note on energetics of this oxidation.
2. Describe de novo synthesis of palmitic acid. Write role of citrate in this process.
3. Give an account of ketone body metabolism. Add a note on ketosis.
4. Trace the pathways for the synthesis of triglyceride from glycolysis, glycerol and monoacylglycerol.
5. Briefly describe cholesterol biosynthesis. Add a note on its regulation.
6. Describe ways of acetyl-CoA formation and utilization.
7. Write an essay on lipoproteinemias.
8. Describe fate and formation of chylomicrons and VLDL.
9. How sphingolipids are synthesized in the body?
10. Write reactions involved in bio-synthesis of lecithin, cephalin, cardiolipin and phosphatidyl inositol.
11. Explain unsaturated fatty acid oxidation in the body.
12. How eicosanoids are produced in the body? Write drugs that work by blocking their formation.

SHORT QUESTIONS

1. Write fate propionate in humans.
2. Write a note on disorders of fatty acid oxidation.
3. Draw fatty acid synthase multienzyme complex. Label its various parts.
4. Define lipolysis. Explain role of lipoprotein lipase in this process.
5. Name sphingomyelin biosynthetic site. Trace reactions of sphingomyelin formation from palmitic acid.
6. Define lipidoses. Explain with any two examples.
7. Write a note on HDL metabolism.
8. Define dyslipoproteinemias. Classify giving an example for each class.
9. Define fatty liver. Write conditions which cause fatty liver. Suggest ways for its prevention.
10. Explain lipid peroxidation by free radicals. Name free radical scavenger systems present in body.
11. Write normal plasma cholesterol level. In what conditions, it is elevated?

12. Write a note on atherosclerosis.
13. Write a note an α-oxidation and ω-oxidation.
14. Write biochemical defects in the following.
    (*a*) Refsum's disease. (*b*) Zellweger's syndrome. (*c*) Jamaican vomiting sickness.
15. Write note on disorders associated with propionate metabolism.
16. How HMG-CoA is formed and utilized?
17. Write normal plasma ketone body level. Name conditions in which it is elevated. How they are detected in urine?
18. Define lipotropic factors. Give examples.
19. Write briefly about lipoprotein a.
20. Write a note on reverse cholesterol transport.
21. Explain action and importance of hypocholesterolemic drugs.
22. Outline steps involved in conversion of cholesterol to bile acids.

MULTIPLE CHOICE QUESTIONS

1. Fatty acid entry into cytosol requires
   (*a*) Fatty acid binding protein (*b*) Albumin
   (*c*) Fatty acid binding protein and Na^+ (*d*) Na^+
2. Peroxisomal fatty acid oxidation
   (*a*) Produces NADPH (*b*) Generates propionyl-CoA and H_2O_2
   (*c*) Acetyl-CoA and H_2O_2 (*d*) Octanoyl-CoA, acetyl-CoA and H_2O_2
3. Methyl malonic acid uria can occur due to
   (*a*) Mutase deficiency (*b*) Vita B_{12} deficiency
   (*c*) Deficiency of both mutase and vit B_{12} (*d*) Folic acid deficiency
4. NADPH required for fatty acid synthesis is derived from
   (*a*) HMP shunt (*b*) Malic enzyme
   (*c*) Isocitrate dehydrogenase (*d*) All of the above
5. Acetyl-CoA carboxylase is subjected to
   (*a*) Allosteric regulation (*b*) Hormonal regulation
   (*c*) Both allosteric and hormonal regulation (*d*) Covalent modification
6. Acyl-CoA cholesterol acyl transferase catalyzes
   (*a*) Esterification of cholesterol
   (*b*) Esterification of cholesterol with fatty acid
   (*c*) Transfer of fatty acid from cholesterol
   (*d*) Removal of fatty acid from cholesterol

FILL IN THE BLANKS

1. A 70 kg adult lipid store is about ....
2. Grizzly bear derives most of its .... and .... from lipid stores during hibernation.

3. Synthesis and oxidation of fatty acid involves .... bond formation and cleavage respectively.
4. Fatty acid synthesis and oxidation are reciprocally regulated by ....
5. Chronic alcoholism leads to .... development.
6. Aspirin works by inhibiting .... reaction.
7. HDL cholesterol is referred as ....
8. Lipoprotein (a) is a .... present in plasma.

CASES

1. A child was brought to hospital with complaints of nausea, vomiting and weakness. Physical examination showed weak extremities. Muscle biopsy showed more triglycerides. Blood fatty acid level was elevated. However blood glucose level was below normal. Write your diagnosis.
2. A middle aged man consulted cardiologist after experiencing chest pain for several times. His pain worsened when he was engaged in any type of mild exercise. His blood cholesterol and triglyceride levels were elevated. However, his HDL-cholesterol was below normal. Write your diagnosis.

11

CHAPTER

BIOLOGICAL OXIDATION AND RESPIRATORY CHAIN

INTRODUCTION

Energy is essential for living cells to perform vital cellular functions. Living cells obtain energy by burning foodstuffs. The foodstuffs are made up of carbohydrates, fats and proteins. The degradation of foodstuffs is accompanied by production of reduced coenzymes like $FADH_2$, $FMNH_2$, $NADH+H^+$ and $NADPH+H^+$. Since the continuation of metabolic pathways depends on availability of FMN, FAD and NAD^+, the reduced co enzymes must be re-oxidized. The oxidation of $FMNH_2$, $FADH_2$ and $NADH+H^+$ by respiratory O_2 with simultaneous production of H_2O is the final stage of biological oxidation reactions. The oxidation of $FADH_2$ and $NADH+H^+$ by O_2 accompanies release of energy, which is used for the formation of ATP and a small amount of energy is released as heat (Figure 11.1*a*). The $NADPH+H^+$ is re oxidized back by biosynthetic pathways that require reduced $NADP^+$.

The transfer of hydrogen atoms or electrons or reducing equivalents of $FADH_2$ and $NADH+H^+$ to respiratory O_2 is a stepwise process. Specific carrier molecules are arranged in a sequence to carry hydrogen (electrons) atoms from $FADH_2$ and $NADH + H^+$ to O_2. During the transfer of electrons form reduced coenzymes to O_2, the carrier molecules undergo coupled oxidation-reduction reactions because whenever one carrier is oxidized the other carrier is simultaneously reduced. Therefore, the electron transfer in biological systems involves coupled oxidation-reduction reactions. The coupled oxidation and reduction reactions during transfer of electrons is shown briefly in Figure 11.1*b*. Further, each hydrogen carrier itself exist in oxidized form and reduced form ($FAD/FADH_2$, O_2/H_2O). Coupled oxidation-reduction reactions involving transfer of electrons or hydrogen atoms from one compound to another compound also occurs in various metabolisms. Specific enzymes, coenzymes are involved in the electron transfer reactions in living systems.

MEDICAL AND BIOLOGICAL IMPORTANCE

1. Biological oxidation deals with the uses of respiratory O_2 in the body.
2. Several important biological oxidation reactions are directly associated with respiratory O_2.

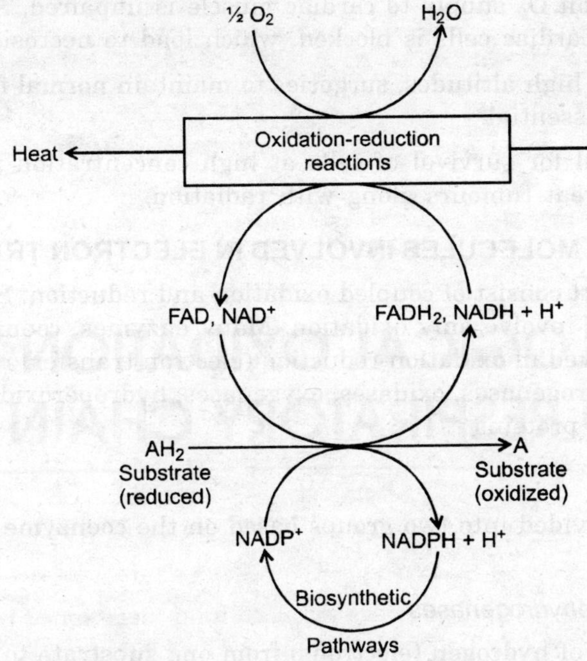

Fig. 11.1 (*a*) **Schematic diagram showing production of reduced coenzymes on oxidation of substrate with subsequent oxidation of them by O_2 and formation of ATP**

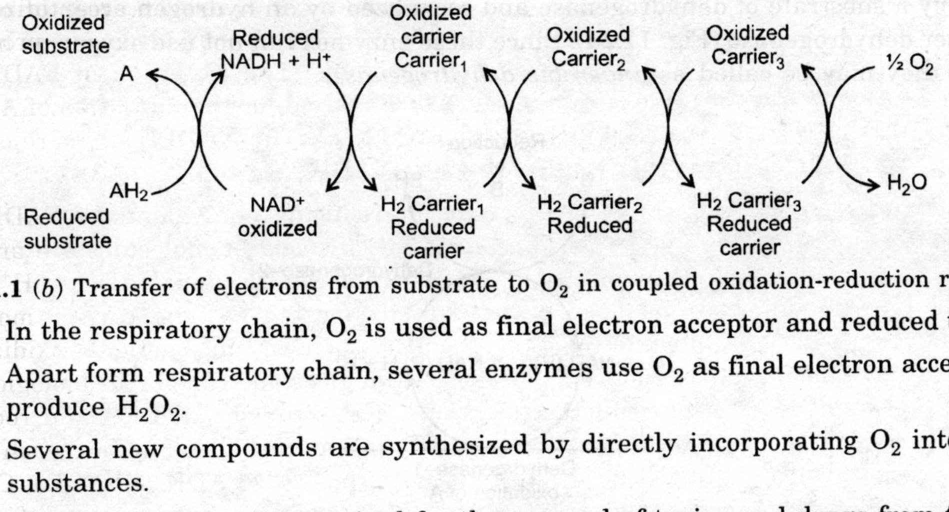

Fig. 11.1 (*b*) **Transfer of electrons from substrate to O_2 in coupled oxidation-reduction reactions**

(*a*) **In the respiratory chain, O_2 is used as final electron acceptor and reduced to water.**

(*b*) **Apart form respiratory chain, several enzymes use O_2 as final electron acceptor and produce H_2O_2.**

(*c*) **Several new compounds are synthesized by directly incorporating O_2 into certain substances.**

(*d*) **Respiratory O_2 is also required for the removal of toxins and drugs from the body.**

(*e*) **Superoxide ion derived from O_2 function as microbicide.**

3. **Biological oxidation provides means for the regeneration of coenzymes, which are used in metabolism.**
4. **It is the final aspect of all energy-producing compounds.**
5. **Transfer of electrons is impaired in certain disease like encephalopathy, lactic acidosis and mitochondrial myopathy.**

6. In myocardial infarction O_2 supply to cardiac muscle is impaired. As a result of this, energy production in cardiac cells is blocked, which lead to necrosis.
7. In some instances like high altitudes, surgeries to maintain normal functioning of body or cells O_2 supply is essential.
8. Though O_2 is essential for survival of cells at high concentration it is toxic to cells. Hence, it is used to treat tumours along with radiation.

ENZYMES AND CARRIER MOLECULES INVOLVED IN ELECTRON TRANSFER

Biological electron transport consist of coupled oxidation and reduction. Sometimes, biological electron transport may involve only oxidation. Many enzymes, coenzymes and several carrier molecules are involved in oxidation-reduction (electron transfer) reactions of biological system. They are dehydrogenases, oxidases, oxygenases, hydroperoxidases, cytochromes, ubiquinone and iron-sulfur proteins.

Dehydrogenases

The dehydrogenases are divided into two groups based on the coenzyme (prosthetic group) they require for activity.

1. Nicotinamide-dependent dehydrogenases

They catalyze the transfer of hydrogen (electrons) from one substrate to another substrate in a coupled oxidation-reduction reaction. They use coenzymes NAD^+ and $NADP^+$ as hydrogen carrier. These coenzymes are loosely associated with apoenzymes. The coenzymes are reduced by a substrate of dehydrogenase and reoxidized by an hydrogen acceptor catalyzed by another dehydrogenase (Fig. 11.2*a*). Since these enzymes can not use oxygen as hydrogen acceptor they may be called as *anaerobic dehydrogenases*.

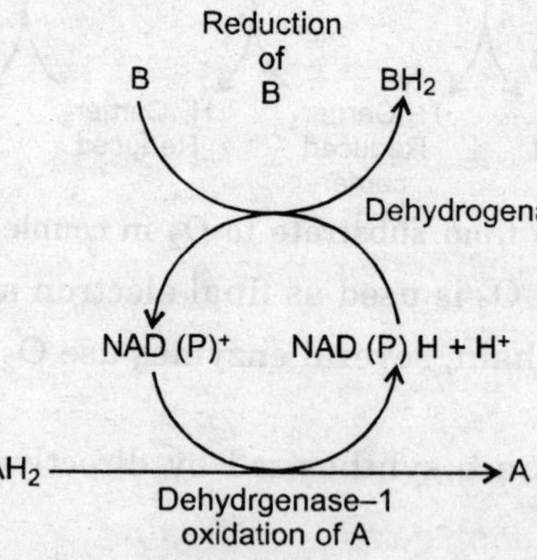

Fig. 11.2 (*a*) Hydrogen transfer from AH_2 to B in a coupled oxidation-reduction using NAD $(P)^+$ as carrier

The mechanism of oxidation of substrates by these enzymes involves removal of pair of hydrogen atoms from substrate. From the pair of hydrogens, an hydride ion (H^-) having two electrons is attached to nicotinamide and remaining hydrogen is released as free proton (H^+). Likewise reduction of substrates by these enzymes involves transfer of hydrogens from nicotinamide. Mechanism is shown in Figure 11.2*b*.

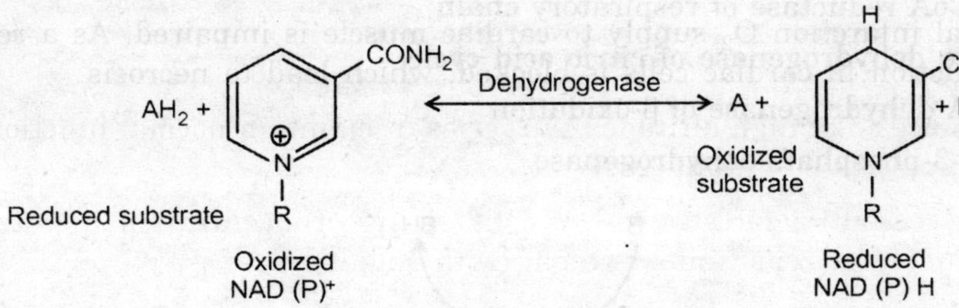

Fig. 11.2 (*b*) Mechanism of oxidation-reduction of a substrate by NAD $(P)^+$ dependent dehydrogenase

Examples:

1. NAD^+ dependent dehydrogenases of various oxidative pathways of carbohydrates, fats and proteins.
   (*a*) Glyceraldehyde-3-phosphate dehydrogenase
   (*b*) Lactate dehydrogenase
   (*c*) Pyruvate dehydrogenase
   (*d*) Malate dehydrogenase
   (*e*) Hydroxyacyl-CoA dehydrogenase
   (*f*) Glutamate dehydrogenase etc.
2. $NADP^+$ dependent dehydrogenases of various pathways.
   (*a*) Glucose-6-phosphate dehydrogenase
   (*b*) Phosphogluconate dehydrogenase
   (*c*) Glutathione reductase
   (*d*) Enoyl reductase
   (*e*) Ketoacyl reductase

2. Riboflavin-dependent dehydrogenases

They catalyze the removal of hydrogen from substrates. They use FMN and FAD as hydrogen carriers. FMN and FAD are tightly bound (prosthetic group) to apo-enzymes. They are of two types.

(*a*) Some of them transfer hydrogen to another substrate in a coupled oxidation and reduction reaction. Since oxygen is not (electron) hydrogen acceptor these are referred as riboflavin dependent anaerobic dehydrogenases (Figure 11.3*a*).

(*b*) Few of the riboflavin-dependent dehydrogenase use oxygen as hydrogen acceptor and produce H_2O_2. Hence, these can be referred as a riboflavin dependent aerobic dehydrogenases (Figure 11.3*a*).

Isoalloxazine ring of riboflavin participates in FMN and FAD dependent hydrogen transfer reactions. Oxidation of a substrate involves reduction of isoalloxazine ring via semiquinone. Likewise reduction of substrates involves oxidation of isoalloxazine (Figure 11.3*b*).

Examples:

(*a*) A Riboflavin-dependent anaerobic dehydrogenases.

1. NADH-CoA reductase of respiratory chain
2. Succinate dehydrogenase of citric acid cycle
3. Acyl-CoA dehydrogenase of β-oxidation
4. Glycerol-3-phosphate dehydrogenase

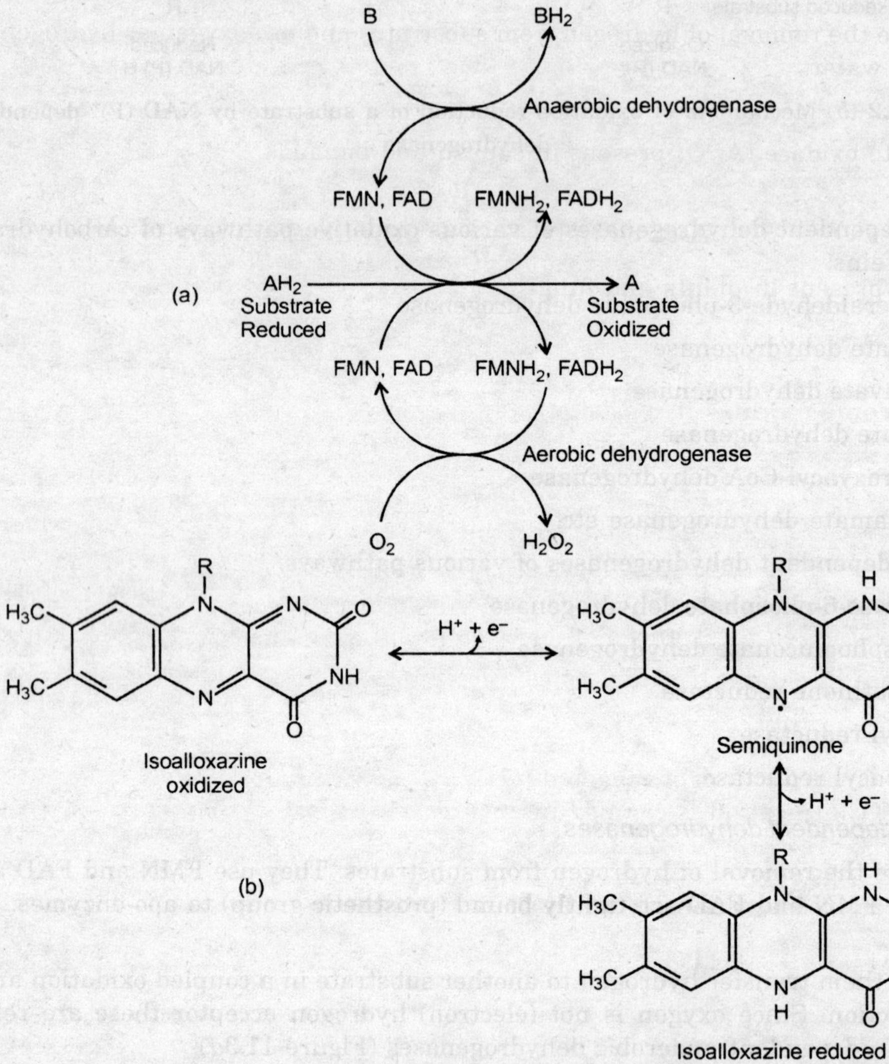

Fig. 11.3 (*a*) Hydrogen transfer from AH_2 to B and O_2 using FMN, FAD as carriers by anaerobic and aerobic dehydrogenases
(*b*) Oxidation-reduction of isoalloxazine of FMN, FAD via semiquinone

(*b*) **FMN and FAD dependent aerobic dehydrogenases or aerobic oxidases.**

1. Aminoacid oxidases of aminoacid catabolism present in liver and kidney. FMN is required by L-aminoacid oxidase and FAD is required by D-aminoacid oxidase.
2. Glucose oxidase an FAD requiring enzyme present in mold.

$$\text{Glucose} \xrightarrow[\text{FAD}]{\text{Glucose oxidase}} \text{Gluconicacid} + H_2O_2$$

Other enzymes are galactose oxidase, xanthine oxidase and aldehyde oxidase etc. The latter two enzymes contain metal ions molybdenum and iron in addition to FAD.

OXIDASES

They catalyze the removal of hydrogen from substrates and use oxygen as hydrogen acceptor and produce water.

Examples

1. Ascorbate oxidase (A. O) present in squash and bananas.

$$\text{Ascorbicacid} \xrightarrow[\text{A.O}]{O_2 \searrow \nearrow H_2O} \text{Dehydro ascorbicacid}$$

2. Laccase present in plants and fungi.

$$\text{Dihydroxy benzene} \xrightarrow[O_2 \nearrow \searrow H_2O]{} \text{quinones}$$

3. **Cytochrome oxidase** It consist of two subunits cytochrome a and cytochrome a_3. Each subunit contain haem iron and copper. It is the terminal component of respiratory chain. It is bound to mitochondrial membrane. Metal ions also participates in oxidation and reduction. It catalyzes unusual four electron reaction as shown below.

$$\text{Cytochrome } a_3(4Fe^{2+}) + O_2 + 4H^+ \longrightarrow \text{Cytocrome } a_3(4Fe^{3+}) + 2H_2O$$

Out of the two subunits only cytochrome a_3 can directly react with oxygen. Cytochrome oxidase catalyzes the transfer of electrons from cytochrome c to molecular oxygen.

4. Tyrosinase of potato. It catalyzes conversion of dihydroxy phenylalanine to quinones.

Oxygenases

They catalyze incorporation of oxygen directly into substrate molecules. They are two types. This type of O_2 utilization is cyanide insensitive (resistant).

(a) Dioxygenases

These catalyze incorporation of two atoms of oxygen into substrate.

$$X \xrightarrow{O_2} XO_2$$

Examples

1. Homogentisate dioxygenase
2. Cyclooxygenase
3. Hydroxy anthranilate dioxygenase
4. Tryptophan dioxygenase

(b) Mono oxygenases

They catalyze incorporation of one atom of oxygen into substrate. The other atom of oxygen is reduced to water. These enzymes are loosely referred as hydroxylases and (or) mixed function oxidases.

$$R-H \xrightarrow[\downarrow]{H_2, O_2} R\text{-}OH + H_2O$$

Examples

1. Kynurenine hydroxylase
2. Tryptophan hydroxylase
3. Phenylalanine hydroxylase
4. Cytochrome P_{450} hydroxylases

Hydroperoxidases

These enzymes catalyze breakdown of H_2O_2 which is produced in the body during reduction of oxygen to water. Reactions of oxidases also produce H_2O_2.

Examples

1. **Catalase** It is present in liver, kidney, bone marrow and blood. Peroxisomes are rich in catalase. It is a heme protein.

$$2H_2O_2 \xrightarrow{\text{Catalase}} 2H_2O + O_2$$

2. **Peroxidase** It is present in milk, leucocytes and plateletes. It is a heme protein. Other tissues also contain this enzyme. It is also called as myeloperoxidase. It converts H_2O_2 to water in presence of hydrogen donor. It is present in peroxisomes.

$$H_2O_2 + H_2 \xrightarrow{\text{Peroxidase}} 2H_2O$$

3. **Glutathione peroxidase** It is present in RBC. It is involved in the removal of H_2O_2 present in RBC. It contains selenium. Glutathione serve as hydrogen donor.

$$H_2O_2 + 2G\text{-}SH \xrightarrow[\text{Peroxidase}]{\text{Glutathione}} 2H_2O + G\text{-}S\text{-}S\text{-}G$$

CYTOCHROMES

The cytochromes are b, c_1 and c. They are components of electron transport chain present in mitochondria. They are heme proteins. Cytochrome c is a peripheral protein. Cytochrome b and c_1 are integral membrane proteins and they are constituents of cytochrome reductase complex. They are involved in transfer of electrons from ubiquinone to cytochrome oxidase. The iron of the cytochromes participates in oxidation-reduction reactions. The iron oscillates between Fe^{2+} and Fe^{3+} states. There are three types of cytochrome b. They are cyt b_{560}, cyt b_{562} and cyt b_{566}.

Cytochromes other than the components of respiratory chain are

Cytochrome P_{450}

It is so named because its complex with carbon monoxide absorbs light at 450 nm. It is a heme protein. It is prosthetic group of monooxygenases or hydroxylases. Cyt P_{450} directly interacts with oxygen. The iron of heme participates in oxidation-reduction reaction. There are two types of cytochrome P_{450} dependent monooxygenases or hydroxylases. They are

1. Microsomal cytochrome P_{450} hydroxylase

It is present in microsomes of liver. It requires NADPH as hydrogen donor. It also contains flavoproteins. It is involved in hydroxylation of several drugs (Figure 11.4*a*) Cyt P_{450}-

hydroxylase is inducible. Hydroxylation of drug by this enzyme system decreases its toxicity. Cyt P_{450}-hydroxylase is responsible for the formation of carcinogens from pre-carcinogens present in food. Sometimes hydroxylation converts prodrug to active drug.

2. Mitochondrial cytochrome P_{450} hydroxylase

It is present in mitochondria of liver, adrenal cortex, testes, ovaries and kidneys. It requires NADPH, flavoproteins and iron-sulfur proteins. In adrenal cortex cyt P_{450} hydroxylase is responsible for hydroxylation of steroid hormones. It is responsible for hydroxylation of bile acids in liver, steroid hormones in testes and ovaries. In kidneys it is responsible for hydroxylation of Vit D (Figure 11.4B).

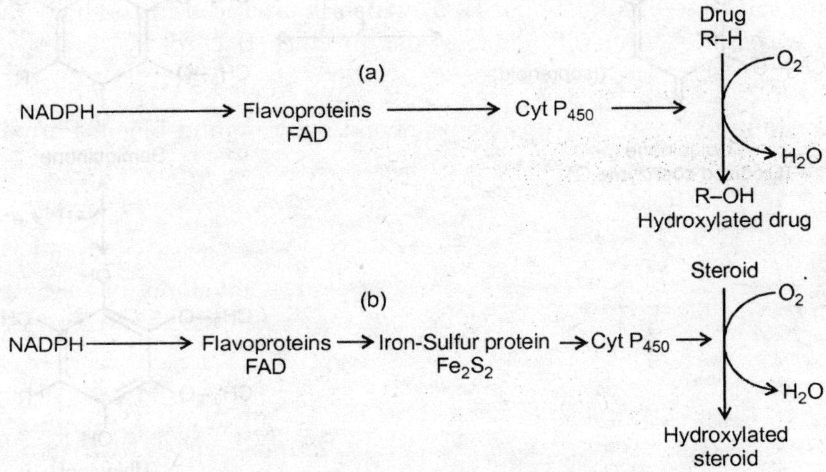

Fig. 11.4 (*a*) Microsomal Cyt P_{450} hydroxylase
(*b*) Mitochondrial Cyt P_{450} hydroxylase

Cytochrome b_5

It is also a heme protein. It is present in liver. It can not directly interact with O_2. It also requires NAD(P)H, flavoproteins. It is involved in the formation of mono unsaturated fatty acids. Cytb_5 dependent enzyme is known as fatty acyl-CoA desaturase.

Ubiquinone or Coenzyme Q (CoQ)

It is a constituent of mitochondrial lipids. It is a component of respiratory chain. It is the only non-protein component of electron transport chain. Because of its ubiquitous nature it is called as ubiquinone. It is a mobile electron carrier of respiratory chain. It collects electrons from NADH and $FADH_2$ and transfers to cytochromes. It participates in coupled oxidation reduction reactions of respiratory chain via semiquinone intermediate (Figure 11.5).

Iron-sulfur proteins

They are proteins containing iron-sulfur centers. Iron and sulfur are present as clusters in these proteins. Iron of these proteins is referred as non-heme iron(NHI). Iron is complexed with organic sulfur and inorganic sulfur. Organic sulfur is contributed by the cysteine residue of protein (Fig. 11.6). Iron and sulfur are present in equimolar amounts. They participate in one electron transfer reactions. Iron oscillates between Fe^{2+} and Fe^{3+}. The oxidized center accept one electron ($Fe^{3+} \xrightarrow{e^-} Fe^{2+}$) and get reduced.

In mammals, several flavin containing iron sulfur proteins are present in the respiratory chain. They transfer electrons from NADH-CoQ reductase and succinate-CoQ reductase to ubiquinone. NADH-CoQ reductase contain 4 Fe_4S_4 centers per molecule of FMN. FAD containing succinate-CoQ reductase has 2 Fe_2 S_2 centers. Adrenodoxin in adrenal cortex contain Fe_2 S_2 center. In plants, ferodoxins contain four iron atoms and four sulfur atoms (Fe_4S_4).

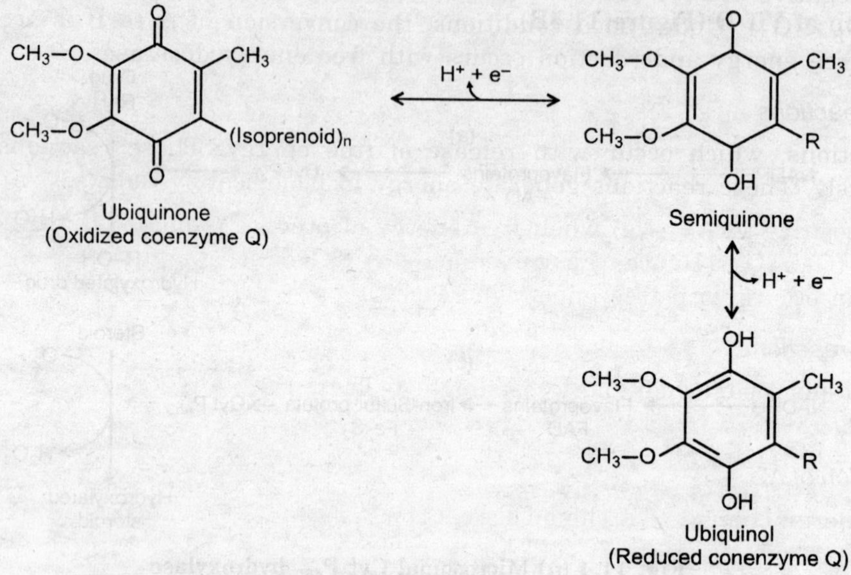

Fig. 11.5 Oxidation-reduction of ubiquinone via semiquinone

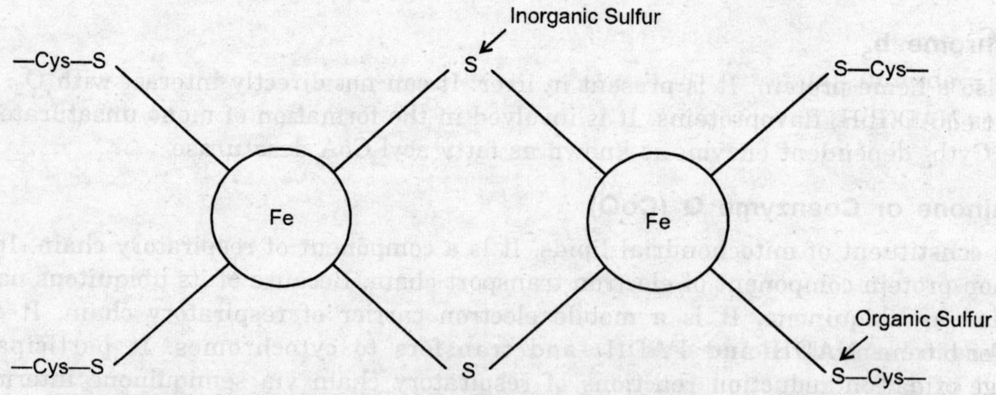

Fig. 11.6 An iron sulfur centre of protein containing two iron atoms and two sulfur atoms (Fe_2Se_2)

Free energy, exergonic and endergonic reactions

Since the transfer of electrons from reduced co enzymes to O_2 involves release of energy and formation of ATP, the energy aspect of chemical reactions has to be explored at this stage.

Free energy

It is the potential energy of a substance. Free energy of a substance is represented by G (Gibbs) and it is difficult to measure G directly.

In any chemical reaction the free energy content of reactant and product are not same. Hence, the free energy change ΔG when a substance A is converted to B can be obtained as $\Delta G = G_B\text{-}G_A$.

Where G_A and G_B are free energy of A and B, respectively.

ΔG is negative ($\Delta G = -ve$) when free energy of product is less than the free energy of reactant ($G_B < G_A$). Under such conditions, the conversion of A to B is accompanied by release of free energy and reaction occurs with free energy decrease.

Exergonic reactions

Those reactions, which occur with release of free energy. These reactions takes place spontaneously. These reactions generate energy in biological systems.

ΔG is positive ($\Delta G = +ve$) when free energy of product is higher than the free energy of reactant ($G_B > G_A$). Hence, the conversion of A to B takes place when energy is supplied and reaction occurs with free energy increase.

Endergonic reactions

These reactions occur when energy is supplied. These reactions consume energy in biological systems.

Determination of ΔG

The free energy change of a chemical reaction A $\longrightarrow$ B is determined by equation.

$$\Delta G = \Delta G^1 + RT \ln \frac{[B]}{[A]}$$

ΔG^1 = standard free energy change when concentrations of A and B are 1M

T = absolute temperature, R = Gas constant

At equilibrium $\Delta G = 0$

Then $$\Delta G^1 = -RT \frac{\ln[B]}{[A]}$$

$$= -RT \ln K_{eq} \text{ (Equilibrium constant } K_{eq} = \frac{[B]}{[A]})$$

For biochemical reactions, ΔG^{01} is used instead of ΔG^1. ΔG^{01} is the standard free energy change of a reactions at p^H 7.0.

High energy compounds

The hydrolysis of these compounds is accompanied by release of large amount of free energy. Since ATP is a high energy compound, the energy released during transfer of electrons from reduced coenzymes to O_2 is conserved in the form of ATP. The energy released when an high energy compound is hydrolyzed is not due to bond that is hydrolyzed. It is due to large difference in the free energy content of reactant and product.

ΔG^{01} for the hydrolysis of ATP is given below

$$ATP \longrightarrow ADP + P_i$$

$$\Delta G^{01} = -7.3 \text{ Kcal/mol } (-30 \text{ KJ/mole})$$

ADP is also energy rich compound because ΔG^{01} for ADP hydrolysis is –7.3 Kcal/mol.

By convention, high energy bond is shown with ~ (squiggle) symbol. So, the ATP is written as

High energy bond

Adenine-Ribose-[P]~[P]~[P]

ΔG^{01} for hydrolysis of other compounds is less. For example, when glucose-6-phosphate is hydrolysed only 3.3 Kcal/mol of energy is released (ΔG^{01} = -3.3 Kcal/mol).

Significance of ATP

1. It is involved in the transfer of energy in the cells. It is often called as *energy currency* of the cell.
2. In the cells, the energy released in an exergonic reaction is used to form ATP and energy required for an endergonic reactions is supplied by hydrolysing ATP. Therefore, in biological systems ATP serve as link between the exergonic and endergonic reactions (Fig. 11.7).
3. Energy of ATP hydrolysis is also used for muscle contraction, transport of ions and molecules across cell membrane, motility of sperm cells etc.

Other nucleoside triphosphates like GTP, UTP, CTP, TTP, dATP, dGTP and dTTP are also high energy compounds. The electronic structure of these compounds is responsible for the release of large free energy on hydrolysis.

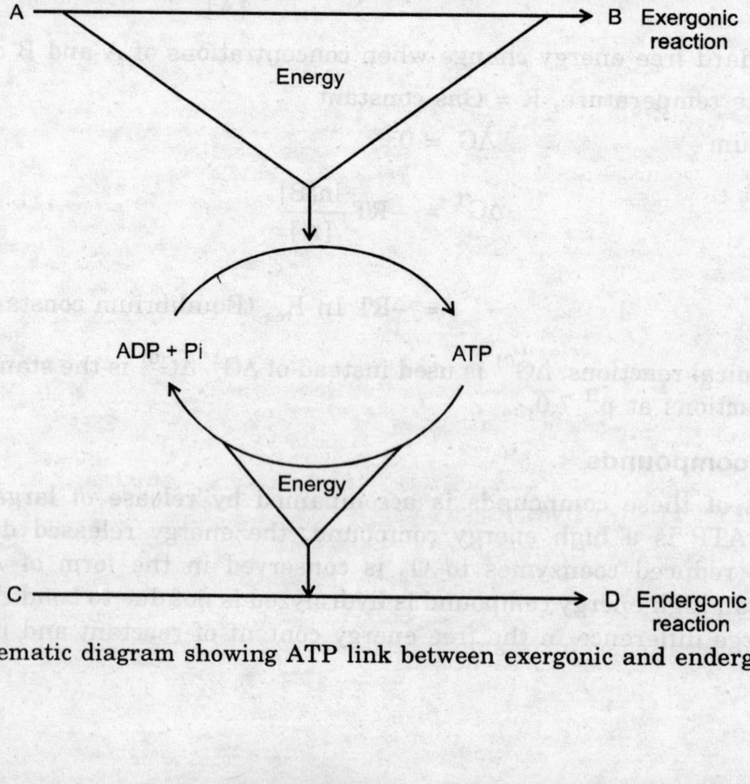

Fig. 11.7 Schematic diagram showing ATP link between exergonic and endergonic reactions

Other high energy compounds are

Phospho creatine

It is present in the skeletal muscle. It is involved in the transfer and storage of energy in muscle. The free energy of hydrolysis of phosphocreatine is 10.3 Kcal/mol ($\Delta G^{0\prime}$ = –10.3 Kcal/mol).

Thioesters

They are formed from the condensation of coenzyme A, a thiol with carboxylic acids. They are also high energy compounds. For example, hydrolysis of acetyl-CoA to acetic acid and water is accomanied by release of 7.5 Kcal/mol of energy (Figure 11.8*a*).

Enolphosphates

They are esters of enol with phosphoric acids. Phosphoenol pyruvate is an example for enol phosphate ester. The free energy released on hydrolysis of this high energy compound is –14.8 Kcal/mol (Figure 11.8*b*).

Acyl phosphates

They are mixed anhydrides. The two acids involved in the mixed anhydride formation are carboxylic acid and phosphoric acid. An example for a high energy mixed anhydride is 1, 3-bisphosphoglycerate. Hydrolysis of 1, 3-bisphospholgycerate is accompanied release of –11.8 Kcal/mol of energy (Figure 11.8*c*).

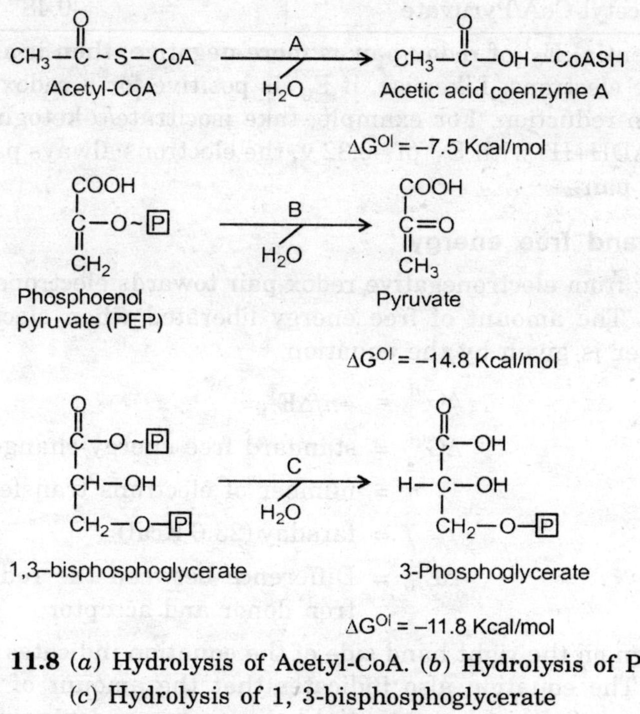

Fig. 11.8 (*a*) Hydrolysis of Acetyl-CoA. (*b*) Hydrolysis of PEP (*c*) Hydrolysis of 1, 3-bisphosphoglycerate

Redox potential

It is an electrochemical concept related to redox reactions.

Redox reactions

The oxidation-reduction reactions are called as redox reactions. The oxidant (acceptor) and reductant (donor) of a redox reaction are known as *redox pair* or *redox couple*. For example, NAD (oxidized form)/NADH (reduced form) constitutes a redox couple.

Redox potential

It is defined as electro motive force (e.m.f.) of a redox pair when oxidant and reductant are present in 1M concentration. The symbol used to indicate redox potential is E_0^1 and units are volts. It indicates the tendency of a redox pair to gain or give electron. The redox potentials of biologically important redox pairs are measured at pH 7.0 by taking hydrogen electrode as standard (reference).

Redox potentials of some redox pairs

Redox pair	Redox potential (E_0^1) in volts
O_2/H_2O	+0.82
Cytochrome c	+0.25
$FAD/FADH_2$	–0.18
$NAD^+/NADH+H^+$	–0.32
α-ketoglutarate/isocitrate	–0.38
Acetyl-CoA/Pyruvate	–0.48

If the redox potential E_0^1 of redox pair is more negative, then it always undergo oxidation or tend to loose electrons. Likewise, if E_0^1 is positive for a redox pair then, it accepts electrons or undergo reduction. For example, take isocitrate/α-ketoglutarate with E_0^1 of –0.38 v and $NAD^+/NADH+H^+$ with E_0^1 of –0.32 v, the electrons always pass from former redox pair to latter redox pair.

Electron transfer and free energy

When electrons flow from electronegative redox pair towards electropositive redox pair free energy is liberated. The amount of free energy liberated when electrons move from one redox pair to another is given by the equation.

$$\Delta G^{01} = -nf\Delta E^1{}_0$$

ΔG^{01} = standard free energy change in calories

n = number of electrons transferred

f = faraday (23.6 Kcal)

$\Delta E^1{}_0$ = Difference between the redox potentials of electron donor and acceptor

The negative sign on the right hand side of the equation indicates release of free energy into surroundings. The equation also indicates that the amount of free energy liberated depends on difference of the redox potential between two redox pairs. So, when electrons flow from NAD to O_2 large amount of free energy is released because of the more redox potential difference between two redox pairs. By sustituting redox potentials of $NAD/NADH_2$ and O_2/H_2O in the above equation, we get

$$\Delta G^{0'} = -2 \times 23.6 \times (-0.32 - 0.82)$$
$$= -56.2 \text{ Kcal}$$

Since only 7.5 Kcal of energy is required for the formation of one molecule of ATP from ADP and Pi, during the transfer of electrons from NAD to O_2, three ATP are generated and remaining energy is released as heat. In addition, this equation can be used to know redox potential difference required for ATP formation in the respiratory chain. Approximately 0.15 volts of redox potential difference is required for one ATP formation.

ELECTRON TRANSPORT CHAIN (ETC) OR RESPIRATORY CHAIN

It is present in inner mitochondrial membrane. Electron transport chain consist of various electron transport or electron carrier molecules. The electron transport molecules are arranged in a sequence. They carry or transfer electrons from reduced coenzymes like NADH, $FADH_2$ to final electron acceptor O_2. The electron transport molecules are called as *components* of respiratory chain. Some of them are proteins and non-protein carriers also present.

The position of a particular component in the respiratory chain depends on its redox potential. The components of respiratory chain are arranged in the order of increasing redox potential. Starting components have negative redox potential and terminal components have positive redox potential. Therefore, in the respiratory chain, electrons flow from negative to positive (Figure 11.9).

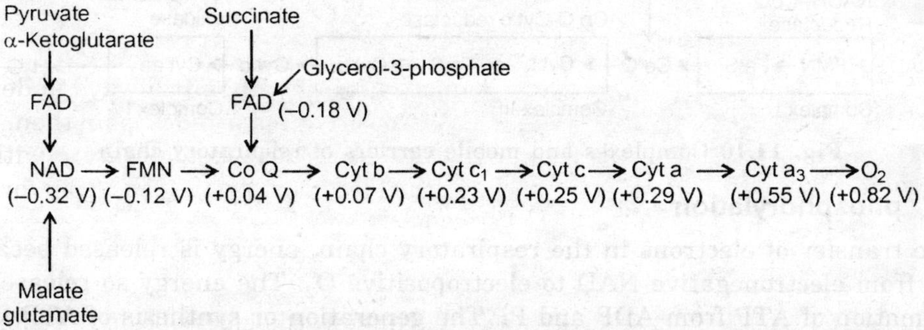

Fig. 11.9 Electron flow in the respiratory chain. Redox potential of each component of electron transport chain is given in parenthesis

In the respiratory chain, electrons flow from NAD to cytochromes via CoQ and then from cytochromes to molecular O_2. CoQ also collects electrons from FAD. The transfer of electrons from substrates to NAD and FAD is catalyzed by dehydrogenases. At the electronegative end of respiratory chain, NAD linked deydrogenases like malate and glutamate dehydrogenases catalyze transfer of electrons from substrate to NAD directly but electrons from substrates like pyruvate, and α-ketoglutarate are transferred via FAD (Figure 11.9). In contrast some FAD linked dehydrogenases like succinate and glycerol-3-phosphate dehydrogenases catalyze transfer of electrons from substrate to CoQ of respiratory chain because their redox potentials are more positive.

Many components of respiratory chain are present as complexes rather than single entities. On NAD, CoQ and cytochrome c are present as individual components rest of the components of respiratory chain are present as complexes. The repiratory chain consist of four complexes and three mobile carriers. The complexes are complex I, II, III and VI and mobile carriers are NAD, CoQ, cytochrome c and O_2. All the complexes are integral membrane proteins. Each complex is involved in oxidation and each complex accepts electrons from mobile electron carrier and pass electrons to another mobile electron carrier (Figure 11.10).

Complex I is NADH-CoQ reductase or NADH dehydrogenase. FMN and Fe:S clusters are prosthetic groups of this enzyme. Electrons collected by NAD are transferred to CoQ by NADH-CoQ reductase via FMN and Fe:S cluser. So NAD is oxidized. Complex II is the succinate-CoQ reductase. It also contains FAD and iron sulfur clusters. Complex II transfers electrons from succinate and glycerol-3-phosphate to CoQ via FAD and Fe:S. Complex III is CoQ-cyt c reductase or cytochrome reductase. It also contains Fe:S cluster. Complex III transfers electrons from CoQ to cytochrome c via cyt b, c, and Fe:S cluster. As a result of this CoQ get oxidized. Complex IV is cytochrome oxidase. It transfers the electrons from cyt c to final electron acceptor O_2 so cyt c is oxidized (Figure 11.10).

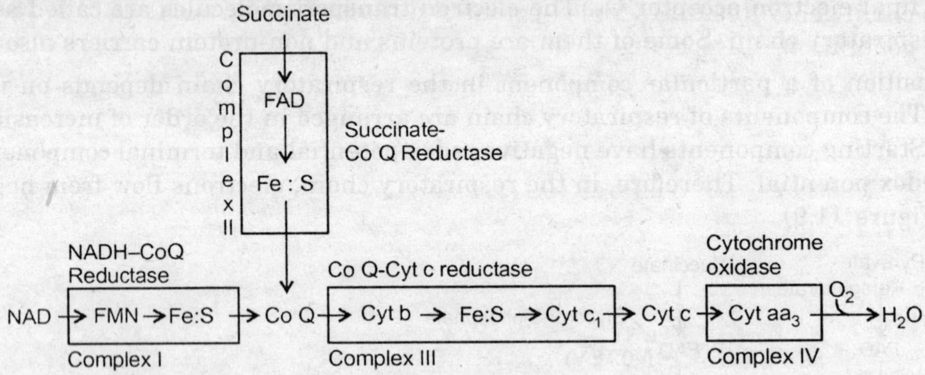

Fig. 11.10 Complexes and mobile carriers of respiratory chain

Oxidative phosphorylation

During the transfer of electrons in the respiratory chain, energy is released because electrons flow from electronegative NAD to electropositive O_2. The energy so released is used for the formation of ATP from ADP and Pi. The generation or synthesis of ATP from ADP and phosphate (Pi) while electrons flow in the respiratory chain is called as oxidative phosphorylation. This process accounts for over 85% of high energy phosphates or ATP produced in the body. Oxidative phosphorylation is the combination of oxidation and phosphorylation. The two processes are coupled to each other and in normal cells one does not usually occur without the other. The word oxidation is used because the transfer of electrons from substrate to oxygen causes oxidation of substrate or when mobile carrier is oxidized then only electrons flow occurs in the respiratory chain.

ATP synthesis

Formation of ATP from ADP and phosphate using energy released when electrons flow in the respiratory chain is catalysed by membrane bound enzyme known as ATP synthase or F_0 F_1 ATPase. It is often referred as another complex V of respiratory chain. It is an integral membrane protein of inner mitocondrial membrane. ATP synthase is oriented vectorially in the inner mitochondrial membrane. It extends from outside of inner mitochondrial membrane to matrix of mitochondria. It is present in the knob-like structure present on the cristae of inner mitochondrial membrane.

ATP synthase consist of two subunits. They are F_0 and F_1 subunits. The spherical part or head of knob is F_1 subunit. It is made up of five polypeptide chains (Figure 11.11*a*). This subunit has catalytic activity. It catalyzes the hydrolysis of ATP *in vitro*. The base of the know is F_0 subunit of ATP synthase. It is embedded in the membrane. It is channel for proton movement (Figure 11.11*a*). When protons move through F_0 subunit from outside to inside of inner mitochondrial membrane F_1 subunit catalyzes the formation of ATP from ADP and Pi using free energy released. The stalk of knob also consist of several proteins. Antibiotic oligomycin binds to stalk and inhibits oxidative phosphorylation.

Sites of phosphorylation or ATP synthesis in the respiratory chain

ATP synthesis takes place only at specific points of respiratory chain like any energy yielding degradative pathways like glycolysis, β-oxidation etc. ATP synthesis in respiratory chain requires a redox potential difference of approximately 0.15 volts. Each complex of respiratory chain generates 0.15 v redox potential difference while electrons flow from NAD to O_2. ATP generation is associated with three complexes of electron transport chain and it is always coupled to the flow of electrons through the complexes. The three complexes that generate ATP from ADP and Pi are complex I, complex III, and complex IV (Figure 11.11*b*).

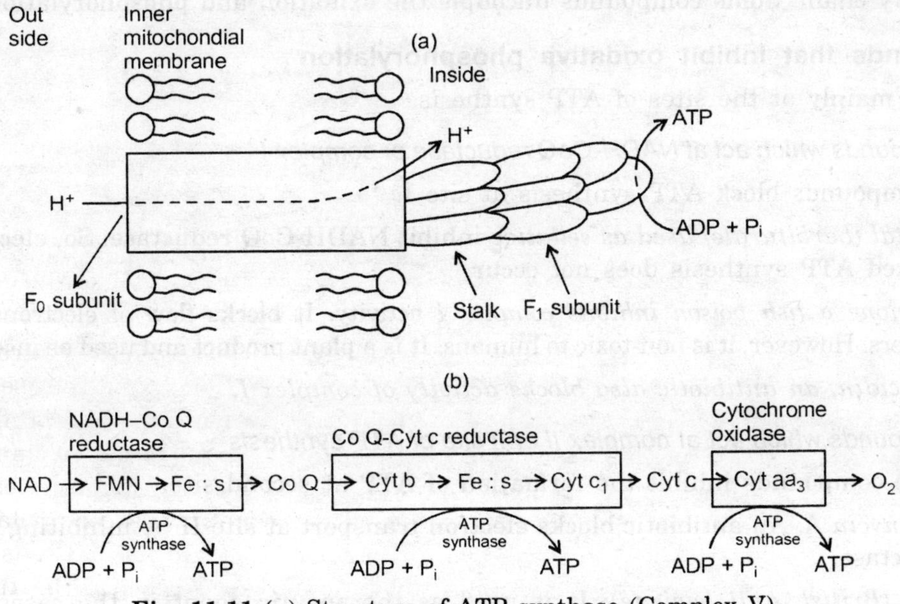

Fig. 11.11 (*a*) Structure of ATP synthase (Complex V)
(*b*) Sites of ATP formation in respiratory chain

P:O ratio

When electrons flow in the respiratory chain from NAD to O_2 formation of ATP occurs and at the same time O_2 is reduced to H_2O. The relationship between ATP generation and oxygen consumption is expressed as P:O ratio. It is defined as ratio of number of ATP synthesized per atom of oxygen consumed when electrons flow in the respiratory chain from substrate to O_2. When a substrate like malate is oxidized by NAD linked malate dehydrogenase NADH is produced. Oxidation of this NADH in respiratory chain is accompanied by formation of 3 ATP molecules and one oxygen atom is reduced of water and the P:O ratio is 3.

So, oxidation of a substrate by NAD linked dehydrogenase generates 3 ATP molecules. Likewise, oxidation of a substrate by Flavoprotein (FAD) dehydrogenase generates 2 ATP molecules per atom of oxygen consumed, i.e., P:O ratio is 2. The difference in the P:O ratio is due to by passing the complex I of the respiratory chain. Synthesis of ATP in respiratory chain when a substrate is oxidized is known as oxidative phosphorylation at respiratory chain level.

Substrate level phosphorylation

It is another process for production of high energy compounds like ATP and GTP. Enol phosphate or thioesters are produced in metabolic particular degradative pathways and they are subsequently utilized to generate ATP.

For example in glycolysis phosphoenol pyruvate is produced and it is subsequently used to generate ATP.

Inhibitors of respiratory Chain

Several drugs, poisons and toxins work by inhibiting activities of respiratory chain complexes. They block oxidative phosphorylation or ATP synthesis or flow of electrons in the respiratory chain. Some compounds uncouple the oxidation and phosphorylation.

Compounds that inhibit oxidative phosphorylation

They act mainly at the sites of ATP synthesis.

(a) Compounds which act at NADH-CoQ reductase or complex I

These compounds block ATP synthesis at site I.

1. *Amytal (barbiturate) used as sedative* inhibit NADH-CoQ reductase. So, electron flow is blocked ATP synthesis does not occur.
2. *Rotenone a fish poison inhibits complex I* activity. It blocks flow of electrons from Fe:S clusters. However, it is non-toxic to humans. It is a plant product and used as insecticide also.
3. *Piericidin, an antibiotic also blocks activity of complex I.*

(b) Compounds which act at complex II or II site of ATP synthesis

These compounds inhibit the formation of ATP at second site.

1. *Antimycin A:* An antibiotic blocks electron transport at site II by inhibiting cytochrome reductase.
2. *BAL (British anti lewisite):* It is used as therapeutic agent in the cases of arsenic poisoning. It inhibits activity of cytochrome reductase.

(c) Compounds which act at site III by inhibiting activity of cytochrome oxidase.

1. **Cyanide (CN)** A powerful poison that inhibit cytochrome oxidase by combining with cytochrome a_3. Cyanide may arise from cyanogenic substance.
2. **Carbon monoxide (CO)** It inhibits activity of cytochrome oxidase. Carbon monoxide is a pollutant present in automobile exhaust.
3. **Hydrogen sulfide (H_2S)** It inhibits cytochrome oxidase. H_2S toxicity occurs during oil drilling operations. It is toxic as cyanide. It is a part of natural gas.
4. **Azide** Sodium azide also inhibits cytochrome oxidase activity.

Other inhibitors of oxidative phosphorylation

1. **Carboxin** It inhibits oxidative phosphorylation by blocking the transfer of electrons from succinate to CoQ.
2. **Atractyloside** It inhibits oxidative phosphorylation by blocking movement of ATP and ADP across inner mitochondrial membrane.
3. **Oligomycin** It interacts with stalk of knob structure and completely blocks oxidation and phosphorylation.
4. **Rutamycin** It blocks phosphorylation without uncoupling.

Uncouplers

These compounds dissociates or uncouples oxidation in respiratory chain from phosphorylation. So, the oxidation takes place without ATP synthesis.

Examples: (1) 2, 4-dinitrophenol (2) Dinitrocresol (3) Salicylanilides (4) Pentachlorophenol (5) CCCP (Carbonylcyanide chloromethoxy phenyl hydrazone). (6) FCCP (Carbanoyl cyanide p. trifluoromethoxy phenyl hydrazone).

Regulation of oxidative phosphorylation

Oxidative phosphorylation in the respiratory chain is subjected to regulation like any metabolic pathway. The rate of oxidative phosphorylation depends on availability of substrates like ADP, P_i, NADH, $FADH_2$, and O_2. When cell has enough ATP the oxidative phosphorylation occurs at lower rate because of non availability of ADP. When the cell is deficient in ATP, ADP availability is more so rate of oxidative phosphorylation is more. The rate of oxidative phosphorylation also depends on the availability of P_i. Therefore, the energy generation in the mitochondria is perfectly tuned to energy demand. The dependence of oxidative phosphorylation on the availability of ADP is known as *respiratory control*.

Mechanism of oxidative phosphorylation

Three models have been proposed to explain ATP synthesis during the transfer of electrons in the respiratory chain. They are

1. The chemical coupling model

According to this model, when electrons are transferred in the respiratory chain, an high energy intermediate is formed. The hydrolysis of this high energy compound is accompanied by the formation of ATP. No such high energy intermediate has been found so far.

2. The conformational coupling model

This model proposes the existence of two conformational states to the inner mitochondrial membrane components. The energy released when electrons flow in the respiratory chain causes conformational change in these components and converts low energy molecules to high energy form. When they return to normal low energy state from high energy state the energy released is used for ATP synthesis. Due to lack of experimental support this model has not been accepted.

3. The chemiosmotic coupling model

According to this model, when electrons flow in the respiratory chain, protons (H^+) are pumped from matrix of mitochondria to outside of inner mitochondrial membrane. As a result of this a proton gradient is generated across inner mitochondrial membrane. The proton gradient in turn leads to potential difference across inner mitochondrial membrane. The electrochemical gradient (low pH and positive charge on outside and high pH and negative charge inside) thus generated drives the mechanism responsible for ATP synthesis. The protons that are ejected by electron transport flows back into matrix of mitochondria through the F_0 subunit of ATP synthase driven by proton gradient. The free energy released as protons flows back into matrix through the F_0 subunit is used by F_1 subunit for ATP synthesis from ADP and P_i (Figure 11.12). This model is supported by many experimental evidences.

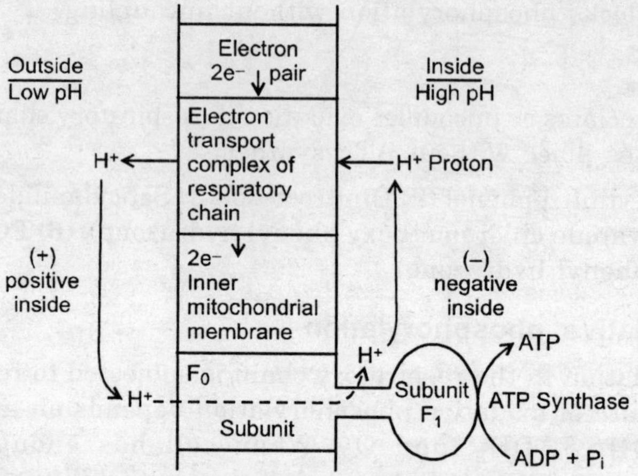

Fig. 11.12 A chemiosmotic model

When a pair of electrons flow from NAD to O_2 in the respiratory chain nearly 10 to 12 protons are pumped out. But only 6 to 8 protons are pumped out when electrons flow from FAD to O_2. Since there are three complexes in the respiratory chain, each complex may extrude 3 to 4 protons when electrons flow from NAD to O_2. This proton extrusion at each complex generates a pH gradient of about 0.05 units across inner mitochondrial membrane. This pH gradient causes development of 0.15 volts potential difference at each complex (Figure 11.12). As discussed earlier, this much potential difference is sufficient for ATP synthase. Thus, flow of a pair of electrons through a complex of respiratory chain is accompanied by one molecule of ATP formation. Since respiratory chain consist of complex I, complex III, and complex IV (from NAD to O_2), three ATPs are formed when electrons flow from NAD to O_2.

Mechanism of ATP synthase catalyzed ATP synthesis

Earlier I mentioned in chemiosmotic hypothesis that energy released during proton translocation is used for ATP synthesis. To understand mechanism of ion translocation coupled ATP synthesis in molecular terms knowledge of ATP synthase structure is needed.

E. Coli ATP synthase is large enzyme complex with molecular weight of 5,20,000 Kda. Its membrane extrinsic F_1 portion is composed of several subunits. It contains three α, three β and one γ, δ and ε sub units. It is designated as $\alpha_3\ \beta_3\ \gamma_1\ \delta_1\ \varepsilon_1$. Membrane embedded F_0 portion is composed of one a, two b, and twelve c subunits. Two slender stalks link F_1 to F_0. The central stalk is formed by γ subunit and part of ε subunit. The ion channel is formed by twelve *c* and *a* subunit of F_0. β subunits of F_1 portion contains catalytic and binding sites (Fig. 11.13).

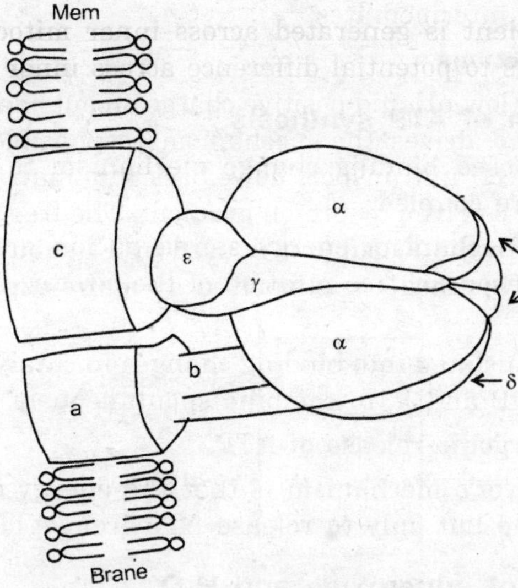

Fig. 11.13 F_1F_0-ATP synthase of *E.Coli*.

ATP synthase is a mechano electrochemical enzyme. Ion translocation generates torsion in the F_1 ATP synthase. Torsion in the γ subunit is generated by rotation of the c-rotor of F_0 portion. Binding of protons to c subunits disturbs electrostatic equilibrium at *a* and *c* interface causing c-rotor to rotate. Due to interaction with β sub units rotation of γ sub unit is constrained. The energy from discharge of proton gradient through F_0 is accumulated as torsional energy in γ sub unit of F_1 portion. Thus the energy of proton gradient is stored as torsional energy in the γ sub unit. The torsional energy stored is released upon reaching threshold strain i.e. after four ion translocations. The released torsional energy causes conformational change in β sub units and thereby causing binding of ADP and P_1, which leads to ATP synthesis. ATP release occurs when β sub units returns to native conformation upon interaction with ε sub unit. Since ATP synthesis is related to torsional energy this mechanism is known as torsional mechanism. Unlike binding change, mechanism torsional mechanism involves irreversible mode of ATP synthesis. ATP synthase enzyme is referred as molecular machine due to rotation of sub unit γ by c-rotor in response to ion translocation.

Respirasome

Recent research indicates that complexes of respiratory chain are not randomly distributed in inner mitochondrial membrane. They assemble in to supra molecular structures. Complex-I, III and IV assemble into super complexes and forms network of super complexes known as respirasome. Two large super complexes and one small super complexe constitutes respirasome (Fig. 11.14). Each large super complex consists of complex-I, dimeric complex-III and two complex-IV dimmers. Hence, it is designated as I_1. III_2, IV_4. Smaller super complex is made up of two complex-IV dimmers and one complex-III dimmer. It is designated as III_2 and IV_4. Further dimmers of ATP synthase also exist in mitochondria.

Functional importance of super complexes

Some of the advantages of super complexes over independent complexes are

(*a*) Substrate channeling

(*b*) Catalytic enhancement

(*c*) Sequestration of reactive intermediates

(*d*) Rapid intramolecular reactions

Binding change mechanism of ATP synthesis

In 1973, Paul D. Boyer proposed binding change mechanism to explain how the proton current and ATP synthesis are coupled.

1. In the binding change, mechanism energy stored as ion gradient across membrane containing F_0 domain is used for free rotation of the c-rotor, the γ shaft and ε subunit attached to c-rotor.
2. This free rotation gets translated into binding changes in catalytic sides in the β subunit of F_1 domain causing ADP and P_i to combine spontaneously to form ATP.
3. This is followed by endergonic release of ATP.
4. The novel element in Boyer's mechanism is that the energy of proton gradient is not used in the synthesis step but only to release ATP from ATP synthase.

Production and utilization of superoxide and H_2O_2

Production of superoxide and H_2O_2

They are produced as by products during reduction of O_2 to water. The reduction of O_2 to H_2O is a multi-step process. Initially oxygen reacts with one electron, superoxide is produced. If oxygen reacts with two electrons hydrogen peroxide is formed. When oxygen reacts with four electrons water is formed (Figure 11.13*a*). Superoxide may also formed from cytochrome P_{450} dependent reactions. Similarly, hydrogen peroxide may also formed from oxidases as mentioned earlier. The superoxide and hydrogen peroxide are toxic to cells. As such superoxide may not be harmful to cell but it generates free radicals like $\dot{O}H$, $\dot{O}R$ etc., which are extremely toxic to cells. Superoxide, $\dot{O}H$, $\dot{O}R$, H_2O_2 are collectively called as reactive oxygen species (ROS).

Fate of superoxide and H_2O_2

For the survival of cells superoxide and H_2O_2 must be destroyed. Superoxide is eliminated by superoxide dismutase an enzyme present in the cytosol of erythrocytes, liver, brain etc. This enzyme contains two metal ions Cu and Zn. Hydrogen peroxide is destroyed by catalase and peroxidase (Figure 11.13*b*).

Role of super oxide and H_2O_2 in phagocytosis

In some cells, superoxide and H_2O_2 are produced as a part of their normal function. For example, macrophages contribute to defense against infectious agents by phagocytosis. These cells engulf bacteria when enters into body. This engulf is followed by respiratory burst, i.e., a rapid increase in oxygen uptake. Under such conditions, O_2 consumption may increase to about 50 folds. Much of this oxygen is used to generate super oxide and hydrogen peroxide. NADPH serves as donor of protons required for super oxide formation. Glucose utilization by HMP shunt, which generates NADPH also increases many folds during phagocytosis. Macrophages contain NADPH oxidase. This enzyme produces superoxide by using NADPH as source of electrons and protons. This superoxide is further reduced to H_2O_2 by superoxide dismutase. The superoxide and H_2O_2 thus produced in turn generate hypochlorite (OCl^-) and hydroxyl ($\dot{O}H$) radicals to kill bacteria (Figure 11.13*c*).

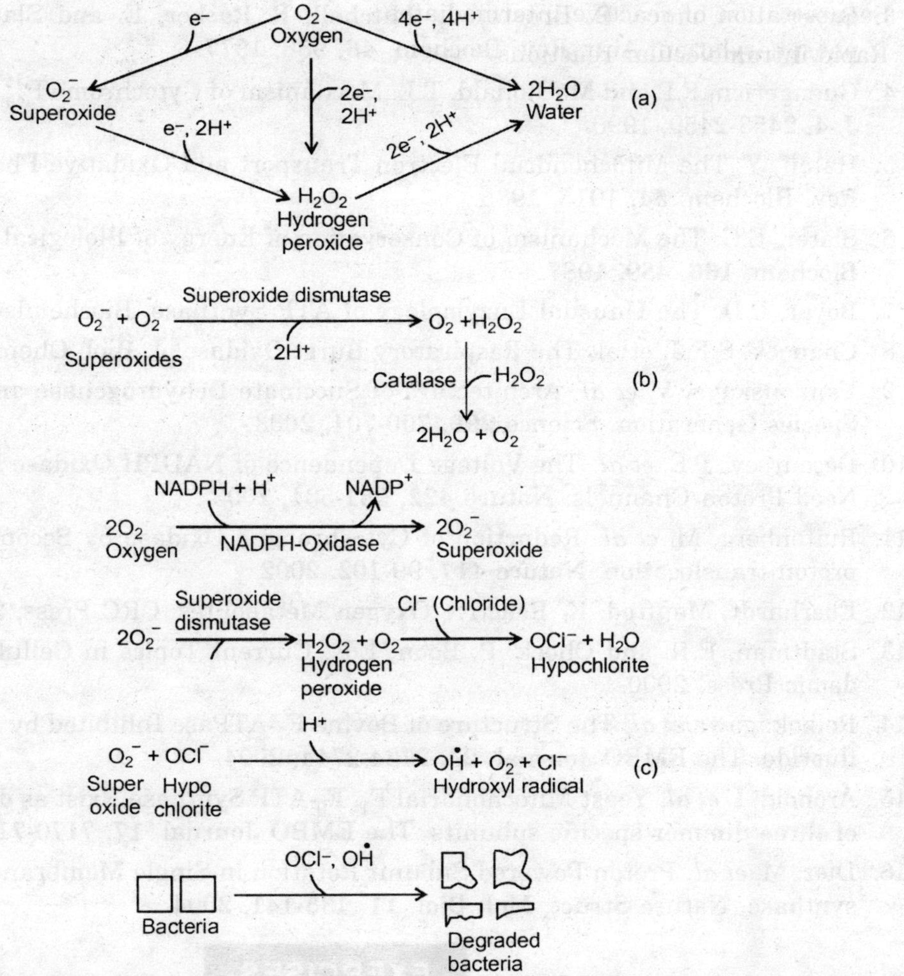

Fig. 11.13 (*a*) Generation of superoxide and hydrogen peroxide. (*b*) Elimination of superoxide and hydrogen peroxide. (*c*) Molecular events of phagocytosis

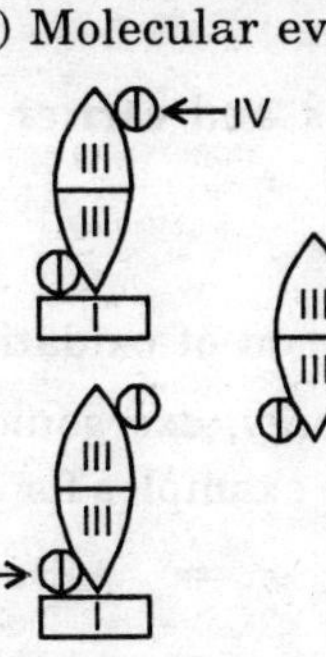

Fig. 11.14 A model respirasome

REFERENCES

1. Morowitz, H.J. Foundation of Bioenergetics. Academic Press, New York, 1978.
2. Boyer, P.D. (Ed.). The Enzymes Vol. 13. 3rd ed. Academic Press, New York, 1976.

3. Boyer, P. Chance, B. Ernster, L. Mitchell, P. Racker, E. and Slater, E.C. Oxidative phosphorylation. Ann. Rev. Biochem. **46**, 966; 1977.
4. Guengericn, F.P and Macdonald, T.L. Mechanism of Cytochrome P_{450} Catalysis. FASEB. J. **4**, 2453-2459, 1990.
5. Hatefi, Y. The Mitochondrial Electron Transport and Oxidative Phosphorylation. Ann. Rev. Biochem. **54**, 1015, 1985.
6. Slater, E.C. The Mechanism of Conservation of Energy of Biological Oxidations. Eur. J. Biochem. **166**, 489, 1987.
7. Boyer, P.D. The Unusual Enzymology of ATP Synthase. Biochemistry. **26**, 8503, 1987.
8. Chanock, S.F.J. et al. The Respiratory Burst Oxidase. J. Biol. Chem. **269**, 24519, 1994.
9. Yankouskaya, V. *et al.* Architecture of Succinate Dehydrogenase and Reactive Oxygen Species Generation. Science **299**, 700-704, 2003.
10. Decoursey, T.E. *et al.* The Voltage Dependence of NADPH Oxidase Reveals Phagocytes Need Proton Channels. Nature **422**, 531-534, 2003.
11. Ruitenberg, M. *et al.* Reduction of Cytochrome c Oxidase by Second Electron leads to proton translocation. Nature **417,** 99-102, 2002.
12. Eberhardt, Manfred. K. Reactive Oxygen Metabolites. CRC Press, 2000.
13. Stadtman, E.R. and Chock. P. Boon, Eds. Current Topics in Cellular regulation. Academic Press, 2000.
14. Reikokagawa *et al.* The Structure of Bovine F_1-ATPase Inhibited by ADP and Beryllium fluoride. The EMBO Journal. **23,** 2734-2744, 2004.
15. Aronold, I. *et al.* Yeast Mitochondrial F_1, F_0-ATP Synthase Exist as dimer. Identification of three dimmer specific subunits. The EMBO Journal. **17**, 7170-7178, 1998.
16. Diez, M. *et al.* Proton Powered Subunit Rotation in Single Membrane Bound F_1, F_0-ATP synthase. Nature Struct. Mol. Biol. **11**, 135-141, 2004.

EXERCISES

ESSAY QUESTIONS

1. Describe various enzymes, coenzymes and carrier molecules involved in biological oxidation-reduction reactions.
2. Describe respiratory chain.
3. Write an essay on models of mechanism of oxidative phosphorylation.
4. Define free energy, standard free energy, exergonic and endergonic reactions and high energy compounds. Explain each one and give examples for high energy compounds. Mention importance of high energy compounds.

SHORT QUESTIONS

1. Write a note on cyt P_{450} hydroxylase system.
2. Define high energy compounds. Explain with examples.
3. Define redox potential. Write its significance.
4. Write components of electron transport chain in the order to electron transfer. Indicate sites of phosphorylation.

5. Define oxidative phosphorylation. Write principle of chemiosmotic hypothesis.
6. How super oxide is formed and utilized in the body?
7. Write enzymes involved in production and utilization of H_2O_2.
8. What is the role H_2O_2 in phagocytosis?
9. Write a note on inhibitors of oxidative phosphorylation.
10. Define reaction oxygen species (ROS). Give examples.
11. Write a note on super complexes of respiratory chain.
12. Define un couplers. Give examples.
13. Write differences between oxidative phosphorylation and substrate level phosphorylation. Give examples.
14. Write equation relating free energy and electron transfer. Write its importance.

MULTIPLE CHOICE QUESTIONS

1. An example for $NADP^+$ dependent dehydrogenase is
   (*a*) Phosphogluconate dehydrogenase. (*b*) Succinate dehydrogenase.
   (*c*) Acyl-CoA dehydrogenase. (*d*) None of these.
2. All of the following statements are correct for oxidases. Except
   (*a*) They catalyze removal of hydrogen from substrates.
   (*b*) They use oxygen as hydrogen acceptor.
   (*c*) They produce H_2O_2.
   (*d*) They produce H_2O.
3. In iron-sulfur proteins
   (*a*) Iron is complexed with organic sulfur.
   (*b*) Iron is complexed with inorganic sulfur.
   (*c*) Iron is complexed with organic and inorganic sulfur.
   (*d*) Iron is complexed with proteins.
4. Which of the following is correct for endergonic reaction.
   (*a*) It occurs with release of energy. (*b*) Its ΔG is negative.
   (*c*) It occurs when energy supplied. (*d*) It occurs with decrease in free energy.
5. Phagocytosis involves
   (*a*) Production of superoxide. (*b*) Production of H_2O_2.
   (*c*) Production of superoxide and H_2O_2. (*d*) None of these.

FILL IN THE BLANKS

1. Excess O_2 is toxic to cells. So it is used in .... treatment.
2. ATP is called as energy .... of the cell.
3. High redox potential indicates tendency of redox pair to .... electrons.
4. P:O ratio is .... when a substance is oxidized by NAD^+ dependent dehydrogenase.
5. An uncoupler .... oxidation in respiratory chain from ....

12

CHAPTER

PROTEIN AND AMINO ACID METABOLISM

MEDICAL AND BIOLOGICAL IMPORTANCE

1. A 70 kg human adult body contains about 12 kg of protein.
2. Body proteins have life times. They undergo degradation and re-synthesis. About 400 gm of body protein is synthesized and degraded per day i.e., about 6 gm of protein is synthesized and broken down per kg body weight per day.
3. Aged proteins, damaged or modified proteins and non-functional proteins of the body undergo degradation. Further degradation is one way of controlling enzyme activity. Hence, continuous re-synthesis and degradation of proteins is a quality control mechanism.
4. Protein degradation may play important role in shaping tissues and organs during pregnancy and development.
5. In starvation, diabetes and tissue injury, protein degradation is more.
6. Protein synthesis and degradation is an integral part of cellular adaptation to changed environment.
7. Plasma free amino acid concentration ranges from 40 to 60 mg%. Excess amino acids can not be stored in the body. First amino group is extracted as ammonia and then carbon skeleton is oxidized to produce energy. In starvation carbon skeletons are used for glucose formation. Carbon skeletons of some amino acids produce acetyl-CoA as end product.
8. Ammonia, which is toxic to cells is converted to urea in the liver. Conversion of ammonia to urea is impaired in some inherited diseases and liver disease.
9. Amino acids are needed for the formation of specialized products like hormones, purines, pyrimidines, porphyrins, vitamins, amines, creatine and glutathione.
10. Amino acid degradation is impaired in several inherited diseases due to lack of enzymes.
11. Amino acid degradation is more in starvation, diabetes and high protein diet.
12. Some cancer cells have high amino acid (aspargine) requirement.

Protein turn over

In all forms of life, proteins once formed may not remain forever. Like intermediates of metabolic path ways, proteins are synthesized and degraded. Hence, body protein is in dynamic state. Continuous synthesis and degradation of protein is called as protein turnover. The rates of protein synthesis and degradation vary according to physiological needs. The rate of protein synthesis is high during growth, lactation and post operative recovery. In starvation, cancer, fever and during morphogenesis rate of degradation of protein is more.

Eventhough, protein turnover involves synthesis as well as degradation of protein, protein degradation, amino acid degradation and formation of non-essential amino acids are detailed in this chapter. Protein synthesis is detailed in chapter-18. Of course conversion of aminoacids to special products is also included in this chapter.

Protein half life

Body proteins have life times. Life time of a protein is expressed in terms of half-life. It is defined as time required for initial amount of protein to be reduced to half. Half life of proteins ranges from minutes to years. For example, lens crystalline have very long half life whereas regulatory enzymes have very short half life. Half life of proteins may be increased or decreased depending on call needs. Half lifes ($T_{1/2}$) of some proteins are given below.

Type of protein	Half life (T½)
Muscle proteins	160 days
Body proteins	80 days
Serum proteins	10 days
Liver proteins	6 days
LDH, cytochromes	>100 hours
HMG-CoA reductase	<2 hours
Oncogene product	<2 hours

Signals for protein breakdown

It is not yet clear what triggers or initiates protein degradation. However, some structural features of proteins which serve as signals for their degradation are identified. They are

1. Ubiquitinization

Ubiquitin is a small protein present in eukaryotes. Ubiquitin attachment to protein serve as signal for degradation of that protein.

2. PEST sequences

PEST sequence proline (P), glutamate (E), serine (S) and threonine (T) rich region of a protein serves as mark for the degradation of the protein.

3. N-terminal amino acids

Amino acids like arginine or lysine, phenyl alanine and aspartate at amino terminal serve as signal for degradation of the protein.

4. Oxidized amino acids

If a protein contains an oxidized amino acid then it undergoes degradation because oxidized amino acid is recognized by protein degrading enzymes.

Protein degradation pathways

Several pathways are involved in the degradation of proteins

1. Ubiquitin dependent pathway

It is a cytosolic pathway for protein degradation. It requires ubiquitin and ATP. Mainly abnormal proteins and short lived proteins are degraded by this pathway.

2. Ubiquitin independent pathway

It is another cytosolic pathway for protein degradation and is not dependent on ubiquitin. Mainly extracellular proteins, membrane proteins and long lived proteins are degraded by this pathway.

3. Receptor dependent pathway

Mainly glycoprotein hormones are degraded by this pathway. The asialated hormone combines with a receptor on cells. They are degraded after internalization.

Enzymes of protein degradation

1. Protease and peptidases

Several intracellular proteases and peptidases are involved in protein degradation. Proteases like tryptase, chymase, elastase, collagenase and calpains hydrolyzes proteins. These endopeptidases cleave internal bonds of proteins forming oligo peptides. Peptidases further degrade oligo peptides to dipeptides. Finally aminoacids are formed by the action of dipeptidases on dipeptides. Aminopeptidase and carboxypeptidase which are exopeptidases are also involved in intracellular protein breakdown.

2. Cathepsins

They are hydrolytic enzymes present in lysosomes. They are responsible for the degradation of glycoprotein hormones and other intracellular proteins.

3. Megapain

It is a high molecular mass protease present in liver, skeletal muscle and reticulocytes. It degrades proteins in presence of ubiquitin.

4. Multicatalytic proteases (Proteosome)

As the name implies they pocess multicatalytic function and present in the cytosol of most of mammalian cells. They can act as trypsin, chymotrypsin etc. These multicatalytic proteases are also involved in intracellular protein break down.

By the combined action of these eznymes or complexes, proteins are hydrolyzed to amino acids.

Other noteworthy functions of intracellular proteases

1. They are involved in post translational modification of proteins particularly in the formation of hormones, kinins and chemotactic peptides.
2. They act as bactericides.
3. They are also involved in inflammation and wound healing.

AMINO ACIDS OF BLOOD PLASMA

Blood plasma contains most of the 20 amino acids. Plasma amino acid level is 40–60 mg%. Plasma amino acid level is not constant throughout the day. It is lowest in the morning and highest in the evening. Further, the concentrations of individual amino acids in the blood are different. For example, glutamine and alanine are present at high concentration where as aspartate is present at low concentration. However, the average half life of a plasma amino acid is about 5 minutes. Amino acids of plasma are rapidly taken up by all tissues.

Source of plasma amino acids

Amino acids in the plasma are mainly derived from endogenous protein breakdown and dietary protein breakdown. Intracellular synthesis may contribute to plasma amino acid pool to some level.

Transport of amino acids into cells

Mostly ATP-dependent active transport is responsible for the entry of amino acids into cells. Several different transport systems, each of which is specific for a particular class of amino acids, are identified in mammalian cells.

Amino acid catabolism

In the adult human body, only 20% of amino acids formed from protein degradation are catabolised to generate energy. The remaining 80% amino acids are used for protein biosynthesis. Further amino acids or proteins consumed excess are also used for energy production. Since most of amino acids formed from protein breakdown are recycled, to maintain normal body functions the diet should contain at least (only) amino acids or proteins (20%) that is used for energy production. In case, if excess is consumed that is also used for energy production because amino acids can not be stored in the body. Under normal conditions, amino acids supply about 5–10% of total body energy. Amino acid catabolism is increased in starvation, diabetes and high protein diet. Intracellular synthesis of some amino acids also occurs. Depending on the cell needs they are utilized. In addition, amino acids are used for the formation of creatine, hormones, glutathione, purines, pyrimidines etc.

Amino acid catabolism occurs in two main stages. First stage is the removal of amino group of amino acids as ammonia. Ammonia is converted to urea and excreted in urine. In the second stage carbon skeletons of amino acids are converted into intermediates of TCA cycle and acetyl-CoA. Then they are either oxidized in TCA cycle for generation of energy or used for glucose synthesis or ketone body formation. Sources and fates of amino acids are shown in Fig. 12.1.

Deamination of amino acids

Since the removal of α-amino group is the first stage of amino acid degradation we shall see now how it occurs. There are several ways for the removal of α-amino group of amino acids. They are (1) Transamination followed by oxidative deamination (2) Oxidative deamination (3) Non-oxidative deamination.

Transamination followed by oxidative deamination

(a) Transamination

Removal of amino group of amino acids by transamination is the first step in the catabolism of most of the aminoacids. The enzymes involved in this process are known as transaminases. They transfer α-amino group to an acceptor mostly to α-keto glutarate. They are named according to substrate whose aminogroup they transfer to α-keto glutarate. For example, (Fig. 12.2a) aspartate transaminase transfer (removes) amino group of asparatate to α-ketoglutarate. This results in formation of oxaloacetate which is α-keto acid of aspartate and glutamate, which is the corresponding amino acid of α-keto glutarate (a keto acid).

Transaminases are present in mitochondria and cytosol of most of the tissues. They contain pyridoxal phosphate as prosthetic group. Though there are more than ten transaminases most important among them are aspartate amino transferase (transaminase) and alanine amino transferase. So, by the action of transaminases α-amino groups of most of the amino acids are transferred to α-ketoglutarate to form glutamate. Thus glutamate serves as a collecting point of α-amino groups.

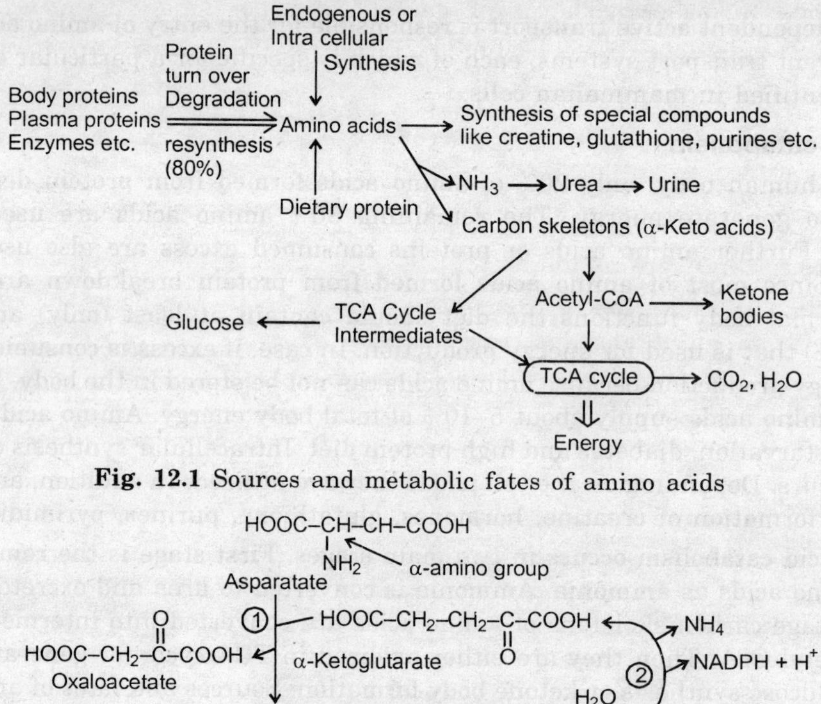

Fig. 12.1 Sources and metabolic fates of amino acids

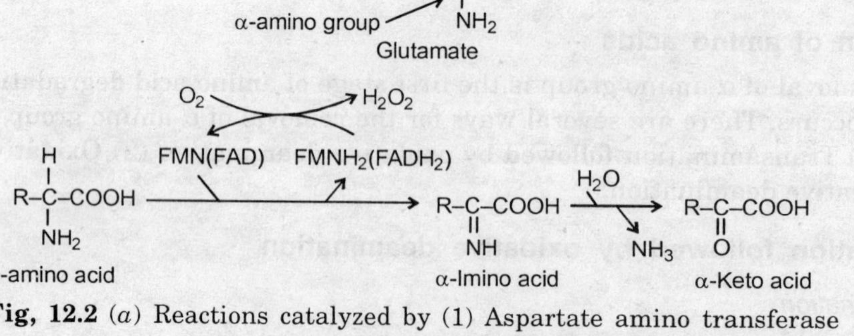

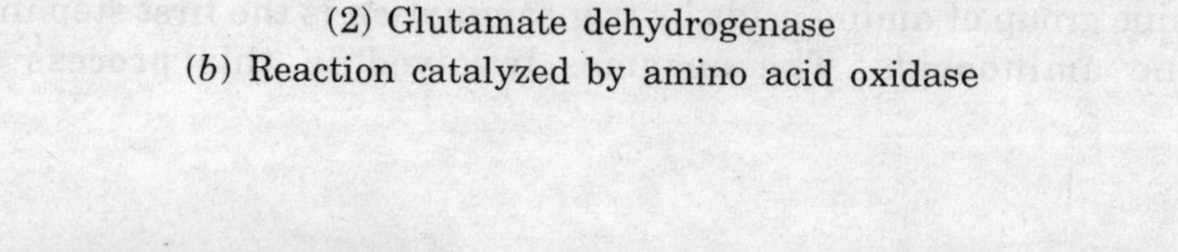

Fig, 12.2 (*a*) Reactions catalyzed by (1) Aspartate amino transferase
(2) Glutamate dehydrogenase
(*b*) Reaction catalyzed by amino acid oxidase

(b) Oxidative deamination

Amino groups that are collected by glutamate are removed as ammonia by enzyme glutamate dehydrogenase in presence of NAD or $NADP^+$. Glutamate dehydrogenase catalyzes oxidative deamination of glutamate to yield α-ketoglutarate and ammonia (Fig. 12.2a). The enzyme is present in mitochondria and cytosol of liver. It is an allosteric enzyme. ATP and GTP are allosteric inhibitors whereas ADP and GDP are allosteric activators.

Thus, the combined action of transaminases and glutamate dehydrogenase results in the net removal of amino groups of most amino acids as ammonia.

Oxidative deamination

Amino acids undergo NAD^+ independent oxidative deamination also. Amino acid oxidases are the enzymes which catalyzes this type of oxidative deamination. They are of two types and dependent on FMN or FAD. They are D-amino acid oxidase and L-amino acid oxidase. Since the activity of L-amino acid oxidase is low its contribution to ammonia production is less.

D-amino acid oxidase

It is present in liver and kidney. It cannot deaminate many amino acids. It uses FAD as cofactor. It can deaminate glycine.

L-amino acid oxidase

It is also present in liver and kidney. It cannot deaminate glycine and dicarboxylic acids. It is dependent on FMN.

The reaction mechanism of these oxidases involves first oxidation of aminoacid to iminoacid. FMN (FAD) are reduced. Next imino acid undergo hydrolytic loss of ammonia to produce α-keto acid (Fig. 12.2b).

Non-oxidative deamination

Non-oxidative deamination of amino acids is catalyzed by specific enzymes. Some of them are given below (Fig. 12.3).

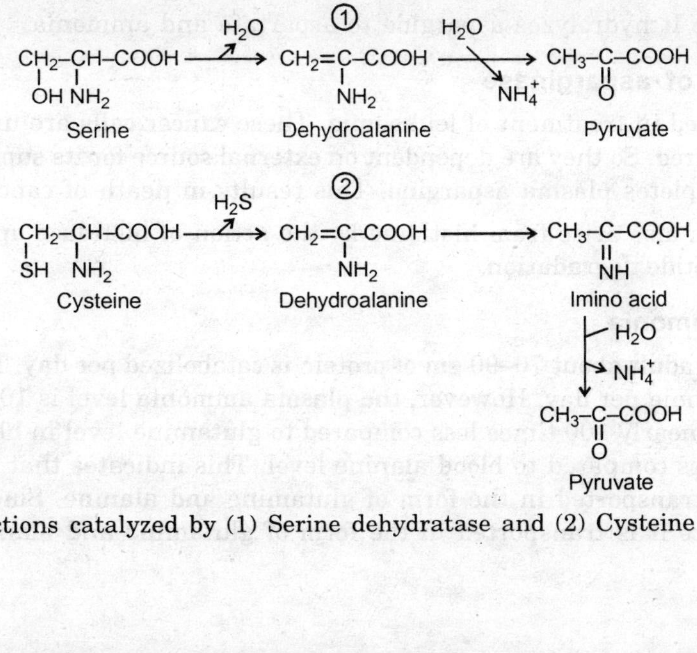

Fig. 12.3 Reactions catalyzed by (1) Serine dehydratase and (2) Cysteine de Sulfhydrase

1. Serine dehydratase

It catalyzes nonoxidative deamination of serine to pyruvate. The reaction mechanism involves dehydration of serine to dehydro alanine followed by hydrolytic loss of ammonia. It requires pyridoxal phosphate as cofactor.

2. Cysteine desulfhydrase

It is present in bacteria and requires pyridoxal phosphate as cofactor. It catalyzes conversion of cysteine to pyruvate. No such desulfhydrase is found in animal tissue. The reaction mechanism involves desulfuration of cysteine to dehydroalanine followed by hydrolytic loss of ammonia from aminoacid. Dehydroalanine tautomerizes to iminoacid.

3. Threonine dehydratase catalyzes non-oxidative deamination of threonine

All the above enzymes are involved in the removal of α-amino group nitrogen as ammonia. Now we shall see removal of amide nitrogen of glutamine and aspargine.

Removal of amide nitrogen of glutamine and aspargine

Specific deamidinases removes amide nitrogen of glutamine and aspargine as ammonia. They are glutaminase and asparginase (Fig. 12.4).

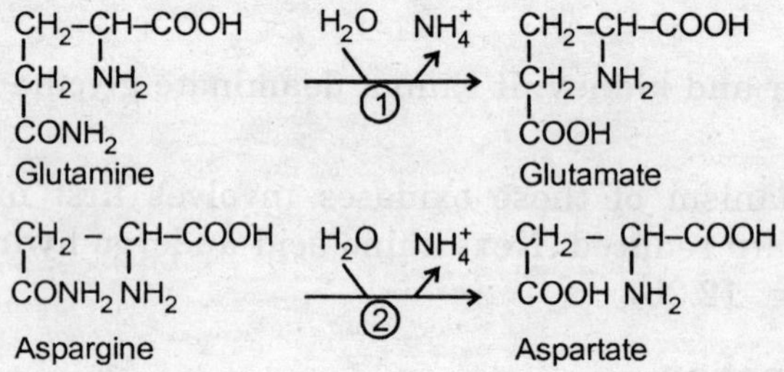

Fig. 12.4 Reactions catalyzed by (1) glutaminase (2) Asparginase

1. **Glutaminase** It is present in kidney. It hydrolyzes glutamine to glutamate and ammonia.
2. **Asparginase** It hydrolyzes aspargine to aspartate and ammonia.

Medical aspect of asparginase

Asparginase is used in treatment of leukaemia. These cancer cells are unable to synthesize aspargine as required. So they are dependent on external source for its supply. Administration of asparginase depletes plasma aspargine. This results in death of cancer cells.

Ammonia can also arise from histidine by the action of histidase and from purine and pyrimidine nucleotide degradation.

Transport of ammonia

In a 70 kg human adult about 70–90 gm of protein is catabolized per day. This produces about 15-20 gm of ammonia per day. However, the plasma ammonia level is 10-20 μg/100 ml. This ammonia level is nearly 100 times less compared to glutamine level in blood (10 mg/100 ml) and manyfolds less compared to blood alanine level. This indicates that ammonia produced in the tissues is transported in the form of glutamine and alanine. Since free ammonia is toxic even in trace it is transported in the form of glutamine and alanine.

Transport of ammonia as glutamine

From the brain and other peripheral organs except muscle ammonia released from amino acids is transported to liver and kidney as amide nitrogen of glutamine.

Formation of glutamine

A widely distributed glutamine synthetase catalyzes the formation of glutamine from glutamate and ammonia in ATP dependent reaction (Fig. 12.5*a*). Glutamine so formed enters circulation.

Transport of ammonia as alanine

Since glutamine synthetase activity is low in skeletal muscle ammonia released from deamination of amino acids is transported in the form alanine to liver. In the muscle by the reversal of glutamate dehydrogenase reaction glutamate is formed from α-keto glutarate and ammonia. Transamination by transaminase converts pyruvate to alanine. Alanine reaches liver through circulation where it is converted to pyruvate by another transaminase (Fig. 12.5*b*). When the pyruvate enters muscle as lactate cycle is completed. Thus, operation of this cycle causes net transfer of ammonia from muscle to liver.

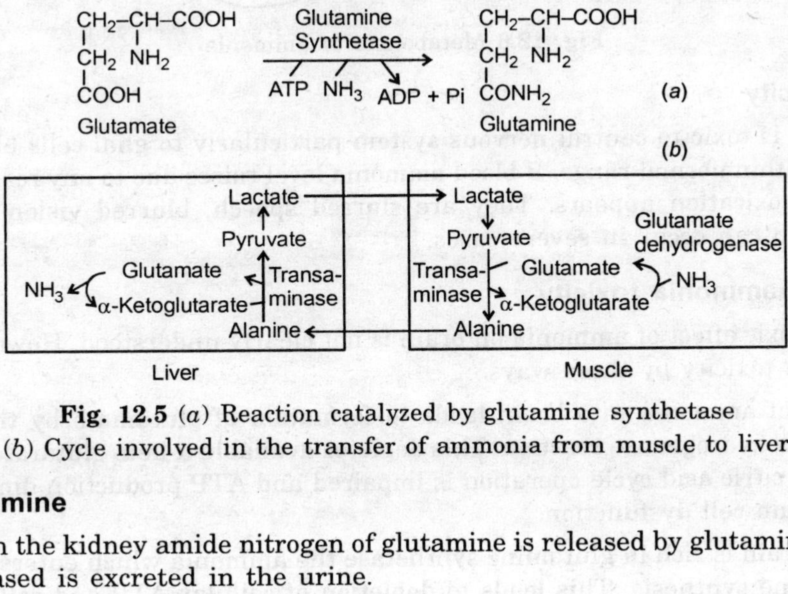

Fig. 12.5 (*a*) Reaction catalyzed by glutamine synthetase
(*b*) Cycle involved in the transfer of ammonia from muscle to liver

Fate of glutamine

1. **Kidney** In the kidney amide nitrogen of glutamine is released by glutaminase. Ammonia thus released is excreted in the urine.
2. **Intestine** Intestine uses glutamine as a fuel. Ammonia is released from glutamine by the action of glutaminase and enters liver through portal circulation.

Role of liver in ammonia metabolism

Under normal conditions liver maintains blood ammonia level within limits by rapidly converting it into urea as we see later. Further ammonia produced from glutamine by the action of glutaminase and deamination of amino acids is converted to urea. Usually portal blood contains high level of ammonia because of the production of ammonia by intestine from glutamine and dietary protein catabolism. However, the ammonia level in systemic blood is many times lower than portal blood. It indicates removal of ammonia from the circulation rapidly. Ammonia metabolism is shown in Fig. 12.6.

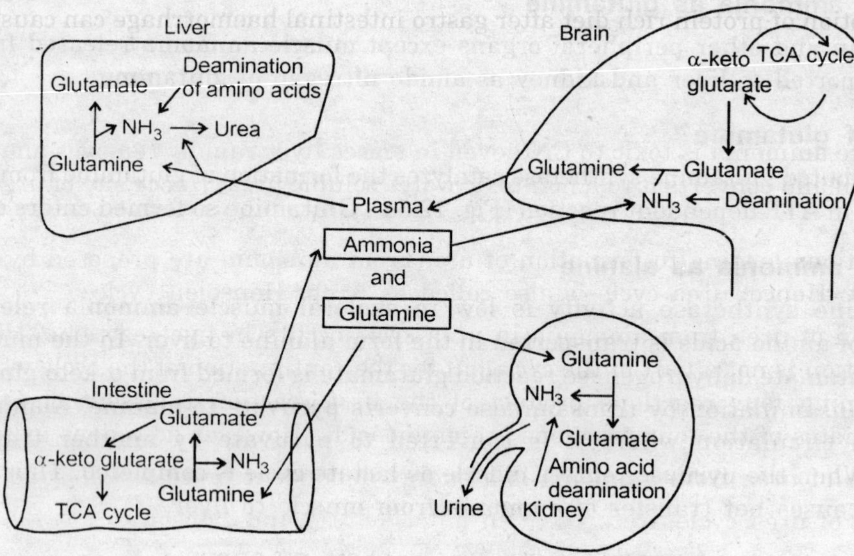

Fig. 12.6 Metabolism of ammonia

Ammonia toxicity

Since ammonia is toxic to central nervous system particularly to glial cells blood ammonia level must be within normal range. If blood ammonia level raises due to any reason symptoms of ammonia intoxication appears. They are slurred speech, blurred vision and tremors. Coma and death can occur in severe cases.

Mechanism of ammonia toxicity

Mechanism of toxic effect of ammonia on brain is not clearly understood. However ammonia can cause brain toxicity by three ways.

1. The entry of ammonia into brain leads to formation of glutamate by the reversal of glutamate dehydrogenase reaction. This depletes available α-keto glutarate in the brain. As a result citric acid cycle operation is impaired and ATP production diminishes. This leads to brain cell dysfunction.
2. Since the brain is rich in glutamine synthetase the ammonia which enters brain is used for glutamine synthesis. This leads to depletion of cellular ATP and cell dysfunction.
3. Since glutamate is considered as neurotransmitter the toxice effect of ammonia may be due to over stimulation of nerve cells by glutamate formed from ammonia and α-keto glutarate by the action of glutamate dehydrogenase.

Causes for ammonia toxicity

1. If hepatic function is impaired plasma ammonia rises to toxic level. Liver function can impair in cases of poisoning due to carbon tetra chloride, heavy metals and viral infections.
2. If collateral communication is developed between portal vein and systematic blood plasma ammonia rises to toxic level. In cirrhosis collateral communication develops between portal vein and systematic blood.

3. Consumption of protein rich diet after gastro intestinal haemorrhage can cause ammonia toxicity.

Urea cycle

1. **Site** Since ammonia is toxic to CNS even in traces liver rapidly removes ammonia from circulation and converts it to a non-toxic water soluble urea. Hence site of urea synthesis is liver.
2. The reactions leading to formation of urea from ammonia are proposed by Krebs and Henseleit. Hence, urea cycle is also called as Krebs-Henseleit cycle.
3. Formation of urea from ammonia in urea cycle occurs in five reactions. However the first reaction is not a part of the cycle but for the continuation of the cycle which consist of remaining four reactions product of the first reaction is essential. Further, the intermediates of the four reactions are aminoacids. However no codons exist for them.
4. Synthesis of urea from ammonia is a energy dependent process.
5. Enzymes of urea cycle are present in mitochondria and cytosol.
6. First two reactions of urea formation occurs in mitochondria and remaining reactions occur in cytosol.

REACTION SEQUENCE OF UREA FORMATION

For the synthesis of urea only one ammonia molecule is used as such. Aspartate serves as donor of another molecule of ammonia. HCO_3^- serves as source of CO_2 required for urea formation.

Formation of carbamoyl phosphate

1. First reaction leading to urea formation is condensation of ammonia and HCO_3^- at the expense of two high-energy bonds to form carbamoyl phosphate. The reaction is catalyzed by mitochondrial carbamoyl phosphate synthetase-I. The enzyme requires N-acetyl glutamate and Mg^{2+}. N-acetyl glutamate is synthesized from acetyl-CoA and glutamate in the liver. 2ATP molecules are hydrolyzed to 2 ADP and 2Pi in the first reaction. Of the $2P_i$ one P_i is consumed in the reaction. Since the product of the reaction carbamoyl phosphate is high energy compound its formation thermodynamically pulls subsequent reactions of urea cycle towards urea formation.

Reactions of urea cycle

2. Now the first reaction of urea cycle is catalyzed by ornithine transcarbamoylase. It condenses carbamoyl phosphate and ornithine to form citrulline. This enzyme is present in mitochondria.

   Since the subsequent reactions of urea cycle occurs in cytosol, citrulline formed eners cytosol through specific transporter present in inner mitochondrial membrane.

3. Arginino succinate synthetase present in cytosol catalyzes second reaction of urea cycle. It condenses citrulline and aspartate at the expense of two high energy bonds to form argininosuccinate. One high energy bond is consumed by the hydrolys is of ATP to AMP and PP_i. Further hydrolysis of PPi to 2Pi by pyrophosphatase leads to consumption of another high energy bond.

4. In the third reaction of urea cycle argininosuccinate is cleaved by argininosuccinase to arginine and fumarate.

5. Regeneration of ornithine and formation of urea from arginine is the final reaction of urea cycle. This reaction is catalyzed by arginase.

The ornithine so formed enters mitochondria through specific transporter present in inner mitochondrial membrane to start reactions of urea cycle once again. Reaction of urea formation are shown in Fig. 12.7.

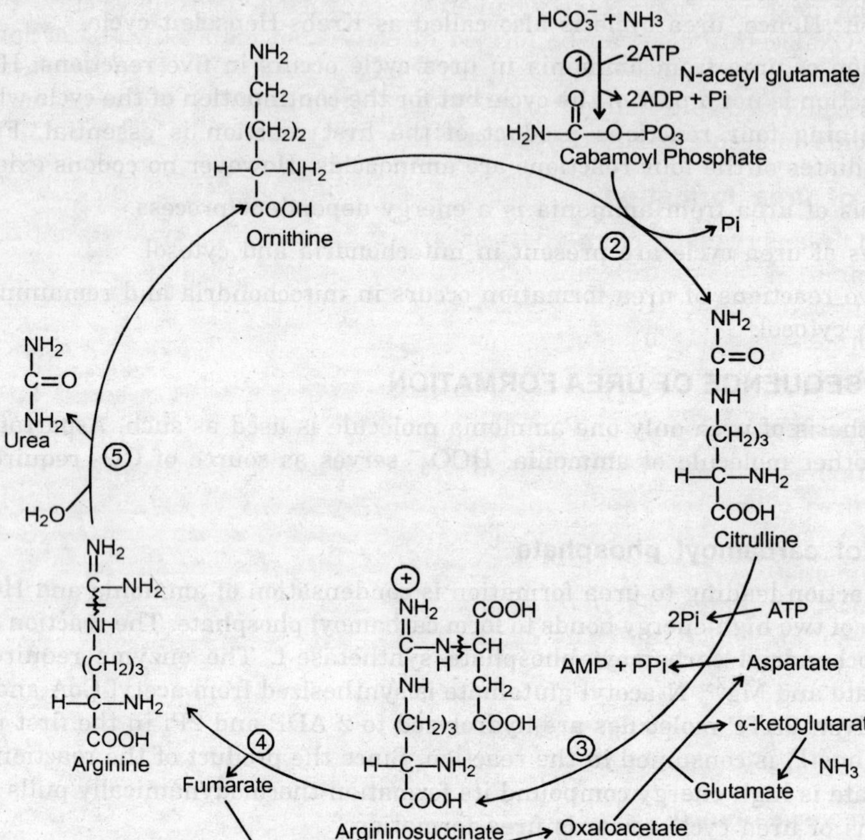

Fig. 12.7 Reactions of urea formatin and formation of aspartate from fumarate ~~~ indicates cleavage

Overall equation for urea formation

$$NH_3 + HCO^-_3 + \text{Aspartate} + 4ATP \longrightarrow \text{Urea} + \text{Fumarate} + 4ADP + 4Pi$$

Fate of urea

Urea has no physiological function. Hence it is transported to kidneys where it is excreted in urine. It is major end product of protein catabolism in humans. About 10-25 gm of urea is excreted in urine per day which makes up to 80-90% of total nitrogen excreted per day. However, blood also contains some urea.

Blood urea

Normal blood urea level is 16-36 mg/100 ml.

Fate of fumarate

Fumarate is recycled in urea cycle by converting it to aspartate. First fumarate is converted to malate by fumarase which is present in cytosol. Malic enzyme generates pyruvate from malate in the next reaction. Next pyruvate is converted to oxalo acetate by pyruvate carboxylase. Oxalocetate also can be formed directly from malate by the action of malate dehydrogenase. Finally aspartate is generated from oxaloacetate by transamination in which glutamate is converted to α-ketoglutarate. Thus operation of this system cause net supply of one ammonia molecule to urea synthesis (Fig. 12.7).

Regulation of urea formation

Formation of urea is regulated by activity of carbamoyl phosphate synthetase-I. This enzyme catalyzes committed step in urea synthesis. N-acetylglutamate regulates this enzyme activity. It is an allosteric activator. High protein in take leads to more N-acetylglutamate formation. Thus high protein in take influences urea formation. In starvation also urea synthesis is more mostly due to increased protein breakdown.

Medical Importance

Urea formation is impaired in several inherited diseases. They are due to deficiency of enzymes of urea cycle. The rate of incidence of urea cycle disorders is one in 2500. Most of these inherited diseases are due to defective genes and are fatal. Since the urea cycle converts ammonia to urea these disorders of urea cycle cause ammonia intoxication. Some common clinical symptoms seen in these diseases are vomiting, irritability, lethargy, seizures, mental retardation, coma and early death. They are

1. Hyper ammonemia Type I

It is due to deficiency of enzyme carbamoyl phosphate synthetase-I. Mental retardation is the main symptom of this condition.

2. Hyper ammonemia Type II

It is most common among others. It is due to deficiency of enzyme ornithine trans carbamoylase. So, in this condition carbamoyl phosphate accumulates and diverted to pyrimidine formation. This results in excretion of oroticacid and uracil in urine. Glutamate also accumulates in this condition.

3. Citrullinemia

This condition is due to the absence of enzyme argininosuccinate synthetase. Hence citrulline accumulates in blood and excreted in urine.

4. Argininosuccinicaciduria

Argininosuccinase is absent in this condition. So, argininosuccinate accumulates in blood and excreted in urine.

5. Hyper argininemia

This condition is due to low arginase activity. Hence, arginine accumulates and excreted in urine. However some urea may be excreted in urine due to kidney arginase.

6. N-acetyl glutamate synthetase deficiency

It is a rare disorder. N-acetyl glutamate synthetase is involved in formation of N-acetyl glutamate from acetyl-CoA and glutamate. Hyper ammonemia and aminoacid uria occurs in this condition. Since carbamoyl glutamate is an analog of acetyl glutamate administration of carbamoyl glutamate can lower symptoms.

Urea production may be decreased in liver diseases

Treatment

Treatment of urea cycle disorders involves removal of excess ammonia from blood and reduction of dietary nitrogen load. Peritonial dialysis is employed to clear ammonia from blood. Administration of compounds which can increase nitrogen excretion is another line of treatment. Benzoic acid and phenyl acetate are two such compounds used in the treatment.

Metabolic fates of carbon skeletons of Amino acids

Initial deamination of aminoacids produces carbon skeletons of amino acids. The carbon skeletons of twenty aminoacids are converted to seven compounds. These seven compounds are ultimately used for the formation of carbohydrates or fat like substances (Fig. 12.8). Depending on the cell needs they may be used for energy production. Hence, amino acids are classified based on the metabolic fate of their carbon skeletons also. They are

1. Glucogenic amino acids

The carbon skeletons of these aminoacids are converted to either glucose or intermediates of TCA cycle. The products may be pyruvate, oxaloacetate, α-ketoglutarate, succinate and fumarate. Glycine, alanine, valine, serine, threonine, cysteine, methionine, aspartate (aspargine), glutamate (glutamine), histidine, arginine and proline are glucogenic amino acids. Note that all non-essential amino acids are glucogenic.

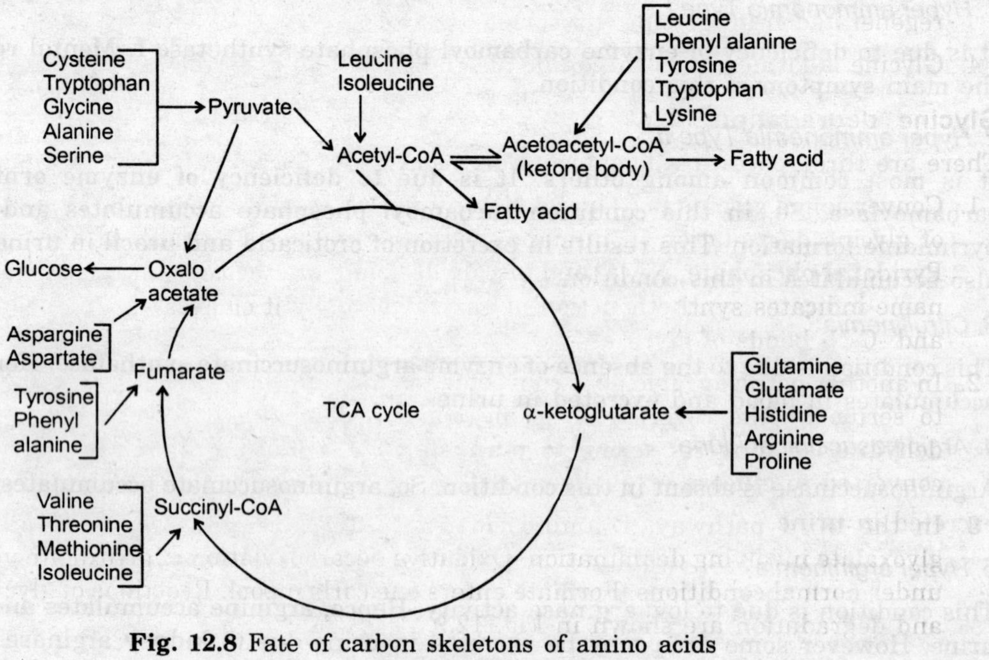

Fig. 12.8 Fate of carbon skeletons of amino acids

2. Ketogenic amino acids

The carbon skeletons of these aminoacids gives rise to fat like substances or intermediates of fatty acid catabolism. The products may be aceto acetyl-CoA and acetyl-CoA. Leucine is the only ketogenic aminoacid. Isoleucine, phenylalanine, tyrosine, tryptophan and lysine are also ketogenic amino acids.

3. Glucogenic and ketogenic amino acids

The carbon skeletons of these amino acids are converted to glucose or intermediates of TCA cycle and fat like substance. The products may be pyruvate, succinate, fumarate and acetyl-CoA. Isoleucine, phenylalanine, tyrosine, tryptophan and lysine are glucogenic and ketogenic amino acids.

METABOLISM OF INDIVIDUAL AMINOACIDS

Glycine Metabolism

It is a non-essential amino acid and is synthesized by living cells.

Glycine synthesis

Glycine is synthesized by four ways.

1. Glycine is formed from serine in a reaction catalyzed by serine trans hydroxy-methylase. Pyridoxal phosphate and tetrahydrofolate are two cofactors required. This enzyme catalyzes -c-c-bond cleavage in the forward reaction and -c-c-bond formation in backward reaction.
2. Glycine may be formed from glyoxalate by transamination. Glyoxalate may arise from serine via ethanolamine. In plants glyoxalate come from isocitrate by the action of isocitratase.
3. **Glycine-choline cycle** In this cycle glycine is synthesized from choline. Choline is regenerated from glycine via serine.
4. Glycine is formed from threonine also by the action of serine trans hydroxy methylase.

Glycine degradation

There are three pathways for glycine degradation.

1. Conversion of glycine to CO_2 and NH_4 by glycine synthase complex is the major pathway of glycine degradation in humans, birds and reptiles. It occurs in liver mitochondria. Pyridoxal phosphate, NAD^+ and tetrahydrofolate are the cofactors required. Though the name indicates synthetic action of enzyme actually it cleaves glycine by splitting –c-c- and -C-N- bonds of glycine.
2. In another pathway, glycine is converted to pyruvate via serine. First glycine is converted to serine by the reversal of serine trans hydroxy methylase reaction. Later serine dehydratase converts serine to pyruvate by eliminating ammonia. Pyruvate may be converted to glucose or oxidized in TCA cycle via acetyl-CoA.
3. In the third pathway, D-aminoacid oxidase or glycine oxidase converts glycine to glyoxalate involving deamination. Oxidative decarboxylation of glyoxalate yields formate under normal conditions. Formate enters one carbon pool. Reactions of glycine synthesis and degradation are shown in Fig. 12.9.

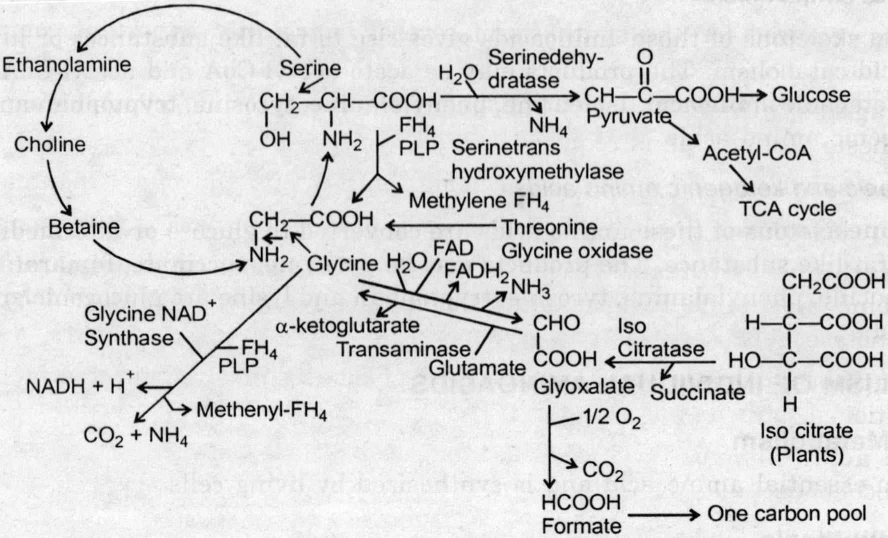

Fig. 12.9 Reactions of synthesis and breakdown of glycine. ↑ indicates —C—C—bond cleaved by serine trans hydroxy methylase and —C—C—bond and —C—N— bond cleavage by glycine synthase

Medical importance

Glycine metabolism is defective in some inherited diseases. They are due to production of defective enzymes (proteins) by defective genes. Inherited diseases of amino acid metabolism are referred as inborn errors of amino acid metabolism. Some of the known diseases of glycine metabolism are

1. Glycin uria

It is a rare genetic disorder of glycine metabolism. It is characterized by excess urinary excretion of glycine. However, plasma glycine level is normal. It is due to defect in reabsorption of glycine by renal tubules. Defective reabsorption is due to non-functional renal transporter of glycine.

2. Primary hyper oxaluria

It is characterized by excretion of large amounts of oxalate (15-60 mg/day) in urine irrespective of dietary oxalate. The conversion of glyoxalate to formate is blocked in this condition. Therefore, glyoxalate is oxidized to oxalate, which is excreted in urine. Excess oxalate combines with calcium to form calcium oxalate crystals in urine, which can deposit in kidney and urinary tract. So, the symptoms are bilateral urolithiasis (stones in both ureters), nephrocalcinosis (stones in kidney) and recurrent urinary tract infections. Death occurs in childhood or early adult life due to renal failure or hypertension.

3. Non-ketotic hyperglycinemia

It is fatal condition. Death occurs in infancy. It is due to defective glycine synthase. Characteristic symptoms are severe mental retardation and excess glycine in blood and urine.

Biological Importance

Glycine is required for the synthesis of several biologically important compounds. It is required for

1. **Collagen synthesis** Majority of body glycine is present in collagen. For other protein synthesis also glycine is required.
2. **Heme synthesis** First reaction of heme synthesis uses glycine (Chapter-22).
3. **Purine synthesis** Entire glycine molecule is used for purine ring formation (Chapter-15).
4. **Glutathione synthesis** Glycine is part of glutathione. It combines with glutamate-cysteine dippeptide to form glutathione. The reaction is catalyzed by glutathione synthetase. ATP serve as energy donor.
5. **Creatine synthesis** Reaction in which glycine is involved in creatine formation is mentioned later in this chapter.
6. **Bile acids formation** Glycine is required for the formation of glycocholic acid and glycochenodeoxy cholic acid.
7. **Hippuric acid synthesis** The reaction in which glycine involved in hippuric acid synthesis is mentioned in Chapter-27.
8. In addition glycine is required for serine and glucose formation as detailed above.
9. Glycine contributes one carbon groups (N-5, 10 methenyl FH_4, formate).
10. Glycine act as inhibitory neurotransmitter.

Metabolism of Alanine

Alanine is a non-essential amino acid.

Alanine synthesis

Alanine is synthesized by three ways.

1. By the action of alanine transaminase pyruvate is converted to alanine (Fig. 12.10*a*).
2. Alanine is produced during breakdown of tryptophan.
3. Alanine is synthesized from cysteine (detailed later).

Degradation

Alanine is converted to pyruvate by reversible reaction of alanine transaminase (Fig. 12.10*a*).

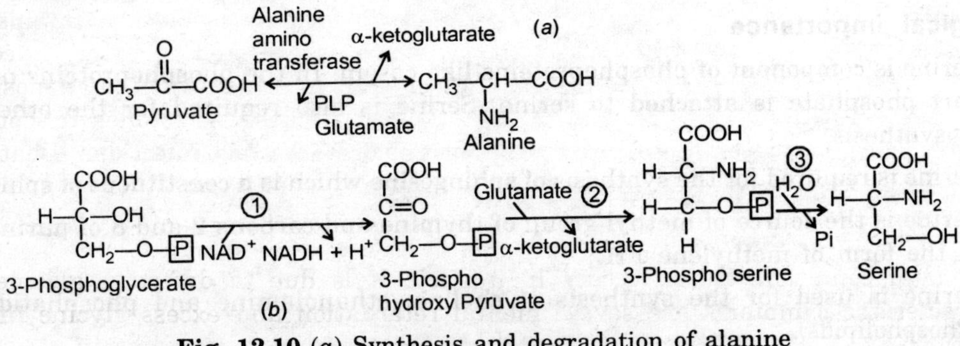

Fig. 12.10 (*a*) Synthesis and degradation of alanine
(*b*) Synthesis of serine from 3-phosphoglycerate

Medical and biological importance

1. Alanine is present in the blood at high concentration about 5 mg/100 ml.
2. Alanine transfers amino group nitrogen of amino acids from muscle to liver where it is converted to urea.
3. Alanine is also involved in the transfer of fuel from liver to muscle. In the liver, carbon skeleton of alanine is used for glucose synthesis. Muscle uses glucose from circulation for energy production (glucose-alanine cycle).
4. Alanine is component of several proteins. Collegen is rich in alanine.

Serine metabolism

Serine is a non-essential aminoacid.

Serine synthesis

Two pathways are responsible for the serine synthesis.

I. The major pathway of serine synthesis starts with 3-phosphoglycerate which is an intermediate of glycolysis (Fig. 12.10*b*).

Reaction sequence

1. Dehydrogenation of 3-phosphoglycerate by 3-phosphoglycerate dehydrogenase to 3-phosphohydroxy pyruvate is the first reaction of serine formation. NAD^+ is the hydrogen acceptor.
2. Transamination by transminase which converts product of the first reaction to 2-phosphoserine is the second reaction.
3. Finally serine is forced from phosphoserine after hydrolysis of phosphate by phosphatase.

II. In another minor pathway serine is formed from glycine by the reversal of serine trans hydroxy methylase reaction.

Degradation of serine

Serine is converted to pyruvate in a major route.

1. Serine dehydratase coverts serine to pyruvate which involves non-oxidative deamination. Pyridoxal phosphate is required.
2. Serine is converted to CO_2 and NH_4 via glycine in a minor route.

Biological importance

1. Serine is component of phosphoproteins like casein. In the phosphoproteins nonprotein part phosphate is attached to serine. Serine is also required for the other protein biosynthesis.
2. Serine is required for the synthesis of sphingosine which is a constituent of sphingolipids.
3. Serine is the source of methyl group of thymine and carbons 2 and 8 of purine nucleus in the form of methylene FH_4.
4. Serine is used for the synthesis of choline, ethanolamine and phosphatidyl serine (Phospholipids).

5. Serine is required for the catabolism of methionine.
6. **Active site.** Serine is the active site of several serine proteases like trypsin, chymotrypsin, cathepsinG etc.
7. **Regulatory site.** Serine is the regulatory site of enzymes like phosphorylase, HMG-CoA reductase etc. whose activity is altered by phosphorylation or dephosphorylation of hydroxyl groups of serine residue.
8. Serine is converted to glucose in times of need.
9. In E. coli serine is required for tryptophan formation.
10. In some bacteria serine is used for cysteine synthesis.

Threonine Metabolism

It is an essential amino acid. So it is not synthesized in humans. However in bacteria it is synthesized from aspartate.

Threonine degradation

It has three degradative pathways.

I. Conversion of threonine to propionyl-CoA is one of the three degradative routes. In this pathway first threonine is converted to α-keto butyrate by threonine dehydratase. Oxidative decarboxylation of α-keto butyrate by a dehydrogenase yield propionyl-CoA (Fig. 12.11).

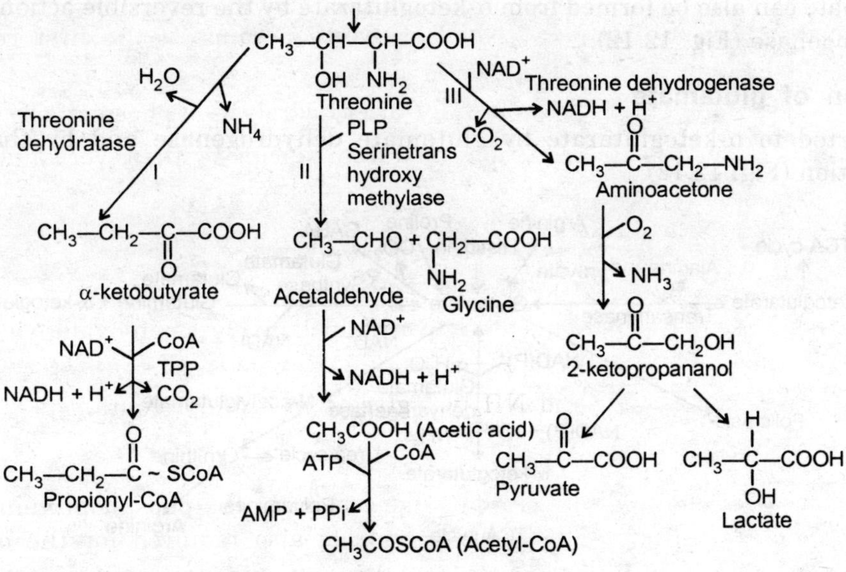

Fig. 12.11 Catabolic routes of threonine

II. Threonine may be converted to glycine and acetyl-CoA by the second degradative route. In this pathway, first serine transhydroxy methylase cleaves threonine to glycine and acetaldehyde. Unlike the conversion of serine to glycine this cleavage is not dependent on tetrahydrofolate (Fig. 12.11). Since acetaldehyde is toxic acetaldehyde is rapidly converted to acetyl-CoA after it is oxidized to acetate. Degradation of glycine is discussed above. Evidence for occurrence of this pathway is lacking still.

III. Conversion of threonine to pyruvate and lactate is the third degradative route of threonine. First threonine dehydrogenase converts threonine to aminoacetone which involves dehydrogenation and decarboxylation. NAD^+ is reduced and CO_2 is released. Amino acetone is converted to either pyruvate or lactate via 2-keto-propananol (Fig. 12.11).

Biological Importance

1. Glycine is a catabolic product of threonine.
2. In certain proteins threonine is present as O-phosphothreonine.
3. Threonine is used for glucose synthesis.
4. In plants and bacteria threonine is used for isoleucine synthesis.

Glutamate Metabolism

It is a non-essential aminoacid.

Synthesis of glutamate

Glutamate is synthesized by several ways.

1. Glutamate is formed from α-ketoglutarate by transamination as mentioned earlier.
2. Catabolism of arginine, histidine and proline produce glutamate.
3. Glutamate is synthesized from glutamine and α-ketoglutarate. Glutamate synthase catalyzes this reaction in presence of NADH.
4. Glutamate can also be formed from α-ketoglutarate by the reversible action of glutamate dehydrogenase (Fig. 12.12).

Degradation of glutamate

It is converted to α-ketoglutarate by glutamate dehydrogenase and by the reversal of transamination (Fig. 12.12).

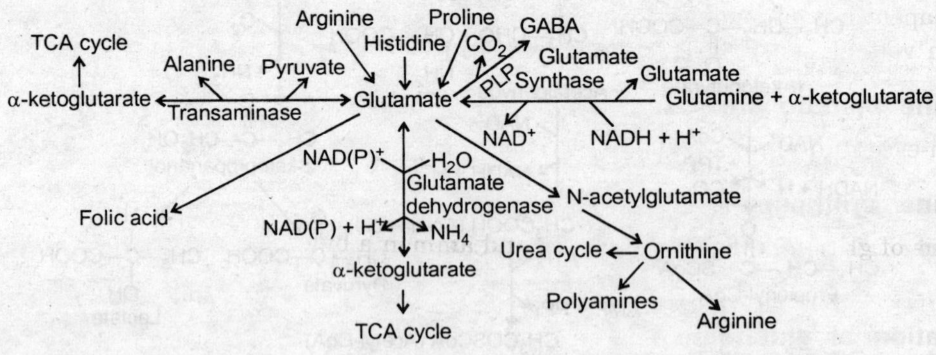

Fig. 12.12 Synthesis and degradation of glutamate and conversion of glutamate to special substances

Biological Importance

Glutamate plays central role in aminoacid metabolism. It supplies amino group required for the synthesis of non-essential amino acids. It has opposite function also. It act as collecting point of aminogroups of aminoacids during catabolism of aminoacids.

1. Glutamate is required for glutathione synthesis.
2. It is required for glutamine synthesis.
3. It is required for synthesis of N-acetyl glutamate which is a cofactor required for the activity of carbamoyl phosphate synthetase-I. N-acetyl glutamate is needed for arginine and ornithine synthesis.
4. **γ-amino butyric acid (GABA)** Decarboxylation of glutamate by pyridoxal phosphate (PLP) dependent glutamate decarboxylase yields γ-amino butyric acid. The enzyme is present in grey matter. GABA is an inhibitory neuro transmitter and present in synaptic vesicles. It acts by hyper polarizing post synaptic membrane. When released GABA binds to receptors which are ligand gated channels present in post synaptic membrane. This leads to opening of gated channels to Cl^-. As a result more Cl^- enters post synaptic membrane and causes hyper polarization which inhibits impulse transmission. GABA receptors are inducible. Alcohol acts by increasing GABA receptors. GABA is a component of homocarnosine a dipeptide present in brain.
5. **γ-carboxylation.** Glutamate of several proteins undergoes γ-carboxylation. γ-carboxylation of glutamate is crucial for blood clotting and bone development.
6. In bacteria it is required for the synthesis of arginine, ornithine and histidine. In humans glutamate is used for proline biosynthesis.
7. Glutamate residues are part of folic acid (stored) in liver.
8. Glutamate act as neurotransmitter.
9. Glucose can be synthesized from glutamate (glucogenic action).
10. Glutamate constitutes active site of matalloproteases like carboxypeptidase.

Medical Importance

1. Anti-epileptic drugs like valproic acid may act by increasing the level of GABA in brain. It increases GABA level either by inhibiting action of enzymes which degrade GABA or by increasing GABA synthesis.
2. In vit B_6 deficiency diminished GABA synthesis results in seizures.
3. Gapapentin is antiepileptic drug. It increases GABA levels in epilepsy patients. It interacts with voltage sensitive calcium channels.

Glutamine metabolism

It is non-essential amino acid.

Glutamine synthesis

Synthesis of glutamine from glutamate and ammonia by glutamine synthetase was detailed earlier.

Degradation of glutamine

It has three degradative routes.

1. In kidney glutaminase hydrolyzes glutamine. See above for details.
2. Glutamine undergoes transamination to α-ketoglutaramic acid. Further, hydrolysis of this compound yields α-ketoglutarate and ammonia.
3. Glutamine is degraded after it is converted to glutamate by glutamate synthase.

Biological Importance

Glutamine plays key role in amino acid (nitrogen) metabolism.

I. Amide nitrogen of glutamine is source of NH_2 groups in biosynthetic reactions of
   1. Purine nucleotides.
   2. Pyrimidine nucleotides.
   3. Amino sugars.
   4. NAD.

II. Glutamine is required for the synthesis of glutamate and aspargine.

III. In bacteria glutamine is required for the synthesis of histidine and tryptophan.

IV. Glutamine is involved in detoxification of indoleacetic acid.

Medical Importance

1. Glutamine concentration in blood is high about 10 mg/100 ml. As mentioned earlier, glutamine transports ammonia from various tissues to kidney and liver for disposal.
2. Phenyl acetyl glutamine, which is a conjugate of glutamine with phenyl acetate is found in urine of phenyl ketonuria patients. Indoleacetyl glutamine is found in urine of Hartnup's disease patients.
3. Glutamine takes part in acid base balance by contributing ammonia in kidney.
4. Glutaminase is a potential anti-cancer drug.

Formation and fates of glutamine are shown in Fig. 12.13.

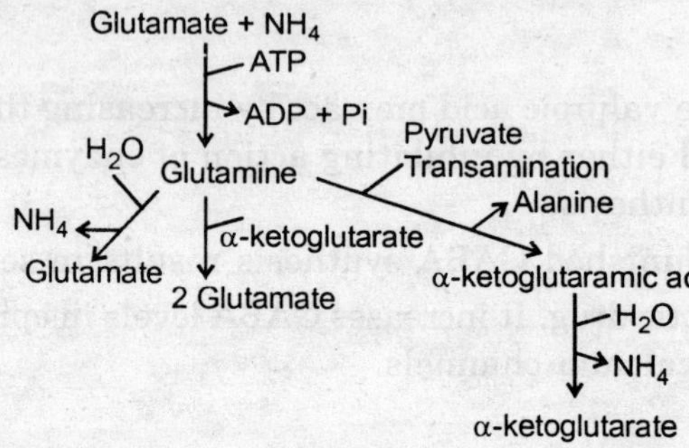

Fig. 12.13 Formation and fates of glutamine

Metabolism of aspartate

It is a non-essential amino acid.

Synthesis of aspartate

Aspartate is formed

1. From oxaloacetate by reversal of transamination reaction.
2. From aspargine by the action of asparginase.

Degradation

It is converted to oxaloacetate by transamination.

Biological Importance

1. Aspartate is required for biosynthetic reactions of purine and pyrimidine nucleotides.
2. Aspartate collects aminogroup of amino acids and supplies this to urea synthesis.
3. It is required for aspargine synthesis.
4. **β-alanine.** Decarboxylation of aspartate by aspartate decarboxylase produces β-alanine. It is a constituent of vitamin pantothenic acid.
5. In bacteria, it is required for threonine, methionine, isoleucine and lysine synthesis.
6. N-acetyl aspartate (NAA) is a neurotransmitter and related to an individuals intellectual level.
7. It is required for protein synthesis. Since it is glucogenic amino acid glucose can be formed from aspartate.
8. It is a component of malate–aspartate shuttle.
9. Aspartate is active site of pepsin.

Aspargine metabolism

It is a non-essential amino acid. It is synthesized from aspartate and ammonia by aspargine synthetase in ATP dependent reaction. Asparginase degrades aspargine to aspartate and ammonia. Aspargine has no important function. However, cancer cells require large amounts of this amino acids.

Arginine Metabolism

It is a semi-essential amino acid.

Arginine synthesis

1. It is formed from arginino succinate as a part of urea cycle. Since arginine is converted to ornithine, it may not be available for protein synthesis. Hence, growing humans must obtain it from diet. For adults, arginine is not an essential amino acid because urea cycle generates enough of arginine.
2. In plants and bacteria, arginine is synthesized from glutamate.

Arginine degradation

In mammals, it is converted to glutamate.

Sequence of reactions

1. Arginine is converted to ornithine by arginase.
2. Ornithine undergoes transamination involving δ-NH_2 group to glutamic semialdehyde. The reaction is catalyzed by ornithine δ-amino transferase.
3. Oxidation of glutamic semialdehyde produces glutamate. The reaction is catalyzed by NAD^+-dependent dehydrogenase (Fig. 12.14).

Medical Importance

Hyperornithinemia It is due to deficiency of ornithine-δ-aminotransferase. Symptoms are atrophy of choroid and retina. If not treated, it leads to loss of vision (blindness).

Biological Importance

1. Arginine is required for creatine synthesis.
2. **Synthesis of nitricoxide (NO) gas** This wonder gas is produced from arginine.
3. **Polyamine synthesis** Arginine supplies ornithine for polyamine biosynthesis.
4. **Synthesis of GABA** In a minor pathway ornithine formed from arginine is used for GABA production in brain.
5. Arginine is converted to glucose.
6. Histones are rich in arginine.

NITRIC OXIDE (NO)

Nitric Oxide Synthase (NOS) a dioxygenase catalyzes the formation of NO from arginine in a NADPH and O_2-dependent reaction. The dioxygenase is present in several tissues like blood vessels, macrophages, penis, brain etc. It incorporates one atom of oxygen into N to form NO and another molecule is incorporated into arginine to form citrulline (Fig. 12.14). Several isoenzymes of this enzyme have been identified. After O_2 and CO_2, NO is the only gaseous molecule recognized in the body. However, it has several pharmacological actions which are not shown by O_2 and CO_2.

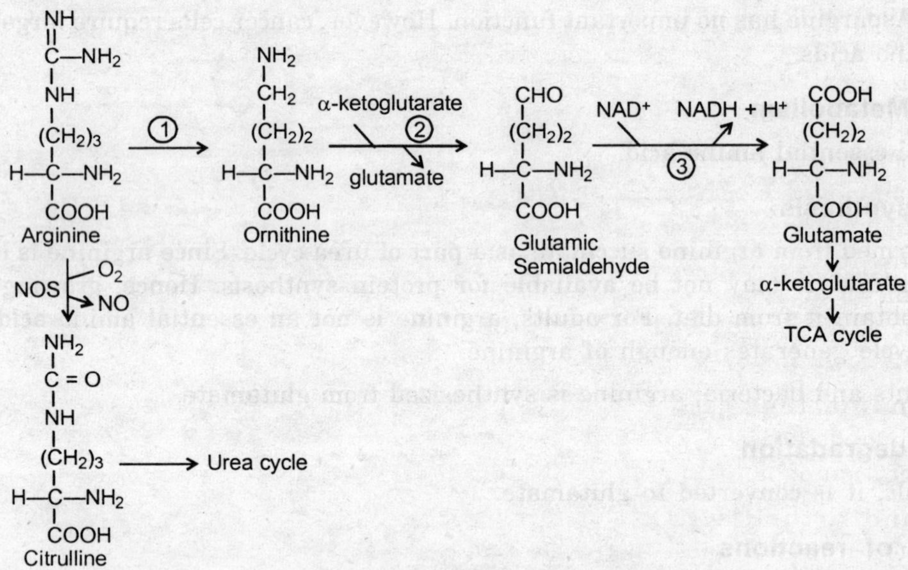

Fig. 12.14 Metabolism of arginine

Iso enzymes of NOS

A family of nitric oxide synthase (NOS) iso enzymes are identified. They are endothelial NOS designated as eNOS, neuronal NOS designated as nNOS and inducible NOS designated as iNOS. In addition to NO, NOS also generates super oxide O^{-}_2. Nitric oxide and its metabolites mediates oxidation, nitration and nitrosation of DNA bases, amino acids and lipids. These nitrated products initiate signalling pathways ranging from regulation of vascular tone to development of learning and memory.

Biological Importance

Like prostaglandins, nitric oxide has wide range of biological functions.

1. It dilates blood vessels.
2. It causes smooth muscle relaxation.
3. It inhibits platelet aggregation.
4. It is involved in the regulation of blood pressure.
5. It is essential for penile erection.
6. It is a neurotransmitter in the brain and in autonomic nervous system.

Medical Importance

1. Viagra increases sexual power of men by affecting nitric oxide metabolism.
2. Glyceryl trinitrate used in the treatment of angina pectoris works by effecting nitric oxide metabolism. It increases NO production.
3. Nitroprusside used to treat hypertension also works by affecting nitric oxide metabolism.
4. **NO and inflammation** The iNOS is induced by inflammatory substances like cytokines. It is the principle enzyme involved in inflammation. In macrophages, iNOS derived NO and O_2^- form potent peroxynitrite ($ONOO^-$), which contributes to cytotoxic action of macro phages in inflammation and immune defence.

   Link between NO and cyclooxygenase pathway in inflammation is established recently. In inflammatory conditions, both iNOs and COX-2 are induced. There is an NO mediated induction of COX-2 leading to increased production of pro inflammatory prostaglandins resulting in exacerbated inflammatory condition. COX-2 activation by NO contributes ischemic brain injury, cerebral ischemia and renal volume depletion. iNOS inhibitors are useful in treating such conditions due to dual inhibition of NO and PG. NO derived from iNOS is involved in promotion of chronic gut inflammation.
5. **NO and immune response** NO is an important modulator of immune response. In some lymphoid tissues NO increases intensity of immune response due to induction of proliferation or induction of apoptosis.
6. **NO and arthritis** In arthritis, there is production of cytotoxic peroxynitrite ($ONOO^-$) from NO and super oxide radicals generated by NOS.
7. **NO and myocarditis** Infections induce iNOS expression in cardiac myocytes. NO produced then inhibits pathogenic viral replication. Patients with acute myocarditis has less NO thus unable to clear the viral burden completely.
8. NO has roles in shock, sepsis, haemorrhage and anti-tumour activity of some cytokines like IL-2.

Polyamines

As the name implies they are molecules containing many amines. They are spermidine and spermine. Since they are identified first in semen they are named accordingly. However, later they are identified in many tissues.

Synthesis of polyamines

Polyamines are synthesized from ornithine and S-adenosylmethylthio propylamine, which serve as donor of amine groups.

Synthesis of S-adenosylmethylthio propylamine. It is synthesized from S-adenosylmethionine. A pyruvate containing decarboxylase catalyzes conversion of S-adenosylmethionine to S-adenosylmethylthio propylamine. The reaction is shown in Fig. 12.15.

Reaction sequence of polyamine synthesis

Ornithine is formed from arginine by arginase as detailed earlier

1. Decarboxylation of ornithine by ornithine decarboxylase (ODC) generates putrescine. ODC has very short half life (5 minutes) and it is site of action of many antitumor drugs.
2. Now transfer of propylamine from S-adenosyl methyl thiopropylamine to putrescine produces spermidine. The reaction is catalyzed by spermidine synthase.
3. Further transfer of propylamine from S-adenosyl methyl thiopropylamine to spermidine produces spermine. The reaction is catalyzed by spermine synthase (Fig. 12.15).

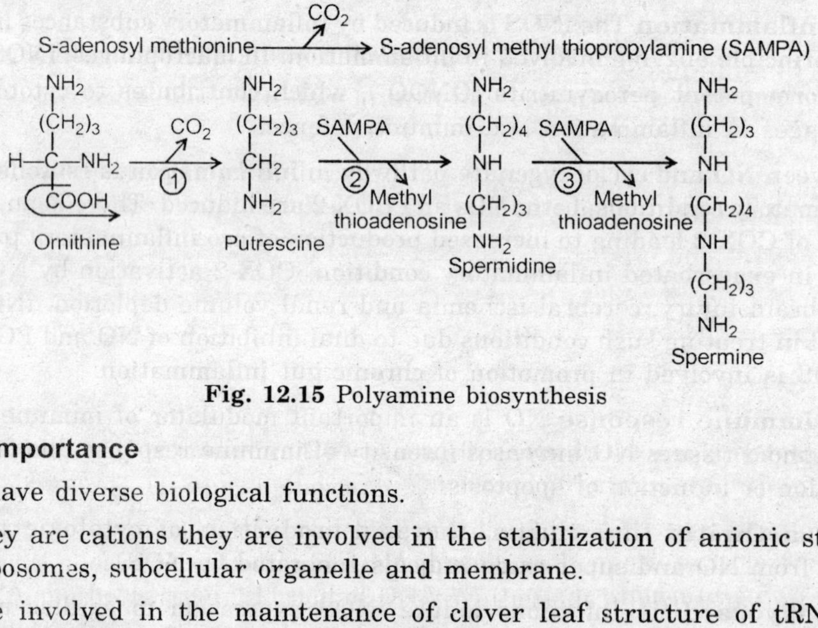

Fig. 12.15 Polyamine biosynthesis

Biological Importance

Polyamines have diverse biological functions.

1. Since they are cations they are involved in the stabilization of anionic structures like DNA, ribosomes, subcellular organelle and membrane.
2. They are involved in the maintenance of clover leaf structure of tRNA. They are required for packing of bacteriophage DNA.
3. They stimulate nucleic acid and protein biosynthesis.
4. They are required for cell growth or cell division.

Medical Importance

1. Since polyamines are required for cell division, inhibitors of polyamine biosynthesis are used as anti cancer drugs. Most of them blocks the action of ornithine decarboxylase. DFMO (difluoromethyl ornithine) is an inhibitor of this enzyme, which is used as anti tumour agent. As such DFMO is inactive. Initial actions of ODC on this molecule

produces active irreversible inhibitor, which covalently bind to active site of enzyme molecule and rendering enzyme inactive (referred as suicide inhibition).

DFMO is also used to cure certain protozoal and parasitic infections. DFMO is effective against African sleeping sickness causing protozoan and pneumonia causing protozoan in AIDS patients. Malarial parasite is also susceptible to DFMO action.

2. Excretion of polyamines in urine is increased in most of the cancers.
3. Polyamine concentration is more in cancer cells.
4. Presence of spermidine is used to identify sperm in suspected rape victims.

Histidine metabolism

It is a semi-essential amino acid.

Synthesis of histidine

1. Growing humans synthesize this aminoacid at low rate. So they need dietary histidine to maintain nitrogen balance.
2. Adult humans mostly derive this amino acid from endogenous sources.
3. Bacteria synthesize this amino acid from PRPP and glutamate.

Degradation of histidine

In the body, histidine is converted to α-ketoglutarate in a sequence of five reactions. They are:

1. Unlike most of the amino acids aminogroup of histidine is removed by non-oxidative deamination as ammonia. Reaction is catalyzed by histidine ammonia lyase (Histidase). Urocanic acid is the product of this reaction (Fig. 12.16).
2. Hydration of urocanic acid by hydratase or urocanase is the next reaction. 4-Imidazolone-5-propionate is the product of this reaction.
3. Cleavage of ring by hydrolase converts imidazolone propionate to formiminoglutamate (FIGLU).
4. Formiminogroup generated in the above reaction is transferred to tetrahydrofolate (FH_4) by glutamate-formiminotransferase. As a result, formimino-FH_4 and glutamate are formed. Formimino-FH_4 serve as donor of one carbon in biosynthetic reactions which we shall see later.
5. Finally α-ketoglutarate is formed from glutamate by transamination.

Biological Importance

1. Histidine produces histamine in several tissues.
2. Histidine is a component of ergothionine in liver and R.B.C.
3. Histidine is a component of carnosine and anserine of muscle.
4. Histidine is a component of homocarnosine in brain.
5. Histidine is preseursor of glucose and glutamate.
6. Histidine contributes one carbon group.
7. Histidine constitutes catalytic site of Zn^{2+} metalloenzymes.

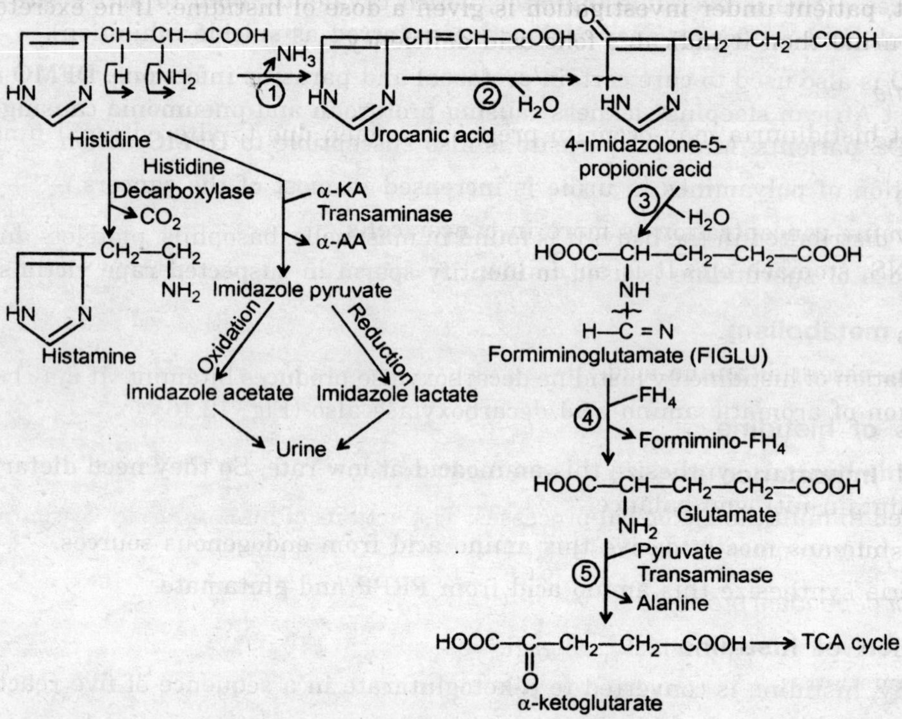

Fig. 12.16 Histidine catabolism and histamine formation ~~~ indicates cleavage Alternate catabolic route for histidine in histidinemia is also shown

Medical Importance

Histidine metabolism is defective in some diseases.

1. Histidinemia

It is due to deficiency of histidine ammonia lyase. Lack of this enzyme results in accumulation of histidine in blood and excretion in urine. Main symptoms are mental retardation and impairment of speech. The urine of the affected individuals also contain imidazole pyruvate, imidazole lactate and imidazole acetate because histidine is catabolized by a alternate route (Fig. 12.16).

2. Imidazole aminoacid uria

This condition is characterized by excretion of imidazoles in urine due to renal transport defect.

3. Urocanic aciduria

It is due to defective urocanase. Large amount of urocanic acid is excreted in urine.

4. FIGLU excretion test

It is a test for folic acid deficiency. Since folic acid is needed for reaction 4 of histidine catabolism, in folicacid deficiency this reaction is blocked. As a result FIGLU accumulates and excreted in urine.

In this test, patient under investigation is given a dose of histidine. If he excretes more of FIGLU in urine then it indicates folic acid deficiency.

5. Histidinuria

A transient histidinuria may occur in pregnant women due to altered renal function.

Histamine

It is widely distributed in the body. It is found in mast cells, basophils, platelets, lungs, blood vessels, CNS, stomach etc. It is an amine.

Synthesis

Decarboxylation of histidine by histidine decarboxylase produces hitamine. It may be produced by the action of aromatic amino acid decarboxylase also (Fig. 12.16).

Biological Importance

It is involved in multiple biological processes. The actions of histamine are mediated through three types of receptors. They are H-1, H-2 and H-3 receptors.

H-1 receptor dependent processes

1. It is involved in anaphylactic, allergic reactions. It is released at the site of injury and inflammation.
2. It is a vasodilator and lowers blood pressure (hypotensive).
3. It causes constriction of bronchi.
4. It causes contraction of smooth muscle.

H-2 receptor dependent process

1. It increases acid production in stomach by activating ATP dependent proton pump present in parietal cells.

H-3 receptor dependent process

1. In the brain, it acts as neurotransmitter and act as awakening amine.

Medical Importance

1. Cimetidine and rantidine etc., used in duodenal and peptic ulcer treatment inhibit acid secretion by binding H-2 receptors.
2. Anti-allergic drugs or anti-histamines like diphenyl hydramine, chlorphenaramine work by binding H-1 receptors.
3. Augmented histamine test is used to assess gastric function.

Proline Metabolism

It is a non-essential amino acid.

Synthesis of proline

Proline is synthesized from glutamate.

Reaction sequence

1. Glutamate kinase phosphorylates glutamate to glutamate-5-phosphate in ATP dependent reaction.
2. Reduction of glutamate-5-phosphate by NADPH-dependent reductase forms glutamate-γ-semialdehyde. Non-enzymatic head to tail condensation of the glutamate semialdehyde produces Δ^1-pyrroline-5-carboxylic acid.
3. Reduction of Δ^1-pyrroline-5-carboxylic acid by NADPH dependent reductase yields proline (Fig. 12.17A).

Degradation of Proline

Proline is converted to glutamate.

Reaction sequence

1. Proline dehydrogenase catalyzes dehydrogenation of proline to Δ^1-pyrroline-5-carboxylic acid. NAD^+ is hydrogen acceptor.

   Glutamate γ-semialdehyde is formed from Δ^1-pyrroline-5-carboxylic acid non-enzymatically.
2. A specific NAD^+ dependent dehydrogenase converts glutamate-γ-semialdehyde to glutamate (Fig. 12.17B).

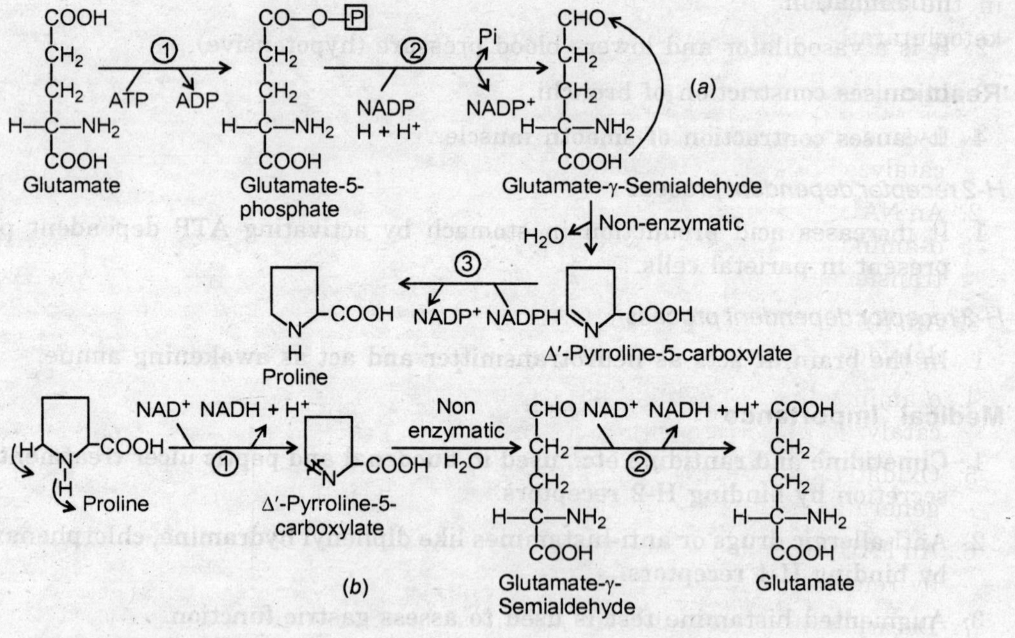

Fig. 12.17 (*a*) Proline synthesis (*b*) Proline degradation

Biological Importance

1. Proline and hydroxy proline are major components of collagen and elastin.
2. Glucose may be be formed from proline.

Medical Importance

1. **Hyper prolinemia Type-I** It is due to lack of proline dehydrogenase. This causes accumulation of proline in blood. Symptoms are mental retardation and renal damage.
2. **Hyper prolinemia Type-II** It is due to lack of second dehydrogenase that converts glutamate-γ-semialdehyde to glutamate. Main symptom is mental retardation.
3. **Hereditary prolin uria** It is due to renal transport defect. This leads to excretion of proline in urine.
4. Hydroxy proline excretion in urine is more in patients undergoing the chemotherapy for tumors.
5. Urinary hydroxy proline may serve as index of connective tissue turnover.
6. In bone metastasis cases also urinary hydroxy proline is more.

Lysine Metabolism

It is an essential amino acid. So, humans are unable to synthesize this amino acid. However, in bacteria it is synthesized from aspartate.

Lysine degradation

Lysine is degraded to one molecule of aceto acetyl-CoA and two molecules of CO_2 by mitochondrial enzymes. Unlike other amino acids, lysine does not undergo transamination in the beginning of catabolism. However, initially ε-aminogroup is transferred to α-ketoglutarate by different mechanism. Later α-aminogroup is removed by transamination.

Reaction sequence

1. Lysine first condenses with α-ketoglutarate to produce saccharopine. The reaction is catalyzed by NADPH-dependent sasccharopine dehydrogenase.
2. An NAD^+-dependent saccharopine dehydrogenase cleaves saccharopine to glutamate and α-aminoadipic acid semialdehyde. The combined action of first two enzymes causes net transfer of ε-amino group of lysine to α-ketoglutarate.
3. An $NADP^+$-dependent aminoadipic acid semialdehyde dehydrogenase oxidizes semial dehydde group to acid group. So α-amino adipic acid is the product.
4. α-aminoadipic acid undergoes transamination to α-keto adipic acid. The reaction is catalyzed by a transaminase and involves transfer of α-amino group.
5. Oxidative decarboxylation of α-keto adipic acid by α-keto acid dehydrogenase complex generates glutaryl-CoA. The enzyme is similar to pyruvate dehydrogenase.
6. An FAD-dependent glutaryl-CoA dehydrogenase converts glutaryl-CoA to glutaconyl-CoA by removing hydrogens from α, β carbons.
7. Decarboxylation of glutaconyl-CoA produces crotonyl-CoA. Further catabolism of crotonyl-CoA is accomplished by enzymes of β-oxidation.
8. Addition of water by hydratase generates β-hydroxy butyryl-CoA from crotonyl-CoA.
9. Dehydrogenation of β-hydroxybutyryl-CoA by NAD^+ dependent dehydrogenase yields acetoacetyl-CoA.

   Reaction sequence of lysine degradation is shown in Fig. 12.18.

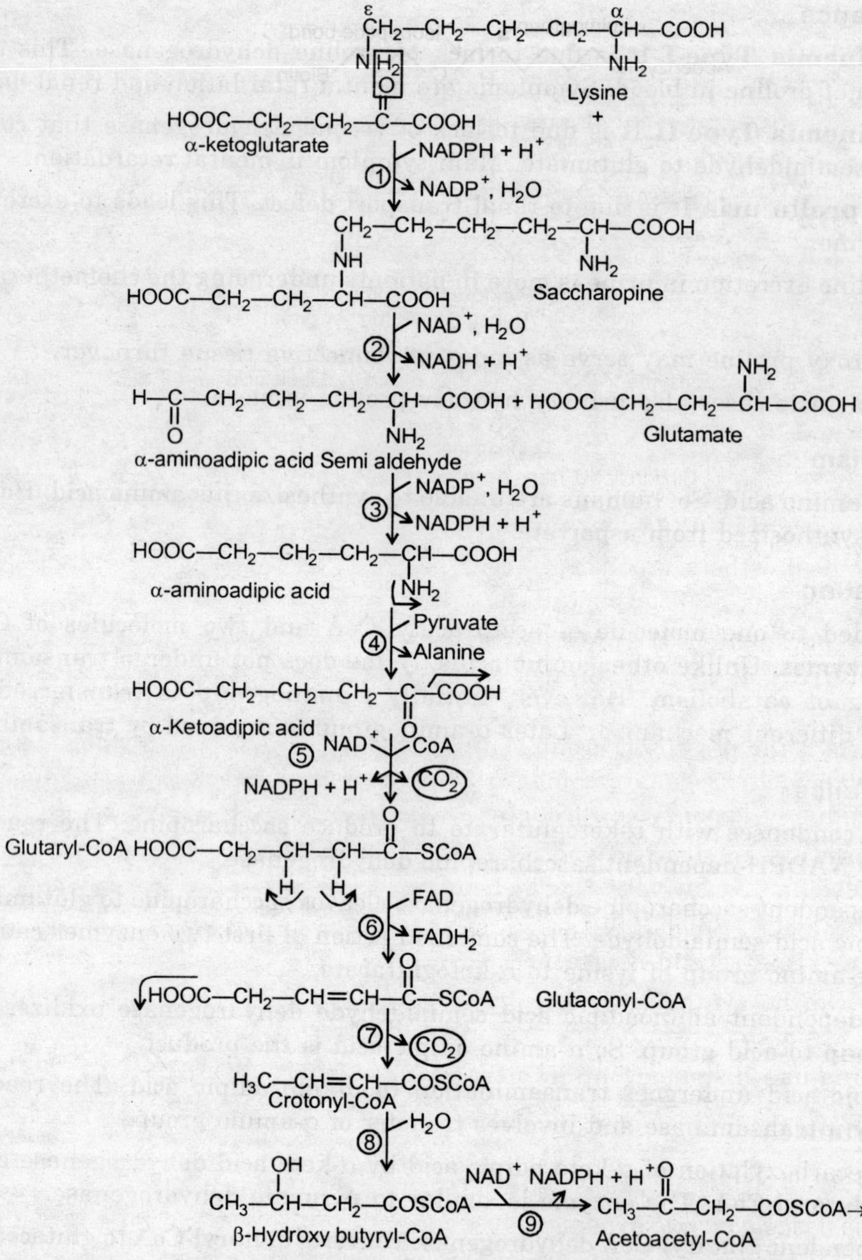

Fig. 12.18 Reaction sequence of lysine degradation

Biological Importance

1. Lysine and hydroxy lysine are component of collagen and elastin. They are involved in cross linking process that converts tropocollagen to collagen.
2. Lysine is required for the synthesis of carnitine.
3. **ε-Amino group** Some prosthetic groups are attached to apoenzymes through ε-amino groups of lysine (Fig. 12.9).

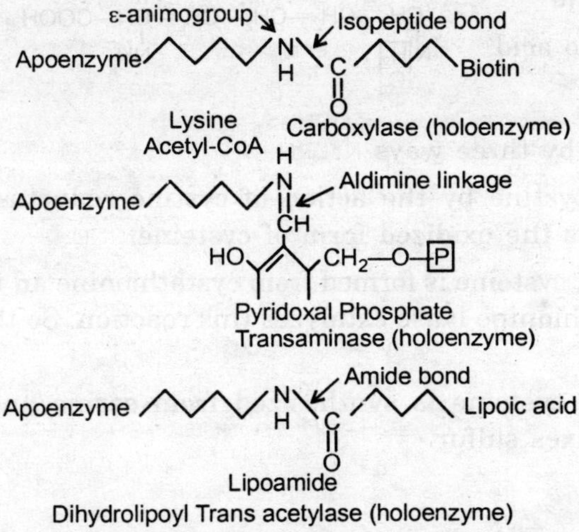

Fig. 12.19 Linkages of ε-amino group of Lysine

(*a*) Biotin is the prosthetic group of acetyl-CoA carboxylase. It is attached to ε-aminogroup of lysine residue of apoenzyme through an isopeptide (amide) linkage.

(*b*) Pyridoxal phosphate is the prosthetic group of transaminase. It is covalently attached to protein part of enzyme through an aldimine linkage involving ε-aminogroup of lysyl residue.

(*c*) Lipoic acid is the prosthetic group of dihydrolipoyl transacetylase which is a member of pyruvate dehydrogenase complex. It is covalently attached to ε-aminogroup of lysyl residue of apoenzyme through an isopeptide bond.

4. **Enzyme function** In some enzymes ε-amino group influences binding of substrate to enzyme molecule. Negatively charged substrate combines with enzymes through positively charged ε-aminogroup.
5. In rhodopsin, 11-*cis*-retinal is attached to opsin through ε-aminogroup of lysine.
6. Fatty acids can be synthesized from lysine and cadavarine is formed from lysine in intestine.
7. Basic proteins like histones contain more of lysine.

Medical Importance

Lysine degradation is defective in some diseases.

1. Hyper lysinemia associated with hyperammonemia

It is due to defective $NADP^+$-dependent saccharopine dehydrogenase. So conversion of lysine to saccharopine is impaired in affected individuals. When these individuals consume protein plasma lysine level raises. In the liver arginase is inhibited by raised plasma lysine. This leads to hyperammonemia.

2. Hyper lysinemia

It is due to defective NAD^+-dependent saccharopine dehydrogenase. So saccharopine is not cleaved in affected people. Both lysine and saccharopine accumulates in blood and mental retardation may be seen.

Metabolism of cysteine

It is non-essential amino acid.

Synthesis of cysteine

Cysteine is synthesized by three ways.

1. It is formed from cystine by the action of cystine reductase. NADH is the donor of hydrogen. Cystine is the oxidized form of cysteine.
2. In mammalian liver, cysteine is formed from cystathionine an intermediate of methionine degradation. Cystathionine lyase catalyzes this reaction. So the sulfur of cysteine comes from methionine.
3. In microorganisms, cysteine is synthesized from serine and H_2S. A PLP dependent cysteine synthase fixes sulfur.

Cysteine degradation

In mammals cysteine is degraded by two pathways. A third pathway of cysteine degradation is present in bacteria.

1. Dioxygenase pathway.

In mammals it is the principal route of cysteine degradation. Cysteine dioxygenase converts cysteine to cysteines sulfinate by incorporating two atoms of oxygen in presence of NAD (P) H and Fe^{2+}. The cysteine sulfinate has three metabolic fates. In mammalian liver, major portion is converted to taurine. This is detailed in biological importance of cysteine. Other minor alternative fates are

(*a*) A direct desulfination of cysteine sulfinate produces alanine and sulfite.

(*b*) Cysteine sulfinate undergoes transamination to form sulfinyl pyruvate. This is followed by desulfination catalyzed by desulfinase, which converts cysteine sulfinate to pyruvate.

2. Transaminase pathway

A transaminase present in mammalian liver and kidney produces mercaptopyruvate from cysteine by the transfer of α-amino group. The mercaptopyruvate is converted to mercaptolactate in a reaction catalyzed by dehydrogenase. The product mercaptolactate is excreted in urine.

Desulfuration of mercaptopyruvate

Alternately mercapto pyruvate undergoes desulfuration by several routes.

1. In one route, sulfur transferase catalyzes the transfer of mercapto pyruvate sulfur to an acceptor to yield pyruvate and H_2S.
2. In the other routes, rhodanase can transfer mercapto pyruvate sulfur to cyanide to form thiocyanate.
3. Sulfur of mercapto pyruvate may be transferred to sulfite to form thiosulfate. Rhodanase is responsible for this transfer also.

Thiosulfate and thiocyanate thus formed are excreted in urine.

4. In bacteria, cysteine is converted to pyruvate by cysteine desulfhydrase.

In Fig. 12.20 cysteine metabolism is shown.

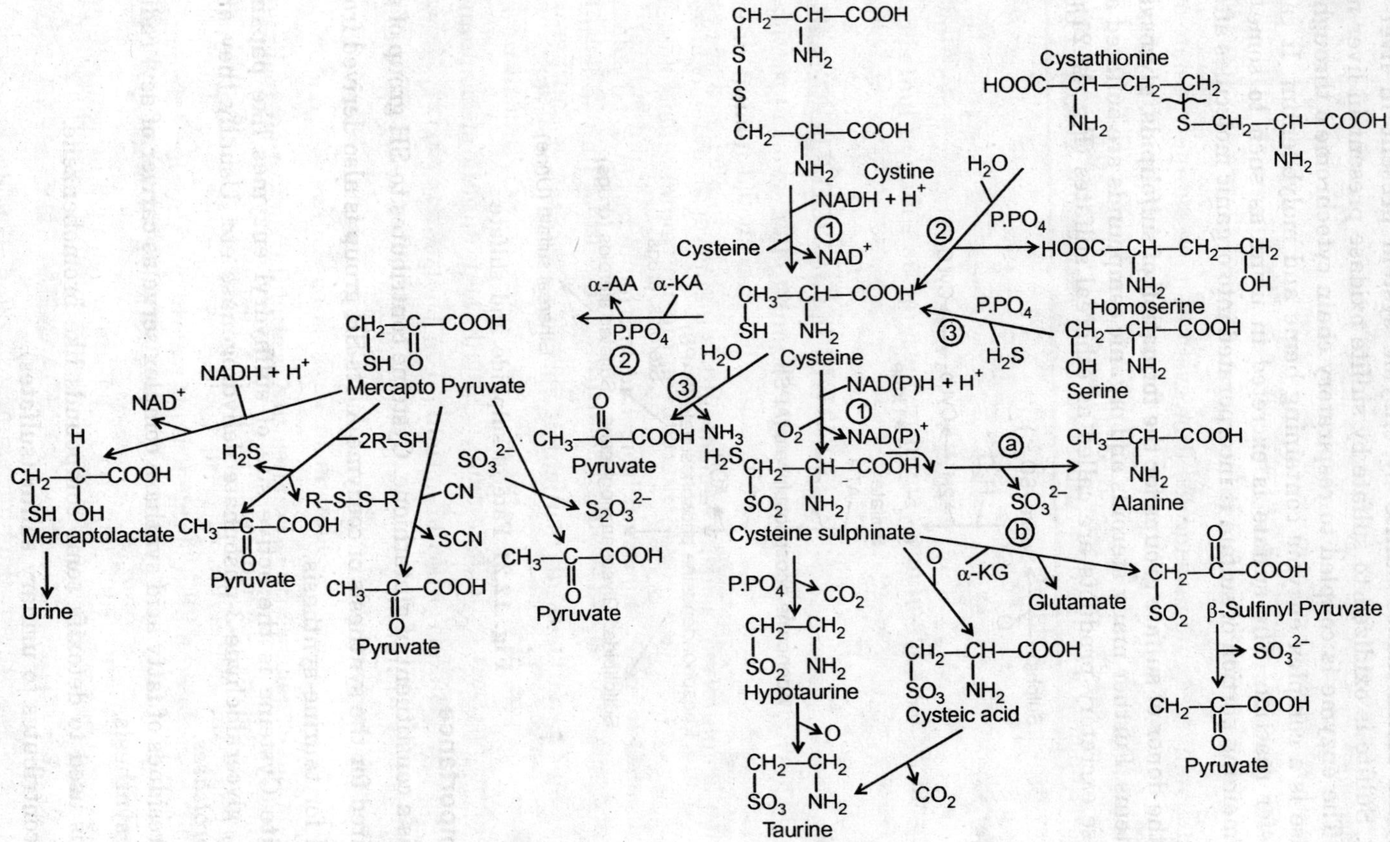

Fig. 12.20 Synthesis and degradation of cysteine. Taurine synthesis is also shown

Fate of sulphide and sulfate

Sulphide may be converted to sulfite by enzyme system present in liver and kidney mitochondria. Sulfite is oxidized to sulfate by sulfite oxidase present in liver mitochondria of mammals. The enzyme is coupled to respiratory chain cytochrome c through cytochrome b_5. The oxidase is a complex enzyme containing heme and molybdenum. It catalyzes two-electron transfer reaction. The sulfate is excreted in urine as such to some extent (Fig. 12.21). The remaining portion of sulfate is incorporated into organic molecules after activation to PAPS.

PAPS is the donor of sulfate groups for the formation of sulfolipids, glycosaminoglycans and some proteins. Further many steroids and organic compounds are sulfated and excreted in urine. These excretory products are called as ethereal sulfates (Fig. 12.21).

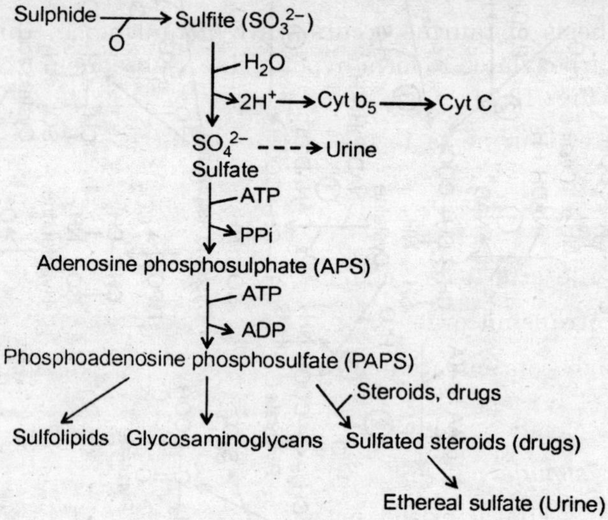

Fig. 12.21 Fate of sulphide and sulfate

Biological Importance

1. Cysteine is a constituent of glutathione. Cysteine contributes to-SH group of glutathione.
2. It is required for the synthesis of coezyme A. Its-SH group is also derived from cysteine.
3. It is used for taurine synthesis.
4. **Active site** Cysteine is the active site of sulfhydryl enzymes like papain, calpains, cathepsin, glyceraldehyde-3-phosphate dehydrogenase etc. Usually they are called as *cysteine proteases*.
5. Cysteine residues of fatty acid synthase complex serve as carrier of acyl radicals during fatty acid synthesis.
6. Cysteine is used to detoxify some compounds like bromobenzene.
7. Cysteine contributes to urinary sulfur (sulfates).
8. Cysteine is sulfate source in the body. Sulfate of cysteine is used for the synthesis of sulfolipids, glycosaminoglycans, proteins and sulfation of steroids and organic compounds.

9. **Proteins structure and function** Cysteine has major role in formation of protein structure and function. Inter or intrachain disulfide bonds of proteins are derived from cysteine residues. The disulfide linkages are crucial for protein function. For example, Insulin act as hormone only when disulfide bonds are intact.
10. Cystine may be formed non-enzymatically from two cysteine molecules.
11. Glucose may be synthesized from cysteine.
12. Cysteine residues of thioredoxin participates in electron transfer or in redox reaction.

Synthesis of taurine

Cysteine sulfinic acid an intermediate of cysteine catabolism is used for the synthesis of taurine. Taurine is formed from cysteine sulfinic acid by two ways.

1. In the liver, synthesis of taurine occurs via hypotaurine. In this route first cysteine sulfinic acid is decarboxylated to form hypotaurine. Subsequent oxidation of hypotaurine produces taurine (Fig. 12.21).
2. On the other route, taurine is formed from cysteic acid after decarboxylation (Fig. 12.21).

Biological Importance

1. It is required for bile acid (tauro cholate) formation.
2. Taurine is a neurotransmitter.
3. It is present in high concentration in cells. The reason is yet to be known.

Medical Importance

1. Cystine-lysin uria or cystinuria

This inherited disease is characterized by excretion of large amounts of cystine, lysine, arginine and ornithine in urine. It is due to renal transport defect. Since cystine is insoluble it forms stones in kidney, ureters and bladder in the affected patients.

2. Cystionsis

It is also an inherited but serious disease. Deposits of crystals of cysteine in the lysosomes of many tissues are found in this disease. Lysosomal dysfunction may be repsonsible for the disease. The patients may die at early age due to renal failure.

3. Sulfituria

It is due to defective sulfite oxidase. This give rise to excretion of more sulfite and thiosulfite in urine. In the affected people neurological functions are impaired.

Metabolism of Methionine

It is an essential amino acid. So, humans lack enzymes that can synthesize this amino acid. However, in plants and some bacteria methionine is synthesized from aspartate and sulfur of methionine comes from cysteine.

Methionine degradation

Methionine is degraded to propionyl-CoA via homocysteine (Fig. 12.22).

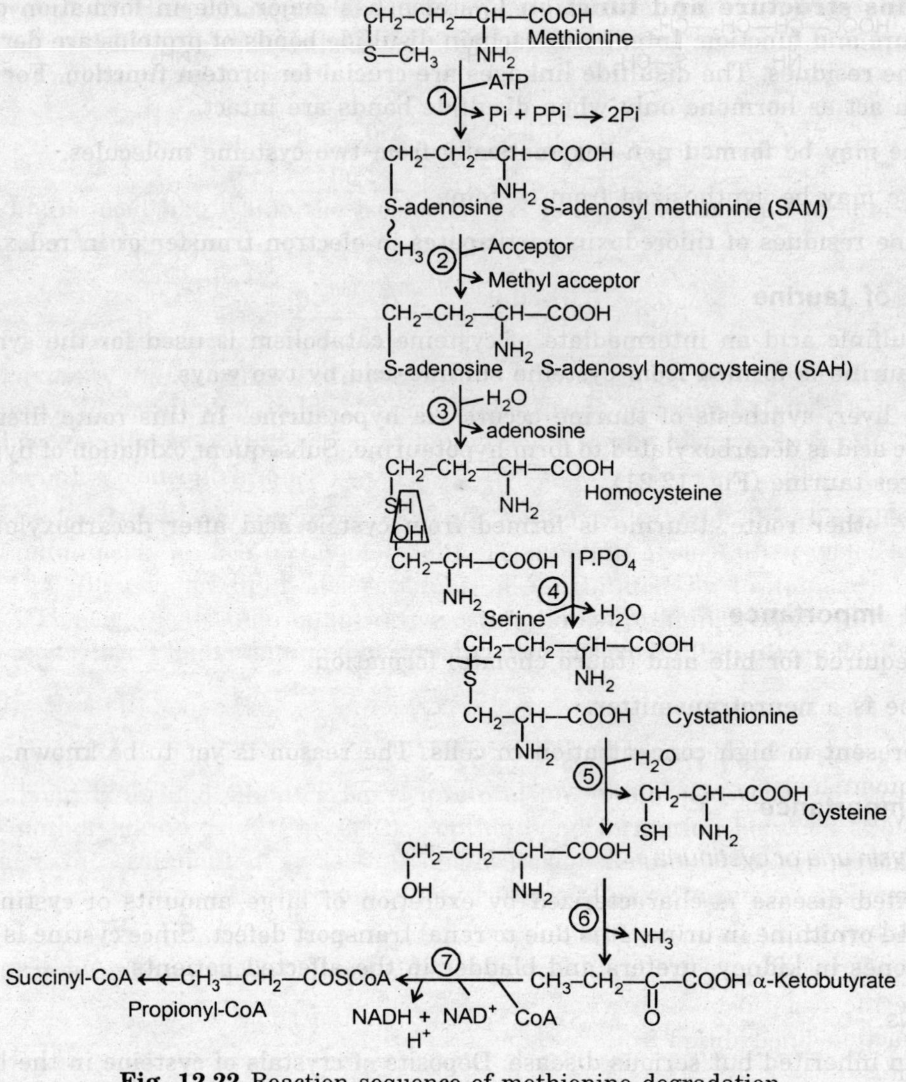

Fig. 12.22 Reaction sequence of methionine degradation

Reaction sequence

1. Formation of S-adenosyl methionine (SAM) or active methionine is the first reaction leading to methionine breakdown. The reaction is catalyzed by S-adenosyl methionine synthase. The reaction deserves special mention. First methionine reacts with ATP to form S-adenosylmethionine and triphosphate. Next, triphosphate is hydrolyzed to pyrophosphate and Pi by enzyme. Further hydrolysis of pyrophosphate by pyrophosphatase makes reaction thermodynamically favourable. So for the formation of S-adenosylmethionine total three high energy bonds are utilized. That is why the sulfonium ion of S-adenosylmethionine is highly reactive and a high energy compound and it function as methyl donor (Fig. 12.23*a*).
2. Transfer of methyl group to an acceptor results in the formation of S-adenosyl homocysteine (SAH) in the next reaction. Methyl transferase catalyzes this reaction.

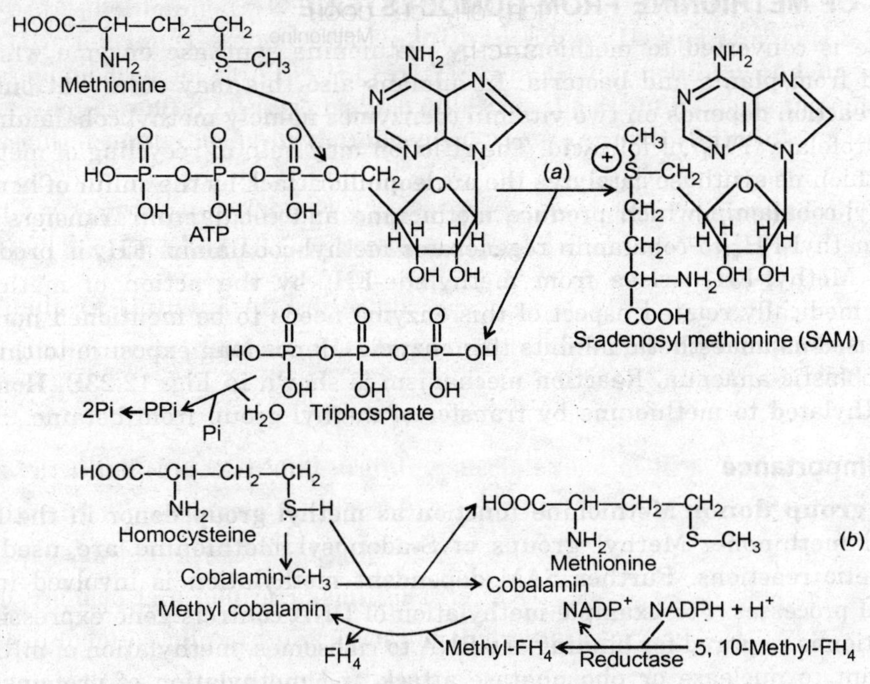

Fig. 12.23 (*a*) Reaction mechanism of S-adenosyl methionine synthase
(*b*) Methionine synthase catalyzed reaction

3. Subsequent hydrolysis of S-adenosyl homocysteine by hydrolase yields adenosine and homocysteine.

   Some amount of homo cysteine may be converted into methionine. However, most of the homocysteine is converted to propionyl- CoA via homo serine after conserving sulfur as cysteine.

4. In the next step cystathionine synthase catalyzes the condensation of homo cysteine with serine to form cystathionine. The reaction is pyridoxal phosphate dependent. In this reaction, C—S bond is formed between carbon of serine and -SH group of homo cysteine.

5. Another pyridoxal phosphate (PLP) dependent cystathioninase hydrolyzes cystathionine to homo serine and cysteine. The carbon skeleton of cysteine is derived from serine and –SH is derived from homo cysteine. Thus, the methionine sulfur is the source for cysteine sulfur. So, if diet contain adequate methionine there is no need for additional cysteine.

6. A deaminase converts homoserine to α-ketobutyrate by removing α-aminogroup as ammonia.

7. Oxidative decarboxylation of α-keto butyrate by α-ketobutyrate dehydrogenase complex yields propionyl-CoA. The reaction is similar to the reaction catalyzed by pyruvate dehydrogenase complex.

Reactions involved in the conversion of propionyl-CoA to succinyl-CoA are detailed earlier in Chapter-10.

SYNTHESIS OF METHIONINE FROM HOMOCYSTEINE

Homocysteine is converted to methionine by methionine synthase enzyme which is well characterized from plants and bacteria. In humans also this may occur but only to some extent. The reaction depends on two vitamin coenzymes namely methyl cobalamin of vit B_{12} and tetrahydrofolate (FH_4) of folicacid. The reaction may help in recycling of methionine in humans. Methionine synthase catalyzes the nucleophilic attack by the sulfur of homocysteine on the methyl-cobalamin which produce methionine and cobalamin. Transfers of methyl group from methyl-FH_4 to cobalamin regenerates methyl-cobalamin. FH_4 is produced from methyl-FH_4. Methyl-FH_4 arises from methylene-FH_4 by the action of methylene-FH_4 reductase. A medically related aspect of this enzyme needs to be mentioned here. Nitrous oxide (N_2O) used as anaesthetic inhibits this enzyme. Hence long exposure to this gas may cause megaloblastic anaemia. Reaction mechanism is shown in Fig. 12.23B. Homocysteine can be remethylated to methionine by transfer of methyl group from betaine.

Biological Importance

1. **Methyl group donor** Methionine function as methyl group donor in the form of S-adenosyl methinone. Methyl groups of S-adenosyl methionine are used in many biosynthetic reactions. Further SAM dependent methylation is involved in multiple biological processes. For example methylation of DNA controls gene expression, t-RNA methylation is required for binding of t-RNA to ribosomes, methylation of mRNA makes it resistant to nuclease or phosphatase attack and methylation of proteins regulates protein turnover by blocking ubiquitinization. Methylation of lysine and argininine residues of histones is associated with occurrence of certain phases of cell cycle. Removal of certain toxic substances involves methylation. In some bacteria methylation of some residues of peptides produce methylated chemotactic peptide (MCP). Now we shall see how methylation takes place.

Transmethylation

It is a process in which methyl group of S-adenosyl methionine is transferred to an acceptor. Usually transferases catalyze the transfer of methyl group and SAH is formed from SAM at the end.

Transmethylation examples

1. Norepinephrine ⟶ Epinephrine
2. Guanidoacetate ⟶ Creatine
3. Ethanolamine ⟶ Choline
4. Acetyl serotonin ⟶ Melatonin
5. Carnosine ⟶ Anserine
6. Nicotinamide ⟶ Methyl nicotinamide
7. Histidine of myosin ⟶ Methyl histidine of myosin
8. DNA bases ⟶ Methylated DNA bases
9. RNA bases ⟶ Methylated RNA bases
10. Proteins ⟶ Methylated proteins

11. Lysine, arginine residues of histones ⟶ Methylated lysine, arginine residues of histones
12. Pyridine (toxin) ⟶ Methyl pyridine
13. Peptides ⟶ Methylated Chemotactic Peptides (MCP)

2. In plants, S-adenosyl methionine is precursor of ethylene, which is required for plant growth and development. Ripening of fruits is also depends on ethylene.
3. S-adenosyl methionine is the source of propylamine required for polyamine synthesis.
4. **Protein synthesis** Methionine is required for synthesis of proteins. N-formyl methionine is starting amino acid for protein biosynthesis in prokaryotes.
5. Methionine is precursor for cysteine.
6. Methionine is also precursor for glucose.
7. Methionine is a constituent of important peptides like enkaphalin and chemotactic peptide.

Medical Importance

Methionine metabolism is defective in some inherited disease.

1. Hyper methioninemia

It is an inherited disease. It is due to defective S-adenosyl methionine synthase. This leads to accumulation of methionine in blood. Severe clinical abnormalities are not observed in this disease.

2. Homocystinuria and homocystinemia

Are the conditions associated with high levels of homocystine, an oxidized product of homocysteine in blood and urine. These symptoms may be due to

(*a*) **Deficiency of cystathionine synthase.** Symptoms are occular abnormalities like dislocation of lens, thrombosis, mental retardation, osteoporosis etc. Block in the conversion of homocysteine of cystathionine causes accumulation of homocysteine in blood.

(*b*) **Deficiency of methylene FH_4 reductase** which is involved in methionine synthesis from homocysteine. This leads to accumulation of homocysteine in blood.

(*c*) **Deficiency of methyl cobalamin** which is required for the synthesis of methionine from homocysteine.

(*d*) Failure of conversion of vit B_{12} to methyl cobalamin. This also blocks conversion of homocysteine to methionine.

3. Cystathioninuria

It is due to deficiency of cystathioninase. So, the condition is characterized by increased excretion of cystathionine in urine due to raised cystathionine in blood.

Metabolism of valine and isoleucine

They are essential amino acids. They are not synthesized in humans. However, in plants and bacteria valine is synthesized from pyruvate and isoleucine is synthesized from aspartate.

Degradation of valine and isoleucine

Degradation of valine and isoleucine occurs in many tissues like liver, kidney etc. Both these amino acids are converted to propionyl-CoA. Hence they are detailed together. Valine is degraded to two CO_2 molecules and one molecule of propionyl-CoA. Isoleucine produces one acetyl-CoA, one CO_2 and one proinonyl-CoA on breakdown (Fig.12.24).

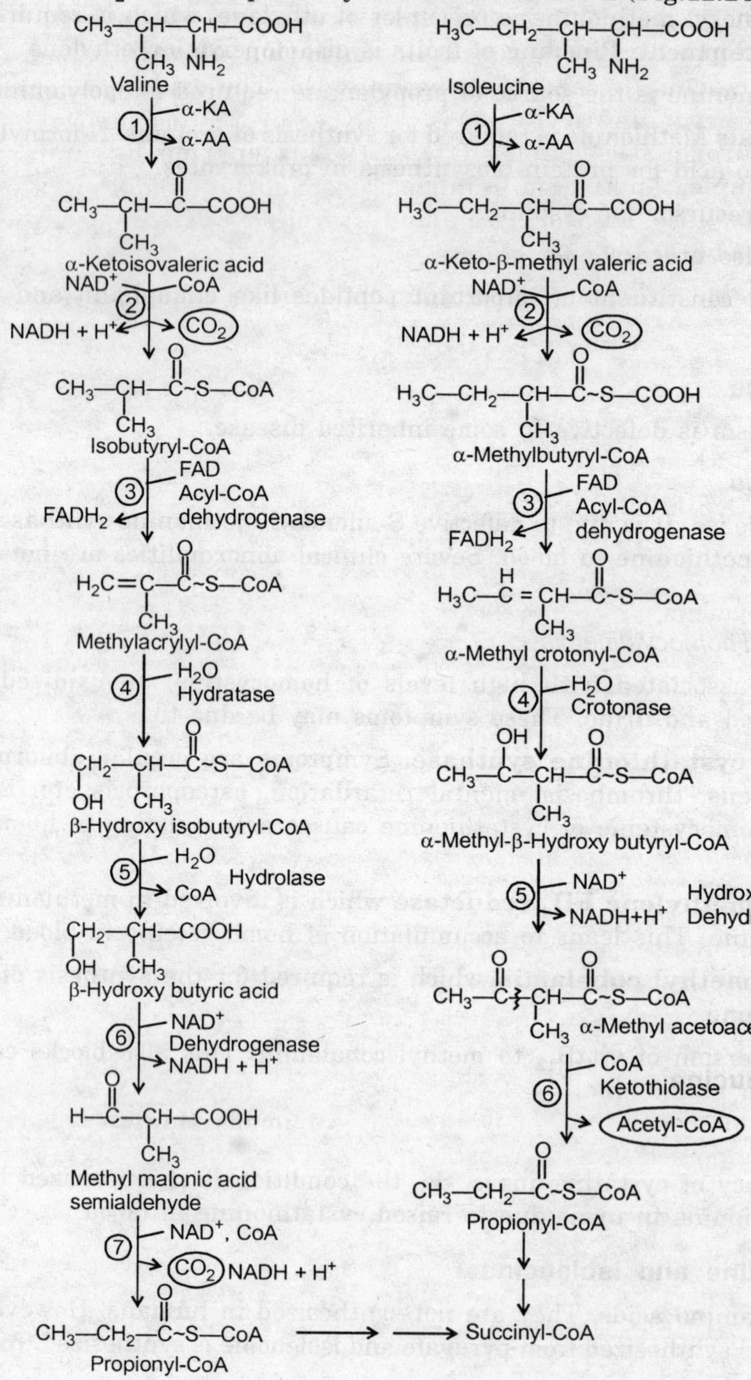

Fig. 12.24 Degradative reactions of valine and isoleucine

Initial transamination followed by oxidative decarboxylation produces isobutyryl-CoA from valine (steps 1,2) and α-methyl butyryl-CoA from isoleucine (steps 1,2) respectively. Further catabolism of these CoAs involves reactions which (may) are analogous to β-oxidation reactions.

In the cytosol of several mammalian tissues a branched chain amino acid transaminase (step1) catalyzes the transamination of valine and isoleucine to corresponding keto acids. It can act on leucine also. The oxidative decarboxylation of α-keto acids to corresponding acyl-CoAs is catalyzed by a mitochondrial branched chain α-keto acid dehydrogenase complex (step 2). This enzyme is similar to pyruvate dehydrogenase complex and bound to inner mitochondrial membrane. Its subunits are α-ketoacid decarboxylase, transacylase and dihydrolipoyl dehydrogenase. This enzyme also act on α-ketoacid of leucine.

Now α-methyl butyryl-CoA of isoleucine undergoes a sequence of dehydrogenation, hydration, dehydrogenation and thiolysis reactions to yield acetyl-CoA and propinoyl-CoA (steps 3 to 6). These reactions are identical to β-oxidation reactions. In contrast isobutyryl-CoA of valine undergoes a sequence of dehydrogenation, hydration, hydrolysis, dehydrogenation and oxidative decarboxylation reactions to yield propionyl-CoA (steps 3 to 7). These reactions are different from β-oxidation reaction.

The conversion of propionyl-CoA to succinyl-CoA is described in Chapter-10.

Biological Importance

1. Valine and isoleucine are required for protein synthesis
2. Valine is precursor of pantothenic acid.
3. Valine and isoleucine are precursors of glucose.
4. Isoleucine is precursor of ketone bodies or fatty acids.

Medical Importance

Valine catabolism is defective in an inherited disease.

Hypervalinemia

It is a rare disease. It is characterized by raised plasma and urine valine level. It is due to impaired valine catabolism. Defective transamination is suspected. Symptoms include vomiting and mental retardation.

Metabolism of leucine

It is an essential amino acid. It is not synthesized by humans. However, plants and bacteria synthesizes this amino acid from pyruvate.

Degradation of leucine

Tissues like liver, kidney and heart convert leucine into acetoacetyl-CoA and acetyl-CoA. Since aceto acetyl-CoA can be converted to acetyl-CoA end product of leucine breakdown is acetyl-CoA. Hence, it is the only ketogenic amino acid in the body (Fig. 12.25).

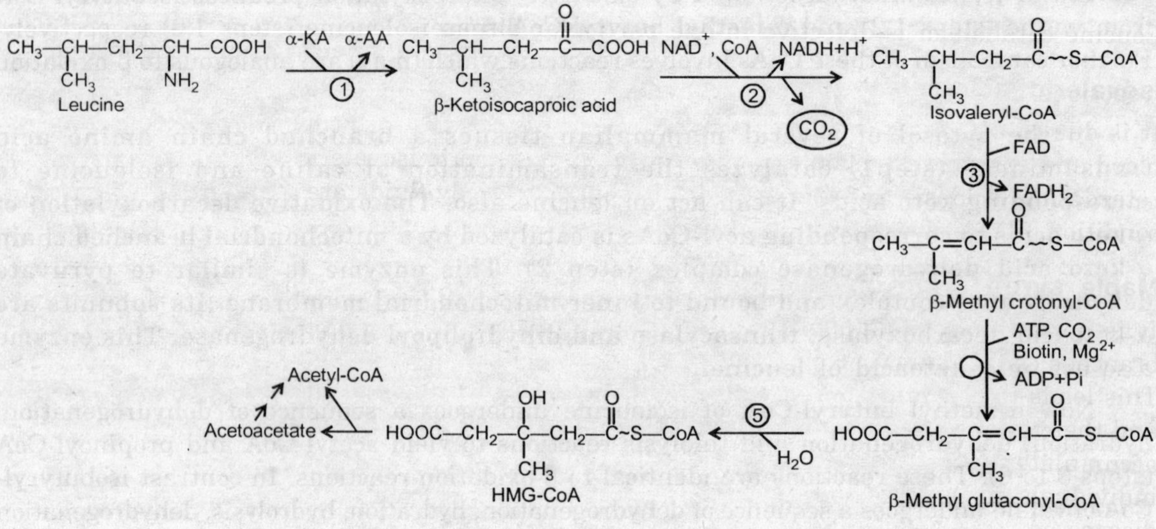

Fig. 12.25 Leucine degradation reaction sequence

Reaction sequence

1. Like valine and isoleucine, leucine first undergoes transamination to corresponding keto acid. The reaction is catalyzed by branched chain amino acid transaminase. This takes place in the cytosol and product is α-keto isocaproic acid.
2. Subsequent oxidative decarboxylation of α-ketoisocaproic acid by mitochondrial branched chain α-keto acid dehydrogenase complex yields isovaleryl-CoA. The enzyme also acts on α-keto acid derivatives of valine and isoleucine also as mentioned.
3. In the next step isovaleryl-CoA undergoes dehydrogenation catalyzed by isovaleryl-CoA dehydrogenase. The reaction is similar to FAD dependent acyl-CoA dehydrogenase reaction of β-oxidation. β-methyl crotonyl-CoA is the product of this reaction.
4. Biotin dependent carboxylation of methyl crotonyl-CoA occurs in this reaction which is rare in degradative pathways. The reaction is catalyzed by methyl crotonyl CoA carboxylase, ATP and Mg^{2+} are required and β-methyl glutaconyl-CoA is the product.
5. Formation of HMG-CoA from β-methyl glutaconyl-CoA by enzyme hydratase is the final reaction of the pathway specific to leucine catabolism.

HMG-CoA lyase an enzyme of ketogenesis present in liver, kidney and heart mitochondria cleaves HMG-CoA to aceto acetate and acetyl-CoA as detailed in chapter-10. The conversion of acetoacetate to acetyl-CoA is also explained in chapter-10.

Biological Importance

1. Leucine is required for protein formation.
2. HMG-CoA of leucine is precursor for cholesterol.
3. Acetyl-CoA of leucine is used for fatty acid and ketone body formation.

Medical Importance

Leucine catabolism is defective in one particular disease.

Isovaleric acidemia

It is due to defective isovaleryl-CoA dehydrogenase. Hence, isovaleryl-CoA accumulates in blood and excreted in urine and sweat after conversion to isovaleric acid. Vomiting, mental retardation, acidosis and cheesy odor of breath and body fluids are usual symptoms of this condition. Excessive consumption of protein may cause coma.

Maple syrup urine disease

It is a rare and fatal inherited disease associated with defective catabolism of all three branched chain aminoacids. It is due to deficiency of branched chain α-keto acid dehydrogenase. This leads to accumulation of valine, leucine and isoleucine and their α-keto acids in blood and their excretion in urine. Hydroxy acids, which are reduced products of α-keto acids also accumulates in blood and are excreted in urine. Due to α-hydroxy acids urine of affected individuals gives characteristic maple syrup or burnt sugar smell and hence the name of the disease as maple syrup urine disease.

Affected infants appear normal at birth but disease may appear during second week and death may occur within weeks if not treated. Main symptoms are mental problems and vomiting.

Intermittent branched chain ketonuria

It is a variant of maple syrup urine disease. Branched chain α-keto acid dehydrogenase is only partially active in affected individuals. However, these individuals utilizes all three branched amino acids reach adulthood and excrete methabolites in urine occasionally.

Metabolism of phenyl alanine and Tyrosine

Phenyl alanine is an essential amino acid. Since tyrosine is a hydroxylated phenyl alanine it is non essential amino acid. In plants and bacteria, phenyl alanine and tyrosine are synthesized from erythrose-4-phosphate and phosphoenolpyruvate.

Degradation of phenyl alanine and tyrosine

Phenyl alanine and tyrosine are degraded to fumarate and aceto acetate. Since degradation of phenylalanine involves first its conversion to tyrosine, a single pathway is responsible for the degradation of both phenylalanine and tyrosine (Fig. 12.26).

Reaction sequence

1. **Conversion of phenylalanine to tyrosine or tyrosine synthesis** First reaction of phenylalanine catabolism is its hydroxylation to tyrosine, which requires a cofactor which is not encountered earlier. A tetra hydrobiopterin (THB) requiring phenylalanine hydroxylase catalyzes this hydroxylation. The enzyme is present in liver and it is a monooxygenase. THB serve as immediate hydrogen source and is converted to dihydrobioprotein (DHB). An NADPH dependent dihydrobiopterin (DHB) reductase converts DHB to THB using NADPH as hydrogen source. Since tyrosine is synthesized from phenylalanine if diet contains tyrosine it can spare phenyl alanine requirement. However, tyrosine can not replace (reduce) phenylalanine requirement for protein synthesis.

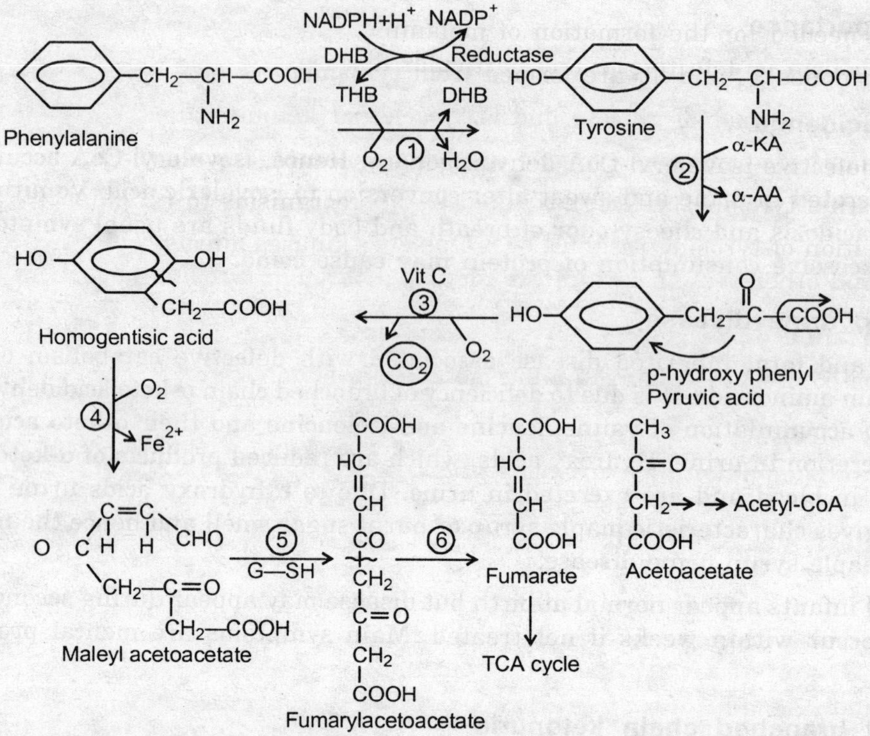

Fig. 12.26 Reaction sequence of phenylalanine and tyrosine degradation ~~~~ indicates cleavage.

2. Now catabolism of tyrosine begins with transamination. p-hydroxy phenyl pyruvic acid is produced from tyrosine by the action of tyrosine transaminase in this reaction. It is an inducible enzyme in liver. Tyrosine and gluco corticoids induces this enzyme.
3. p-hydroxy phenyl pyruvate hydroxylase a copper containing dioxygenase converts p-hydroxy phenyl pyruvic acid to homogentisic acid in a complex reaction involving hydroxylation of benzene ring, decarboxylation and shifting of side chain. Vit c presence also required for this reaction.
4. In this reaction, benzene ring of homogentisic acid is cleaved by another dioxygenase called as homogentisic acid oxidase to form maleyl aceto acetate. The enzyme is nonheme iron (NHI) containing metalloprotein.
5. A glutathione dependent maleyl aceto acetate *cis-trans* isomerase isomerizes maleyl aceto acetate to fumaryl aceto acetate.
6. Finally fumarate and aceto acetate are formed from fumaryl aceto acetate by the action of an hydrolase.

Thus, four atoms of phenylalanine are released as fumarate, one carbon is released as CO_2 and remaining four atoms are released as aceto acetate. Fumarate may undergo further catabolism in TCA cycle. The conversion of aceto acetate to acetyl-CoA is detailed in chapter-10.

Biological importance

1. Tyrosine is required for the synthesis of adrenal hormones like epinephrine, norepinephrine and dopamine.

2. Tyrosine is needed for the formation of melanin.
3. Thyroid hormones T_3 and T_4 are formed from tyrosine.
4. Tyrosine is a precursor of glucose and fatty acids or ketone bodies.
5. For the formation of proteins tyrosine and phenylalanine are required.
6. In the intestine tyrosine is decarboxylated by microorgnisms to tyramine.
7. Phosphorylation of tyrosine residues of proteins by kinases affects cell growth. Actions of insulin and other growth factors are mediated through tyrosine phosphorylation.

Medical Importance

In several inherited diseases phenylalanine metabolism is defective.

1. Phenyl ketonuria (PKU)

It is due to lack of phenylalanine hydroxylase. So, affected individuals are unable to convert phenylalnine to tyrosine and this leads to accumulation of phenylalanine in blood. Increased blood phenylalanine is a useful index in the diagnosis of this disease. Further phenylalnine is channeled to other pathways. As a result other catabolites of phenylalanine are produced. They are phenyl pyruvate, phenyl lactate and phenyl acetate. Phenyl acetate is further conjugated with glutamine to form phenyl acetyl glutamine. All these catabolites are excreted in urine. Conversion of phenylalanine to other catabolites is shown in Fig. 12.27. Since the affected individuals excrete phenyl ketone (phenyl pyruvate) in the urine the condition is named as phenyl ketonuria.

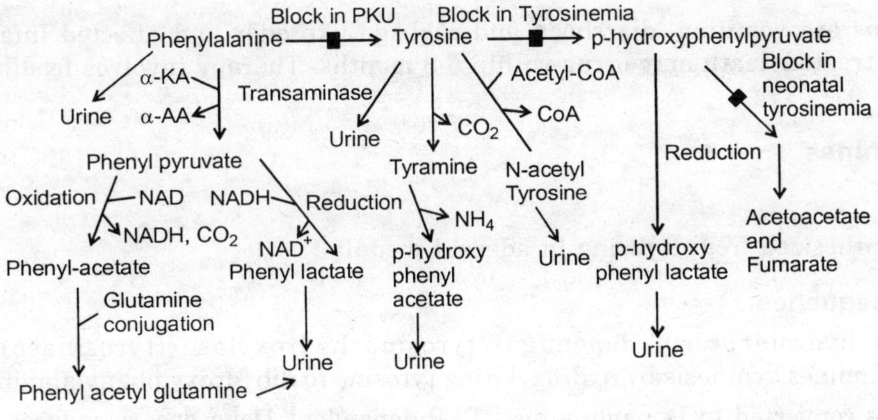

Fig. 12.27 Alternative catabolic pathways of phenylalanine, tyrosine and p-hydroxy phenyl pyruvate in PKU, tyrosinemia and neonatal tyrosinemia respectively

Symptoms are mental retardation and convulsions. Therapy involves feeding protein hydrolysates low in phenyl alanine.

2. Tyrosinemia

It is due to defective tyrosine transaminase. So conversion of tyrosine to p-hydroxyphenyl pyruvate is impaired in the affected people. This leads to accumulation of tyrosine in blood. Through the alternate routes tyrosine is converted to p-hydroxyphenyl acetate and N-acetyl tyrosine (Fig. 12.27) and they are excreted in urine along with tyrosine.

Symptoms are mental retardation, skin and eye lesions. Treatment involves feeding diet low in tyrosine.

3. Neonatal tyrosinemia

It is due to defective p-hydroxyphenyl pyruvate hydroxylase. As a result p-hydroxy phenyl pyruvate is not converted to homogentisate and it accumulates in the blood and excreted in urine either as such or after its conversion to ρ-hydroxy phenyl acetate (Fig. 12.27). Tyrosine accumulation in blood and excretion in urine along with N-acetyl tyrosine is also observed in affected individuals. Treatment involves feeding diet low in protein.

4. Alkaptonuria

It is due to absence of homogentisic acid oxidase. Deficiency of this enzyme leads to accumulations of homogentisic acid in blood and it is excreted in urine. Further the urine turns dark on standing in air. This is characteristic feature of this condition. When exposed to air homogentisic acid present in urine is oxidized to quinone by atmospheric O_2. This undergoes polymerization to produce black pigment which is responsible for the dark color that develops on standing.

Symptoms in the later stage are pigmentation of connective tissue which is known as ochronosis and arthritis.

5. Tyrosinosis

It is characterized by elevated plasma tyrosine level. Other catabolites of tyrosine are also present in excess in plasma. It may be due to defective maleyl aceto acetate isomerase or fumarylaceto acetate hydrolase.

Symptoms are vomiting, diarrhoea and cabbage like odor and affected infants fail to grow. If not treated death may occur within 6-8 months. Therapy involves feeding tyrosine low diet.

Catecholamines

Synthesis

They are synthesized from tyrosine in adernal medulla.

Reaction sequence

1. A tetra hydrobiopterin dependent tyrosine hydroxylase (tyrosinase) initiates catecholamines synthesis by hydroxylating tyrosine to dihydroxy phenylalanine (DOPA).
2. DOPA is converted to Dopamine by a PLP dependent Dopa decarboxylase.
3. A copper containing hydroxylase hydroxylates side chain β-carbon of dopamine in presence of vitc to produce nor epinephrine (noradenaline).
4. Methylation of nor epinephrine by N-methyl transferase using SAM as methyl donor produces epinephrine (adrenaline). Reactions are shown in Fig. 12.28.

Biological Importance

Epinephrine and nor epinephrine are adrenal medullary hormones. They are involved in several biological processes. They mediate their action through 4 types of adrenergic receptors. They are α_1, α_2, β_1 and β_2 receptors. Epinephrine actions are mostly mediated through α-receptors whereas nor epinephrine actions are mediated through β-receptors.

1. They rises blood pressure by acting on heart and blood vessels.
2. They cause relaxation of smooth muscle of soft tissues.
3. Epinephrine increases glycogenolysis and lipolysis as described in chapters-9 and 10.
4. Nor epinephrine is involved in sympathetic nerve impulse transmission. It is a inhibitory neurotransmitter.
5. Dopamine is a neurotransmitter present in substantia nigra of brain. It is a inhibitory neurotransmitter.

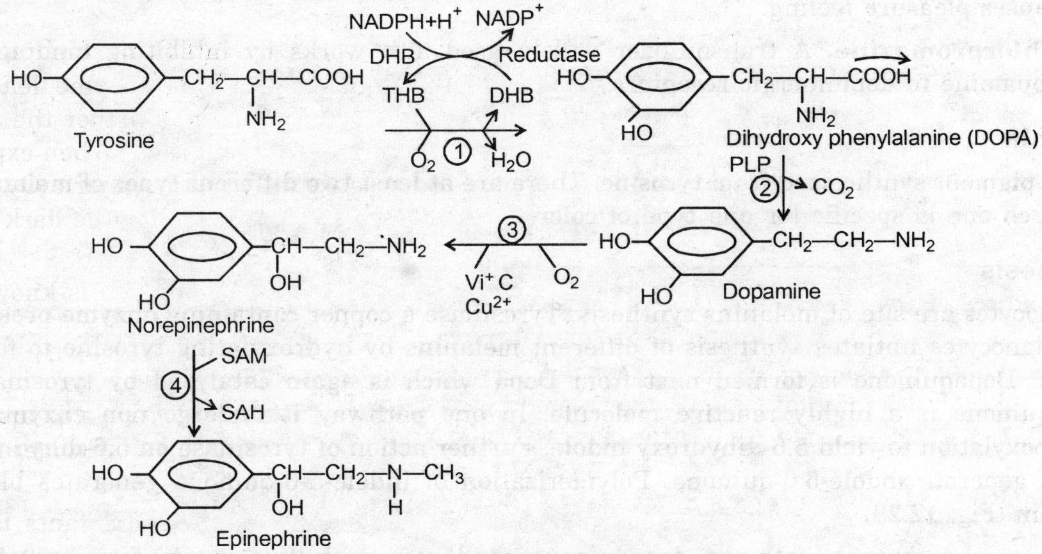

Fig. 12.28 Catecholamine biosynthesis

Medical Importance

Catecholamine metabolism is defective in several diseases. Some antihypertensive drugs and psychoactive substances work by interfering with catecholamine metabolism.

1. **Pheochromo cytomas.** Tumors of adrenal medulla are called as pheochromocytomas. Over production of catecholamines occurs in such tumors of adrenal medulla. Affected individuals suffers intermittent hypertension and this may progress into permanent hypertension. Further urine of these patients contain more of catecholamines and catabolic products of catacholamines like vanilmandelic acid (VMA).
2. **Neuroblastoma.** It is another malignant condition of adrenal medulla associated with increased production of catecholamines. It is seen in children.
3. Methyl dopa and carbidopa are antihypertensive drugs. They work by inhibiting the action of Dopa decarboxylase.
4. Phentolamine hydrochloride and metaprolol are also antihypertensive drugs. They are referred as adrenergic inhibitors. They work by inhibiting binding of catecholamines to adrenergic receptors.
5. **Parkinson's disease.** People over 50 years of age are affected by this disease. It is due to decreased production of dopamine in the brain. Symptoms are tremors, expressionless face and slow voluntary movements.

6. **Schizophrenia.** It is another neurological disease in which disturbances in behaviour, emotions and thinking are found. Negative thinking like social withdrawl is most common in affected individuals. Circumstancial evidence indicates involvement of dopamine in this disease. Dopamine production is more in the brain. This causes excess firing of dopaminergic neurons which may be responsible for some of the symptoms.
7. **Cocaine.** A habitual drug causes pleasure sensation or hallucinations by inhibiting uptake of dopamine at nerve endings. Since dopamine is a inhibitory neurotransmitter when its uptake is blocked nerve impulses pass uninterrupted (continuously) and this causes pleasure feeling.
8. **Chlorpromazine.** A transquilizer widely used also works by inhibiting binding of dopamine to dopminergic receptors.

Melanin

It is a pigment synthesized from tyrosine. There are at least two different types of melanins and each one is specific for one type of color.

Synthesis

Melanocytes are site of melanins synthesis. Tyrosinase a copper containing enzyme present in melanocytes initiates synthesis of different melanins by hydroxylating tyrosine to form DOPA. Dopaquinone is formed next from Dopa which is again catalyzed by tyrosinase. Dopaquinone is a highly reactive molecule. In one pathway it undergo non enzymatic decarboxylation to yield 5,6-dihydroxy indole. Further action of tyrosinase on 5,6-dihydroxy indole generate indole-5,6-quinone. Polymerization of indole-5-6-quinone generates black melanin (Fig. 12.29).

In another branch pathway dopaquinone condenses with cysteine to form cysteinyl dopaquinone. After few steps red melanin is synthesized (Fig. 12.29).

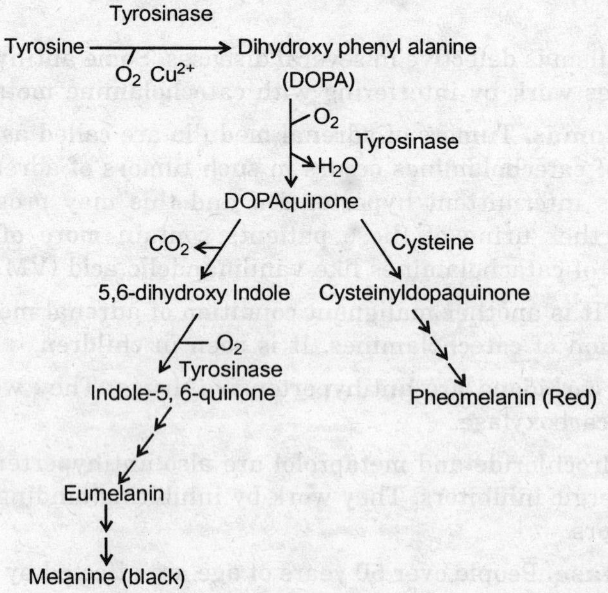

Fig. 12.29 Schematic diagram showing synthesis of black and red melanins from tyrosine

Biological Importance

1. Melanins are found in skin, hair, eye, brain, retina etc. Melanins are tightly bound to proteins. They are responsible for the characteristic color of these tissues.
2. Usually skin color of an individual depends on relative amounts of black and red melanins. This is inturn depends on concentration of melanocytes as well as activities of different pathways. This is the reason for the existence of infinite variations in skin colors.

Medical Importance

Melanin synthesis is defective in an inherited disease.

Albinism

It is due to defective tyrosinase. Affected individuals are referred as albinos. Due to lack of tyrosinase melanin formation is impaired. So pigmentation of tissues is defective. Albinos are susceptible to sun burns and skin cancer on exposure to sun light.

Thyroid Hormones

Thyroid gland synthesizes thyroid hormones from tyrosine and iodine. Thyroglobulin a glycoprotein present in thyroid cells provides tyrosine residues required for hormone synthesis.

Reaction sequence

1. Synthesis of thyroid hormones is initiated by membrane bound heme containing iodide peroxidase. It iodinates tyrosyl residues of thyroglobulin (TG) in presence of H_2O_2 to form monoiodo tyrosine (MIT) and diiodotyrosine (DIT).
2. Condensation of MIT and DIT produces tri-iodotyronine (T_3) and thyroxine (tetraiodotyronine-T_4) which are still bound to thyroglobulin.
3. Proteolysis generates free T_3 and T_4 from thyroglobulin (Fig. 12.30).

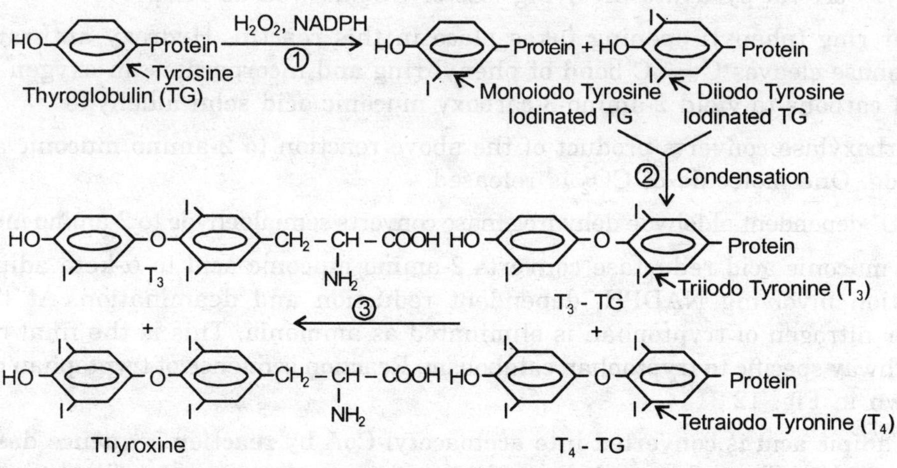

Fig. 12.30 Biosynthesis of thyroid hormones

Biological Importance

1. Thyroxine is a calorigenic agent. It is involved in BMR regulation.

2. Influence of thyroxine on blood sugar level is detailed in chapter-9.
3. Thyroxine is a anabolic hormone. It increases protein synthesis and DNA synthesis.

Tryptophan Metabolism

It is an essential aminoacid. In plants and bacteria, it is synthesized from erythrose-4-phosphate and phosphoenolpyruvate.

Degradation of Tryptophan

Tryptophan is catabolized in liver. A single pathway is responsible for the degradation of tryptophan to small molecules (97%) and synthesis of niacin (3%). One molecule of tryptophan is converted into 2 molecules of NH_3, one molecule of acetoacetyl-CoA, one molecule of acetyl-CoA, 4 molecules of CO_2 and one molecule of formate. Synthesis of niacin we shall learn later.

Reaction sequence

1. Opening of indole ring of tryptophan by tryptophan dioxygenase a heme containing enzyme is the first reaction of tryptophan breakdown. This enzyme cleaves C = C bond of indole ring and incorporates a single oxygen into each of carbons to yeild N-formyl kynurenine. It is an inducible enzyme. Glucocorticoids and tryptophan are its inducers.
2. In the next reaction, formyl group of N-formyl kynurenine is removed as formate by hydrolysis. Enzyme formylase catalyzes this reaction. Formate enters one carbon pool and kynurenine is the product of this reaction.
3. Kynurenine is converted to 3-hydroxy kynurenine by hydroxylation in this reaction. Kynurenine-3-monooxygenase catalyzes this reaction in presence of NADPH and O_2.
4. In the subsequent reaction, 3-hydroxy kynurenine is hydrolysed to 3-hydroxy anthranilic acid and alanine by a pyridoxal phosphate dependent kynureninase. Alanine is converted to acetyl-CoA via pyruvate involving loss of CO_2 as well as NH_4.
5. Another ring (phenyl) opening takes place in this reactin. Hydroxy anthranilate-3,4-dioxygenase cleaves C = C bond of phenyl ring and incorporates an oxygen atom into each of carbons to yield 2-amino-3-carboxy muconic acid semi aldehyde.
6. A decarboxylase converts product of the above reaction to 2-amino muconic acid semi-aldehyde. One molecule of CO_2 is released.
7. An NAD^+ dependent aldehyde dehydrogenase converts semialdehyde to 2-amino muconic cid.
8. Amino muconic acid reductase converts 2-amino muconic acid to α-keto adipic acid in a reaction involving NADPH, dependent reduction and deamination. At this stage, another nitrogen of tryptophan is eliminated as ammonia. This is the final reaction of the pathway specific to tryptophan catabolism. Reaction sequence of tryptophan catabolism is shown in Fig. 12.31.

α-keto adipic acid is converted into acetoacetyl-CoA by reaction sequence described for lysine degradation. Thus, the catabolic pathway of tryptophan merges with lysine catabolic pathway at α-keto adipic acid stage.

Biological Importance

1. Tryptophan is the precursor of niacin.

2. Serotonin is synthesized from tryptophan.
3. Hormone melatonin is formed from tryptophan.

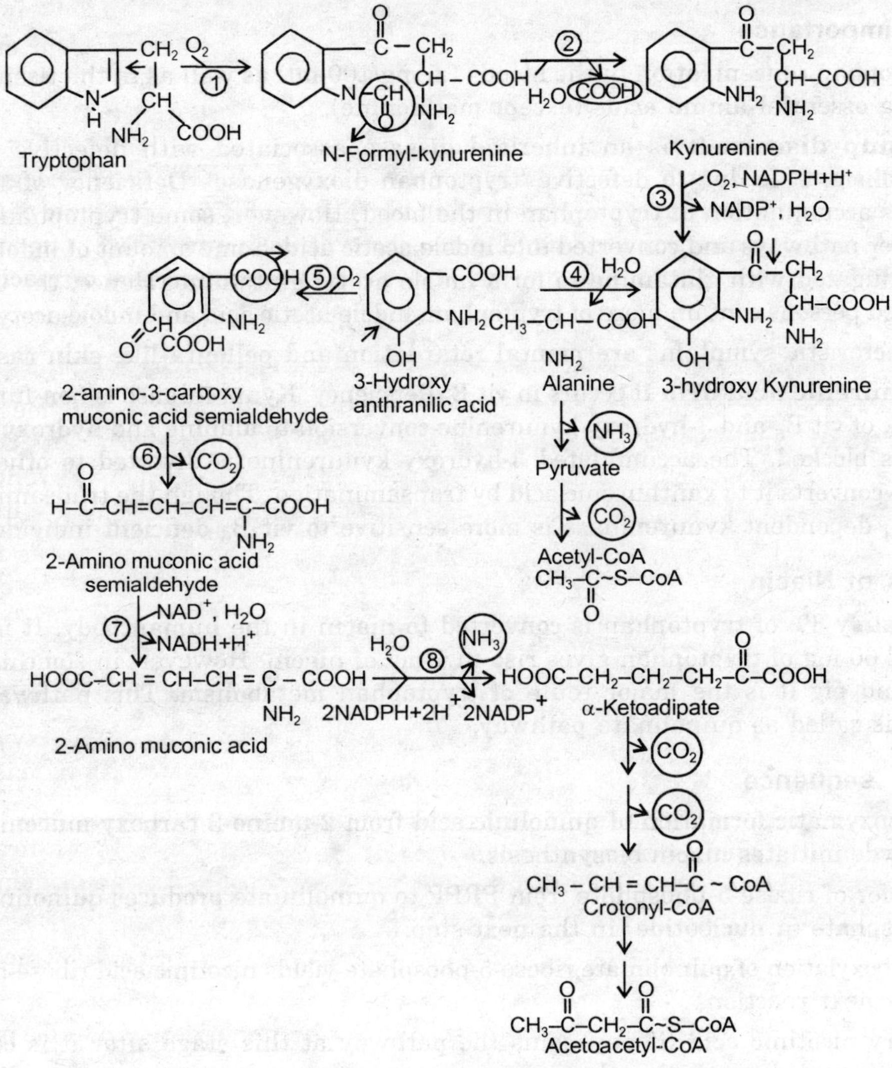

Fig. 12.31 Reaction sequence of tryptophan degradation

4. Non-essential amino acid alanine is synthesized from tryptophan.
5. Tryptophan is a source of one carbon group (formate).
6. In the large intestine, indole and skatole are produced from tryptophan by the action of intestinal flora. The characteristic foul smell of feces is due to these compounds.
7. In plants, hormone indoleacetic acid is synthesized from tryptophan.
8. Tryptophan is a precursor of glucose (alanine) and fat or ketone bodies (acetyl-CoA and aceto acetyl-CoA).

9. Tryptophan is present at low concentrations in cereals and legumes, which are commonly consumed.
10. Tryptophan is required for synthesis of proteins.

Medical importance

1. Tryptophan concentration in the blood (1.5 mg/100 ml) as well as in the tissues is lowest among essential amino acids (except methionine).
2. **Hartnup disease** It is an inherited disease associated with defective tryptophan catabolism. It is due to defective 'tryptophan dioxygenase'. Deficiency of this enzyme causes accumulation of tryptophan in the blood. However, some tryptophan is diverted to other pathways and converted into indole acetic acid. Some amount of indoleacetic acid is conjugated with glutamine to form indole acetyl glutamine. Hence, the urine of the affected persons contain more of tryptophan, indole acetic acid and indole acetylglutamine.

   Characteristic symptoms are mental retardation and pellagra like skin rash.
3. **Xanthurenic acid uria** It occurs in vit B_6 deficiency. Kynureninase is non-functional due to lack of vit B_6 and 3-hydroxy kynurenine conversion to alanine and hydroxy anthranilic acid is blocked. The accumulated 3-hydroxy kynurenine is diverted to other pathway, which converts it to xanthurenic acid by transamination. Though the transaminase is also vit B_6, dependent kynureninase is more sensitive to vit B_6 deficient individuals.

Synthesis of Niacin

Approximately 3% of tryptophan is converted to niacin in the human body. It is estimated that about 60 mg of tryptophan gives rise to 1 mg of niacin. However, in some animals like rat, dog and pig it is the major route of tryptophan metabolism. This pathway of niacin synthesis is called as quinolinate pathway.

Reaction sequence

1. Non-enzymatic formation of quinolinic acid from 2-amino-3-carboxy muconic acid semi aldehyde initiates niacin biosynthesis.
2. Transfer of ribose-5-phosphate from PRPP to quinoliniate produces quinoliniate ribose-5-phosphate (a nucleotide) in the next step.
3. Decarboxylation of quinoliniate ribose-5-phosphate yields nicotinic acid ribose-5-phosphate in the next reaction.

   Dietary nicotinic acid (if any) joins the pathway at this stage after it is converted to nicotinic acid ribose-5-phosphate.
4. Transfer of nucleotide moiety from ATP generates desamido-NAD.
5. Finally transfer of amide nitrogen from glutamine in a ATP-dependent reaction yields NAD (Fig. 12.32).

Medical and biological importance

It is discussed under water soluble vitamins. See chapter-23.

Synthesis of serotonin

Serotonin is synthesized from tryptophan in central nervous system, platelets and mast cells etc.

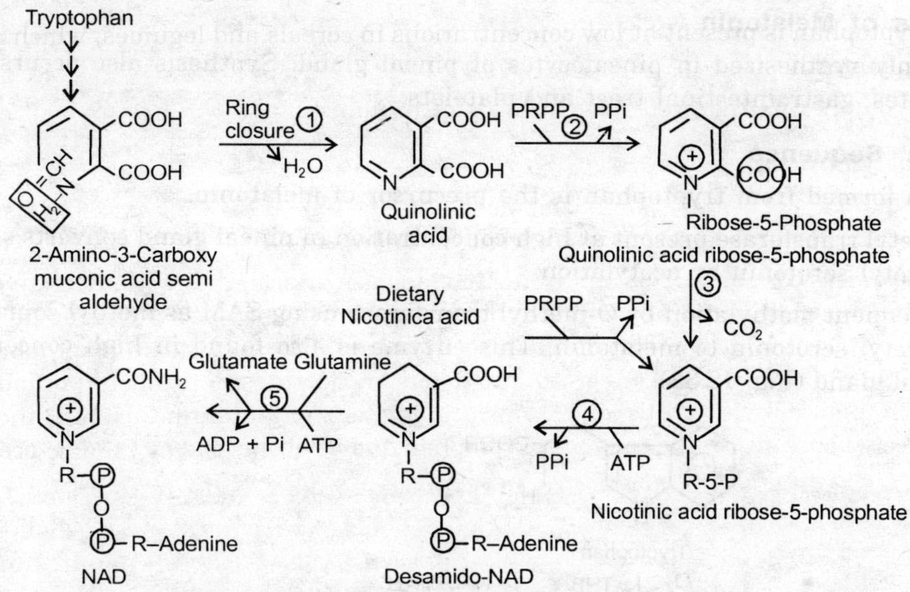

Fig. 12.32 Synthesis of NAD from tryptophan

Reaction sequence

1. A tryptophan hydroxylase, which is similar to phenylalanine hydroxylase catalyzes hydroxylation of tryptophan. NADPH, tetrahydrobiopterin and O_2 are required for this reaction.
2. A vit B_6-dependent decarboxylase converts hydroxy tryptophan to serotonin or 5-hydroxy tryptamine (5-HT) in the subsequent reaction (Fig. 12.33).

Biological Importance

1. Serotonin is a neurotransmitter in the CNS.
2. It is a vaso constrictor.
3. It regulates blood pressure.
4. It stimulates smooth muscle contraction.
5. It regulates peristalysis of gastrointestinal tract.
6. It is present in the venom of toads and wasps.

Medical Importance

1. Blood serotonin level is not constant throughout the day. It undergoes cyclic variations.
2. **Malignant carcinoid (Argentaffinoma)** The disease is characterized by wide spread serotonin producing tumour cells in argentaffin tissue of abdomen. Normally about one percent of tryptophan is converted into serotonin. But in this diseases about 60% of tryptophan is diverted towards serotonin formation. This also results in decreased formation of niacin from tryptophan. So the symptoms are pellagra like rash, diarrhoea and cutaneous vasomotor episodes (flushing) due to excess serotonin. The urine of these individuals contain more 5- hydroxy indole acetic acid (HIAA).
3. **Lysergicacid diethyl amide (LSD)** It is psychoactive hallucinating habitual drug. It work by mimicking the effects of serotonin in the CNS.

Synthesis of Melatonin

It is mainly synthesized in pinealocytes of pineal gland. Synthesis also occurs in retina, erythrocytes, gastrointestinal tract and platelets.

Reaction Sequence

Serotonin formed from tryptophan is the precursor of melatonin.

1. N-acetyl transferase present at high concentration in pineal gland converts serotonin to N–acetyl serotonin by acetylation.
2. Subsequent methylation by O-methyl transferase using SAM as methyl source converts N–acetyl serotonin to melatonin. This enzyme is also found in high concentration in pineal gland (Fig. 12.33).

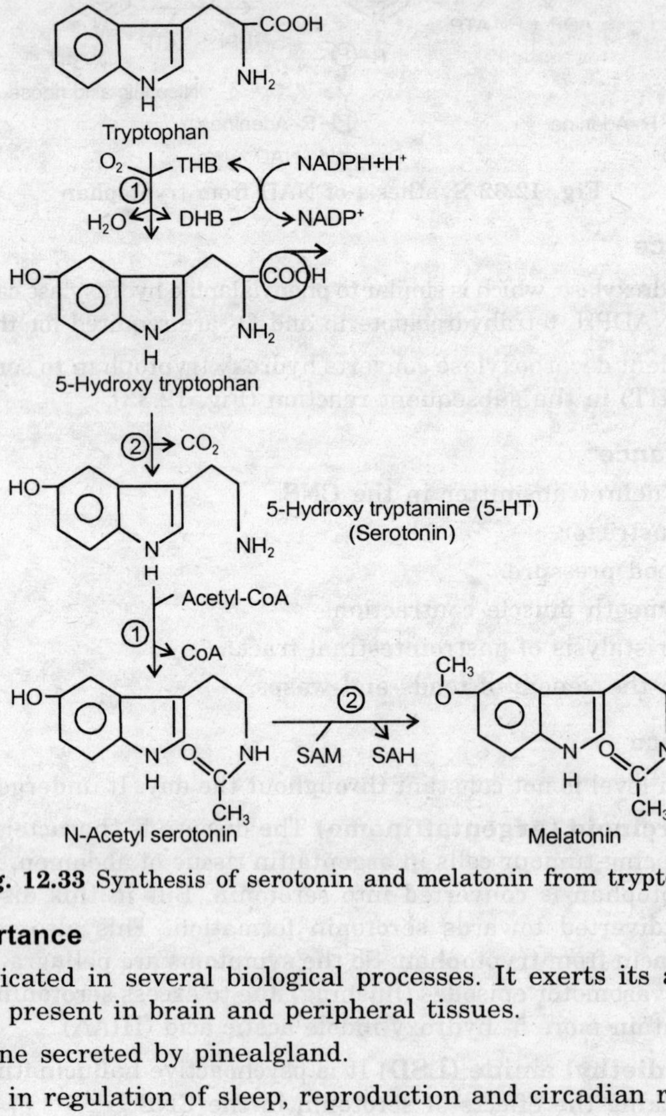

Fig. 12.33 Synthesis of serotonin and melatonin from tryptophan

Biological Importance

Melatonin is implicated in several biological processes. It exerts its action through three types of receptors present in brain and peripheral tissues.

1. It is a hormone secreted by pinealgland.
2. It is involved in regulation of sleep, reproduction and circadian rhythms.

3. It regulates pigmentation of skin.
4. It acts as anti-oxidant and free radical scavenger. The acetyl and methoxy groups are involved in this function.
5. It controls ageing process. It is an anti-ageing agent.

Medical Importance

1. Plasma melatonin level is not constant throughout the day. Usually it is more at night and less during day.
2. Since it is involved in sleep regulation several sleep associated disorders like jet lag, shift work disorder are treated with melatonin.
3. Yoga and meditation induce melatonin secretion. This is the reason for their hypnotic action.
4. Insomnia seen in old people is due to decreased secretion of melatonin.

One carbon metabolism

Several catabolic pathways produce one carbon groups or units. They are used in anabolic pathways. One carbon groups involved in intermediary metabolism are methyl ($-CH_3$), methylene ($-CH_2$-), methenyl (=CH–), formyl (–CHO), formimino (–CHNH), formate (–COOH) and CO_2 or HCO_3^-. Some of these one carbon groups like formyl and formate groups are highly toxic in free form and are deleterious to life. Therefore, in living systems they are attached to certain compounds and they act as carriers of one carbon groups.

Some of the one carbon group carriers identified are tetrahydrofolicacid (FH_4) a reduced form of folic acid, S-adenosylmethionine (SAM), cobalamin and biotin.

1. Folic acid carries $-CH_3$, $-CH_2$, =CH–, –CHNH, –CHO etc.
2. S-adenosyl methionine and cobalamin carries methyl groups.
3. Biotin carries HCO_3^- or CO_2 groups.

One carbon units attachment site

All the above one carbon groups are attached to C, N, S etc. atoms of carriers. Nitrogen 5 and 10 of tetrahydrofolate are involved in the attachment with one carbon units. Further one carbon groups linked to tetrahydrofolate are inter convertible. Sulfur of SAM is the attachment site for methyl groups. Cobalt of cobalamin is the attachment site for methyl groups. For CO_2, N of imidazole of biotin is the site of attachment.

Sources of one carbons linked to FH_4

1. **Serine and glycine** Amino acids serine and glycine are predominant source of one carbons linked to FH_4. As mentioned earlier serine degradation yields N-5, 10 methylene -FH_4 where as glycine breakdown produces N-5, 10 methenyl FH_4.
2. Histidine catabolism yields N-5 formimino FH_4.
3. Tryptophan catabolism yields formate, which is converted to N-10 formyl FH_4 after reacting with FH_4 in a ATP-dependent reaction catalyzed by synthetase (Fig. 12.34). Small amount of formate may arise from glycine breakdown.

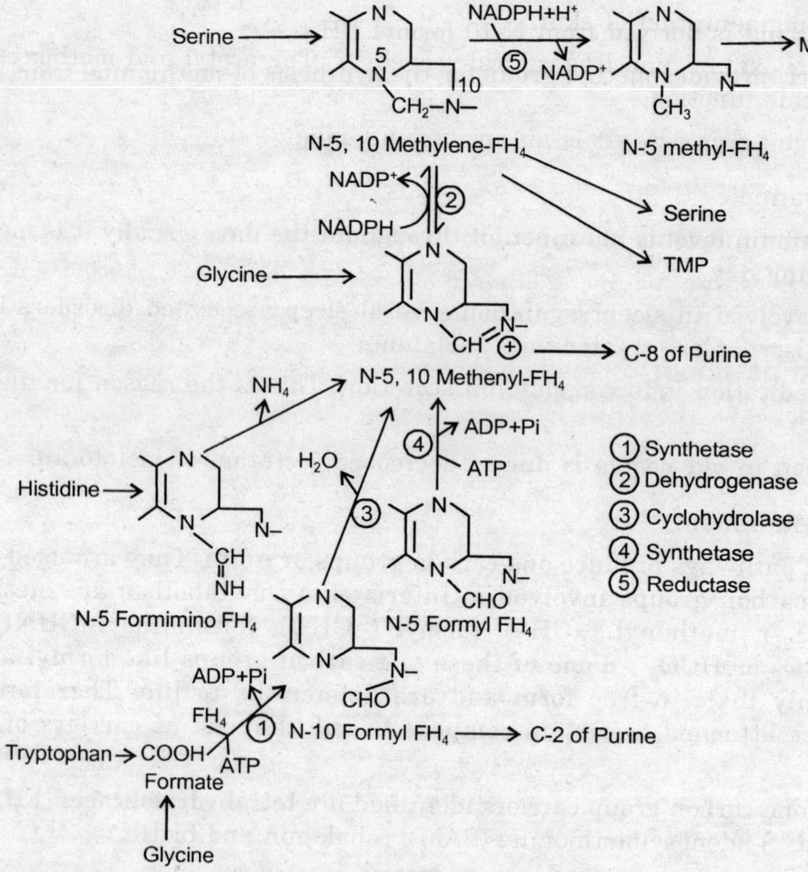

Fig. 12.34 Generation, interconversion and utilization of one carbons linked to FH_4

Inter conversions of one carbons linked to FH_4

One carbons linked to FH_4 undergoes inter conversions.

1. N-5, 10 methylene FH_4 and N-5, 10 methenyl FH_4 are inter convertible. A $NADP^+$ dependent dehydrogenase catalyzes inter conversion.
2. N-10 formyl FH_4 is converted to N-5, 10 methenyl FH_4 by dehydration catalyzed by cyclohydrolase.
3. N-5 formimino FH_4 is converted to N-5, 10 methenyl FH_4 by the loss of NH_3.
4. N-5 formyl FH_4 or folinic acid may be converted to N-5, 10 methenyl FH_4 in a ATP dependent reaction catalysed by synthetase.
5. N-5, 10 methylene FH_4 undergoes conversion to N-5 methyl FH_4 in presence of NADPH catalyzed by reductase.

Utilization of one carbons linked to FH_4

One carbons linked to FH_4 are used in several biosynthetic reactions.

1. N-5, 10 methylene FH_4 one carbon is used in biosynthesis of TMP and serine.
2. N-5, 10 methenyl FH_4 is the source of C-8 of purine ring.

3. C-2 of purine ring is derived from N-10 formyl FH_4.
4. N-5 methyl FH_4 provides methyl group for the synthesis of methionine from homocysterine.

Formation, inter conversion and utilization of one carbons linked to folic acid are shown in Fig. 12.34.

S–adenosyl methionine role in one carbon metabolism

Formation of S-adenosyl methionine and methylation reactions in which SAM acts as methyl donor and importance of methylation in biological processes are detailed earlier.

Methyl cobalamin as donor of methyl group

Mainly it is responsible for the synthesis of methionine from homocysteine. It is the immediate methyl source for methionine synthesis. Cobalamin acquires methyl group from N-5 methyl FH_4.

Role of Biotin in one carbon metabolism

Biotin is prosthetic group of several carboxylases. Carboxylation of substrate by carboxylase involves initial ATP dependent fixation CO_2 to biotin to form N-carboxy biotin. Later CO_2 is transferred to acceptor substrate from N-carboxy biotin to form product. Acetyl -CoA carboxylase, pyruvate carboxylase and propionyl –CoA carboxylase catalyzed reactions involves formation of N-carboxy biotin (Fig. 12.35).

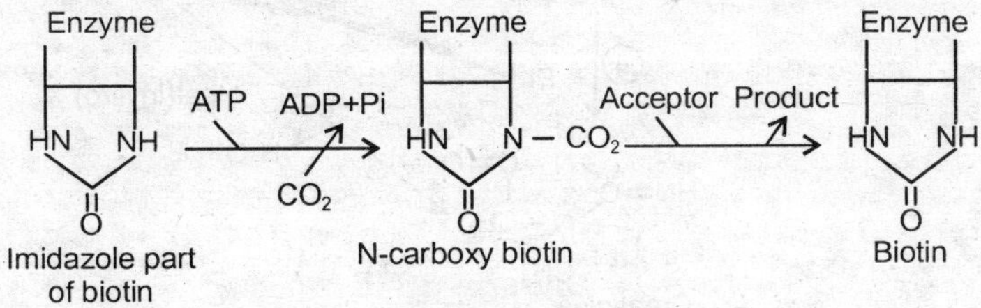

Fig. 12.35 Biotin as carrier of one carbon unit (CO_2)

Creatine metabolism

It is mainly synthesized in tissues other than skeletal muscle like liver, kidney and pancreas. Creatine synthesized in these organs diffuses into blood from which it is rapidly taken up by skeletal muscle. Creatine is present in cardiac muscle and brain also.

Synthesis of creatine

Three amino acids are involved in creatine synthesis. They are arginine, glycine and methionine.

1. The first reaction is the transfer of guanidino group of arginine to glycine to form guanidoacetate (glycocyamine). The reaction is catalyzed by 'trans amidinase present in kidneys.
2. Methylation of guanidoacetate by methyl transferase using SAM as methyl donor yields creatine. This reaction occurs in liver. The rate of creatine synthesis in liver is controlled by feed back mechanism. Blood creatine level controls trans amidinase activity.

Formation of Phosphocreatine

3. In the skeletal muscle creatine is converted to phosphocreatine by creatine phosphokinase. ATP is the phosphate donor (Fig. 12.36).

Formation of creatinine from phosphocreatine

4. Since creatine phosphate is relatively unstable some amount of creatine phosphate is non enzymatically converted to creatinine (Fig. 12.36).

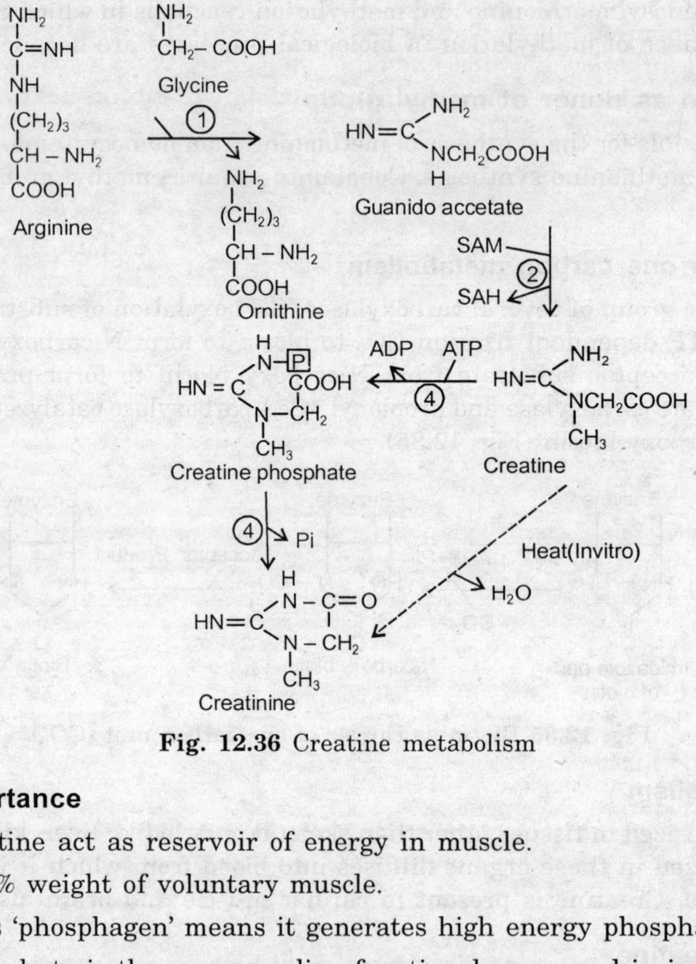

Fig. 12.36 Creatine metabolism

Biological Importance

1. Phospho creatine act as reservoir of energy in muscle.
2. It accounts 1% weight of voluntary muscle.
3. It is called as 'phosphagen' means it generates high energy phosphate bond.
4. Arginine phosphate is the corresponding functional compound in invertebrates.

Medical importance

1. Urine of men contains little of creatine about 50 mg/day.
2. In growing children and in women urine more creatine is found.
3. Pregnant women urine also contain more of creatine.
4. **Creatinuria** Excretion of more of creatine in urine occurs if the muscle mass is reduced as in muscular dystrophy, polymyositis, poliomyelitis, rhematoid arthritis etc. Creatinuria also occurs in catabolic states like starvation, hyper thyroidism, diabetes,

fever and corticosteroid therapy. Myasthenia gravis affected people and athelets undergoing training also excrete creatine in urine.

5. **Urine creatinine** Creatinine formed from phosphocreatine in muscle diffuse from muscle and is excreted in urine as a waste product. About 1-1.5 gm of creatinine is excreted per day. Its excretion depends on muscle mass. Usually more in men and less in women. Creatinine is an hydride of creatine. It can be obtained from creatine in the laboratory by treating with acid at high temperature.
6. **Creatinine clearance** Since creatinine is not reabsorbed by renal tubules and creatinine excretion is not influenced by diet and other endogenous factors clearance studies using creatinine are helpful in assessing kidney function. Creatinine clearance approximately parallels glomerular filtration rate (GFR).

REFERENCES

1. Hilt, W. and Wolf, D.H. Proteosomes destruction as a programme. Trends Biochem. Sci. **21**, 96-101, 1996.
2. Hershko, A. Ubiquitin mediated protein degradation. J. Biol. Chem. **263,** 15237–15240, 1988.
3. Meister, A. Mechanism and regulation of glutamine-dependent carbamoyl phosphate synthetase of *E. Coli.* In Advances in Enzymology and related areas of molecular biology. Vol. 62. Wiley Inter Science, P. 315, 1989.
4. Bru Silow, S.W. Disroders of urea cycle. Hosp. Pract. **10**, 65, 1985.
5. Wellener, D. and Meister, A. A survey of inborn errors of aminoacid metabolism and transport in man. Ann Rev. Biochem. **50**, 911, 1981.
6. Ledley, F.D. Dilella, A.G. and Woo, S.L.C. Molecular biology of phenylalanine hydroxylase and phenyl ketonuria. Trends Genetics, P. 309, Nov. 1985.
7. Lazarus, R.A. Dietrich, R.F. Wallick, D.E. and Benkovic, S.J. On the mechanism of action of phenyl alanine hydroxylase. Biochemistry **20**, 6834-6841, 1981.
8. Pegg, A.E. Polyamine metabolism and its importance in neoplastic growth and as a target for chemotherapy. Cancer Res. **48**, 759-774, 1988.
9. Moncada, S. Feelisch, M., Bune, R. and Higgs, E.A. (Eds.). The biology of NO. Portland Press, London, 1994.
10. Yeaman, S.J. The mammaliam α-Keto acid dehydrogenase. Trends Biochem. Sci. **11**, 293-296, 1986.
11. Humm, A. *et al.* Crystal structure and mechanism of human L-Arginine: Glycine amido transferase a mitochondrial enzyme involved in creatine biosynthesis. The EMBO. J. **16**, 3373-3385, 1997.
12. Kalatzix, V. *et al.* Cystinosin the protein defective in cystinosis is H^+ driven lysosomal cystine transporter. The EMBO.J. **20**, 5940-5949, 2001.
13. Yanofsky, L. Using studies on tryptophan metabolism to answer basic biological questions. J. Biol. Chem. **278**, 10859-10878, 2003.

14. Peter, S. Branched chain amino acids: Biochemistry, Physiophathology and Clinical Science. Raven Press, 1992.
15. Cohen, S.S. A guide to polyamines. Oxford University Press, 1998.
16. Steven Vincent, R. nitric oxide in the nervous system. Academic Press, 1995.
17. Barett, A.J. *et al.* Lysosomal cysteine proteases. Oxford University Press, 1998.
18. LucA.Cynobar. Amino acid metabolism and therapy in health and nutritional diseases. CRC Press, 2003.
19. Zhang, X. *et al.* Tryptophan hydroxylase-2 controls brain serotonin synthesis. Science **305**, 217, 2004.
20. Salvemini, T.R. Billar and Vodovotz, Y. (Eds.). Nitric oxide and inflammation. Birkhauser Verlag, Basal, 2001.
21. Paul, R.S. Baker, *et al.* Red cell membrane and plasma linolenic acid nitration products. Proc. Natl. Acad. Sci. USA **101**, 11577-11582, 2004.
22. Nakai, T. *et al.* structure of p-protein of glycine cleavage system. Implications for non-ketotic hyperglycinemia. The EMBOJ, **24**, 1523-1536, 2005.

EXERCISES

ESSAY QUESTIONS

1. Describe amino acid deamination reactions.
2. Describe urea cycle. Add a note on disorders of urea cycle.
3. Describe metabolism of glycine.
4. Describe metabolism of phenylalanine.
5. Describe metabolism of cysteine. Write fate of its sulfur in the body.
6. Describe metabolic roles of aspartate and glutamate.
7. Describe metabolism of tryptophan. Write its conversion to niacin in the body.
8. Describe lysine metabolism.
9. Give an account of one carbon metabolism in the body.
10. Describe valine and isoleucine metabolism.
11. Describe inherited diseases of amino acid metabolism.
12. How ammonia is formed and disposed in the body ?
13. Describe metabolism of methionine.
14. How SAM is formed and utilized ? Trace SAM degradation route and mention diseases associated with it.
15. Describe creatine metabolism. Add a note on clinical importance of urine creatinine.
16. Write formation of hormones from tyrosine. Mention their functions and associated diseases.
17. How arginine is formed and used in the body ? Write about important compounds derived from arginine.

SHORT QUESTIONS

1. Define protein turnover and protein half life. Name protein break bown signals.

2. Name enzymes of intracellular protein degradation. Write their other important functions.
3. Write normal plasma ammonia level. How it is transported to liver from various organs ?
4. Write glutamine biological importance.
5. How nitric oxide is formed ? Write its biological roles.
6. Write synthesis and biological actions of polyamines.
7. Write formation and functions of histamine.
8. Define transmethylation. Give examples.
9. Write formation and actions of catecholamines.
10. Write formation and biological role of serotonin.
11. Write a note on creatine metabolism.
12. How melatonin is formed? Mention its biological roles.
13. Write about disorders of catecholamine metabolism.
14. How serotonin is formed? Write its functions.
15. Name the biochemical defects in the following.
    (a) Hartnup disease (b) Malignant carcinoid
    (c) Insomnia (d) Schizophrenia
16. How sulfate is formed and utilized? Write disease associated.
17. Write reactions and clinical importance of the following enzymes.
    (a) AST (b) ALT
    (c) Histidase.
18. Explain mechanism of ammonia toxicity.
19. Write briefly about hyperammonemias.
20. How urea cycle is linked to citric acid cycle? Explain.
21. Classify amino acids based on metabolic fate. Give examples.

MULTIPLE CHOICE QUESTIONS

1. Which of the following statement is correct regarding protein degradation.
    (a) Protein degradation is more in well-fed state.
    (b) It is more in starvation.
    (c) It is more in diabetes.
    (d) It is more in starvation and diabetes.
2. All of the following statements are true for amino acids. Except
    (a) They are required for synthesis of hormones.
    (b) They are required for the synthesis of purines.
    (c) They are required for the synthesis of glutathione.
    (d) They are stored when excess.
3. Ubiquitin is a protein required for
    (a) Protein degradation. (b) Amino acid degradation.
    (c) Glycoprotein degradation. (d) Protein synthesis.

4. In plasma
   (*a*) Concentration of glutamine is low.
   (*b*) Concentration of aspartate is high.
   (*c*) Concentration of glutamine is high where as concentration of aspartate is low.
   (*d*) Concentration of glutamine and aspartate is equal.
5. Creatine formation requires
   (*a*) Glycine, Arginine (*b*) Arginine, Methionine
   (*c*) Glycine, arginine and methionine (*d*) Methionine, glycine
6. Schizophrenia is associated with altered
   (*a*) Dopamine metabolism. (*b*) Phenylalanine metabolism.
   (*c*) Tyrosine metabolism. (*d*) Epinephrine metabolism.

FILL IN THE BLANKS

1. Cancer cells require more of ---------------- than any other amino acid.
2. Plasma ammonia level is elevated when function of --------------- is impaired.
3. An example for only ketogenic amino acids is ----------------.
4. ---------------- metabolism is affected by ---------------- used in the treatment of hypertension.
5. Inhibitors of polyamine synthesis are --------------- drugs.
6. Cimetidine used in the treatment of peptic ulcer inhibits acid secretion in stomach by binding to ----------------.

CASES

1. A 4-year-old child was brought to hospital by her parents after noticing blood in urine. Blood urea level was elevated and her urinary oxalate was also higher. Write your diagnosis.
2. A 2-year-old boy was brought to hospital with delayed milestones, hypopigmented skin and eczema. His mother informed that he had seizures in early life. Blood phenylalanine level was elevated and urine gave mousy odor. Write your diagnosis.
3. A mother rushed to pediatric clinic after noticing dark stains on diapers used by baby. Urine of the baby turned dark on standing and gave purple black color on addition of ferric chloride. Write your diagnosis.

13 **CHAPTER**

INTEGRATION OF METABOLISM

MEDICAL AND BIOLOGICAL IMPORTANCE

1. In the body, individual pathways of carbohydrate, lipid and protein metabolism or tissues or organs do not function in isolation. They are interrelated and they interact with each other. They form a community in which one pathway (organ) produce substrate to another pathway (organ). Apart from substrates, hormones and nervous system also act as links between pathways or organs (Fig. 13.1). Since energy is vital for survival of organism as whole these pathways are directed to meet energy requirements under various conditions. The integration of these pathways to generate energy is largely controlled by hormones like insulin, glucagon and catecholamines. They control flow of substrates between pathways mainly by regulating enzyme activity. Changes in the levels of these hormones in plasma allow body to store energy and grow when food is available in plenty or to make stored energy available for utilization when food is not available. These hormones are also responsible for the conversion of body protein to fuel (glucose) when food is in short supply and usually this may be accompanied by weight loss.

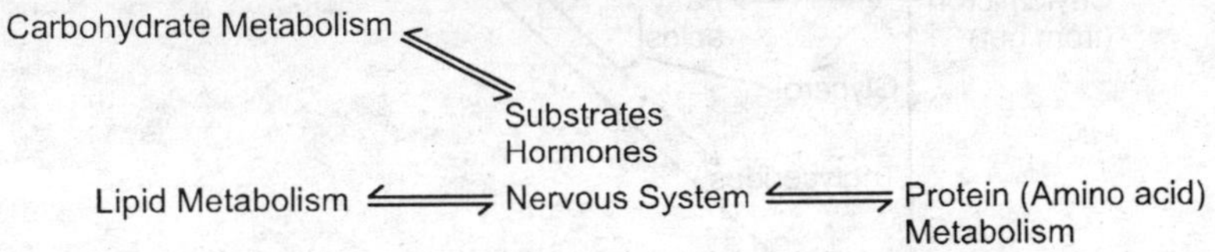

Fig. 13.1 Integration of Metabolism.

2. Integration of carbohydrate, lipid and protein metabolisms can occur in well-fed state, obesity, starvation, diabetes mellitus and in other conditions like stress, injury, surgery etc.
3. Since the pathways of carbohydrate, protein and lipid metabolisms are inter connected, the disorders of one metabolism can affect other metabolism.

INTEGRATION OF CARBOHYDRATE, LIPID AND PROTEIN METABOLISM IN WELL-FED STATE

In the well-fed condition, liver is flooded with monosaccharides, fatty acids, triglycerides and amino acids. Further, in well-fed state-blood-glucose level is more. As result of this, hormone insulin is secreted by pancreas and secretion of glucagon, catecholamines is inhibited. Therefore, in well-fed condition, blood contains more nutrients and insulin. Insulin regulates flow of substrates between various pathways by controlling enzyme activities in liver, adipose tissue and muscle.

Metabolic changes in liver in well fed state

Insulin affects carbohydrate and lipid metabolisms in liver in well-fed state.

Carbohydrate Metabolism

1. Since insulin raises the levels of regulatory enzymes of glycolysis like phospho fructokinase and pyruvate kinase glycolysis is increased. As a result of this, more glucose is converted to acetyl – CoA.
2. Gluconeogenesis is decreased because activities of enzymes of gluconeogenesis like pyruvate carboxylase, fructose-1, 6-bisphosphatase decreases in presence of insulin.
3. Glucose utilization through HMP shunt increases because insulin raises glucose-6-phosphate dehydrogenase and phosphogluconate dehydrogenase levels. This results in more NADPH production.
4. Glycogenesis is more in liver because insulin increases activity of glycogen synthase by decreasing cAMP level (Fig. 13.2).

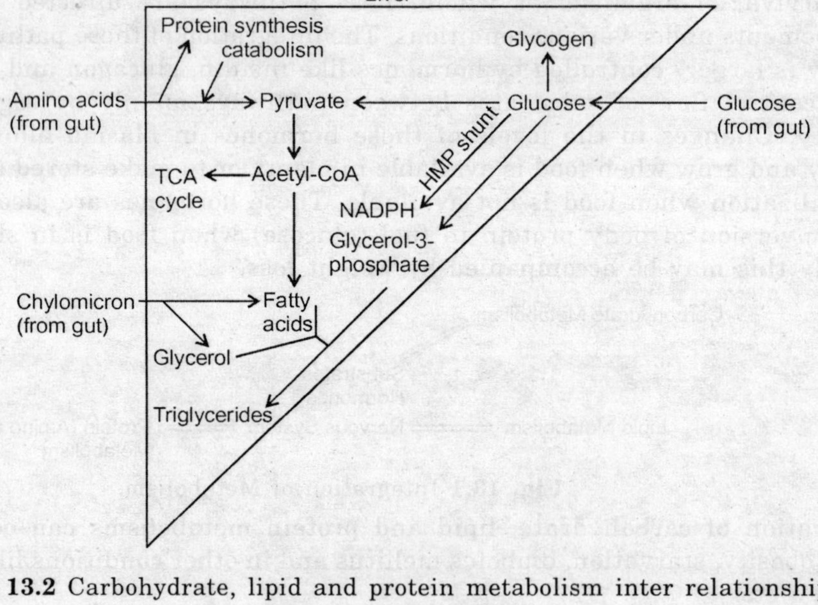

Fig. 13.2 Carbohydrate, lipid and protein metabolism inter relationships in fed state in liver

Lipid Metabolism

1. Fatty acid biosynthesis in liver increases because of availability of substrates like acetyl-CoA and NADPH. In addition, insulin favours fatty acid biosynthesis by keeping acetyl-CoA carboxylase in active form.

2. Triglyceride formation is more because excess glucose is converted to glycerol-3-phosphate through glycolysis. Triglyceride synthesis takes place by using glycerol-3-phosphate and fatty acids produced (Fig. 13.2).

Amino acid Metabolism

1. Since plenty of amino acids are available in fed state, new protein synthesis occurs to replace old proteins and to support growth.
2. Excess amino acids are degraded to acetyl-CoA (pyruvate) or intermediates of TCA cycle because they can not be stored in the body. The acetyl-CoA is used for fatty acid biosynthesis (Fig. 13.2).

Metabolic changes in adipose tissue in well fed state

Carbohydrate metabolism

In well-fed state, insulin enhances glucose uptake by adipose tissue. This glucose is used to generate NADPH through HMP shunt and glycerol-3-phosphate through glycolysis.

Lipid Metabolism

1. More of glycerides are produced by using available NADPH, glycerol-3-phosphate and acetyl-CoA.
2. Triglyceride break down is slowed down because insulin dephosphorylates hormone sensitive lipase by decreasing cAMP levels.

Metabolic changes in skeletal muscle in well-fed state

Since insulin increases uptake of glucose by skeletal muscle glycogen formation is more. Some glucose is also used for energy production. Amino acid uptake increases in skeletal muscle following a meal. New protein is synthesized to replace old proteins by using the amino acids.

OBESITY

As carbohydrate, lipid and protein metabolisms are interrelated in well-fed state, if a person remains in that state for long in such a way that the stored fat is never used for energy production then fat accumulates in the body. The continuous accumulation of fat leads to obesity. So, in obesity there is an increase in adipose tissue fat. It mainly comes from excess of food or calories consumed or over normal intake. It is also called as disorder of lipid metabolism because it is due to excessive fat in adipose tissue. Obesity may also be due to endocrine dysfunction. A person is said to be obsese if the weight is 20% over the mean weight for age and sex.

Obesity is good example of disease of life style. An increased risk of this disease is seen in most adults who have body mass index (BMI) of 25.0 Kg/m^2 or above. Obesity reached epidemic proportions in the USA and threatens to become global epidemic. According to WHO classification 54% of US adults are overweight a BMI > 30 Kg/m^2. Increasing trends of obesity are reported from USA, UK, Europe, Canada, Brazil, India, East Germany, Thailand, Mauritius and Australia.

Intake of excess food leads of flooding of liver with nutrients like glucose, amino acids and lipids. In the liver, the excess glucose is converted to fat. Further the excess amino acids are also converted to fat after converting to acetyl-CoA via pyruvate. This fat together with dietary fat is transported to adipose tissue from liver via VLDL where it accumulates (Fig. 13.3).

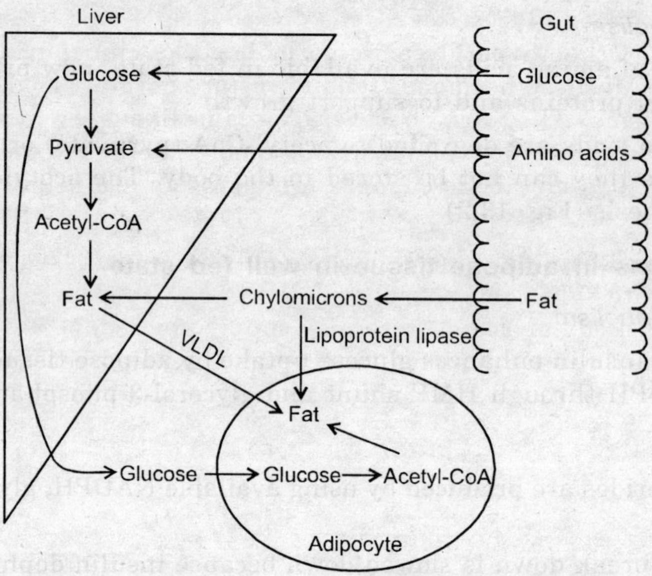

Fig. 13.3 Metabolic interrelationship in obesity

Dangers of obesity

It decreases life span of affected individual. it may lead to several health problems like

(*a*) Cardiovascular diseases
(*b*) Hypertension
(*c*) Adult onset diabetes
(*d*) Psychological problems

Usually, it is a problem of affluent countries, but it affects rich Indians also.

Treatment

Since obesity is the result of imbalance between energy intake and expenditure, the excess weight can be reduced by consuming less food. Increase in physical activity can help in removing excess fat because energy expenditure increases proportionately with increase in activity. Excess fat tissue can be removed surgically. Several beauty clinics are engaged in India in slimming or trimming of obese people.

A puzzling fact about obesity is the failure of these attempts in reducing fat in obsese people. The reason for this is may be more of adipocytes in affected people.

Anti-obesity therapy involving induction of apoptosis in adipose tissue is currently under investigation.

STARVATION

Acute lack of food is called as starvation. Other name to this condition is fasting. It ultimately leads to death. In the third world countries people below poverty line or during famine are exposed to starvation. Politicians, trade union leaders and social activists adopt this to achieve goals.

Metabolic changes in starvation

In starvation, blood glucose level falls due to lack of food. It stimulates pancreas to produce glucagon. Other hyperglycemic hormones like epinephrine and glucocorticoids are also secreted. All these hormones tend to restore normal blood glucose level through different mechanisms. They act on several organs like liver, adipose tissue, skeletal muscle etc. They regulate flow of substrates among metabolic pathways by controlling enzyme activities. The metabolic changes in starvation are usually opposite to changes in well-fed state.

In the liver and skeletal muscle, glycogenolysis is increased because glucagon and epinephrine activates glycogen phosphorylase via cAMP. Hence, the blood glucose level returns to normal. Body glycogen store may supply glucose for few days (1 or two days). Once the glycogen stores are depleted fat moves out from adipose tissue because hormone sensitive lipase is activated by glucagon through cAMP.

At this stage of starvation, except brain rest of the tissues use fatty acids for energy production. Since the brain can not oxidize fatty acids glucose is produced in the liver from glucogenic amino acids, which are derived from tissue protein. Lactate and glycerol are also used for glucose formation. As a result of this, the blood glucose level remains normal and brain uses glucose for energy production. It is estimated that 100 gm of protein can generate 57 gm of glucose. At the same time ketone body formation in liver is increased due to utilization of fatty acid for energy production. To spare body protein a metabolic adjustment occurs in brain at this stage of starvation (2 to 3 weeks of fasting) and brain start using ketone bodies for energy production (Fig. 13.4). After several weeks of fasting or starvation, utilization of muscle protein for glucose production declines because of less demand of glucose by brain. The utilization of fatty acids by peripheral tissues and ketone body utilization by brain continues till the body fat is depleted.

In the final phase of starvation, *i.e.,* when the body fat is exhausted, the energy demand of body must be met entirely from muscle protein. So for the survival of individual muscle protein breakdown occurs at increased rate and the individual becomes physically inactive, which ultimately leads to death.

Biochemical and Clinical symptoms of starvation

1. Hypoglycemia
2. Raised plasma free fatty acid level
3. Increased gluconeogenesis
4. Ketoacidosis
5. Muscle wasting
6. Physical inactivity
7. Coma
8. Ultimately death

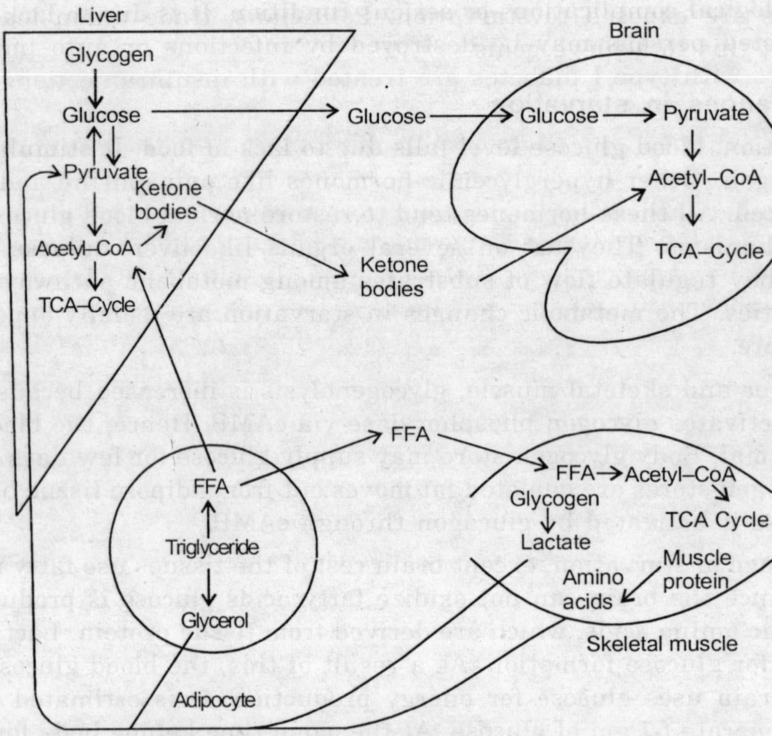

Fig. 13.4 Metabolic interplay among tissues in starvation

DIABETES MELLITUS

Diabetes mellitus is the major health problem affecting people all over the world. It is one of the most extensively investigated human disease. Diabetes mellitus is a Greek word. In Greek diabetes means siphon and mellitus means sweet. Since affected people excrete large quantities of urine with sweet taste the condition is named as diabetes mellitus.

Diabetes Mellitus is defined as condition that occurs due to absence of insulin or presence of factors that oppose insulin resulting in elevated glucose levels in blood and urine.

The incidence of diabetes in general population is about 2 to 3%. It is familial disease hence susceptibility to diabetes depends on genetic composition. Incidence of diabetes also depends on life style and dietary habits or type of food consumed. Diabetes is increasing globally. WHO predicts that in about 25 years the number of diabetics in India increases from current 23 million to about 57 million. As early as 2005, every third diabetic in world will be Indian. There are two types of diabetes.

1. Juvenile (onset) diabetes or insulin-dependent diabetes (IDDM) or Type I diabetes

It occurs early in life. It accounts for about 10-20% of diabetic cases. Affected individuals are usually thin or lean or under nourished. It appears usually in childhood or puberty. The age of affected people is always below 30 years. It is sudden in onset and leads to pathological complications or serious condition. It is due to lack of insulin. The β-cells of affected persons may be destroyed by infections or auto immune diseases. Hence, patients with type I diabetes are treated with insulin injections.

2. Adult (onset) diabetes or non-insulin dependent diabetes (NIDDM) or type II diabetes

It appears late in life usually after 30 years. It accounts for 80-90% of diabetic cases. It occurs gradually and milder condition and pathological complications are less. Affected persons are usually obese. It is a genetic disorder. Insulin production may be normal in the affected persons but number of insulin receptors are less. So, affected individuals are insulin resistant, *i.e.,* insulin injections are not helpful. Treatment of patients with Type II diabetes involves use of oral hypoglycemic sulfonyl urea drugs. Further, weight reduction and dietary modifications are helpful in controlling the disease.

In addition to the two types of diabetes other types of diabetes are recognized by WHO. They are 1. Maturity onset diabetes of young (MODY) 2. Malnutrition related diabetes mellitus (MRDM). 3. Gestational diabetes mellitus (GDM) 4. Impaired glucose tolerance diabetes mellitus (IGTDM). 5. Diabetes mellitus associated with other conditions like pancreatic disease, genetic diseases, drug or chemicals induced.

Maturity onset diabetes of young (MODY)

It is due to the mutations in genes. Five genes are known to cause MODY. Mutations in these genes produce proteins with altered functions. They are

(a) Glucokinase gene mutation

Mutations of glucokinase gene leads to deficiency of this enzyme. Patients affected with this condition have moderate fasting hyperglycemia from birth.

(b) Transcription factor gene mutations

Mutations, in genes of transcription factors like hepatocyte nuclear factor–1α (HNF–1α), HNF – 4α, HNF – 1β and insulin promoter factor – 1 (IPF – 1) lead to MODY. However these patients have normal fasting glucose in childhood but develop hyperglycemia in early adulthood.

Biochemical and clinical symptoms

Acute cases of diabetes are associated with

1. Hyperglycemia
2. Glycosuria and polyuria
3. Increased hunger (polydipsia)
4. Increased thirst (polyphagia)
5. Ketosis is usually present in type I diabetes and rare in type II diabetic cases
6. In uncontrolled cases ketoacidosis
7. Weight loss
8. Delayed wound healing
9. Coma and death may occur if untreated

Chronic effects of diabetes mellitus

In long standing or chronic cases of diabetes in addition to the above symptoms atherosclerosis, coronary artery disease, diabetic neuropathy, diabetic nephropathy and diabetic cataract (retinopathy) develops. Hypertension may also develop in some diabetic cases. Because of involvement of many diseases, diabetes is called as *syndrome*. In diabetic neuropathy, there is general loss of peripheral sensation particularly of lower limbs. The delayed wound healing and loss of sensation in lower limbs are responsible for development of diabetic foot and amputation. Diabetic nephropathy is due to thickening of capillary basement membrane and increased permeability of capillaries. It is responsible for renal failure in diabetic cases. Diabetic cataract is the leading cause of blindness in diabetics. It occurs due to accumulation of sorbitol in lens. Sorbitol is formed from glucose by reduction catalyzed by aldose reductase. Inhibitors of this enzyme may be helpful in preventing development of cataract. How hyperglycemia leads to other diseases in diabetes in unclear.

Metabolic changes in diabetes mellitus

Some of metabolic changes in diabetes are similar to starvation. Main differences between diabetes and starvation are blood glucose and insulin levels. In starvation, blood glucose level remain normal whereas in diabetes it is elevated. The insulin level is normal in starvation and in diabetes insulin action is minimal. Since insulin is antagonist to glucagon, in diabetes glucagon actions are unopposed. Initially glucagon level in the blood raises and returns to normal later.

Carbohydrate metabolism

In diabetes the blood glucose level increases because of decreased utilization of glucose by peripheral tissues. Due to lack of insulin peripheral tissues like adipose tissue and skeletal muscle are unable to take up glucose. So glucose conversion to fat and glycogen is blocked in adipose tissue and skeletal muscle respectively. In addition, glucagon stimulates gluconeogenesis and glycogenolysis in liver which contributes to blood glucose (Fig. 13.5). Therefore, blood glucose level raises (hyperglycemia) and when the blood sugar level exceeds renal threshold value glucose is excreted in urine (glycosuria).

Mechanism of hyperglycemia induced diabetic complications

Earlier, it was mentioned that how hyperglycemia leads to complications in diabetes is unclear. However, research carried out recently provided mechanism by which elevated levels of glucose disturb cellular properties.

1. Persistent hyperglycemia in chronic diabetes induce oxidative stress, which leads to increased generations of reactive oxygen species in mitochondria.
2. This results in variety of harmful oxidative products, which are known to complicate diabetic pathology.
3. Some of the biochemical mechanisms involved in hyperglycemia induced organ damage are A. Activation of proteinkinase – C isoforms. B. Increased glycation end product C. Increased flux of glucose into aldose reductase (sorbitol) pathway. D. Increased hexosamine synthesis.

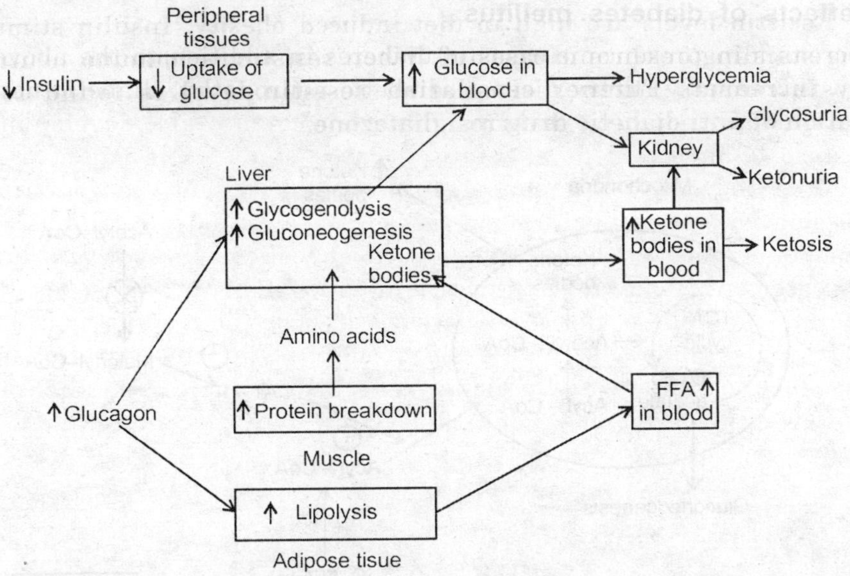

Fig. 13.5 Metabolic interplay in diabetes that leads to biochemical symptoms

Lipid metabolism

Since glucose is not available for utilization most of the tissues except brain use fatty acids for energy production. Glucagon stimulates lipolysis in adipose tissue by activating hormone sensitive lipase via cAMP. As a result of this, plasma free fatty acid level raises and more fatty acids enter liver for utilization. In the liver fatty acid oxidation is increased because more acyl-CoA are transported into mitochondria by CAT-I. Usually in fed state the activity of CAT-I is inhibited by malonyl-CoA. In diabetes malonyl-CoA synthesis is blocked. So CAT-I activity is more and more acyl-CoAs are transported into mitochondria (Fig. 13.6). Therefore, fatty acid oxidation is more in liver in diabetes and starvation. Moreover the excess acetyl-CoA arising from increased fatty acid oxidation is used for ketone body formation instead of its oxidation in TCA cycle in the hepatocyte mitochondria. In starvation and diabetes the TCA cycle in liver is unable to utilize excess acetyl-CoA because oxaloacetate which is an intermediate of TCA cycle is diverted to gluconeogenesis (Fig. 13.6). Non-availability of oxaloacetate limits TCA cycle capacity to oxidize acetyl-CoA. When ketone body formation is increased it leads to ketosis and ultimately ketoacidosis. The mobilization of adipose tissue fat and ketogenesis are far greater in diabetes than in starvation. So, ketoacidosis is more severe in diabetes than in starvation. Triglyceride metabolism is also affected in diabetes. Plasma triglyceride level is more in diabetes and reason for this is unclear.

Molecular link between diabetes and obesity

Earlier I mentioned that obesity leads to type 2 diabetes mellitus. For long time the molecular link between these remained mystery despite strong clinical link. However, recently researchers identified some molecules which are suspected as link between obesity and diabetes.

A unique molecule termed as resistin (resistance to insulin) is involved in mediating insulin resistance in diet induced obesity. The resistin is a protein molecule produced by adipocyte. Resistin levels are high in diet induced obesity. Insulin stimulated glucose uptake decreases in presence of resistin. When resistin is immuno neutralized insulin sensitivity increased. Further circulating resistin level is found to decrease on administration of anti-diabetic drug rosigliatazone.

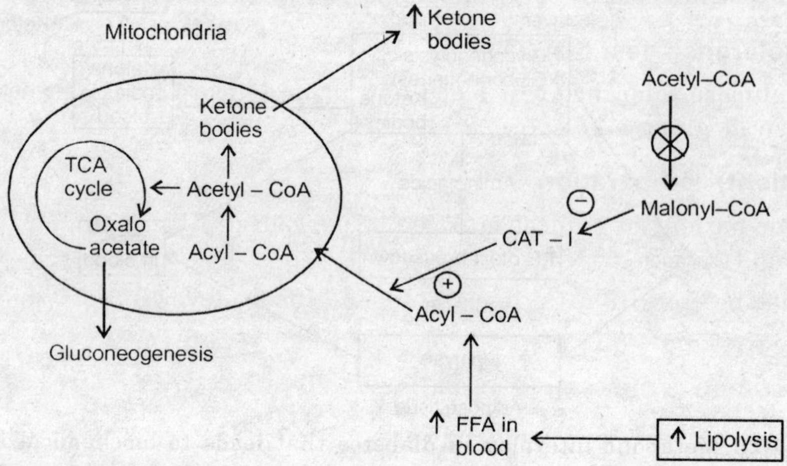

Fig. 13.6 Relationship between fatty acid oxidation and ketone body formation in diabetes

In addition to resistin, other adipocytokines are also involved in development of obesity-related insulin resistance. They are adiponectin, leptin, phasminogen activating inhibitor type–1, TNF–α, Peroxisome proliferator activating receptor–γ, (PPAR–γ) etc. Adiponectin promotes clearance of free fatty acids from plasma and expression of fatty acids transport protein.

Peroxisome proliferator activating receptors (PPARS) are family of nuclear receptors. They are PPAR – α, PPAR – δ and PPAR–γ. They are activated by fatty acids and their derivatives.

PPAR – γ is involved in regulation of adipocyte differentiation and insulin signalling. Mutation in PPAR – γ is found to predispose people to obesity.

Disregulated production of these adipocytokines is associated with development of obesity-related insulin resistance. Adiponectin appears to be a critical link between obesity, diabetes and atherosclerosis.

GLUCOSE TOLERANCE TEST (GTT)

1. It is a test commonly performed in hospitals biochemistry laboratory to know the status of carbohydrate metabolism and extent of its integration with other metabolisms in an individual under normal and disease conditions.
2. The word glucose tolerance refers to body ability to oxidize or metabolize a given test dose of glucose. The response of blood glucose level and urine glucose to the test dose of glucose is the degree of measure of glucose tolerance. If the blood glucose level and urine glucose are maintained within normal range after a test dose of glucose is given then it is known as or considered as normal glucose tolerance or response. Depending on physiological or pathological conditions glucose tolerance increases, impairs and decreases.

3. Depending on route of administration of test dose glucose it is named as (*a*) Oral glucose tolerance test (OGTT) (*b*) Intravenous glucose tolerance test (IVGTT).
4. Since free glucose is not a part of our normal diet glucose tolerance test is considered as artificial test devised by man for diagnostic (prognostic) purposes.

Oral glucose tolerance test (OGTT)

In this type of glucose tolerance test blood and urine glucose levels are evaluated after an oral test dose of glucose.

Individual (patient) preparation

1. Individual or patient or subject must be in post absorptive state, *i.e.*, overnight (12 hour) fasting.
2. Subject must be free from taking any blood glucose level influencing drugs.
3. Subject must take adequate carbohydrate in diet for three days prior to the test.
4. Fasting blood and urine samples of patient (individual) are collected to know fasting blood glucose level and urine glucose.

OGTT procedure

The patient (individual) is given a oral test dose of 75 mg of glucose dissolved in 200 ml water. Alternatively patient may be given 1 gm of glucose per kg body weight dissolved in 200 ml water. Thereafter blood and urine samples are collected at every 30 minutes interval for 2 hours and 30 minutes. The blood samples glucose level is determined. Glucose in urine samples is detected using Benedict's qualitative test. The OGTT curve (graph) is obtained by plotting blood glucose levels against time.

Normal OGTT curve

An individual with normal glucose tolerance generates normal OGTT curve (Fig. 13.7). The individuals fasting blood glucose level remains within 60-90 mg% range (O–Toluidine method). After oral test load of glucose blood glucose level reaches peak in one hour (110–130 mg%) and it does not exceed renal threshold for glucose which is about 180 mg%. Thereafter blood glucose levels falls and reaches normal fasting level at the end of 2 hours. Further more, none of the urine samples collected during test period show glucose as blood glucose level remained within renal threshold value.

Abnormal OGTT curves

They are obtained when an individuals glucose tolerance is decreased, impaired and increased.

(a) Decreased glucose tolerance

It occurs in diabetes mellitus. The fasting blood glucose level is always above (130 mg%) and usually influenced by severity of diabetes mellitus. In mild diabetes, the fasting blood glucose level is less than 150 mg% whereas in severe diabetes it is higher than 180 mg%. Further aft·· test dose of glucose increase in blood glucose level is higher than normal individua. ıd blood glucose level does not return to normal level even after 2 hours which is characteristic of diabetes. Moreover, one of the urine samples show glucose in mild diabetes but all of the urine samples gives positive Benedict's test in the case of severe diabetes. Decreased glucose tolerance occurs in other conditions like (I) Liver disease (II) Hyperthyroidism (III) Hyper Pituitarism (IV) Cushing's syndrome (V) Arseniasis (VI) Pregnancy (VII) Old Age.

(b) Impaired glucose tolerance (IGT)

It is an unusual OGTT curve observed recently in several countries due to changed life styles and urbanization (industrialization). Fasting blood glucose of an individual with impaired glucose tolerance is above 90 mg% but below 130 mg%. Further, the blood glucose level does not return to fasting level even after 2 hours and usually it is higher than 140 mg% but below 200 mg% (Fig. 13.7).

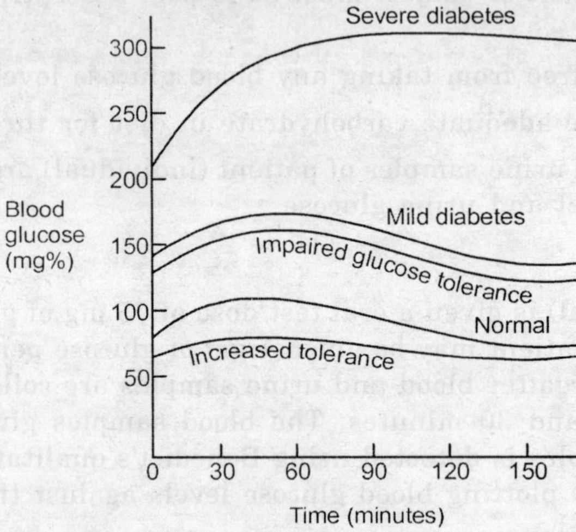

Fig. 13.7 Oral glucose tolerance test

(c) Increased glucose tolerance

A flat OGTT curve is observed when an individual glucose tolerance is increased (Fig. 13.7). It occurs in (*i*) Hypopituitarism (*ii*) Addison's disease (*iii*) Hypothyroidism (*iv*) Intestinal malaborption (*v*) Impaired glucose reabsorption in kidney (renal glycosuria).

Medical importance

1. OGTT is used in diagnosis of diabetes mellitus.
2. OGTT is also useful in differential diagnosis.
3. IGT is considered as risk factor for diabetes and coronary artery disease. As age advances, features of IGT curve may change to diabetic form. Hence individuals with IGT needs careful follow up. IGT is found increasing in young people due to urbanization and sedentary life style. IGT is found to be less prevalent in low economic (income) group.

Intravenous glucose tolerance test (IVGTT)

1. This type of GTT is performed in patients whose gastrointestinal tract is unable to absorb glucose properly.

2. Patient preparation is same as OGTT.
3. After an overnight fasting, a test dose of glucose 0.5 gm/kg body weight prepared as 25% solution with distilled water is given in three minute time. Mid injection time is taken as 0 time. Blood samples are collected at 10 minutes intervals for one hour.
4. In a normal individual, the blood glucose level reaches peak in few minutes after glucose load is given then start decreasing by 20 to 30 minutes and returns to normal by 45 to 60 minutes.
5. In case of decreased glucose tolerance blood glucose level does not return to normal after usual one hour.
6. Further in IVGTT glucose tolerance of a person is expressed as t-half. It is defined as a time in minutes required for peak blood glucose to get reduced to half. A t-half value below 45 indicates normal glucose tolerance. In diabetics t-half value is more than 60.

REFERENCES

1. Gordon, E.S. Metabolic aspects of obesity. Adv. Metab. Disorders **4**, 229, 1970.
2. Herzog, D.B. and Copeland, P.M. Eating disorders. N. Engl. J. Med. **313**, 295, 1985.
3. Brownlee, M. and Cerami, A. Biochemistry of complications of diabetes mellitus. Ann. Rev. Biochem. **50**, 385, 1981.
4. Youg, V.R. and Scrim Shaw, N.S. The physiology of starvation. Sci. Am **225(4)**, 14, 1971.
5. Kerndt, P.R. Fasting. History, pathophysiology and complications. West J. Med. **137**, 379, 1982.
6. Meguid, M.M. Uncomplicated and stressed starvation. Surg. Clin. North America. **66**, 529, 1981.
7. Polonsky, K.S. Dynamics of insulin secretion in obesity and diabetes. Int. J. Obesity, **24**, S29-S31, 2000.
8. Kolonin, M.G. *et al.* Reversal of obesity by targeted ablation of adipose tissue. Nature Medicine. **10**, 625-632, 2004.
9. Sharma, A.M. Adipose tissue. A mediator of cardiovascular risk. Int. J. Obesity, **26**, S5-S7, 2002.
10. Eisenberth, G.S. Polonsky, K.S. and Buse, J.E. Type-I diabetes mellitus. Williams text book of Endocrinology Larsen *et al.* (Eds.) 10th ed. Saunder, 2003.
11. Tseng, C.H. *et al.* Long term arsenic exposure and incidence of non-insulin dependent diabetes mellitus. Environ. Health Perspect. **108**, 847-851, 2000.
12. Nourooz – Zadeh, J. *et al.* Relationship between plasma measure of oxidative stress and metabolic control in non-insulin dependant diabetes mellitus, Diabetologia, **40**, 647-654, 1997.
13. Giuglino, D; Ceriello, A and Paolisso, G. oxidative stress and diabetic complications in diabetics. Diabetic Care **19**, 257-267, 1996.

14. Sinclair, J.A. Free radical mechanisms and vascular complifications of diabetes mellitus. Diabet. Rev. **2**, 7-10, 1993.

15. Brazil, M. Metabolic syndrome outside the site, a lateral approach to phosphotase inhibition. Nat. Rev. Drug. Dis. **3**, 736, 2004.

16. Fukuhara, A. *et al.* Visfatin: A protein secreted by viscreral fat that mimics effect of insulin. Science. **307,** 426-430, 2005.

EXERCISES

ESSAY QUESTIONS

1. Give an account of metabolic changes that occur in liver, adipose tissue and skeletal muscle under well fed conditions.
2. Describe diabetes mellitus.
3. Define obesity and starvation. Write metobolic changes that occur in these conditions. Add a note on dangers of these conditions.

SHORT QUESTIONS

1. Write a note on obesity.
2. Define starvation. What are biochemical and clinical symptoms of starvation?
3. Write briefly on metabolic changes that occur in liver during starvation.
4. Explain reason for ketoacidosis in diabetes and starvation.
5. Define diabetes mellitus. Write about types of diabetes mellitus.
6. Write a notes on oral glucose tolerance test (OGTT).
7. Write about biochemical and clinical symptoms of diabetics.
8. Explain changes occur in diabetes in carbohydrate metabolism.

CASES

1. A 40-year-old man started experiencing excessive thirst, polyuria and loss of weight for past couple of weeks. However his appetite was normal. His skin was dry and eye balls sunk. His blood glucose level was very high and urine gave brick red color with Benedict's test. Write your diagnosis.
2. During hunger strike by a major political party, a volunteer was brought to hospital in coma. His blood glucose, pH and bicarbonate levels were 55 mg%, 7.30 and 18 meq/L respectively. Urine gave positive Rothera's test. Write your diagnosis.

14 CHAPTER

NUCLEOTIDES

Occurrence

Nucleotides are present in all types of cells.

MEDICAL AND BIOLOGICAL IMPORTANCE

1. Nucleotides are high energy compounds.
2. Nucleotides are required for formation of co-enzymes of some members of vitamins B complex group.
3. Some nucleotides are called as 'second messenger' because many hormones exert their action through nucleotides.
4. Some nucleotides act as carrier or donor of activated sugars, sulphates and nitrogenous compounds.
5. Some nucleotides are involved in signal transduction.
6. Some nucleotides are involved in regulation of metabolic pathways.
7. Nucleotides act as alarmones. They regulate cell metabolism and alarms cell when all is not well in cell.
8. Synthetic analogs of nucleosides and nitrogenous bases are anticancer and antiviral agents.
9. Some nitrogenous bases are CNS stimulants.
10. Some bases act as anti-oxidants.
11. Some nucleotide analogs are mutagens.
12. Nucleosides also act as carriers of groups or compounds.
13. Nucleotides are building blocks of nucleic acids.
14. Purines play major role in cardiovascular biology in normal and pathological conditions. They are involved in cardiac aging, angiogenesis, hypertension etc. Purino receptors are identified in cardiovascular system.
15. Cyclic nucleotide cAMP is involved in regeneration of nervous tissues that are injured.
16. Some nucleotides are involved in regulation of ion channel activity. For example,

ATP sensitive K^+ channel couple cell metabolism to either cell excitability or potassium secretion.

17. Purine nucleotides support rotation of γ-subunit of ATP synthase of electron transport chain. Extra ring in purines is indispensable for the operation of molecular motor.

Chemical nature of nucleotides

Hydrolysis of nucleotides produce nitrogen bases, sugars and phosphate.

Nitrogenous bases. Nucleotides contain two types of nitrogenous bases. They are purine bases and pyrimidine bases.

Purine bases

They are derived from parent compound purine. Purine contains heterocyclic ring system. Fusion of pyrimidine ring with imidazole yields purine ring (Fig. 14.1). The carbon (c) and nitrogen (N) atoms of purine ring are numberered in anti-clockwise direction (Fig. 14.1).

The purines present in nucleotides are adenine and guanine. The structures of adenine and guanine along with their systematic names are shown in Fig. 14.1.

Other purine bases are hypoxanthine and xanthine. They are intermediates in the formation of adenine and guanine nucleotides. Uric acid is another purine base. It is the end product of purine nucleotide catabolism. The structures of these bases are shown in Fig. 14.1.

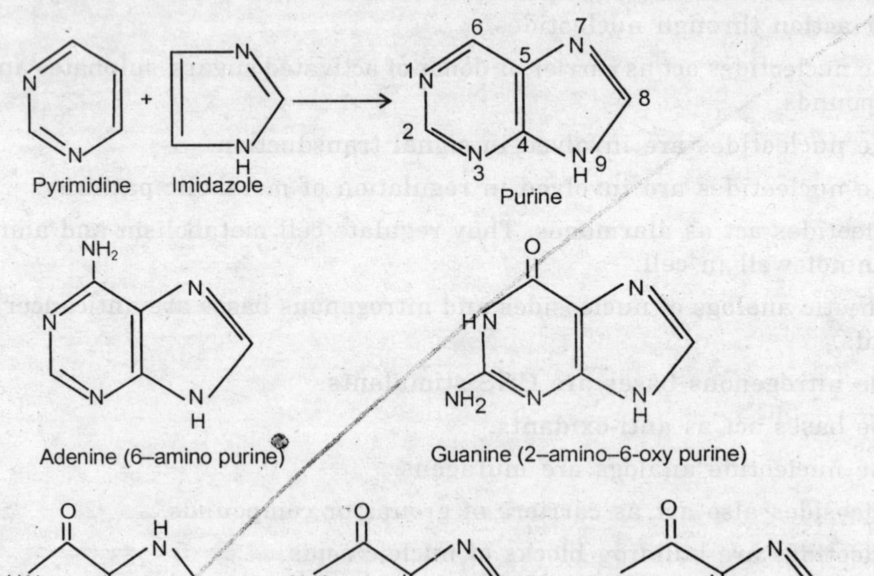

Fig. 14.1 Structures of purine bases

Physicochemical properties of purine bases

1. Purine bases are sparingly soluble in water. Uric acid and xanthine tend to crystalize at physiological pH at high concentration.
2. Purine bases absorb light in UV region at 260 nm. This property is used for detection and quantitation of purine nucleotides.
3. Purine bases are capable of forming hydrogen bonds.
4. Purine bases like guanine exhibit keto-enol tautomerism at body pH. The ketoform predominates. However, small amount of enol form is present (Fig. 14.2).
5. Purine bases exhibit amino-imino tautomerism at body pH. However, amino form predominates (Fig. 14.2).

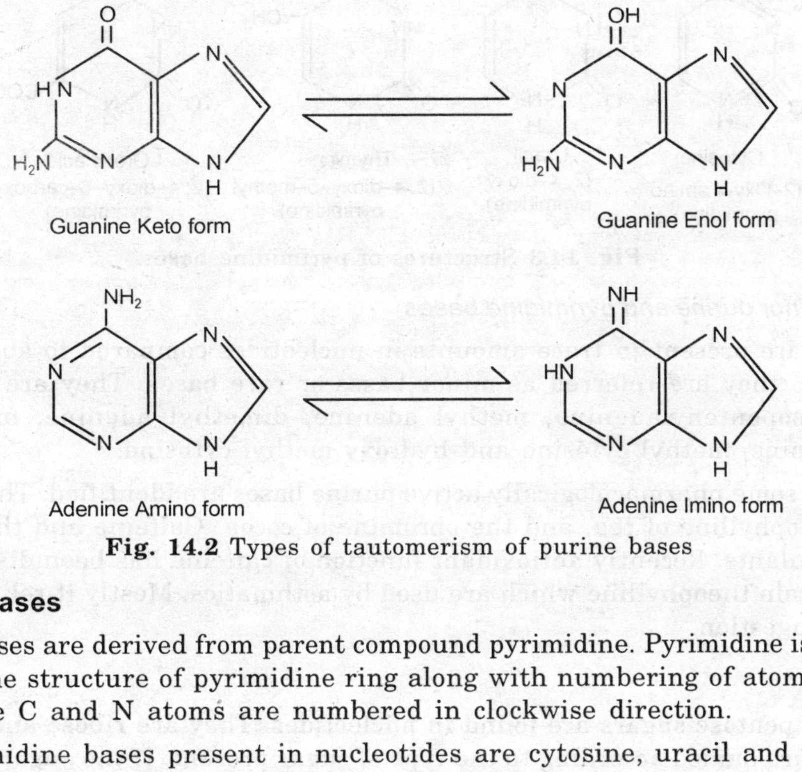

Fig. 14.2 Types of tautomerism of purine bases

Pyrimidine bases

Pyrimidine bases are derived from parent compound pyrimidine. Pyrimidine is a heterocylic compound. The structure of pyrimidine ring along with numbering of atoms is shown in Fig. 14.3. The C and N atoms are numbered in clockwise direction.

The pyrimidine bases present in nucleotides are cytosine, uracil and thymine. The structures of these pyrimidines along with their systematic names are shown in Fig. 14.3.

Other pyrimidine bases are orotic acid and dihydroorotic acid. They are intermediates in the formation of pyrimidine nucleotides.

Physicochemical properties of pyrimidine bases

1. Pyrimidine bases are soluble in water at body pH.
2. Pyrimidine bases also absorb UV light at 260 nm. This property is used to detect and estimate pyrimidine nucleotides.
3. They are capable of forming hydrogen bonds.

4. They too exhibit keto-enol tautomerism as well as amino-imino tautomerism like purine bases.

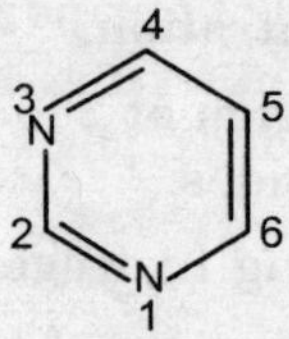

Pyrimidine

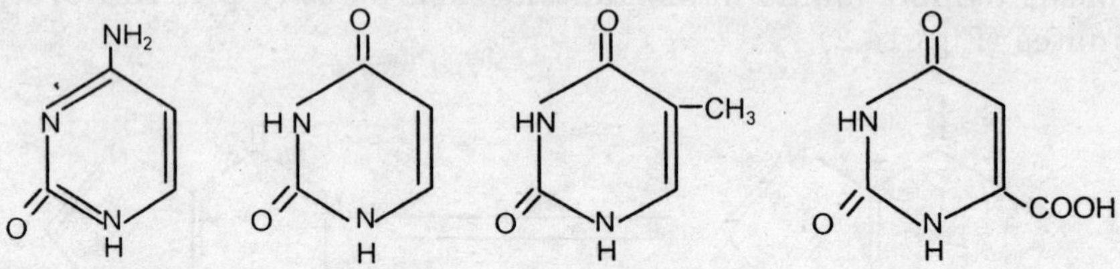

Cytosine (2–Oxy-4 amino pyrimidine) | Uracil (2, 4–dioxy pyrimidine) | Thymine (2, 4–dioxy–5–methyl pyrimidine) | Orotic acid (2, 4–dioxy–6–carboxy pyrimidine)

Fig. 14.3 Structures of pyrimidine bases

Unusual or minor purine and pyrimidine bases

These bases are present in trace amounts in nucleotides compared to above mentioned bases. Hence, they are referred as minor bases or rare bases. They are dihydrouracil, thiouracil, isopentenyladenine, methyl adenine, dimethyl adenine, methylguanine, dimethylguanine, methyl cytosine and hydroxy methyl cytosine.

In plants some pharmacologically active purine bases are identified. They are caffeine of coffee, theophylline of tea, and the obromine of cocoa. Caffeine and theophylline act as CNS stimulants. Recently antioxidant function of caffeine has been discovered. Some inhalers contain theophylline which are used by asthmatics. Mostly it relieves nasal and bronchial congestion.

Sugars

Two types of pentose sugars are found in nucleotides. They are ribose and deoxy ribose. Nucleotides are named according to the type of sugar present. If the sugar is deoxyribose then nucleotide is named as deoxyribonucleotide. Similarly, if the sugar is ribose then nucleotide is named as ribonucleotide.

Some characteristic features of sugar present in nucleotides

1. Normally it is a 5-numbered furanose ring.
2. Only D-isomer is present.
3. Configuration around first carbon atom is 'β'-form.
4. As mentioned earlier in deoxyribose, only hydrogen is present instead of OH group of 2 carbon atom of furanose ring (Fig. 14.4).

Nucleosides

A nucleoside is composed of purine and pyrimidine base and sugar. In the case of purine nucleosides, the sugar is attached to N-9 of purine ring where as in pyrimidine nucleosides the sugar is attached to N-1 of pyrimidine ring (Fig. 14.4). So, the type of linkage is N-glycosidic and sugar can be ribose or deoxyribose.

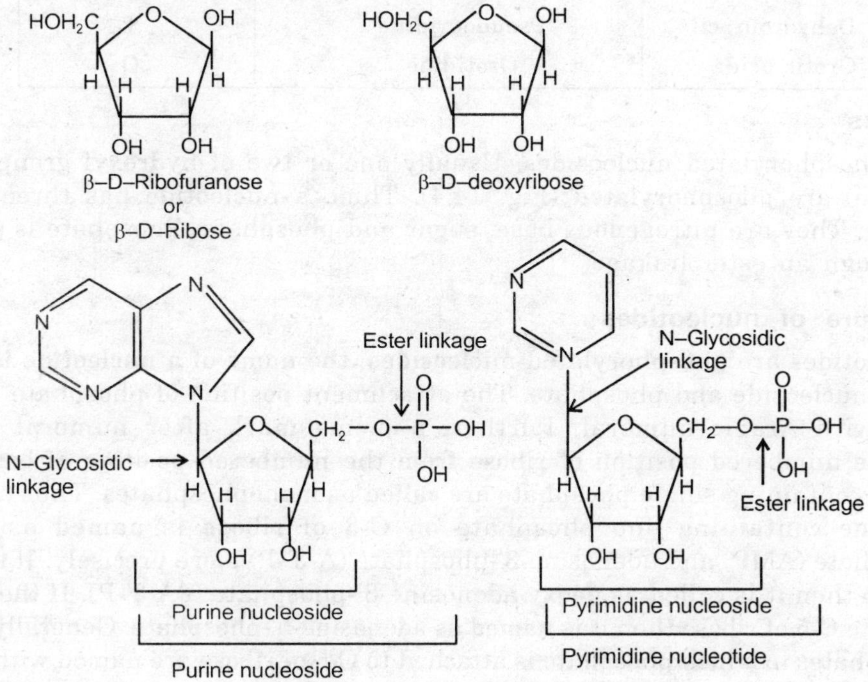

Fig. 14.4 Structures of ribose, deoxyribose; purine and pyrimidine nucleosides and their corresponding nucleotides

NOMENCLATURE OF NUCLEOSIDES

Nucleosides are named as derivatives of bases. For example, adenine linked to ribose is called as adenosine. Capital letter A is used to indicate adenine containing nucleoside. If adenine is linked to deoxyribose then it is named as deoxy adenosine and it is abbreviated as dA. Names and abbreviation of purine and pyrimidine nucleosides are given in Table 14.1.

Table 14.1 Nomenclature of bases and nucleosides

Base	Nucleosides	Abbreviation
Adenine	Adenosine	A
	Deoxyadenosine	dA
Guanine	Guanosine	G
	Deoxyguanosine	dG
Hypoxanthine	Inosine	I
Xanthine	Xanthosine	X

(Contd.)

Cytosine	Cytidine	C
	Deoxycytidine	dC
Thymine	Ribothymidine	T
	Deoxythymidine	dT
Uracil	Uridine	U
Dehydrouracil	Pseudouridine	Ψ
Orotic acid	Orotidine	O

Nucleotides

They are phosphorylated nucleosides. Usually one or two of hydroxyl groups of ribose (deoxyribose) are phosphorylated (Fig. 14.4). Thus, a nucleotide has three structural components. They are nitrogenous base, sugar and phosphate. Phosphate is attached to ribose through an ester linkage.

Nomenclature of nucleotides

Since nucleotides are phosphorylated nucleosides, the name of a nucleotide is composed of name of nucleoside and phosphate. The attachment position of phosphate to ribose is indicated with Arabic numeral. Further, a prime mark after numeral is used to differentiate numbered position of ribose from the numbered position of base. Usually nucleotides containing single phosphate are called as monophosphates. Thus a nucleotide of adenosine containing one phosphate on C-3 of ribose is named as adenosine monophosphate (AMP) and adenosine-3'-phosphate (A-3'-P) more precisely. If the sugar is deoxyribose then it is called as deoxy adenosine-3'-phosphate (dA-3'-P). If the phosphate is attached to C-5 of ribose then it is named as adenosine-5'-phosphate. Generally nucleotide mono phosphates in which phosphate is attached to C-5 of ribose are named without primed numeral. Hence, adenosine-5'-phosphate is called as *adenosine monophosphate* (Fig. 14.5).

Because of phosphate nucleotides are acidic in nature. Hence they are named by adding word 'lic acid' to the name of the base or nucleoside. For example nucleotide of adenine is called as adenylic acid. Nucleotide of uracil is named as uridylic acid. Names and abbreviations of nucleotides are given in Table 14.2.

Table 14.2 Nomenclature of nucleotides

Name	Alternate name	Abbreviation
Adenosine monophosphate	Adenylic acid	AMP
Deoxy adenosine monophosphate	Deoxyadenylic acid	dAMP
Guanosine monophosphate	Guanylic acid	GMP
Deoxy guanosine monophosphate	Deoxy guanylic acid	dGMP
Cytidine monophosphate	Cytidylic acid	CMP
Deoxy cytidine monophosphate	Deoxy cytidylic acid	dCMP
Deoxy thymidine monophosphate	Deoxy thymidylic acid	dTMP
Uridine monophosphate	Uridylic acid	UMP
Inosine monophosphate	Inosinic acid	IMP
Orotidine monophospahate	Orotidylic acid	OMP

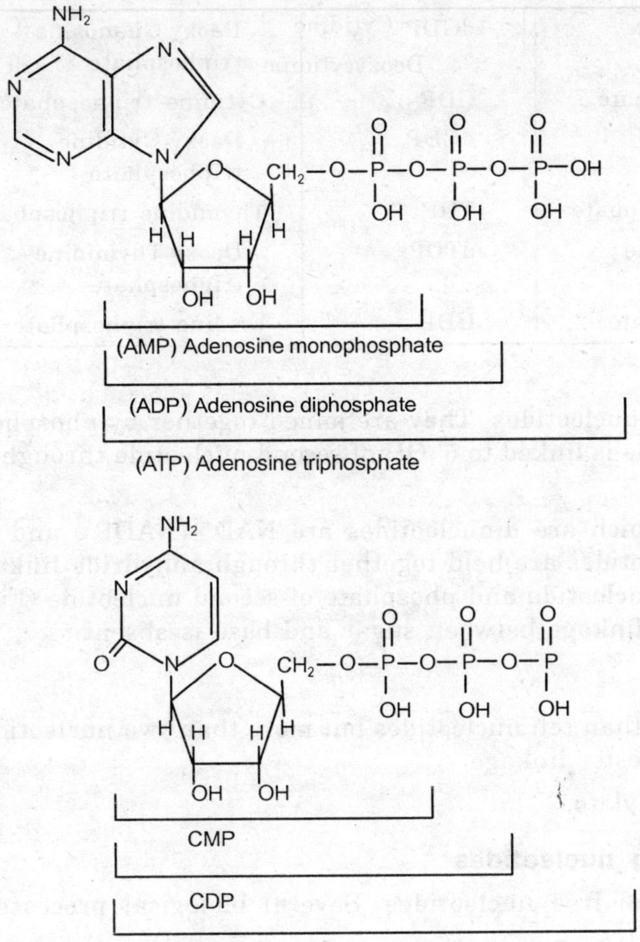

Fig. 14.5 Structures of nucleoside mono, di and triphosphate of adenine and cytosine

Nucleoside di and triphosphates

They are nucleosides in which two or three phosphate groups are attached to C-5 or C-3 of ribose. Since they are phosphorylated nucleosides they are nucleotides also. For example, adenosine with two phosphates attached to ribose is called as adenosine diphosphate (ADP) (Fig. 14.5). Likewise adenosine triphosphate (ATP) (Fig. 14.5). Names and abbreviations of some nucleoside di and tri phosphates are given in Table 14.3. Phosphates are in acid anhydride forms. The high energy nature of nucleoside di and triphosphates is described in chapter-11.

Table 14.3 Some nucleoside di and triphosphates

Name of diphosphate	Abbreviation	Name of triphosphate	Abbreviation
Adenosine diphosphate	ADP	Adenosine triphosphate	ATP
Deoxy Adenosine diphosphate	dADP	Deoxy Adenosine triphosphate	dATP
Guanosine diphosphate	GDP	Guanosine triphosphate	GTP

(Contd.)

Deoxy Guanosine diphosphate	dGDP	Deoxy Guanosine triphosphate	dGTP
Cytidine diphosphate	CDP	Cytidine triphosphate	CTP
Deoxy Cytidine diphosphate	dCDP	Deoxy Cytidine triphosphate	dCTP
Thymidine diphosphate	TDP	Thymidine triphosphate	TTP
Deoxy Thymidine diphosphate	dTDP	Deoxy Thymidine triphosphate	dTTP
Uridine diphosphate	UDP	Uridine triphosphate	UTP

Dinucleotides

They consist of two nucleotides. They are joined together by phosphodiester linkage. 3'-OH of first nucleotide is linked to 5'-OH of second nucleotide through the phosphodiester linkage (Fig. 14.6).

Two co-enzymes, which are dinucleotides are NAD^+ ($NADP^+$) and FAD. But in these dinucleotides, nucleotides are held together through anhydride linkage formed between phosphate of first nucleotide and phosphate of second nucleotide (Fig. 14.6). Further in FAD the glycosidic linkage between sugar and base is absent.

Oligonucleotides

They consist of less than ten nucleotides but more than two nucleotides. Nucleotides are joined by phosphodiester linkage.

Example: oligo adenylate.

Naturally occurring nucleotides

Cells contain several free nucleotides. Several biological processes depends on free nucleotides.

Adenine nucleotides and their functions

1. ATP is energy currency of cell. In mammalian cells, its concentration is about 1 mM/L.
2. Oxidative phosphorylation of respiratory chain requires ADP. ADP is a high energy compound.
3. ATP, ADP and AMP are allosteric effectors of several enzymes.
4. Several hormones exerts their action through cyclic AMP or cAMP (Fig. 14.7).
5. Phosphoadenosine phosphosulfate (PAPS) is the donor of sulfate groups in many biosynthetic reactions (Fig. 14.7).
6. Adenine nucleotides are constituents of FAD and NAD^+, $NADP^+$ (Fig. 14.6), co-enzyme A and vitamin B_{12} co-enzyme.
7. Diadenosine triphosphate and diadenosine poly phosphate are neurotransmitters and affect platelet aggregation and blood pressure.
8. Oligoadenylate is mediator for interferon action.
9. ATP is required for protein biosynthesis.

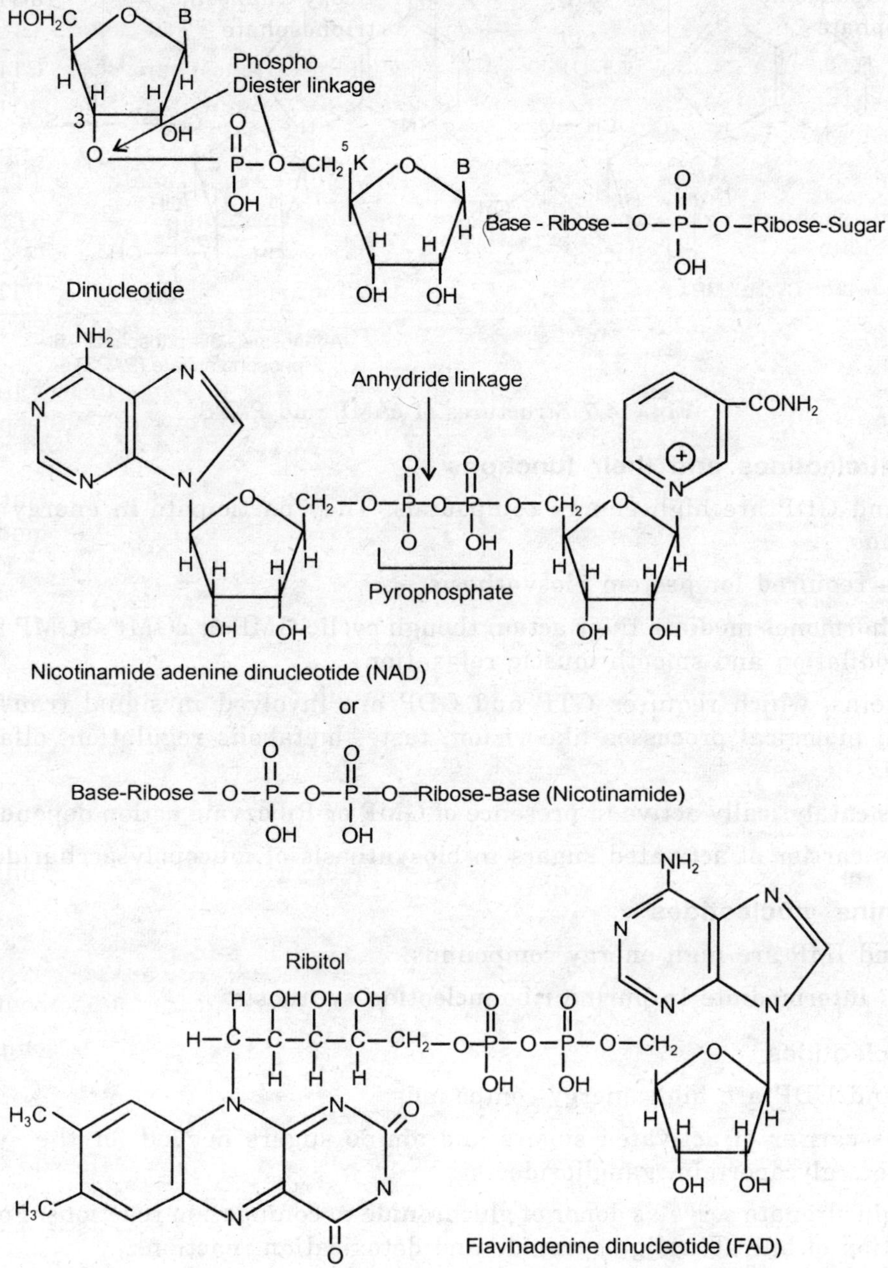

Fig. 14.6 Structures of dinucleotides

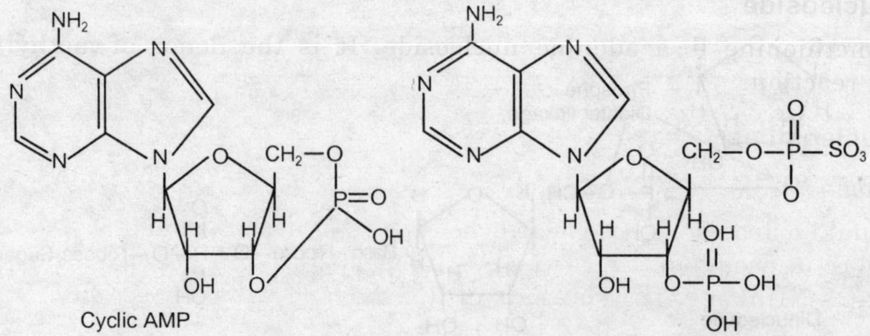

Cyclic AMP

Adenosine - 3′ - phosphate - 5′ - phospho sulfate (PAPS)

Fig. 14.7 Structures of cAMP and PAPS

Guanine nucleotides and their functions

1. GTP and GDP are high energy compounds. They participate in energy-dependent reactions.
2. GTP is required for protein biosynthesis.
3. Many hormones mediate their action though cyclic GMP or cGMP. cGMP is involved in vasodilation and smooth muscle relaxation.
4. G-proteins, which requires GTP and GDP are involved in signal transduction of several biological processes like vision, taste, metabolic regulation, olfaction, and cancer.
5. RNA is catalytically active in presence of GMP or Ribozyme action depends on GMP.
6. GDP is carrier of activated sugars in biosynthesis of mucopolysaccharides.

Hypoxanthine nucleotides

1. IDP and IMP are high energy compounds.
2. IMP is intermediate in purine ribonucleotide synthesis.

Uracil nucleotides

1. UTP and UDP are high energy compounds.
2. UDP is carrier of activated sugars and amino sugars needed for the synthesis of glycogen, glycoportein, gangliosides etc.
3. UDP-glucuronate serve as donor of glucuronide in conjugation reactions. For example, formation of bilirubin diglucuronide and detoxication reactions.

Cytosine nucleotides

1. CTP and CDP are high energy compounds.
2. CDP-choline serve as donor of choline in biosynthesis of phospholipid.
3. CMP-NANA is donor of NANA in biosynthesis of gangliosides.
4. Cyclic CMP also exist in cells.

Adenine nucleoside

S-adenosyl methionine is a adenine nucleoside. It is the donor of methyl groups in biosynthesis reactions.

Unusual nucleosides

1. Pseudouridine

In this unusual nucleoside, ribose is attached to C-5 of uracil instead of N-1, which is not common. Hence in pseudouridine —C—C— linkage is present between uracil and ribose instead of —C—N inkage. It is present in RNA, which we shall see later.

2. Ribothymidine

This unusual nucleoside of thymine contains ribose and it is present in RNA, which is not common as we learn later.

Purine and pyrimidine analogs

Several synthetic analogs of purines and pyrimidines are used as anti-cancer agents. Their actions are detailed in next chapter.

Purine analogs

1. Mercaptopurine
2. Thioguanine
3. 2-Aminopurine
4. Allopurinol
5. Azathiopurine. A modified mercaptopurine. It is an immune suppressive agent.

Pyrimidine analogs

1. 5-Flurouracil

Nucleoside analogs

Nucleoside analogs containing modified bases or sugars are used as anti-cancer agents, anti-viral agents and mutagens.

1. **Deazauridine** It is nucleoside with unnatural base. It is anti-cancer drug.
2. **6-Azauridine** Another nucleoside with unnatural base. An anti-cancer agent.
3. **Adenine arabinoside (Ara-A)** It is a nucleoside with abnormal pentose. It acts as anti-cancer agent as well as anti-viral agent.
4. **Arabinosyl cytosine (Ara-C)** It is a cytosine arabinoside used in cancer treatment.
5. **AZT (3'-azido-3'-deoxy thymidine) or Azido thymidine** It is used in treatment of AIDS. It can prevent progression of the disease if given at an early stage.
6. **Dideoxy cytidine** It is used in viral infections.
7. **Bromodeoxy uridine** It is a mutagen.
8. **Iododeoxy uridine** It is an anti-viral agent.
9. **Fluorodeoxy uridine** It is anti-cancer agent.

REFERENCES

1. Hartman, S.C. Purines and pyrimidines in metabolic pathways, Greenberg (Ed.). Vol. 4. Academic Press, New York, 1970.
2. Holley, R.W. The nucleotide sequence of nucleic acids, Sci. Am. **214**, 30, 1966.
3. Hutchinson, D.W. Nucleotides and coenzymes. J. Wiley, New York, 1964.
4. Jost, J.P. and Ricken Berg, H.V. Cyclic AMP. Ann. Rev. Biochem. **40**, 741, 1971.
5. Zemeenick, P.C. Diadenosine tetra phophate. Its role in cellular metabolism Anal. Biochem. **134**, 1-10, 1983.
6. Naim, M., Seifert, R. Numberg, M. Grunbaum, L. and Schultz, G. Some taste substances are direct activators of G-proteins. Biochem. J. **297**, 451-454, 1994.
7. Joanne, S. Ingwell, ATP and the heart, Kluwar academic publisher, 2002.
8. Keneeth Alan Jacobson. Purines in cellular signalling: targets for new drugs. Springer Verlag, NY, 1990.
9. Amir pelleg. Effect of extracellular adenosine and ATP on cardiomyocytes. Vol.6. Landes Bioscience, 1999.
10. Geoffrey Burnstock. (Ed.). Cardiovascular biology of purines, Vol. 209, Kluwer Academic Publisher, 1998.
11. Dimple, H.Bhatt *et al.* cAMP induced repair of zebra fish spinal circuits. Science. **305**, 254-258, 2004.
12. Noji, H. *et al.* Purine but not pyrimidine nucleotides support rotation of F_0-ATPase, J. Biol. Chem. **276**, 25480-25486, 2001.

EXERCISES

ESSAY QUESTIONS

1. Give an account of naturally occurring nucleotides.
2. Define nucleoside, nucleotide. Give purine and pyrimidine based example for each. Write functions of nucleotides and nucleosides.

SHORT QUESTIONS

1. Name purine and pyrimidine bases found in nucleic acids.
2. Write structures of purine and pyrimidine bases indicating numbers of carbon and nitrogen atoms.
3. Write composition of nucleoside, nucleotide, dinucleotide and oligonucleotide.
4. Wrtie function of adenine nucleotides.
5. Write briefly about unusual nucleosides.
6. Name pyrimidine nucleoside analogs. Write their clinical importance.
7. Write cAMP and PAPS structures label components.
8. Write on nucleoside and nucleotide triphosphates.

15
CHAPTER

NUCLEOTIDE METABOLISM

MEDICAL AND BIOLOGICAL IMPORTANCE

1. Deoxyribonucleotides are required for DNA synthesis.
2. Ribonucleotides are required for RNA synthesis.
3. Biosynthesis of purine and pyrimidine nucleotides is essential for DNA replication (cell division) and growth of all types of mammalian cells, bacteria and virus. If the supply of nucleotides is blocked cell division (viral replication) and growth is halted. So, compounds, which can block nucleotide biosynthesis effectively halt growth of cells, bacteria and virus. Indeed, many anti-tumor, anti-bacterial and anti-viral agents currently used are inhibitors of nucleotide (nucleic acid) biosynthesis.
4. Nucleotide metabolism is defective in diseases like gout, orotic aciduria, immunodeficiency syndrome and Lesch-Nyhan syndrome.
5. Nucleotides are required for few co-enzymes formation.
6. Several roles of nucleotides are detailed in Chapter 14.
7. Nucleotide metabolism in malarial parasite differs from its human host. These differences in metabolic pathways between parasites and host are used for development of new anti-malarial agents, which can help in tackling of malaria a worst courage of mankind.
8. *Giardia lamblia,* which causes giardiasis in humans and *trichomonas fetus* that causes embryonic death in cows are unable to synthesize purines via *de novo* pathways. They rely mainly on salvage pathways. Hence, enzymes in salvage pathways are potential targets of therapeutic agents for the treatment of diseases caused by these parasites.

Biosynthesis of Nucleotides

There are two types of pathways for nucleotide biosynthesis.

1. *De novo* pathways
2. Salvage pathways

De novo pathways for nucleotide biosynthesis

1. Purine and pyrimidine nucleotides are synthesized by two separate pathways present in cytosol of most of the cells. They are
   (*a*) *De novo* pathway for purine nucleotide biosynthesis, and
   (*b*) *De novo* pathway for pyrimidine nucleotide biosynthesis.
2. Both purine and pyrimidine nucleotide biosynthetic pathways are energy intensive processes.
3. Both pathways are linked to HMP shunt as well as glycolysis.

De novo purine nucleotide biosynthesis

1. Liver is the major site of purine nucleotide biosynthesis.
2. Purine nucleotide biosynthesis involves construction of purine ring on ribose-5-phosphate. So, intermediates of purine nucleotide biosynthesis are bound to ribose-5-phosphate (Fig. 15.1).
3. Formation of purine ring on ribose-5-phosphate proceeds in two phases.
   (*a*) In the first phase, nitrogen atom is attached to ribose-5-phsophate on which imidazole ring is formed.
   (*b*) In the second phase, remaining part of purine ring is constructed around the imidazole and nitrogen atom that initiated the synthesis becomes N-9 of purine ring.

Reaction sequence

1. Formation of phosphoribosyl pyrophosphate (PRPP) from ribose-5-phosphate is the first reaction of *de novo* pathway for purine nucleotide biosynthesis. The reaction is catalyzed by PRPP synthetase in presence of ATP and Mg^{2+}. AMP is formed in this reaction from ATP. One high energy bond is consumed in this reaction.
2. In this reaction, NH_2 of glutamine (amide) displaces PP_i from PRPP to yield β-5-phospho ribosyl-1-amine. PP_i is hyrolyzed to P_i. The former reaction is catalyzed by phosphoribosyl-1-amido transferase and pyrophosphatase catalyzes latter reaction. One high energy bond is consumed in this reaction. Construction of purine ring requires nine additional reactions.
3. β-5-phosphoribosyl-1-amine reacts with carboxyl group of glycine to form 5-phosphoribosyl glycinamide in a ATP-dependent reaction catalyzed by glycinamide kino synthetase. One high energy, bond is utilized.
4. The 5-phosphoribosyl glycinamide is formylated in this reaction by transformylase to 5-phosphoribosyl-N-formyl glycinamide.
5. In this reaction, carbonyl oxygen of amide is replaced with $-NH_2$ of (amide) of glutamine to form amidine. The reaction is catalyzed by ATP dependent 5-phosphoribosyl-N-formyl glycinamidine synthetase. One high energy, bond is utilized.
6. In this step, 5-phosphoribosyl aminoimidazole synthetase catalyzes imidazole ring formation in an intramolecular ATP-dependent reaction by eliminating water between amide group and N-formyl group. One high energy, bond is consumed.

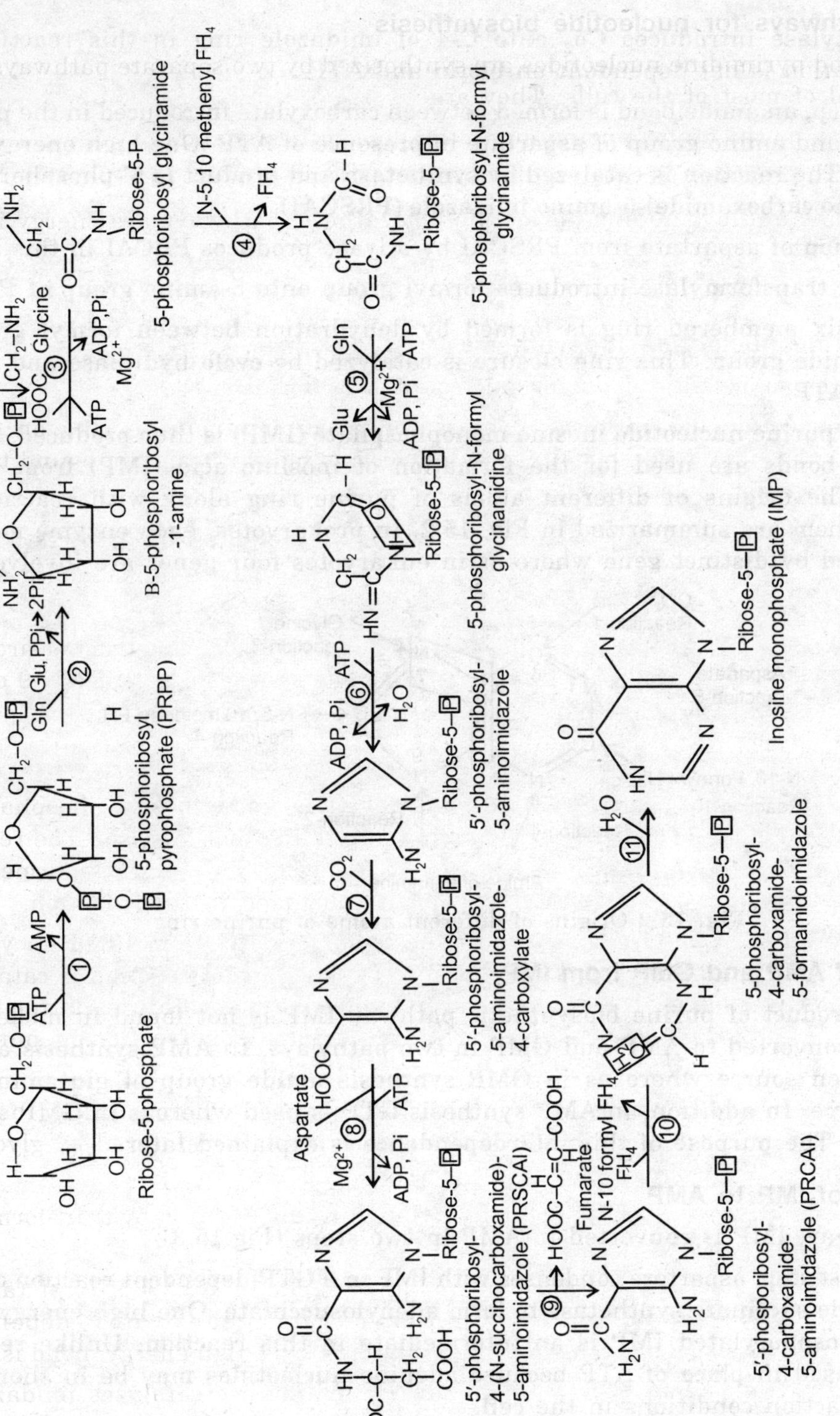

Fig. 15.1 *De novo* purine nucleotide biosynthesis reaction sequence

7. A carboxylase introduces Co_2 onto C-4 of imidazole ring in this reaction. This carboxylation is not dependent on biotin and ATP.
8. In this step, an amide bond is formed between carboxylate introduced in the preceding reaction and amino group of aspartate in presence of ATP. One high energy bond is utilized. The reaction is catalyzed by synthetase and product is 5′-phosphoribosyl-4-(N-succino carboxamide)-5-amino imidazole (PRSCAI).
9. Elimination of aspartate from PRSCAI by a lyase produces PRCAI in this reaction.
10. A second transformylase introduces formyl group onto 5-amino group of PRCAI.
11. Finally six membered ring is formed by dehydration between formyl group and carboxamide group. This ring closure is catalyzed by cyclo hydrolase and does not require ATP.

The first purine nucleotide inosine monophosphate (IMP) is thus produced. Total six high energy bonds are used for the formation of inosinic acid (IMP) from ribose-5-phosphate. The origins of different atoms of purine ring along with reactions that contributes them are summarized in Fig. 15.2. In prokaryotes, each enzyme mentioned above is coded by distinct gene where as in eukaryotes four genes are involved.

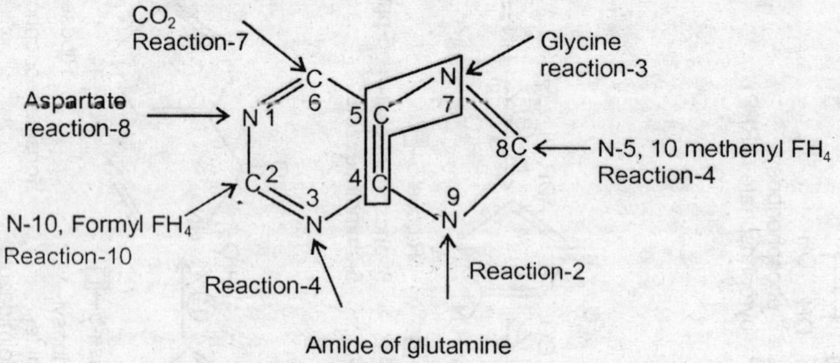

Fig. 15.2 Origins of different atoms of purine ring

Formation of AMP and GMP from IMP

The initial product of purine biosynthetic pathway IMP is not found in nucleic acids. Hence, it is converted to AMP and GMP in two pathways. In AMP synthesis aspartate is the nitrogen source where as in GMP synthesis amide group of glutamine is the nitrogen source. In addition, in AMP synthesis GTP is used whereas in GMP synthesis ATP is used. The purpose of this interdependence is explained later.

Conversion of IMP to AMP

In one pathway, IMP is converted to AMP in two steps (Fig.15.3).

1. In the first step, aspartate condenses with IMP in a GTP-dependent reaction catalyzed by adenylo succinate synthetase to form adenylosuccinate. One high energy, bond is used. Phosphorylated IMP is an intermediate in this reaction. Unlike reaction-8. GTP is used in place of ATP because adenine nucleotides may be in short supply under reaction conditions in the cell.
2. In this step, fumarate is released from adenylosuccinate by adenylosuccinase forming AMP. The reaction is similar to reaction-9 of purine biosynthesis.

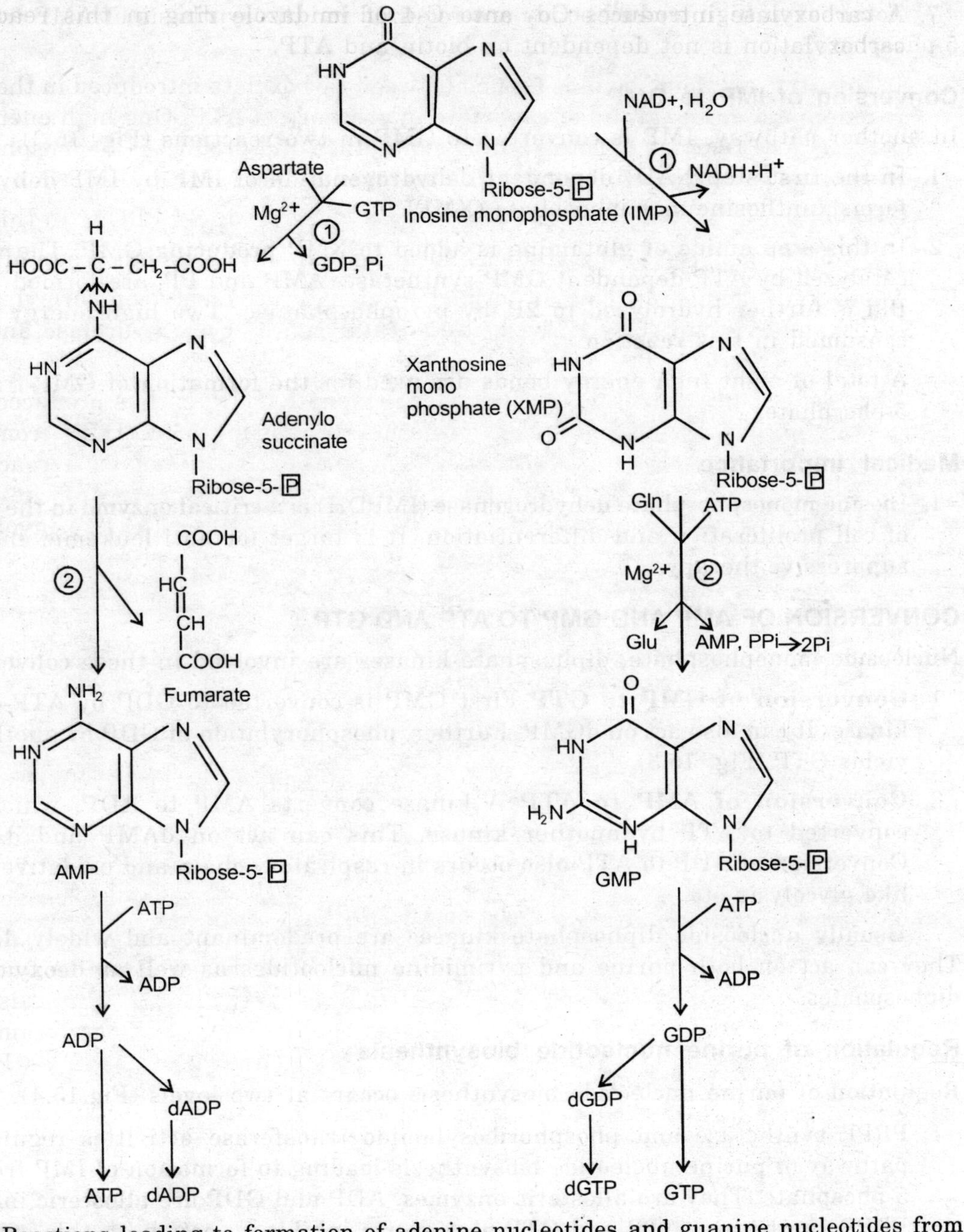

Fig. 15.3 Reactions leading to formation of adenine nucleotides and guanine nucleotides from IMP

Adenylosuccinate synthetase (ADSS) exist in two isoforms. They are ADSS-1 and ADSS-2. ADSS-1 is basic isozyme. It has higher K_m for IMP and lower K_m for aspartate. It is susceptible for inhibition by fructose-1, 6-bisphosphate. ADSS-2 is acidic isozyme and strongly inhibited by nucleotides. Hence, ADSS-2 is involved in *denovo* synthesis of AMP and ADSS-1 is part of purine nucleotide cycle.

Total seven high energy bonds are required for the synthesis of AMP from ribose-5-phosphate.

Conversion of IMP to GMP

In another pathway, IMP is converted to GMP in two reactions (Fig. 15.3).

1. In the first step NAD^+ dependent dehydrogenation of IMP by IMP dehydrogenase forms xanthosine monophosphate (XMP).
2. In this step amide of glutamine is added to XMP producing GMP. The reaction is catalyzed by ATP-dependent GMP synthetase. AMP and PP_i are formed from ATP. PPi is further hydrolyzed to $2P_i$ by pyrophosphatase. Two high energy bonds are consumed in this reaction.

   A total of eight high energy bonds are used for the formation of GMP from ribose-5-phosphate.

Medical importance

1. Inosine monosphosphate dehydrogenase (IMPDH) is a critical enzyme in the regulation of cell proliferation and differentiation. It is target for anti leukemic and immuno suppressive therapy.

CONVERSION OF AMP AND GMP TO ATP AND GTP

Nucleoside monophosphate, diphosphate kinases are involved in these conversions.

1. **Conversion of GMP to GTP** First GMP is converted to GDP by ATP-dependent kinase. It can also act on dGMP. Further, phosphorylation of GDP by another kinase yields GTP (Fig. 15.3).
2. **Conversion of AMP to ATP** A kinase converts AMP to ADP, which is later converted to ATP by another kinase. This can act on dAMP and dADP also. Conversion of ADP to ATP also occurs in respiratory chain and oxidative pathways like glycolysis etc.

   Usually nucleoside diphosphate kinases are predominant and widely distributed. They can act on both purine and pyrimidine nucleotides as well as deoxy nucleotide diphosphates.

Regulation of purine nucleotide biosynthesis

Regulation of purine nucleotide biosynthesis occurs at two levels (Fig.15.4).

1. PRPP synthetase and phosphoribosylamido transferase activities regulates main pathway of purine nucleotide biosynthesis leading to formation of IMP from ribose-5-phosphate. They are allosteric enzymes. ADP and GDP are allosteric inhibitors of PRPP synthetase. ATP and GTP also exerts inhibitory action on this enzyme. The enzyme has separate binding sites for ADP and GDP. In RBC, 2,3-BPG inhibits this enzyme. IMP, GMP and AMP are allosteric inhibitors of amido transferase. The enzyme has separate binding sties for IMP, GMP and AMP. In presence of AMP, GMP or IMP the enzyme is converted to inactive form. PRPP is positive effector. In presence of PRPP, enzyme is converted to active form. However, amido transferase has minor regulatory role only in mammals.

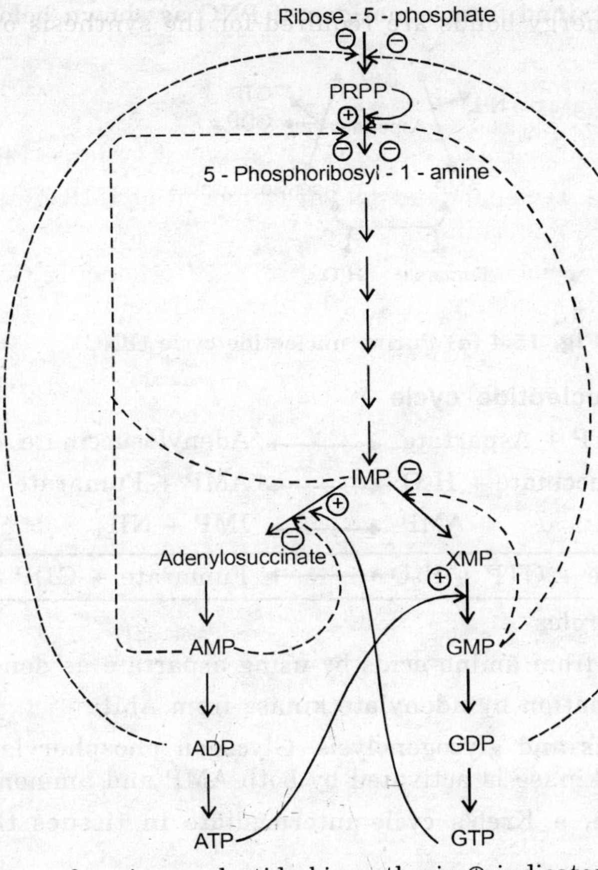

Fig. 15.4 Regulation of purine nucleotide biosynthesis ⊕ indicates activations, ⊖ inhibition

2. Branching pathways leading to formation of AMP and GMP from IMP are subjected to two types of regulation.
   (*a*) One is the regulation of branched pathways by their respective end product below the branch point. So, AMP controls its own biosynthesis from IMP by competitively inhibiting the activity of adenylosuccinate synthetase. Likewise GMP controls its own formation from IMP by allosterically inhibiting the activity of IMP dehydrogenase.
   (*b*) Another way of regulation of branched pathways is achieved by ATP and GTP. As mentioned earlier synthesis of AMP from IMP requires GTP and synthesis of GMP from IMP requires ATP. So excess ATP promotes GMP production and excess GTP promotes AMP production. This inverse relation balances production of ATP and GTP from IMP.

Purine nucleotide cycle (PNC)

It is active in muscle, brain, kidney, liver and pancreatic cells. ADSS, Adenylosuccinate and adenylate (adenosine) deaminase constitutes this cycle. (Fig. 15.4*a*). Net reaction of this cycle is given below.

$$\text{Aspartate} + \text{GTP} + H_2O \rightleftharpoons \text{Fumarate} + NH_3 + \text{GDP} + P_i$$

This equation is obtained from equations of PNC as shown below.

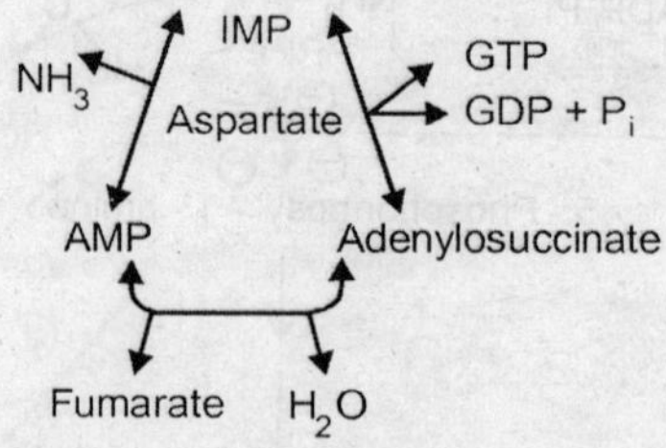

Fig. 15.4 (*a*) Purine nucleotide cycle (PNC)

Reactions of Purine nucleotide cycle

1. IMP + GTP + Aspartate $\longleftrightarrow$ Adenylosuccinate + GDP + P_i
2. Adenylosuccinate + H_2O $\longleftrightarrow$ AMP + Fumarate
3. AMP $\longleftrightarrow$ IMP + NH_3

1 + 2 + 3: Aspartate + GTP + H_2O $\longleftrightarrow$ Fumarate + GDP + P_i + NH_3

The PNC has following roles

1. Releasing ammonia from amino acids by using aspartate as donor.
2. Favouring ATP formation by adenylate kinase from AMP.
3. Regulating glycolysis and glycogenolysis. Glycogen phosphorylase is activated by IMP. Phosphofructokinase is activated by both AMP and ammonia.
4. Supplying fumarate, a Kreb's cycle intermediate in tissues that lack pyruvate carboxylase.

Pyrimidine nucleotide biosynthesis *De novo*

Since pyrimidine ring is a part of purine ring one might expect that biosynthesis of these rings may occur in a similar way. However, biosynthetic pattern of pyrimidine nucleotides differs from purine nucleotide biosynthesis. In pyrimidine nucleotide, biosynthesis the heterocyclic pyrimidine ring is constructed first from aspartate and carbamoyl phosphate and ribose-5-phosphate is added later. Hence, the intermediates of the pathway are not attached to ribose-5-phosphate.

Site

Cytosol of liver cells and most of the other cells have enzymes of pyrimidine nucleotide formation. HMP shunt provides ribose-5-phosphate and NADPH.

Reaction sequence

In prokaryotes, each enzyme of *de novo* pathway for pyrimidine nucleotide biosynthesis is coded by distinct gene. In mammals, two multicatalytic proteins and an unicatalytic protein coded by three distinct genes are responsible for the biosynthesis of pyrimidine nucleotides. First three reactions are catalyzed by single multicatalytic protein, 4th reaction is catalyzed unicatalytic protein and 5,6 reactions are catalyzed by another single multicatalytic polypeptide (Fig. 15.5).

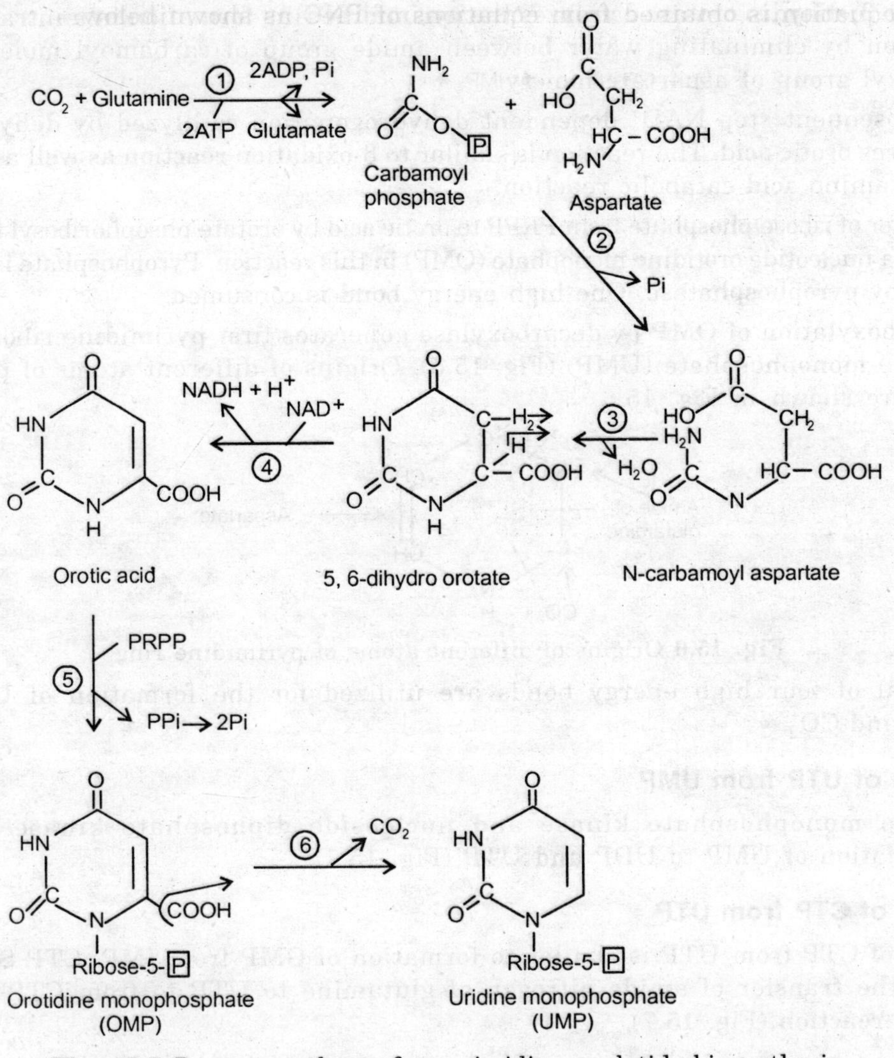

Fig. 15.5 *De novo* pathway for pyrimidine nuclotide biosynthesis

1. Formation of carbamoyl phosphate from glutamine and CO_2 is the first reaction of pyrimidine nucleotide biosynthesis. The reaction is catalyzed by carbamoyl phosphate synthetase-II (CPS-II), which is different from urea cycle CPS-I. Unlike CPS-I, CPS-II does not require N-acetyl glutamate. However two high energy bonds are utilized for carbamoyl phosphate formation here also. Carbamoyl group is activated at the expense of 2 ATPs for acyl group transfer that occurs in the next reaction. The carbamoyl phosphate carries amide nitrogen of glutamine and carbon of CO_2 into pyrimidine ring.
2. Formation of carbamoylaspartate is the first step uniquely committed to pyrimidine nucleotide biosynthesis. Aspartate transcarbamoylase catalyzes this reaction in which α–amino group of aspartate reacts with carbamoyl group of carbamoyl phosphate to form carbamoyl aspartate.

3. In step 3, dihydro orotase catalyzes the pyrimidine ring formation in a intra molecular reaction by eliminating water between amide group of carbamoyl moiety and β–carboxyl group of aspartate moiety.
4. In subsequent step NAD^+ dependent dehydrogenation catalyzed by dehydrogenase produces orotic acid. The reaction is similar to β-oxidation reaction as well as branched chain amino acid catabolic reaction.
5. Transfer of ribose phosphate from PRPP to orotic acid by orotate phsophoribosyl transferase yields a nucleotide orotidine monophate (OMP) in this reaction. Pyrophosphate is converted to Pi by pyrophosphatase. One high energy bond is consumed.
6. Decarboxylation of OMP by decarboxylase generates first pyrimidine ribonucleotide uridine monophosphate (UMP) (Fig. 15.5). Origins of different atoms of pyrimidine ring are shown in Fig. 15.6.

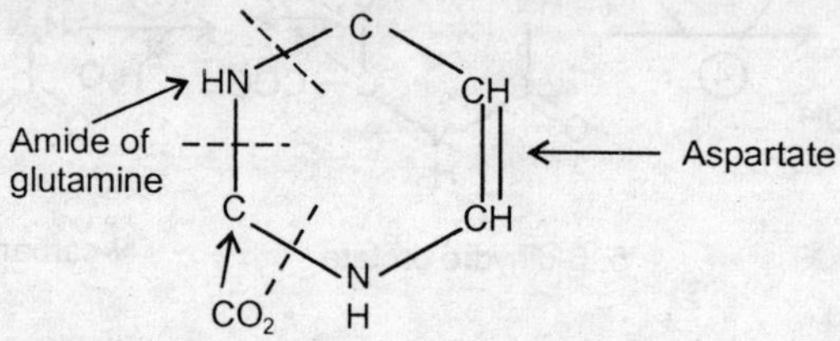

Fig. 15.6 Origins of different atoms of pyrimidine ring

A total of four high energy bonds are utilized for the formation of UMP from aspartate and CO_2.

Formation of UTP from UMP

Nucleoside monophosphate kinase and nucleoside diphosphate kinase catalyzes phosphorylation of UMP to UDP and UTP (Fig. 15.7).

Synthesis of CTP from UTP

Synthesis of CTP from UTP is similar to formation of GMP from IMP. CTP Synthetase catalyzes the transfer of amide nitrogen of glutamine to UTP to from CTP in a ATP dependent reaction (Fig. 15.7).

Synthesis of a dTTP from CTP

Synthesis of a dTTP from CTP occurs in two routes via dUMP. Depending on the organism or cell, one pathway predominates.

1. In one route, first CTP is converted to CDP by hydrolysis catalyzed by nucleotidase. Ribonucleotide reductase converts CDP to dCDP. This reaction is again described in the later part of this chapter. Further hydrolysis by a nucleotidase converts dCDP to dCMP. Deamination of dCMP by amino hydrolase yields dUMP. Thymidylate synthase catalyzes the formation of dTMP from dUMP by transferring one carbon group from N-5, 10-methylene FH_4. This one carbon group transfer reaction deserves special mention. The enzyme transfers methylene group to C-5 of dUMP and methylene group is subsequently reduced to methyl group of thymine by FH_4. This results in the formation of FH_2 unlike other one carbon transfer reaction of FH_4 where FH_4 is produced. For the continuation of one carbon metabolism, FH_2 must be reduced back to FH_4. This is brought about by dihydrofolate reductase using NADPH as hydrogen donor. Many anti-cancer drugs and antibiotics work by inhibiting

this conversion. As mentioned in Chapter 12, the transfer of one carbon from serine by serine transhydroxy methylase generates N-5,10 methylene FH_4. Finally dTTP is formed from dTMP by two successive phosphorylations catalyzed by nucleoside monosphosphate and diphosphate kinase respectively (Fig.15.7).

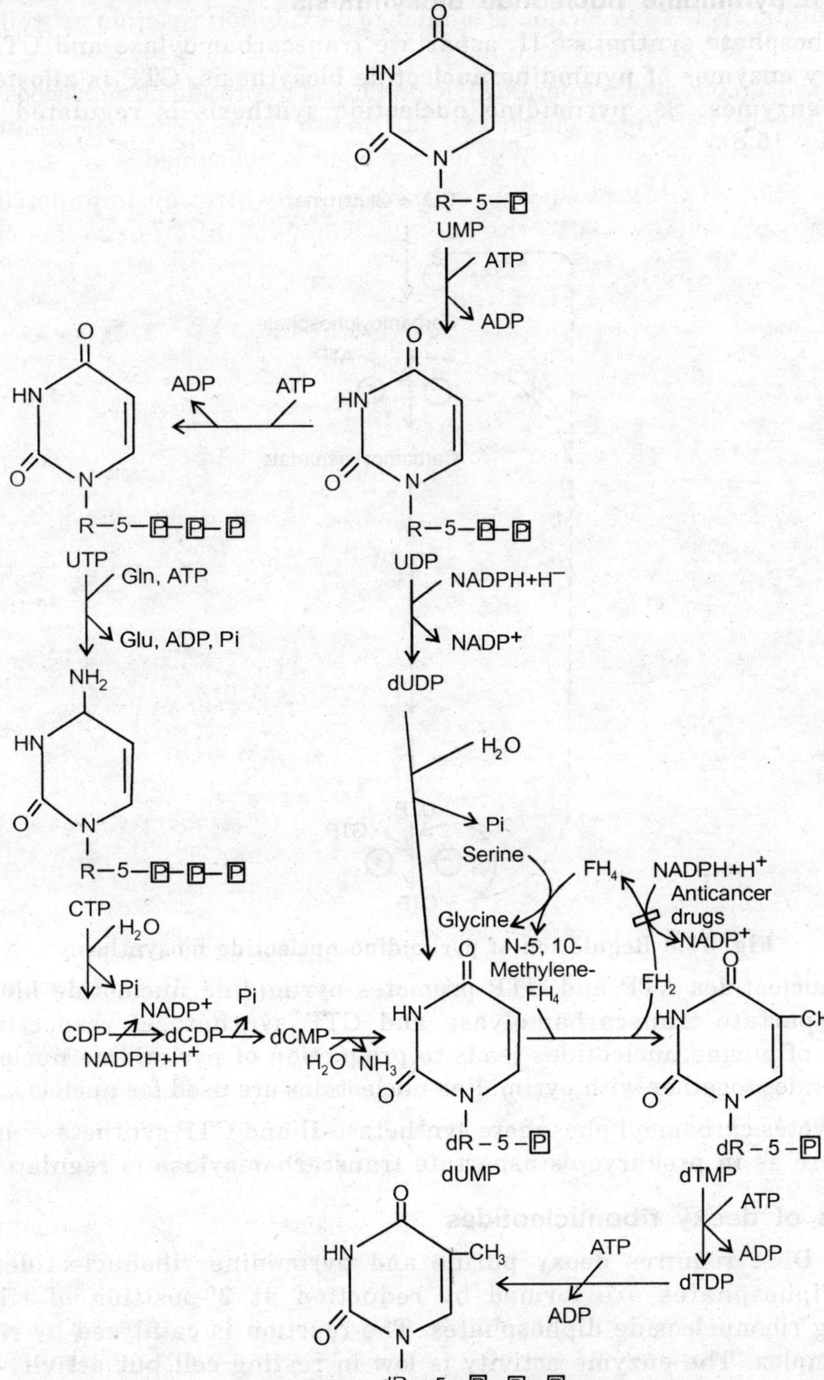

Fig. 15.7 Synthesis of CTP and dTTP from UMP

2. In the other route UDP is converted to dUDP by ribonucleotide reductase. dUMP is formed from dUDP by hydrolysis catalyzed by nucleotidase. Now synthesis of dTTP from dUMP occurs by reactions described for above route.

Regulation of pyrimidine nucleotide biosynthesis

Carbamoyl phosphate synthetase-II, aspartate transcarbamoylase and CTP synthetase are regulatory enzymes of pyrimdine nucleotide biosythesis. CTP is allosteric inhibitor of all three enzymes. So, pyrimidine nucleotide synthesis is regulated by allosteric inhibition (Fig. 15.8).

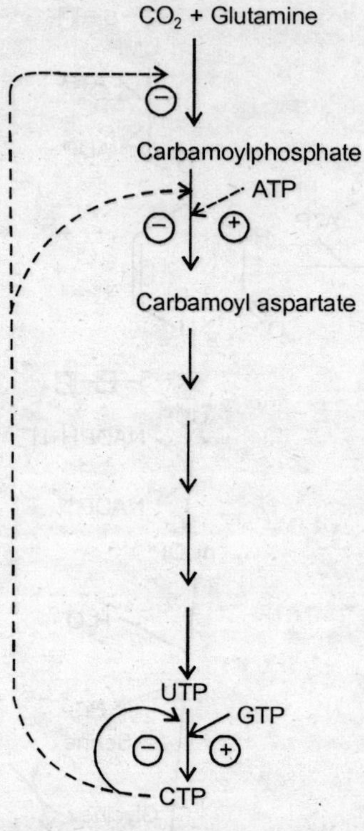

Fig. 15.8 Regulation of pyrimidine nucleotide biosynthesis

Purine nucleotides ATP and GTP promotes pyrimidine nucleotide biosynthesis by activating aspartate transcarbamolyase and CTP synthetase, respectively. Hence, accumulation of purine nucleotides leads to production of pyrimidine nucleotides. Then purine nucleotides together with pyrimidine nucleotides are used for nucleic acid synthesis.

In eukaryotes carbamoyl phosphate synthetase-II and CTP synthetase are regulatory enzymes where as in prokaryotes aspartate transcarbamoylase is regulatory enzyme.

Biosynthesis of deoxy ribonucleotides

Synthesis of DNA requires deoxy purine and pyrimidine ribonucleotides. Deoxyribo nucleoside diphosphates are formed by reduction at 2′-position of ribose ring of corresponding ribonucleoside diphosphates. The reaction is catalyzed by ribonucleotide reductase complex. The enzyme activity is low in resting cell but activity increases in S-phase of cell cycle. The enzyme has broad substrate specificity. It can convert ADP,

GDP, CDP and UDP to corresponding dADP, dGDP, dCDP and dUDP. For the conversion of ribonucleoside diphosphates to corresponding deoxy ribonucleoside diphosphates the enzyme requires a small protein thioredoxin as electron donor. Thioredoxin contain two cysteine residues. The -SH groups of two cysteine residues participates in oxidation-reduction reaction. Lipoic acid serve as electron source *in vitro*. Ribonucleotide reduction by ribonucleotide reductase oxidizes thioredoxin. Reduced thioredoxin is regenerated by thioredoxin reductase using NADPH as hydrogen donor. Thioredoxin reductase is a flavoprotein contains FAD. So electrons flow from NADPH to FAD then to thioredoxin during reduction of ribonucleoside diphosphates (Fig. 15.9). HMP shunt provides NADPH required for reduction of ribonucleoside diphosphates.

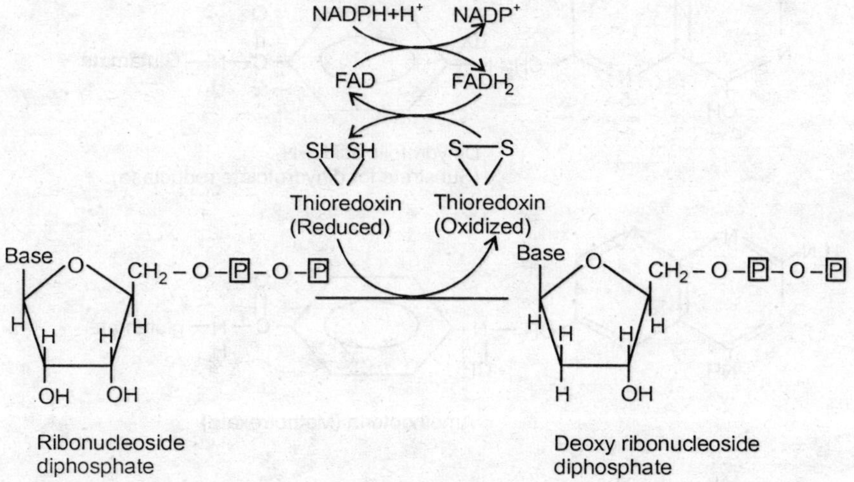

Fig. 15.9 Reactions catalyzed by ribonucleotide reductase and thioredoxin reductase

Ribonucleotide reductase is a allosteric enzyme. Several nucleoside triphosphates controls activity of the enzyme through unknown mechanism and this may be the reason for broad substrate specificity of the enzyme. Some known activators of this enzyme are ATP, dGTP, TTP and inhibitors are dATP, ATP, TTP etc. Activation and inhibition of this enzyme by a particular nucleoside triphosphate depends on substrate.

In *E. Coli*, ribonucleotide reductase glutathione serve as electron donor instead of thioredoxin.

Medical importance

Bacterial growth, viral growth and tumor growth requires nucleic acid synthesis. This in turn depends on nucleotide biosynthesis. Hence, inhibitors of nucleotide biosynthesis are potential antibacterial, antiviral and anti-tumor (cancer) agents. Since normal cell growth also requires nucleic acid biosynthesis these agents cause side or toxic affects. However, the severity of toxic effects varies from one drug to another drug. Rapidly dividing epithelial cells of gastrointestinal tract, bone marrow stem cells and hair follicles are affected most by these agents. Hence, symptoms like decreased blood count, gastrointestinal disturbances and hair loss may occur in individuals undergoing treatment with these agents. Some commonly used inhibitors of nucleotide biosynthesis are given below.

Anti folates or folic acid analogs

Folic acid analogs used in cancer chemotherapy are amethopterin and aminopterin (Fig. 15.10). They inhibit dihydrofolate reductase, which converts dihydrofolate to tetrahydrofolate. This blocks regeneration of FH_4 (Fig. 15.7) and rapidly dividing cells exhaust their FH_4 stores faster than normal cells. Thus, further multiplication or growth of cancer cells is halted and remission of cancer occurs. These antifolates are used in treatment of leukemia and chorio carcinoma.

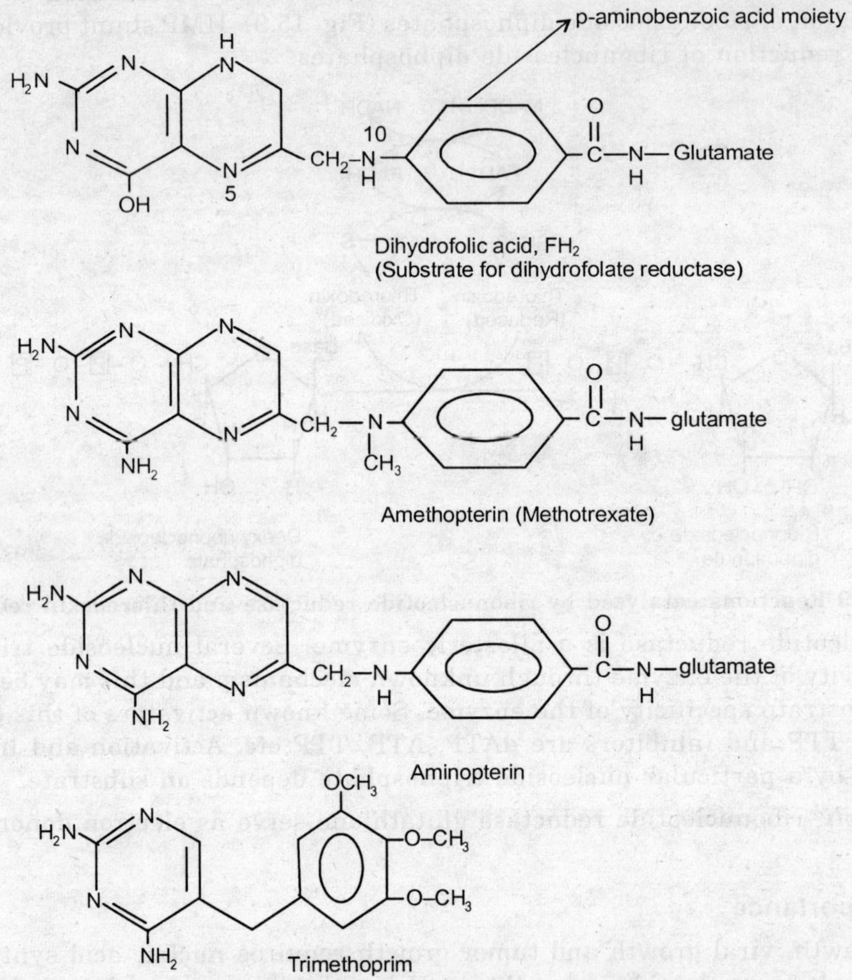

Fig. 15.10 Folic acid and its analogs

Trimethoprim

It is an antibiotic. It is an inhibitor of bacterial dihydrofolate reductase and used to treat bacterial infections. It is inactive against mammalian dihydrofolate reductase and hence it is tolerated well (Fig. 15.10).

Sulfa drugs

They are antibiotics. Most of them are structural analogs of p-amino benzoic acid part of folic acid. Sulfanilamide is one such a drug. It works by blocking formation of folic acid, which is required for purine nucleotide biosynthesis. Bacterial growth is impaired due to lack of nucleotides. Since humans obtain folic acid from diet purine nucleotide synthesis in humans is not affected.

Glutamine antagonists (anti-metabolites)

Since glutamine is required for purine nucleotide biosynthesis (N-3, 9 of purine ring and 2-amino group of GMP) and pyrimidine nucleotide biosynthesis (N-1 of pyrimidine ring) antagonists of glutamine are anti-cancer agents. They are azaserine (produced by streptomyces) and acivicin a synthetic analog of glutamine. They block DNA synthesis by antagonizing metabolic role of glutamine. They are irreversible inhibitors of amidotranferases that catalyze ATP dependent transfer of amide of glutamine to an acceptor. Structures of glutamine, azaserine and acivicin are shown in Fig. 15.11.

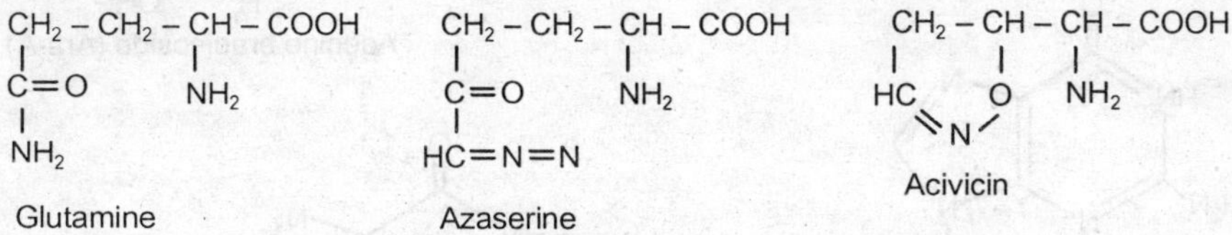

Fig. 15.11 Glutamine and its analogs

PURINE ANALOGS

1.6-Mercaptopurine

It is an anti-cancer agent and used in leukemia. It requires initial activation to become clinically active. It forms 6-thio IMP in the body. Since it can not be converted to either GMP or AMP it accumulates and inhibits phosphoribosylamido transferase. This blocks AMP and GMP formation also. Further it may be incorporated into DNA and RNA. DNA containing nucleotide of mercaptopurine develops strand breaks and transcription of a RNA is blocked. Thus, the cell growth is halted and cancer remission occurs.

Xanthine oxidase may inactivate 6-mercaptopurine. It converts 6-mercaptopurine to 6-mercaptouric acid. The latter compound is excreted in urine. So to increase potency of 6-mercaptopurine allopurinol is also given simultaneously (so called *cock tail drug therapy* or *combination chemotherapy*).

Purine nucleoside analogs

Purine nucleoside analogs inhibit nucleic acid synthesis rather than nucleotide biosynthesis. So they are mentioned later under inhibitors of replication.

1. **Adenine arabinoside (Ara-A)** It is an anti-viral agent. It is widely used in the treatment of viral encephalitis. In the body it is converted to nucleoside triphosphate and inhibits DNA polymerase of virus.
2. **Acyclovir (acyclo guanosine)** It is also an anti-viral agent and used in treatment of herpes simplex virus infections. It is also converted to nucleoside triphosphate in the body and interfers with viral DNA replication.

3. **2′–3′-dideoxy inosine (DDI)** It is an anti-viral agent. It is incorporated into new DNA after conversion to triphosphate. This blocks elongation of replicative new DNA due to lack of 3′-OH terminus.

Structures of purine and its nucleoside analgos are shown in Fig. 15.12.

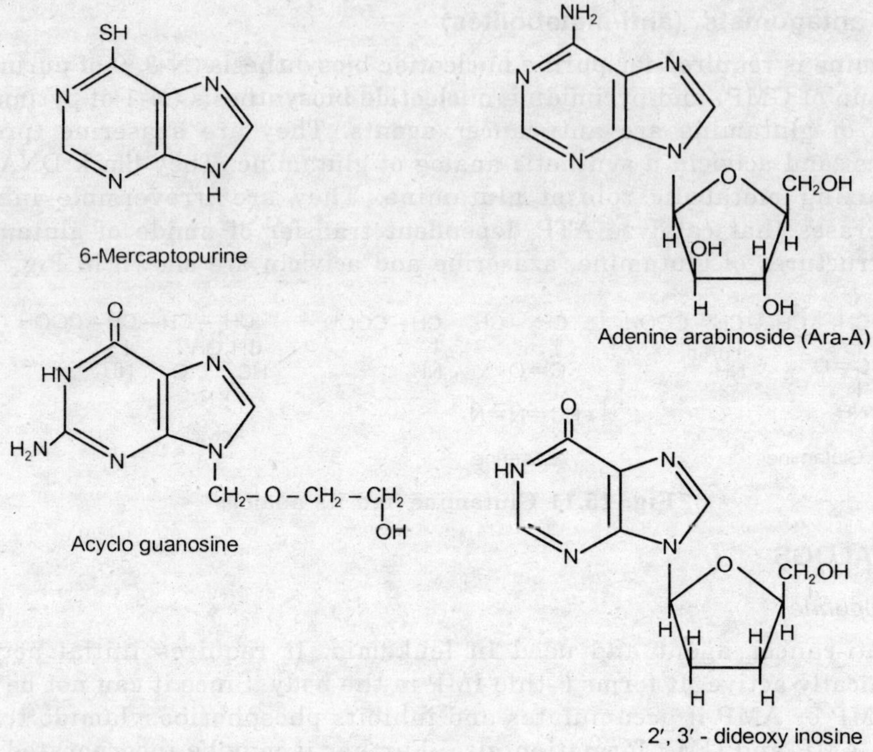

Fig. 15.12 Structures of some purine and its nucleoside analogs

Pyrimidine analogs

1. 5-Fluorouracil

It is converted to fluoro deoxy uridine monophosphate (dFUMP) by salvage pathway enzymes Fig. 15.13. dFUMP competes with dUMP to bind at active site of thymidylate synthase and forms irreversible enzyme-dFUMP-FH_4 ternary complex. Prior to forming ternary complex dFUMP undergoes part of reaction and for this reason dFUMP is referred as suicide substrate. Release of free enzyme from complex is thus blocked. This reduces the availability of d TMP and dTTP for DNA synthesis. This blocks cell division and thus tumor growth. Further, dFUMP is converted to dFUTP and may be incorporated into DNA and RNA.

Pyrimidine nucleoside analogs

1. **5-Fluorodeoxy uridine (dFU)** It is an anti-tumor agent. It is a nucleoside of fluorouracil. Its action is due to its conversion to fluorodeoxy uridine monophosphate (d FUMP) in the body (see above).
2. **De azauridine** It is an anti-tumor agent. It is a nucleoside containing altered uracil base. It inhibits ribonucleotide reductase after phosphorylation.

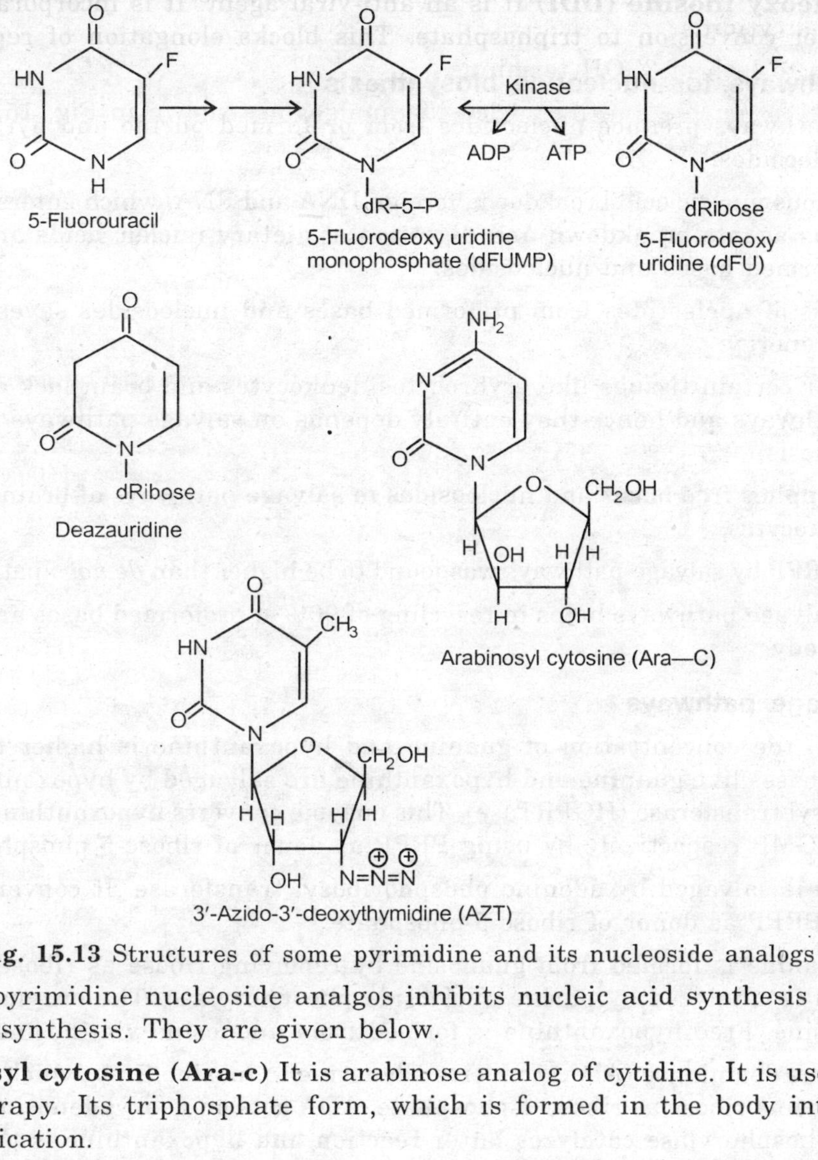

Fig. 15.13 Structures of some pyrimidine and its nucleoside analogs

Some of pyrimidine nucleoside analgos inhibits nucleic acid synthesis rather than nucleotide biosynthesis. They are given below.

1. **Arabinosyl cytosine (Ara-c)** It is arabinose analog of cytidine. It is used in cancer chemotherapy. Its triphosphate form, which is formed in the body interfers with DNA replication.
2. **3′-Azido-3′ deoxy thymidine (AZT) or Azothymidine** It is used in the treatment of AIDS. It inhibits HIV reverse transcriptase after its conversion to triphosphate.

Structures of pyrimidine and its nucleoside analogs are given in Fig. 15.13.

Orotic acid uria

It is an inherited disease in which pyrimidine nucleotide biosynthesis is defective. The condition is characterized by accumulation of orotic acid in the blood and its increased excretion in urine. Growth retardation and anemia are seen in affected individual. It is due to deficiency of orotate phosphoribosyl transferase and orotidylate decarboxylase. Orotic aciduria also occurs with allopurinol treatment. The reason for this is explained in later part of this chapter. A mild orotic acid uria occurs in deficiency of ornithine transcarbamolyase. Remission of anaemia occurs on administration of uridine and cytidine.

Salvage pathways for nucleotide biosynthesis

1. These pathways produce nucleotides from preformed purine and pyrimidine bases and nucleosides.
2. Endogenous nucleic acid breakdown, foreign DNA and RNA, which enters body through infectious agents breakdown and digestion of dietary nucleic acids are the sources for preformed bases and nucleosides.
3. Synthesis of nucleotides from preformed bases and nucleosides saves considerable cellular energy.
4. Moreover certain tissues like eryhrocytes, leukocytes and brain lack enzymes of *de novo* pathways and hence they entirely depends on salvage pathways for nucleotide biosynthesis.
5. Liver supplies free bases and nucleosides to salvage pathways of brain, erythrocytes and leukocytes.
6. Use of PRPP by salvage pathways was found to be higher than *de novo* pathways in man.
7. These salvage pathways helps in recycling of 90% of preformed bases and nucleosides in the body.

Purine salvage pathways

In the blood, the concentration of guanine and hypoxanthine is higher than adenine. Free purine bases like guanine and hypoxanthine are salvaged by hypoxanthine-guanine phosphoribosyl transferase (HGPRTase). This enzyme converts hypoxanthine and guanine to IMP and GMP respectively by using PRPP as donor of ribose-5-phosphate.

Adenine is salvaged by adenine phosphoribosyl transferase. It converts adenine to AMP using PRPP as donor of ribose-5-phosphate.

Free guanine is formed from guanosine by removing ribose as ribose-1-phosphate. The reaction is catalyzed by purine nucleoside phosphorylase. The enzyme also acts on deoxyguanosine. Free hypoxanthine is formed from adenosine via inosine.

Adenosine deaminase (ADA) converts adenosine to inosine first, which is followed by release of inosine ribose as ribose-1-phosphate. ADA acts on deoxyadenosine also. Purine nucleoside phosphorylase catalyzes latter reaction and hypoxanthine is the product.

Adenosine nucleosidase catalyzes the formation of adenine from adenosine by removing ribose as ribose-1-phosphate.

Alternatively, purine nucleosides are salvaged by distinct kinases which, phosphorylates nucleosides. Adenosine kinase catalyzes conversion of adenosine to AMP. Deoxy adenosine and deoxyguanosine are salvaged by deoxy adenosine kinase.

Energy aspect of purine salvage pathways

Only two high-energy bonds are required fro the conversion of free bases to nucleoside mono phosphates (one high energy bond for PRPP formation and another high energy bond by way of PP hydrolysis).

One high energy bond is used for the formation of nucleoside monophosphates from nucleosides.

Purine salvage pathways are summarized in Fig. 15.14.

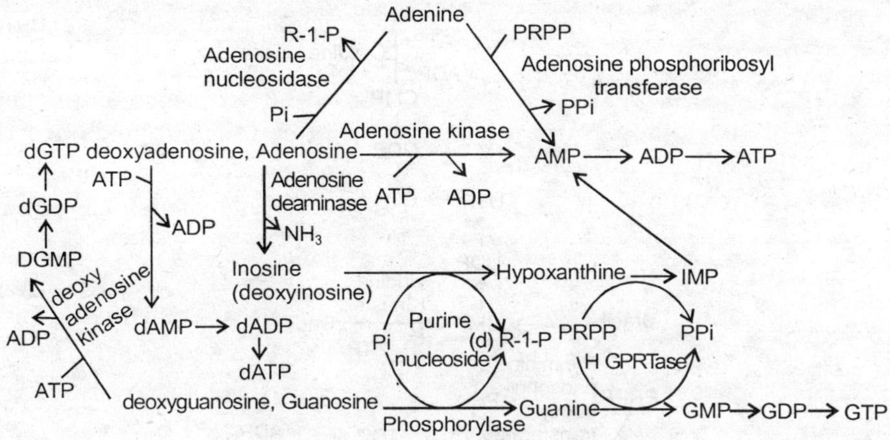

Fig. 15.14 Purine salvage pathways

Pyrimidine salvage pathways

Free pyrimidine bases are salvaged by pyrimidine phosphoribosyl transferase. It catalyses conversion of uracil or thymine to UMP and TMP using PRPP as donor of ribose phosphate. It also acts on 5-fluorouracil and orotate. Thymine is salvaged by thymidine phosphorylase. It catalyzes conversion of thymine to deoxy thymidine by incorporating deoxy ribose. It is a reversible reaction.

Pyrimidine nucleosides are salvaged by distinct pyrimidine nucleoside kinases. They phosphorylate nucleosides using ATP as phosphate donor. Cytidine and deoxy cytidine are phsophorylated by cytidine kinase and deoxy cytidine kinase, respectively. Likewise deoxy thymidine is phosphorylated by thymidine kinase a well distributed enzyme of pyrimidine salvage pathway. Uridine is phosphorylated by uridine kinase. Pyrimidine salvage pathways are summarized in Fig. 15.15.

Medical importance

Salvage pathways are affected in some diseases or syndromes.

1. Immuno deficiency disease

It may be due to

(*a*) Lack of adenosine deaminase (ADA). It leads to accumulation of deoxy adenosine and increased production of dATP from deoxy adenosine by salvage pathway. Since ATP is an effective inhibitor of ribonucleotide reductase synthesis of other deoxy nucleoside triphosphates is blocked. T-lymphocytes as well as B-lymphocytes do not mature due to impaired DNA synthesis. Affected individuals are more prone to infections. This condition is usually called as *severe combined immunodeficiency disease* (SCIDD).

(*b*) Deficiency of purine nucleoside phosphorylase. It is a milder form only **T-lymphocyte** production is impaired. Lack of this enzyme leads to accumulation of deoxy **guanosine** and dGTP. This blocks conversion of CDP to dCDP by ribonucleotide reductase. So, dCTP required for a DNA synthesis is not available and proliferation of T-cells is impaired.

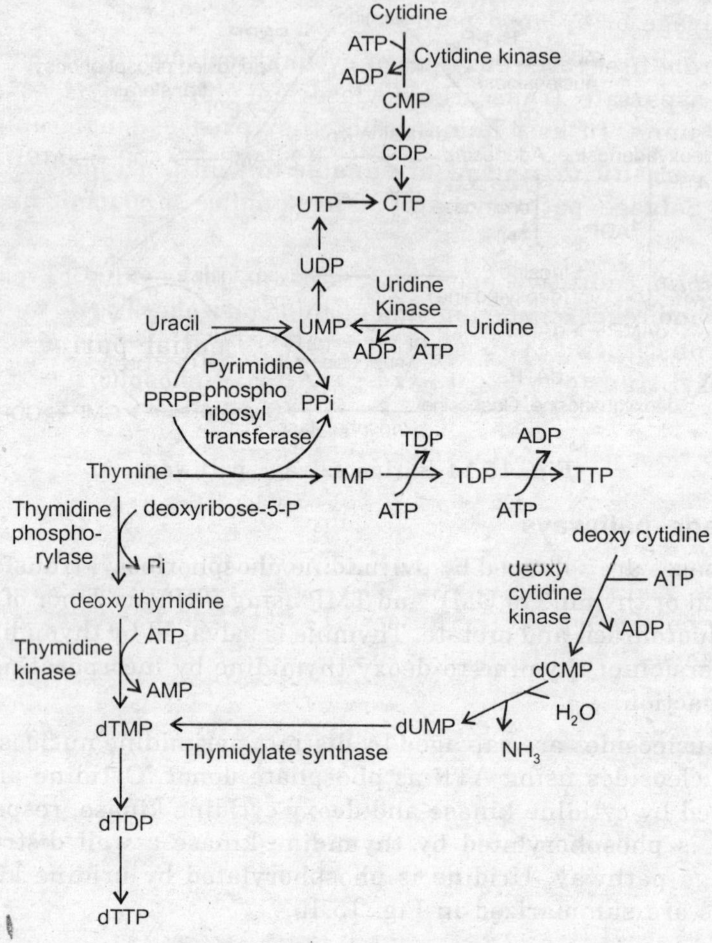

Fig. 15.15 Pyrimidine salvage pathways

2. Lesch-Nyhan syndrome

It is due to lack of HGPRT ase. Lack of this enzyme leads to accumulation of PRPP and decreased IMP or GMP levels. Since PRPP is a positive effector of amidotransferase purine nucleotide synthesis is promoted. In addition, low levels of IMP or GMP also promotes purine nucleotide biosynthesis because feed back inhibition of amidotransferase by GMP or IMP is decreased.

Symptoms are hyperuricemia, mental retardation, self mutilation and anaemia. Uric acid excretion is more in urine.

Nucleotide metabolism of malarial parasite *P. faliciparum*

Nucleotide metabolism is one area where differences exist between the pathways of *P. falcipuram* and those of human host.

1. *P. Falcipuram* synthesizes purines by the salvage pathway and pyrimidines by *denovo* pathways. AMP and GMP are synthesized from IMP which is formed from hypoxanthine by HGPRTase catalyzed reaction.
2. In human cells, purines are synthesized by *de novo* and pyrimidines are synthesized by either salvage or *de novo* pathways.
3. In *P. falcipuram* first three enzymes of pyrimidine biosynthesis carbamoyl phosphate synthetase, aspartate transcarbamoylase and dihydrorotase exist as a separate independent units. In host human cells, they exist as single unit.

Many other parasitic organisms are unable to synthesize purine nucleotides via *de novo* pathways. Salvage pathways are main supplies of purine nucleotides in these parasites.

1. *Giardia lamblia* causative agent of giardiasis lacks *de novo* pathways of purine biosynthesis and relies on adenine and guanine phosphoribosyl transferases (APRTase, GPRTase) constituting two separate and essential purine salvage pathways. Phosphoribosyl transferases catalyzes transfer of phosphoribosyl group from PRPP to purine base.
2. *Trichomones fetus* which causes embryonic death and infertility in cows depends primarily on a single enzyme of salvage pathway HGPRTase for its purine needs.

Medical importance

Malarial parasite developed resistance to several drugs that are currently used. Hence new drugs must be developed. The differences in metabolic pathways between parasite and host may be used for development of new drugs. Enzymes in salvage pathways are potential targets of new therapeutic agents.

Digestion of dietary nucleic acids

Earlier I mentioned that salvage pathways converts free bases and nucleosides of dietary nucleic acid origin to nucleotides. Hence, digestion of dietary nucleic acids is detailed here (Fig. 15.16).

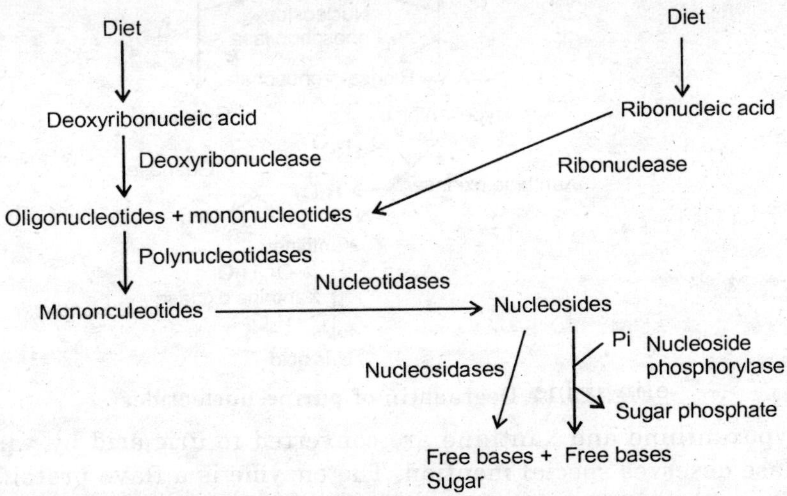

Fig. 15.16 Digestion of dietary nucleic acids

Pancreatic deoxy ribonuclease (DNAs) and ribonuclease (RNAs) initiates digestion of dietary nucleic acids in the duodenum. They are endonucleases and hence deoxyribonuclease converts deoxy ribonucleic acids to deoxy oligonucleotides and deoxy monoribonucleotides where as ribonuclease converts ribonucleic acids to oligo ribonucleotides and mono ribonucleotides.

Polynucleotidases and nucleotidases present in intestinal secretions converts oligonucleotides to nucleotides and mononucleotides to nucleosides respectively.

Nucleotidases also hydrolyze nucleotides formed from oligonocleotides to nucleosides.

Nucleosides may be absorbed as such or they may be converted to free bases by the action of nucleosidases and reaches liver though portal circulation.

Degradation of Purine nucleotides

Liver is the major organ involved in degradation of purine nucleotides. Lysosomal enzymes converts nucleic acids to nucleotides. Majority of purine nucleotides so produced are AMP and GMP. AMP is converted to IMP by adenylate deaminase present in most of the tissues. Next, nucleotidases convert IMP, AMP and GMP to corresponding nucleosides namely inosine, adenosine and guanosine. By the action of adenosine deaminase adenosine is converted to inosine. Now purine nucleoside phosphorylase converts guanosine to guanine and inosine to hypoxanthine by transferring ribose. Deamination of guanine by guanase produces xanthine (Fig. 15.17).

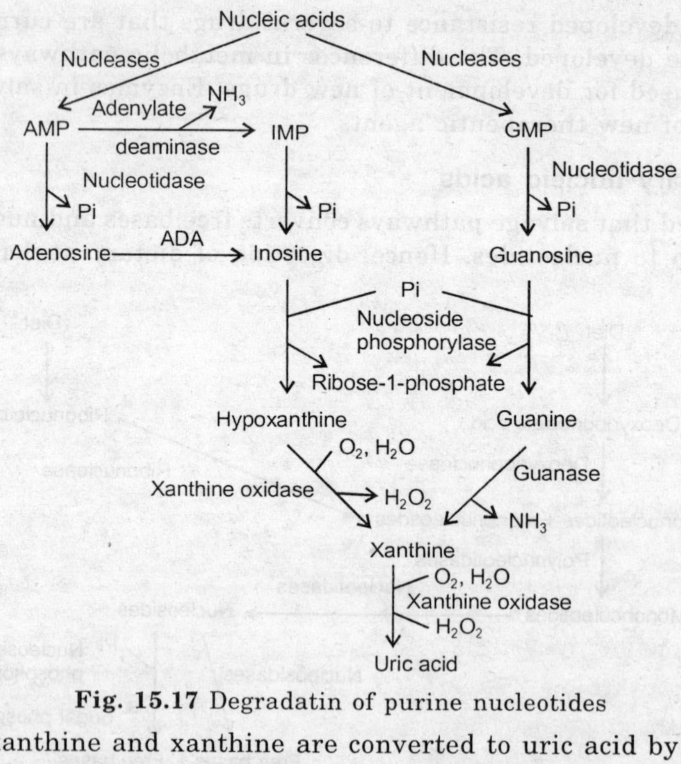

Fig. 15.17 Degradatin of purine nucleotides

Finally hypoxanthine and xanthine are converted to uric acid by xanthine oxidase. Xanthine oxidase deserves special mention. The enzyme is a flavo protein contains FAD and molybdenum (Mo). It is concentrated in liver and intestine. It contains two iron sulfur clusters. Enzyme produces highly toxic H_2O_2 along with products which is removed by catalase. Further role of xanthine oxidase is given later.

Medical Importance

Catabolism of purine nucleotides is abnormal in some diseases. Hence normal fate of uric acid which is end product of purine catabolism is given below.

Fate of uric acid

Uric acid produced in different tissues diffuses into circulation and carried to kidneys for elimination. Uric acid daily production is about 500-600mg. However, most of it is removed by kidney. Daily output is about 0.3-0.5 gm/day on normal diet. The normal blood uric acid level is below 6 mg/100ml. So one can expect that impaired renal function may lead to accumulation of uric acid in blood.

Gout

It is common disease associated with excessive purine catabolism. It is characterized by hyperuricemia and excessive excretion of uric acid in urine. It is more common in men (95%). Incidence rate is 3 in 1000.

Clinical symptoms

Since uric acid is less soluble in the body fluid aqueous environment excessive uric acid leads to formation and deposition of urate crystals in joints, cartilage of fingers, big toe and other soft tissues. 'Tophi' is the name given to urate deposits. Deposition of urate in joints leads to gouty arthritic attacks.

Hyperuricemia or gout is due to

(*a*) Over production of uric acid.

(*b*) Impaired excretion of uric acid.

1. **Primary gout** It is due to excessive formation of purine nucleotides and their degradation. It is an inherited disease. It occurs due to

   (*a*) Deficiency of HGPRT ase (Lesch-Nyhan syndrome).

   (*b*) Increased PRPP synthase activity.

2. **Secondary gout** It can be acquired as well as inherited disease. It occurs as consequence of other diseases, which cause excessive uric acid production. They are

   (*a*) Leukemia, polycythemia. Nucleic acid turnover is more in both these diseases which is responsible for uricemia.

   (*b*) Von-Gierke's disease. In this disease, glucose-6-phosphate accumulates due to lack of glucose-6-phosphatase, which is diverted to HMP shunt. As a result more pentose phosphates are produced. This leads to accumulation of PRPP and increased purine nucleotide biosynthesis.

   (*c*) Increased glutathione reductase activity.

3. **Renal gout** If the hyperuricemia is due to impaired excretion of uric acid by kidney then it is called as renal gout. It occurs due to

   (*a*) Defective uric acid transport in renal tubules.

   (*b*) Glomerulonephritis.

Treatment

Since many symptoms of gout are related to excessive uric acid in body drugs used in treatment of gout work by lowering uric acid production or level.

Hypoxanthine analog

Allopurinol is the drug used in the treatment of gout. It is a hypoxanthine analog which is substrate for xanthine oxidase. Since allopurinol is structurally similar to hypoxanthine one might expect that it inhibits xanthine oxidase by binding at active site. However situation is different *in vivo*. Indeed, uric acid production decreases in allopurinol administered patients due to irreversible inactivation of xanthine oxidase by alloxanthine (Fig. 15.18). Xanthine oxidase converts allopurinol to alloxanthine by hydroxylation. Hence, allopurinol can be considered as prodrug. It is converted to active drug by xanthine oxidase, which subsequently inactivate the enzyme and thus uric acid production is decreased. This type of enzyme inactivation is often referred as suicide inhibition.

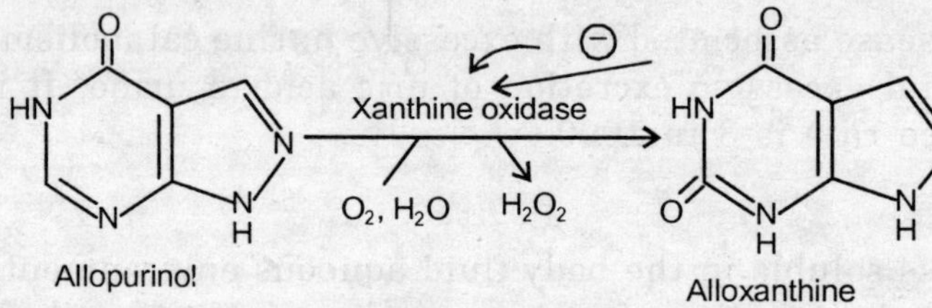

Fig. 15.18 Conversion of allopurinol to alloxanthine by xanthine oxidase

Sulfin pyrazone and proben acid

These drugs lower uric acid level by increasing its excretion by kidney. They interfers with tubular reabsorption of uric acid. They are uricosuric drugs.

Xanthinuria

It is an inherited disease and characterized by hypouricemia and increased excretion of hypoxanthine and xanthine in urine. Hepatic or intestinal xanthine oxidase is deficient. In severe cases, xanthine lithiasis may occur due to deposition of xanthine crystals in kidney.

Degradation of pyrimidine nucleotides

Liver is the major organ involved in breakdown of pyrimidine nucleotides. Since pyrimidine ring is part of purine ring one might expect that pyrimidine nucleotide degradation is similar to purine nucleotide degradation. However, the degradative pattern of pyrimidine nucleotides differs from purine nucleotide degradation. Pyrimidine nucleotide are degraded to amino acids β-alanine and β-amino isobutyric acid (BAIB) by cleaving pyrimidine ring.

Catabolism of pyrimidine nucleotides proceeds in three phases depending on organism (Fig. 15.19). Nucleases convert nucleic acids to pyrimidine nucleotides.

1. In the first phase, pyrimidine nucleotides undergoes dephosphorylation, deamination and glycosidic bond cleavage reactions to yield free bases.
2. In the second phase, uracil and thymine undergo sequence of reduction (unusual in degradative phase) hydration and deamination reactions to yield β-alanine and β-amino isobutyric acid.

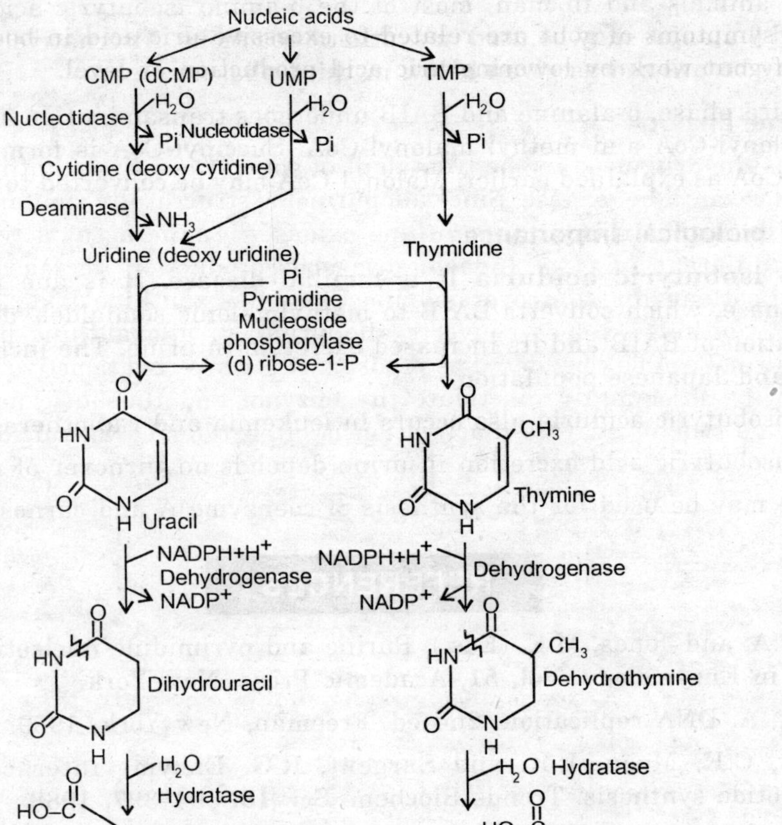

Fig. 15.19 Reactions of pyrimidine nucleotide catabolism ~~~ indicates cleavage

In many animals and in man, most of the β-amino isobutyric acid is excreted in urine and β-alanine may be used in synthetic reactions. Alternatively, β-alanine and BAIB may be utilized as given below in third phase.

3. In the third phase, β-alanine and BAIB undergoes transamination and activation to yield malonyl-CoA and methyl malonyl-CoA. Succinyl-CoA is formed from methyl malonyl-CoA as explained earlier. Malonyl-CoA may be converted to CO_2 ultimately.

Medical and biological Importance

1. **β-Amino isobutyric aciduria** It is familial disease. It is due to deficiency of transaminase, which converts BAIB to methylmalonic semialdehyde. This leads to accumulation of BAIB and its increased excretion in urine. The incidence is 25% in Chinese and Japanese population.
2. β-amino isobutyric aciduria also occurs in leukemia and radiotherapy.
3. β-amino isobutyric acid excretion in urine depends on turnover of nucleic acids.
4. β-alanine may be used for the synthesis of coenzyme A and carnosine.

REFERENCES

1. Hoffee, P.A. and Jones, M.E. (Eds.). Purine and pyrimidine nucleotide metabolism. Methods in Enzymology. Vol. 51, Academic Press, New York.
2. Kornberg, A. DNA replication. 2nd ed. Freeman, New York, 1989.
3. Mathews, C.K. Moen, L.K. and Sargent, R.G. Enzyme interactions in deoxy ribonucleotide synthesis. Trends Biochem. Sci. **13**, 394–397, 1988.
4. Reichard, P. and Ehrenberg, A. Ribonucleotide reductase, Science **221**, 514, 1983.
5. Murray, A.W. The biological significance of purine salvage. Ann. Rev. Biochem. **40**, 811, 1971.
6. Wilson, J.M. HGPRTase deficiency. New Engl. J. Med. **309**, 900, 1983.
7. Kelly, W.N. and Smith I.H. Hereditary orotic acid uria. In Stanbury, J.B; Wyngarden, J.B. and Frederickson, D.S. (Eds.) The metabolic basis of inherited diseases. 4 ed. Mc Graw-Hill, New York, 1978.
8. Lo, B. Hyperuricemia and gout. West J. Med **142**, 104, 1985.
9. Goldstein, Barry, M. and Krzysztof, P. (Eds.). Inosine monophosphate (IMP) dehydrogenase; A major therapeutic target. American Chemical Society, 2003.
10. Chang, M.C.Y. *et al.* Turning on ribonucleotide reductase by light initiated amino acid radical generation. Proc. Natl. Acad. Sci. USA **101**, 6882-6887, 2004.
11. Barsott, C. *et al.* Purine and pyrimidine salvage in whole rat brain. J. Biol. Chem. **277**, 9865-9869, 2002.
12. Craig, S.P. and Eukin, A.E. Purine phosphoribosyl transferases. J. Biol. Chem. **275**, 20231-20234, 2000.
13. Sarver, A.E. and Weng, C.C. The adenine phosphoribosyl transferase from *giardia lamblia.* J. Biol. Chem. **277**, 39973-39980, 2002.

14. Borza, T. *et al.* Variations in the response of mouse isoenzymes of adenylosuccinate synthatase to inhibitors of physiological relevance. J. Biol. Chem. **278**, 6673-6679, 2003.

15. Genini, D. *et al.* Nucleotide requirements for *in vitro* activation of apoptosis protein activating factor – 1 (Apaf-1) mediated caspase pathway. J. Biol. Chem. **275**, 29-34, 2000.

16. Scott, G.S. *et al.* Uric acid protects against secondary damage after spinal cord injury. Proc. Natl. Acad. Sci. USA. **102**, 3483-3488, 2005.

17. Graphen Giesser, E. *et al.* External ATP triggers Ca^{2+} signals suited for synchronization of pancreatic β-cells. J. Endocrimol. **185**, 69-79, 2005.

EXERCISES

ESSAY QUESTIONS

1. Describe de novo pathway of purine nucleotide biosyntheis. Add a note on energy consumed in this process.
2. Trace the pathway for the formation of UMP from CO_2 and aspartate. Add a note on regulation of this pathway.
3. Write an essay on drugs that work by acting at various stages of purine and pyrimidine nucleotide biosynthesis.
4. Trace the pathway for the formation of AMP and GMP from ribose –5-phosphate. How this pathway is regulated?

SHORT QUESTIONS

1. Write purine ring. Label origins of its carbon and nitrogen atoms.
2. Write a note on ribonucleotide reductase.
3. Write salient features of salvage pathways. How purine bases are salvaged ?
4. Trace purine nucleotide degradation reactions.
5. Define gout. Name conditions which cause gout.
6. Write biochemical defect in (*a*) severe combined immuno deficiency syndrome (SCID) (*b*) Lesch-Nyhan syndrome.
7. Write normal plasma uric acid level. In what diseases it is elevated ? How drugs used to lower this level work? Explain.
8. Write briefly on digestion of nucleic acids.
9. Write a note on antimetabolites.

MULTIPLE CHOICE QUESTIONS

1. Inhibition of dihydrofolate reductase by aminopterin.

   (*a*) Prevents growth of cancer cells.

   (*b*) Promotes cancer cell growth.

   (*c*) Leads to remission of cancer due to lack of FH_4.

   (*d*) Is an example for enzyme inhibition.

2. Glutamine antagonists work as anticancer agents
   (*a*) By inhibiting amido transferases.
   (*b*) By blocking purine nucleotide formation.
   (*c*) By inhibiting amido transferases that catalyze transfer of amide of glutamine to an acceptor.
   (*d*) By blocking formation of AMP from IMP.
3. Fluoro deoxy uridine monophosphate (dFUMP) is
   (*a*) Suicide substrate.
   (*b*) Suicide substrate of thymidylate synthase.
   (*c*) Inhibitor of thymidylate synthase.
   (*d*) Formed from uracil.
4. All of the following statements are true for orotic aciduria. Except
   (*a*) Orotic acid is excreted in urine.
   (*b*) Anaemia is a symptom of this disease.
   (*c*) Growth retardation is seen in affected people.
   (*d*) Self mutilation is another symptom of this disease.
5. Hypoxanthine–guanine phosphoribosyl transferase is
   (*a*) An enzyme of purine salvage pathway.
   (*b*) An enzyme of de novo purine nucleotide biosynthesis.
   (*c*) Elevated in immuno-deficiency disease.
   (*d*) Inhibited by xanthine.

FILL IN THE BLANKS

1. De novo pathway of purine nucleotide synthesis is linked to --------------- pathway.
2. --------------- --------------- --------------- lack enzymes of purine nucleotide biosynthesis.
3. DNAs and RNAs are --------------- nucleases present in pancreatic fluid.
4. Inhibition of xanthine oxidase by alloxanthine is referred as --------------- inhibition.
5. BAIB excretion in urine is increased in --------------- and --------------- .

CASES

1. A mother brought 6-month-old boy to the pediatrician for his unusual urge to bite lips, fingers and failure to develop mentally. His blood picture indicated megaloblastic anaemia. Serum uric acid level was elevated and uric acid was found in excess in urine. Write your diagnosis.
2. An 8-month-old child was referred to pediatric clinic for recurrent throat and lung infections since birth. Blood picture showed decreased amounts of immunoglobulins, T and B lymphocytes. Write your diagnosis.

16
CHAPTER

NUCLEIC ACIDS

OCCURRENCE

Two types of nucleic acids are present in all mammalian cells including humans. They are DNA-deoxy ribonucleic acid and RNA-ribonucleic acid. DNA is present in nucleus and mitochondria. RNA is present in nucleus and cytoplasm. Nucleic acids are also present in bacteria, viruses and plants.

MEDICAL AND BIOLOGICAL IMPORTANCE

1. Nucleic acids serve as genetic material of living organisms including humans.
2. Nucleic acids are involved in the storage, transfer and expression of genetic information.
3. Nucleic acids contain all the necessary information required for the formation of individual or organism.
4. Nucleic acids determines physical fitness of an individual to life.
5. Some nucleic acids acts as enzymes and coenzymes. For example, RNA, act as catalyst and RNA is coenzyme for telomerase which seals ends of chromosomes.
6. DNA exhibits structural polymorphism. It assumes several forms depending on certain conditions. Several DNA variants are known.
7. Some RNAs without protein products are found recently in mammals, yeast and bacteria. They are involved in cellular functions.
8. Human Genome Project (HGP) is completed in 2000. It is considered as a major achievement of man after landing on moon. It is useful for finding causes of several diseases whose causes are unknown till. It may also lead to development of new therapeutics as well as diagnostics.

Chemical nature of nucleic acids

Nucleic acids are acidic substances containing nitrogenous bases, sugar and phosphorus. Both DNA and RNA are polynucleotides. They are polymers of nucleotides.

Phosphodiester linkage

In polynucleotides, nucleotides are joined together by phosphodiester linkage. Diester linkage of phosphate joins 3′ OH and 5′ OH belonging two separate sugars (Figure 16.1).

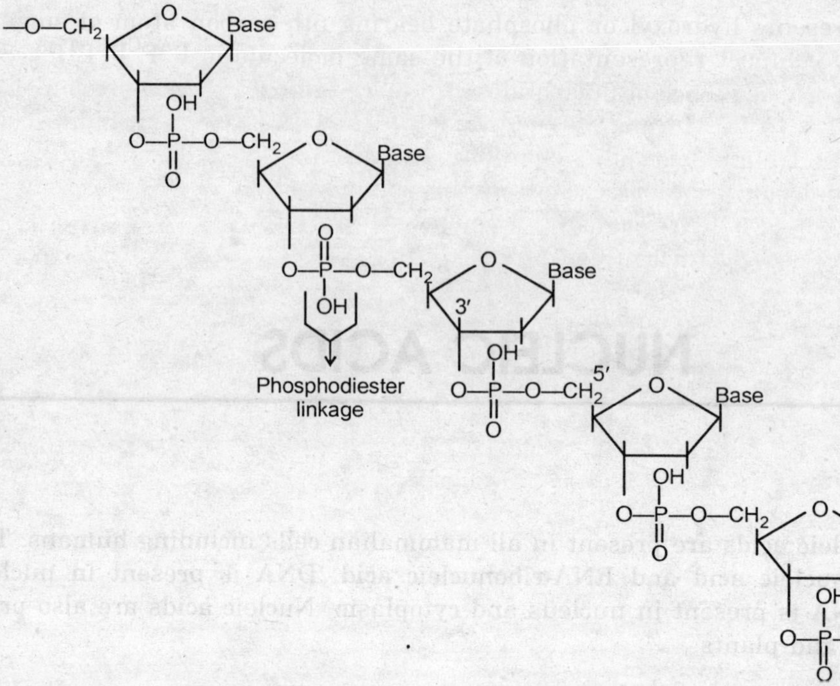

Fig. 16.1 Structure of a polynucleotide segment

Nucleic acid structure

Primary structure of nucleic acids

Nucleotide sequence of a polynucleotide is known as primary structure of nucleic acid. The primary structure confers individuality to polynucleotide chain. Polynucleotide chain has direction. They are represented in 5′ → 3′ direction only. However, the phosphodiester linkage runs in 3′ → 5′ direction. Each poly nucleotide chain has two ends. The 5′ end carrying phosphate is shown on the left hand side and 3′ end carrying unreacted hydroxyl is shown on the right hand side (Figure 16.2a). Primary structures of DNA and RNA exist in single stranded DNA and RNA organisms.

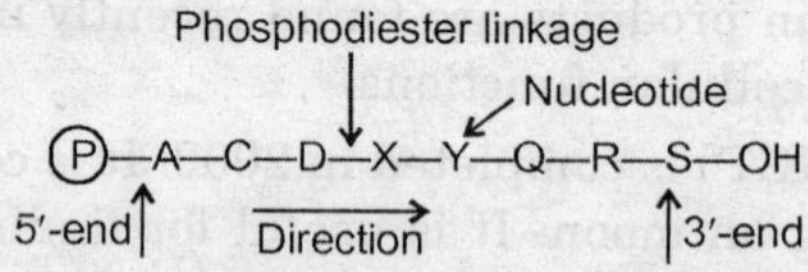

Fig. 16.2 (*a*) Primary structure of nucleic acid. Letters A, C, D, X, Y, Q, R, S are nucleotides

Short-hand representation of polynucleotides

Since polynucleotide consists of various bases, sugars and phosphates writing a segment of polynucleotide showing structures of bases, sugars with attached phosphates is awkward or highly inconvenient. So, short hand or compact representation of polynucleotide has been proposed. In compact nomenclature or polynucleotide letters A, G, C and T represents nitrogenous bases adenine, guanine, cytosine and thymine, respectively. A vertical line represents sugar back bone. The branches of verticle lines with numerals 3′ and 5′ represents hydroxyl bearing carbon atoms of sugar. A branch at the middle of the verticle line represents hydroxyl bearing 3rd carbon atom of sugar. Another branch at the bottom of verticle line represents hydroxyl or phosphate bearing 5th carbon atom of sugar (Figure 16.2b). The more compact representation of the same molecule is $P^AP^CP^GP^TP^A$. Since primary structure is the sequence of nucleotides still more compact representation of the same molecule is ACGTA. In this primary structure, letters A, G, C, T stands for nucleotides and sequence is written from left to right. Therefore, in DNA and RNA, letters A, G, C, T stands for nucleotides and sugar is deoxy ribose if the polynucleotide is a segment of DNA and sugar is ribose if it is a RNA segment. Remember that letters A, C, U, G, T stands for nucleosides in the case of nucleotides.

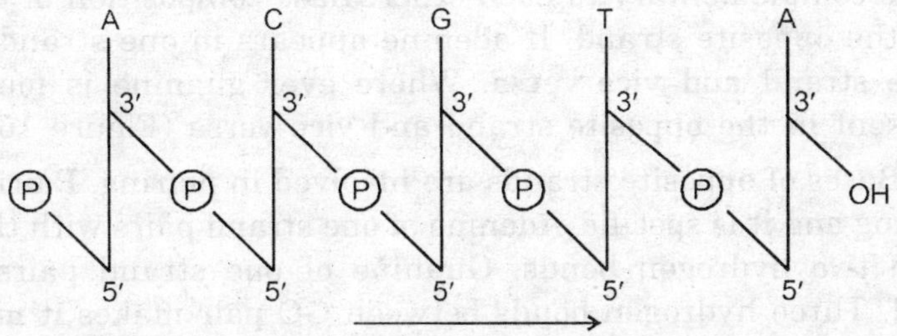

Fig. 16.2 (*b*) Short hand representation of a polynucleotide segment. Note the direction of polynucleotide chain and phosphodiester linkage

Structure of DNA

E. Chargoff and his colleagues extensively studied base composition of DNA. Their studies provided valuable information on the structure of DNA.

Characteristics of DNA base composition

1. In DNA, number of adenine residues is equal to the number of thymine residues *i.e.,* A = T. Further number of guanine residues is equal to number of cytosine residues *i.e.,* G = C. As corollary sum of purine residues is equal to sum of pyrimidine residues A + G = C + T.
2. DNAs from different tissues of same species have same base composition.
3. Base composition of DNA varies from one species to another species.
4. DNAs from closely related species have similar base composition.
5. DNAs of widely different species have different base composition.
6. DNA base composition of a species is not affected by age, nutritional state and environment.

In 1953, J.D. Watson and F.H.C. Crick proposed precise three dimentional model of DNA structure based on model building studies, base composition and X-ray diffraction studies. This model is popularly known as DNA double helix. Using this model, they also suggested a precise mechanism for the transfer of genetic information to daughter cells from parent cells.

Salient features of double helix

1. Two polynucleotide chains are coiled around a central axis in the form of right handed double helix. It represents secondary structure of DNA. It is present in double stranded DNA containing organisms (Figure 16.3a).

2. Each polynucleotide chain is made up of 4 types of nucleotides. They are adenylate, guanylate, thymidylate and cytidylate.
3. Each polynucleotide chain has direction or polarity. Further each polynucleotide chain has 5′ phosphorylated and 3′ hydroxyl end.
4. The back bone of each strand consist of alternating sugar and phosphates. The bases projects inwards and they are perpendicular to the central axis (Figure 16.3c).
5. The two strands run in opposite direction, i.e., they are anti-parallel.
6. The strands are complementary to each other. Base composition of one strand is complementary to the opposite strand. If adenine appears in one strand thymine is found in the opposite strand and vice versa. Where ever guanine is found in one strand cytosine is present in the opposite strand and vice versa (Figure 16.3a).
7. **Base pairing** Bases of opposite strands are involved in pairing. Pairing occurs through hydrogen bonding and it is specific. Adenine of one strand pairs with thymine of opposite strand through two hydrogen bonds. Guanine of one strand pairs with cytosine of opposite strand. Three hydrogen bonds between GC pair makes it more stronger than AT pair (Figures 16.3b).

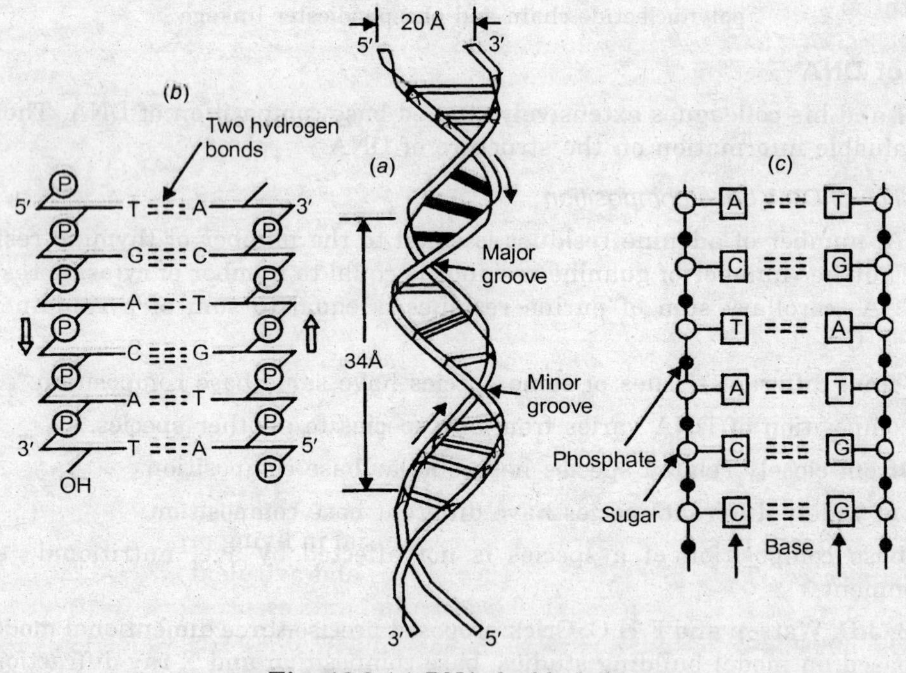

Fig. 16.3 (*a*) DNA double helix

(*b*) Base pairing among complementary bases of opposite strands

(*c*) Alternating sugar and phosphate form back bone of strnad. Bases project inwards and perpendicular to central axis

8. Complementarity of strands and base pairing are the outstanding features of Watson-Crick model. Specific base pairing immediately suggests a copying mechanism for DNA.
9. The large number of hydrogen bonds along entire length of DNA makes DNA molecule highly stable.

10. Major and minor grooves are present on double helix. They arise because glycosidic bonds of base pairs are not opposite to each other.
11. The base pairs are stacked and 3.4 Å apart. The pitch of the helix (One turn) is 34 A^{o} and accommodates ten base pairs.
12. Apart from hydrogen bonding, the double helix is stabilized by hydrophobic attraction between bases.
13. The width of double helix is 20 Å.
14. Watson-Crick model is known as B-DNA. Majority of the nuclear DNA is in B-form.

Functions of DNA

1. DNA is the genetic material of living systems. It is super chip ever made by man present in living systems.
2. DNA contains all the information required for the formation of an individual or organism.
3. The genetic information in DNA is converted to characteristic features of living organisms like colour of the skin and eye, height, intelligence, ability to metabolize particular substance, ability to with stand stress, susceptibility to disease and unable to produce or synthesize certain substances etc.
4. All the above phenotype characters of living organisms are intimately related to functions of proteins. Thus, DNA is the source of information for the synthesis of all cellular proteins. The segment of DNA that contains information for a protein is known as *gene.*
5. DNA is transmitted from parent to off spring and hence DNA flows from one generation to other in a given species. Further, DNA provides information inherited by daughter cells from parent cells.
6. The amount of DNA per cell is proportional to the complexity of the organism and hence to the amount of genetic information. The amount of DNA in mammalian cell is 1000 times more than bacteria. Likewise, bacteria contains more DNA than virus and plasmids.
7. The amount of DNA in any given species or cell is constant and is not affected by nutritional or metabolic states.

DNA as the gene

Studies on bacterial transformation carried out by Avery and his colleagues provided first experimental evidence to prove DNA is genetic material in living organisms. They used two types of pneumococci. They are virulent (pathogenic) and avirulent (non-pathogenic) types. DNA isolated from heat killed virulent organism when introduced into avirulent organism it transformed avirulent organism into virulent organism. Deoxy ribonuclease treatment of DNA isolated prior to introduction destroyed transforming capacity of DNA. These observations indicated that DNA is a genetic material.

Other forms of DNA

Most of the DNA in the genome is in B-form. Other forms of DNA are

1. **A-DNA** When DNA fibre is dehydrated it acquires another form. It is known as A-DNA. It is shorter than B-DNA. The base pairs are not perpendicular to the axis they are tilted by 19°. In A and B forms, glycosidic bonds are in 'anti' conformation.

2. **Z-DNA** It is left handed double helix. A small stretch of Z-DNA can occur in B-DNA. Z-DNA is due to the presence of dinucleotides like CG CG CG containing alternate purine and pyrimidine bases. In Z-DNA, glycosidic bonds are in syn conformation.

Eukaryotic DNA

In non-dividing eukaryotic cell DNA exist as nucleoprotein called *chromatin*. Chromatin consist of DNA and basic proteins histones. This organizes into 23 pairs of chromosomes before cell division. Each chromosome represents one DNA molecule. The chromosomal DNA has length of about 30-60 mm. Such long molecule is present in nucleus whose dimension is less than 5 microns (5 u) (1 u = 10^{-3} mm). So, DNA molecule is tightly packed such that it can be accommodated within nuclear limit. Histones are used for packing of DNA. Five types of histones are used for packing of DNA. They are H1, H2A, H2B, H3 and H4.

Nucleosomes

Whole DNA is not packed as single coil instead it is present as small coils known as nucleosomes. Each nucleosome consist of histone octamer, which is made up of two units of H2A, H2B, H3 and H4 histones and DNA. Usually DNA is coiled around octamer, and approximately it takes two turns around histone octamer. Each nucleosome is joined by linker DNA and HI type of histones (Figure 16.4a). The nucleosomes along with linker DNAs appears as beads on a string under electron microscope (Figure 16.4b). Further coiling of nucleosomes forms chromatin fibre. Thus, long thread likc DNA molecule is folded into chromosomes.

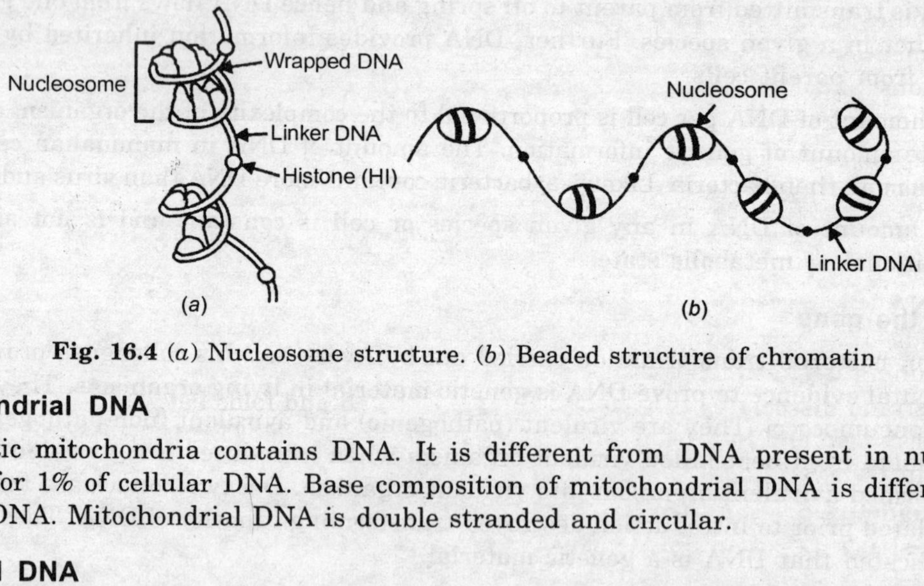

Fig. 16.4 (*a*) Nucleosome structure. (*b*) Beaded structure of chromatin

Mitochondrial DNA

Eukaryotic mitochondria contains DNA. It is different from DNA present in nucleus. It account for 1% of cellular DNA. Base composition of mitochondrial DNA is different from nuclear DNA. Mitochondrial DNA is double stranded and circular.

Bacterial DNA

Bacteria like *E. Coli* contains single molecule of double stranded DNA. *E. Coli* DNA is 1.4 mm long which is 700 times bigger than the size of bacteria. Hence in bacteria also DNA is tightly packed or folded. In *E. Coli* the two ends of DNA are joined to form circular DNA. Histones are not used for packing of bacterial DNA because they are absent in bacteria. Super coiling of circular DNA allows its containment with in nuclear zone. Super-coiled DNA may be in association with some proteins, which stabilizes super coil (Figure 16.5a).

Viral DNA

Viruses are extremely small particles. They are composed of a piece of DNA, which is surrounded by protein coat called *capsid*. Viral DNA may be single stranded or double stranded. Adeno virus (cold virus), Herpes virus and Pox virus are examples for double stranded viruses. Parvo virus is a example for single strand DNA virus (Figure 16.5b).

Plasmids

They exist in bacteria as circular DNA molecules. Plasmid DNA is different from bacterial DNA. They are present in anti-biotic resistant bacteria. They contain genes for inactivation of anti-biotics. pBR 322 of *E. Coli* is an example for plasmid. Plasmids are used as vectors in genetic engineering (Figure 16.5c).

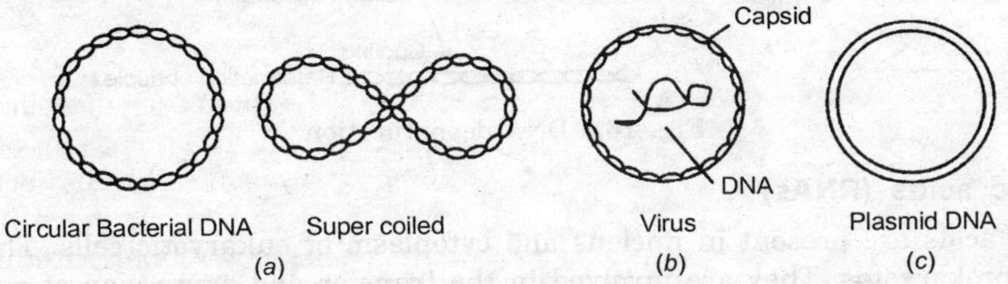

Fig. 16.5 (*a*) Bacterial DNA (*b*) Virus (*c*) Plasmid

DNA structural polymorphism or DNA variants

Recent studies have established existence of several forms of DNA structures not just A, B and Z as mentioned earlier. The helical structure of DNA assumes various forms depending on conditions. Some DNA structures show minor differences from Watson-Crick model while many of them are completely different in essential features such as handedness, base pairing and number of strands. DNA variants are identified by one letter code and currently there are polymorphic DNA structures associated with 21 of 26 letters of English alphabet. Only, F, Q, U, V and Y are not used.

Few unusual and interesting DNA structures are

(*a*) **H-DNA** It is an intramolecular triple helical structure of DNA. It is made up of three strands. It is formed at low P^H conditions. This type of structure is formed in DNA containing long stretches of polypurine and polypyrimidine sequences. The pyrimidine rich strand dissociates from complementary strand and folds back on itself to lie in the major groove and hydrogen bonded to purine rich strand. This type of structures plays role in transcriptional control of gene expression.

(*b*) **G-Quadruplex structure** It is made up of four strands. Several four-stranded quadruplex DNA structures occurs in G-rich DNA sequences. They are also known as G-tetrads. In these DNA structures, the four strands are parallely arranged. They are found in telomeric regions of chromosomes.

(*c*) **Holliday junction** This type of DNA structure forms during genetic recombination. One of the strand from each of the duplex DNA molecules exchange to form four ways junction, which is known as Holliday junction.

Thus DNA molecule has chameleon like property assumes various forms depending on environment.

Denaturation of DNA

When DNA molecule is heated it denatures and strands separate. Thermal denaturation of DNA is known as melting of DNA. Melting point of DNA is known as *Tm*. It is a characteristic of given DNA. If the heat denatured DNA is cooled base pairing occurs between strands and reformation of double, stranded molecule takes place. This process is known as *annealing*. It is very useful in genetic engineering particularly in DNA hybridization techniques (Figure 16.6).

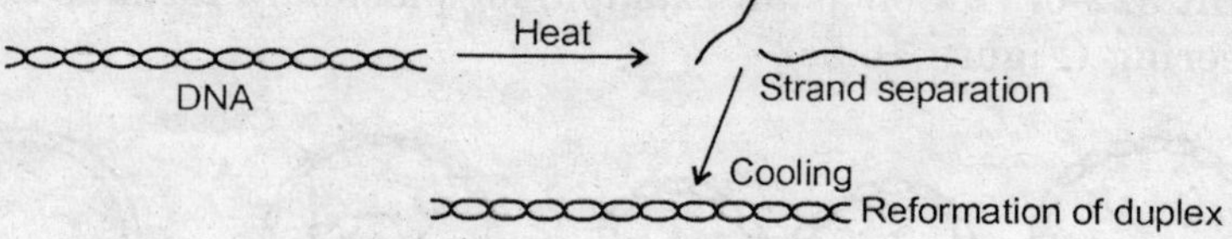

Fig. 16.6 DNA deenaturation

Ribonucleic acids (RNAs)

Ribonucleic acids are present in nucleus and cytoplasm of eukaryotic cells. They are also present in prokaryotes. They are involved in the transfer and expression of genetic information. They act as primers for DNA formation. Some RNA act as enzymes as well as coenzymes. RNA also function as genetic material for viruses.

Chemical nature of ribonucleic acids

Like DNAs, RNAs are also poly nucleotides. In RNA polymer, purine and pyrimidine nucleotides are linked together through phosphodiester linkage. The sugar present in a RNA is ribose.

There are mainly three types of RNAs in all prokaryotic and eukaryotic cells. The three types of RNA are 1. Messenger RNA or m-RNA, 2. Transfer RNA or t-RNA, 3. Ribosmal RNA or r-RNA. They differ from each other by size, function and stability.

Messenger RNA

It accounts for 1-5% of cellular RNA.

Structure

1. Majority of mRNA has primary structure. They are single-stranded linear molecules. They consist of 1000-10,000 nucleotides (Figure 16.7a).
2. mRNA molecules have free or phosphorylated 3' and 5' end.
3. mRNA molecules have different life spans. Their life span ranges from few minutes to days.
4. Eukaryotic mRNA are more stable than prokaryotic mRNA.
5. The mRNA nucleotide sequence is complementary from which it is synthesized or copied.
6. Some eukaryotic mRNA molecules are capped at 5' end. The cap is methylated GTP (m^7 GTP). Some mRNA contain internal methylated nucleotides. Capping protects mRNA from nuclease attack.

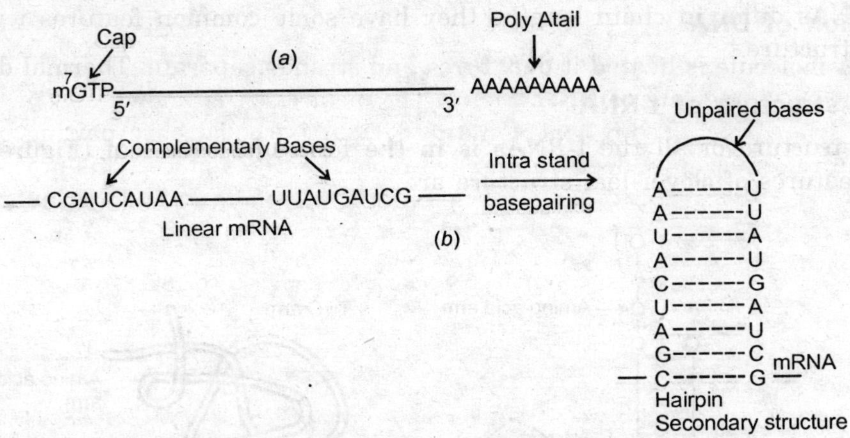

Fig. 16.7 (*a*) Structure of mRNA
(*b*) Secondary structure formation from linear mRNA molecules

7. At 3′ end of most of eukaryotic mRNA, a polymer of adenylate (poly A) is found as tail. Poly A tail protects mRNA from nucleaes attack.
8. In prokaryotes 5′ end of mRNA contains a sequence rich in A and G. Such sequence is known as *Shine-Dalgarno sequence*. It helps attachment of mRNA with ribosome during protein synthesis.
9. Some prokaryotic mRNA has secondary structure. Intrastrand base paring among complementary bases allows folding of liner molecule. As a result hairpin, or loop like secondary structure is formed. (Figure 16.7b).

Functions

1. mRNA is direct carrier of genetic information from the nucleus to the cytoplasm.
2. Usually a molecule of mRNA contains information required for the formation of one protein molecule.
3. Genetic information is present in mRNA in the form of genetic code.
4. Some times single mRNA may contain information for the formation of more than one protein.

Transfer RNA

t-RNA accounts for 10-15% of total cell RNA.

Structure

They are the smallest of all the RNAs. Usually they consist of 50-100 nucleotides. They are single strand molecules. t-RNA molecules contain many unusual bases 7-15 per molecule. They are methylated adenine, guanine, cytosine and thymine, dihydrouracil, pseudo uridine, isopentenyl adenine etc. These unusual bases are important for binding of t-RNA to ribosomes and interaction of t-RNA with aminoacyl-t-RNA synthetases. About half of the nucleotides in t-RNA are involved in intrachain base pairing. As a result, double helical segments are formed in t-RNA. Further some bases are not involved in the base pairing resulting in loops and arms formation in t-RNA. Thus, folding in primary structure generate secondary structure.

Though t-RNAs differ in chain lengths they have some common features with regard to secondary structure.

Secondary structure of t-RNA

Secondary structure of all the t-RNAs is in the form of clover leaf (Figure 16.8a). The important features of clover-leaf structure are

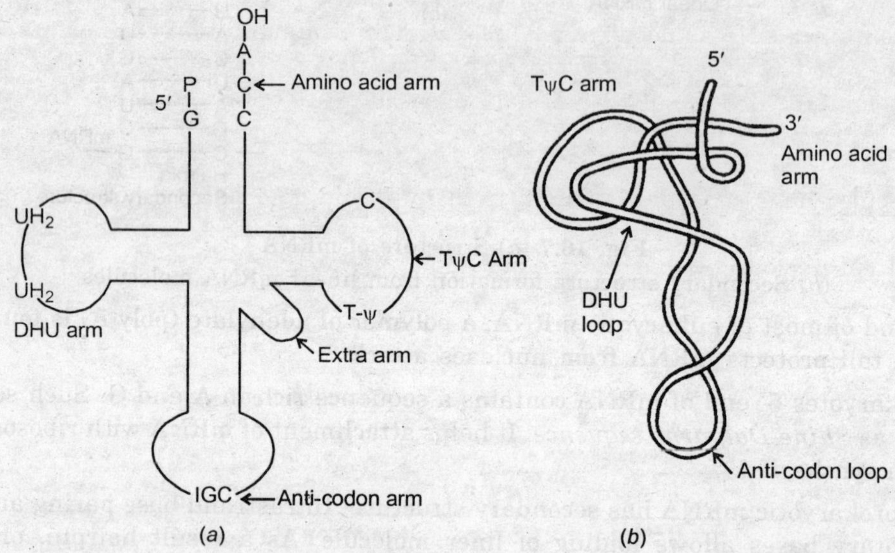

Fig. 16.8 (*a*) Secondary structure of t-RNA (*b*) Tertiary structure of t-RNA

1. An amino acid arm where amino acid is attached to 3′-OH of adenosine moiety of t-RNA. ACC is the common base sequence at this 3′-end.
2. Tφc arm, which contains sequence of ribothymidine-pseudouridine-cytidine. Greek alphabet φ (Psi) stands for pseudo uridine. Thymine and pseudouracil are the two unusual bases found in this arm.
3. An anti-codon arm, which recognizes codon on mRNA.
4. DHU arm, which contains many dihydrouridine (UH_2) residues.
5. The 5′ end of t-RNA is phosphorylated and residue is guanosine.
6. About 75% t-RNA molecules have extra arm. It consist of 3-5 base pairs. It is found between TφC and anti-codon arm.

Tertiary structure of t-RNA

X-ray diffraction analysis indicated complex three-dimentional structure for t-RNA molecule. Three-dimentional structure of t-RNA looks like inverted or tilted L. The anti-codon arm is at the tip of the vertical arm of tilted L. The acceptor arm is at the tip of horizontal arm of tilted L. The D loop and TφC loop are pushed into corner of tilted L (Figure 16.8b).

Functions

1. It is the carrier of amino acids to the site of protein synthesis.

2. There is at least one t-RNA molecule to each of 20 amino acids required for protein synthesis.
3. Eukaryotic t-RNAs are less stable where as prokaryotic RNAs are more stable.

Ribosomal RNA

Ribosomal RNA or r-RNA accounts for 80% of total cellular RNA. It is present in ribosomes. In ribosomes, r-RNA is found in combination with protein. It is known as *ribonucleoprotein*. The length of r-RNA ranges form 100-600 nucleotides. Both prokaryotic and eukaryotic ribosomes contain r-RNA molecules. r-RNAs differ in sedimentation coefficients (S). There are four types of r-RNAs in eukaryotes. They are 5, 5.8, 18 and 28S r-RNA molecules. Prokaryotes contains 3 types of r-RNA molecules. They are 5, 16 and 23S r-RNA molecules.

Structure

r-RNA molecules have secondary structure. Intra strand base pairing between complementary base generates double helical segments or loops. They are known as domains. 16S r-RNA with 1500 nucleotides has four major domains (Figure 16.8c). The three-dimentional tertiary structure of r-RNA is highly complex.

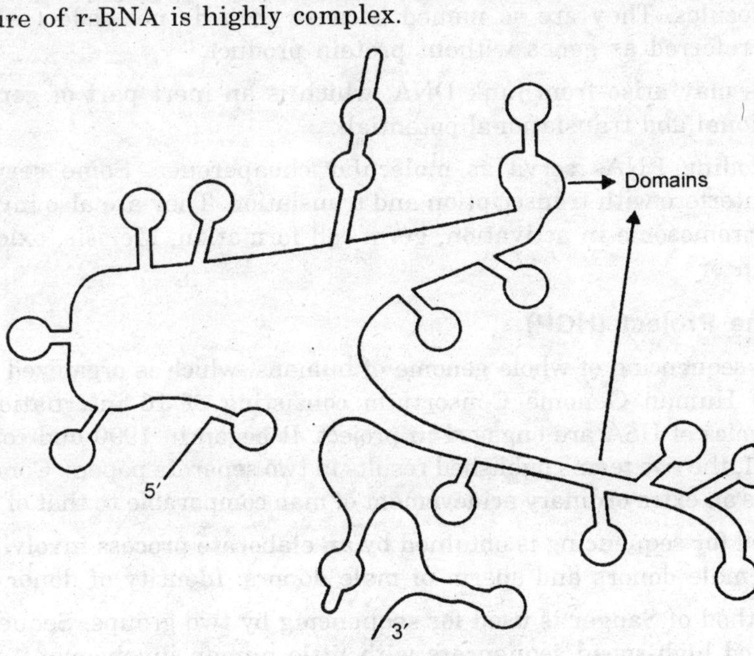

Fig. 16.8 (*c*) Secondary structure of 16S r-RNA

Functions

1. r-RNAs are required for the formation of ribosomes.
2. 16S RNA is involved in initiation of protein synthesis.

Differences between DNA and RNA

DNA	RNA
1. Sugar moiety is deoxy ribose	Sugar moiety is ribose
2. Uracil, a pyrimidine base is usually absent	Thymine, a pyrimidine base is usually absent

(Contd.)

3. Double-stranded molecules	Single stranded molecules
4. Sum of purine bases is equal to sum of pyrimidine bases A + G = C + T	Sum of purine bases is not equal to sum pyrimidine bases A + G # C + T
5. Resistant to hydrolysis by alkali because of absence of hydroxyl group on 2 carbon atom of deoxyribose	Because of presence of hydroxyl group on 2 carbon atom of ribose RNA is easily hydrolyzed by alkali
6. Bases are not modified	Bases are modified
7. No catalytic activity	Some RNA are catalytically active
8. Only one form or type	More than three types
9. Usually not subjected to degradation in cell	Degraded in the cell by nucleases

Non-Coding RNAs

There are another type of RNAs found recently in mammals, yeast and bacteria. They are small RNA molecules. They are so named because they do not code for protein product. They are often referred as genes without protein product.

These RNAs may arise from junk DNA, which is an inert part of genome which is of little transcriptional and translational potential.

Some non-coding RNAs serve as molecular cheaperones. Some serve as anti-sense molecules and interfere with transcription and translation. They are also involved in genomic imprinting, X-chromosome in activation, germ cell formation, Meiosis, oxidative stress and diseases like cancer.

Human Genome Project (HGP)

It is involved in sequencing of whole genome of humans, which is organized as chromosomes. Two groups (*a*) Human Genome Consortium consisting of 16 international centres and (*b*) Celera Genomics of USA are engaged in project. It began in 1990 and completed by 2000. In February 2001, the two teams published results in two separate papers. Completion of human genome project is an extra ordinary achievement of man comparable to that of landing on moon.

Genome used for sequencing is obtained by an elaborate process involving DNA samples from blood of female donors and sperm of male donors. Identity of donor is not disclosed.

Dideoxy method of Sanger is used for sequencing by two groups. Sequencing is done by specially designed high-speed sequencers with little human involvement, which have very high (through) put. Though both groups used dideoxy method for sequencing, they adopted different approach for sequencing. Human genome consortium adopted Top-down approach in which genome is first segregated into smaller segments in a stepwise manner and when pieces are small enough, they are sequenced. After sequencing, these individual pieces are joined together to get chromosome of their origin by back tracking.

Shot-gun procedure or Bottom-up approach is adopted by Celera genomics headed by Venter for sequencing. It is known as whole Genome Shot-gun (WGS) procedure. It involves breaking the genomic DNA into small fragments and sequencing all of them in an unbiased manner. All the sequenced fragments are assembled by matching identifying pairs of sequences among any two fragments.

When sequencing of fragments is completed, its genes or protein coding regions are detected by using computational biology procedures. Total number of genes present in 3.2 billion base pairs containing human genome ranges from 33,000 to 1,50,000. The remaining non-coding DNA is often termed as junk DNA. It is genes-containing array of sequences that determines coordination, communication and functions of the cells which are ultimately responsible for proper health and well being of an individual. Human genome sequence provide some solutions to atleast few medical problems which remained mystery.

Sequencing of human genome allows mapping of disease genes on specific locations on chromosomes. Some disease genes, which are mapped on chromosomes are given below.

Chromosome	**Disease genes**
Chromosome 1	Gaucher's disease, Breast Cancer
Chromosome 3	Alkaptonuria, Myeloid, Leukamia
Chromosome 6	Celiac disease, Hemochromatosis
Chromosome 7	Cystic fibrosis, Split hand/Foot malformation
Chromosome 8	Lipo protein lipase, Cohen syndrome
Chromosome 9	Fanconi anaemia Type C
Chromosome 10	Wolman disease
Chromosome 11	Ataxia telangiectasia, Wilm's tumour
Chromosome 12	Phenyl ketonuria
Chromosome 13	Wilson's disease, Retinoblastoma
Chromosome 14	Alzheirmer disease, Spastic paraplegia
Chromosome 15	Tay-Sach's disease, Bloom syndrome
Chromosome 16	Fanconi anaemia Type A, Inflammatory bowel disease.
Chromosome 18	Niemann–Pick disease, Colorectal cancer.
Chromosome 20	Polymorphic severe combined immuno deficiency
Chromosome X	Duchenne muscular dystrophy, Adreno leukodystrophy
Chromosome Y	Prostate cancer, Adenocarcinoma

Identification of new disease genes may provide starting point for the development of new diagnostic kits. Further genome sequence enables identification culprit genes involved in diseases whose underlying causes are yet to be elucidated.

Sequence information provides molecular details of signal transduction, differential expression of gene products in various tissues during normal growth, uncontrolled growth in tumour tissues. Human genome sequence allows identification of species.

Synthesizing life

1. It is creation of life in the laboratory.
2. It involves integration of chemistry and biochemistry.
3. Methods are recently developed for creating minimal life forms in the laboratory.

4. Synthetic genes or synthetic nucleotide fragments are generated by automated solid phase chemical synthesis.
5. Enzymatic ligation of synthetic genes is used to assemble genes. This results in creation of genome or life.
6. Polio virus with molecular formula of $C_{332,\ 652}\ H_{492,\ 388}\ N_{98,\ 245}\ O_{131,\ 196}\ P_{7501}\ S_{2340}$ has been created recently in laboratory.
7. It replicates in laboratory, which is one of the most important property of any life form.

Several other new life forms will be generated soon and the consequences of these attempts by man may be beneficial to human race.

REFERENCES

1. Freifelder, D. Molecular Biology. 2nd ed. Jones and Bartlett Publishers, Boston, 1987.
2. Watson, J.D. and Crick, F.H.C. Molecular structure of nucleic acids. A structure for DNA. Nature **171**, 737-738, 1953.
3. Saenger, W. Principles of nucleic acid structure. Springer-Verlag, New York, 1984.
4. Schimmel, P. Soll, D. and Abelson, J. Eds. Transfer RNA. Cold spring Harbor Laboratory. New York, 1979.
5. Van Holde, K.E. Chromatin. Springer–Verlag. New York, 1988.
6. Davidson, J.N. The biochemistry of nucleic acids. Academic Press, New York, 1972.
7. Rich, A. and Raj Bhandary, V.L. Transfer RNA: Molecular structure, sequence and properties. Ann. Rev. Biochem. **45**, 805, 1976.
8. Brown, T and Brown, T.W. Genomes. Wiley-Liss, 2002.
9. Gesteland, R.F., Cech, T.R. and Atkins, J.F. (Eds.). The RNA World. Cold Spring Harbor Laboratory, NY, 1999.
10. Watson, J.D.A. passion for DNA: genes, genomes and Society. Cold Spring Harbor Laboratory Press, 2000.
11. Driel, R.V. and Arie, P.O. Nuclear organization, chromatin structure and gene expression. Oxford University Press, NY 1997.
12. Donald M. Crothers, Nucleic acids: structure, properties and functions, University Science Books, 2000.
13. Olby, R. Quiet debut for the double helix. Nature **421**, 402-405, 2003.
14. Parkinson, G.N. Lee M.P.H. and Neidle, S. Crystal structure of parallel quadruplexes from human telomeric DNA. Nature **417**, 876, 2002.
15. Sumen, N.C. DNA in material world. Nature **421**, 427-431, 2003.
16. Ariyoshi, M. *et al.* Crystal structure of the holliday junction DNA in complex with a single RuvAtetramer. Proc. Natl. Acad. Sci. USA **97**, 8257-8262, 2002.
17. Contor, C.R. and Smith C.L. Genomics: the science and technology behind human genome project (E-book). J. Wiley. New York, 2004.
18. Myers, E.W. Sutton, G.G. Smith, H.O. Ademson, D. and Venter, J. Craig. On the sequencing and assembly of human genome. Proc. Natl. Acad. Sci. USA **99**, 4145-4146, 2002.

19. Venter, J.C. *et al.* The sequence of human genome. Science. **291**, 1304-1351, 2001.

20. International human genome sequencing consortium (HGSC). Nature. **409**, 860-921, 2001.

21. Vanderpool, C.K. and Gottesman. S. Non-coding RNAs at the membrane. Nature Structural and Molecular Biology. Vol. 12, April 2005.

EXERCISES

ESSAY QUESTIONS

1. Draw DNA double helix. Describe its main features. Add a note on DNA functions.
2. Define RNA. Classify. Write structure and functions of each one.
3. Briefly describe nucleic acids.

SHORT QUESTIONS

1. Name different types of RNAs. Write main features and functions of mRNA.
2. Name differences between DNA and RNA.
3. Draw clover leaf structure of tRNA. Label its different parts. Mention functions of tRNA.
4. How eukaryotic DNA is organized?
5. Explain the following
   (*a*) DNA as gene
   (*b*) Denaturation of DNA
6. Write about functions of nucleic acids.
7. Write a note on DNA polymorphism.
8. How bacterial DNA is organized.
9. Write differences between prokaryotic and eukaryotic DNA.
10. Define plasmid. Give example. Write its importance.
11. Write a note on nucleosome.
12. Explain Ribosomal RNA. How it differs from other RNAs?
13. Write a note on unusual bases of RNAs.

MULTIPLE CHOICE QUESTIONS

1. Each polynucleotide chain
   (*a*) Has direction.
   (*b*) Has 5′ and 3′ end.
   (*c*) Has direction and two ends.
   (*d*) Has phosphodiester linkages.
2. ATTATA is sequence of a DNA segment. Each letter stands for
   (*a*) Bases.
   (*b*) Nucleosides.
   (*c*) Nucleotides.
   (*d*) Purine and pyrimidine bases.

3. Shine-Dalgarno sequence is present in
   (*a*) Eukaryotic mRNA.
   (*b*) Prokaryotic mRNA.
   (*c*) At 5′ end of prokaryotic mRNA.
   (*d*) At 3′ end of eukaryotic mRNA.
4. Ribosomes are
   (*a*) Nucleic acids.
   (*b*) Proteins.
   (*c*) Ribonucleo proteins.
   (*d*) Nucleosomes.
5. Loops in RNA molecules are
   (*a*) Due to intra strand base pairing.
   (*b*) Due to inter strand base pairing.
   (*c*) Due to intra strand base pairing between complementary bases.
   (*d*) Involved in transfer of genetic information.

FILL IN THE BLANKS

1. In polynucleotides phosphodiester linkage joins 3′-OH and 5′-OH belonging to .... sugars.
2. ACGCATA is sequence of one DNA strand. Then .... is sequence of opposite strand.
3. DNAs from different tissues of same species have .... base composition.
4. When DNA is dehydrated it acquires .... form.
5. An extra arm in tRNA is found between .... and .... arm.

17

CHAPTER

BIOSYNTHESIS OF NUCLEIC ACIDS

Genetic information stored in DNA in the form of nucleotide sequence flows from DNA to DNA, DNA to RNA then from RNA to protein. This genetic information flow is popularly called as *central dogma of molecular genetics*. Usually central dogma of molecular genetics involves three different processes. They are

1. Replication

Synthesis of new DNA or information copying is known as replication. In this process information is transmitted from parent to daughter. The new DNA is identical to parent DNA (Figure 17.1).

2. Transcription

Synthesis of RNA from DNA or information transfer is known as transcription. In this process, information is transferred from DNA to RNA (Figure 17.1).

3. Translation

Synthesis of proteins using information present in RNAs or information decoding is known as translation. In this process, information present in RNA in the form of nucleotide sequence, is converted into sequence of amino acids (Figure 17.1).

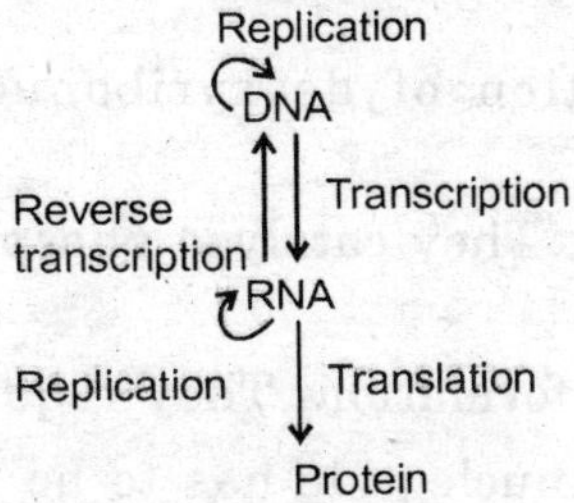

Fig. 17.1 Flow of genetic information in central dogma of molecular genetics

In some viruses RNA function as genetic material. In such viruses replication involves flow of information from RNA to RNA. Further, during their replication genetic information stored in RNA flows to DNA temporarily. This process is known as *reverse transcription*. Therefore these two processes are also included in central dogma in 1970 (Figure 17.1).

MEDICAL AND BIOLOGICAL IMPORTANCE

1. For the transfer of genetic information from parent to offspring synthesis of new DNA is essential.
2. Likewise, new DNA synthesis is essential for cell multiplication.
3. Inhibitors of DNA synthesis are used in the treatment of cancer, bacterial and viral infections.
4. For the transfer of genetic information from the nucleus to cytoplasm new RNA synthesis is essential.
5. Inhibitors of RNA synthesis are used in the treatment of bacterial infections.
6. Some toxins work by blocking RNA synthesis.
7. RNA synthesis is essential for the multiplication of RNA containing viruses (retroviruses).
8. Some RNAs act as enzymes and facilitate their own formation.
9. Some diseases are due to defective DNA repair.

DNA REPLICATION

Major function of replication is to provide genetic information required by daughter cell from parent cell. When cell prepares for division all the cell components must double. During S-phase of cell cycle DNA replication occurs. During this period, concentration of deoxy ribo nucleotides increases to several folds. When cell divides, each daughter cell must contain entire genetic information of parent cell. So, newly formed daughter cell contains an identical copy of parental DNA and its phenotype characters are same as that of parent.

Enzymes of DNA replication

Most of the enzymes of metabolic pathways catalyze single step reactions. But enzymes of replication catalyze multi-step reactions because DNA molecule is not a simple small molecule. Hence, reactions catalyzed by the enzymes of DNA replication are described prior to replication process.

DNA Polymerases

1. They catalyze polymerization of deoxyribonucleotides into nucleic acids or polynucleotides.
2. They contain metal ion Zn^{2+}. They catalyze phosphodiester link formation between nucleotides.
3. They can not initiate chain formation. They require primer with 3'-OH group.
4. They can not decide, which nucleotide has to be incorporated or polymerized.
5. The polymerization by polymerase requires presence of DNA strand. The DNA strand directs polymerization of nucleotides in order according to base pairing rule.
6. The DNA strand that directs polymerization by polymerase is known as template strand. Hence, the polymerases are called as DNA-dependent DNA polymerase or template directed polymerases.

7. A phosphodiester linkage is formed by nucleophilic attack of 3'-OH of primer on innermost phosphate of incoming nucleotide (Fig. 17.2).

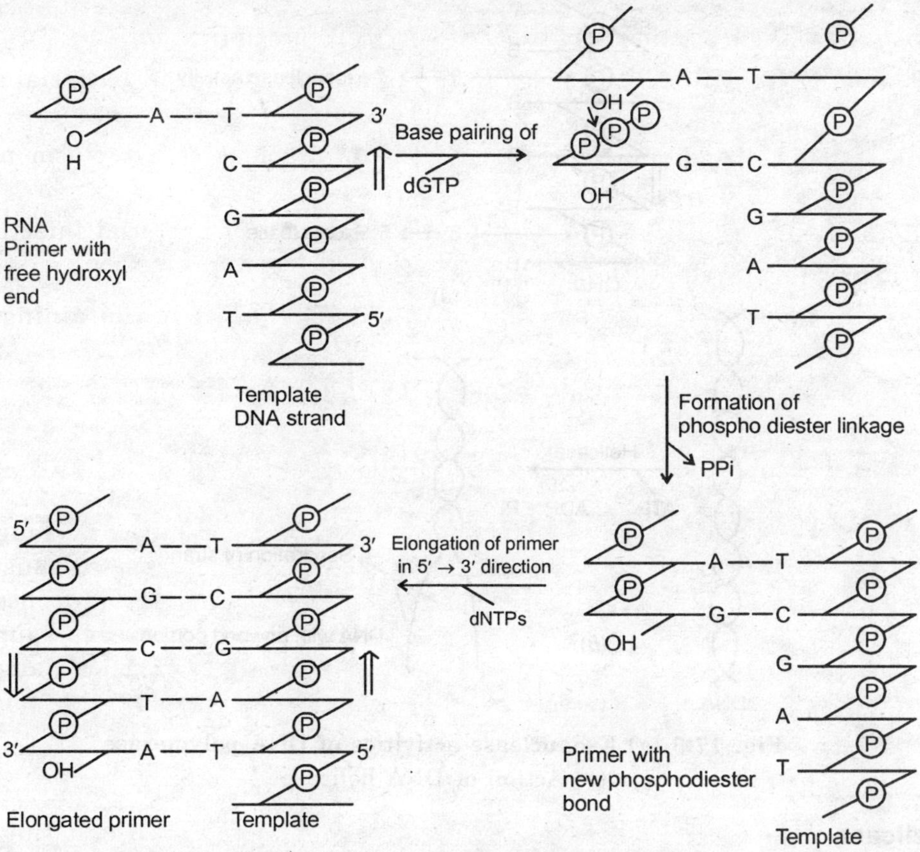

Fig. 17.2 Action of DNA polymerase, dNTPs-deoxy nucleoside tri phosphates

8. After the formation of initial phosphodiester bond, the primer is elongated by further addition of deoxy ribonucleotides.
9. They catalyze polymerization in 5'→ 3' direction.

Some DNA directed–DNA polymerases are

1. *DNA Polymerase I*

It requires DNA primer for polymerization. It is mainly involved in elongation of nascent DNA. It is a minor replication enzyme in prokaryotes. It has 5'→ 3' and 3'→ 5' exonuclease activities also. It removes wrong nucleotide that is incorporated into polymer by using 3'→ 5' exonuclease activity (Fig. 17.3a). This action enhances the accuracy of DNA replication.

2. *DNA Polymerase III*

Major enzyme of DNA replication in prokaryotes. It requires RNA primer.

DNA Ligase

It joins ends of two segments of DNA by catalyzing the formation of phosphodiester bond.

In prokaryotes, NAD^+ is required whereas in eukaryotes ATP is required. The phospho diester linkage formation occurs through ADP deoxyribose intermediate (Fig. 17.4).

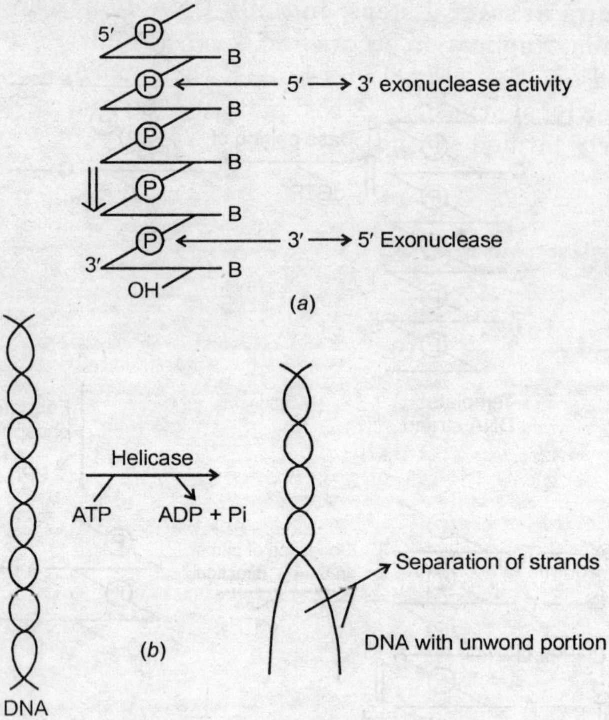

Fig. 17.3 (*a*) Exonuclease activities of DNA polymerase
(*b*) Action of DNA helicase

DNA Helicase

It catalyzes unwinding of DNA double helix. The separation of DNA strands requires energy which is supplied by hydrolyzing ATP (Fig. 17.3b).

DNA Gyrase or DNA topo isomerase II

When DNA unwinds, super coils are formed in DNA. They are removed by DNA gyrase. DNA gyrase removes super coils by creating negative super coils in a ATP-dependent reaction. It can create super coils in a relaxed DNA.

Process of replication

Single DNA molecule of prokaryotes consist of 2×10^9 bases. So, it is too long to be made in single piece. A molecule of DNA polymerase can polymerize about 3000 bases to polynucleotide strand per minute. Hence, formation of entire DNA molecule by single molecule of polymerase starting from 5' end will take weeks. But observed time for replication was 4-8 hours in eukaryotes and less than two hours in prokaryotes. Therefore, to complete DNA replication in that short period the DNA polymerase must act at several places or cell should contain many DNA polymerase molecules. It has been estimated that eukaryotic cells contain 20000 DNA polymerases and prokaryotes contains about 20 DNA polymerases per cell. These polymerases starts replication at several points simultaneously. The segments of DNA that are replicated are called as replicons or replication units. There may be 1000 replicons in a chromosome during cell division. DNA replication occurs in several steps. Initially DNA duplex unwinds at several places to facilitate replication. Replication occurs and several replicons are generated. Replicons are ultimately joined together (Fig. 17.5). Finally the separation of strands generate two DNA molecules. Newly synthesized DNA molecule consist of a strand derived from parent and one newly formed strand.

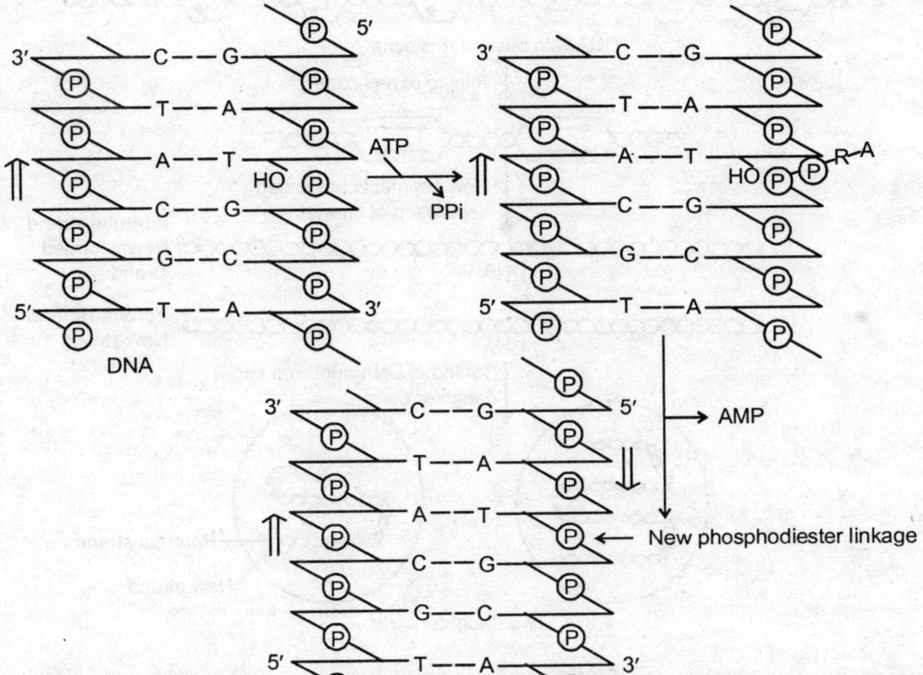

Fig. 17.4 Action of DNA ligase

Semi conservative replication

When a cell divides, one strand of parental DNA pass on to daughter cell unchanged. Remaining strand in each daughter cell is newly synthesized. This is known as semi conservative replication (Fig. 17.5).

Molecular events of replicon

Replication in *E. Coli* starts at a unique origin, proceeds in opposite directions simultaneously and completed in 100 minutes. Replication at a replicon involves unwinding of DNA, initiation, elongation and several protein (s) factors (Fig. 17.6).

1. A sequence of 245 base pairs in *E. Coli* chromosome serves as starting point for replication. It is designated as ori C. It has binding sites for DNA binding proteins.
2. Binding of dna A protein to ori C initiates unwinding of DNA and synthesis of primer RNA.

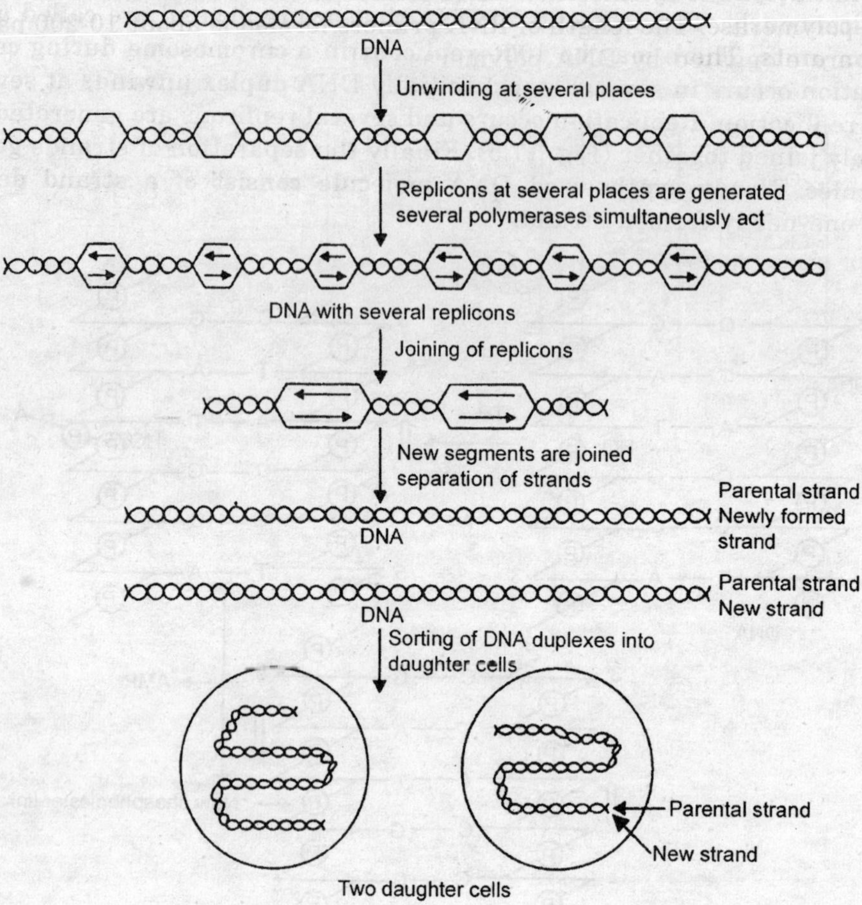

Fig. 17.5 Process of replication. Note in daughter cell out of two stands one strand is derived from parental DNA and another strand is newly formed

3. A complex of dna B and dna C also binds to ori C to open the duplex DNA. dna B is helicase. It can bind to single strand DNA. By the action of helicase DNA unwinding occurs.
4. The unwinding of DNA at ori C causes formation of super coils in DNA molecule which prevents further unwinding of DNA.
5. DNA Gyrase removes super coils by introducing negative super coils to favour replication.
6. Single strand binding proteins (SSBP) binds to single strands of unwound portion of DNA duplex and stabilizes the single strands. In the absence of SSB, proteins strands can rewind.
7. Thus by the action of helicase and DNA binding proteins, SSB proteins a replication fork is created. At this fork, both strands of parental DNA serves as templates for the DNA synthesis.

8. Now to initiate DNA synthesis, a RNA primer is formed by the action of primase, an RNA-polymerase. The length of RNA primers formed is about 10-200 bases. These primers are elongated by DNA polymerase III.

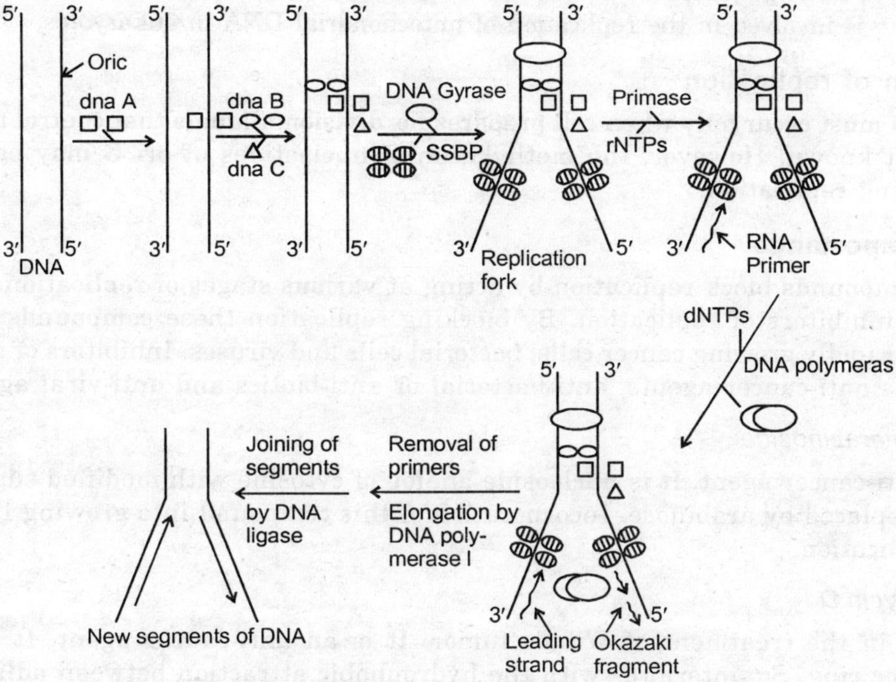

Fig. 17.6 Molecular events of replicon

rNTPs = Ribonucleoside triphosphates. dNTPs = Deoxy nucleoside triphosphates

9. A dimeric DNA-polymerase III holoenzyme synthesizes both strands of DNA at replication fork from RNA primers. Usually one enzyme molecule replicates one strand of DNA.
10. DNA-polymerase III holo enzyme consist of several subunits. They are α, β, γ, δ etc. α -Subunit is catalytic subunit. The β-subunit contributes to high processivity. The DNA polymerase III can polymerize hundreds of nucleotides per second whereas DNA polymerase I can polymerize only 10 nucleotides per second.
11. Since DNA polymerase III can not polymerize nucleotides in 3' → 5' direction, the synthesis of two strands of DNA by this enzyme occurs in some what different manner.
12. One strand of DNA is synthesized continuously and it is known as *leading strand*.
13. Another strand is synthesized discontinuously in the form of okazaki fragments. It is known as *lagging strand*. The length of these segments ranges from 1000 to 2000 bases. They are also synthesized in 5' → 3' direction only.
14. The gaps between okazaki fragments are filled by DNA polymerase I. RNA primers are removed by 5' → 3' exonuclease activity of DNA polymerase I.
15. Finally DNA ligase joins the ends of okazaki fragments.

Enzymes of eukaryotic replication

DNA replication in eukaryotes is a complicated process because of the bound histones. In eukaryotes DNA polymerase α has action similar to that of DNA polymerase III. DNA polymerase β is similar to DNA polymerase - I. Okazaki fragments are small (100-200 nucleotides). DNA polymerase γ is involved in the replication of mitochondrial DNA in eukaryotes.

Regulation of replication

Replication must occur only when cell prepares for division. Signals that control replication are not yet known. However, the methylation of nucleotides of ori C may be one way of controlling replication.

Medical importance

Several compounds block replication by acting at various stages of replication. They are known as inhibitors of replication. By blocking replication these compounds slows the division of rapidly growing cancer cells, bacterial cells and viruses. Inhibitors of replication are used as anti-cancer agents, anti-bacterial or anti-biotics and anti-viral agents.

1. *Cytosine arabinoside*

It is an anti-cancer agent. It is nucleoside analog of cytosine with modified sugar. Usual ribose is replaced by arabinose. Incorporation of this compound into growing DNA chain blocks replication.

2. *Actinomycin D*

It is used in the treatment of Wilm's tumor. It is an anti-cancer agent. It has broad hydrophobic ring. So, interferes with the hydrophobic attraction between adjacent base pairs of DNA. As a result, distortion of DNA occurs and replication is blocked.

3. *Bleomycin*

It is an antibiotic. It breaks-C-C-bond of ribose in DNA molecule.

4. *Acyclovir*

It is another nucleoside analog used in viral infection caused by herpes virus. It is an analog of guanosine in which pentose is replaced with three carbon sugar. It is converted to triphosphate *in vivo,* which inhibits viral DNA polymerase.

5. *Replication origins and cancer*

Large number of replication origins in eukaryotes are puzzling molecular biologists for long time. Recent research suggests that large number of replication origins allows completion of replication before cell enter 'M' phase. During G_1 phase of cell cycle replication origins are prepared to fire and subsequently activated in S-phase. If DNA replication is not completed in 'S' phase gross chromosomal rearrangements may occur. Therefore, reduction in replication origins alters progression of S-phase, mitosis and chromosomal translocations. Since gross chromosomal rearrangements are associated with cancer development, large number of replication origins are necessary for normal cell division. Thus, large number of replication origins prevents a normal cell turning into cancer cell. In future diagnostic tests that can predict a cell to become cancer cell based on replication origins may be developed.

6. *DNA topoisomerase inhibitors*

Many drugs used for treatment of parasitic diseases like leishmaniasis (Kala-Azar), trypanosomiasis (Sleeping sickness) are inhibitors of topoisomerases of parasites. Some DNA topoisomerase inhibitors are used as anti-bacterial and anti-cancer drugs. Leishmaniass and trypanosomiasis caused by protozoan parasites *leishmania donovani* and *trypanosoma brucei* affects millions of people worldwide. They developed resistance to most of currently used drugs. DNA topoismerase is target for development of new drugs. Some examples of topoisomerase inhibitors with potent anti-trypanosomal activity are pentamidine, berenil, samorine etc. anilino acridines have potent anti-leishmanial activity.

DNA repair

Even though the replication takes place at high accuracy an error can occur for every 30,000 bases. Such errors in replication produce damaged DNA or DNA with altered base composition. Further, damage to DNA may result from the action of physical, chemical and environmental agents. Maintenance of the integrity of DNA molecule is very important for the survival of species or organisms. Therefore, species evolved mechanisms for the removal of damaged DNA. The damaged DNA is either removed or replaced with normal DNA. There are two types of DNA-repair mechanisms. They are

1. *Excision repair*

It is more common and universal mechanism for DNA repair. The damaged DNA is recognized by an endonuclease known as excinuclease. It cuts the damaged strand at two sites and removes it. The gap so generated is elongated by DNA polymerase I. The new strand is joined by the action of ligase (Fig. 17.7).

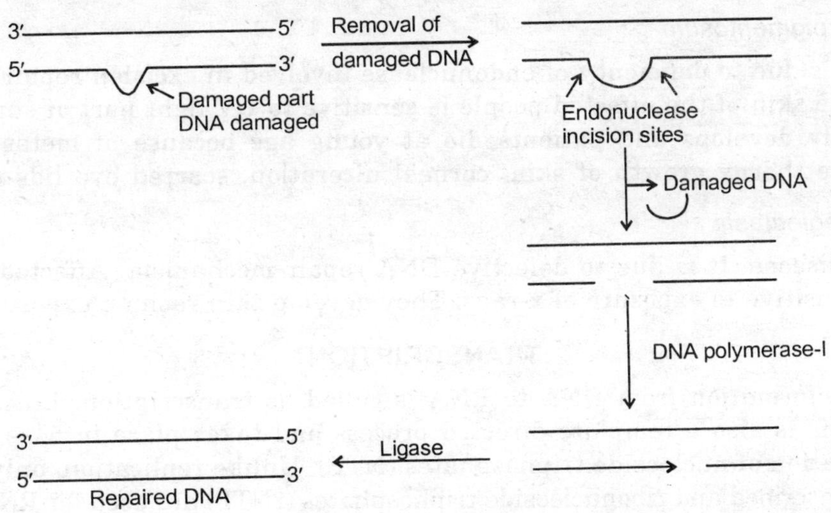

Fig. 17.7 Excision repair mechanism

2. *Enzymatic photo reactivation*

It is a direct repair mechanism. Exposure of DNA to UV light causes formation of thymine dimer between two adjacent thymine bases. When it is exposed to visible light a photolyase binds to damanged DNA and cleaves covalent bonds between thymine dimer (Fig. 17.8).

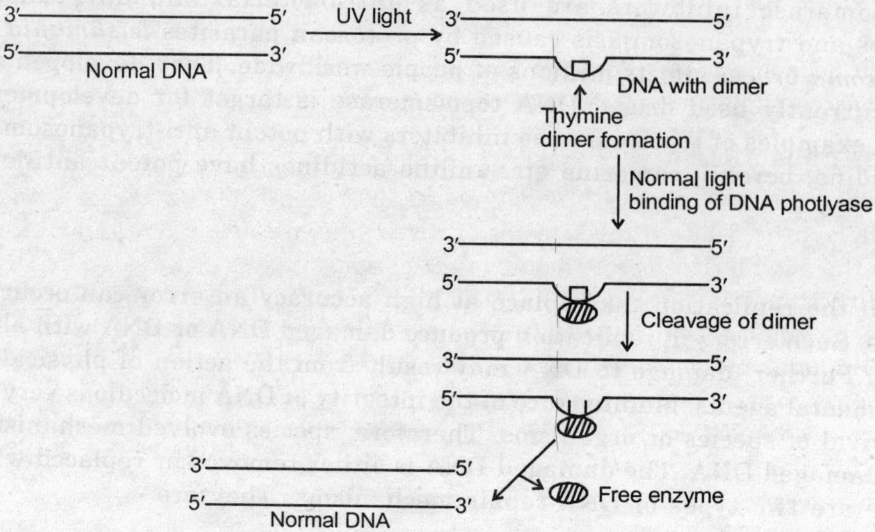

Fig. 17.8 Thymine dimer removal by photolyase

Medical importance

When DNA-repair mechanisms are defective due to absence of enzymes of DNA repair this leads to diseases. These diseases are inherited *i.e.,* they are due to defective genes.

1. Xeroderma pigmentosum

This disease is due to deficiency of endonuclease involved in excision repair. It is a rare condition. The skin of the affected people is sensitive to UV light part of sun light. Skin cancer usually develops and patients die at young age because of metastasis. Other symptoms are thorny growth of skin, corneal ulceration, scarred eye lids etc.

2. Ataxia telangiectasia

It is a rare disease. It is due to defective DNA repair mechanism. Affected individuals are highly sensitive to exposure of x-rays. They develop skin rash on exposure to x-rays.

TRANSCRIPTION

Transfer of information from DNA to RNA is called as transcription. Like replication, RNA synthesis is also a template directed process and takes place in 5' → 3' direction by polymerization of nucleoside triphosphates (NTP). Unlike replication, only one strand of DNA is transcribed and ribonucleoside triphosphates (rNTP) are used for RNA synthesis.

Synthesis of RNA is quite similar in prokaryotes and eukaryotes but enzymes and signals are different. The strand of DNA that is transcribed into RNA is called as template or sense strand whereas other strand is called as *coding* or *anti-sense strand.* The sequence of RNA is complementary to the sequence of template strand and it is same as that of coding strand except for U replacing T (Fig. 17.9).

5′______G C A C C T G C A T C A G C A T C A G C A T C A G C A T T C G A A C G______3′ Coding strand

3′______C G T G G A C G T A G T C G T A G T C G T A G T C G T A A G C T T G C______5′ Template

C C U G C A U C A G C A U C A G C A U C A G C A U U

5′ Nascent RNA 3′

Fig. 17.9 Sequence of nascent RNA is complementory to tempalte strand. Sequence of nascent RNA is same as that of coding strand except for U replacing T

Enzymes of transcription

In prokaryotes, DNA directed RNA polymerase is the major enzyme of transcription. It catalyzes the synthesis of all three types of RNAs like mRNA, tRNA and rRNA in *E. Coli.* It catalyzes the polymerization of ribonucleotide triphosphates as directed by DNA template in 5' → 3' direction (Fig. 17.10). Unlike DNA polymerases it does not require primer and can initiate polymerization. It does not possess nuclease activity also. It requires Zn^{2+} and Mn^{2+}. Holoenzyme consists of five subunits. They are $\alpha\alpha$ $\beta\beta'$ and σ. The coenzyme consists of only four subunits $\alpha\alpha$ $\beta\beta'$ (Fig. 17.10) σ factor is found separately. The 2 α subunits are required for chain initiation and keeps all factors together. β subunit is responsible for elongation and β' is required for DNA binding. σ Factor aids in recognition of promoter and it is a regulatory factor. It can alter the specificity of RNA polymerase.

In eukaryotes, different RNA polymerases catalyzes formation of different RNAs. DNA-dependent RNA polymerase I synthesizes rRNA. DNA-directed RNA polymerase II synthesizes mRNA. RNA polymerase III catalyzes the formation of tRNA.

Mechanism of transcription

RNA synthesis involves initiation, elongation and termination (Fig. 17.11).

Initiation

1. Initiation of RNA synthesis involves binding of RNA polymerase to the template strand. Certain regions of DNA serves as initiation signals. They are known as *promoter sites.*
2. RNA polymerase identifies promoter by search process. σ factor is essential for this search process.
3. Holoenzyme binds to the template at the promoter site.
4. When RNA polymerase binds to promoter site unwinding of DNA occurs and sets the stage for first phosphodiester linkage formation.
5. RNA polymerase has two binding sites one site is specific for purine nucleotides like ATP or GTP as directed by template strand and used for initiation. Another site is common for any four nucleotides like ATP, GTP, UTP and CTP.
6. In this case, ATP binds to purine nucleotide site and UTP binds to another site because of sequence TA in the template strand at the starts site.
7. When once nucleotides are bound phosphodiester linkage is formed by the nucleophilic attack of 3′-OH of first nucleotide (ATP) on to inner most phosphate of second nucleotide (UTP) and thus chain growth is initiated.
8. After these initial events of RNA formation at 5′ end, the σ factor is released.

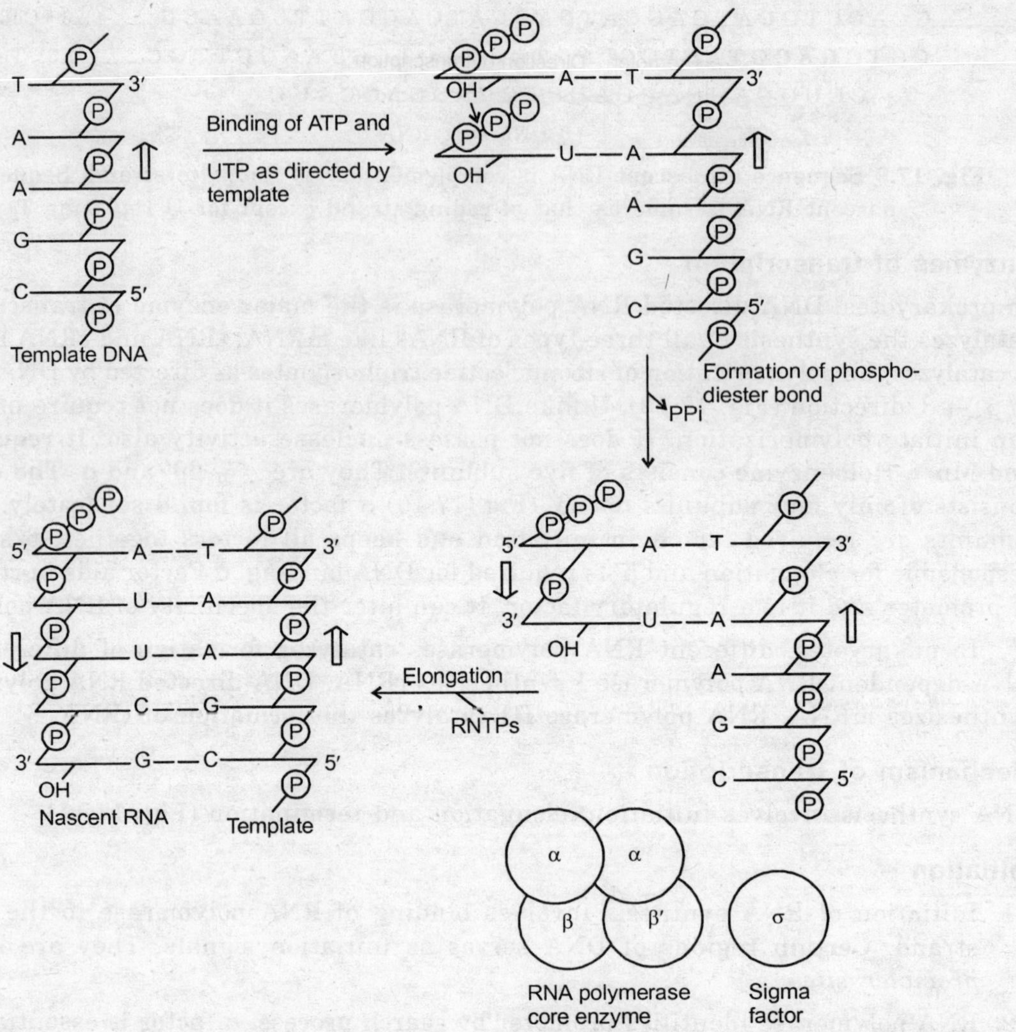

Fig. 17.10 Action of RNA polymerase. Note that nascent RNA is base paired to template RNTPs = Ribonucleoside triphosphates. Structure of RNA polymerase is shown separately

Elongation

9. Elongation of RNA molecule occurs in 5′ → 3′ direction as the RNA polymerase polymerizes rNTPs anti-parallel to template strand.
10. As RNA polymerase progress along the DNA molecule unwinding of DNA takes place ahead of 3′ end of nascent RNA. The growing RNA or nascent RNA is base paired to template strand.
11. The rewinding of parental DNA promotes dissociation of nascent RNA from template strand during elongation.

Termination

12. Certain regions of DNA serves as termination signals and they are involved in termination of RNA synthesis.

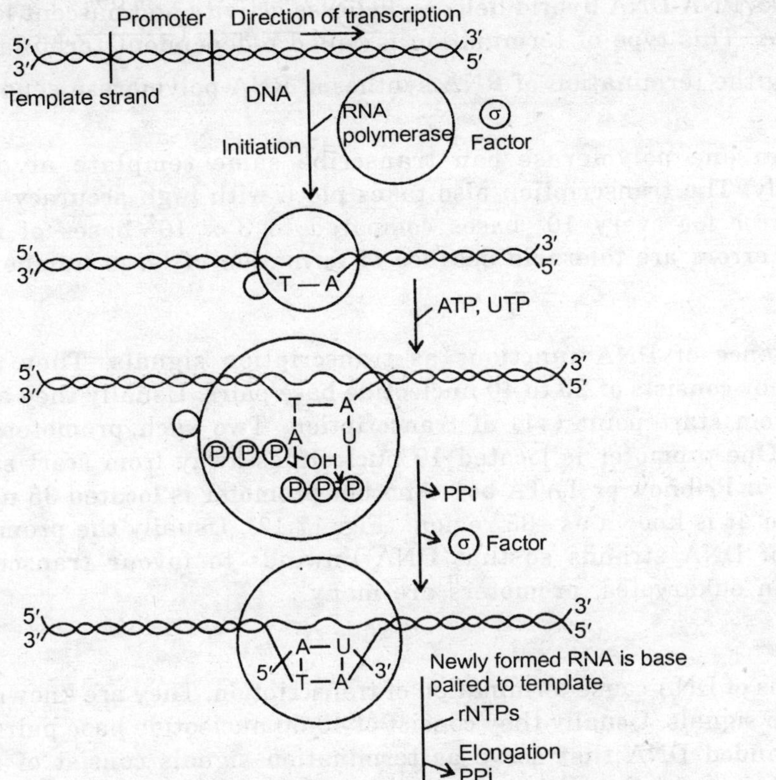

Fig. 17.11 Mechanism of transcription. Template strand is shown with thin line

13. When termination signal is read by RNA polymerase hair-pin loop is formed in the nascent RNA.

14. A terminator protein known as Rho (ρ) recognizes the hair-pin loop in nascent RNA and breaks RNA-DNA hybrid helix by helicase activity and nascent RNA is separated from DNA. This type of termination is called ρ-dependent termination.
15. Following the termination of RNA synthesis, RNA polymerase separates from DNA molecule.

More than one polymerase can transcribe same template at different places simultaneously. The transcription also takes place with high accuracy. However, there can be an error for every 10^4 bases compared to 3×10^4 bases of replication. The transcription errors are tolerable because of formation of large number of copies.

Promoters

Specific sequence of DNA functions as transcription signals. They are referred as promoters. They consists of 20 to 40 nucleotide base pairs. Usually they are located away (upstream) from start point (+1) of transcription. Two such promoters are known in prokaryotes. One promoter is located 10 nucleotides away from start site. It is known as –10 region or Pribnow or TATA box. Another promoter is located 35 nucleotides away from start site. It is known as –35 region. (Fig. 17.12). Usually the promoters facilitates dissociation of DNA strands so that DNA unwinds to favour transcription by RNA polymerase. In eukaryotes, promoters are many.

Terminators

Specific regions of DNA cause termination of transcription. They are known as terminators or termination signals. Usually they consist of 40-50 nucleotide base pairs. The segments of double stranded DNA that serve as termination signals consist of inverted repeat sequences rich in GC followed by AT rich region. They are also known as palindromes. In this region of DNA, the sequence of one strand is same as the sequence on the complementary strand when read in $5' \rightarrow 3'$ direction and hence the name palindrome (Fig. 17.12). Transcription of this region by RNA polymerase generates hair pin (loop) structure followed by uracil rich sequence at the 3′ and of nascent RNA (Fig. 17.12). The presence of U-U-U-U sequence at the stem of hair pin (loop) facilitates unwinding of nascent RNA from DNA because of weak attraction between AU pair. This leads to termination of transcription.. This type of termination of RNA synthesis is often called as ρ-*independent termination*.

RNA-dependent RNA polymerase (RdRP)

1. It occurs in several eukaryotic cells. It uses single stranded RNA templates as substrates and generates complementary RNA strand.
2. It is involved in a number of regulation process like post transcriptional gene slicing or RNA editing, mRNA amplification, anti-sense RNA synthesis to remove excess or defective RNA molecules from the cell.
3. It is insensitive to α-amanitin and rifampicin.

Medical importance

Synthesis of RNA is blocked by several compounds. They block transcription by acting at different levels of transcription. They are often called as inhibitors of transcription. Some antibiotics and toxins work by inhibiting transcription.

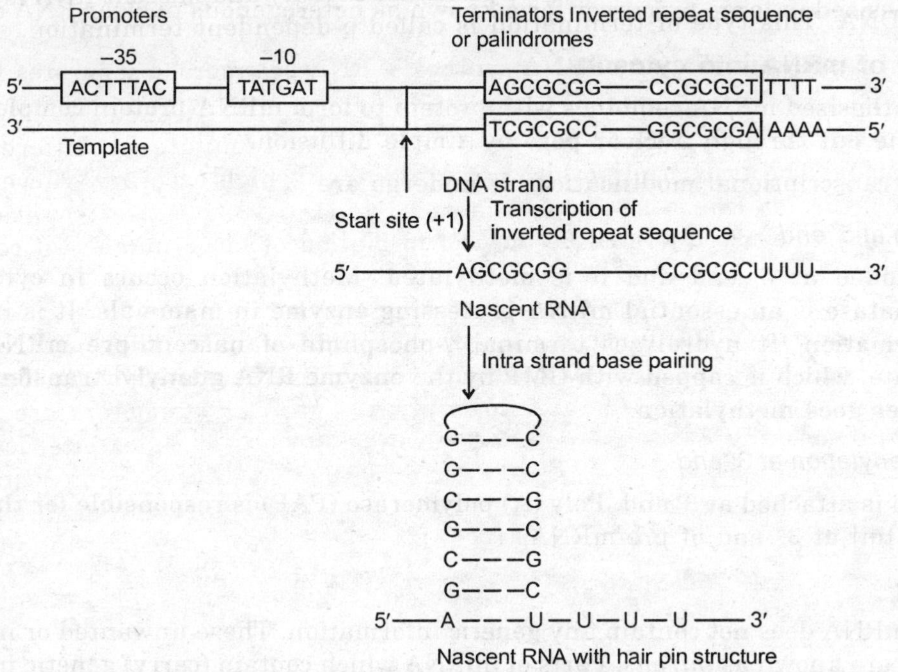

Fig. 17.12 Promoters and terminator regions of DNA. Formation of hair pin loop occurs when palindrome is transcribed

1. *∝-Amanitin*

It is produced by particular variety of mushrooms. It inhibits RNA polymerase III. Prokaryotic enzymes are not affected by this poison. It is responsible for mushroom poisoning cases all over the world. It causes pain in gastrointestinal tract, vomitting, diarrhoea and nausae.

2. *Rifamycin and Rifampicin*

They are antibiotics. They block transcription by inhibiting first phosphodiester bond formation.

3. *Aflatoxin*

A fungus that grows on moist ground nut produces aflatoxin, which inhibit transcription.

4. *Actinomycin D*

It inhibits transcription by preventing unwinding of DNA.

Post transcriptional modifications

All three types of RNAs are synthesized in precursor forms in eukaryotes. These precursors are converted to functional RNA molecules by post-trasncriptional modifications. Usually, these modifications takes place in nucleus. Some prokaryotic RNAs also undergo these modifications.

Messenger RNA

It is synthesized in large precursor form known as heterogenous nuclear RNA or hnRNA.

Transport of mRNA into cytosol

Newly synthesized mRNA combines with protein to form mRNA-protein complex (mRNP) which come out through nuclear pore by simple diffusion.

The post transcriptional modifications it undergo are

1. *Capping at 5′ end*

GDP is added at 5' end and it is methylated. Methylation occurs in cytosol. RNA Triphosphatase is an essential mRNA processing enzyme in mammals. It is involved in 5' cap formation. It hydrolyzes terminal γ-phosphate of nascent pre mRNA to form diphosphate, which is capped with GMP by the enzyme RNA guanylyl transferase. Later GMP under goes methylation.

2. *Poly adenylation at 3′ end*

Poly A tail is attached at 3' end. Poly (A) polymerase (PAP) is responsible for the addition of poly A tail at 3" end of pre-mRNA.

3. *Splicing*

Parts of hnRNA does not contain any genetic information. These unwanted or intervening sequences are known as *introns*. Parts of hnRNA which contain (carry) genetic information are known as *exons* (Fig. 17.13). Splicing removes introns and joins exons to form functional mRNA. Splicing requires special proteins and small nuclear RNA's or SnRNAs. Usually SnRNAs consist of about 100 nucleotides. The base composition of SnRNA is complementary to the ends of introns. This helps SnRNA and introns to base pair and this leads to loop formation. As a result, adjacent exons come together (Fig. 17.13). Finally removal of intron loop and joining of exons takes place (Fig. 17.13).

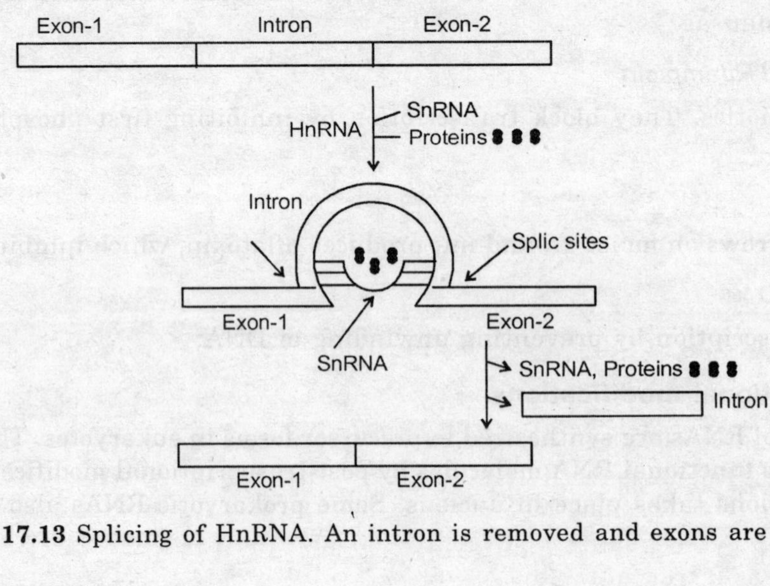

Fig. 17.13 Splicing of HnRNA. An intron is removed and exons are joined

Transfer RNA

It is synthesized in large precursor form. It may contain nucleotide sequence for more than one tRNA. Ribonucleases removes extra nucleotide sequence. Other modifications of tRNA are

1. Characteristic CCA sequence is added at 3′ end.
2. Psudouridylate and ribothymidylate are formed.

Ribosomal RNA

Ribosomal RNAs are synthesized in large precursor form known as pre rRNA. In eukaryotes, four rRNA molecules 5, 5.8, 18 and 28S are generated from single 45S precursor molecule by nuclease digestion.

RETROVIRUSES

Medical importance

RNA is genetic material of these viruses. Most of tumor producing viruses are retroviruses. Rous Sarcoma virus, leukaemia virus and AIDS virus are few examples for retroviruses. They contain oncogenes. In these viruses, genetic information flows from RNA to DNA then to RNA and to protein. Retroviruses are used in gene therapy.

Replication of retroviruses

1. There is a unique mechanism for replication of retroviruses.
2. The replication is carried out by reverse transcriptase present in these viruses.
3. Reverse transcriptase is RNA directed DNA polymerase. It has other activities like ribonuclease activity and DNA directed DNA polymerase activity.
4. Usually the retrovirus lack complete machinery required for replication. So they replicate only after they enter a host.
5. In the host cell, retroviral RNA is used as template to form single stranded DNA by reverse transcriptase (Fig. 17.14).
6. Then the same enzyme cleaves RNA from RNA – DNA hybrid and leaving single stranded DNA, which serves as template for the formation of double stranded DNA that is again carried out by reverse transriptase (Fig. 17.14).
7. The double stranded DNA contains information of native RNA hence it is known as *provirus* and it is integrated into host DNA.
8. Transcription of host DNA containing provirus produces genetic material of RNA viruses (Fig. 17.14).
9. Finally viral proteins are formed when viral RNA is translated.
10. Assembly of viral proteins with RNA generates new virus particles.

Ribozymes

Catalytically or enzymatically active RNAs are known as ribozymes. RNA of ciliated protozoa tetra hymena is catalytically active. It is synthesized in large precursor form known as pre-rRNA. It consist of an intron and two exons. Functional rRNA is generated from precursor by self splicing. Pre-rRNA is also referred as self splicing RNA. Self-splicing removes intron and joins exons. It has nuclease (hydrolytic) activity and ligase or trans esterification activity. Self-nuclease activity removes introns where as transesterification activity joins exons. GMP is required for catalytic activity. GMP binds to specific region of pre-rRNA. Various steps involved in generation of rRNA from pre-rRNA are out lined in Fig. 17.15.

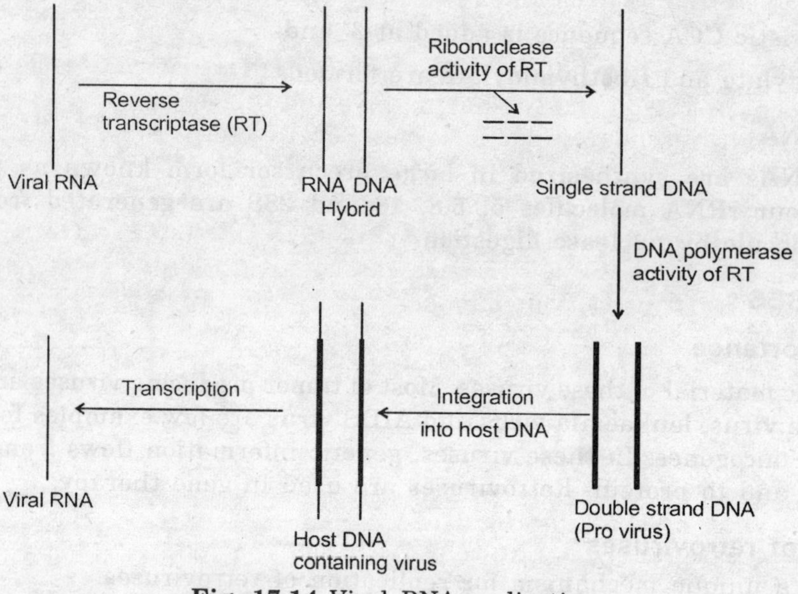

Fig. 17.14 Viral RNA replication

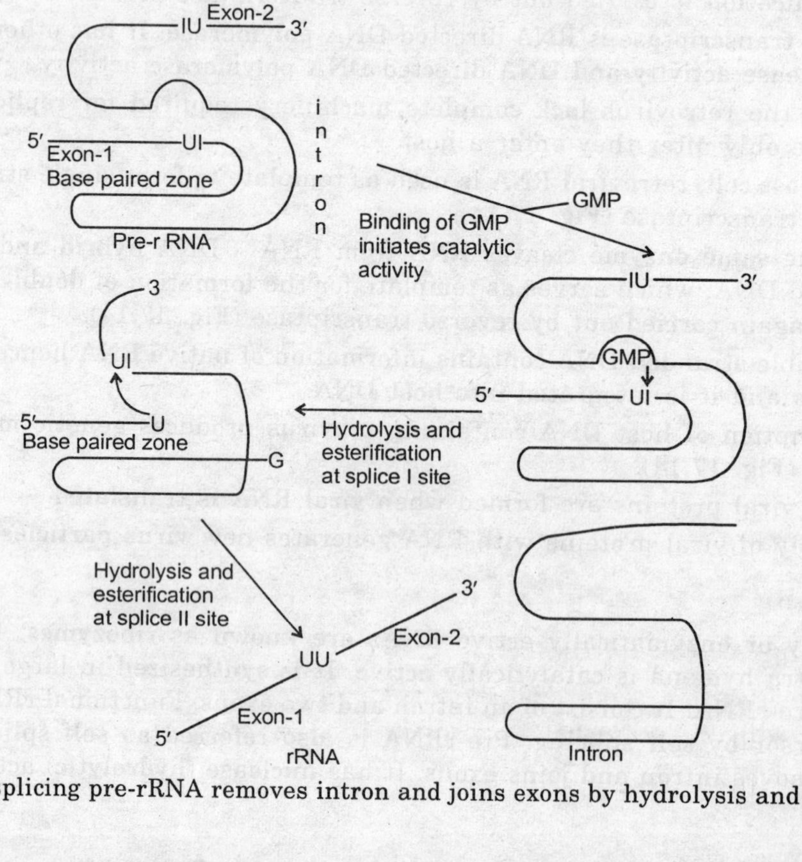

Fig. 17.15 Self splicing pre-rRNA removes intron and joins exons by hydrolysis and esterification

RESTRICTION ENDO NUCLEASES OR RESTRICTION ENZYMES

These enzymes cut both DNA strands at specific sites. They are present in prokaryotes and absent in eukaryotes. They can not cut DNA of cell of their origin. They hydrolyze only foreign DNA molecules. Methylation protects DNA from attack of restriction endonucleases. Since they restrict the entry of foreign DNA into host DNA by cutting foreign DNA they are referred as restriction enzymes.

They show extreme structural specificity towards DNA molecules upon which they act. Only a segment or region of DNA having inverted repeat sequences or palindromic sequences is cleaved by restriction endonucleases. Several restriction enzymes are isolated from bacteria and viruses. They differ in structural requirement, cleavage site and produces DNA fragments with characteristic ends. For example, action of restriction endonuclease of *E. Coli* which is known as *Eco.* RI on DNA produces DNA fragments with sticky or cohesive ends. These cohesive ends can base pair with complementary strand (Fig. 17.16*a*). In contrast restriction endonuclease of Para influenza, which is known as *HpaI action* on DNA produces DNA fragments with blunt ends (Fig. 17.16*b*).

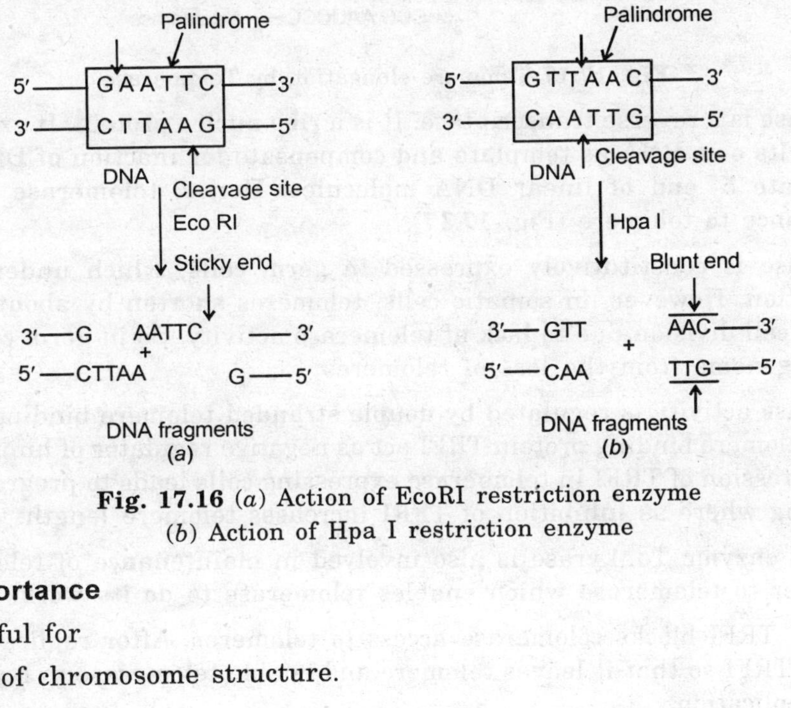

Fig. 17.16 (*a*) Action of EcoRI restriction enzyme
(*b*) Action of Hpa I restriction enzyme

Medical importance

They are useful for

(*a*) Analysis of chromosome structure.

(*b*) Isolation of genes.

(*c*) DNA sequencing.

(*d*) Recombinant DNA technology.

(*e*) RFLP (Restricted Fragment Length Polymorphism).

Telomere, Telomerase and Cancer

1. **Telomere** is chromosomal end. It is composed of short G-rich randomly repeated sequence, which is extended to form single stranded over hang.

2. $(TTAGGG)_n$ is characteristic repeat found in telomeres. DNA replication mechanism can not replicate single-stranded telomeres. So, telomeric DNA is lost with each cell division when telomere erode to critical size cell cease to divide and die. Thus, telomere serveas, replicometer which count cell division and ultimately triggers replicative senescence or cell aging. Further, telomeres prevent chromosomal fusion and offer genomic integrity and stability (Fig. 17.17).

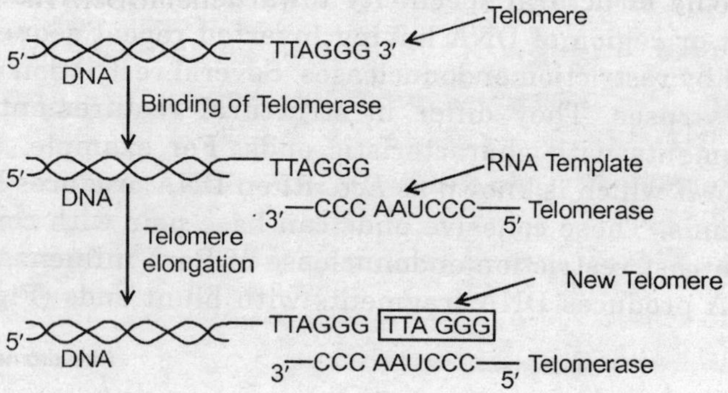

Fig. 17.17 Telomere elongation by Telomerase

3. Telomerase is a reverse transcriptase. It is a ribo nucleo protein. It extends telomere by using its own RNA as template and compensate for inaction of DNA polymerase to replicate 5′ end of linear DNA molecules. Hence, telomerase is involved in maintenance to telomere (Fig. 17.17).
4. Telomerase is constitutively expressed in germ cells, which undergo continuous proliferation. However, in somatic cells, telomeres shorten by about 50 base pairs per each cell division due to lack of telomerase activity. So in germ cells telomerase protects genome from the loss of telomeres.
5. Telomerase activity is regulated by double stranded telomere binding proteins The human telomere binding protein TRFI act as negative regulator of human telomerase. Over expression of TRFI in telomerase expressing cells leads to progressive telomere shortening where as inhibition of TFRI increases telomere length.
6. A second enzyme Tankyrase is also involved in maintenance of telomere. It serve as partner to telomerase which enables telomerase to do its work.
7. Normally TRFI blocks telomerase access to telomeres. After replication tankyrase modifies TRFI so that it leaves telomere and enable telomerase to replace DNA lost during replication.
8. Thus, telomerase activity is developmentally connected in cell cycle dependant manner, which involves either telemore shortening, stability or even elongation.
9. Immortal eukaryotic cells or cancer cells or virus transformed cells that pocess unlimited proliferation capacity exhibit high telomerase activity. Expression of telomerase allows cells to repair their or elongate telomeres. As a result, cell division continues, cells proliferate and ultimately immortalization of cells occurs, which is characteristic of cancer cells.

REFERENCES

1. Kornberg, A. and Baker. DNA replication. 2nd ed. Freeman, New York, 1991.
2. Watson, J.D. Hopkins, N.H. Steitz, J.A. and Weiner, A.M. Molecular biology of the gene, 4th ed. Benjamin/Cummings, California, 1986.
3. Allewell, N. Why does DNA bend? Trends Biochem. Sci. **13**, 193-195, 1988.
4. Sancar, A. and Sancar, G.B. DNA repair enzymes. Ann. Rev. Biochem. **57**, 29-68, 1988.
5. Cozzarelli, N.R. The mechanism of action of inhibitors of DNA synthesis. Ann. Rev. Biochem. **46**, 641, 1977.
6. Varmus, H. Retroviruses. Science **240**, 1427-1435, 1988.
7. Mills, D.R. Kraner, F.R. and Spiegelmen, S. Complete sequence of replicating RNA molecule. Science **180**, 816, 1973.
8. Katz, R.A. and Stalka, M.A. The retroviral enzymes. Ann. Rev. Biochem. **63**, 133-173, 1994.
9. Cech, T.R. The chemistry of self splicing RNA and RNA enzymes. Science **236**, 1532-1539, 1987.
10. Kim, H. *et al.* Regulation of poly (A) polymerase. The EMBO. J. **22**, 5208-5219, 2003.
11. Chengala, A. *et al.* Structure and mechanism of RNA triphosphatase component of mammalian mRNA capping enzyme. The EMBO. J. **20**, 2575-2580, 2001.
12. Shav–Tal *et al.* Dynamics of single mRNP in nucleus of living cells. Science **304**, 1797-1800, 2004.
13. Nakono, S-I, Chadelawada, D.M. and Bevilacqua, P.C. General acid-base catalysis in the mechanism of Hepatitis delta virus ribozyme. Science **287**, 1493-1497, 2000.
14. Anja-Katrin Bielinsky. Replication origins: why do we need so many. Cell cycle. **2**, 310-315, 2003.
15. Martin-Cordero, C. *et al.* Curcumin as DNA topoisomerase poison. J. Enzyme inhib. Med. Chem. **18**, 505-509, 2003.
16. Peter J. Unrau and David P. Bastal. An oxo-carbenium ion intermediate of ribozyme reaction indicated by kinetic isotope effects. Proc. Natl. Acad. Sci. USA **100**, 15393-15397, 2003.
17. Albert's, B. DNA replication and recombination. Nature **421,** 431–435, 2003.
18. Bielinsky, A.K. and Gerbi, S.A. Where it all starts: eukaryotic origins of DNA replication. J. Cell Sci. **114**, 643-651, 2001.
19. Bell, S.P. and Dutea, A. DNA replication in eukaryotic cells. Ann. Rev. Biochem. **71**, 333-374, 2002.
20. Smiraldo, P.G. Telomerase: Amystery by name alone. IUBMB Life. **56**, 573-574, 2004.
21. Jennifer, A.D. Ribozyme catalysis: Not different just worse. Nat. Structu. Mol. Biol. **12**, 395-402, 2005.

EXERCISES

ESSAY QUESTIONS

1. Define replication. Describe various stages of replication.
2. Define transcription. Describe mechanism of transcription.
3. Write an essay on enzymes of nucleic acid biosynthesis. Mention their importance.
4. Explain central dogma of molecular biology. Write on factors associated with nucleic acids biosynthesis.
5. Define retroviruses, ribozymes, restriction enzymes. Give examples. Explain retroviral replication mechanism.

SHORT QUESTIONS

1. Write a note on inhibitors of replication.
2. Explain DNA repair mechanisms.
3. Define promoters and palindromes. Explain their role in transcription.
4. Define hnRNA. How it is converted to mRNA?
5. Explain retroviral replication process.
6. What are restriction enzymes? Explain their action with examples.
7. Write a note on post transcriptional modifications.
8. Define promoters, terminators. Give examples. Explain their role in nucleic acid formation.
9. Write biochemical defects in the following diseases:
   (*a*) Xeroderma pigmentosum
   (*b*) Ataxia talengiectasia.
10. Write briefly on inhibitors of transcription.
11. Write reactions and clinically important inhibitors of DNA and RNA polymerases.
12. Outline process of replication.
13. Write about okazaki fragments.
14. Explain importance of non-coding RNA.
15. Write clinical importance of DNA topoisomerase inhibitors.

MULTIPLE CHOICE QUESTIONS

1. Inhibitors of replication are used as
   (*a*) Anti-cancer agents.
   (*b*) Anti-viral agents.
   (*c*) Anti-bacterial agents.
   (*d*) Anti-cancer, anti-viral and anti-bacterial agents.
2. DNA polymerases
   (*a*) Are involved in nucleic acid synthesis.
   (*b*) Are template directed enzymes.
   (*c*) Act in $3' \rightarrow 5'$ direction.
   (*d*) Initiates chain formation.

3. All of the following statements are correct regarding xeroderma pigmentosum. Except
   (*a*) Thorny growth of skin is a symptom of this disease.
   (*b*) Skin of affected person is in sensitive to UV light.
   (*c*) Corneal ulceration is seen in affected people.
   (*d*) Patients of this disease die at young age.
4. Rifampicin blocks transcription
   (*a*) By inhibiting first phophodiester bond formation.
   (*b*) By binding with σ factor.
   (*c*) By preventing unwinding of DNA.
   (*d*) By forming loops in DNA-RNA hybrid.
5. RFLP is used for
   (*a*) Analysis of chromosome structure.
   (*b*) DNA estimation.
   (*c*) Production of antibodies.
   (*d*) Synthesis of nucleic acids.

FILL IN THE BLANKS

1. Synthesis of DNA is essential for cell -------------.
2. Synthesis of RNA is essential for ------------ of genetic in formation from ------------ to -------------.
3. DNA gyrase catalyzes ------------ dependent reaction.
4. Catalytic RNA requires ------------ for catalytic activity.
5. ------------ is genetic material in retroviruses.

18
CHAPTER

PROTEIN BIOSYNTHESIS

MEDICAL AND BIOLOGICAL IMPORTANCE

1. Protein biosynthesis deals with mechanism of polypeptide chain formation in living organisms.
2. Usually polypeptide chain is formed from N-terminal amino acid.
3. Genetic code aids decoding of information present in the sequence of nucleotides into amino acid sequence of a protein.
4. Alterations in genetic code causes formation of a protein with altered amino acid sequence.
5. Various abnormal haemoglobins (Hb variants) are due to changes in the genetic code.
6. Sometimes, alteration in genetic code causes cancer in susceptible individuals.
7. Accuracy of protein biosynthesis decreases in old age.
8. Polypeptide chain formation is a energy intensive process.
9. Several antibiotics and toxins work by blocking protein biosynthesis.
10. Ribosomes and some translational factors act as Chaperones.
11. Ribosomal RNAs are useful in study of phylogeny and biological diversity.

Protein biosynthesis is a process by which information present in nucleotide sequence of mRNA is converted into amino acid sequence of a protein. Other name given to this process is translation. Since mRNA as such has no affinity towards amino acids, the conversion of information present in the nucleotide sequence of mRNA into amino acid sequence of a protein requires an adaptor molecule. This adaptor molecule must be able to identify specific nucleotide sequence on mRNA and an amino acid. The tRNA serves as adaptor molecule by recognizing specific nucleotide sequence on mRNA through anti codon arm and corresponding amino acid through amino acid arm.

Genetic code

In the nucleotide, sequence of mRNA code words are present for amino acids. These code words are collectively referred as genetic code. Since the code words on mRNA originates from genes or DNA they are called as *genetic code*. Hence, genetic information or gene is nothing but code words for amino acids. Genetic code is presented in Table 18.1.

Table 18.1 Genetic code

FIRST NUCLEOTIDE		Second Nucleotide G		A		C		U		THIRD NUCLEOTIDE
	G	GGG		GAG	Glu	GCG		GUG		G
		GGA	Gly	GAA		GCA	Ala	GUA	Val	A
		GGC		GAC	Asp	GCC		GUC		C
		GGW		GAU		GCU		GUU		U
	A	AAG	Arg	AAG	Lys	ACG		AUG	Met	G
		AGA		AAA		ACA	Thr	AUA		A
		AGC	Ser	AAC	Asn	ACC		AUC	Ileu	C
		AGU		AAU		ACU		AUU		U
	C	CGG		CAG	Gln	CCG		CUG		G
		CGA	Arg	CAA		CCA	Pro	CUA	Leu	A
		CGC		CAC	His	CCC		CUC		C
		CGU		CAU		CCU		CUU		U
	U	UGG	Try	UAG	Ter	UCG		UUG	Leu	G
		UGA	Ter	UAA		UCA	Ser	UUA		A
		UGC	Cys	UAC	Tyr	UCC		UUC	Phe	C
		UUU		UAU		UCU		UUU		U

Characteristics of genetic code

1. It is triplet code. Each amino acid is coded by sequence of three nucleotides. It is known as *codon*. For example, UUU codes for phenylalanine, GGG codes for glycine and CCC codes for proline.
2. Some codons function as initiation codons for protein synthesis. For example, AUG in prokaryotes initiates polypeptide chain formation.
3. Some codons do not code for any amino acid and they cause termination of polypeptide chain formation. They are called as *nonsense codons* or *termination codons*. They are UAA, UAG or UGA.
4. A given codon codes only one amino acid. But an amino acid is indicated or coded by more than one codon.

   Existence of more than one code word for an amino acid is known as degeneracy of genetic code. For example, arginine is coded by six codons.

5. The genetic code is universal. Codon of a given amino acid is identical in all species.
6. For a given codon on mRNA, an anti-codon is present on tRNA. Codon and anti-codon always read from $5' \rightarrow 3'$ direction. Further, codon and anticodons are anti-parallel and complementary in base composition. They interact with each other through base pairing.
7. Genetic code is commaless. Once reading of codons on mRNA begins it is continued until a termination codon is reached.
8. For proper function of codon, only first two nucleotides are essential the third nucleotide is flexible, i.e., even if third nucleotide is changed in a codon, that codon indicates same aminoacid. For example, three codons for a alanine GCA, GCC and GCU interacts with alanine anticodon IGC. This is known as *wobble phenomenon*. Thus, the base pairing of third nucleotide of codon with anti-codon is less specific.

Ribosomes

They are complexes of RNA and protein. Non-covalent forces or bonds keeps them together. They are called as ribonucleo proteins because they are rich in ribonucleic acids. They are very large molecules compared to proteins. They are present in both prokaryotes and eukaryotes. They are classified based on their sedimentation coefficients (S).

Prokaryotic ribosome

It is a 70S ribosome. It consist of two subunits one larger 50S subunit and smaller 30S subunit. Two rRNAs are present in 50S subunit. They are 23S and 5S. About 34 proteins are present in 50S subunit. The 30S subunit has one 16S rRNA and 21 proteins (Figure 18.1).

Eukaryotic ribosome

It is a 80S ribosome. It contains larger 60S subunit and smaller 40S subunit. The 60S subunit contains three rRNAs. They are 28S, 5.8S and 5S RNAs. The 40S subunit contains one 18S RNA molecule. Eukaryotic ribosome may contain 70-90 proteins (Figure 18.1).

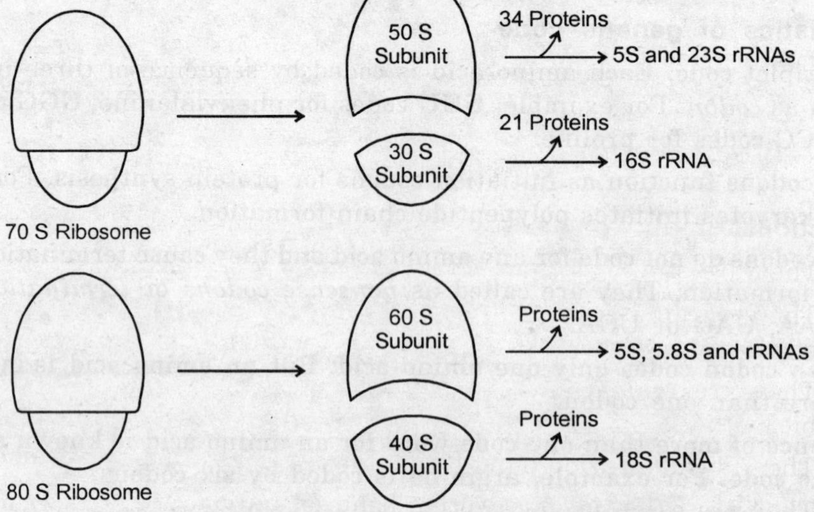

Fig. 18.1 Ribosomes and their composition

Formation of ribosome

Information required for the formation of ribosome is present in the primary structure of protein. Association of submits into ribosome requires presence of Mg^{2+}. In addition, ribosomal subunits undergo dissociation, easily.

Structure of ribosomes

Like proteins ribosomes have characteristic three-dimensional structure. An outline of 70S ribosome is shown in Figure 18.2*a*.

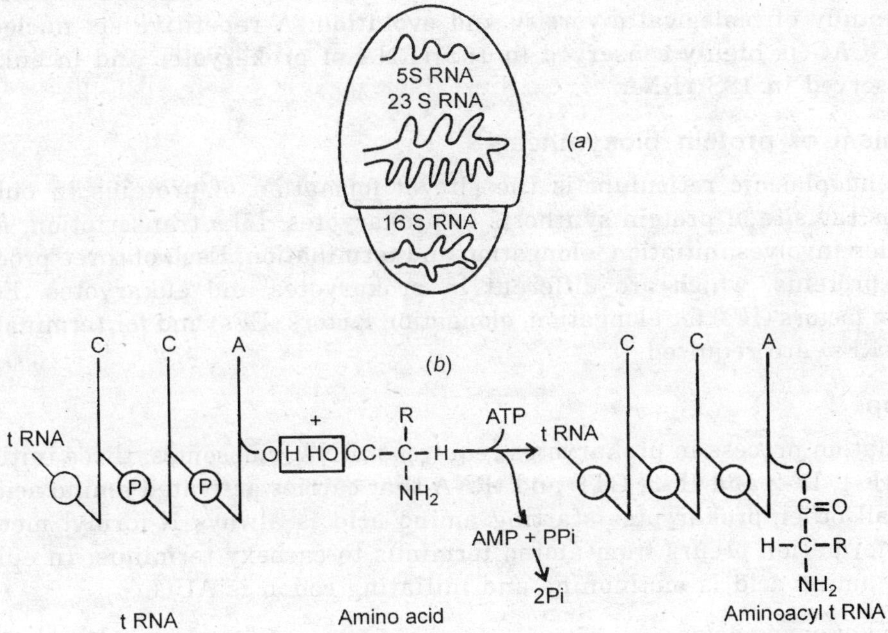

$$\text{Methionine} + \text{tRNA f} \xrightarrow[\text{tRNA Synthetase}]{\text{MethionineAminoacyl}} \text{Met} - \text{t RNA f} \qquad (c)$$

$$N^{10}\text{–formyl tetrahydrofolatc} + \text{Met} - \text{tRNA f} \xrightarrow{\text{Transformylase}} \text{f Met} - \text{tRNA} + \text{tetra hydrofolate}$$

Fig. 18.2 (*a*) Structure of 70S Ribosome
(*b*) Formation of aminoacyl-tRNA
(*c*) Formation of initiating tRNA

Functions of ribosomes

1. They are site of protein biosynthesis.
2. They coordinate interaction between aminoacyl tRNAs, mRNA and various factors of protein biosynthesis.
3. They are required for selection of specific region on mRNA to initiate protein biosynthesis.
4. They favour peptide bond formaiton by facilitating codon and anti-codon pairing.
5. They are essential for peptide bond formation.

6. **Ribosome as Chaperone.** Ribosomes assist protein folding in wide variety of systems very effectively. The peptidyl transferase centre modulates folding of proteins. Ribosome is general chaperone for preventing aggregation of unstable ribosomal proteins until they become associated with RNA.
7. **Ribosomal RNA, bio diversity and evolution.** Ribosomal RNAs are essential components of all living organisms, which are functionally and evolutionarily conserved. Hence, they are useful in phylogeny and biodiversity studies. The universal phylogenetic tree of life has been proposed based on small subunit rRNA gene sequences. Among several small subunits RNAs 16S rRNA has been extensively used for study of biological diversity and evolution. A repetitive six nucleotide pattern CAGCAG is highly conserved in 16S rRNA of prokaryotes and in eukaryotes, it is conserved in 18S rRNA.

Mechanism of protein biosynthesis

Rough endoplasmic reticulum is the site of formation of proteins in eukaryotes and cytosol is the site of protein synthesis in prokaryotes. Like transcription, mechanism of translation involves initiation, elongation and termination. Each of three processes require several proteins, which are different in prokaryotes and eukaryotes. For initiation, initiation factors (IFs) for elongation, elongation factors (EFs) and for termination releasing factors (RFs) are required.

Initiation

The initiation process in prokaryotes requires mRNA, ribosomes, three initiation protein factors IF-1, IF-2 and IF-3, GTP and tRNA that carries activated amino acids. In *E. Coli* and in all other prokaryotes starting amino acid is always N-formyl methionine. The protein formation occurs from amino terminus to carboxy terminus. In eukaryotes, the starting amino acid is methionine and initiating codon is AUG.

Activation of amino acids

For protein synthesis, initial activation of amino acid is required. This activation is essential because energy is required for peptide bond formation. Activation involves esterification of amino acid with tRNA. In the cytosol amino acid is esterified to corresponding tRNA by enzyme aminoacyl- tRNA synthetase at the expense of ATP. The aminoacyl group is attached to either free 2′ or 3′ hydroxyl group of terminal A residue of tRNA molecule present at 3′-end of tRNA. The formation of amino acyl-t RNA is accompanied by hydrolysis of ATP to AMP and PP_i. Further, hydrolysis of PP_i to $2P_i$ by pyrophosphatase makes the reaction irreversible (Figure 18.2b). In the cytosol 20 different aminoacids are esterified to their corresponding tRNAs by 20 different amino acyl-tRNA synthetases each of which is specific for one amino acid and corresponding t-RNA.

Formation of N-formyl methionine-tRNA

It occurs in two steps. First methionine is esterified to N-formyl methionine carrying tRNA, which is designated as tRNAf by methionine amino acyl-tRNA synthetase. In the second reaction a formyl group is transferred to the methionine from N^{10}-formyl tetra hydrofolate by specific transformylase enzyme (Figure 18.2c). Met -tRNAm is another tRNA used for inserting methionine in the interior.

INITIATION PROCESS

Initiation process occurs in three steps

1. The first step is the binding of three initiation factors to free 30S subunit. IF-3 binds to free 30S subunit. IF-2 as such cannot bind to 30S subunit. It combines with GTP forms IF-2-GTP complex. IF-1 and IF-2 with bound GTP joins 30S subunit containing IF-3.
2. The 30S subunit with attached three factors is ready to accept mRNA and initiating tRNA. Attachment of mRNA to 30S subunit is aided by 16S ribosomal RNA and purine rich Shine-Dalgarno sequence near 5′ end. The messenger RNA is attached to 30S subunit near 5′ end of the message. Now the initiating tRNA recognize AUG codon and joins 30S-mRNA complex through codon-anticodon base pairing to form 30S initiation complex. Formation of 30S initiation complex is accompanied by the release of IF-3. Once IF-3 is released the initiation complex develops high affinity for 50S subunit and binds to one available from the pool.
3. The 50S subunit has two sites. They are an aminoacid (A) site and peptidyl (P) site. The P site accommodates tRNA containing growing polypeptide chain and A site accommodates incoming aminoacyl tRNA. Usually anti-codons of tRNAs present in P site and A site base pairs with codons on mRNA. The 50S subunit joins 30S initiation complex. The bound GTP is hydrolyzed and IF-1, IF-2 and GDP are released. Product of this step is 70S initiation complex (Figure 18.3). In the 70S initiation complex fmet-t RNAf occupies P site and the A site is vacant. Only initiating tRNA binds to P site all other aminoacyl tRNA bind to A site.

Elongation

Now the polypeptide chain is elongated by covalent attachment of successive amino acids from amino terminus to carboxy terminus. tRNAs carries amino acid to ribosomes. In addition to aminoacyl-tRNAs elongation requires three elongation factors EF-Tu, EF-Ts and EF-G and GTP. Elongation process occurs in three steps.

1. *Binding of amino acyl-tRNA to A site*

Second codon next to initiation codon on mRNA dictates nature of incoming amino acyl-tRNA. The incoming amino acyl-tRNA can not combine with 70S initiation complex directly. So, it forms complex with EF-Tu-GTP. This complex carrying appropriate amino acyl-tRNA as dictated by second codon on mRNA base pairs with codon on mRNA and occupies A site of 70S initiation complex. This is accompanied by hydrolysis of GTP to GDP and Pi and resulting ET-Tu-GDP complex dissociates from ribosomes. For the next elongation step, EF-Tu-GTP is required hence a second elongation factor EF-Ts regenerates EF-Tu-GTP complex from EF-Tu-GDP complex. First EF-Ts reacts with EF-Tu-GDP complex displace GDP and forms EF-Tu-EF-Ts complex. Now GTP reacts with this complex replaces EF-Ts and forms EF-Tu-GTP complex. All these events are shown in Figure 18.3.

2. *Peptide bond formation*

Two amino acyl-tRNAs on the two sites of ribosome sets the stage for first peptide bond formation. The peptidyl transferase activity of 50S ribosomal subunit catalyzes the peptide bond formation between two amino acids. This process is also known as trans peptidation, because the peptide bond formation involves transfer of fmet from tRNA located in the P site to α-amino group of amino acyl-tRNA in the A site. Nucleophilic attack of α-amino group of incoming amino acyl-tRNA on carboxyl group of fmet of met-tRNA generates peptide bond. As a result, a dipeptide is generated on tRNA of A site leaving empty tRNA f on P site (Figure 18.4).

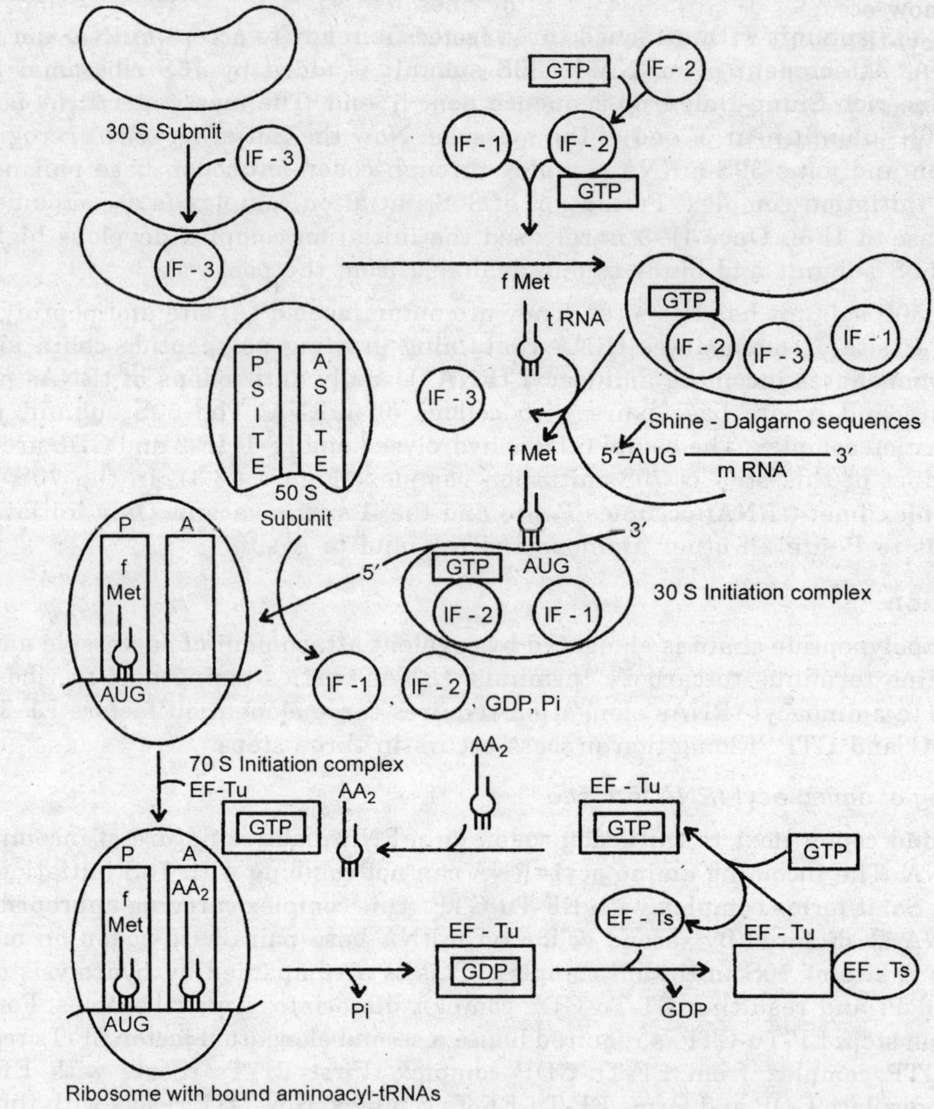

Fig. 18.3 Initiation and binding of aminoacyl–tRNA to A site

3. *Translocation*

The second in coming aminoacyl tRNA can bind to A site of ribosome only when dipeptidyl tRNA is shifted to P site from A site of ribosome. Elongation factor EF-G and GTP are involved in the transfer of dipeptidyl tRNA from A site to P site. Initially, the EF-G binds to a GTP and then forms complex with ribosome. This causes release of free tRNA from P site and transfer of dipeptidyl tRNA from A site to P site. As peptidyl tRNA moves to P site the mRNA also moves by three nucleotides. At this stage, initiation AUG codon comes out of ribosome, second codon with attached dipeptidyl-tRNA is on P site of ribosome and third codon is exposed in the A site. This process is accompained by hydrolysis of GTP to GDP and P_i and release of EF-G. The growing polypeptide chain or dipeptidyl t RNA now occupies P site and A site of ribosome is ready to receive second, incoming amino acyl-tRNA. EF-G, GTP complex is formed from EF-G and GTP and this can be used again. The elongation process is repeated several times adding one amino acid each time until a stop codon is encountered in the A site. Through out the process the polypeptide chain is attached to tRNA carrying the last amino acid added (Figure 18.4).

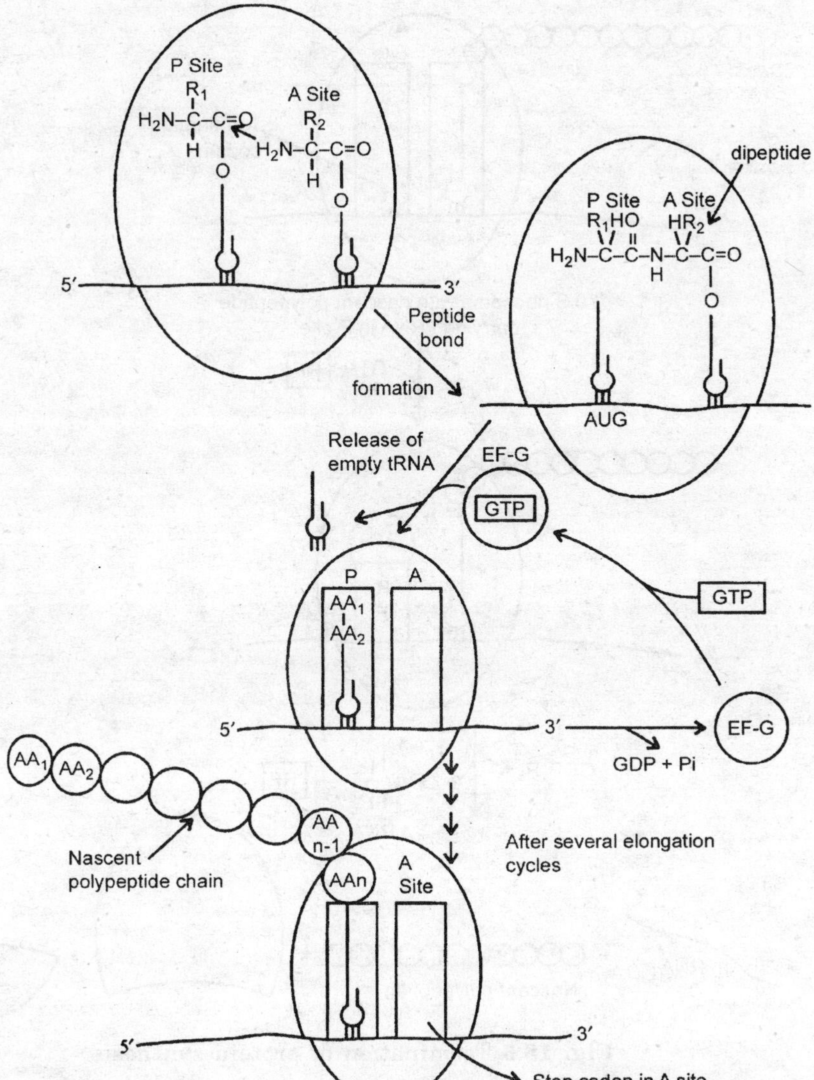

Fig. 18.4 Peptide bond formation, translocation and several elongation cycles of protein synthesis

Termination

Appearance of termination codon in A site signals termination and release of newly synthesized polypeptide chain from tRNA. It requires releasing factors (RFs) and GTP. Usually there is no tRNA, which can recognize termination codon on A site. But it is recognized by releasing factors. There are three releasing factors. They are RF-1, RF-2 and RF-3 and they are capable of recognizing termination codon on A site and they bind where tRNA would bind. Peptidyl transferase activity of ribosomes is responsible for the release of polypeptide synthesized from tRNA. Hydrolysis of GTP releases mRNA, tRNA and RF from ribosomes (Figure 18.5). Now the 70S ribosome is unstable and dissociates to 50S and 30S subunits.

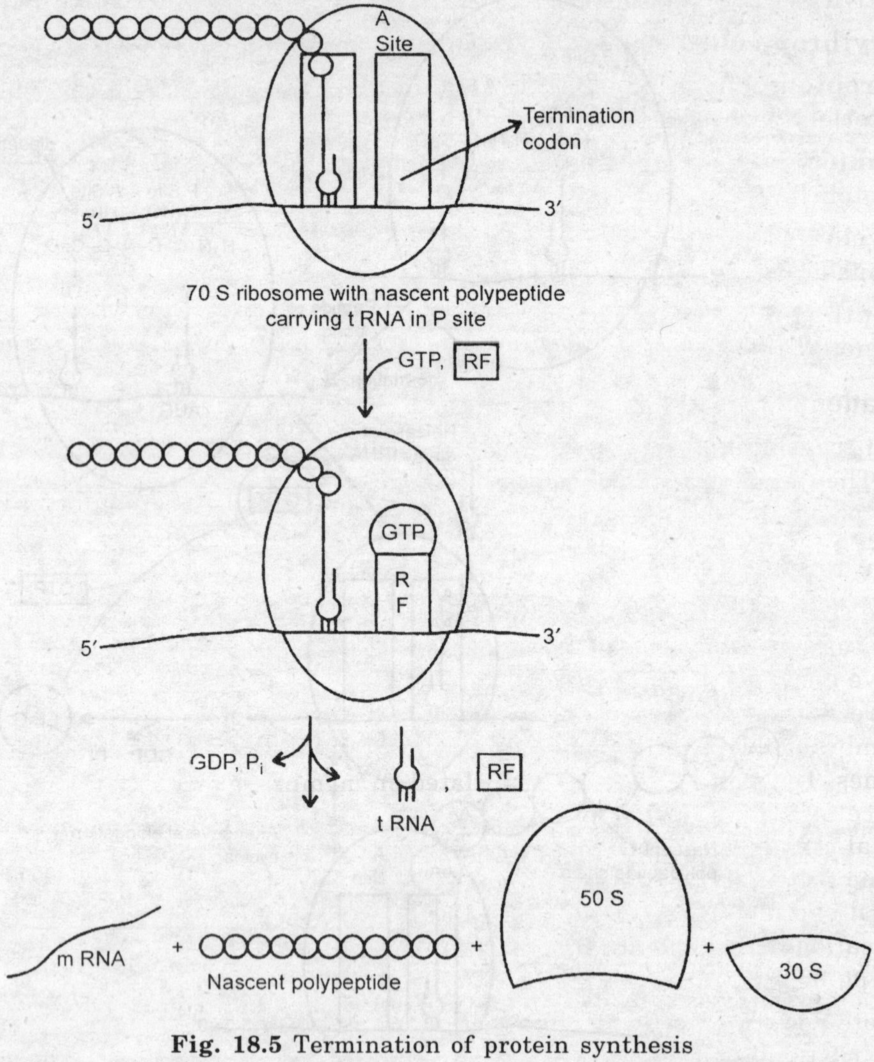

Fig. 18.5 Termination of protein synthesis

Medical importance

Many antibiotics and toxins work by inhibiting protein biosynthesis. They act at different stages of protein biosynthesis. Antibiotics block protein biosynthesis in prokaryotes. Usually eukaryotic protein synthesis is not affected by these antibiotics.

1. **Puromycin** It is derived from mold. It has structure very similar to that of 3′ end of aminoacyl-tRNA. So, it get incorporated into growing polypeptide chain by replacing incoming aminoacyl tRNA. As a result peptidyl puromycin is formed. Further addition of amino acids to peptidyl puromycin is blocked. Hence it is discharged from ribosome and protein synthesis is terminated.
2. **Tetracyclins** They inhibit protein synthesis by preventing the binding of aminoacyl-tRNA to A site.
3. **Chloramphenicol** It inhibits protein biosynthesis by blocking peptidyl transferase activity of 50S subunit.
4. **Erythromycin** It binds to 50S subunit and inhibits translocation step.
5. **Streptomycin** It binds to 30S subunit and cause misreading of genetic code. It also interfers with binding of initiating tRNA to ribosome.
6. **Tunicamycin** It prevents attachments of oligosaccharide side chains to certain glyco proteins.
7. **Cyclo heximide** It inhibits protein biosynthesis in eukaryotes by blocking peptidyl transferase activity of 60S eukaryotic ribosome.
8. **Diptheria toxin** It is produced by bacteria that cause diptheria in children. It inhibits protein synthesis in eukaryotes. It inactivates elongation factor of eukaryotes.

Translational factors as chaperones

Several translational factors also possess chaperone activity. They are IF-2, EF-Tu and EF-G. They assist co-translational folding. They are ancestral chaperones dedicated to folding of nascent polypeptides before the evolution of general chaperones.

Protein targeting

Now we shall examine how proteins are transported to various locations in the cell from the site of synthesis where they function as cytosolic enzyme, membrane components, digestive enzymes, hormones etc. Proteins have intrinsic signals or molecular addresses that directs their transport and localization in the cell. Secretary proteins are translated on membrane bound ribosomes where as cytosolic proteins are synthesized on free ribosomes. The mRNAs that are translated on membrane bound ribosomes contain unique sequence of codons upstream of initiating codon. These sequence of codons are known as signal codons. Translation of signal sequence results in unique amino acid sequence on amino terminal end of nascent polypeptide. The unique amino acid sequence is known as signal peptide. These signals has all information for targeting proteins to organelles, translocation across membrane or assembly into membranes. Different signals exist for each type of protein targeting.

Protein sorting pathway of secretary proteins begins with synthesis of signal peptide by free ribosomes in cytosol. A signal recognition particle (SRP), which is composed of RNA and protein binds to signal peptide when it emerges from ribosome and forms complex. As a result, translation is arrested and complex moves to endoplasmic reticulum (ER). SRP receptor or docking protein present on the cytosolic surface of ER is recognized by the complex and binds to receptor. This is followed by release of translational arrest and release of SRP and docking protein. A ribosome receptor, translocon of endoplasmic reticulum aids passage of peptide chain through lipid bilayer and synthesis proceeds on membrane-bound ribosomes. After completion of synthesis signal, peptide is cleaved by signal peptidase and mature protein is released into ER. In Figure 18.6 steps of secretary protein sorting pathway are shown.

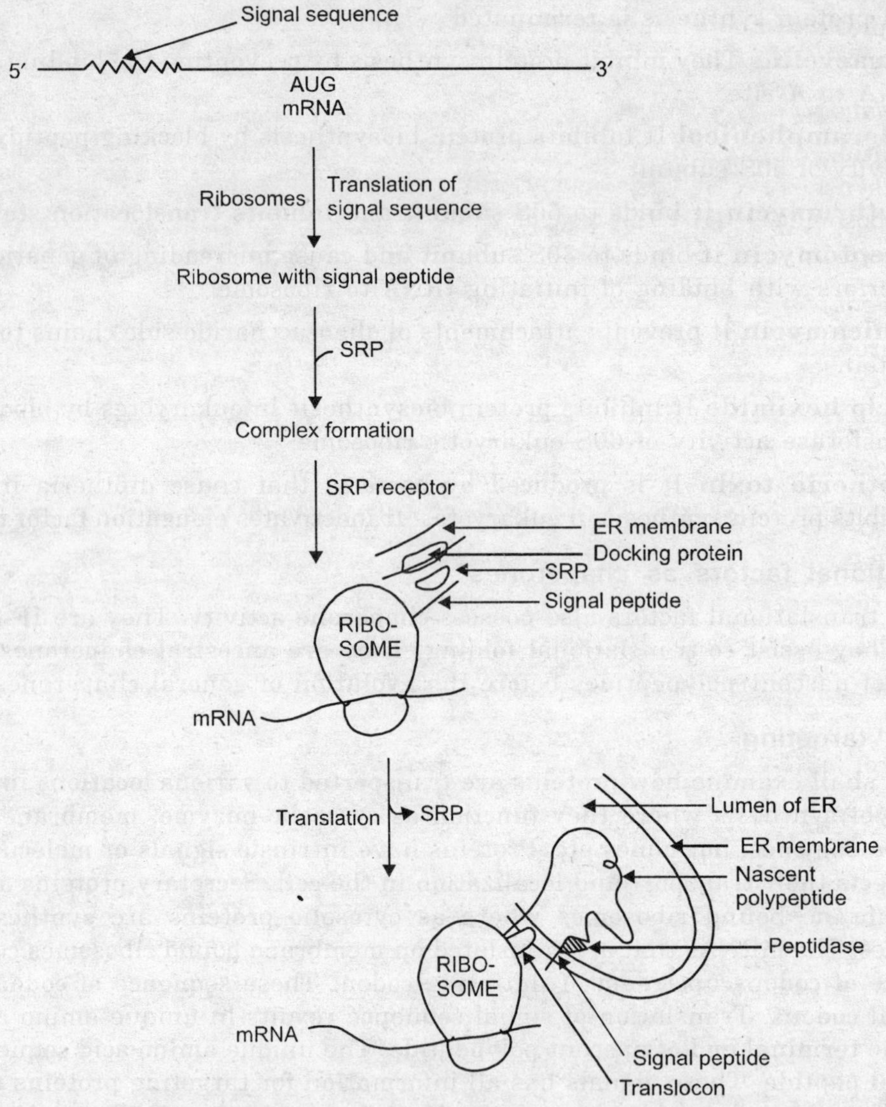

Fig. 18.6 Secretary protein sorting pathway

Post-translational modifications

Majority of proteins, which emerges from the ribosome are not biologically active proteins. Post-translational modifications convert these into functional proteins. Usually protein may attain proper conformation by the time it is released from the ribsome. Some of the post-translational modifications are

1. *Phosphorylation*

The hydroxyl groups of serine and tyrosine residues of some proteins are phosphorylated after they leave ribosome. Specific enzymes catalyzes this phosphorylation. For example, casein has many phosphate groups, which are attached to hydroxyl group of serine after it comes out of ribosomes. Phosphorylation converts inactive enzymes to active enzymes like phosphorylase. Sometimes, phosphorylation of certain proteins is harmful to cells. For example, phosphorylation of tyrosine residues of certain proteins converts normal cells to cancer cells.

2. *Glycosylation*

The formation of glyco proteins occurs in two stages. First the protein part of glyco protein is synthesized on ribosomes. Later, carbohydrate is covalently attached to protein outside ribosome. Usually the carbohydrate is attached to aspargine or serine residues of proteins.

3. *Attachment of prosthetic groups*

Initially protein part of conjugated protein is synthesized on ribosome. Prosthetic groups are attached to proteins after they leaves ribosomes. For example, heme group is attached later to hemeproteins.

4. *Hydroxylation*

Proline and lysine residues of collagen subunits are hydroxylated after they leaves ribosomes.

5. *Disulfide bond formation*

In some proteins, inter or intrachain disulfide bonds are formed after proteins leaves ribosome. In the case of oligomeric proteins, interchain disulfide bonds are formed.

6. *Methylation*

In some proteins, lysine residues are methylated after they leaves ribosomes. For example, muscle proteins and cytochrome c.

7. *Carboxylation*

Carboxyl groups are added to glutamic and aspartic acid residues of some proteins after they leaves ribosome. For example, γ-carboxylation of glutamyl residues of blood clotting factors like prothrombin.

8. *Removal of initiating amino acid*

The initiating amino acid is removed in some proteins as soon as they comes out of ribosome.

9. *Proteolytic modifications*

Some proteins that are going to be exported from the cell undergo proteolytic modification. For example, some hormones and enzymes.

10. *Iodination*

Iodination of tyrosine residues of thyroglobulin occurs outside of ribosomes.

11. *Palmitoylation*

It is the covalent attachment of lipid moieties to proteins that is found in prokaryotes and eukaryotes. Palmitic acid is the lipid post translationally attached to intergral and peripheral membrane proteins. Palmitic acid is attached in the form of palmitoyl-CoA. The reaction is catalyzed by protein palmitoyl acyl transferase (PPAT). Two types of palmitoylation is known. They are S-Palmitoylation and N-Palmitoylation.

S-Palmitoylation

If palmitate residue is attached to –SH group of cysteine of protein through thioester linkage then it is known as S-Palmitoylation.

N-Palmitoylation

In which palmitate is attached to amino terminal cysteine of the protein through amide linkage.

Functions of palmitoylation

Functions of palmitoylation depends on protein that is being considered.

(*a*) Palmitoylation increases hydrophobicity of proteins and this facilitates their association with membrane.

(*b*) Palmitoylation has role in protein targeting. For example targeting of proteins to axons and dendrites in neurons is influenced by palmitoylation. Palmitoylation facilitates transport of newly synthesized chemokine receptor to plasma membrane.

(*c*) Palmitoylation is involved in modulation of protein-protein interaction. For example, palmitoylation is crucial for binding of erythrocyte membrane protein 4.2 to anion exchanger band 3.

(*d*) Enzyme activity is regulated by palmitoylation. For example, carbamoyl phosphate synthetase-I activity is inhibited by palmitoylation of active site –SH group. Methyl malonyl semi aldehyde dehydrogenase is another enzme whose activity is regulated by palmitoylation.

(*e*) Palmitoylation influences protein partitioning into domains.

Mutations

Mutation is change in the nucleotide sequence of a gene. Single nucleotide or more than one nucleotide of the gene is changed.

Medical importance

Mutations in genes results in nonfunctional protein production and cancer development.

Single point mutations

In which a single nucleotide (base) of gene is changed. They may be

Transitions

In which a purine base is changed to another purine base or a pyrimidine base is changed to another pyrimidine bases.

$$A \leftrightarrow G \quad C \leftrightarrow T$$

Transversions

In which a purine base is changed to either of pyrimidine bases or a pyrimidine base is changed to either of purine bases.

$$A \rightarrow C \text{ or } T; G \rightarrow C \text{ or } T; C \rightarrow A \text{ or } G; T \rightarrow A \text{ or } G$$

If the gene-containing single-point mutation is transcribed into mRNA, then mRNA molecule contains changed bases in codons. Single nucleotide (base) changes in the codons of mRNA produces altered protein when it is translated. Some times normal protein may be produced because of the degeneracy of genetic code.

Some single point mutations are:

I. Missense mutation

In which a wrong amino acid is incorporated into protein due to changed base in codon. Wrong amino acid in protein may not affect function of protein, can partially affect function of protein, abolish protein function. Hence, missense mutation is further subdivided into

1. *Acceptable missense mutation*

Haemoglobin Hikari is an example for acceptable missense mutation. It is due to alteration of codon on mRNA. Alteration of third nuclcotide in codon AAA converts it to new codon AAU (AAA→AAU), which codes aspargine instead of usual lysine. As a result in **61** position of β chain aspargine is incorporated in place of lysine and abnormal haemoglobin Hb Hikari is produced. But function of this abnormal Hb is normal (not affected). Composition of Hb Hikari is shown as $\alpha_2\ \beta_2^{61\text{Lys}\rightarrow\text{Asn}}$.

2. *Partially acceptable missense mutation*

HbS is an example for partially acceptable missense mutation. In HbS normal amino acid at 6 position of β chain glutamic acid is replaced by valine due to alteration of codon from GAA to GUA (GAA→GUA). However, HbS is partially functional. HbS is shown as $\alpha_2\ \beta_2^{\ 6\text{glu}\rightarrow\text{val}}$.

3. *Unacceptable missense mutation*

HbM (Boston) is an example for this type of mutation. In HbM, histidine at 58 position of α chain is replaced by tyrosine due to alteration of codon from CAC to UAC (CAC→UAC). HbM is functionally not active. HbM is written as $\alpha_2^{58\text{His}\rightarrow\text{Tyr}}\beta_2$.

II. Nonsense mutation

In which a normal codon is converted to termination (nonsense) codon due to change of base in codon. HbMckees Rocks is an example for nonsense mutation. In this abnormal Hb, the β-chain is shortened to 144 residues due to alteration of codon UAA, which codes Tyr to UAG. Alteration of third nucleotide in codon coverts UAA to termination codon UAG. As a result, Hb synthesis is prematurely terminated.

Frame shift mutations

Deletion or insertion of one or more of nucleotides in the codons (genes) of mRNA generates proteins with altered amino acide pattern when it is translated. Usually these mutations leads to addition or deletion of amino acids.

1. *Deletion mutation*

Abnormal haemoglobin, Hb Wayne is an example for deletion mutation. It is due to deletion of a nucleotide at 3′ end of 138 codon in mRNA for α chain. As a result, the α-chain is elongated beyond its normal length and the α-chain of Hb Wayne contains 146 amino acids instead of normal 141 residues.

2. *Insertion mutation*

Abnormal haemoglobin Hb Cranston is an example for insertion mutation. It is due to insertion of two nucleotides at the 5' end of 145 codon in mRNA for β chain. As a result, β chain is elongated beyond its normal length and β chain of Hb Cranston contains 157 amino acids instead of normal 146 amino acids.

Mutation and cancer

Mutation in genes often leads to cancer. Cancer causing genes are called as *oncogenes*. Oncogene identified for bladder carcinoma differs from normal gene in only one nucleotide substitution. Likewise, retroviruses can convert normal gene to on-cogene.

REFERENCES

1. Woese, C.R. The genetic code. Harper and Row, New York, 1967.
2. Wittmann, H.G. Architecture of prokaryotic ribosomes. Ann. Rev. Biochem. **52**, 35-65, 1983.
3. Schimmel, P. Aminoacyl t-RNA synthetases. Ann. Rev. Biogchem. **56**, 125-158 , 1987.
4. Bermek. (Ed.). Mechanism of protein synthesis. Springer-Verlag, New York, 1985.
5. Maitre, V.E.A Stryer, A. and Chanduri, A. Initiation factors in protein synthesis. Ann. Rev. Biochem. **51**, 869-900, 1982.
6. Jiminez, A. Inhibitors of translation. Trends Biochem. Sci. **1**, 28-29, 1976.
7. Nierhaus, K.H. and Wilson, D.N. (Eds.). Protein synthesis and ribosome structure: translating the Genome. J. Wiley. New York, 2004.
8. Franklin, W.R. Molecular Biology. WCB/Mc. Grew Hill, 1999.
9. Mark, P. and Alexander, G. Genes and signals. Cold Spring Harbour Laboratory Press, NY, 2002.
10. Benjamin, M. Abell, *et al.* Signal recognition particle mediates post translational targeting in Eukaryotes. The EMBO Journal **23**, 2755-2764, 2004.
11. Zhou, W. *et al.* Isolation and Identification of short nucleotide sequences that affects translation initiation in *S. Cerevisiae.* Proc. Natl. Acad. Sci. (USA). **100**, 4457-4462, 2003.
12. Salazar, J.C. *et al.* A truncated aminoacyl-tRNA synthatase modifies RNA. Proc. Natl. Acd. Sci. (USA). **101,** 7536-7541, 2004.
13. Yusupou, M.M. *et al.* Crystal structure of the ribosome at 5.5Å resolution, Science. **292,** 883-896, 2001.
14. Caldas, T. *et al.* Chaperone properties of bacterial elongation factor EFG and initiation factor IF-2. J. Biol. Chem. **275**, 855-860, 2000.
15. Ogle, J.M. *et al.* Recognition of cognate transfer RNA by 30S ribosomal sub unit. Science. **292**, 982-987, 2001.

16. Holden, P. *et al.* Secretion of a oligomeri cartilage matrix protein is affected by signal peptide. J. Biol. Chem. **280**, 17172-17179, 2005.

17. Rosenfield, N. *et al.* Gene regulation at single cell level. Science. **307**, 1962-1965, 2005.

EXERCISES

ESSAY QUESTIONS

1. Define translation. Describe translation process in prokaryotes.
2. Write an essay on genetic code and mutations.
3. Describe structure of ribosomes. Write their role in protein biosynthesis.
4. Write about inhibition of translation and post-translation modifications.

SHORT QUESTIONS

1. Define genetic code. Write its characteristics.
2. Explain structure and functions of ribosomes.
3. Explain post-translation modifications of proteins with examples.
4. Define mutation. Name different types of mutations. Give an example for each.
5. Write a note on frame shift mutations.
6. Define transition and transversion mutations. Write consequences of these on protein translated.
7. Write briefly on single point mutations.
8. How nascent polypeptide is terminated?
9. Write about translational factors.
10. Explain initiation process of translation.
11. How amino acids are activated? Write its importance.
12. Draw ribosome structure. Label its parts.
13. Explain elongation step of protein synthesis.
14. Writ importance of P and A sites in translation.

MULTIPLE CHOICE QUESTIONS

1. Polypeptide chain formation occurs.

   (*a*) From amino terminus to carboxy terminus.

   (*b*) From amino terminus.

   (*c*) From carboxy terminus.

   (*d*) During starvation.

2. Aminoacyl-tRNA synthesis involves

   (*a*) Formation of ester bond.

   (*b*) Consumption of two high energy bonds.

(*c*) Formation of ester bond and utilization of two high energy bonds.

(*d*) None of the above.

3. Diphtheria toxin inhibits protein synthesis

(*a*) By inactivating initiation factor.

(*b*) By inactivating elongation factor.

(*c*) By preventing peptide bond formation.

(*d*) By combining with ribosomes.

4. Mutations in genes

(*a*) Results in nonfunctional protein production.

(*b*) May cause cancer.

(*c*) Produces non-functional proteins and cancer.

(*d*) May be due to DNA damage.

5. Which of the following statement is correct regarding Hemoglobin Wayne ?

(*a*) It is an example for single point mutation.

(*b*) It contains 146 aminoacids in α-chain.

(*c*) Its α-chain contains 146 aminoacids instead of normal 141 residues.

(*d*) Its β-chain contains only 140 aminoacids.

FILL IN THE BLANKS

1. Protein biosynthesis is .... intensive process.
2. tRNA serve as .... molecule in protein biosynthesis.
3. ....are essential for release of nascent polypeptide chain.
4. In transition a purine base is changed to another .... base.
5. Initiating amino acid of nascent protein is .... as soon as it comes out of ribosome.

19
CHAPTER

REGULATION OF GENE EXPRESSION

MEDICAL AND BIOLOGICAL IMPORTANCE

1. Gene expression is subjected to regulation throughout the life span of prokaryotic and eukaryotic cells.
2. Total DNA or whole genome is never expressed at any given time.
3. Expression of genes is turned on or turned off depending on biological needs, developmental stage or time, environmental (external) and nutritional factors. For example, when cell prepares for division only genes that have role in cell division are expressed like genes which code replication enzymes and genes that code proteins which are essential for proper cell division. After cell divides expression of these genes is turned off and expression of genes that are involved in various house keeping activities or maintenance of cell is turned on. Further, the extent of expression of genes that are involved in various cellular processes also differs. For example, enzymes of glycolysis and TCA cycle are expressed several times where as enzymes of gluconeogenesis are expressed only when needed. When cell completes its life span apoptosis occurs due to expression of certain genes associated with it.
4. Development of human embryo to infant involves turning on or tuning off of several genes. Growth of infant into adult involves excessive expression of genes that are essential for growth. Once growth is completed, these genes are turned off. Old age occurs due to decreased expression of vital genes.
5. Gene expression is tissue specific and species specific. Even though all eukaryotic cells contain same information, its expression depends on tissue. For example, insulin is expressed in pancreas but not in other tissues. Similarly, urea cycle enzymes are expressed in liver only.
6. Evolution of species involves turning on or turning off of certain genes.
7. Depending on environmental or nutritional factors, expression of certain genes is increased or decreased. For example, expression of key enzymes of gluconeogenesis is increased in starvation like wise when toxic substances are consumed expression of certain genes increases to destroy these toxic substances. In contrast when a particular substance is present in cellular environment at definite concentration

expression of certain genes is diminished. For example, enzymes of gluconeogenesis are not expressed in well-fed state.

8. In prokaryotes also, genes are turned-on or-off depending on situation. When bacteria is present in a medium lacking specific amino acid expression of certain genes increases. In contrast when bacteria is present in a medium rich in specific amino acid expression of genes, which are involved in its synthesis decreases.
9. In eukaryotes, gene expression is affected by hormones. Proper understanding of hormonal regulation of gene expression is essential for development of drugs or treatment. Vitamins also regulates gene expression in eukaryotes.
10. Cancer is due to altered gene expression.
11. Antisense molecules can block gene expression, which is the basis for antisense therapy.
12. Peptide nucleic acids and locked nucleic acids are used to block gene expression.
13. Maintenance of proper intracellular metal level involves turning on or off of gene expression.

We shall first examine gene expression in prokaryotes then proceed to eukaryotic gene regulation. Gene regulation in prokaryotes is well known at molecular level. However, gene regulation in eukaryotes at molecular level is not known completely in several processes.

GENE REGULATION BY INDUCTION AND REPRESSION

Induction

Increased expression of genes in response to an inducer is called as induction. Increased expression of genes results in increased concentration of enzymes because enzymes are gene products. Hence, these enzymes are often called as *inducible enzymes*. Under normal conditions, these enzymes are present in small amounts but their concentration raises to many folds in presence of inducer due to increased expression of genes.

Repression

Diminished expression of genes in presence of repressor is called as repression. Decreased expression of genes results in low amounts of enzymes in cells. These enzymes are known as repressible enzymes.

Lac operon Model

To explain gene regulation by induction and repression, Jacob and Monod proposed operon model. This model explains regulation of gene expression at transcriptional and translational levels. Since this model was proposed to explain lactose metabolism in *E. Coli* it is named as Lac operon. Operon consist of structural genes, operator gene and promoter gene (site). They are located adjacent to each other on *E. Coli* DNA. There are three structural genes. They are z, y and a and they are located adjacent to each other. These structural genes codes for β- galactosidase, permease and transacetylase respectively. Further on the *E. Coli* DNA adjacent to promoter gene regulatory gene (i) is located. It regulates operon. It codes a regulatory protein known as repressor. When the regulatory gene is transcribed mRNA is generated which is turn gives rise to repressor on translation. The repressor molecule binds to operator gene and prevents the transcription of structural genes by RNA polymerase. As a result the enzymes involved in lactose, catabolism are not formed or repressed. Thus, in the absence of lactose repression of genes (enzymes) occurs (Figure 19.1).

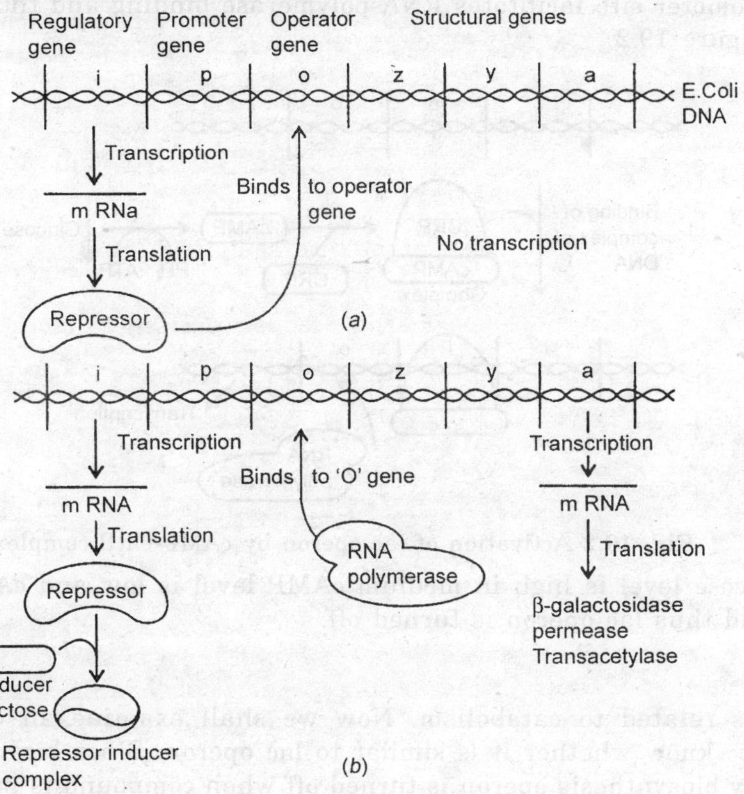

Fig. 19.1 Induction and repression of lac operon
(*a*) In the absence of lactose (*b*) In the presence of lactose

In the presence of lactose, enzymes of lactose metabolism are induced. When present lactose (inducer) binds to repressor molecule and forms inducer-repressor complex. This complex can not bind at operator gene. So, formation of inducer-repressor complex prevents repressor to bind with operator gene. As a result, operator gene becomes free. Now RNA polymerase binds to free operator gene and structural genes are transcribed to corresponding mRNAs. From these three mRNAs enzymes required for utilization of lactose are synthesized and cells use lactose as carbon or energy source (Figure 19.1). Thus, in presence of lactose induction of genes occurs.

Regulation of Lac operon by glucose and cAMP

When *E. Coli* is grown in medium containing glucose and lactose, lac operon is turned off and cells use exclusively glucose. When glucose is exhausted lac operon is turned on or activated. So, lac operon is subjected to glucose regulation. The inhibitory action of glucose on lac operon is called as catabolite repression. We shall learn about mechanism involved in regulation of lac operon by glucose. cAMP has different function in *E. Coli*. Its intracellular level is inversely related to glucose concentration in medium. Its level in *E. Coli* is high when glucose level is low in the medium. High cAMP level activates lac operon through catabolite repressor protein (CRP). This protein has DNA binding region. When cAMP binds to CRP this protein undergoes conformational change and its affinity for promoter site on *E. Coli* DNA increases. The binding of cAMP-CRP complex to DNA on promoter site facilitates RNA polymerase binding and thus transcription of lac operon (Figure 19.2).

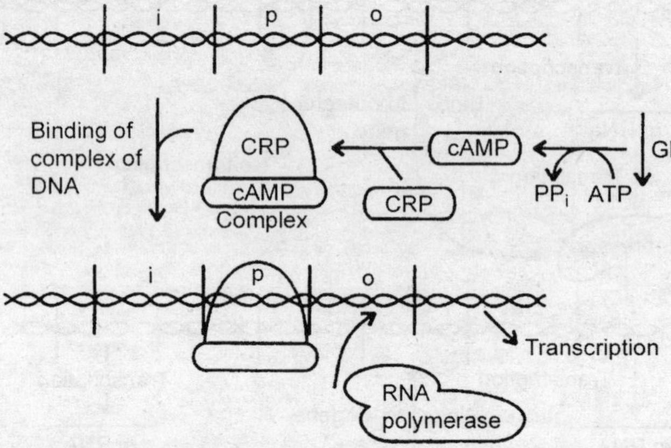

Fig. 19.2 Activation of lac operon by cAMP-CRP complex

When glucose level is high in medium cAMP level is low and cAMP-CRP complex dissociates and thus lac operon is turned off.

Try operon

Lac operon is related to catabolism. Now we shall examine an operon related to biosynthesis to know whether it is similar to lac operon. Since biosynthesis consumes energy usually biosynthesis operon is turned off when compound is present in medium. We shall examine biosynthesis operon related to synthesis of tryptophan to know how tryptophan in medium can turn off its own synthesis. Since the operon is related to tryptophan metabolism it is called as tryptophan operon or try operon.

Try operon consist of five structural gens, promoter gene and operator gene. Regulatory gene, which controls try operon codes for aporepressor. When tryptophan is present in medium it acts as corepressor and binds to aporepressor to form holo repressor, which binds to operator gene. This prevents binding of RNA polymerase and transcription of five structural genes, which code for enzymes of tryptophan biosynthesis. Repression of try opron by tryptophan is shown in Figure 19.3.

When tryptophan is absent operator site is free and transcription of structural genes occurs and tryptophan is synthesized.

Metal operon

Metal ions are essential at low concentrations but are toxic at high concentrations. Hence, intracellular level of these metals must be finely adjusted to avoid metal deprivation or metal toxicity. Regulatory mechanisms exist in cells to retain only essential amounts of metal while toxic levels are avoided.

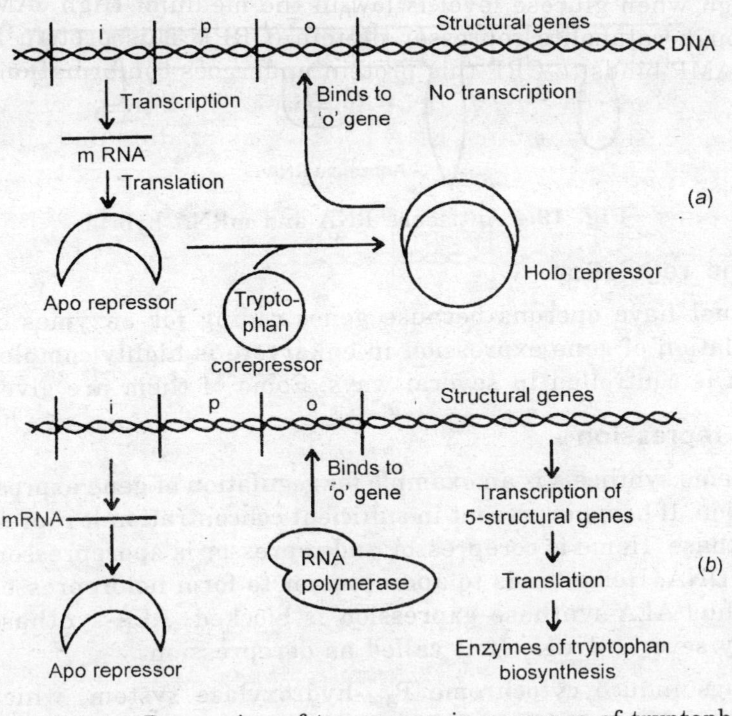

Fig. 19.3 (*a*) Repression of try operon in presence of tryptophan

(*b*) Expression of try operon in the absence of tryptophan

Metal operons present in cells are responsible for maintenance of safe intracellular level of essential metal ions. These operons are regulated at the level of transcription initiation or translational level by transacting regulatory proteins. Mettallo-regulatory proteins senses the intracellular level of specific metal ions and mediate transcriptional or translational response. Metal operons consists of structural gene, regulatory gene and operator/promoter sites.

Znt operon

1. It is related to removal of excess zinc from the cell.
2. It consists of znt A gene, which is zinc, efflux gene and znt R.
3. Znt R gene product act as direct zinc sensor. The c-terminal of znt R recognizes zinc.
4. Znt A product is zinc specific transporter.
5. Increased intracellular level of zinc induces expression of zinc efflux gene.
6. The concentration of zinc in cell brought down by transporting excess zinc to outside of cell.
7. This is followed by repression of znt A gene.

Regulation of gene expression by anti-sense RNA

Several prokaryotic genes are regulated by anti-sense RNA. Antisense RNA is transcription product of anti-sense strand of DNA. It can pair with mRNA and blocks its translation. Pairing of antisense RNA with a mRNA is shown in Figure 19.4.

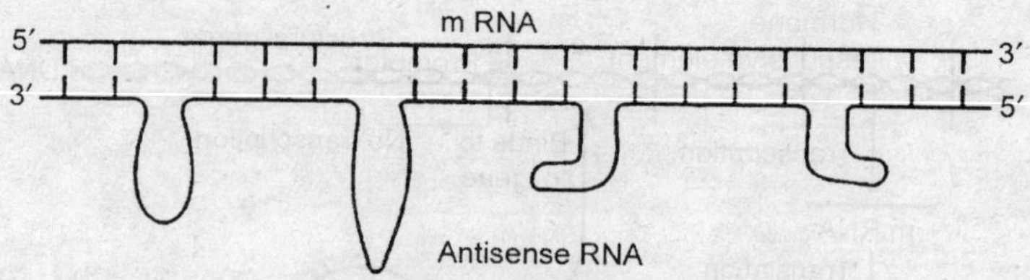

Fig. 19.4 Antisense RNA and mRNA hybrid

Eukaryotic gene regulation

Eukaryotes do not have operons because genes coding for enzymes of a pathway are scattered. Regulation of gene expression in eukaryote is highly complex. In eukaryotes, gene expression is controlled in several ways. Some of them are given below.

Induction and repression

1. Control of heme synthesis is an example for regulation of gene expression by induction and repression. If heme is present in sufficient concentration it represses the synthesis of ALA-synthase. Heme is corepressor and repressor is aporepressor which alone can not bind to DNA. Heme binds to aporepressor to form holorepressor, which binds to DNA and thus ALA-synthase expression is blocked. ALA-synthase is subjected to induction by several drugs. It is called as derepression.
2. Several drugs induce cytochrome P_{450}-hydroxylase system, which detoxify these drugs.
3. Several enzymes of amino acid metabolism are inducible. For example, high protein diet increases expression of enzymes of urea cycle to several folds. Likewise, tyrosine rich diet increases expression of tyrosine transaminase to several folds.

Methylation

Methylation of DNA is one way of controlling gene expression in eukaryotes. Methylation of bases blocks their expression. This types of gene regulation was observed during development.

Gene amplification

Amplification of genes is one more way of controlling gene expression in eukaryotes. Under certain conditions, single copy genes are amplified to many folds. Cancer cells drug resistance is due to gene amplification. For example, exposure to methotrexate causes amplification of dihydrofolate reductase gene. Replication of gene several times lead to amplification.

Regulation of gene expression by hormones and vitamins

Many steroid hormones, retinoic acid and vitamin D exert their action by affecting gene expression. They induce synthesis of enzymes and proteins in target cells. They form complex with receptor after entering target cell. These complexes migrate to nucleaus where they bind to specific sequence of DNA known as *hormone responsive element* (HRE) or enhancer. This leads to activation of promoters and binding of RNA polymerase to DNA and thus transcription (Figure 19.5) The enhancers as such to do not affect promoter activity. Silencers, which suppress expression of genes are also identified in eukaryotes.

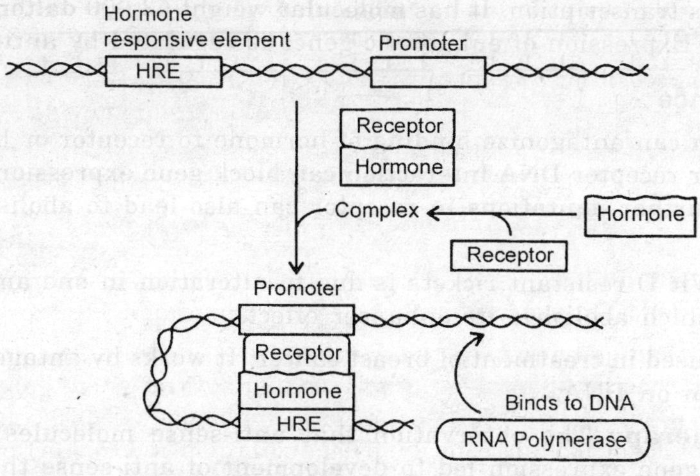

Fig. 19.5 Schematic diagram showing gene activation by hormones

Zinc finger proteins

The mechanism by which binding of receptor-hormone (vitamin) complex causes activation of transcription is known at *molecular level* in some cases. The receptors has three regions, a DNA binding region, hormone binding region and variable region. These receptors are called as *zinc-finger proteins* (transcriptional factors) because they contain zinc finger motifs.

DNA binding region of these receptors contain tandemely repeated 2-40 domains (motifs). Each motif consists of 30 amino acids and zinc atom. A pair of cysteine residues, a pair of histidine residues and other hydrophobic amino acids are present in each motif. Zinc is held by two cysteine residues and two histidine residues through coordinate linkages to form zinc finger (Figure 19.6). The three-dimentional structure of each zinc finger consist of two anti-parallel β-strands and a short stretch of α-helix. Zinc finger motifs bind to major groove of DNA and holds on strand of DNA releasing another strand for transcription. Several proteins containing zinc finger motifs are purified and well characterized. Some zinc finger proteins have four cysteine residues rather than two cysteine and two histidine residues.

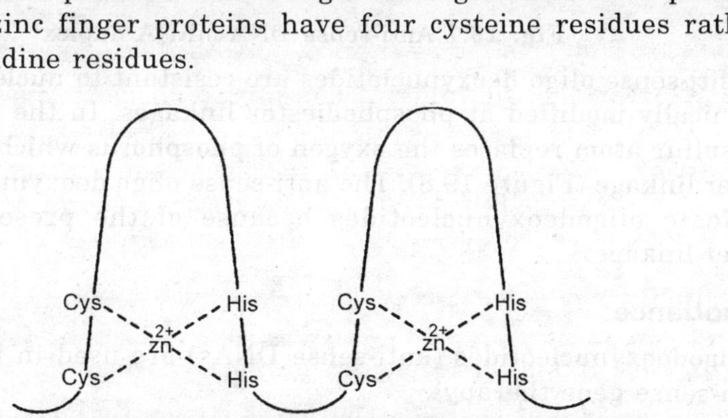

Fig. 19.6 Two zinc finger motifs of steroid hormone binding receptor (zinc finger protein)

Other noteworthy DNA binding protein is tumour suppressor protein p^{53}. When DNA is damaged, the expression of this particular protein increases several folds. It binds to

DNA and regulates transcription. It has molecular weight 53,000 daltons and hence it is designated as p^{53}. Expression of eukaryotic genes is regulated by anti-sense RNA also.

Medical importance

Compounds, which can antagonize binding of hormone to receptor or hormone receptor complex to DNA or receptor DNA interaction can block gene expression and can abolish hormone effect. Further, mutations in receptor can also lead to abolishion of hormone effect.

1. One form of Vit D resistant rickets is due to alteration in one amino acid residue of receptor, which abolishes its enhancer effect.
2. Tamoxifen is used in treatment of breast cancer. It works by antagonizing oestrogen receptor action on DNA.
3. **Antisense therapy** The observation that anti-sense molecules are involved in regulation of gene expression led to development of anti-sense therapy.
4. Tumour suppressor protein p^{53}, is anti-cancer agent. It prevents development of cancer in normal people.

Antisense technology

This technology deals with development and use of anti-sense molecules in chemotherapy. Short segments of a anti-sense DNA consisting of 15-20 nucleotides are used to specifically block expression of a given gene. Anti-sense DNA molecules are not natural ones. They are synthesized from deoxy ribonucleotides *in vitro.* So, chemically anti-sense DNA is anti-oligo deoxynucleotide and often termed as *anti-sense oligodeoxy nucleotide*.

When introduced into human body, anti-sense oligodeoxy nucleotide binds to heparin binding sites of cell membrane and are internalized. In side the cell, it forms mRNA-DNA hybrid and thus blocks gene expression (Figure 19.7). Inside the cell, they are not hydrolyzed by nucleases.

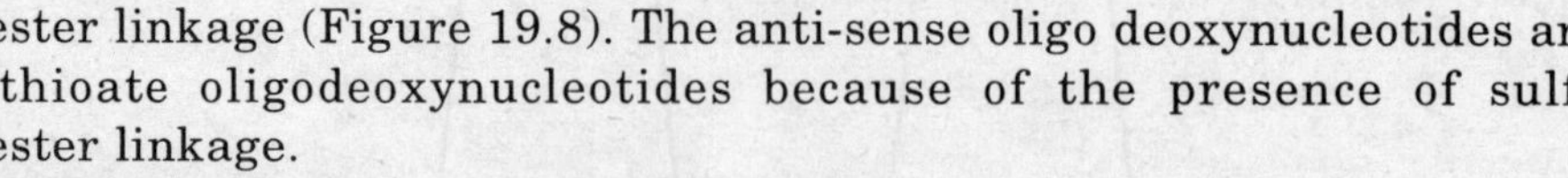

Fig. 19.7 Anti-sense DNA-mRNA duplex

Usually anti-sense oligo deoxynucletides are resistant to nuclease digestion because they are chemically modified at phosphodiester linkages. In the anti-sense oligo deoxy nucleotide a sulfur atom replaces the oxygen of phosphorus which is not a part of usual phosphodiester linkage (Figure 19.8). The anti-sense oligo deoxynucleotides are called as phosphorothioate oligodeoxynucleotides because of the presence of sulfur in the phosphodiester linkage.

Medical importance

Anti-sense oligodeoxynucleotides (anti-sense DNAs) are used in the treatment of some diseases (anti-sense gene therapy).

1. They are used as anti-cancer or anti-neoplastic agents in the treatment of acute myelogenous leukaemia.
2. They are also used as anti-viral agents in the treatment of AIDS.

3. Anti-sense genes are used to treat inherited diseases like β-thalassemia also. In β-thalassemia, accumulation of α-chain in RBC triggers their destruction, which leads to anaemia. Introducing anti-sense gene for α-chain gene results in inhibition of expression of α-chain gene and thus production of α-chains.
4. Most of the cancers can be controlled by introducing anti-sense genes for cancer genes after identifying oncogenes or proto oncogenes.

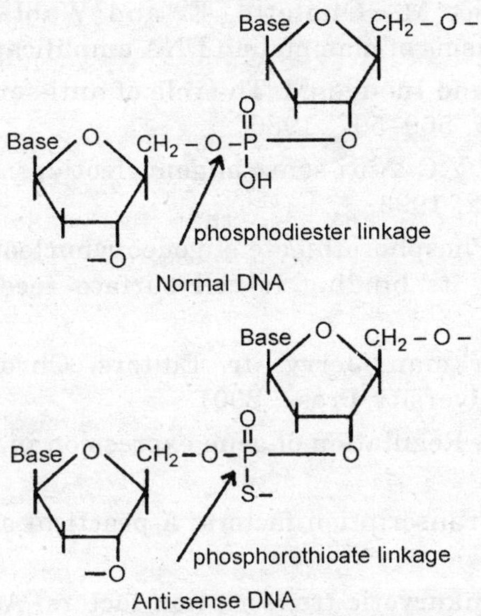

Fig. 19.8 Structures of anti-sense DNA and normal DNA segments

Peptide nucleic acid (PNA) based anti-genomic inhibition

1. Phosphorothioate linked DNA oligonucleotides (S-DNA) are anti-sense molecules developed in mid 1980s.
2. Peptide nucleic acids (PNAs) are new class of anti-sense molecules developed recently.
3. PNAs have higher affinity for RNA and forms more stable complex with RNA than S-DNA/RNA complex.
4. PNAs are highly resistant to enzymatic degradation than S-DNA. Some PNAs selectively inhibit replication of templates carrying mutated pathogenic genes.
5. PNAs are useful in targeting short sequences of RNA.
6. They are also useful in treating diseases involving single nucleotide polymorphism (SNP).

Locked nucleic acids (LNAs)

1. They are another class of oligonucleotide molecules developed recently.
2. They are bicyclic DNA analogs. They exhibit high affinity towards complementary RNA as well as DNA. They form duplex with RNA and DNA.
3. They are used in blocking gene expressions.

REFERENCES

1. Jacob, F. and Monod. Genetic regulatory mechanism in the synthesis of proteins. J. Mol. Biol. **3**, 318–356, 1961.
2. Beato, M. Gene regulation by steroid hormones. Cell. **56**, 335–344, 1989.
3. Klug, A. and Rhodes, D. Zinc fingers. Sci. Am. **200 (2),** 32, 1993.
4. Stark, C.R., Debatisse, M., Gimlotto, E. and Wabl, G.M. Recent progress in understanding mechanisms of mammalian DNA amplification. Cell. **57**, 901–908, 1989.
5. Green, P.J., Pines, O. and Inouye, M. The role of anti-sense RNA in gene regulation. Ann. Rev. Biochem. **55**, 569–597, 1986.
6. Stein, C.A. and Chang, Y.C. Anti-sense oligonucleotides: Is the bullet really magical. Science **261,** 1004–1012, 1993.
7. Guvakova, M.A. *et al.* Phosphorothioate oligodeoxynucleotides bind to basic fibroblast growth factors inhibit its binding to cell surface receptors. J. Biol. Chem. **270**, 2620–2627, 1995.
8. Elgin, Sarah, C., Workman, Jerry. Jr. Editors. Chromatin structure and gene expression. Oxford University Press, 2001.
9. Lin, E. and Lynch, A.S. Regulation of gene expression in *E. Coli.* Chapman and Hall, England, 1996.
10. David, S. Latchman. Transcription factors: A practical approach. Oxford University Press, 1999.
11. Latchman, David S. Eukaryotic transcription factors. Academic Press, 2003.
12. Wagner, Rolf. Transcription regulation in prokaryotes. Oxford University Press, 2000.
13. Kaladimos, C.G. *et al.* Structure and flexibility adaptation in non-specific and specific protein-DNA complex. Science. **305**, 386–389, 2004.
14. Christopher Janson. Ed. Peptide nucleic acids, morpholinos and related anti-sense molecules. Eurekah Bioscience, 2003.
15. Clawson, G.A. *et al.* Inhibition of papilloma progression by anti-sense oligonucleotides targeted to HPV 11 E6/E7 RNA. Gene therapy, 1st July, 2004.
16. Crempton, D.J. *et al.* The arginine fingers of bacteriophage gene helicase Proc. Natl. Acad. Sci. USA **101**, 4373–4378, 2004.

EXERCISES

ESSAY QUESTION

1. Define induction and repression. Explain salient features of lac operon model with help of a figure.

SHORT QUESTIONS

1. Write a note on try operon. How it differs from lac operon?
2. Write a note on zinc fingers.
3. Define anti-sense molecules. Write their applications. How they differ from normal DNA?

20

CHAPTER

RECOMBINANT DNA TECHNOLOGY

MEDICAL AND BIOLOGICAL IMPORTANCE

1. It is called as technology because recombinant DNA is man's creation. It is not present in nature.
2. This chapter deals with techniques based on recombinant DNA. These technique are used to improve health care mainly. Of course they are widely used in forensic science also.
3. This technology is used to improve agriculture, food industry and live stock production also.
4. Biotechnology is the name given to another branch of science in which recombinant DNA technology is an integral part.
5. It is a major break through that is achieved nearly after two centuries of biological research. A new class of vaccines DNA vaccines are produced using this technology.
6. Using this technology genes are manipulated (engineered) to produce important biological materials, which is otherwise not possible.
7. Insertion of genes of one species into the genetic material of other species is made possible by this technology. So, human gene product can be produced in plants (transgenic plants) and vice versa.
8. This technology is used for commercial production of vaccines, cytokines, hormones, proteins etc.
9. Gene therapy, which offers treatment for some incurable inherited diseases is another off shoot of this technology.
10. This technology paved way for the development and production of transgenic animals. Sheep dolly is created recently by cloning.
11. This technology may lead to creation of man in laboratory without the sperm or oocytes or ovarian follicles (germ cells).
12. Cells can be immortalized and non-existant species can be created by using this technology.

Recombinant DNA

It is not found in life forms and it is not a natural DNA. It is a man made DNA. Recombinant DNA is prepared by combining DNA from two different sources or species. Other names given to recombinant DNA are cloned DNA and chimeric DNA. Organisms containing recombinant DNA are often called as *clones*.

Recombinant DNA Technology

As mentioned earlier, it refers to several techniques in which recombinant DNA is involved either directly or indirectly. Popular name for recombinant DNA technology is genetic engineering because genes (organisms) are engineered in such way that they produce only desired product in bulk quantities as in factories or they perform a specific function.

Plasmids are used to carry desired gene (foreign DNA). Plasmids are double stranded DNA molecules present in anti-biotic resistant bacteria. They contain genes for the inactivation of anti-biotics and hence they confer anti-biotic resistance to bacteria.

Bacteriophages, retroviruses are also used to carry foreign DNA in some techniques. They often termed as vectors.

Different steps of recombinant DNA technology that is used to obtain a gene product are given below.

1. Plasmid is cut with restriction endo nuclease to produce DNA with sticky (cohesive) ends. The plasmid with sticky ends can combine with any DNA, which has similar sticky ends.
2. A desired gene with same sticky ends is obtained from human DNA by cutting human DNA with same restriction endo nuclease (EcoRI).
3. Two fragments are annealed and covalently linked by DNA ligase to produce recombinant DNA.
4. The recombinant DNA thus generated is inserted into bacteria by a process called as *tranformation*.
5. Bacterial colonies containing recombinant DNA as well as normal bacteria are grown on agar medium.
6. Clones are transferred on to nitro cellulose disc by placing nitro cellulose disc that fits inside the plate on top of the clones.
7. By treating with SDS, DNA of clones is liberated. The DNA is then denatured and made single stranded by treatment with alkali.
8. At this stage, recombinant DNA is identified by using cDNA probe. cDNA is a single stranded molecule. It can be prepared from radiolabelled P^{32} nucleoside triphosphates using DNA polymerase. cDNA also can be prepared from mRNA using reverse transcriptase. This type of cDNA synthesis is possible when amino acid sequence of gene product is known. Usually base composition of cDNA probe is complementary to base composition of desired gene. So, cDNA hybridizes with desired gene. DNA probes are also used in other techiques like southern blotting, DNA finger printing, in situ hybridization etc.
9. After washing excess probe, the disc is dried and exposed to X-ray film.

10. When the X-Ray film is developed a faint image of disc containing dark spots is seen. Dark spots corresponds to colonies containing recombinant DNA.
11. Finally colonies containing recombinant DNA are separated by comparing images with original plate and cultured.
12. In the culture medium gene product accumulates due to expression of inserted human gene by bacteria.

All the steps are shown in Figure 20.1.

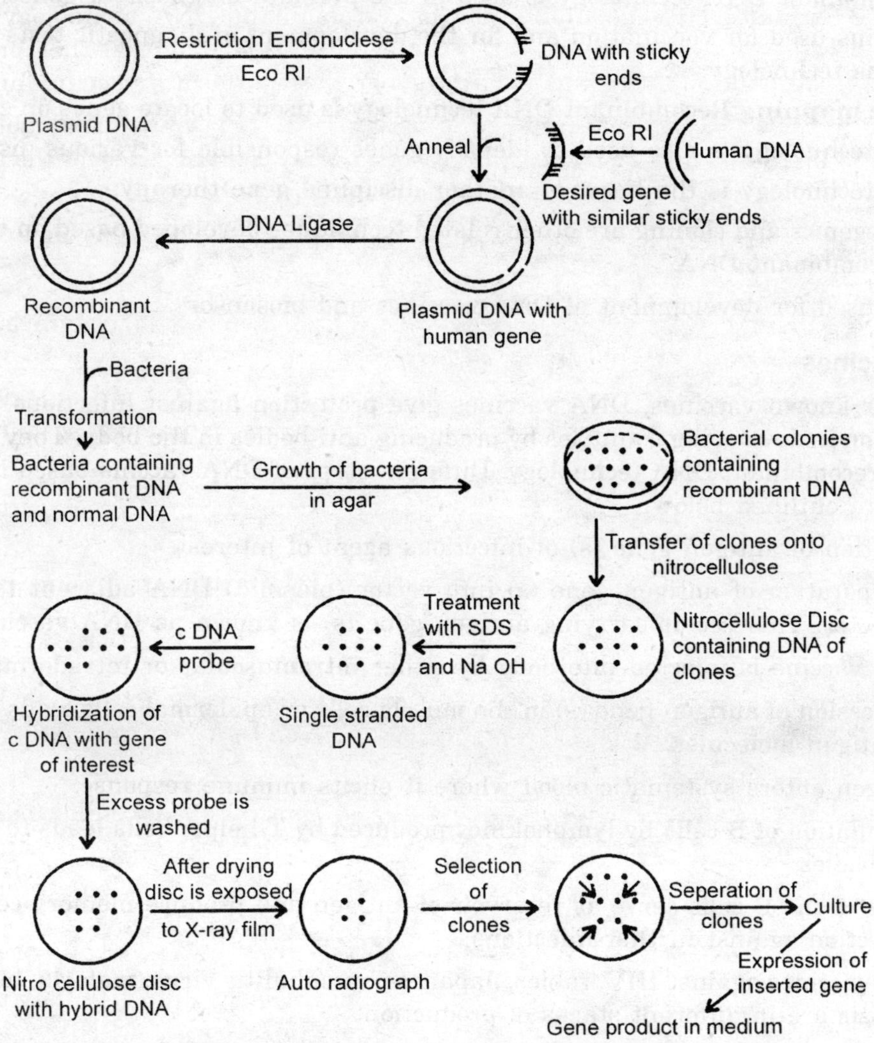

Fig. 20.1 Steps of recombinant DNA technology used for obtaining gene product

Medical and biological importance

1. Recombinant DNA technology is widely used in medicine, pharmaceutical or biotechnology industries and in agriculture.

2. Hormone insulin is produced in bulk quantities by using this technology and used in treatment of insulin-dependent diabetics. Other important proteins produced using this technology are growth hormones, interferon etc. Interferon is a cytokine produced in the body to protect from viral infections.
3. Blood clotting factor VIII and tissue plasminogen activator (t-PA) are also produced by this technology. T-PA is used in treatment of thrombosis where as blood clotting factor VIII is used in treatment of haemophilia.
4. Recombinant DNA technology is used in the prenatal diagnosis of genetic diseases.
5. Proteins used for vaccination and for the development of diagnostic tests are obtained by this technology.
6. **Gene mapping** Recombinant DNA technology is used to locate genes on chromosomes.
7. This technology is also used to identify genes responsible for various diseases.
8. This technology is the heart of another discipline gene therapy.
9. Transgenics and cloning are other related techniques developed based on the principles of recombinant DNA.
10. It is used for development of DNA vaccines and biosensors.

DNA vaccines

Like other known vaccines, DNA vaccines give protection against infectious diseases that are common in developing countries by producing anti-bodies in the body. They are produced by using recombinant DNA technology. Different steps of DNA vaccine-based immunization process are outlined below.

1. Selection of antigen gene (s) of infectious agent of interest.
2. Incorporation of antigen gene (s) into vector (plasmid) DNA adjacent to appropriate promoter. This vector carrying antigen gene (s) is known as DNA vaccine.
3. DNA vaccine is injected into body by either intramuscular or intradermal route.
4. Expression of antigen gene (s) in the muscle cells or epidermal cells leads to production of antigen molecules.
5. Antigen enters systematic blood where it elicits immune response.
6. Stimulation of B cells by lymphokines produced by T-helper cells leads to production of anti-bodies.
7. Some of the B cells serve as reservoir of antigen and produce memory cells that gives protection against further infections.

DNA vaccines against HIV, rabies, Japanese encephalitis virus, malaria, hepatitis B and tuberculosis are in different stages of production.

Bio sensors

Many naturally occurring biological macromolecules have tendency to recognize each other and react to form new molecule or complex or hybrid. For example, an enzyme recognizes its substrate among many molecules and reacts to form product. Similarly an antigen binds to specific anti-body to form antigen antibody complex and a single strand DNA forms double helix when it finds a complementary strand. A biosensor is designed by combining this property of biomolecules with chemistry and electronics. Usually a biosensor consist of (*a*) **Biological recognition component** Which detects target substance in a sample by selective binding. It may be an enzyme, gene, antibody and bound to supporting material.

(*b*) **Tranduction (translation) or amplification component** Which converts (translates) reaction between bio-recognition molecule and target molecule in a sample into measurable or detectable signal.

By recombinant DNA technology enzymes, genes or antibodies that are used as bio-recognition component of biosensor are obtained in large quantities. For example, heroin is detected by biosensor in which heroin esterase and morphine dehydrogenase obtained through recombinant DNA technology are bio-recognition component.

Biosensors are used to detect genes, mutations, insects, microorganisms, toxins or pollutants etc. A portable biosensor that measures blood glucose instantly is used by diabetics in several parts of the world. In near future, an individual may find out what is wrong in his health at home by using appropriate portable bio sensor. Like wise he may be able to check quality of air, food or water he consumes with the help of biosensors.

Gene therapy

Some inherited diseases due to deficiency of a particular gene or gene product are fatal and generally proper treatment is not available. Gene therapy offers chance of correcting such fatal diseases. Gene therapy is the use of genes to correct genetic disease or use of genes as therapeutic agents.

Various steps involved in gene therapy are given below.

1. Preparation of recombinant DNA consisting of vector and gene of interest.
2. Introduction of vector into host cells.
3. Integration of vector into genome.
4. Expression of gene in the host.
5. Production of gene product in the host.
6. Deficiency of protein (gene) is corrected.

Vectors used in gene therapy

Retroviruses particularly murine leukemia virus (MLV) is used as gene carrier. When virus infect host cell, the recombinant retroviral RNA is reverse transcribed and integrated randomly into host cell DNA.

Eventhough, the gene therapy was initially developed for the treatment of inherited diseases, now it is used in treatment of cancer, neurological diseases and infectious diseases.

Cystic fibrosis, severe combined immunodeficiency disease (SCID), familial hyper cholesterolemia, hemophilia and Duchenne muscular dystrophy (DMD) are genetic diseases treated by using gene therapy.

Acquired diseases treated with gene therapy are cancer, cardiovascular diseases, Alzhemer's disease, Parkinson's disease and AIDS.

Gene therapy protocols for correction of some disorders are given below. Protocols varies from one disease to another disease.

Steps of SCID gene therapy

1. A retroviral vector carrying adenosine deaminase (ADA) cDNA is prepared.
2. T cells are isolated from patient.
3. T cells are cultured.
4. T cells are transfected with retroviral vector. Vector is integrated into T-cell genome.
5. T cells containing ADA gene are cultured.
6. Finally T-cells containing ADA gene are infused into patient blood.

Steps of familial hyper cholesterolemia gene therapy

1. Preparation of retroviral vector carrying LDL receptor gene.
2. Hepatocytes are isolated from patients liver.
3. Transfection of hepatocytes with virus carrying LDL receptor gene.
4. Introduction of modified hepatocytes into portal blood of patient.

Cystic fibrosis gene therapy protocol differs from the above examples. It involves direct introduction of viral vectors containing cystic fibrosis transmembrane regulator (CFTR) gene into nasal or bronchial epithelitum where it is expressed after integration into host DNA.

Cancer gene therapy involves introduction of tumor cells containing genes for cytokines into patient. An alternative cancer gene therapy involves introduction of tumor suppressor gene into patient.

Some gene therapy protocols are used in genetic immunization or DNA vaccines.

Transgenics

It deals with genetically engineered higher organisms. Transgenic animals are those animals, which have a piece of foreign DNA stably integrated into their genome (DNA). These transgenic animals exhibit a property, which is characteristics of foreign DNA in addition to their normal features.

Steps involved in production of transgenic goat that produces human gene product in milk are given below.

1. Human gene of interest is inserted into vector next to a goat promoter gene. Promotor gene is essential for the expression of human gene in goat.
2. Several copies of clones are produced *in vitro.*
3. Under microscope, clones are injected into fertilized eggs or embryos.
4. Modified embryos are implanted into reproductive tract of foster mothers.
5. Some of the baby goats born are transgenic, i.e., human gene is integrated into baby goat genome.
6. Using northern blot, expression of gene in baby goat is ascertained.
7. Finally, human gene product is expressed in milk of transgenic goat.

Various steps of transgenic animal production are given Figure 20.2. Other transgenic animals created are large mice. They are produced by injecting rat growth hormone into fertilized mouse eggs.

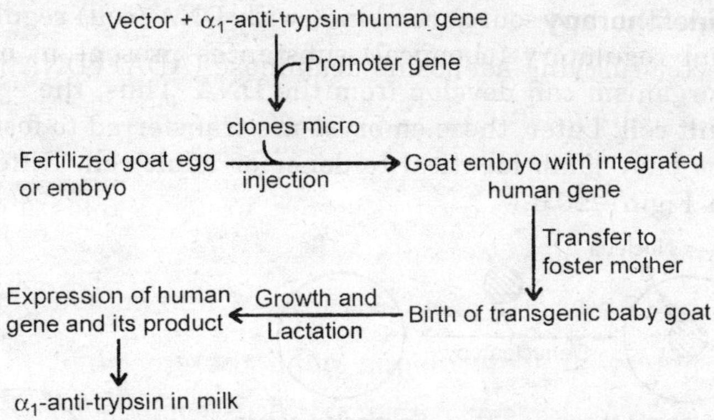

Fig. 20.2 Steps of transgenic animal production

Transgenic plants are also produced by using recombinant DNA technology. They are used as bioreactors for the production of antigens (vaccines) and antibodies.

Edible vaccines

Edible vaccines are edible plant parts containing antigens of infectious agents. They are produced by genetically engineered transgenic plants. Different steps of edible vaccine-based immunization process are outlined below.

1. For production of edible vaccine, a plant whose products are consumed as such (raw) and stable to cooking condition is selected. Banana, cucumber and tomato can be good choice.
2. Selection of antigen gene (s) of infectious agent of interest.
3. Insertion of antigen gene into vector adjacent to a promoter.
4. Integration of vector with host DNA leads to conversion of normal host into transgenic plant.
5. Expression of antigen in edible part of transgenic plant.
6. Feeding of edible part containing antigen elicits immune response by stimulating mucosal immune system.
7. Antibodies are produced in the body at mucosal surfaces of gut and respiratory tract.
8. Individual is protected from future infections.

Banana containing vaccine against *E. Coli* infections is available in the form of infant food in some parts of the World for vaccination of children. Potatoes containing vaccines against cholera, diarrhoea and tobacco containing vaccine against hepatitis B are at different stages of development in several countries.

Cloning

It is a process that gives rise to genetically identical organisms. Cloning of higher organisms leads to duplicity or creation of identical twins. It is a asexual reproduction (replication) of mammals. In simple words cloning refers to making or producing ones own copy (xerox).

In mammalian cloning, DNA of adult cell is injected into oocyte or unfertilized egg cell whose DNA was removed. So, in this process, DNAs from two different sources are not combined instead DNA from one source combines with DNA (cell) regulating substances of other cell. The special regulatory (chemical) substances present in oocyte reprogramme DNA, so that whole organism can develop from the DNA. Thus, the egg cell develops into embryo instead of adult cell. Later, these embryos are transferred to foster mothers. Finally foster mother delivers baby lamb identical to donor or adult cell. Different steps of sheep cloning are shown in Figure 20.3.

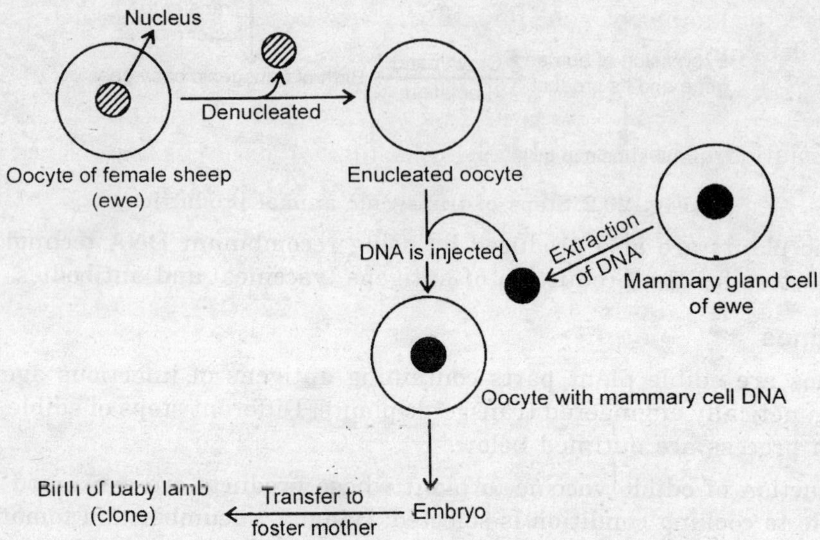

Fig. 20.3 Steps of sheep cloning

Gene targeting

1. It is modified form of the cloning technique. It involves modification or manipulation of somatic cell DNA before it is injected into enucleated oocyte.
2. Further gene targeting involves homologous recombination of targeted gene and host DNA where as integration of trans gene in the host genome in transgenic is a non-homologous recombination.
3. Somatic cell is first transformed, (transfected) with gene (DNA) of interest, which is meant for gene targeting. The rest of the technique is identical to that of cloning.

   Gene targeting is used for both gene knock out and gene knock in.

(*a*) **Gene knock out** It involves targeted inactivation of gene. Mutations are introduced into somatic cell DNA to make gene inactive. Then this DNA is expressed in oocyte. Clones produced lacks gene that is inactivated.

(b) **Gene knock in** It involves targeted insertion of gene. A gene of interest is inserted into somatic DNA before it is injected into enucleated oocyte. Gene is expressed in clones.

Applications

1. Gene targeting is done in mice, sheep and fly.
2. Gene targeting is used to study genetics of human diseases and gene therapy.

3. In gene therepy, inactive copy of gene is replaced with functional gene.
4. Gene targeting can be applied in any animal species.
5. Gene targeting in animals allows selective breeding of animals for generation.
6. Gene targeting is used to establish function of gene or gene product like enzyme or hormone etc.
7. In pharmaceutical industry, gene targeting is used to over express proteins of therapeutic value in milch animals.

Stem cells

1. In 1998, isolation of human-stem cells by using two different approaches is published.
2. These cells are able to differentiate into all types of cells or tissues. Further, they can be maintained as undifferentiated cells in culture and are able to reproduce themselves throughout life span of organisms.
3. Stem cells exist in growing and adult humans. Stem cells are isolated from embryo, cord blood, bone marrow, liver, brain etc.
4. Only embryonic stem cells are able to differentiate into any cell type. Others produce only narrow range of cells.
5. Generally developmental potential of a stem cell is restricted to differentiate cell of the tissue in which it is present.

Applications

Stem cells have many potential uses in medicine and molecular biology.

1. They are used for replacement of lost or degenerated tissue.
2. They are useful in delivering therapeutic gene products directly into the tissue. Genetically engineered stem cells express therapeutic genes in tissue of choice.
3. They are used in gene therapy. For example, neural stem cells are used for gene therapy of tumor growth suppression.
4. They are useful for exploring normal process of tissue development.

Hybridoma technology

It is used to produce mono-clonal antibodies. Mono-clonal antibodies are antibodies produced by one cell line (clone) and they are directed against one specific antigen. Lymphocytes in the body are polyclonal (multiple cell lines) and they can produce many types of antibodies (polyclonal) against antigens. Separation of single cell line that produce only one antibody from the mixture of polyclonal cells is a hard task. Hybridoma technology involves preparation of hybridoma (hybrid) cells to produce monoclonal antibodies.

Hybridomas

A simple method of producing single cell line of polyclonal cells involves fusion of two cell populations. Fusion generates hybrid cells with desired properties. These hybridoma cells produce mono-clonal antibodies.

Different steps of hybridoma technology are given below.

1. A mouse is immunized with an antigen.
2. Spleen of the mouse is removed after several weeks. During this period, antibodies producing cells are formed in sufficient amounts in the spleen.
3. B-Lymphocytes are removed from spleen and fused with myeloma cells in presence of polyethyleneglycol (PEG). Myeloma cells are used for funsion because lymphocytes obtained after immunization are incapable of continous growth in culture. Therefore, fusion of lymphocytes with myeloma cells leads to immortalization (infinite life span) of cells. More over the myeloma cells lack HGPRTase which is used as genetic marker to identify fused cells.
4. Fused cells are allowed to grow in medium containing HAT (hypoxanthine, aminopterin and thymine).
5. Spleen cells die in the medium because they are not immortalized and myeloma cells also die because they can not survive in HAT medium due to lack of HGPRTase.
6. Only hybridoma cells formed by the fusion of lymphocytes with myeloma cells proliferate because they are immortal and contain HGPRTase of lymphocytes. Thus, the hybridoma cells are obtained. Further, the DNA of hybridoma cells is derived from myeloma cells and lymphocytes.
7. The hybridoma cells are screened for mono-clonal cells by using antibodies.
8. Finally mono-clonal cells are obtained and cultured to produce mono-clonal antibodies.

Steps of hybridoma technology are shown in Figure 20.4.

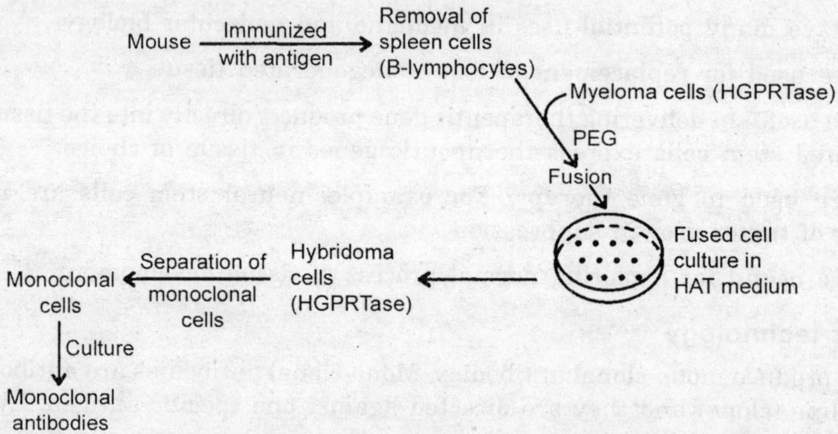

Fig. 20.4 Steps of hybridoma technology

Medical and biological importance

1. Mono-clonal antibodies are used to identify small amounts of antigen in the body.
2. They are used in drug delivery (magic bullets).
3. Some toxins are removed from circulation by using mono-clonal antibodies.
4. In cancer therapy, mono-clonal antibodies are made to carry a toxin, which can kill cancer cells after binding to cancer cells.

5. In some organ transplantations, mono-clonal antibodies are used.
6. Mono-clonal antibodies are used to purify enzymes.
7. They are used in isolation of specific antigens from mixture of proteins.
8. They are used in immunodiagnostics to determine infectious agents in the body.
9. They may be used to subclassify blood groups and tumor or cancer cells.

Hybridization techniques

These techniques are based on the tendency of two DNA strands to form duplex. Inter strand hydrogen bonding between complementary sequences favours duplex formation. A DNA strand and RNA strand containing complementary sequences also can form duplex. Usually two DNA strands involved in duplex formation comes from two different sources. In the case of DNA-RNA duplex also DNA and RNA may have different origins. Thus, duplex formed are hybrids. Hence, the name hybridization techniques. Some hybridization techniques are given below.

Southern blot

It is technique used to detect specific DNA fragment from mixture of DNA fragments. A cDNA probe of gene of interest is used in this technique. This probe hybridizes with the gene of interest thus leading to its identification. Different steps of southern blot are given below.

1. Chromosal DNA is purified and cleaved by restriction endo nuclease. A mixture of DNA fragments are obtained.
2. The fragments are separated by agarose gel electrophoresis. The gel is prepared from agarose in a suitable buffer. The DNA fragments are loaded into a well at one end of the gel and electrophoresid. Under conditions of experiment DNA fragments carry net negative charge and hence they move towards anode. Since the gel act as molecular sieve movements of DNA fragments towards anode depends on their sizes. Small fragments move faster where as big fragments get retarded. Thus, the DNA fragments are separated according to size.
3. The DNA in the separated fragments is denatured and made single stranded by soaking gel first in a HCl then in NaOH.
4. DNA is transferred to nitrocellulose in this step. This is carried out first by placing nitrocellulose sheet on the gel. Next the buffer in the gel is removed with help of several blotting papers. The blotting paper when placed on nitrocellulose sheet draws DNA also with buffer. DNA sticks to nitrocellulose and only the buffer passes through nitrocellulose and absorbed by blotting paper. Thus a perfect nitrocellulose print of the gel is obtained.
5. Now nitrocellulose sheet is incubated with buffer containing cDNA probe. cDNA probe is P^{32} radiolabelled.
6. cDNA probe hybridizes with gene of interest and excess probe is washed off.
7. Nitro cellulose sheet is dried and placed next to x-ray film. The fragments to which cDNA probe is bound appears as bands on film when it is developed.

   Different steps of southern blot are shown in Figure 20.5.

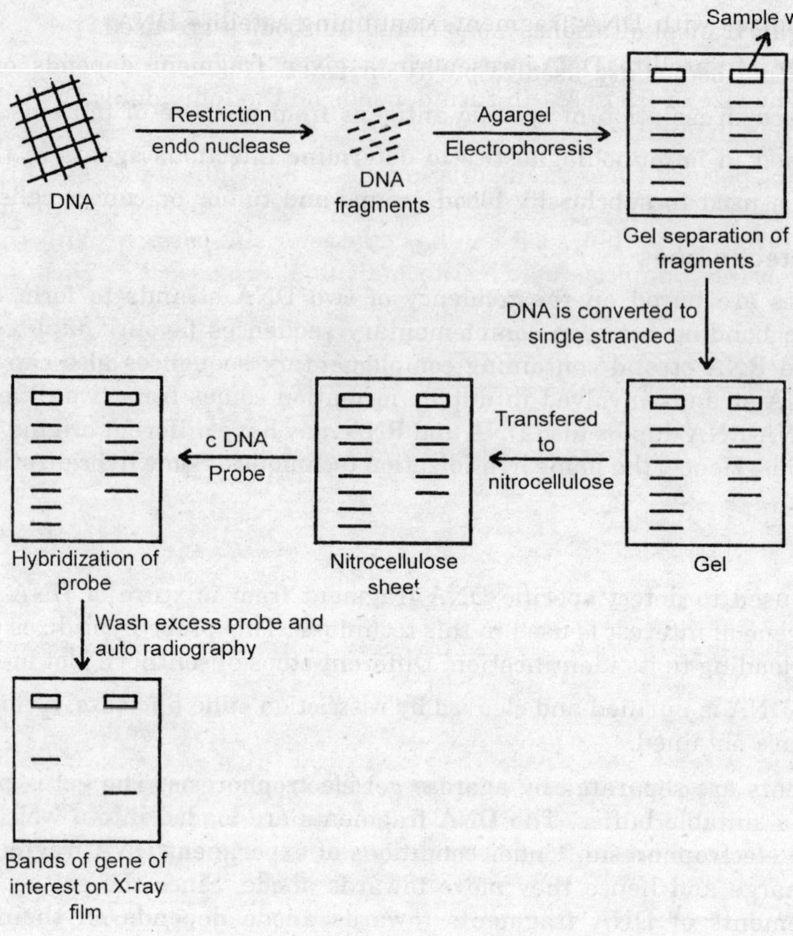

Fig. 20.5 Steps of southern blot

DNA finger printing

Use of finger prints in crime detection (forensic science) is well known. Like finger prints, DNA of an individual is characteristic of that individual. In other words, DNA make up of every human is different. DNA finger printing is a technique used to identify an individual from DNA obtained from blood or semen or piece of tissue.

The technique is based on identification of tandem repeats of satellite DNA. Satellite DNA consist of repetitive sequence. For example, satellite DNA of fruit fly consist of repetitive sequence ACA AA CT. The length of repetitive sequence or satellite DNA varies and depends on the organism or individual. In addition, satellite DNA is repeated several times (10^7) and present on all chromosomes of genome (Figure 20.6).

Various steps of DNA finger printing are given below.

1. DNA of suspect is cleaved with restriction endonuclease, which does not cut satellite DNA.
2. The fragments are separated on agarose gel electrophoresis and southern blotted.
3. Satellite DNA is identified by radiolabelled satellite DNA probe.

4. Probe hybridizes with DNA fragments containing satellite DNA.
5. The number of satellite DNA present in a given fragment depends on the size of fragment. The size of fragment in turn depends on the individuals DNA. It varies from individual to individual.
6. Southern-blot pattern thus obtained is unique to individuals just like finger print and it is called as *DNA finger print*. In Figure 20.6, DNA finger prints of four unrelated people are given. Note that each one has characteristic pattern. With the help of this DNA finger print, sample is matched to individual or suspect.

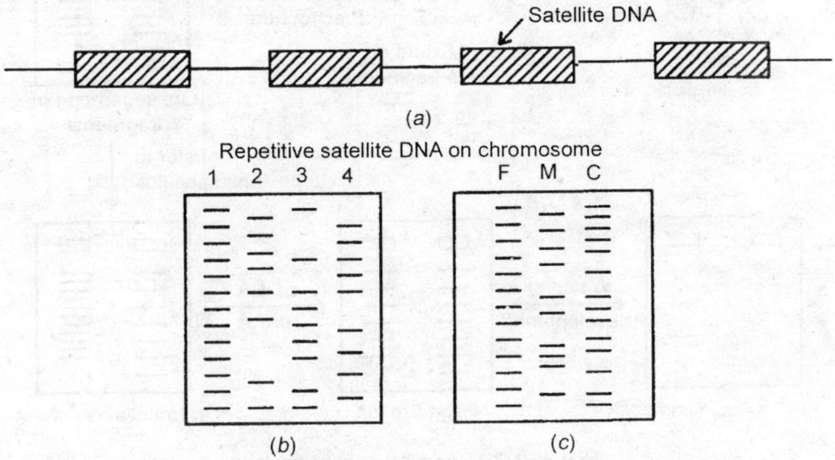

Fig. 20.6 (*a*) Tandemly repeated repetitive sequence
(*b*) DNA finger prints of four unrelated people
(*c*) DNA finger prints of father (F), mother (M) and child (C)

DNA finger printing and parental dispute

Since half of the child DNA comes from parental DNA, DNA finger prints are used to establish parentage of child by matching childs DNA finger prints with parental DNA finger prints (Figure 20.6).

In situ hybridization (ISH)

It is a technique used to detect the presence of a particular DNA or RNA in cells. It is also used to identify cells expressing particular mRNA. A radiolablled DNA (RNA) probe which hybridizes with gene of interest is used in this technique. This technique is also used to detect the presence of foreign DNA or viral RNA in cells. Steps of this technique are given below.

1. Fixation of DNA or cells.
2. Denaturation of DNA to separate strands.
3. Addition of radiolabelled probe. Excess probe is removed by washing.
4. Visualization of hybrid.

Fluoroscent *in situ* hybridization (FISH)

In this technique, fluroscent probe is used instead of radiolabelled probe. Hence, fluoroscent signal at the site of hybridization reveals presence of gene of interest. It is mainly used to identify chromosomes, regions of chromosomes and of course individual genes.

Northern blot

It is conceptually similar to southern blot. It is mainly used to detect specific RNA fragment from mixture of RNA fragmetns. Steps of northern blot are given below (Figure 20.7).

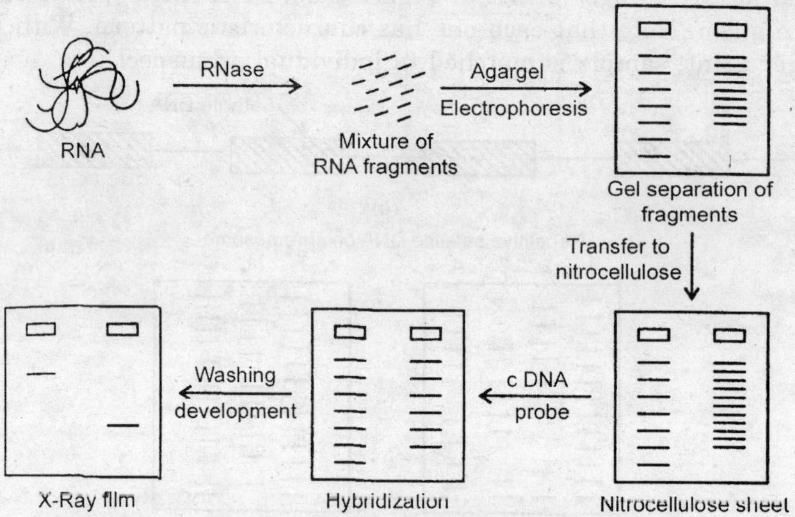

Fig. 20.7 Steps of northern blot

1. Mixture of RNA fragments are obtained from RNA by action of ribonuclease (RNAs).
2. Fragments are separated by agar-gel electrophoresis.
3. Nitrocellulose print of fragments are obtained.
4. cDNA probe is added and excess probe is washed.
5. Visualization of hybrid on X-Ray film as band.

Western blot

It is also similar to southern blot in many ways except in the nature of probe used. In this blotting technique, radiolabelled (polyclonal) or (monoclonal) is used as probe.

This technique is used to identify a specific protein from mixture of proteins. Steps of western blot are given below (Figure 20.8).

1. Protein mixture containing desired protein is subjected to elctrophoresis to separate proteins.
2. Nitro cellulose print is obtained.
3. Antibody probe (radiolabelled) is added.
4. Visualization of antigen-antibody complex on X-Ray film.

DNA chip technology

This technology also based on principle of hybridization. Most of the above blotting techniques are useful in single DNA or gene experiments. But life of any organism is result of co-ordinated interaction of thousands of millions of genes and their products in highly complex manner. Using DNA chip technology, data of millions of genes is obtained. Various steps of DNA chip technology are given below.

1. **DNA chip.** A DNA chip contains an array of DNA samples or genes or synthetic oligonucleotides. Hence, DNA micro array is the alternate name for DNA chip.

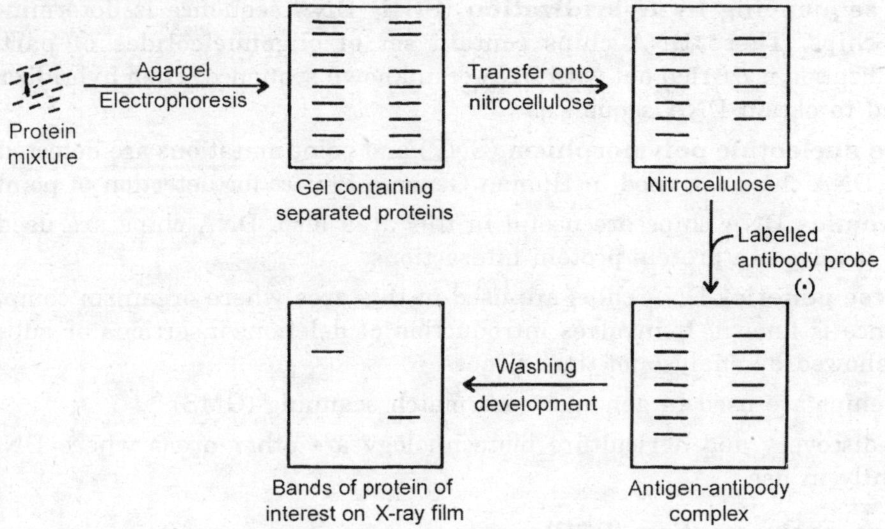

Fig. 20.8 Steps of western blot

DNA chip preparation

DNA chips are prepared by two ways

(*a*) **Photolithography** DNA samples are fixed on solid support with the help of high speed robotics.

(*b*) **Inkjet spotting (printing)** DNA samples or genes of interest are fixed on solid support by inkjet delivery.

2. Fluoroscently labelled cDNA probes of genes of interest are prepared. Number of cDNA probes depends on number of genes of interest.
3. Incubation of cDNA probe with DNA of micro array.
4. cDNA probe hybridizes with corresponding DNA sequences and forms duplex.
5. Fluoroscent tags of hybridized duplexes are excited by laser.
6. A digital image of the array is obtained by using microscope fitted with camera. Then it is fed to computer and data is analysed using special programme.

Applications

DNA chips play a role in the field of genomics similar to that of semi conductors role in electronics. DNA chip technology replaces many gel or filter based assays that are currently in use. DNA chips have many number of applications which will increase in future.

1. **Functional genomics** In the functional genomics area, DNA chips are used for measurement of expression level of genes or expression patterns of genes. A limited number of genes involved in a pathway may be selected.
2. **Diagnostics and genetic mapping** DNA chips are used for diagnositcs. For example, diagnostic chips are prepared to detect mutant alleles in cystic fibrosis and beta globin genes. DNA chips are also used for genotyping of hepatitis C virus in blood samples.
3. **DNA sequencing by hybridization (SBH)** DNA sequence is determined by using DNA chips. These DNA chips contain set of oligonucleotides of particular size. Hybridization is carried out with DNA of unknown sequence. Then hybridization pattern is used to obtain DNA sequence.
4. **Single nucleotide polymorphism (SNP)** and point mutations are detected using DNA chips. DNA chips are used in Human Genome Project for detection of point mutations.
5. **Proteomics** DNA chips are useful in this area also. DNA chips are used to identify genes involved in protein-protein interactions.
6. **Reverse genetics** DNA chips are used in this area where organism complete genome sequence is known. It involves introduction of deletions/insertions or substitutions at will followed by analysis of their fitness.
7. DNA chips are used in genomic miss match scanning (GMS).
8. Drug discovery and agriculture biotechnology are other areas where DNA chips are currently in use.

Polymerase chain reaction (PCR)

1. It is an *in vitro* DNA replication technique.
2. Heat stable DNA polymerase is used for replication.
3. Heat stable Taq DNA polymerase is obtained from thermophilic bacteria (*thermus aquaticus*).
4. Thermophilic bacteria are those bacteria that inhabit hot springs (hot climate). Their enzymes have remarkable properties like stable to extreme temperature (heat).
5. Since Taq DNA polymerase is stable to heat its catalytic activity is not affected when DNA denaturation is carried out at high temperature in this technique.
6. In this technique DNA replication takes place in cyclic manner. Each cycle doubles the DNA amount. The product of the first cycle becomes the template of the next cycle. Thus the initial DNA amount is amplified to several times. Twenty cycles of PCR can amplify particular DNA segment to 10^5 or more times.
7. Replication of DNA by Taq DNA polymerase requires primers. Two oligonucleotide primers are synthesized by using appropriate methods. These primers bind to DNA that is to be amplified (replicated) at specific sequences on opposite strands.

   Steps of PCR are shown in Figure 20.9.

Medical and biological importance

1. PCR amplifies DNA rapidly and selectively.
2. Very small amount (50-100 bp) of DNA from single cell or sperm cell or hair follicle can be amplified to large quantities by PCR.

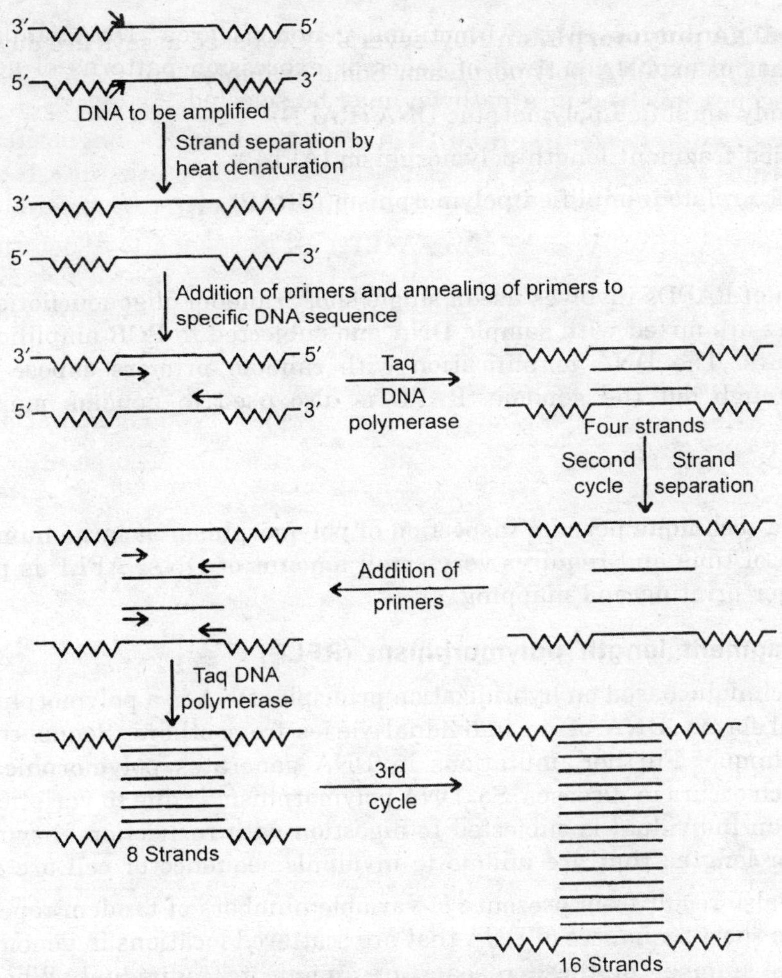

Fig. 20.9 Polymerase chain reaction (3 cycles)

3. PCR is used to detect infectious agents in the body because infenctions are due to presence of (viral or bacterial) foreign DNA.
4. PCR is used for prenatal diagnosis of genetic diseases, which are due to alterations in DNA like sickle cell anemia, hemophilia etc.
5. PCR is used to detect certain cancers like leukemia, thyroid cancer etc.
6. PCR is used for tissue typing which is essential for organ transplantation.
7. In the forensic work amplification of little DNA recovered from the suspect or from the crime site by PCR allows generation of sufficient DNA for finger printing.
8. DNA recovered from archaelogical materials (sites) is amplified by PCR and used to study evolution or civilization.
9. PCR can be used to create extinct animals like dinosaurs by amplifing DNA recovered from fossile materials.
10. Reverse transcriptase polymerase chain reaction (RT-PCR) is used to amplify RNA.

11. **PCR and DNA polymorphism** Now several PCR based assays are developed to detect DNA variations or DNA polymorphism. Some examples are

    (*a*) Randomly amplified polymorphic DNA (RAPD)

    (*b*) Amplified fragment length polymorphism (AFLP)

    (*c*) Sequence related amplified polymorphism (SRAP) etc.

RAPD

The generation of RAPDs involves use of single short random oligoneucliotides. When these random primers are mixed with sample DNA and subjected to PCR amplification of several fragments occurs. The DNA amplification with random primers expose polymorphisms distributed through out the genome. RAPD is also used in genome mapping and gene tagging.

AFLP

This PCR-based technique permits inspection of polymorphism at large number of loci with in short period of time and requires very small amount of DNA. AFLP is potentially used in genome finger printing and mapping.

Restriction fragment length polymorphism (RFLP)

It is another technique based on hybridization principle. DNA is a polymorphic molecule, *i.e.*, exist in several forms. DNA of an individual varies from others. Sequence of DNA of an individual is unique. Further, mutations in DNA generates polymorphic DNA in same individual, which occurs in diseases. So, DNA polymorphism is due to variations in sequence. When DNA of an individual is subjected to digestion with restriction enzyme fragments of varying sizes or lengths that are unique to inviduals sequence or cell are produced.

RFLP may also result from presence of variable numbers of tandem repeates (VNTR) in DNA. These are short sequences of DNA that are scattered locations in genome and repeated in tandem. The number of these repeats are unique to individual. When DNA of two individuals is subjected to digestion with restriction enzymes fragments that vary in length and number are generated. Therefore, RFLP of two individuals results from the differences in the location and number of cleavage sites. Differences in DNA of two individual may be due to evolutionary changes.

RFLP is similar to southern blotting in many aspects. Initial step of RFLP involves digestion of more DNA samples with restriction enzymes where as in southern blotting only one DNA sample is digested. Rest of the steps of RFLP are those of southern blotting. Hence, in RFLP next step probes are used for hybridization. Probes hybridizes with fragment containing complementary sequences. Then polymorphisms are detected by presence or absence of bands after hybridization.

Applications

1. RFLP is used as a diagnostic test of inherited disease. For example, HbS: In HbS gene there is loss of one restriction site for restriction enzyme due to mutation where as normal HbA gene has two cleavage sites. So, RFLP of sickle-cell anemia patient shows two bands where as in RFLP of normal individual three bands appear.
2. RFLP is also used to identify chromosomal difference.

3. RFLP is used for isolation and sequencing of closely related genes.
4. RFLP is combination with PCR is used to detect DNA variations.

Bioinformatics

1. It is the combination of IT (Information Technology) and Life Sciences like Biochemistry, Molecular Biology, Biotechnology etc.
2. It is defined as application of information technology and science for organisation management, mining and use of life sciences.
3. Main application areas of bioinformatics are genomics, proteomics, pharmacogenomics, chemiinformatics etc.
4. One of the earliest application are a of bioinformatics is in drug design process. Bioinformatics revolutionized traditional approach of drug discovery from target discovery and screening to discovery and development of therapeutic agents whose role in prevention of cure of a disease is well validated. Further, drugs so designed have less failures.
5. Following steps of bioinformatics based method of designing drug that is an enzyme inhibitor.
   (*a*) Selection of chemical fragments from molecular library.
   (*b*) Assembly of chemical fragments in a piece-wise manner into possible inhibitor molecule.
   (*c*) Using docking algorithm all the possible inhibitor molecules are screened to select highly potent inhibitor which precisely fits in the binding cavity of enzyme.
6. Knowledge of genome sequence allows structure activity based drug designing. Following are steps of drug designing process, which involves genome sequence knowledge.
   (*a*) Determination of protein sequence using DNA sequence.
   (*b*) Prediction algorithms are used to visualise structure adopted by the protein molecule.
   (*c*) Using docking algorithm a molecule that binds and alters protein function is identified as a drug.

REFERENCES

1. Wu, K., Grossman, L. and Moldave, K. (Eds.). Recombinant DNA methodology. Academic Press, New York, 1989.
2. Berger, S.L. and Kimmal, A.R. Methods in Enzymology, Vol. **152**, Academic Press, California, 1987.
3. Kantoff, P.W. Prospects for gene therapy for immuno deficiency disease. Ann. Rev. Immunol, **6**, 58–94, 1988.
4. Agarwal, S. and Jang, J. GEM 91. An anti-sense oligo nucleotide phosphorothioate as a therapeutic agent for AIDS. Anti-sense Res. Dev. **2**, 261–266, 1992.
5. Rangarajan, P.N. and Padmanabhan, G. Gene therapy: principles, practice, problems and prospects. Curr. Sci. **71 (5)**, 360–367, 1996.
6. Marx, J.L. DNA finger printing takes witness stand. Science **240**, 1616–1618, 1988.

7. Mullus, K.B. The unusual origin of polymerase chain reaction. Sci. Am. P. 56, April 1990.
8. Meada, M.H. Dairy Gene. The Sciences. New York Academy of Sciences, New York, P. 21, October 1997.
9. Michel, K. and Schmidtke. J. DNA finger printing. BIOS Scientific Pub. USA, Canada, 1994.
10. Schena, Mark, (Ed.) DNA micro arrays: A practical appraoch, Oxford University Press, 1999.
11. Siebert, P. (Ed.). The PCR technique. RT-PCR. Eaton Publishing, MA, USA, 1998.
12. Mcpherson, M-J and Moller, S.G. PCR, Springer-Verlag Talos, 2000.
13. Dieffenbach, Carl. W. and Gabriel, S.D. PCR primer: A Laboratory manual. Cold Spring Harbor Laboratory Press, NY, 2003.
14. K. Shah *et al.* Molecular imaging of gene therapy for cancer. Gene Therapy. **11,** 1175–1187, 2004.
15. Li, G. and Quiors. Sequence related amplified polymorphism (SRAP) a new marker system based on simple PCR reaction: its application to mapping and gene tagging in Brassica. Theor. Appl. Genet. **103**, 455–461, 2001.
16. vander wurff. A.W.G. Chan, Y.L. vanstraalan, N.M. and Schouten. J. TE-AFLP; Combining rapidity and robustness in DNA finger printing. Nucleic acids Research. **28**, 105–109, 2000.
17. Song, H. *et al.* Neural stem cells from adult hippo campus develop essential properties of functional CNS neurons. Nature **417**, 39–44, 2002.
18. Gage, F.H. Mammalian neural stem cells. Science. **287**, 1433–1438, 2000.
19. Lesk, A.M. (Ed.). Introduction to Bioinformatics. Oxford University Press, New York, 2002.
20. Isner, J.M. Myocardial gene therapy. Nature. **415**, 234–239, 2002.
21. Austin, C.P. *et al.* The knockout mouse project. Nature Genetics. **36**, 921–924, 2004.
22. Kubota, C. *et al.* Serial bull cloning by somatic cell nuclear transfer. Nature Biotechnology. **22**, 693–694, 2004.
23. Susan M. Rhind *et al.* Human cloning: can it be made safe. Nat. Rev. Geneti. **4**, 855–864, 2003.
24. Rebeca J. Morris *et al.* Capturing and profiling adult hair follicle stem cells. Nature Biotechnology. **22**, 411–417, 2004.
25. Arekawa, T. *et al.* Efficacy of food plant based oral cholera toxin B sub unit vaccine. Nature. Biotechnol. **16**, 292–297, 1998.
26. Karatzas, C.N. Designer milk from transgenic clones. Nature. Biotechnol. **21**, 138–139, 2003.
27. Nishimura, E. K. *et al.* Mechanism of hair graying: Incomplete melanocyte stem cell maintenance in the Niche. Science. **307**, 720-724, 2005.

EXERCISES

ESSAY QUESTIONS

1. Define recombinant DNA. Explain steps of recombinant DNA technology used for production of human gene products in a biotechnology company.

2. Give an account of gene therapy.
3. Describe production and application of hybridomas.
4. Describe hybridization techniques.
5. Describe polymerase chain reaction (PCR).

Short questions

1. Write steps involved in production of transgenic animals.
2. Define cloning. Write steps necessary for production of cloned sheep.
3. Write a note on DNA vaccines.
4. Define edible vaccines. Write steps of edible vaccination.
5. Write a biosensor working principle. Name components of a biosensor and write their applications.
6. Explain western blot technique. Write its significance.
7. Write recombinant DNA technology applications.

Fill in the blanks

1. Recombinant DNA technology may lead to creation of .... species.
2. cDNA probe is .... molecule prepared from ^{32}P labelled nucleoside triphosphates.
3. Cloning is a .... reproduction of mammals.
4. .... cells are immortal.
5. ACAAACT is repetitive sequence of fruit fly ....

21
CHAPTER

CANCER AND AIDS

MEDICAL AND BIOLOGICAL IMPORTANCE

1. Cancer is a major health problem affecting humans throughout the world. Several types of cancers affecting major organs like lung, brain, kidney, colon, breast, oesophagus and stomach have been identified.
2. Rate of incidence of cancer of particular organ in particular population depends on several factors like age, sex, dietary habits, environment, geographical location, genetic make up, culture, physical exercise etc. For example in India oral cancer is common in betal nut chewing regions and in reverse smokers. Stomach cancer is more in Japanese and Chinese people. Colon cancer is common in advanced countries and lung cancer is common in smokers. Old people are more prone to any type of cancer. Brain cancer and blood cancer are common in children. Men above 50 are prone to prostate cancer. Women above 45 are prone to breast, ovarian and cervical cancers.
3. Rate of incidence of cancer of particular organ varies from developed countries to developing countries. (Table 21.1). Lung and colorectal cancers are high in developed countries while stomach and cervical cancer are more in developing countries. Further in India pharyngeal cancers are high in Western India where as stomach cancers are more common in Southern India.

Nearly 10 million new cases of cancer are diagnosed globally every year. It is estimated that by 2020 ten million persons would die of cancer every year World wide.

Table 21.1 Cancer incidence rate in developed and developing Countries

Cancer site	Developed countries	Developing countries
Lung	62	24
Colon and rectum	20-45	2-8
Stomach	10	60
Cervix	14	30
Prostate	30	10
Mouth and pharynx	13	25

4. Nuclear architecture is altered in cancer cells. New anticancer drugs that revert these changes may be developed. Like wise new tumour marker based on nuclear structural changes may be used in cancer diagnosis.
5. Extensive research carried out for the last two decades on various types of cancer led to development of proper treatment for at least some types of cancers. However, it greatly expanded our knowledge on molecular mechanism of cancer.
6. AIDS is another major health problem that surfaced around second half 20th century. According to WHO (World Health Organization) estimation about 20 million people are affected by AIDS. At least about 5-10000 people get infected for every 24 hours. Spread of this infectious disease also depends on several factors. In developing countries it is spreading faster due to prevalent socioeconomic conditions.
7. Though the various facets of cancer and AIDS are being probed thoroughly for the last two decades proper cure is not in sight particularly for AIDS.

CANCER

Growth of all types of cells is controlled in the body. If the growth of cell is not controlled they continue to proliferate which leads to malignancy. So cancer is malignant growth (un controlled growth) of cells. Malignant growth of cell is also called as tumour. Cancer of a particular organ or tissue develops when the cells of that organ have lost growth control. In addition cancer cells has other abilities a) Invasion b) Metastasis. Cancer cells are carried to other parts of the body by circulation where they develop further. So, Cancer of one organ if not detected can spread to other organs (Figure 21.1).

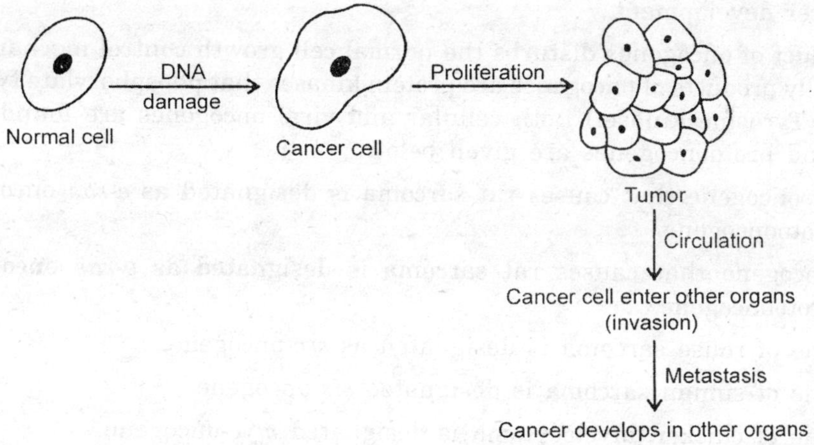

Fig. 21.1 Cancer development from normal cell.

Nomenclature and classification of Cancers

Generally cancers are named according to the organ affected. However they are classified based on the three embryonic germ layers from which tissue or organ is derived.

1. Carcinomas

Are the cancer of cells or organs derived from either ectoderm or endoderm. Cancers of epithelial tissues, nervous tissues, glands etc. are named as carcinomas.

Example:

(*a*) **Adenocarcinoma:** Cancer of gland.

(*b*) **Squamous cell carcinoma:** Cancer of squamous cells of epithelial tissues.

(*c*) **Gliomas:** Cancer of brain nervous tissues.

2. Sarcomas

Are cancers of tissues of mesodermal origin. Generally cancers of bone, cartilage, connective tissue, muscle etc are called as sarcomas.

Examples:

(a) **Osteosarcoma:** Bone cancer.

(*b*) **Fibrosarcoma:** Connective tissue cancer.

Cancer is primarily due to DNA damage or damage of genes. DNA damage may result from the action of biological, chemical, physical and environmental agents on DNA. Incidence of cancer also depends on the genetic make up of an individual.

Cancer genes

Oncogenes. Are genes responsible for development of cancer.

Proto oncogenes. They are precursors of oncogenes. They are converted to oncogenes by activation.

Tumour suppressor genes. They are present in normal healthy people. Products of them prevent cancer development.

The product of oncogenes disturbs the normal cell growth control mechanism leading to cancer. Usually products of oncogenes are protein kinases that phosphorylate tyrosine residues of proteins. (Tyrosine kinase.) Both cellular and viral oncogenes are found. Examples for oncogenes and protooncogenes are given below.

1. Cellular oncogene that causes rat sarcoma is designated as *c-ras* oncogene. Likewise *c-ras* protooncogene.
2. Viral oncogene that causes rat sarcoma is designated as *v-ras* oncogene. Likewise *v-ras* protooncogene.
3. Oncogene of rouse sarcoma is designated as *src*-oncogene.
4. Oncogene of simian sarcoma is designated *sis*-oncogene.
5. Oncogene of chicken myelocytoma is designated *myc*-oncogene.

Carcinogenesis

By several ways carcinogenesis occurs in humans and other animals. Usually they are named according causative agent or factor. Different types of carcinogenesis are given below:

1. **Biological agents that cause cancer or biological (viral) carcinogenesis.** Some DNA and RNA viruses are carcinogenic and hence they are called as oncogenic viruses. When normal cells are cultured with oncogenic viruses, the normal cells are transformed into cancer (tumour) cells. Oncogenes of the viruses are responsible for the development of cancer.

Examples

1. Hepatitis B virus cause liver cancer in humans.
2. Retro viruses also cause cancer in humans.

2. **Chemical carcinogens or mutagens or chemical carcinogenesis.** Many chemical substances cause mutations in DNA. They are called mutagens. Sometimes this mutation in DNA may convert normal cell to cancer cell. Then they are called as carcinogens.

Examples

1. Cigarette smoke causes lung cancer in humans.
2. Aflatoxins are carcinogens.
3. Nitrosamine, Benzapyrins and asbestos also cause cancer.

3. **Physical agents that cause cancer or physical carcinogenesis.** Exposure to radiation may damage DNA. UV light exposure causes mutation in DNA of skin cells. Mutant DNA mediates carcinogenesis by activation of oncogenes which leads to development of cancer of skin or multiple tumours of skin.

Cancer due to genetic factors:

Some genes in DNA are associated with development of cancer in susceptible individuals. Examples:

1. Retinoblastoma, cancer of eye develops in people carrying RBI gene.
2. Wilm's tumour, kidney cancer develops in children having gene WTI.

Activation of protooncogene to oncogene

By several ways activation of protooncogene to oncogene can occur. Some of them are given below.

(*a*) **Point mutation.** Point mutation converts protooncogene to oncogene. Human bladder carcinoma is due to point mutation. Mutation may be due to error during replication.

(*b*) **Gene amplification.** Amplification of oncogenes results in the formation of products of these genes by several folds. This in turn converts normal cells to cancer cells.

(*c*) Chromosomal translocation, promoter/enhancer insertion also leads to activation of protooncogene to oncogene.

Mechanism of action of oncogenes or Mechanism of carcinogenesis

The product of oncogene converts normal cell to cancer cell by several ways.

1. The product of *c-ras* oncogene is a less active GTPase. This leads to prolonged activation of adenylate cyclase and hence activities of cAMP dependent proteinkinase. As a result cellular metabolism is altered and normal cell is transformed into cancer cell.
2. *Myc*-oncogene product is DNA binding protein or transcription factor (TF). It regulates expression of cell cycle genes. As a result cell cycle is altered.
3. *Src*-oncogene product is tyrosinekinase. It phosphorylates cyclins and cyclin dependent kinases of cell cycle. This results in cell cycle alteration.
4. Some oncogene products are polypeptide growth factors that affect cell cycle and mitosis.

Mechanism of virus mediated carcinogenesis

1. Several human tumour viruses induce immortalization of human tissue cells. It is followed by malignant conversion which involves several steps.
2. Human papilloma viruses (HPV), human T-lymphocyte virus (HTLV) possess defined oncogenes that stimulate proliferation of human cells.
3. Human papilloma virus causes cervical cancer. Cancer of cervix is the number one cancer in Indian women. In India about 100,000 women develop this cancer every year.
4. Human T-lymphocyte virus causes T-lymphocyte leukemia.
5. The oncogenes of HPV are E6 and E7. They are able to immortalize keratinocytes. They contain all necessary information for immortalization.
6. The E7 protein releases transcription factor which activates genes engaged in cell cycle progression.
7. The E6 protein binds P^{53} and abolishes its tumour suppressive and Trans activational properties. It also promotes ubiquitinisation of P^{53} and its subsequent proteolysis.
8. Thus E6 and E7 are able to immortalize cells independently and both genes cooperate effectively in immortalization of cells.

Metabolism of carcinogen

Metabolism of carcinogen after entering the body is mainly directed towards producing metabolites which can be excreted. The enzyme systems of phase-I and phase-II reactions of metabolism of xenobiotics are mainly responsible for the formation of excretory metabolites. Sometimes these compounds lead to tumour formation. If it leads to formation of malignant tumour then it is known as Cancer. Cytochrome P_{450} enzymes of phase-I are involved in the formation of a carcinogen.

Mechanism of a carcinogen mediated carcinogenesis

1. Carcinogenesis by a carcinogen involves several steps.
2. First step is the induction of molecular lesion.
3. Second step is the fixation of molecular lesion by DNA replication.
4. The ultimate carcinogenic forms of carcinogens are highly reactive electrophiles which are reactive towards DNA.
5. They bind covalently with DNA to produce DNA adduct.
6. This type of DNA modification is major driving force for cancer development.

Nuclear structure of Cancer cells

1. In cancer cells nuclear architecture is altered. These alterations are characteristics of tumour type.
2. Components of nuclear matrix play a role in organization of chromosomes and nuclear components. Protein composition of nuclear matrix is altered in cancer cells.
3. Oncogenes induce tumor-specific nuclear changes and these in turn changes gene regulation.
4. In cancer cells chromosomal territories and gene loci are changed.

5. Structural changes in tumour cells lead to changes in nucleoli and perinuclear compartment.
6. These changes can be used as potential tumour markers and targets for anti-cancer drugs.

Treatment of cancer

Several types of treatments are available for cancer management. Some are given below. Cancer gene therapy is explained in earlier chapter.

1. Chemotherapy

Compounds that block replication of cells and anti metabolites that block nucleotide biosynthesis are used as anticancer agents or in chemotherapy of cancer.

(*a*) **Mercapto purine.** It is a purine analog used in the treatment of luekaemia. It is converted into nucleotide *in vivo* and incorporated into nucleic acids and interferes with replication.

(*b*) **Fluoro uracil.** It is a pyrimidine analog and used in the treatment of colorectal cancer. *In vivo* it is converted fluorodeoxy uridine phosphate and inhibits replication.

(*c*) **Methotrexate.** It is a folic acid analog and used in the treatment of chorio carcinoma.

(*d*) **Azaserine.** It is a glutamine analog used in cancer treatment. It blocks nucleic acid biosynthesis (replication) by inhibiting glutamine dependent metabolic reactions.

(*e*) **Acivicin.** Another glutamine analog used as anticancer agent. It is a competitive inhibitor of glutamine utilizing enzyme.

Methotrexate, azaserine and acivicin are anti metabolites used in cancer treatment. They are called as anti metabolites because they block nucleic acid synthesis by anatgonizing metabolic role of glutamine.

2. Radiotherapy

Radiation can break phosphodiester linkages of DNA and interferes with replication process. As a result growth of cancer cells can come down. Based on this principle radiation is used to treat tumours.

3. Surgery

It is the treatment of choice in the advanced stages of cancer. Cancer (tumour) tissue is removed by surgery. Usually surgery is performed with operataing microscope.

4. Photo chemotherapy

It is a newly introduced treatment for cancer. It uses a photosensitive drug and laser light to destroy cancer cells.

5. Suicide Gene Therapy (Molecular surgery)

It is a kind of gene therapy used in the treatment of solid tumours where therapeutic gene is targeted at tumour cells killing cells which expressing it. It is also known as molecular surgery. The suicide genes are enzymes which activates low toxic prodrug to toxic potent drug. Herpes simplex thymidine kinase (HSTK) and cytosine deaminase (CD) are two such enzymes. HSTK converts non-toxic anti-viral drug ganciclovir to toxic form by phosphorylation.

CD converts non-toxic fluorocytosine into toxic fluorouracil. Vectors carrying genes of these enzymes are injected directly into tumour. It is followed by intratumoural injection of prodrug.

Tumour Markers

Cancer (tumour or malignant) cells produce abnormal substances. Usually these substances are not produced by normal cells. The abnormal substances produced by the cancer cells are enzymes, hormones and proteins. These substances are released into blood by cancer cells. As a result their level in blood rises. Measurement of these substances in blood or serum provides useful information about cancer. Hence, they are called as tumour markers, Nowadays measurement of tumour markers in blood is an integral part of oncology. Tumour marker measurement is used in

(*a*) Detection of cancer.

(*b*) Diagnosis of cancer.

(*c*) Prognosis of cancer.

(*d*) Determination of cancer stage.

(*e*) Determination of location of cancer in the body.

(*f*) Determination of organ involved in cancer.

(*g*) Cancer therapy.

Some clinically important tumour markers are

1. **α-Feto protein(AFP).** It is a plasma protein and usually absent in normal people plasma. It is tumour marker for liver cancer and germ cell cancer.
2. **Calcitonin.** It is a hormone. It is tumour marker for thyroid cancer.
3. **Carcino embryonic antigen (CEA).** It is a protein and it is tumour marker for lung cancer, breast cancer, colon cancer and pancreas cancer.
4. **Human chorionic gonodotropin (HCG).** It is tropic hormone. It is tumour marker for germ cell cancer and trophoblast cancer.
5. **Acid phosphatase.** It is tumour marker for prostate cancer.
6. **High mobility group chromosomal proteins (HMGCP).** They are family of non-histone chromosomal proteins that serve as architectural elements in chromatin . In normal tissues these proteins are expressed at very low levels. Their level is elevated in many human cancers. This small molecular weight proteins' expression is increased in neoplastic transformation of cells and metastatic of tumour progression. They can serve as novel diagnostic tumour markers.

Disadvantages of tumour markers

1. These tumour markers usually detect cancer at advanced stage. So they are of little help in saving lives.
2. A given marker is useful in the detection of only one type of cancer.
3. Sometimes measurement of more than one type of tumour marker may be helpful or required.

AIDS

It is the abbreviated form of Acquired Immuno Deficiency Syndrome. It is an acquired disease. It is an infectious disease. In this disease body immune or defense system weakens. It is named as syndrome because full blown disease makes up many diseases.

AIDS is caused by a virus called as Human Immuno Deficiency Virus type-I (HIV-I). It is a retrovirus, It consists of RNA which is surrounded by two types of proteins. The RNA core is enveloped in membrane lipid bilayer containing glycoproteins (Figure 21.2). When HIV infects humans it infects T-cells of lymphocytes which form an important part of immune system. The lymphocytes (T-cells) fight diseases by killing disease causing agents. The cell surface of T-cells contains a glycoprotein receptor known as CD-4 receptor. The T-cells are also called as CD-4 cells because of this. AIDS virus attacks CD-4 cells and kills them. So when a person is infected with HIV for prolonged period his CD-4 cell count decreases and he is susceptible to infections.

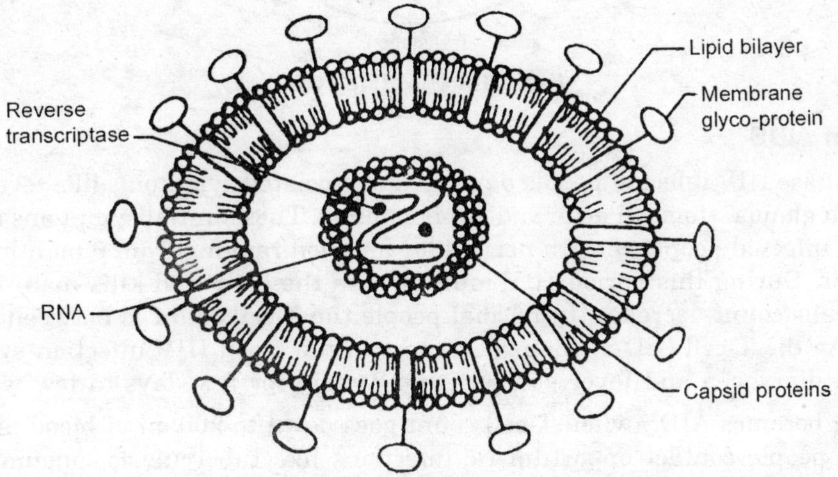

Fig. 21.2 Structure of AIDS virus

HIV Life cycle

1. HIV genetic material is single stranded RNA.
2. When HIV enters into body, it gets attached to T-cell through CD-4 receptor.
3. Then HIV internalizes in the cell after fusing with membrane of CD-4 cell. Its contents are released into the CD-4 cell.
4. The genetic material of HIV is transformed into DNA by reverse transcriptase.
5. The HIV DNA is integrated into host DNA.
6. Expression of HIV RNA and translation of RNA produces proproteins in the CD-4 cell.
7. Pro proteins are processed by protease (HIV) to perfect proteins of HIV.
8. Assembling of RNA and HIV proteins into new HIV particles.
9. Newly formed HIV comes out of CD-4 cell by killing it or when CD-4 cell dies.

Various events involved in HIV life cycle are shown in Figure 21.3.

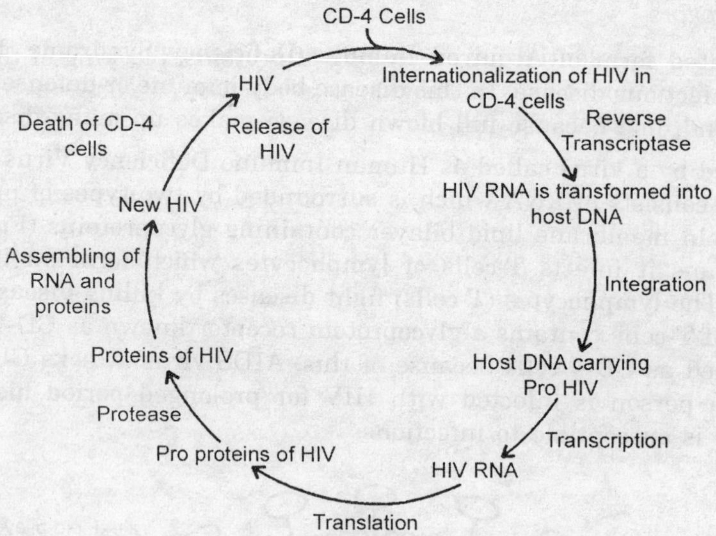

Fig. 21.3 HIV Life cycle

Symptoms of AIDS

In the early phase HIV infected people develop flu associated symptoms like fever, headache, swollen lymph glands, stomach ache and swollen joints. These initial symptoms subside after few days and infected people remain normal for a period ranging from 6 months to 10 years or even longer. During this period HIV multiplies in the body and kills many T-cells. As a result CD-4 cells count decrease. In normal people the T-cell count is between 500 to 1500/ ml of blood. As the T-cell (CD-4) count decreases in the blood HIV infection symptoms like night sweats, diarrhoea and fever surfaces and remain for few days to few weeks.

HIV infection becomes AIDS when T-cell count goes down to 200/ml of blood. At this stage, HIV infected people contact opportunistic infections like tuberculosis, pneumonia, weight loss, tumours and fungal infections. Recovery from these conditions is slow and requires extensive treatment.

Laboratory Diagnosis

When a person is infected with HIV antibodies to HIV are produced in the body like in any other infection. So the presence of HIV antibodies in the blood indicates infection. Most of the AIDS detection tests are based on identification of HIV antibodies in the blood. Enzyme linked immunosorptive assay (ELISA) and western blot technique are used to detect HIV antibodies in blood. Some AIDS detection tests are based on genetic material of HIV.

AIDS Therapy

Currently AIDS treatment involves use of two classes of drugs. They are

(a) Inhibitors of reverse transcriptase

Since reverse transcriptase is important for replication of HIV blocking reverse transcriptase action can control HIV proliferation. Some of the reverse transcriptase inhibitors used as drugs are AZT, ddI, ddc, d4T and 3TC.

(b) Protease inhibitors

Since HIV protease is essential for processing of proteins, blocking of this enzyme also can arrest HIV proliferation. Some of HIV protease inhibitors used as drug are indinavir, saquinavir, ritonavir and nelfinavir.

HIV AND CANCER

In India, HIV-1 is mostly responsible for AIDS. HIV-2 is common in West Africa and found in India also. Both HIV-1 and HIV-2 are not directly oncogenic. However, Kaposi's sarcoma of AIDS patients is largely an attribute of HIV.

Kaposi's sarcoma (KS) is a rare tumour found only in men over sixty years in certain Eastern European and Mediterranean population. However, risk of KS in HIV infected adult male homosexuals less than sixty years old is some ten thousand fold higher than that of their counterparts in general population. With AIDS, endemic KS has become most common of all tumours in Sub Saharan Africa. The epidemology of KS before and after AIDS suggested a transmissible agent may underlie tumour. Human herpes virus-8 (HHV-8) or KS-associated herpes virus (KSHV) is discovered as responsible for KS in humans. KSHV DNA is found in KS biopsies alone and in HIV positive patients. Both KSHV and HIV infections are independent and highly risk factors in the development of KS in AIDS patients. The risk of KS in KSHV positive patients's increases with decreasing CD-4 T lymphocytes as occurs in AIDS. It is believed that Tat protein of HIV-1 has role in KS pathogenesis. It acts synergistically with cellular growth factors. However, KS commonly occurs in KSHV patients with HIV-1 than with HIV-2 infection. In HIV positive patient KSHV is also associated with lympho proliferative disease.

Burkitt's lymphoma (BL) and Non-Hodgkin lymphoma (NHL) are two lymphomas frequently seen in AIDS cases. NHL in AIDS occurs in brain and BL in gut. Incidence of any cancer increases in AIDS patients due to immune suppression. The immune suppression induced by HIV accelerates progression of malignancy. Liver cancer, skin cancer, testicular cancer and treatocarcinoma are more in AIDS patients. Hence, cancers associated with AIDS are probably opportunistic neoplasms like opportunistic infections.

REFERENCES

1. Weinberg, R.A. A molecular basis of cancer. Sci. Am. **249(5)**, 126-142, 1983.
2. Boyle, P. Nutritional factors and cancer. In Human Nutrition and Dietetics. Garrow, J.S. and James, W.P.T. (Eds.) 9th ed. Churchill Livingstone, Edinburgh, 1993.
3. Lavecchia, C. Bidoli, E. and Barra, L. Types of Cigarettes and cancer of upper digestive and respiratory tract. Cancer causes control. **1**, 69-74, 1990.
4. Dwyer, M.J. Biomedical aspect of HIV and AIDS. Curr. Sci. **69(10)**, 823-827, 1995.
5. Wlodawer, A. and Ericikson, J.W. Structure based inhibitors of HIV-1 proteases. Ann. Rev. Biochem. **62,** 543-585, 1993.
6. Roberts, N.A. Drug resistance patterns of saquinavir and other HIV protease inhibitors. AIDS, **9,** 527-532, 1995.
7. J. Cohen, HIV/AIDS in Asia, Science, June, 2004.

8. HIV/AIDS in India, Science, April 2004.
9. Ryan, K.M. and Vousden, K. Cancer: Pinning a change on P^{53}. Nature **419,** 795-797,2002.
10. Mikail, V. Blagosklonny. Cell immortality and Hall marks of cancer. Cell cycle. **2,** 296-299, 2003.
11. Kristi, G. Bache. *et al.* Defective down regulation of receptor tyrosine kinases in cancer. The EMBO Journal. **23,** 2707-2714, 2004.
12. Donald, W.K. *et al.* (Eds.) 6th ed. Cancer medicine, BC Decker, 2003.
13. Veldwij, K.M.R. *et al.* Suicide gene therapy of Sarcoma cell lines using recombinant adeno associated virus vectors. Cancer gene therapy. **11,** 577-580, 2004.
14. Bandura, J.L. and Calvi, B.R. Duplication of genome in normal and cancer cell cycle. Cancer Biol. Ther. **1,** 8-13, 2002.
15. Zink, D. *et al.* Nuclear structure in cancer cells. Nat. Rev. Cancer. **4,** 677-687, 2004.
16. Parkin, D.M. *et al.* Estimating world cancer burden. Int. J., Cancer. **4,** 153-156, 2001.
17. Mathew, A. Cancer registration with emphasis on Indian Scenario. In 'Basic information for cancer registry documentation' (Ed. Mathew. A.), Regional Cancer Centre, Trivendrum, pp11-17, 2003.
18. Davis, M.I. *et al.* Crystal structure of prostate specific antigen a tumor marker and peptidase. Proc. Natl. Acad. Sci. USA. **102**, 5881-5986, 2005.

EXERCISES

SHORT QUESTIONS

1. Define oncogenes, protooncogenes and tumour suppressor genes. Give examples for chemical carcinogens. Explain how they cause cancer.
2. What are tumour markers ? Give an example and its clinical importance.
3. Expand HIV. Write a note on HIV life cycle.
4. Write symptoms and treatments available for AIDS.

22
CHAPTER

PORPHYRIN AND HAEMOGLOBIN METABOLISM

MEDICAL AND BIOLOGICAL IMPORTANCE

1. Porphyrins are present in biological fluids like blood, bile, urine and feces of animals and invertebrates. They are also found in plants and bacteria.
2. Porphyrins are components of hemeproteins of animals and invertebrates. Heme is metalloporphyrin. It contains metal iron in the centre of porphyrin ring. Hence heme proteins are referred as metalloporphyrinoproteins.
3. Hemeproteins like hemoglobin and myoglobin are involved in O_2 transport in animals and vertebrates.
4. In invertebrates erythrocruorins which are also hemeproteins are responsible for the O_2 transport.
5. Hemeproteins like cytochromes and cytochrome oxidase are components of respiratory chain and involved in electron transport.
6. Cytochrome P_{450} which is involved in detoxification of drugs is a hemeprotein.
7. Some hemeproteins are involved in metabolism. For example tryptophan dioxygenase an enzyme of tryptophan catabolism is a metelloprophyrinoprotein and cyclooxygenase an enzyme of prostaglandin synthesis is a hemeprotein.
8. Hemeproteins like catalase and peroxidase are involved in the removal of H_2O_2.
9. In plants porphyrins are components of chlorophyll and phycobilins.
10. In bacteria porphyrins are components of cyanocobalamin.
11. A group of inherited diseases known as porphyrias are due to abnormalities in heme (porphyrin) biosynthesis. Lead poisoning also blocks porphyrin biosynthesis.
12. A common disease jaundice is due to excessive catabolism of porphyrins or heme containing compounds. Hepatitis and cancer of pancreas also can cause jaundice.
13. A group of inherited diseases known as hemoglobinopathies are due to abnormalities in production of hemoglobin.
14. Carbon monoxide a poisonous gas present in automobile exhaust works by combining with hemoglobin.

15. Photosensitive property of porphyrins is used in cancer photochemotherapy.
16. Bilirubin end product of heme catabolism act as antioxidant.
17. Hemoglobin is a source of protein for malarial parasite during malaria. Enzymes of hemoglobin degradation pathway are exploited for new drug design.

Porphyrins Chemistry

Porphyrins are derived from a parent compound porphin. Porphin is a tetrapyrrole and it is a cyclic compound. In porphin, 4 pyrroles are linked through methenyl (—CH=) bridges. Four pyrrole rings of porphin are shown with Roman numbers I, II, III and IV. Methenyl bridges are indicated by Greek numbers α, β, γ and δ. Substituent positions of I, II, III and IV rings are indicated with Indo-Arabic numbers 1, 2, 3, 4, 5, 6 and 7, 8 respectively (Fig. 22.1). The eight numbered substituent positions corresponds to eight hydrogen atoms of pyrrole rings.

Short hand representation of Porphyrins

Naturally occurring porphyrins contain various side chains in place of 8 hydrogen atoms. They differ only in side chains attached to four pyrrole rings. Hence Fischer proposed a short hand form for porphyrins in which only substitutions are particularly shown. In this short hand form as shown in Fig. 22.1 each pyrrole ring with numbered substituent positions is shown as bracket. The four brackets are indicated with Roman numbers and they are joined by eliminating the methenyl bridges to form cross shape.

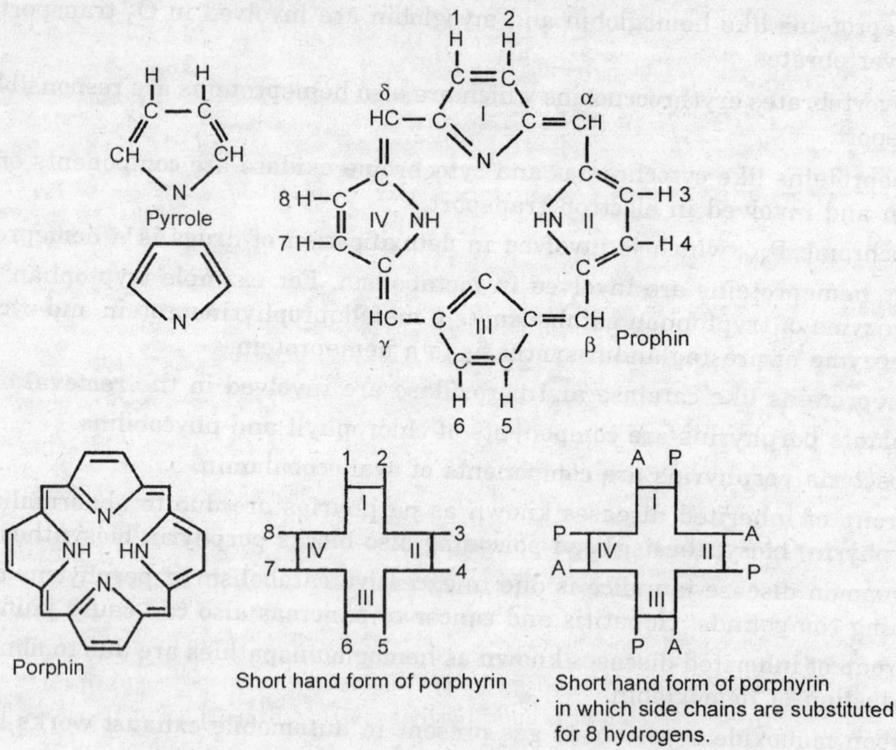

Fig. 22.1 Structures of pyrrole, porphin and porphyrin

Porphyrins Isomers

Porphyrins are intermediates of heme biosynthesis. Each porphyrin can exist in many isomeric forms which depends on kinds of side chains and arrangement of side chains. For example a porphyrin like uroporphyrin with two type of side chains acetate (A), propionate (P) can exist in four isomeric forms or four types. They are type I, type II, type III and type IV. In uroporphyrin I side chains are arranged symmetrically. In other types side chains A, P are arranged asymmetrically (Fig. 22.2). In nature I and III type porphyrins are more. However type III is predominant and more important for heme biosynthesis.

Protoporphyrin with three types of side chain can exist in fifteen isomeric forms. In protoporphyrins two pyrrole rings contain methyl (M) and propionate (P) side chains. Other two pyrrole rings contain methyl (M) and Vinyl (V) side chains. Heme of hemoglobin contains protoporphyrin IX (Fig. 22.2).

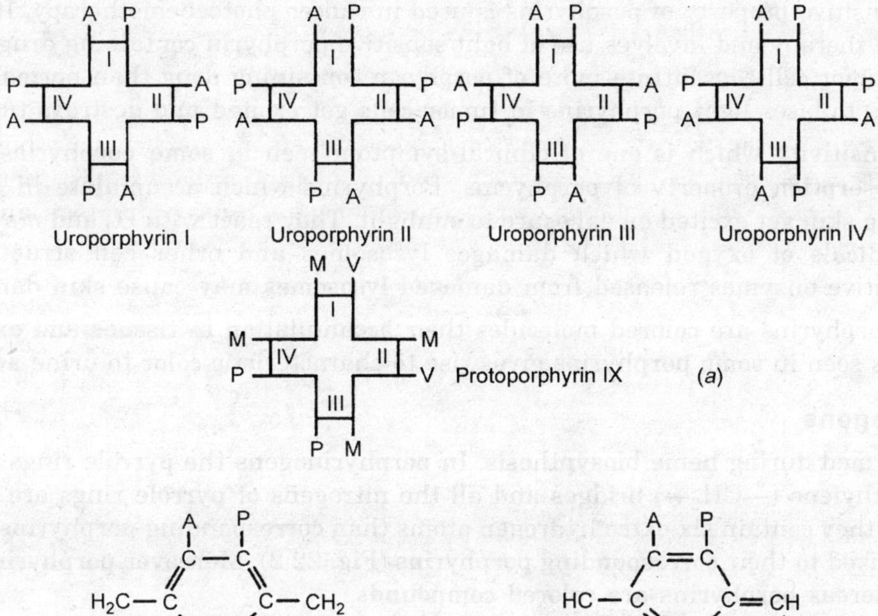

Fig. 22.2 (*a*) Short hand forms of uroporphyrin and protoporphyrin.
(*b*) Conversion of uroporphyrinogen III to uroporphyrin III.

Properties of Porphyrins

1. **Solubility.** If a prophyrin has polar side chains then it is more soluble in aqueous

environment of blood. If a porphyrin has nonpolar side chains then it is less soluble in blood.

2. **Light absorption.** All porphyrins absorb light maximally at 400 nm. Porphyrins also can absorb light in the visible region. When porphyrin combines with metal its absorption changes. For example protoporphyrin IX absorbs light at 645 nm whereas heme which is the combination of protoporphyrin IX and iron absorb light at 545 nm. Light absorption properties of porphyrins are used for their identification.
3. **Fluoroescence.** Porphyrins show fluoroescence in organic solvents when they are exposed to UV-light. This property is used to detect porphyrins in biological fluids.
4. All porphyrins are colored compounds.

Medical Importance

1. Photosensitive property of porphyrins is used in cancer photochemotherapy. It is a combination therapy and involves use of light sensitive porphyrin containing drug and laser light. Tumor cell concentrate more of porphyrin containing drug than normal cells. On exposure to laser light porphyrins in tumor cells get excited and destroys tumor cells.
2. Photosensitivity which is one of clinical symptom seen in some porphyrias is due to light absorption property of porphyrins. Porphyrins which accumulate in areas surrounding skin get excited on exposure to sunlight. They react with O_2 and may generate free radicals of oxygen which damages lysosomes and other cell structures. The degradative enzymes released from damaged lysosomes may cause skin damage.
3. Since porphyrins are colored molecules their accumulation in tissues and excretion in urine as seen in some porphyrias gives rise to characteristic color to urine and tissues.

Porphyrinogens

They are formed during heme biosynthesis. In porphyrinogens the pyrrole rings are linked through methylene ($—CH_2—$) bridges and all the nitrogens of pyrrole rings are hydrogenated. Hence they contain six extra hydrogen atoms than corresponding porphyrins. They can be auto oxidized to their corresponding porphyrins (Fig. 22.2). Moreover porphyrinogens are colorless whereas porphyrins are colored compounds.

Heme biosynthesis

Heme is synthesized by most of the cells except mature erythrocytes. However bonemarrow and liver are chief organs involved in heme production. Bonemarrow produces about 80% and rest is produced by liver.

Reaction Sequence

In heme synthesis first and last three reactions occurs in mitochondria and intermediate reactions takes place in cytosol. Amino acid glycine and succinyl-CoA of citric acid cycle are starting materials for the heme formation (Fig. 22.3).

1. Formation of δ-aminolevulinic acid (ALA) from succinyl-CoA and glycine is the first reaction of heme biosynthesis and involves —C—C— bond formation. The reaction is catalyzed by aminolevulinic acid synthase or ALA synthase which takes place in two steps. The first step of reaction is mediated by pyridoxal phosphate the prosthetic group of ALA synthase. It forms a Schiff base with glycine which then condenses with succinyl-

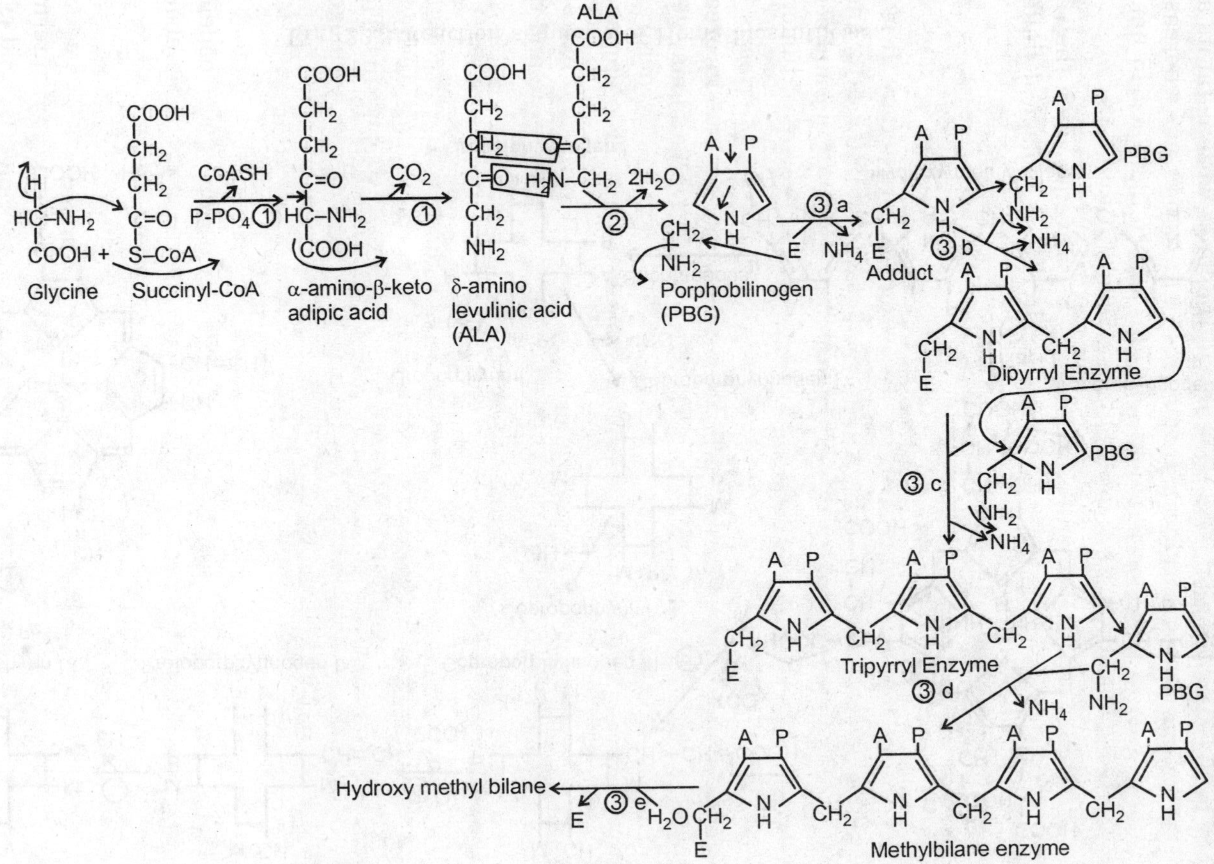

Fig. 22.3 Reaction sequence of Heme biosynthesis. Arrow mark indicates newly formed —C—C— and —C—N— linkages.

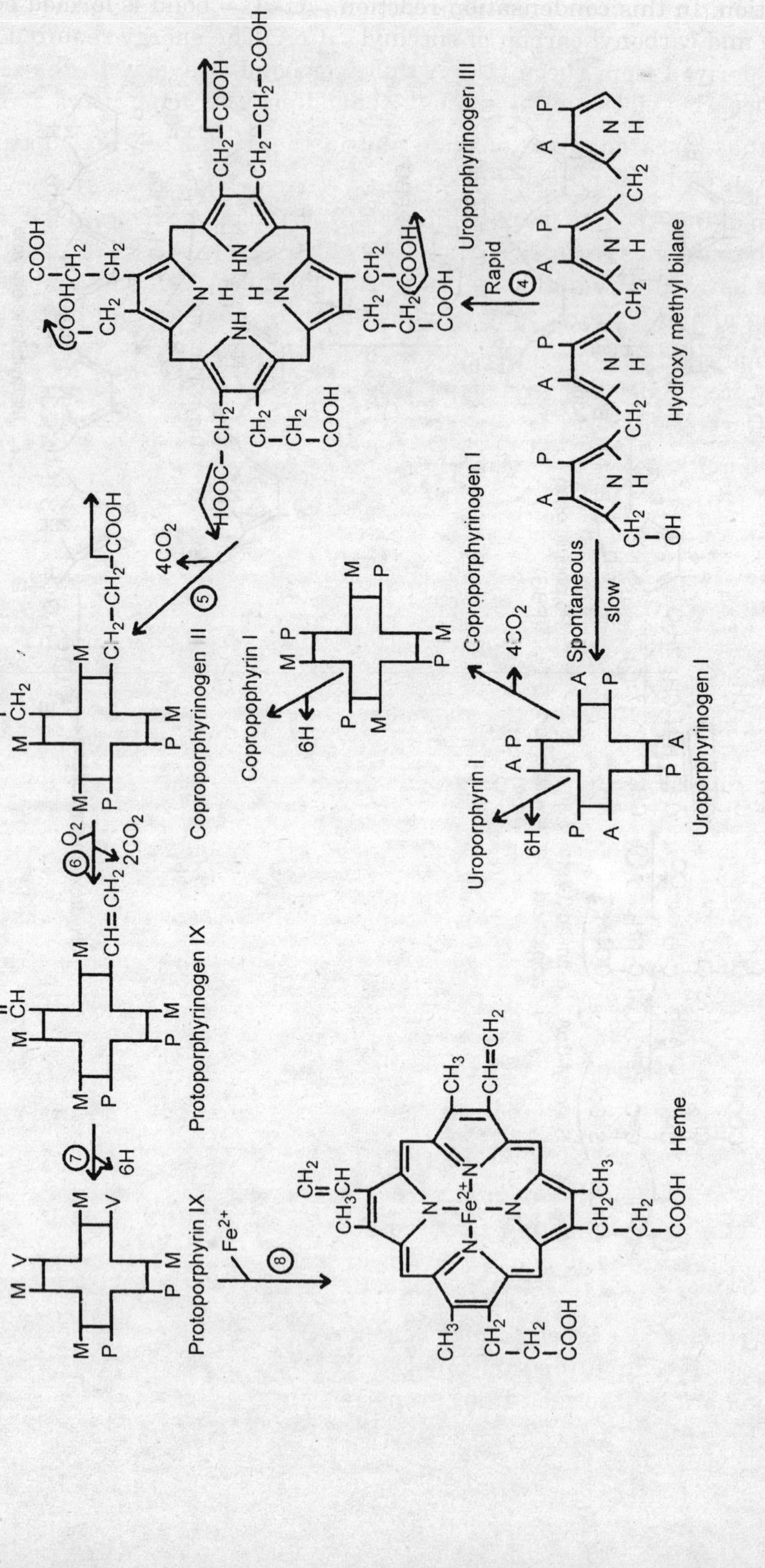

Fig. 22.3 Reaction sequence of Heme biosynthesis.

CoA to yield enzyme bound α-amino-β-keto adipic acid. Mg^{2+} ions are also required for condensation. In this condensation reaction —C—C— bond is formed between α-carbon of glycine and carbonyl carbon of succinyl —CoA. The energy required for this reaction is mostly derived from succinyl-CoA thioester bond cleavage. In the second step of the reaction decarboxylation of α-amino-β-Keto adipic acid generates δ-aminolevulinic acid.

ALA synthase is a adaptive enzyme and in the liver it is rate limiting enzyme. The enzyme is present in mitochondria.

2. Formation of first pyrrole porphobilinogen (PBG) from two molecules of δ-amino levulinic acid in the cytosol is the next reaction which involves —C—C bond and C-N- bond formation between two aminolevulinic acid molecules. The reaction is catalyzed by -SH containing amino levulinic acid dehydratase. The enzyme contains Zn^{2+} also.

   The enzyme catalyzes pyrrole ring formation in a intermolecular reaction by eliminating two water molecules from two ALA molecules. Removal of a water molecule between β Carbon of first ALA and γ-carbon of second ALA generate —C—C— bond. Elimination of other water molecule between γ-carbon of first ALA and amino group of second ALA produces —C—N— bond. The pyrrole ring thus formed has acetate (A) and propionate (P) side chains.

   Since the enzyme has -SH group it is inhibited by metals. Hence more ALA is excreted in urine in lead poisoning. The transport of ALA from mitochondria to cytosol is blocked by hemin. Other name given to this enzyme is porphobilinogen synthase.

3. In this reaction 4PBG molecules undergoes head to tail condensation to yield a linear tetra pyrrole. The reaction is multistep process and catalyzed by uroporphyrinogen synthase I.

   (*a*) Free PBG molecule can not initiate condensation. Hence initially enzyme forms covalent adduct by displacing amino group of first PBG as NH_4.

   (*b*) Now first head to tail condensation between covalent adduct (enzyme bound PBG) and second PBG generates an enzyme bound dipyrrole. A carbon bridge connects two pyrroles. The amino group of second PBG is released as NH_4.

   (*c*) Subsequent condensation of enzyme bound dipyrrole with third PBG yields tripyrrole. The amino group of third PBG is released as NH_4.

   (*d*) Finally enzyme bound tetrapyrrole (methyl bilane enzyme) is formed by condensation of tripyrrole with 4th PBG molecule. The amino group of 4th PBG is lost as NH_4.

   (*e*) Hydrolysis of methyl bilane enzyme yields free enzyme and hydroxy methyl bilane.

   The uroporphyrinogen I synthase is also called as porphobilinogen deaminase.

4. Formation of porphyrin skeleton occurs in this reaction. First hydroxy methyl bilane formed in the above reaction undergoes cyclization with simultaneous flipping of last pyrrole to uroporphyrinogen III in presence of uro porphyrinogen III cosynthase.

   Alternatively hydroxy methyl bilane undergoes spontaneous cyclization to uroporphyrinogen I. Since former reaction is a rapid process most of hydroxymethyl bilane is converted to uroporphyrinogen III rather than uroporphyrinogen I. In bacteria cobalamins are synthesized from uroporphyrinogen III.

5. In this reaction all the acetate side chains of uroporphyrinogen III undergoes decarboxylation to methyl groups. The reaction is catalyzed by uroporphyrinogen decarboxylase and coproporphyrinogen III is the product.

   The enzyme also can convert uroporphyrinogen I to coproporphyrinogen I if available. However only coproporphyrinogen III enters mitochondria.

6. In mitochondria coproporphyrinogen III is converted to protoporphyrinogen IX by enzyme coproporphyrinogen III oxidase in presence of molecular oxygen. The enzyme catalyzes decarboxylation as well as oxidation of two propionic acid side chains of I and II pyrroles of coproporphyrinogen III to form protoporphyrinogen IX.

7. Protoporphyrinogen IX is oxidized to protoporphyrin IX by protoporphyrinogen oxidase in presence of molecular oxygen.

8. Finally incorporation of Fe^{2+} into protoporphyrin IX by heme synthase yields heme. In heme Fe^{2+} occupies the centre of the planer structure. Lead is an inhibitor of heme synthase. Hence in lead poisoning protoporphyrin is excreted in urine and feces.

   In plants protoporphyrin is used for chlorphyll and phycobilin formation.

Regulation of Heme biosynthesis

ALA synthase activity controls heme biosynthesis in liver. In the liver ALA synthase activity is controlled by (1) Feedback inhibition (2) Repression, derepression (Induction). Heme the end product of the pathway is allosteric inhibitor of ALA synthase. In the regulation of ALA synthase by repression heme act as corepressor and combines with aporepressor to form holorepressor which prevents expression of ALA synthase gene.

De repression of ALA synthase in presence of drugs like barbiturates and steroids occurs due to diversion or increased utilization of heme for cyt P_{450} hydroxylase system.

In developing erythrocytes of bonemarrow heme synthesis is a one time process and heme synthesis stops as RBC maturation occurs.

Medical Importance

Body fluids like blood and bile contains microgram quantities of porphyrins. Small amounts of porphyrins and its precursors are excreted in urine and feces. Under normal conditions 0-30 µg of uroporphyrin and 80-200 µg of coproporphyrin are excreted in urine per day. About 0.5 mg of coproporphyrin and small amount of protoporphyrin are excreted in feces per day. In men values are slightly higher. Further the excretion of protophyrin is influenced by meat.

Porphyrin precursors are also excreted in urine. Under normal conditions 2 mg of PBG and 1-7 mg of ALA are excreted in urine per day.

Porphyrias

They are diseases of heme biosynthesis characterized by increased excretion of porphyrins or porphyrin precursors in urine and feces. Accumulation of porphyrins or porphyrin precursors in plasma and tissues also occurs. They may be inherited (autosomal) and acquired.

There are several types of inherited porphyrias and they are classified into 2 groups based on organ or cells that are affected. They are 1. Erythropoietic porphyrias 2. Hepatic porphyrias. The erythropoietic porphyrias are (*a*) Congenital or hereditary erythropoietic porphyria (*b*) Erythropoietic protoporphyria. The hepatic porphyrias are (*a*) Acute intermittent porphyria (*b*) Variegate porphyria (*c*) Hereditary coproporphyria (*d*) Porphyria cutanea tarda.

Congenital or hereditary erythropoietic porphyria

It is due to deficiency of uroporphyrinogen III cosynthase. This leads to accumulation and excretion of large amounts of uroporphyrinogen I and coproporphyrinogen I in urine. Further high levels of uroporphyrin - I in erythrocytes leads to premature destruction. The urine of the affected individuals turns red on standing due to formation of red uro and coproporphyrins from uroporphyringen I and coproporphyrinogen I by the action of atmospheric O_2.

Clinical symptoms are photosensitivity, pink bones and teeth, hemolytic anaemia and cutaneous lesions.

Erythropoietic Protoporphyria

In this condition ferrochelatase enzyme is partially active. Hence affected individuals plasma and erythrocytes contain excess of protoporphyrin IX and there is increased excretion of protoporphyrin IX in feces. However, excretion of porphyrin or its precursors in urine is normal in the patients.

Photosensitivity (solar uriticaria) is main clinical symptom. Cirrhosis of liver and anaemia also may develop later.

Acute intermittent Porphyria (AIP)

It is due to partial deficiency of uroporphyrinogen I synthase. This leads to accumulation of PBG and ALA in liver, plasma and other organs and hence affected individuals excretes large amounts of PBG and ALA in urine. The urine of these patients turns dark on standing due to polymerization of PBG and ALA to porphobilin and porphyrins.

Clinical symptoms are abdominal pain, smooth muscle spasms, neuropsychiatric symptoms, hypertension, constipation and hyper cholesterolemia but no photosensitivity. Abdominal pain and neuro psychiatric problems are due to toxic effect of accumulated PBG and ALA on nerves and CNS. The disease usually occurs after puberty. Barbiturates, steroids and alcohol aggrevates condition.

Variegate Porphyria (VP)

It is due to deficiency of protoporphyrinogen oxidase. ALA synthase may be more active due to lack of sufficient heme. Hence patients of this disease excrete large quantities of PBG, ALA, uro and coproporphyrins in urine. The urine may be colored due to excretion of uro and coproporphyrins. Fecal excretion of uro and coproporphyrins is more.

Photosensitivity is constant clinical symptom. Other symptoms may vary and hence the name. Alcohol and other drugs can aggrevate the condition.

Hereditary Coproporphyria (HCP)

It is due to partial deficiency of coproporphyrinogen III oxidase. This leads to excretion of large amounts of coproporphyrinogen III in urine and feces. PBG excretion in urine is also increased in this condition. The urine may contain red pigment coproporphyrin which is formed on exposure to light.

Clinical symptoms are photosensitivity and those of AIP.

Porphyria Cutanea tarda (PCT)

It is due to partial deficiency of uroporphyrinogen decarboxylase. This leads to excretion of large quantities of uroporphyrin I and III in urine. Hence urine of these patients appears pinkish to brown. PBG excretion was also found to be increased.

Photosensitivity is the major clinical symptom of this disease. It is the most common porphyria. It appears during 4-6 decades of life. Hepato cellular damage from alcoholism etc. is characteristic of this condition.

Acquired or toxic porphyria

Certain poisons (toxins) and drugs cause this type of porphyria. Some toxins which can cause porphyria are heavy metal like lead, alcohol and hexachlorobenzene. Lead inhibits ALA dehydratase and heme synthase of heme biosynthesis. Hence in lead poisoning ALA excretion is highest in urine. Excretion of porphyrins in urine also goes up to 10 mg per day in lead poisoning. Automobile exhaust is a common source for lead in environment. Drugs which can cause porphyria are steroids, oral contraceptives, barbiturates and pesticides.

Hemoglobin formation

Heme activates synthesis of globin in nucleated reticulocytes of bone marrow cells. In a human adult approximately 8 gm of globin is synthesized per day. In other words about 15% of amino acids from daily protein intake are used for globin synthesis. The two chains of globin are formed independently at same rate. Hemin and protoporphyrin IX also increase globin synthesis. The heme and globin combination generates hemoglobin which is also called as metalloporphyrinoprotein.

The red color of the blood is due to hemoglobin in erythrocytes. The normal hemoglobin (Hb) concentration in blood is 12-15 gm/100 ml. Several forms of hemoglobin are identified in normal blood. They are HbA, HbF, HbA_2, and HbA_{1C}.

Adult hemoglobin or HbA

It is the major hemoglobin present in adult blood and in the blood of children over 6 months of age. It accounts more than 90% of total hemoglobin.

Structure of HbA

Human hemoglobin has molecular weight of 64,400 daltons. It contains 4 heme prosthetic groups and globin. About 574 amino acids are present in globin and globin part contains 4 polypeptide chains of two types. Each polypeptide chain is attached to one heme prosthetic group. Two types of polypeptide chains are α and β. About 141 aminoacids are present in α-chain and 146 aminoacids residues are present in β-chain.

Thus hemoglobin is a tetramer consisting of two types of four polypeptide chains and designated as $\alpha_2 \beta_2$. Overall shape of tetrameric protein is spherical.

Each subunit contains 8 α-helical regions. They are designated as A, B, C, D, E, F, G and H. In each subunit hydrophobic residues are present in interior whereas hydrophilic residues are present on outer surface. This makes subunit soluble in water but its interior is impermeable to water. In each subunit heme moiety is buried in hydrophobic interior. Heme group is attached through Fe to imidazole N of histidine of F α-helical region (Figure 22.4).

In hemoglobin molecule the interaction between subunits is unique. Unlike subunits *i.e.* $\alpha_1 - \beta_1$ and $\alpha_2 - \beta_2$ interact extensively and they are mainly hydrophobic, hydrogen bonds and salt bridges. In contrast there are only polar type interactions between like subunits *i.e.* $\alpha_1 - \alpha_2$ and $\beta_1 - \beta_2$ (Figure 22.4).

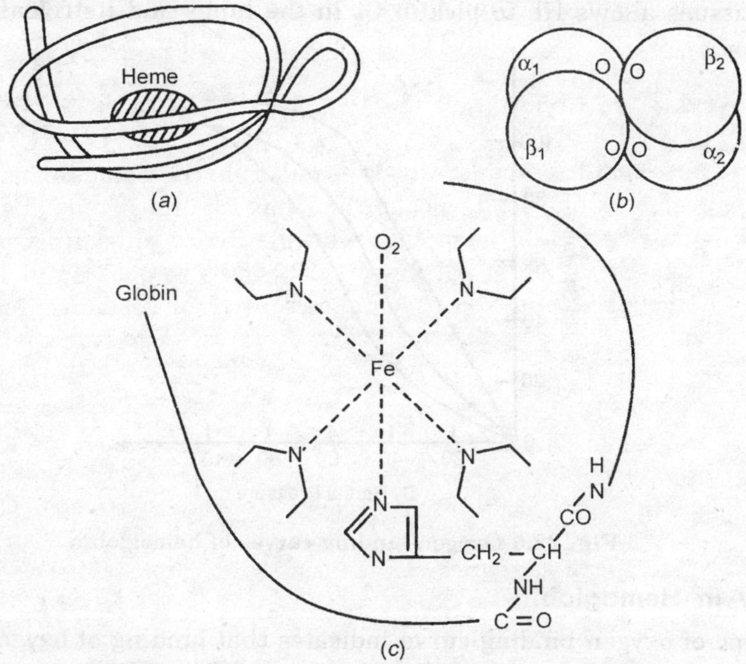

Fig. 22.4 (*a*) Structure of hemoglobin subunit.
(*b*) Schematic diagram showing arrangement of Hb subunits.
(*c*) Attachments of hemeiron. Broken lines indicates coordinate bonds.

Medical Importance

1. Hemoglobin transports oxygen from lungs (gills) to tissues. One gram of Hb carries 1.34 ml of oxygen (O_2) from the lungs to tissues. About 20 ml of O_2 is carried by 100 ml of blood (15 × 1.34) and hence oxygen carrying capacity of blood is 20% (v/v).

   One Hb molecule carries $4O_2$ molecules. Each heme moiety combines with one O_2 molecule. In each subunit of Hb O_2 binds to Fe on the opposite side of histidine ligand (Figure 22.4). Hb with bound O_2 is called as oxyhemoglobin (HbO_2).
2. Hb also transports CO_2 from tissues to lungs.
3. Hb is the major blood buffer.
4. In anaemia and asthma O_2 carrying capacity of blood is decreased due to low Hb and low respiratory rate respectively.
5. In congestive heart failure Hb remain unsaturated due to defective circulation.

Oxygen Binding Curves

Binding of oxygen by Hb deserves special mention. Several factors influences oxygen binding by Hb. The plot of oxygen tension (partial pressure) against percentage saturation yields sigmoidal curve (Figure 22.5). The sigmoidal curve indicates that oxygen binding by Hb depends on partial pressure of O_2. The curve also explains how Hb transports O_2 from the lungs to tissues. Since O_2 partial pressure is more in lungs Hb binds to lot of O_2 in lungs. When oxyhemoglobin reaches tissues where its oxygen binding capacity is less due to low O_2 partial pressure the O_2 is released. Thus the differential O_2 partial pressure that exist in lungs and tissues allows Hb to pickup O_2 in the lungs and its release in the tissues.

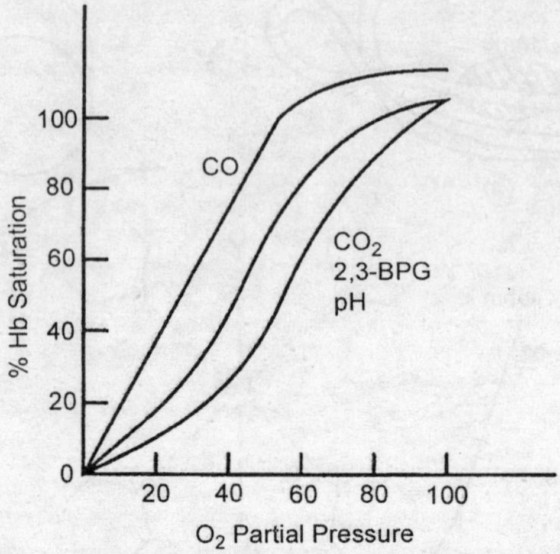

Fig. 22.5 Oxygen binding curves of hemoglobin

Cooperativity in Hemoglobin

Sigmoidal shape of oxygen binding curve indicates that binding of oxygen by Hb is slow at low O_2 tension and it increases rapidly after a particular O_2 tension and then reaches maximum. It is due to cooperative binding of O_2 by Hb like substrate binding by allosteric enzyme (see also allosteric enzymes in Chapter 4). The mechanism of cooperative binding of O_2 by Hb has been studied extensively. The quaternary structure (conformation) of oxyhemoglobin was found to be different from hemoglobin or deoxyhemoglobin. The conformation of deoxyhemoglobin is referred as tense (T) form in which all four subunits are circles and it has less affinity for O_2. The conformation of oxyhemoglobin is referred as relaxed (R) form in which all subunits are squares and it has high affinity for O_2.

In the cooperative oxygen binding by Hb when O_2 binds to one of subunits of T form conformation of that subunit is altered. This in turn alters inter subunit interaction. This leads to formation of high affinity R form and hence further binding of O_2 to other subunits is rapid (Figure 22.6). Thus in cooperative O_2 binding by Hb binding of one O_2 to a subunit increases affinities of other subunits for O_2.

Effect of binding of O_2 to Fe of heme

As mentioned above binding of O_2 to heme of subunit converts T form to R form. Now we shall examine how binding of O_2 to heme leads to this conformational change. In the absence of O_2 the iron is held outside the plane of heme by coordination of iron to imidazole of histidine. When oxygen binds to iron, iron is drawn into plane of heme and this also pulls imidazole ring of histidine (Figure 22.7). This small movement of histidine is transmitted to other groups of subunit through hydrogen bonding network and causes subunit to assume high affinity form. This change in the subunit alters its interactions with adjacent subunits and this in turn induces them to change into high affinity form.

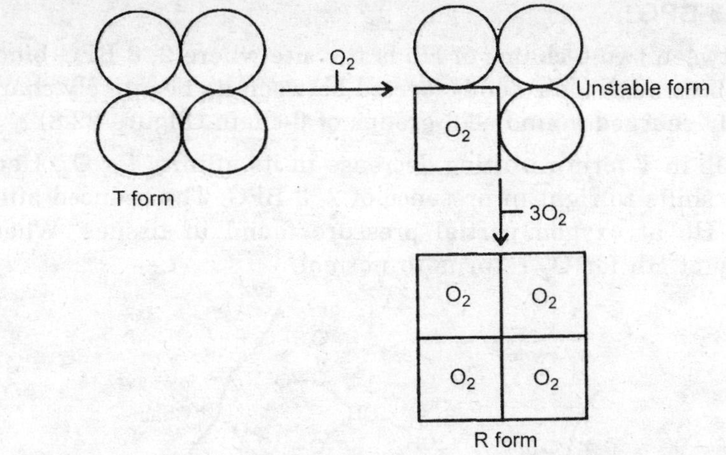

Fig. 22.6 Schematic diagram showing cooperativity in hemoglobin

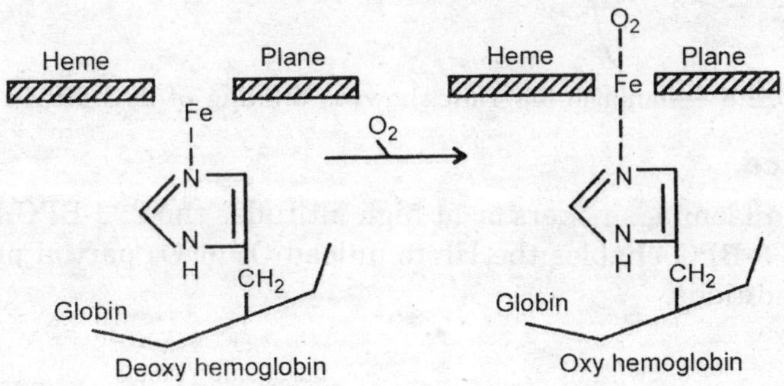

Fig. 22.7 Effect of oxygen binding on histidine residues of hemoglobin

Effect of CO_2, 2, 3-BPG and pH

In presence of CO_2, 2, 3-BPG and at low pH the oxygen binding curve of Hb shifts to right. However the curve remains in sigmoidal shape [Figure 22.5].

Effect of CO_2

CO_2 combines with terminal amino groups of Hb to form carbamino hemoglobin (carbamate). This stabilizes the Hb in T form resulting decrease in its affinity for O_2. Hence the oxygen binding curve of Hb shifts to right.

$$Hb - NH_2 + CO_2 \leftrightarrow Hb - NH - COO + H^+$$

The above reaction is rapid and reversible.

Carbamino Hb is involved in the transport of CO_2 from tissues to lungs.

Effect of 2, 3 – BPG

As mentioned in Chapter – 9, 2, 3 – BPG is synthesized in erythrocytes from 1, 3 BPG. The concentration of 2, 3-BPG in RBC is almost equal to Hb concentration. 2, 3-BPG binds to deoxy Hb and stabilizes it in T form. This results in decrease in affinity of Hb for O_2. Hence oxygen binding curve of Hb shifts to right.

Binding Site of 2, 3-BPG

A cavity present between two β-chains of Hb is the site where 2, 3-BPG binds Hb. It binds to two β-chains of Hb through ionic bonds formed between its negatively charged phosphate groups and positively charged amino acid groups of β-chain (Figure 22.8).

This stabilizes Hb in T form resulting decrease in its affinity for O_2. Hence the oxygen binding curve of Hb shifts to right in presence of 2, 3-BPG. The reduced affinity facilitates release of O_2 from Hb at oxygen partial pressure found in tissues. When 2, 3-BPG is removed the affinity of Hb for O_2 returns to normal.

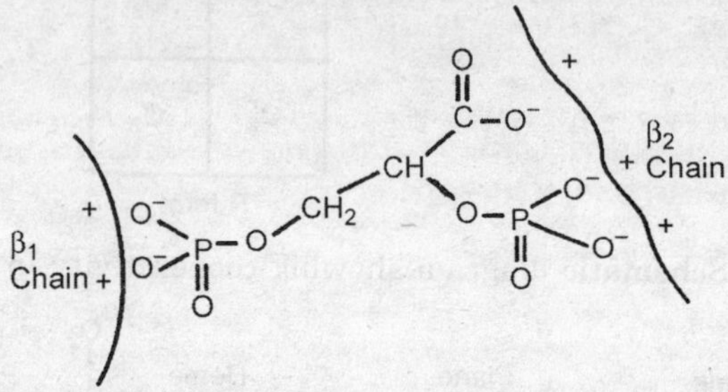

Fig. 22.8 Schematic diagram showing binding of 2, 3–BPG to Hb

Medical Importance

In chronic hypoxia, anaemia, smokers or at high altitudes the 2, 3-BPG level increases. This elevated levels of 2, 3-BPG enables the Hb to unload O_2 at O_2 partial pressure prevalent in tissues in these conditions.

Effect of pH

Increase in hydrogen ion concentration results in decrease in affinity of Hb for O_2. Hence oxygen binding curve shifts to right at low pH. This is called as Bohr effect. It is due to stabilization of Hb in T form. In presence of excess H^+ ionizable groups of Hb are protonated which enables them to stabilize Hb in T form by forming ionic bonds.

Medical Importance

1. A low pH in rapidly contracting skeletal muscle enables HbO_2 to unload O_2 rapidly. In some circulatory defects also the pH is low in tissues. This low pH enables Hb O_2 to unload O_2 rapidly.
2. Further the release of O_2 from HbO_2 is accompanied by uptake of H^+. This helps in removing excess H^+ from tissues by Hb.

Foetal Hemoglobin (HbF)

It is main Hb found in foetus and in new born. It contains two α-chains and two γ-chains and hence it is designated as $\alpha_2\gamma_2$. It binds O_2 more tightly which makes it suitable for foetal environment. Soon after the birth the synthesis of γ-chain diminishes and synthesis of β chain begins. By sixth month β-chain replaces γ-chain completely and hence blood of new born of more than six months age contains HbA.

Hereditary Persistence of Foetal Hemoglobin (HPFH)

It is a relatively benign condition where production of HbF continues in adult life. It is reported from some North Indian states. Any major hematological abnormality is usually absent.

HEMOGLOBIN A_2 (HbA_2)

It accounts 2% of total hemoglobin. It contains two α-chains and two δ-chains and hence it is designated as $\alpha_2\delta_2$. Its function is unknown.

Glycosylated hemoglobin (HbA_{1C})

In this form of hemoglobin glucose residues are attached to $-NH_2$ groups of N-terminal valine of β-chains. Hence it is designated as α_2, (β-N-glucose)$_2$. It is formed by non-enzymatic attachment of glucose. The rate of formation of glycosylated Hb depends on blood glucose level.

The formation glycosylated Hb is slow and irreversible. Initially glucose reacts with free amino group to form Schiff base. Later the Schiff base undergoes Amadori rearrangement to a stable ketoamine (Figure 22.9).

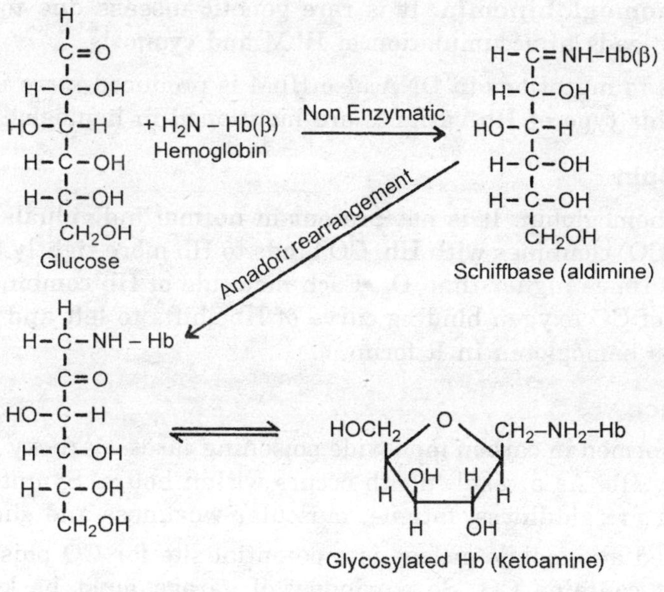

Fig. 22.9 Formation of glycosylated hemoglobin.

Medical Importance

1. Glycosylated Hb in normal blood accounts for 4-7% of total Hb.
2. Ion exchange chromatographic methods are used to estimate glycated Hb in blood.
3. In diabetics glycosylated Hb may account for upto 20% of total Hb.
4. Since the half life of RBC is 60 days the blood glycosylated Hb level reflects patients blood glucose level over the past two months. If the patient takes insulin (medication) as directed then his blood glycated Hb level is normal. If he is careless about medication

then his blood glycosylated Hb level is two or three times higher than normal. Thus glycated Hb measurement can be used to monitor diabetic patient.

5. Glycosylated Hb measurement in blood also can be used to know whether a given drug is effective in controlling blood sugar over a period of time.

Methemoglobin (HbM)

It accounts for 1-2% of total Hb. In this hemoglobin iron is present in ferric state and hence it is unable to transport oxygen.

Medical Importance

In normal individuals the HbM is converted to HbA by HbM reductase using NADH or NADPH as source of hydrogen. Vitamin E also reduces HbM to HbA. However it uses G-SH as hydrogen donor.

HbM level is changed in some diseases. Some of the conditions are given below.

1. **Acquired methemoglobinemia.** Toxic chemicals, analgesics, antipyretics and some anaesthetics cause methemoglobinemia by preventing the conversion of HbM to Hb A or favouring formation of more HbM.
2. **Familial methemoglobinemia.** It is rare genetic disease due to deficiency of HbM reductase. This leads to accumulation of HbM and cyanosis.
3. **Mutation.** Due to mutations in DNA also HbM is produced more in some individuals. Examples for this type of Hb variants are mentioned in hemoglobinopathies.

Carboxy Hemoglobin

It is an unnatural hemoglobin. It is not present in normal individuals. It is formed when carbon monooxide (CO) combines with Hb. CO binds to Hb more tightly than O_2 and affinity of Hb for CO is 210 times higher than O_2. Each molecule of Hb combines with 4 molecules of CO. In presence of CO oxygen binding curve of Hb shifts to left and assumes hyperbolic shape. CO stabilizes hemoglobin in R form.

Medical Importance

1. Carboxy Hb is formed in carbon monoxide poisoning cases. Carboxy Hb formation blocks O_2 transport by Hb. As a result death occurs within hours. Symptoms of carbon monoxide poisoning are giddiness, fatigue, muscular weakness and shortness of breath.

   Poorly ventilated automobile garage is a potential site for CO poisoning because automobile exhaust contains CO. So a window of garage must be kept open always to prevent CO poisoning.
2. Carboxy Hb content is more in the blood of smokers (4-8%).

Hemoglobinopathies

These are group of inherted diseases in which either hemoglobin composition or hemoglobin synthesis is altered. Hemoglobin with altered composition is called as hemoglobin variant or mutant hemoglobin or abnormal Hb. More than 300 hemoglobin variants have been identified. Some of the variants are most common within particular racial groups. Some of them are concentrated in particular geographical regions. Therefore most of the hemoglobin variants are designated by the place name of its discovery.

In India hemoglobinopathies constitutes bulk of non communicable genetic diseases. They cause high degree of morbidity, moderate to severe hemolytic anemia among susceptible people like infants, children, adolescent girls, pregnant women etc. A vast number of hemoglobin variants are found in India. The abnormal hemoglobin found in India are HbD, HbE, HbH, HbJ, HbK, HbL, HbM, HbQ, HbS etc. Distribution of hemoglobin variants in different states of India is given below.

S.No.	State	Hemoglobin variant
1.	Andhra Pradesh	HbS
2.	Kerala	HbS
3.	Karnataka	HbS, HbQ, HbK
4.	Tamilnadu	HbS, HbE, HbK
5.	Maharashtra	HbS, HbD, HbQ, HbJ, HbE
6.	Orissa	HbS, HbD, HbE
7.	Madhya Pradesh	HbS, HbD
8.	Gujarat	HbS, HbD, HbM, HbJ, HbL
9.	Bihar	HbS
10.	Uttar Pradesh	HbS, HbD, HbE
11.	West Bengal	HbS, HbD, HbJ, HbK, HbE
12.	Rajasthan	HbS, HbD
13.	Nagaland	HbE
14.	Arunachal Pradesh	HbE, HbS

Most commonly found abnormal hemoglobins in India are HbS, HbE, HbD. Further HbS is widely distributed in all over India.

In most of abnormal Hbs only composition of globin is altered. Prosthetic group heme remains unchanged. In majority of hemoglobin variants only one amino acid in a chain is replaced by another amino acid.

Hemoglobinopathies or appearance of abnormal Hbs are due to mutations in DNA (Chapter 18). Some Hb variants are due to point mutations and some of them are due to frame shift mutations. Usually Hb variant appears in homozygotes carrying two defective genes. In heterozygotes both normal and mutant hemoglobin appears because normal and defective or mutant gene are present.

Sickle cell hemoglobin (HbS)

It is most common and most severe abnormal Hb. It is due to point mutation in DNA and sickle cell hemoglobin differs from normal Hb in single amino acid of β-chain. Glutamate at position six of β-chain is replaced by valine in HbS and hence it is designated as $\alpha_2\beta_2^{6glu\rightarrow val}$. This alteration make HbS more positive hence it can be separated easily from HbA by electrophoresis (Figure 22.10).

The alteration in β-chain of Hb affects shape of erythrocyte. Erythrocytes containing HbS exhibit normal binding of O_2 in the lungs and as long as HbS is in the oxygenated form they have normal shape. When HbS undergoes deoxygenation presence of valine on the surface of subunit results in sticky patch which causes aggregation of subunits into long fibres. The long fibres deform erythrocyte membrane and induces characteristic sickle shape (Figure 22.10).

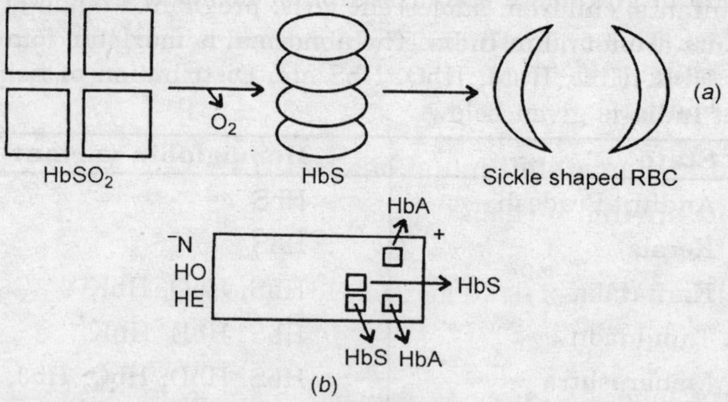

Fig. 22.10 (*a*) Formation of sickle shaped RBC due to HbS.
(*b*) Electrophoretic pattern of HbS and HbA in normal individuals (N), homozygotes (HO) and heterozygotes (HE)

The sickle shaped erythrocytes have decreased life span and hence removed from circulation rapidly. This leads to decreased Hb in blood and anaemia. Thus sickle cell hemoglobin causes sickle cell anaemia in homozygotes and sickle cell traits in heterozygotes. Other symptoms are dizziness, weakness and shortness of breath on exercise.

Hemoglobin E

1. This abnormal hemoglobin is β chain mutant. Glutamate at position 26 of β chain is replaced by lysine. Hence it is designated as $\alpha_2\beta_2^{26Glu \rightarrow Lys}$.
2. About 50 millions people of South East Asia carry the gene for HbE. It is prevalent in India, Bangladesh, Indonesia, Malaysia, Myanmar, Singapore and Thailand.
3. In India this abnormal hemoglobin is prevalent in Eastern states i.e. West Bengal, Assam, Arunachal Pradesh, Nagaland, Manipur, Tripura and Meghalaya. It occurs sporadically in other regions of India.
4. In homozygotes condition is known as HbE disease where as in heterozygotes it is known as HbE triat.
5. Clinical symptoms are mild or without anaemia, microcytosis and hypochromic erythrocytes.

Other noteworthy hemoglobins with a altered amino acid in one of the chain are

(*a*) HbI Philadelphia in which lysine is replaced by glutamate at 16th position of α-chain. It is designated as $\alpha_2^{16lys \rightarrow glu}\beta_2$.

(*b*) Hb Punjab in which glutamate at 121 position in β-chain is replaced by glycine end hence it is designated as $\alpha_2\beta_2^{121glu \rightarrow gly}$. This hemoglobin variant is known as HbD. In hemozygotes condition is known as HbD disease. It is also found in Jammu and Kashmir, Uttar Pradesh, Orissa and Maharashtra.

(*c*) HbM Boston in which histidine at 58 position in α-chain is replaced by tyrosine and hence it is designated as $\alpha_2^{58\,his \rightarrow tyr}\beta_2$. The phenolic group of tyrosine stabilizes heme iron in ferric state. Another example for HbM is HbM Milwaukee in which valine is replaced by glutamate at 67 position of β-chain. It is designated as $\alpha_2\beta_2^{67val\rightarrow glu}$. Gamma carboxyl group of glutamate stabilizes iron of heme in ferric state.

(*d*) **Hb KoyaDora.** This type of hemoglobin variant is found in tribal population of East Godavari districts of Andhra Pradesh. It is due to single point mutation. It is a α-chain termination mutant.

Hb Variants due to frame shift mutations in DNA

1. **Hb Constant spring.** α-chain contains 31 amino acids extra at C-terminus in this abnormal Hb.
2. **Hb Gun Hill.** In β-chain of this abnormal Hb amino acid residues from 93 to 97 are deleted.

Thalassemias

They are group of inherited diseases in which total synthesis of one of globin chain is defective. Anaemia is most common symptom. Since most of affected individuals are of mediterranean origin the term thalassemia (mediterranean anaemia) was applied to these diseases. The thalassemias are classified into α and β type based on the chain affected.

α-Thalassemia

Synthesis of α-chain of globin is affected in this condition. This leads to decreased formation of HbA ($\alpha_2\beta_2$) and HbF ($\alpha_2\gamma_2$). The free γ and β chain may form abnormal Hb like Hb Barts (γ_4) and HbH (β_4). The formation of abnormal Hb triggers hemolysis and anemia develops.

In India there are reports of the α-Thalassemia. It is also known as HbH disease due to presence of hemoglobin variants HbH in affected individuals. The prevalence of α-Thalassemia in India varies from one sub-geographical area to another. In Orrisa it is around 70% and 11% in Andhra Pradesh. The exact molecule nature of α-Thalassemia in India is not known. However it all due to deletion.

β-Thalassemia

Synthesis of β-chain of globin is affected in this condition. This leads to decreased formation of HbA. However HbF formation is normal. Since α-chains can not form tetramer they produce large inclusion bodies. This triggers hemolysis and cause anaemia. In homozygotes anaemia is most notable and it is called as Cooley's anaemia (β-thalassemia major). In heterozygotes the condition is often referred as β-thalassemia minor.

β-Thalassemia Major (TM) is the commonest genetic disease in India with prevalence of 1-17% in general population. It usually occurs in infancy. In India there are over 25 million carriers of the disease and eight thousand thalassemia babies are born every year. It is also known as HbC disease. It is characterized by ineffective erythropoiesis, bone marrow expansion and rapid destruction of erythrocytes which is the major cause for anaemia. Due to anaemia frequent blood transfusions are required to maintain life. Hemosiderosis is later complication of the disease. If left untreated affected children die of heart failure in early childhood. Bone marrow transplantation is the only proper treatment for the disease.

Thalassemia intermedia

This thalassemia results from complete absence of both beta and delta chain synthesis. More of gamma chain is produced. It is milder than beta thalassemia. Heterozygous forms are common and resembles beta thalassemia triat.

Hemoglobin Degradation

Hemoglobin is released from aged erythrocytes by the reticuloendothelial cells of spleen and liver. Further Hb released in vascular system is transported to liver by haptoglobin which is a γ-globin that can bind two Hb molecules. In the liver hemoglobin is split to heme and globin. About 6-10 gm of hemoglobin are degraded per day. Heme derived from other heme containing proteins is also transported to liver bound to hemopexin. Globin may be reused either as such or degraded to amino acids which may be recycled (Fig. 22.11).

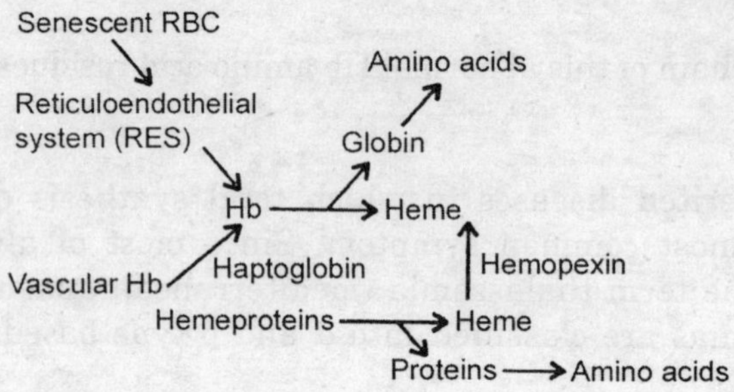

Fig. 22.11 Formation of heme from hemoglobin and other proteins

Heme catabolism

In the liver heme is degraded to bilirubin by reticuloendothelial cells. About 35 mg of bilirubin is formed from 1 gm of hemoglobin. The conversion of heme to bilirubin occurs in microsomes. By the time the heme reaches microsomes it is converted to hemin which is reduced to heme with NADPH. Now the first reaction of heme catabolism is initiated by heme oxygenase a complex enzyme system present in microsomes. In presence of NADPH oxygen is added to α-methenyl bridge of heme to form hydroxy heme. In the second step bridge carbon is removed as CO by adding another oxygen and hydroxy heme is converted to verdohemin. These changes in heme molecule decreases affinity of iron for heme and hence ferrous iron dissociates and free tetra pyrrole is released as biliverdin which is green in color and has linear structure.

The biliverdin is then converted to bilirubin by reducing γ-methenyl bridge to methylene bridge. The reaction is catalyzed by biliverdin reductase a cytosolic enzyme and requires NADPH as hydrogen donor. In mammals bilirubin is the end product of heme catabolism where as in birds and amphibia biliverdin is the end product (Fig. 22.12).

Medical Importance

1. Bilirubin is a powerful antioxidant like ascorbic acid. It is effective against soluble peroxides. Like vitamin E bilirubin is a good anti-oxidant in membranes.
2. However free bilirubin has high affinity for membrane lipids which can interfere with function of nervous system.
3. Heme oxygenase exist in two isoforms. Heme oxygenase-I and hemeoxygenase-II. Hemoxygenase-I is inducible enzyme. In diabetes hemeoxygenase activity is modified. It interacts with NO which may change vascular function in retina.

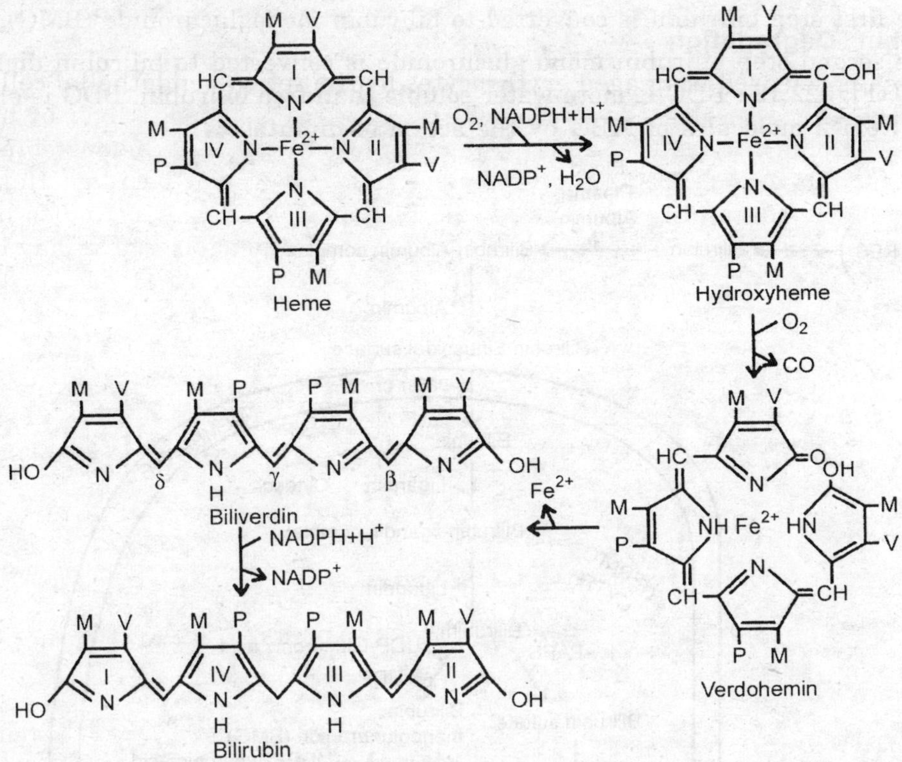

Fig. 22.12 Conversion of heme to bilirubin

Bilirubin Metabolism

Bilirubin produced in reticulo endothelial cells is released into blood. Since bilirubin is water insoluble, in the blood plasma bilirubin is bound to albumin. Under normal conditions about 250-350 mg of bilirubin is produced. About 70-80% of this is derived from heme of hemoglobin and remaining 20-30% arises from other heme containing proteins. In the plasma one gram of albumin can bind 4 mg of bilirubin. Further metabolism of bilirubin occurs mainly in liver which is detailed below.

Uptake of bilirubin by hepatocytes

In liver bilirubin is removed from albumin and taken up by hepatocytes. Uptake of free bilirubin by hepatocytes is mediated by a carrier protein of liver cells. At the sinusoidal surfaces of hepatocyte carrier protein combines with free bilirubin and transports bilirubin into cytosol of hepatocyte. The carrier protein can facilitate bilirubin transport on both directions depending on biliriubin concentration (Fig. 22.13). In the cytosol bilirubin binds to two binding proteins ligandin and z or y protein. These proteins carry bilirubin to smooth endoplasmic reticulum where it is conjugated.

Conversion of bilirubin to bilirubin diglucuronide and bilirubin sulfate

It involves conjugation of bilirubin with glucuronic acid. UDP-glucuronic acid (UDPG) is the source of glucuronic acid. UDP-glucuronyl transferase catalyzes this conjugation. It occurs in two steps.

1. In the first step bilirubin is converted to bilirubin monoglucuronide (BMG).
2. In the second step bilirubin mono glucuronide is converted to bilirubin diglucuronide (BDG) (Fig. 22.13). BDG is more water soluble than free bilirubin. BDG is also synthesized from 2 molecules of MBG by the action of dimutase.

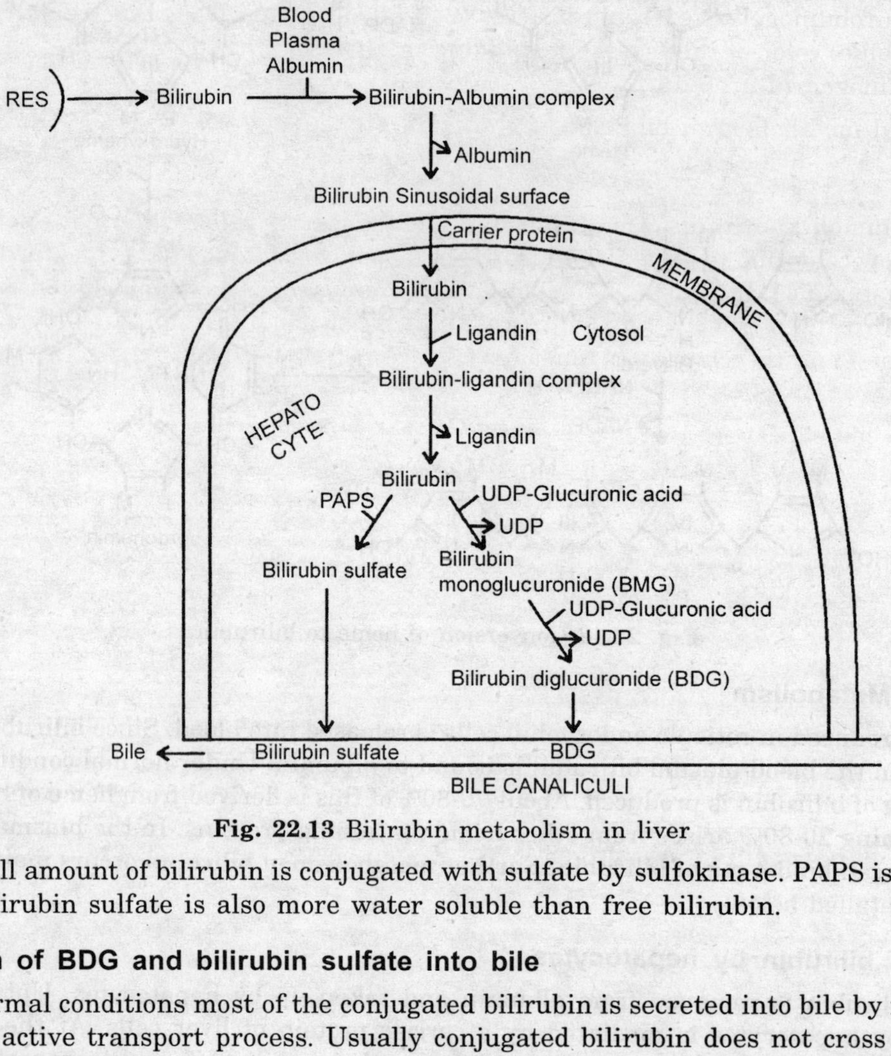

Fig. 22.13 Bilirubin metabolism in liver

A small amount of bilirubin is conjugated with sulfate by sulfokinase. PAPS is the sulfate donor. Bilirubin sulfate is also more water soluble than free bilirubin.

Secretion of BDG and bilirubin sulfate into bile

Under normal conditions most of the conjugated bilirubin is secreted into bile by mechanism involving active transport process. Usually conjugated bilirubin does not cross hepatocyte cytoplasmic membrane.

Intestinal Metabolism of Bilirubin

1. In terminal part of ileum and in large intestine bilirubin diglucuronide is hydrolyzed by bacterial glucuronidase to bilirubin and glucuronide. Likewise bilirubin sulfate is hydrolyzed by bacterial sulfatase to bilirubin and sulfate.
2. Bilirubin formed undergoes series of reduction reactions catalyzed by bacterial enzymes.
3. Reduction of methenyl bridges and vinyl groups of pyrrole rings yields mesobilirubinogen.
4. Further reduction of I and II pyrrole rings of mesobilirubinogen generates urobilinogen (stercobilinogen).

5. A small fraction of urobilinogen is reabsorbed and reexcreted through the bile by liver. This is known as enterohepatic urobilinogen cycle. However a small part enters circulation and is excreted in urine (<4 mg/day). One exposure to atmospheric O_2 this urobilinogen is oxidized to urobilin which is responsible for yellow color of urine.
6. Most of urobilinogen is excreted in feces (240 mg/day) and it is responsible for brown orange (blue) color of the feces. On standing in air feces turns to dark due to oxidation of urobilinogen to urobilin by O_2.

Intestinal metabolism of bilirubin is shown in Fig. 22.14.

Jaundice

It is most common known disease of bilirubin metabolism in which skin and sclera of eye acquires yellow color due to excessive bilirubin in blood. Normal blood plasma bilirubin level is 1 mg/dl. In jaundice the plasma bilirubin level is high. Hence excess bilirubin diffuses into tissues and turns them yellow. Further, excess bilirubin leads to a condition known as hyper bilirubinemia. Thus the characteristic signs of jaudice are hyperbilirubinemia and yellow colored skin and sclera.

Based on clinical causes jaundice is classified into pre hepatic jaundice, hepatic jaundice and post hepatic jaundice. However jaundice (Icterus) may be due to several underlying diseases.

Pre hepatic or hemolytic jaundice

It is due to excessive breakdown of erythrocytes. This leads to increased production of bilirubin. But liver cells are unable to conjugate all bilirubin formed. Hence unconjugated bilirubin level of plasma is elevated. Excessive breakdown of RBC occurs in hemglobinopathies, hereditary spherocytosis, incompatible blood transfusion and in malaria. Administration of sulfonamides, aspirin and primaquine can cause excessive breakdown of RBC in glucose-6-phosphate dehydrogenase deficiency. Aniline dyes and nitrites can cause methemoglobinemia and hemolysis.

Hepatic or hepatocellular jaundice

It is due to damaged hepatocytes. Poisons like chloroform, carbon tetrachloride, phosphorus, antibiotics, amanita mushroom poison and hepatitis virus can damage parenchymal cells of liver. In cirrhosis also liver cell damage occurs. Damaged hepatocytes are unable to perform functions. So in hepatic jaundice liver cells are unable to conjugate or secrete bilirubin though the production of bilirubin is as usual. If conjugation of bilirubin is impaired unconjugated bilirubin in plasma is elevated . If secretion of conjugated bilirubin is impaired conjugated bilirubin in plasma is elevated. Therefore in hepatic jaundice appreciable amounts of conjugated as well as unconjugated bilirubin are present in plasma.

Post hepatic or obstructive jaundice

It is due to obstruction of bile duct. Gall stones and cancer of head of pancreas can cause obstruction of bile duct. Due to blockage of bile duct conjugated bilirubin secreted by liver returns to blood. Hence in obstructive jaundice conjugated bilirubin in plasma is elevated. Cholestatic jaundice is term used to indicate all forms of extrahepatic or post hepatic obstructive jaundice.

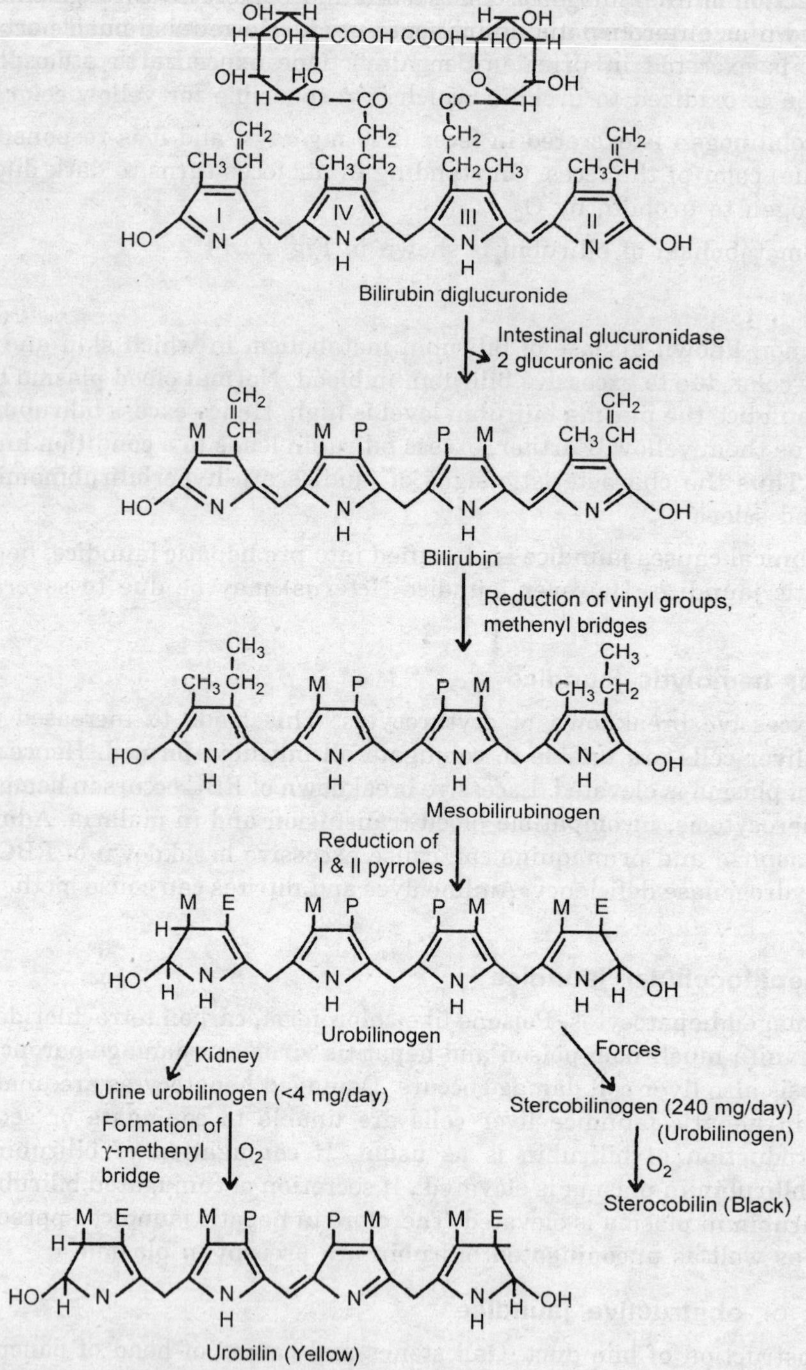

Fig. 22.14 Intestinal metabolism of bilirubin

Vanden Bergh reaction and Jaundice

Since bilirubin level is elevated in all forms of jaundice measurement of serum bilirubin is useful in the diagnosis and management of jaundice. Vanden Bergh devised a method based on Ehrlichs reaction for measurement of bilirubin in plasma. It involves coupling of diazotized sulphanilic acid (diazo reagent) and bilirubin to produce a reddish purple azo compound. It consists of two parts (*a*) Direct Vanden Bergh reaction and (*b*) Indirect Vanden Bergh reaction.

Direct Vanden Bergh Reaction

Since conjugated bilirubin is soluble in water it reacts directly with diazo reagent to produce purple color. This is called as direct Vanden Bergh reaction. So direct Vanden Bergh reaction measures only conjugated bilirubin.

In direct Vanden Bergh Reaction

Since unconjugated bilirubin is less soluble in water it reacts with diazo reagent only in presence of methanol to produce purple color. This is called as indirect Vanden Bergh reaction. So in direct Vanden Bergh reaction measures only unconjugated bilirubin.

Vanden Bergh reaction is useful in differential diagnosis of jaundice. Normal serum gives indirect Vanden Bergh reaction because of more of unconjugated bilirubin and it does not give a direct Vanden Bergh reaction. Hemolytic jaundice serum also gives indirect Vanden Bergh reaction because of more of unconjugated bilirubin. However with obstructive jaundice serum direct Vanden Bergh reaction is obtained because of more of conjugated bilirubin. Similarly with a hepatic jaundice serum also direct Vanden Bergh reaction can be obtained.

Urine bilirubin in Jaundice

Normal urine does not contain bilirubin because normal blood contains water insoluble unconjugated bilirubin which can not be filtered at glomerulus. Bilirubin is excreted in urine in hepatic and obstructive jaundice because conjugated bilirubin level in plasma is above renal threshold value in these conditions. However bilirubin is absent in urine in hemolytic jaundice. Excretion of bilirubin urine is called as choluria. So hepatic and obstructive jaundice are called as choluric jaundice where as hemolytic jaundice is called as acholuric jaundice.

Urine Urobilinogen in Jaundice

About 4 mg of urobilinogen is excreted in urine per day. The excretion of urobilinogen depends on amount of bilirubin entering intestine which in turn depends on amount of bilirubin formed. In obstructive jaundice urobilinogen is not found in urine because bilirubin can not enter intestine. In hemolytic jaundice urine urobilinogen is more because of increased production of bilirubin.

Urine bilirubin and Urobilinogen in Jaundice

Combination of urine bilirubin and urobilinogen is useful in differential diagnosis of jaundice. Presence of bilirubin in urine without urobilinogen suggests obstructive jaundice. Absence of bilirubin in urine with increased urobilinogen suggest hemolytic jaundice.

Vanden Bergh reaction, serum and urine bilirubin and urine and fecal urobilinogen in normal and jaundice persons are given in Table 22.1.

Table 22.1 Vanden Bergh reaction, Serum and urine bilirubin and urine and fecal urobilinogen in normal and jaundice persons.

	Van den Bergh reaction	Serum bilirubin	Urine bilirubin	Urine urobilinogen	Fecal urobilinogen
Normal	Indirect	Free (unconjugated) bilirubin : 0.2-0.7 mg/dl Conjugated bilirubin 0.1-0.4 mg/dl	Absent	4mg/day	240mg/day
Hemolytic jaundice	Indirect	Increased free bilirubin	Absent	Increased	Increased
Hepatic jaundice	Direct	Both free and conjugated bilirubin are increased	Present	Decreased	Decreased
Obstructive jaundice	Direct	Increased conjugated bilirubin	Present	Absent	Absent (traces)

In addition to various types of jaundice plasma bilirubin level is elevated (hyperbilirubinemia) in some genetic or acquired diseases. There are two types of hyper bilirubinemias. They are given below.

Unconjugated hyperbilirubinemlas

In which unconjugated bilirubin is more in plasma. Some of them are given below.

(a) Neonatal physiologic jaundice

It is a transient condition seen in newborns or neonates. The newborns immature hepatic system is unable to metabolize bilirubin produced from excessive breakdown of RBC. This leads to excessive unconjugated bilirubin in plasma. Further UDP-glucuronyl transferase is less active and synthesis of UDP-glucuronic acid is impaired in affected newborns. Excessive bilirubin binds membrane lipids of nervous system causes encephalopathy or kernicterus. Photo therapy and phenobarbitol administration may increase hepatic excretion of unconjugated bilirubin.

(b) Crigler-Najjer Syndrome Type I

It is a rare inherited disease and it is fatal within first 15 months of life. Serum bilirubin is more than 20 mg/dl. The unconjugated hyper bilirubinema is due to absence of UDP-glucuronyl transferase. Phototherapy is helpful.

(c) Crigler-Najjer Syndrome Type II

It is mild and rare inherited disease. Serum bilirubin is below 20 mg/dl and mostly it is unconjugated type. Unconjugated hyperbilirubinemia is due to lack of UDP-glucuronyl transferase that adds second glucuronic acid to bilirubin monglucuronic acid. Phenobarbitol treatment is helpful.

(d) Gilbert's disease

Unconjugated hyperbilirubinemia in this disease is due to defect in uptake of bilirubin by parenchymal cells of liver. UPD-glucuronyl transferase is also less active in this disease.

Conjugated hyperbilirubinemias

In which conjugated bilirubin is more in plasma. Some of them are given below.

(a) Dubin-Johnson syndrome or chronic idiopathic jaundice

It is a rare inherited disease. It can occur in adult life or in childhood. Conjugated hyperbilirubinemia is due to defect in the secretion of bilirubin into bile. Parenchymal cells contain an unidentified pigment and are unable to secret other conjugated compounds also.

(b) Rotor's syndrome

Chronic conjugated hyperbilirubinemia is characteristic of this syndrome. Exact cause for this is not known. However live histology is normal. Conjugated hyperbilirubinemia may be due to defective bilirubin transport by hepatocytes.

Hemoglobin degradation in Malarial Parasite (*P. Falciparum*)

Rapidly growing malarial parasite needs amino acids in large amounts. However *de novo* biosynthesis of amino acids in parasite is limited. Hence hemoglobin of host is used as a major amino acids source by parasite.

1. In malarial parasite hemoglobin is digested to amino acids and heme.
2. It begins with uptake of hemoglobin by endocytosis.
3. The endocytic vesicle empty the contents into food vacuole, a specialized lysosome like organelle of parasite.
4. Two aspartic proteases plasmepsin-I and plasmepsin-IV initiates hemoglobin degradation by cleaving susceptible bonds. By the action of these proteases hemoglobin is converted to polypeptides.
5. The polypeptides are further cleaved by falcilysin to peptides.
6. Malarial parasites also contain papain like cysteine proteases which can digest hemoglobin. They are falcipain-1, falcipain-2 and falcipain-3.
7. However these enzymes differ in mode of action. Falcipain-1 is capable of cleaving native hemoglobin while falcipain-2 cleaves denatured hemoglobin.
8. Falcipain-3 is suited well for hydrolysis of hemoglobin at acidic pH of food vacuole.
9. The peptides formed by the action of all these enzymes are transported into cytosol of parasite by a transporter where they are digested by amino peptidases to amino acids.

Medical Importance

1. Malaria disease caused by *plasmodium falciparum* continues to be disease with highest mortality rate.
2. Due to development of resistance of to all currently prescribed drugs treatment of malaria is limited. Hence identification of antimalarial drug targets is crucial.
3. Metabolic pathway of hemoglobin degradation in parasite can be exploited in new drug design.

REFERENCES

1. Dolphin, D. (Ed.). The Porphyrins. Academic Press, New York, 1979.
2. Granick, S. and Beale, S.I. Hemes, Chlorophylls and related compounds. Adv. Enzymology **40**, 33-203, 1978.
3. Dickerson, R.E. and Geis, I. Hemoglobin: Structure, function, evolution and pathology. Benjamin/Cummings, California.
4. Case, D.A. and Karplus, M. Dynamics of ligand binding to heme proteins. J. Mol. Biol. **132**, 343-368, 1979.
5. Pauling, I. Sickle cell anaemia a molecular disease. Science **110,** 543, 1949.
6. Geffner, M.E. Acquired methemoglobinemia. West J. Med. **134**, 7, 1981.
7. Bunn. H.F. Evaluation of glycosylated hemoglobin in diabetes patients. Diabetes **30,** 613, 1981.
8. Weatherall, D.J. *et al.* The hemoglobinopathies. In the metabolic basis of inherited disease. Scriver, C.R. *et al.* (Eds.). 6th ed. McGraw-Hill, New York, 1989.
9. Michael. T. Editor. Transport of bilirubin and its conjugate across hepatocellular membrane domain in conjugated hyperbilirubinemia of Dubin-Johnson syndrome. Landes Bio Science, Texas, 2003.
10. Michael. T. (Ed.). The ABC of Canalicular transport. Landes Bio Science. Texas, 2003.
11. Anguita, E. *et al.* Globin gene activation during heamopoiesis is driven by protein complexes nucleated by GATA-1 and GATA-2. The EMBO Journal **23,** 2841-2852, 2004.
12. Hani Atamma and William H. Frey. A role for heme in Alzheimer's disease : Heme binds amyloid β and has altered metabolism. Proc. Natl. Acad. Sci. USA **101,** 11153-11158, 2004.
13. Cukiernik, M. *et al.* Heme oxygenase in retina in diabetes. Curr. Eye. Res. **27**, 301-308, 2003.
14. Jaronczyk, K. *et al.* The source of heme for vascular heme oxygenase-II. Can. J. Physiol. Pharmacol. **82,** 218-224, 2004.
15. Greenbaum, L. *et al.* Nuclear distribution of porphobilinogen deaminase (PBGD) in glioma cells : A regulatory role in cancer transformation. Brit. J. Can. **86,** 1006-1011, 2002.
16. Schwartz, D.V. *et al.* Differentiation dependent photo dynamic therapy regulated by porphobilinogen deaminase in melanoma. Brit.J. Can. **90,** 1833-1841, 2004.
17. Gladwin, T.M. *et al.* Nitric oxide reactions with hemoglobin. Nat. Med. **9,** 496-500, 2003.
18. Harding, A-H. *et al.* Habitual fish consumption and glycated hemoglobin. Eur. J. Clin. Nutr. **58,** 277-284, 2004.
19. Cosby, K. *et al.* Nitrite reduction to nitric oxide by deoxyhemoglobin vasodilates human circulation. Nat. Med. **9,** 1498-1505, 2003.
20. Huang, C.S. *et al.* Genetic factors related to unconjugated hyperbilirubinemia amongst adults. Pharmacogenet. Genomics. **15**, 43-50, 2005.

EXERCISES

ESSAY QUESTIONS

1. Trace pathway for the synthesis of heme from glycine.
2. Define porphyrias. Classify them. Give example for each of them.
3. Give an account of oxygen binding curves of hemoglobin.
4. Describe hemoglobinopathies.
5. How bilirubin is formed from heme? How it is detoxified in liver?
6. Define jaundice. Classify. Explain each class of jaundice.
7. Write normal plasma bilirubin level. How it is formed? Write its fate. Explain principle of test of its detection in plasma.
8. How heme is synthesized? Write its regulation. Add a note on diseases associated with heme biosynthesis.
9. Write normal hemoglobin level in blood. Describe its structure and function. Add a note on abnormal hemoglobins.

SHORT QUESTIONS

1. What are porphyrus? Write short hand form of porphyrin. Explain the isomerism shown by them.
2. Explain structure and function of hemoglobin (HbA).
3. Write formation and medical importance of glycosylated hemoglobin.
4. Write principle of Van den Bergh reaction. Write its importance in differential diagnosis of jaundice.
5. Write importance of urine bilirubin and urobilinogen in differential diagnosis of jaundice.
6. Write a note on hyperbilirubinemias.
7. Write a note on thalassemias.
8. Define unconjugated hyperbilirubinemias. Write biochemical defects in the following diseases:
   (*a*) Neonatal physiological jaundice
   (*b*) Crigler-Najjer syndrome.
9. Write normal conjugated bilirubin level in plasma. Define conjugated hyperbilirubinemias. Name biochemical defects in the following diseases:
   (*a*) Dubin-Johnson syndrome
   (*b*) Rotor's syndrome.
10. Write a note on urine bilirubin and urobilinogen. Name tests of their detection.
11. Briefly explain bilirubin conjugation.
12. How heme is degraded?
13. Write a note on foetal hemoglobin and carboxyhemoglobin.
14. Write biochemical defect in
    (*a*) Erythropoietic Porphyria
    (*b*) Coproporphyria
    (*c*) Acquired porphyria.

MULTIPLE CHOICE QUESTIONS

1. All the following statements are correct regarding heme catabolism. Except
   (*a*) Porphyrin ring is cleaved. (*b*) Bilirubin is end product.
   (*c*) Release of carbon of porphyrin as CO. (*d*) Occurs in intestine.
2. Protoporphyrin IX conversion to heme involves
   (*a*) Incorporation of iron.
   (*b*) Incorporation of iron by ferro chelatase.
   (*c*) Oxidation of side chains of I and II rings.
   (*d*) Reduction of side chains of III and IV rings.
3. Which of the following statement is correct regarding ALA synthase.
   (*a*) Heme is the allosteric inhibitor. (*b*) Heme act as inducer.
   (*c*) Its synthesis is repressed by steroids. (*d*) It is present in cytosol.
4. Single hemoglobin molecule binds
   (*a*) Two O_2 molecules. (*b*) One O_2 molecule.
   (*c*) Four O_2 molecules. (*d*) Six O_2 molecules.
5. Subunit composition of foetal hemoglobin is
   (*a*) $\alpha_2\beta_2$ (*b*) $\alpha_2\gamma_2$
   (*c*) $\alpha_2\delta_2$ (*d*) $\alpha_2\varepsilon_2$

FILL IN THE BLANKS

1. Heme proteins are referred as .... proteins.
2. Cancer photochemotherapy involves use of .... property of porphyrins.
3. Porphyrinogens are converted to porphyrins by ....
4. Secretion of conjugated bilirubin involves .... process.
5. In intestine bilirubin undergoes series of .... reactions.

CASES

1. An automobiles garage worker who suddenly developed shortness of breath, severe muscle weakness, fatigue and giddiness was rushed to hospital. His carboxy hemoglobin level was elevated. Write your diagnosis.
2. A college student came to hospital with complaint of recurrent abdominal pain. On questioning he informed that pain increases on eating oil rich foods. Clinical examination showed yellow colored sclera. His serum total bilirubin, conjugated and unconjugated bilirubin levels were 8 mg% 6 mg% and 2 mg% respectively. Urine gave positive for bilirubin. However urobilinogen was not found in urine. Write your diagnosis.

23
CHAPTER

VITAMINS

INTRODUCTION

Vitamins are defined as small organic molecules present in diet which are required in small amounts. Most of the vitamins are not synthesized in the body and hence they must be supplied in the diet. However few vitamins are synthesized in the body. Though most of them are present in diet as such some are present as precursors. The precursor forms of vitamins are called as provitamins. In the body these provitamins are converted to vitamins.

Vitamins are divided into two groups. They are fat soluble vitamins and water soluble vitamins.

Fat Soluble Vitamins

They are vitamins A, D, E and K. They have some common properties. They are: 1. Fat soluble. 2. Require bile salts for absorption. 3. Stored in liver. 4. Stable to normal cooking conditions. 5. Excreted in feces.

Water Soluble Vitamins

They are members of vitamin B complex and Vitamin C. Their common properties are 1. Water solubility. 2. Except Vitamin B_{12} others are not stored. 3. Unstable to normal cooking conditions. 4. Excreted in urine.

MEDICAL AND BIOLOGICAL IMPORTANCE

1. Vitamins are essential for growth, maintenance and reproduction. However, they are not used for energy production.
2. Fat soluble vitamins are required for normal and colour vision, blood clotting, bone formation and maintenance of membrane structure.
3. Most of the water soluble vitamins function as coenzymes or prosthetic groups of several enzymes involved in carbohydrate, lipid and amino acid metabolism etc.
4. Vitamins A and D act as steroid hormones.
5. Pregnant and lactating women require higher amounts of vitamins. During post operative recovery also vitamin requirement is more.

6. Lack of vitamin in the diet produce characteristic deficiency symptoms. Since intestinal flora synthesizes some vitamins prolonged use of antibiotics also produce vitamin deficiency.
7. Deficiency of fat soluble vitamins produce night blindness, skeletal deformation, haemorrhages and hemolysis.
8. Deficiency of water soluble vitamins produce beriberi, glossitis, pellagra, microcytic anaemia, megaloblastic anaemia and scurvy.
9. Since most of the water soluble vitamins are components of enzymes their deficiency leads to blocks in metabolic reactions. This in turn causes characteristic biochemical symptoms. For example pyridoxine deficiency is characterized by xanthurenicaciduria and vitamin B_{12} deficiency is characterized by methyl malonic aciduria.
10. Some drugs and compounds present in natural sources act as antivitamins. So they induce vitamin deficiency. For example isonicotinic acid hydrazide (INH) used in tuberculosis cause pyridoxine deficiency. Avidin present in egg white binds to water soluble vitamin biotin and prevents its absorption. This leads to biotin deficiency.
11. Some vitamin analogs are used as drugs. For example folic acid analogs are used as anticancer agents and antibiotics. Likewise vit K analog dicoumarol is used as anticoagulant to prevent thromboembolism.
12. Moderate consumption of some vitamins is found to decrease occurrence or severity of some diseases. For example carotenes, Vitamin E and Vitamin D consumption at moderate level reduces incidence of cancer and cardiovascular diseases. Consumption of vitamin C in significant amounts reduces severity of cold. They slow down ageing process also. However, excessive consumption of fat soluble vitamins leads to toxicity.
13. Malabsorption syndromes or gastroenteritis or dysentery may impair absorption of vitamins. This may lead to vitamin deficiency.
14. Since bile is required for the absorption of fat soluble vitamins in obstructive jaundice, Steathorrea, sprue (celiac disease) etc. their absorption is impaired. This leads to vitamin deficiency.
15. Vit B_{12}, Folic acid and Vit B_6 are beneficial to coronary artery disease patients. They lower plasma homocysteine levels.

FAT SOLUBLE VITAMINS

VITAMIN A

Chemistry

The word Vitamin A refers to group of compounds which exhibit Vitamin A activity. They are retinol (Vitamin A alcohol), retinal (Vitamin A aldehyde) and retinoic acid (Vitamin A acid). They are also referred as retinoids. Retinal and retinoic acid are formed from retinol. Further retinal and retinol are inter convertible. But retinoic acid cannot be converted to either retinal or retinol.

The three forms of Vitamin A are derivatives of a 20 carbon compound which is composed of β–ionine ring (methyl substituted cyclohexenylring) and side chain containing two isoprene units with four conjugated double bonds. Due to the presence of double bonds in isoprenoid side chain vitamin A exhibits cis-trans (geometric) isomerism (Figure 23.1). Due to the presence of 4 double bonds vitamin A can be oxidized by air or light slowly.

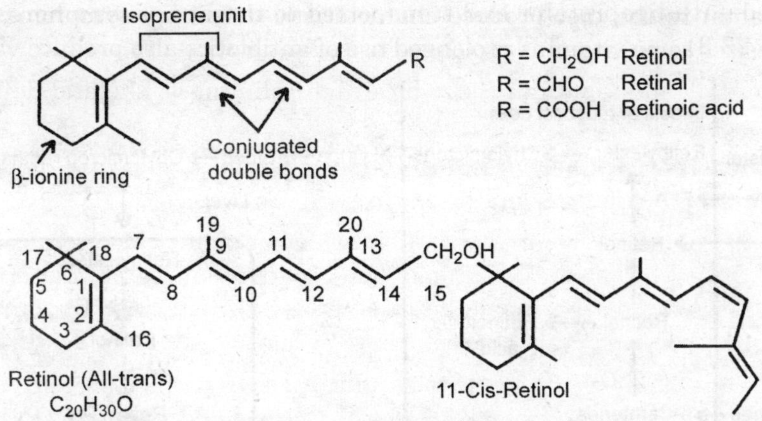

Fig. 23.1 Structures of vit. A. Geometric isomers of vit A are also shown

In nature vitamin A occurs in two forms. In the foods of animal origin it is present as retinolesters. In plant foods it is present in provitamin form which is known as carotenes. There are three types of carotenes present in plants. They are α-carotenes, β-carotenes and γ-carotenes. These carotenes are called as carotenoids. β-carotenes are most potent source of retinol because one molecule of β-carotene yields two molecules of Vitamin A *in vivo* (Figure 23.2). However α, γ-carotenes can yield only one molecule of vitamin A.

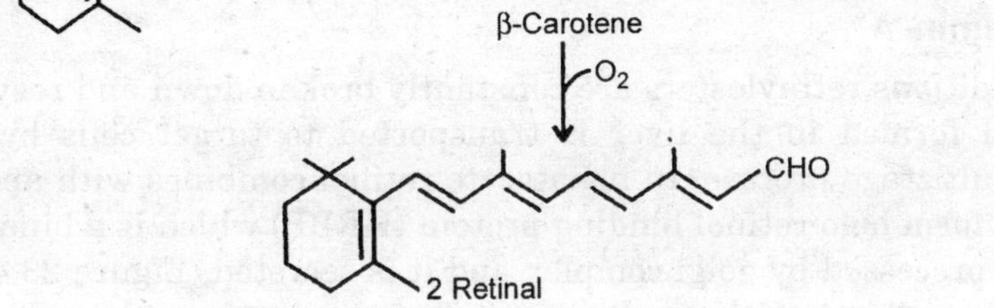

Fig. 23.2 Conversion of β-carotene to retinal

Absorption of Vitamin A

In the intestine pancreatic esterase hydrolyzes retinolesters present in the diet to retinol and free fatty acid in presence of bile salts. Retinol is absorbed by mucosal cells. β-carotenes are also absorbed by mucosal cells. A dioxygenase present in the intestinal mucosal cells cleaves most of the β-carotene of dietary origin to two molecules of retinal in presence of oxygen. The conversion of β-carotene is limited. Six μg of β-carotene is converted to 1μg of retinal. Retinal formed is reduced to retinol by NAD(P)H dependent reductase present in mucosal cells of intestine. The reaction is a reversible one. Retinal can be oxidized to retinoic acid by using NAD^+ or FAD as hydrogen acceptor. Retinoic acid formed is absorbed through portal venous system and transported to target cells after binding with albumin. A part of β-carotene absorbed does not undergo conversion to retinal and it is associated with lipoproteins and transported to target tissues where it is converted to retinal (Figure 23.3).

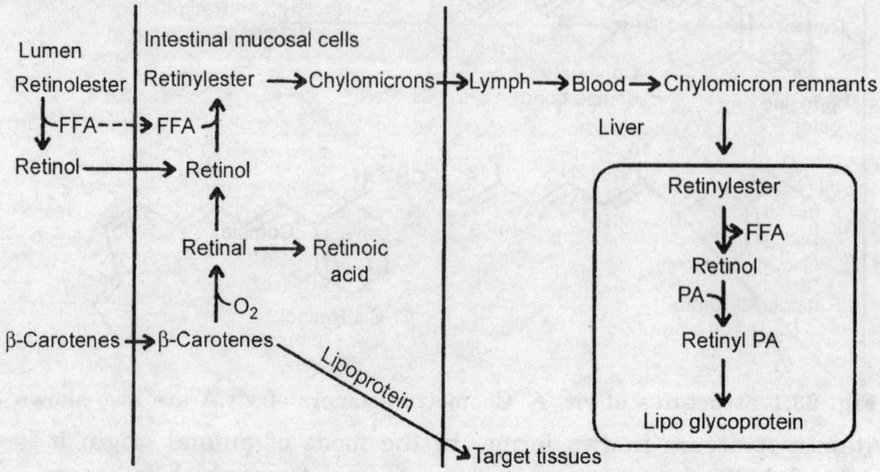

Fig. 23.3 Absorption and fate of dietary vit A. FFA : Free fatty acid. PA : Palmitic acid

In the mucosal cells of intestine the retinol generated from animal and plant sources is esterified with fatty acids and incorporated into chylomicrons which enters blood stream via lymph. In the circulation chylomicron remnants formed from chylomicrons contain virtually all retinyl esters. These chylomicron remnants are taken up by liver. In the liver retinyl esters are liberated from chylomicron remnants and are hydrolysed to retinol and free fatty acid. Retinylester is resynthesized in liver with palmitic acid and stored as lipoglycoprotein in lipocytes of liver (Figure 23.3).

Transport of Vitamin A

Under normal conditions retinylesters are constantly broken down and resynthesized in the liver. Free retinol formed in the liver is transported to target cells by way of protein complex. It is a multistage process. In hepatocyte retinol combines with apo retinol binding protein (APRB) to form holo retinol binding protein (HRBP) which is a binary complex. This binary complex is processed by golgi complex and it is secreted (Figure 23.4). In the plasma the binary complex combines with prealbumin to form ternary complex which reaches target cells. The ternary complex then binds to specific receptor on cell membrane of target tissues and retinol is released into cell. In target cells some of the retinol is converted to retinal and retionic acid. With in cells retinol and retinoic acid combines with cellular retinol binding protein (CRBP) and cellular retinoic acid binding protein (CRABP) respectively. Then these complexes enters nucleus to exert their action (Figure 23.4).

Functions of vitamin A

The three major retinoids retinal, retinol and retinoic acid have unique functions.

1. Retinal is required for normal and color vision.
2. Retinol is required for reproduction and growth. Retinol supports spermatogenesis, oogenesis and placental development.
3. Retinol is required for differentiation and function as steroid hormone.

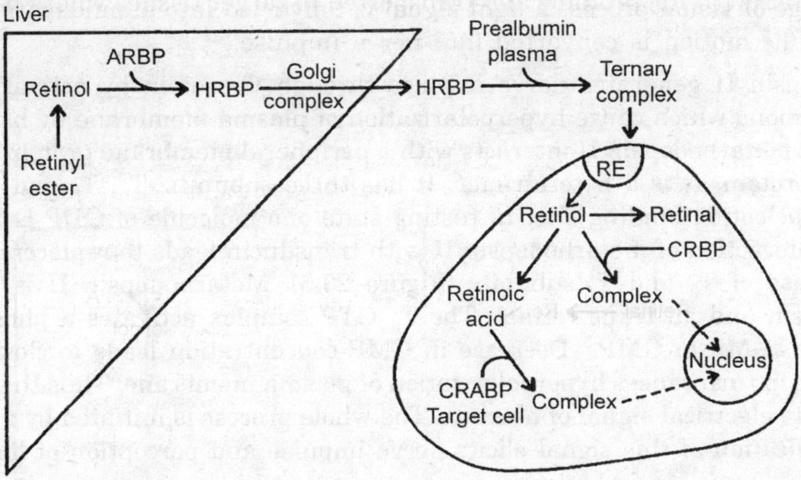

Fig. 23.4 Transport of vit A from liver to target cells. RE : Receptor

4. Retinoic acid is required for the synthesis of glycoproteins or mucopolysaccharides. Retinoyl phosphate act as glycosyl carrier.
5. Retinoic acid also act as steroid hormone. It also promote growth and differentiation but only to some extent.
6. Retinol and retinoic acid are involved in regulation of gene expression.
7. Vitamin A has several other important functions which are not yet clear. Some of them are given below.
   (*a*) Vitamin A is required for integrity of epithelial cells of gastro-intestinal tract, skin, respiratory tract and urinary tract and salivary glands.
   (*b*) Vitamin A is required for maintenance of nervous tissue particularly myelin sheath formation.
   (*c*) Vitamin A is required for tooth formation and bone growth.
   (*d*) **Cancer.** Retinoids are found to prevent chemical carcinogenesis. Synthetic retinoids are found to prevent breast cancer and bladder cancer. β-carotenes function as antioxidants (Free radical scavenger). They eliminate reactive oxygen species.
   (*f*) **Acne and psoriasis.** Vitamin A is useful in treatment of skin disorders like acne and psoriasis.

Retinal and vision

Rods and cones present in the retina are responsible for normal and colour vision. Rods are responsible for vision in dim light where as cones are responsible for visual acuity and color vision. The rods contain visual pigment rhodopsin which is made up of 11-cis retinal and opsin a glycoprotein. Rhodopsin is an integral membrane glycoprotein. 11-cis retinal is attached to apoprotein opsin through ε-amino group of lysine. When photon (light) strikes it undergoes conversion to all trans retinol. At the same time apoprotein dissociates as opsin (Figure 23.5). The conversion of rhodopsin to opsin and all trans retinal occurs through several intermediates whose life span ranges from picoseconds to a minute (Figure 23.6). So in the first stage of visual process a light signal is converted into atomic motion. In the next stage this atomic motion is converted into nerve impulse.

Metarhodopsin II generates nerve impulse through G-protein by activating cascade of enzymatic reactions which cause hyperpolarization of plasma membrane by blocking Na^+ ion channels. First metarhodopsin II interacts with a peripheral membrane protein transducin (T) which is a G-protein. It is a heterotrimer. It has three subunits. T_α, T_β and T_γ. T_α subunit has guanine nucleotide binding site. In resting state one molecule of GDP is bound to T_α of transducin. Interaction of metarhodopsin II with transducin leads to replacement of GDP by GTP and release of T_β and T_γ subunits (Figure 23.5). Metarhodopsin II is hydrolyzed by protease to opsin and all trans retinal. The T_α GTP complex activates a phosphodiesterase which converts cGMP to GMP. Decrease in GMP concentration leads to closing of Na^+ ion channels which in turn causes hyperpolarization of plasma membrane. Thus the light stimulus is converted into electrical signal of neurons. The whole process is initiated by a single photon. Further amplification of this signal elicits nerve impulse and perception of light by brain.

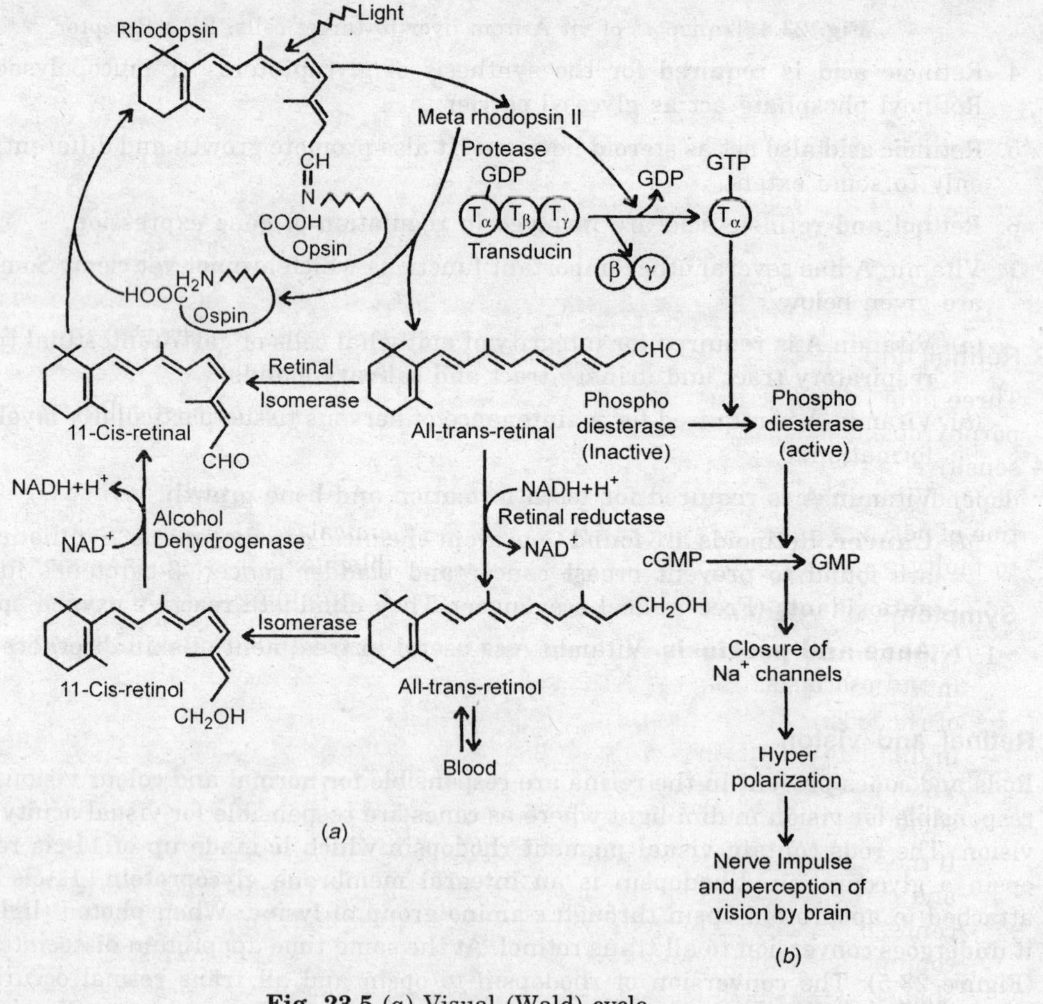

Fig. 23.5 (*a*) Visual (Wald) cycle.
(*b*) Transducin mediated conversion of chemical signal into nerve impulse

The all trans retinal formed is converted to all trans retinol by reductase using NADH as hydrogen donor and pass into blood. A small amount of all trans retinal may be isomerized to 11-cis retinal. However this small amount of 11-cis-retinal is unable to regenerate adequate amount of rhodopsin as required for vision. Hence for the resynthesis of rhodopsin constant supply of Vitamin A is required from the diet. In retina all trans retinol of dietary origin is isomerized by an isomerase to 11-cis-retinol. Finally 11-cis retinal is generated by alcohol dehydrogenase from 11-cis-retinol. The enzyme is present in retina and uses NAD^+ as hydrogen acceptor. Visual pigment rhodopsin is formed from opsin and 11-cis-retinal (Figure 23.5) to complete visual cycle (Wald cycle). If diet does not contain vitamin A the resynthesis of rhodopsin is blocked and perception of vision by brain is delayed.

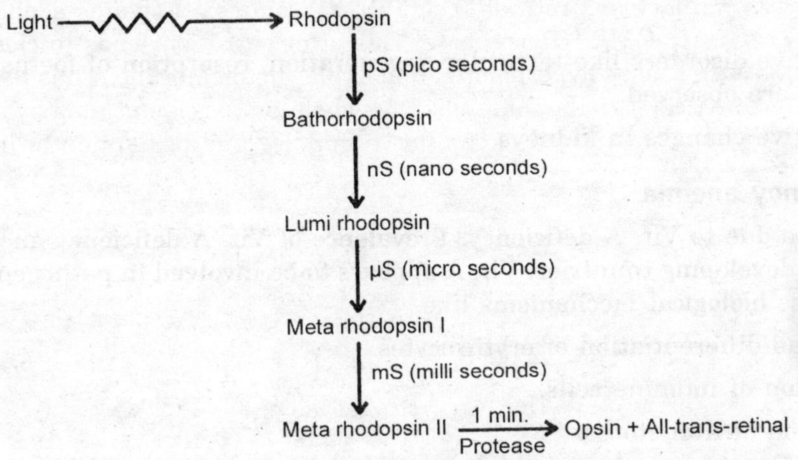

Fig. 23.6 Light induced conversion of rhodopsin to opsin and all-trans-retinal

Retinal and colour vision

Three light sensitive pigments present in cones are responsible for colour vision. They are porphyropsin, iodopsin and cyanopsin. All three pigments contain 11-cis retinal and are sensitive to red, green and blue colours respectively. When the photon (light) strikes retina depending on the colour of the light a particular pigment is bleached. This leads to generation of nerve impulse and perception of colour by brain. Defective apoprotein production due to faulty genes leads to colour blindness.

Symptoms of Vitamin A deficiency

1. **Night blindness or nyctalopia.** In early stages of Vitamin A deficiency the affected individual is not able to see clearly in dim light or night due to block in the resynthesis of rhodopsin. In the later stage of deficiency the affected individual cannot see or read in dim light. Thus loss of night vision (night blindness) is the major initial symptom of Vitamin A deficiency. Night blindness in adults or in preschool children is common in some regions of this country where intake of vitamin A is low.

   If the night blindness is not treated it progresses to xerophthalmia in which conjunctival and corneal epithelium of the eye is keratinised. Due to keratinisation of epithelium conjunctiva is dry, thickens, wrinkled and pigmented. This condition is called as xerosis conjunctiva. Further in affected children of below 6 years age Bitot's spots a triangular shaped white plaques on conjunctiva are seen. Due to keratinisation of epithelium cornea is dry and gives dull appearance (xerosis cornea).

When xerosis of conjuctiva and cornea is not treated it leads to keratomalacia which is characterized by degenerated corneal epithelium. Finally permanent blindness results from corneal perforation or ulceration and scarring.

2. Growth of bone and formation of tooth are defective. Thick and long bones are formed.
3. Nerve growth also affected. Degeneration of myelin sheath occurs.
4. Keratinisation of mucous secreting epithelial cells (hyperkeratosis) lining respiratory tract and reproductive tract occurs. Mucous secretion by salivary and lacrymal glands is also affected.
5. Deposition of keratin in skin (xeroderma) gives rise to characteristic toad skin appearance.
6. Reproductive disorders like testicular degeneration, resorption of foetus or foetal malformation are observed.
7. Degenerative changes in kidneys.

Vit. A deficiency anemia

It is an anemia due to Vit. A deficiency. Prevalence of Vit. A deficiency anemia is high in populations of developing countries. Vit. A appears to be involved in pathogenesis of anemia through diverse biological mechanisms like.

(*a*) Growth and differentiation of erythrocytes.

(*b*) Proliferation of immune cells.

(*c*) Mobilization of iron stores.

Vit. A supplementation reduces severity of anemia.

Sources

(*a*) **Animal sources.** As mentioned earlier it is present as retionolesters is animal foods. Marine fish oils like halibut liver oil, cod liver oil and shark liver oils are excellent sources. Liver of sheep or goat or pig is also excellent source. Butter, egg, and milk are good sources. Freshwater fish contain Vitamin A_2 (dehydroretinol) which is only 40% active.

(*b*) **Plant sources.** In plant foods vitamin A is present as carotenes. Plant oil like red palm oil is excellent source. Other plant sources are

Leafy vegetables. Amarnath leaves, coriander leaves, curry leaves, drumstick leaves, spinach and cabbage are good sources.

Yellow vegetables like carrot, pumpkin and sweet potato and other vegetables like bottle gouard, drum sticks and ripe tomatoes also contain appreciable amounts of vitamin A.

Fruits. Yellow pigmented fruits papaya, mango, jackfruit, banana and oranges also contain vitamin A in good amounts.

Daily requirement (RDA)

Adults (men and women). 750 µg of retinol or 3 mg of carotene (1 CMR) or 2500 I.U. (International units, 1 I.U = 0.3 µg of retinol.)

Vit A toxicity (Hyper vitaminosis)

It occurs when mega doses of Vitamin A (about 10-20 times of RDA) is taken or too many mangos or other vitamin A containing preparation are taken. Signs and symptoms of vitamin A toxicity are weakness, headache, muscle stiffness, increased intracranial pressure and hypertension. Fortunately symptoms disappear within week after stopping excess intake.

Antagonists of vit A

Some chemically unrelated compounds are found to antagonize vitamin A in experimental animals. Some are citral, sodium benzoate and monobromobenzene.

VITAMIN D

Chemistry

The term vitamin D refers to group of two compounds that exhibit vitamin D activity. They are vitamin D_2 also called as ergo calciferol and vitamin D_3 also called as cholecalciferol. These active forms of vitamin D_2 and vitamin D_3 are formed from provitamins which are sterols. The provitamin of vitamin D_2 is ergosterol which is found in ergot and yeast. It is a derivative of cholesterol. The provitamin of vitamin D_3 is 7-dehydrocholesterol which is found in animals. It is also a derivative of cholesterol.

The provitamins are converted to active forms on exposure to ultraviolet light present in sunlight or in any other light. The conversion involves opening of B-ring of steroid nucleus (Figure 23.7). For this reason active forms of vitamin D are not sterols. Since the formation of vitamin D_2 and vitamin D_3 is dependent on sunlight they are referred as sunshine vitamins. However exposure to mercury light also leads to conversion of provitamin to active vitamin. In humans 7-dehydrocholesterol present beneath skin is converted to vitamin D_3 on exposure to sunlight.

Absorption, transport and storage

Dietary vitamin D_2 and vitamin D_3 are absorbed in the small intestine in presence of bile salts. In the intestinal mucosal cells absorbed Vit D is incorporated into chylomicrons and enters circulation via lymph. In the circulation vitamin D dissociates from chylomicrons and binds to specific vitamin D binding protein (DBP) which has higher affinity for vitamin D_3. So a binary complex containing vitamin D and DBP is found in plasma. Further, vitamin D_3 formed in the skin also combines with vitamin D binding protein and forms a binary complex. Different tissues take up vitamin D from DBP and vitamin D complex. Vitamin D is stored in liver and adipose tissue. Vitamin D binding protein can combine with different forms of Vitamin D.

Formation of 1, 25-dihydroxy Cholecalciferol (Calcitriol)

Calcitriol which is the most active form of vitamin D that acts as steroid hormone is formed in kidney. This requires initial hydroxylation of vitamin D_3 at 25-position which takes place in liver. A cytochrome P_{450}-dependent 25-hydroxylase present in endoplasmic reticulum catalyzes the conversion of cholecalciferol to 25-hydroxy cholecalciferol. This combines with DBP and then transported to kidney. A mitochondrial cytochrome P_{450}-dependent α-hydroxylase catalyzes the formation of 1, 25-dihydroxy cholecalciferol or calcitriol from 25-hydroxycholecalciferol (Figure 23.7). Calcitriol is referred as hormone because it is produced in kidney and functions in intestine and bone. Further it is referred as steroid hormone because in intestine it increases protein synthesis by stimulating gene expression like steroid hormone. α-hydroxylase activity is also found in bone, cartilage and placenta.

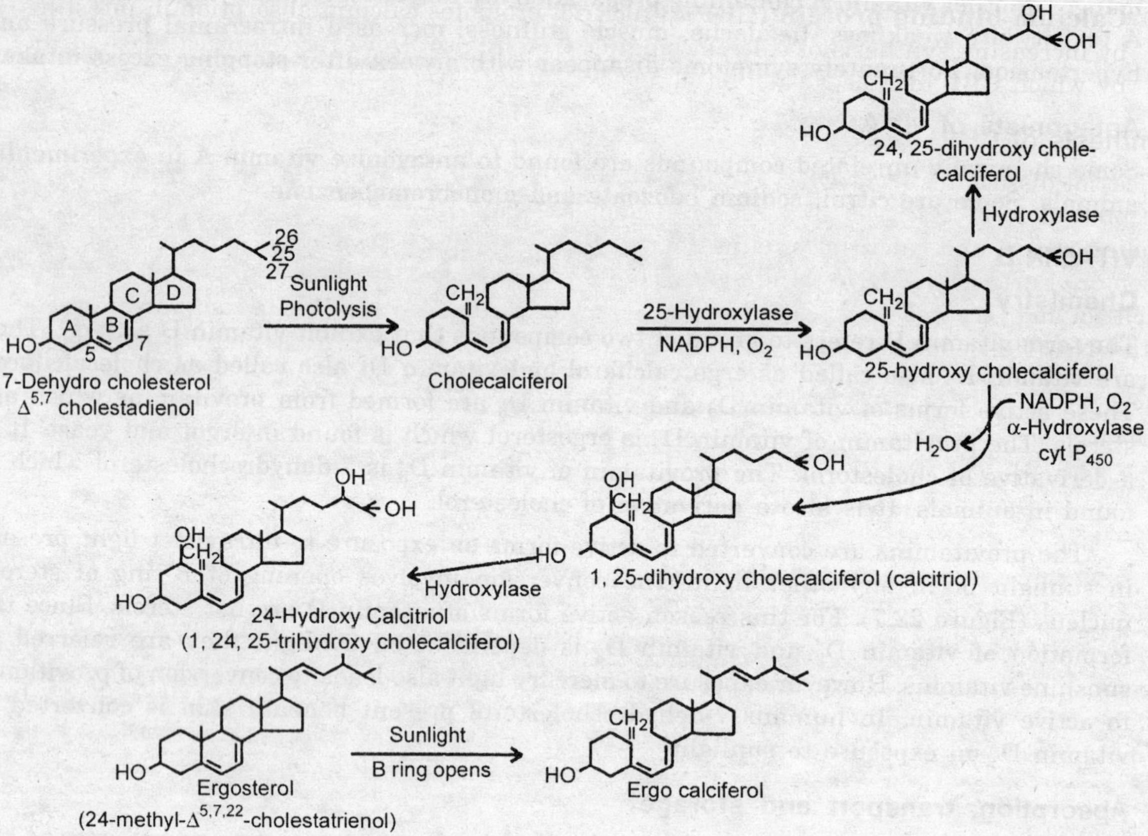

Fig. 23.7 Formation and fate of calcitriol. Conversion of provit D_2 to vit D_2 is also shown

Regulation of vitamin D metabolism

α-hydroxylase activity regulates vitamin D metabolism. Activity of α-hydroxylase depends on plasma calcitriol level. Calcitriol regulates its own biosynthesis by feed back inhibition of α-hydroxylase. Increased plasma calcium and phosphate level also inhibits α-hydroxylase.

α-hydroxylase activity is stimulated by parathyroid hormone (PTH), low plasma calcium and phosphate levels and hormones like estrogen and growth hormone.

Medical Importance

α-hydroxylase activity was found to be low in hypothyroidism and renal diseases.

Functions of calcitriol

1. Major action of calcitriol is to increase absorption of calcium and phosphate in the intestine particularly in duodenum and jejunum.

Absorption of calcium

Calcitriol promotes calcium absorption by two mechanisms.

(*a*) **Active transport.** Calcitriol promotes uptake of calcium by mucosal cells from brush border against concentration gradiant. This process is dependent on oxidative energy.

(*b*) **Calcium binding protein (CBP).** Calcitriol promotes calcium absorption in intestine by increasing synthesis of calcium binding protein also. However the exact mechanism by which CBP increases calcium absorption in intestine is not clear.

Synthesis of CBP

Calcitriol dissociates from DBP and enters intestinal cell where it combines with cytosolic receptor to form calcitriol and receptor complex. This receptor has two regions a DNA binding region and calcitriol binding region. Calcitriol binds to calcitriol binding region of receptor. Further the DNA binding region of receptor consist of zinc finger motifs. The calcitriol and receptor complex enters nucleus where zinc finger motifs of complex interacts with DNA. This leads to transcription and synthesis of calcium binding protein (Figure 23.8).

Lumen

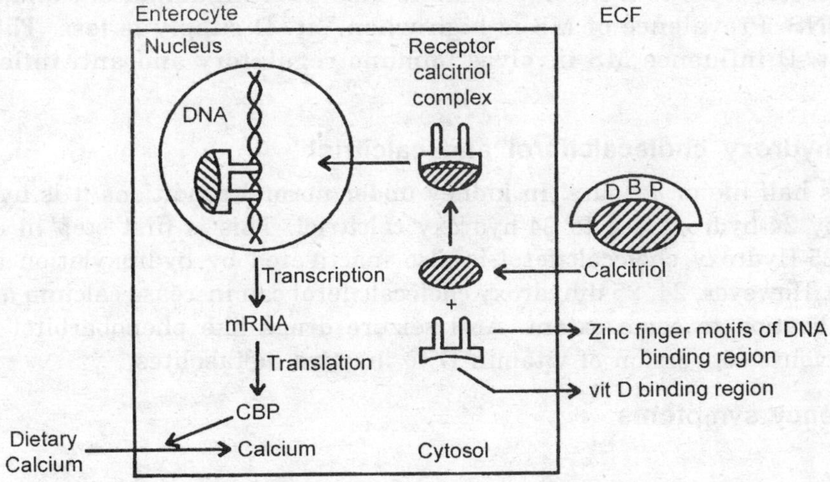

Fig. 23.8 Calcitriol mediated calcium binding protein (CBP) synthesis in enterocyte. DBP-Vit D binding protein

Absorption of Phosphorus

Calcitriol promotes absorption of phosphorus in intestine by different mechanism which is dependent on sodium and glucose.

2. Calcitriol is required for bone formation and mineralisation of bone. It increases synthesis of osteocalcin a calcium binding protein of bone. Osteocalcin is involved in deposition of calcium salts in bone.
3. Calcitriol affects calcium and phosphorus excretion by kidney. It reduces the excretion of calcium and phosphorus.
4. Vitamin D is involved in maintenance of normal muscle tone.
5. **Calcitriol, immune response and tuberculosis**

   (*a*) Calcitriol is an immuno regulatory hormone. It stimulates cell mediated immunity. It plays a vital role in monocyte/macrophage activation. The effects of Vit. D are exerted by the interaction through Vit. D receptor (VDR). VDR is a member of super family of steroid receptors.

(*b*) Calcitriol is one of mediators shown to impair growth of mycobacterium which causes tuberculosis.

(*c*) Vit. D receptor gene exhibits polymorphism. Susceptibility or resistance to pulmonary as well as spinal tuberculosis is linked to VDR polymorphism.

(*d*) Therefore intake of Vit. D may probably regulate immunity to tuberculosis in susceptible people.

(*e*) **Vit. D deficiency and tuberculosis.** VDR polymorphism and Vit. D deficiency are strongly associated with tuberculosis in certain populations.

(*f*) **Vit. D receptor gene polymorphism and cancer.** Vit D receptor gene polymorphism are associated with breast cancer risk.

Multiple sclerosis and Vit. D

Multiple sclerosis (MS) is a chronic immune mediated inflammatory and degenerative disease of CNS. Prevalence of MS is high when Vit. D supply is less. The mechanism by which Vit. D influence MS involves immuno regulatory and anti inflammatory actions.

Fate of 25-hydroxy cholecalciferol and calcitriol

Calcitriol has half life of 3 hours. In kidney under normal conditions it is hydroxylated at 24-position by 24-hydroxylase to 24-hydroxy calcitriol. This is first step in destruction of vitamin D. 25-Hydroxy cholecalciferol is also inactivated by hydroxylation at 24-position (Figure 23.7). However, 24, 25 dihydroxy cholecalciferol can increase calcium absorption and bone mineralization to some extent. Anti seizure drugs like phenobarbitol and diphenyl hydantoin favours conversion of vitamin D to inactive metabolites.

Vit D deficiency symptoms

1. Rickets

In children vitamin D deficiency causes rickets. The disease occurs in children of low income groups whose dietary intake is low. Since vitamin D is required for bone formation its deficiency results in soft bones. Teeth formation is also affected. This leads to deformities in skull, chest, spine, legs and pelvis. Deformities of skull are craniotabes round unossified areas formed in occipital region due to softening of skull bones and development of parietal and frontal eminences (parietal, frontal bossing). Craniotabes is early sign. Chest deformities are pigeon breast due to deformation of sternum and rachitic rosary beading in costachondrial junctions of ribs. Deformities of legs are bow legs due to curvature at junction of lower and upper portions of legs and knees are away : knock knees due to angulation at junction of lower and upper portions of legs and knees are closer. Pelvic and spine deformities develop at later stages.

2. Osteomalacia

Vitamin D deficiency causes osteomalacia in adults. It is seen in pregnant women and women in pardha in India. Skeletal pain is early sign. Deformities of ribs, spine, pelvis and legs are seen.

3. Osteoporosis

Vitamin D deficiency causes osteoporosis in old people. Photolysis of provitamins dcreases with age. This and together with decreased sex hormone production may lead to deficiency. Symptoms are bone pain and porous bones. Bone fractures are common.

Rickets of inherited origin

(*a*) **Vitamin D resistant or independent rickets type I.** It is due to defective conversion of 25-hydroxy cholecalciferol to calcitriol due to defect in hydroxylation.

(*b*) **Vitamin D resistant rickets type II.** The receptor protein of calcitriol is unable to form proper zinc finger motifs due to defect in DNA binding region. This impairs its interaction with DNA and transcription is not stimulated.

Biochemical symptoms in vit D deficiency

Blood calcium and phosphorus levels are low (hypocalcemia and hypophosphatemia).

Sources

Vitamin D is mostly present in foods of animal origin. Marine fish liver oils like halibut liver oil, cod liver oil and shark liver oil are good sources. Sardines, egg yolk and butter contains small amounts. However, milk is a poor source of vitamin D, Mushrooms contain small amounts of vitamin D.

Daily requirement (RDA)

Adults. 200 International units (IU)/day or 5 μg of vitamin D. 400 international units (I.U)/ day or 10 μg of vitamin D_3 per day for pregnant and lactating women. In tropical countries the daily requirement decreases if they are exposed to sunlight.

Toxicity (Hyper vitaminosis)

Ingestion of mega doses of vitamin D results in toxicity of Vit D. Signs and symptoms of vitamin D toxicity are loss of appetite, nausae, thirst, vomiting, polyuria and calcification of lungs, renal tubules and arteries. Muscle wasting also occurs. Demineralisation of bone similar to vitamin D deficiency is seen. Symptoms appear after 1-3 months of excess intake. Discontinuation of vitamin D intake leads to disappearance of symptoms.

VITAMIN E

Chemistry

The term vitamin E refers to group of four (often six) compounds that exhibit vitamin E activity. They are α-tocopherol, β-tocopherol, γ-tocopherol and δ-tocopherol. They are derivatives of tocol or 6-hydroxy chromane ring with phytyl side chain (Figure-23.9). They differ in methyl groups in positions 5, 7, and 8 of chromane ring. α-tocopherol has three methyl groups in positions, 5, 7 and 8 of chromane ring. The chromane ring of β and γ tocopherols contain two methyl groups in 5, 8 and 7, 8 respectively. However δ-tocopherol has one methyl group in position 8 of chromane ring.

Tocopherols are alkaline sensitive and their vitamin activity is destroyed by oxidation. Among all tocopherols α-tocopherol is most potent and widely distributed in nature. Cooking and food processing may destroy vitamin E to some extent.

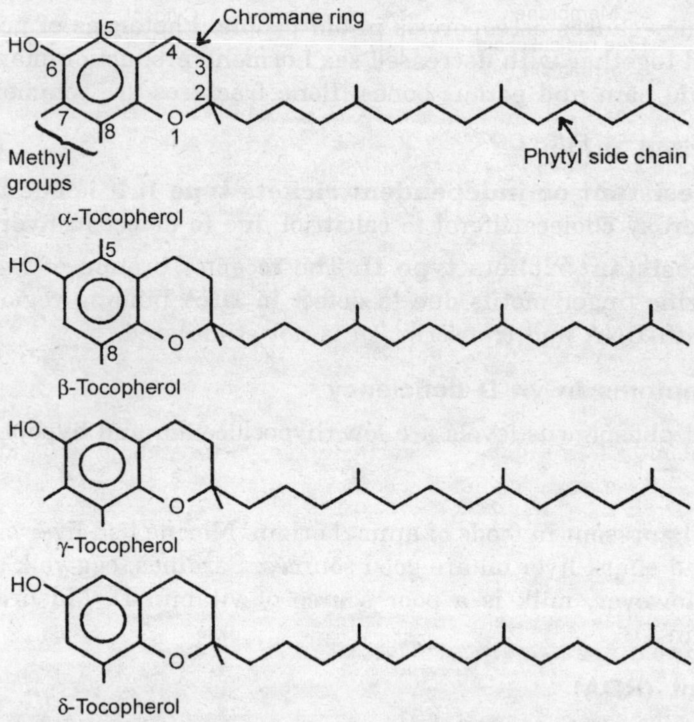

Fig. 23.9 Structures of tocopherols

Absorption, transport and storage

Dietary tocopherols are absorbed in small intestine in presence of bile salts. Absorbed tocopherols are incorporated into chylomicrons in mucosal cells of intestine and enters circulation via lymph. In plasma tocopherols are released from chylomicrons by lipoprotein lipase. Liver takes up half of tocopherol and it is stored. Skeletal muscle and adipose tissue also stores vitamin E. From the liver tocopherols are transported to other tissues in β-lipoprotein.

Functions of Vitamin E

1. α-tocopherol present in cell membrane, membrane of subcellular organelle and in cytosol function as antioxidant or free radical scavenger. It is present in high concentration in tissues which are exposed to high O_2 pressure like erythrocytes, lungs, retina etc. It prevents peroxidation of membrane lipids particularly polyunsaturated fatty acid (PUFA) of membrane phospholipids.

Peroxidation of membrane lipids produce peroxy ($RO\dot{O}$) radicals (Chapter 10) which initiate free radical chain reaction. They react with other membrane lipids and converts them into peroxy radicals (Figure 23.10). This peroxidation of membrane lipids leads to changes in membrane structure and damage. α-tocopherols present in membrane protects membrane lipids from peroxy radicals attack by eliminating them. It act as chain breaking antioxidant.

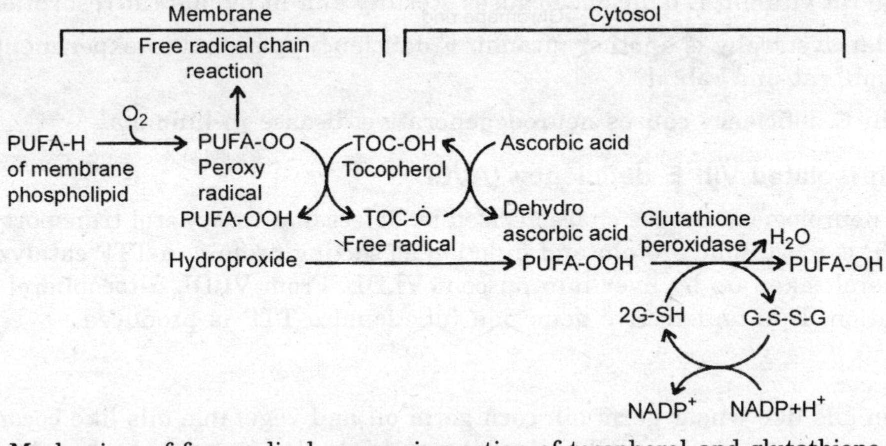

Fig. 23.10 Mechanism of free radical scavenging action of tocopherol and glutathione peroxidase in membrane and cytosol respectively

Mechanism of free radical scavenging action of tocopherol

α-tocopherol converts peroxy radical to hydroperoxide. This produces tocopherol free radical which further reacts with another peroxy radical to form non free radical oxidized product (Figure 23.11). The oxidized product of tocopherol is conjugated with glucuronic acid and excreted in bile. Alternatively free radical of tocopherol may react with ascorbic acid to form tocopherol and dehydroascorbic acid. In the cytosol hydroperoxide is removed by glutathione peroxidase using glutathione. It converts hydroperoxide of PUFA into hydroxy PUFA (Figure 23.10). Since glutathione peroxidase contain selenium vitamin E and selenium act together in the cells in defence against lipid peroxides.

$$\underset{\text{Peroxy radical}}{\text{R-OO}^\bullet} + \underset{\text{Tocopherol}}{\text{TOC-OH}} \longrightarrow \underset{\text{Hydroperoxide}}{\text{R-OOH}} + \underset{\text{Free radical of tocopherol}}{\text{TOC-}\dot{\text{O}}}$$

$$\underset{\text{Peroxy radical}}{\text{R-OO}^\bullet} + \underset{\text{Tocopherol free radical}}{\text{TOC-O}^\bullet} \longrightarrow \underset{\text{Hydroperoxide}}{\text{R-OOH}} + \text{Oxidized product of tocopherol}$$

Fig. 23.11 Elimination of peroxy radicals by tocopherol

2. Vitamin E is required for fertility in experimental animals like rat. It supports spermatogenesis in male rats and foetal growth in female rats.
3. Vitamin E is involved in maintenance of muscle tone in experimental animals.
4. Vitamin E increases synthesis of hemeproteins by increasing synthesis of ALA synthase and ALA dehydratase.
5. Vitamin E prevents dietary vitamin A and carotenes from oxidative damage.

Symptoms of Vitamin E deficiency

1. In adults vitamin E deficiency symptoms are rare. However in infants vitamin E deficiency causes hemolytic anaemia. It is due to increased susceptibility of erythrocytes to hemolysis.

2. In male rat vitamin E deficiency causes sterility and in female rat resorption of foetus.
3. Muscular dystrophy is another vitamin E deficiency symptom in experimental animals like lamb, rat and rabbit.
4. Vitamin E deficiency causes neurodegenerative disease in humans.

Ataxia with isolated Vit. E deficiency (AVED)

It is a rare neurological disease characterized by defect in α-tocopherol transport protein (α-TTP). α-TTP is a cytosolic protein and function as sorting protein. α-TTP catalyzes transfer of α-tocopherol taken up by liver into nascent VLDL. From VLDL α-tocopherol is released into circulation. Due to defective gene non functional α-TTP is produced.

Sources

Cereal germ oils like wheat germ oil, corn germ oil and vegetable oils like coconut oil, sun flower oil, peanut oil, ricebran oil, palm oil, mustard oil, cotton seed oil and soyabean oil are rich sources of vitamin E. Vegetables, fruits and meat are relatively poor sources of vitamin E.

Daily Requirement

Selenium and polyunsaturated fatty acid (PUFA) content influences daily requirement. An adult needs 10 mg of vitamin E per day when PUFA intake is 5 g per day. Vitamin E requirement during pregnancy and lactation is about 12-13 mg/day.

Therapeutic Uses of Vitamin E

Several ailments are treated with large doses of vitamin E. They are cardiovascular diseases, sterility, muscular dystrophy and diabetes. Large dose of vitamin E are also used to protect from aging and to improve athletic performance in running and other related events. However most of these beneficial effects of vitamin E lacks evidence.

1. Modified Vitamin E (α-tocopheryl Succinate, α-TOS) is a proapoptic agent. It induces apoptosis. It is antineoplastic agent.
2. Mixed tocopherols inhibit platelet aggregation in humans.
3. Vitamin E along with selenium are used to prevent prostate cancer.

Toxicity

Because of false claims like large dose of vitamin E improves sexual powers, halts aging process and athletic performance self medication with mega doses of vitamin E leads to toxicity. Symptoms of vitamin E toxicity (though it is rare) are clotting disorders, abnormal lipid profiles and decreased thyroxine level in blood.

VITAMIN K

Chemistry

The term vitamin K refers to group of compounds that exhibits vitamin K activity. They are (*a*) Vitamin K_1 also called as phylloquinone is the major form of vitamin found in plants particularly in green leafy vegetables. (*b*) Vitamin K_2 also known as menaquinone is the vitamin K present in animals and synthesized by intestinal flora. They are derivatives of naphthoquinone and differ in side chain. Phylloquinone contain phytylside chain where as menaquinone contains polyisoprenoid side chain made up of 7 isoprene units (Figure 23.12). Several variants of vitamin K_2 containing more than 7 isoprenoid units in the side chain are also identified.

Menadione is a synthetic analog of vitamin K. It is also called as vitamin K_3. It lacks characteristic side chain present in vitamin K_1 and K_2 (Figure 23.12). It is converted to vitamin K_2 by alkylation in the body.

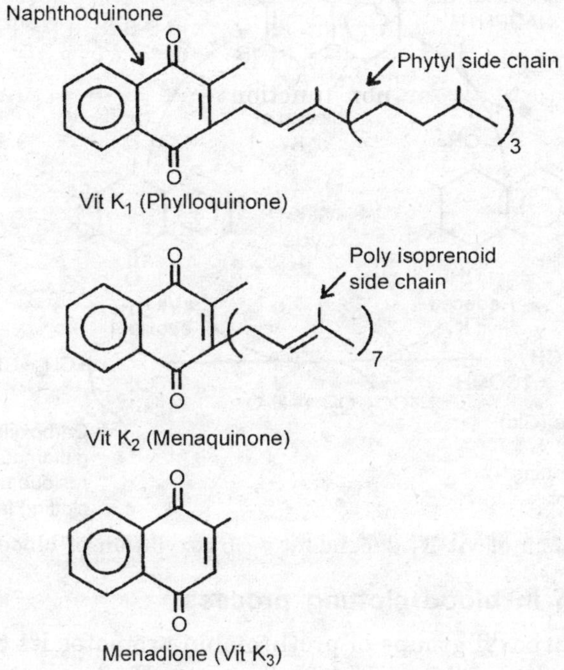

Fig. 23.12 Structures of vitamin K

Absorption and Transport

Vitamin K of dietary origin is absorbed in small intestine in presence of bile salts. In mucosal cells of intestine absorbed vitamin K is incorporated into chylomicrons. It reaches liver after entering circulation through the lymph. Liver distributes vitamin K to other tissues. It rarely accumulates in liver and peripheral tissues.

Functions of Vitamin K

1. Vitamin K is required for the synthesis of blood clotting factors like prothrombin (factor II), proconvertin or cothromboplastin (factor VII), stuarts factor (factor IX) and christamas factor (factor X). It is involved in the post translational modifications of these factors. It is required for the carboxylation of the γ-carbon atom of glutamic residues of these factors. The γ-carboxylation generates calcium binding sites which is essential for blood clotting process.

Mechanism of Vitamin K_1 dependent γ-carboxylation

It occurs in endoplasmic reticulum of liver cells. A carboxylase adds CO_2 to γ-carbon atom of glutamate (Glu) to form γ-carboxylated glutamate (Gla). In this reaction reduced vitamin

K_1 act as a CO substrate and gets converted to vitamin K_1 epoxide. O_2 is also required for this reaction. Reduced vitamin K_1 is regenerated from vitamin K_1 epoxide by an epoxide reductase using R-SH as hydrogen donor. Vitamin K_1 quinone is an intermediate in this conversion process. A monooxygenase which converts reduced vitamin K_1 to epoxide is also identified. However, the function of this conversion is yet to be known (Figure 23.13).

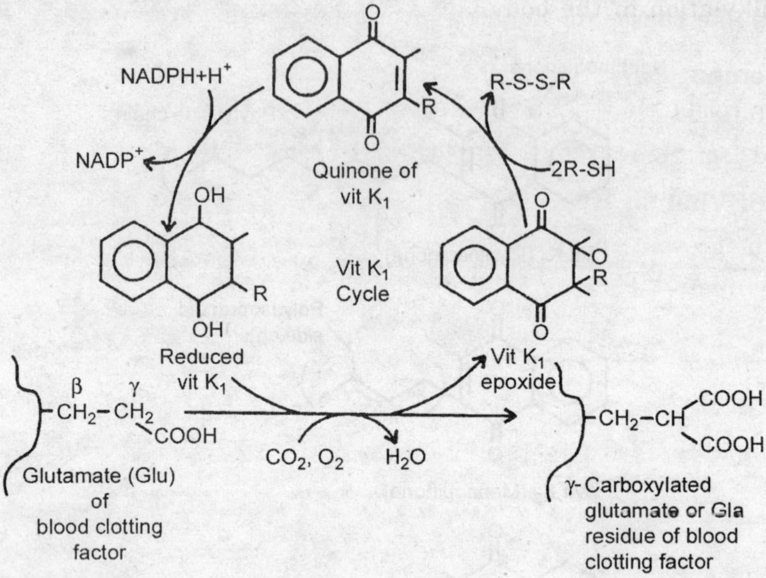

Fig. 23.13 Mechanism of vit K_1 dependent γ-carboxylation of blood clotting factors

Role of γ-carboxylation in blood clotting process

Binding of calcium to γ-carboxyl groups of prothrombin promotes its conversion to thrombin by blood clotting factors during blood clotting process. However the part of prothrombin which is carboxylated is eliminated during activation.

2. Vitamin K is also required for the γ-carboxylation of glutamate residues of another calcium binding protein osteocalcin in bone. This carboxylation is also catalyzed by vitamin K dependent carboxylase.

Deficiency Symptoms of vitamin K

1. Haemorrhage in the new born is most common vitamin K deficiency symptom. It occur in one out of 400 new borns particularly in premature infants. It may be due to low vitamin K storage level or insufficient intestinal flora. In new born vitamin K deficiency gives rise to increased prothrombin time. This leads to uncontrolled bleeding through nose (epitaxis) and gastrointestinal tract. However it can be treated successfully with intra muscular injections of vitamin K.
2. In adults vitamin K deficiency rarely occurs. However prolonged use of antibiotics may cause vitamin K deficiency due to elimination of intestinal flora.

Biochemical Symptoms of vitamin K deficiency

Hypoprothrombinemia is the major symptom. However proconvertin level also found decreased.

Sources

Plant Sources

Cauliflower, Cabbage, spinach, turnip greens, peas and soybean are rich sources. Rice, whole wheat, oats, tomatoes, peaches, banana and potato contain small amounts.

Animal sources

Dairy products like cheese, butter and farm products like eggs and liver are good sources.

Daily Requirement

Adults. 70-140 μg/day.

Pregnancy and lactation : 150-200 μg/ day.

Antagonists of Vitamin K

1. Dicoumarol present in spoiled sweet cloves is a vitamin K antagonist. It is used as anticoagulant to prevent thromboembolism.
2. Warfarin is another antagonist of vitamin K. It is a derivative of dicoumarol (Figure 23.14).

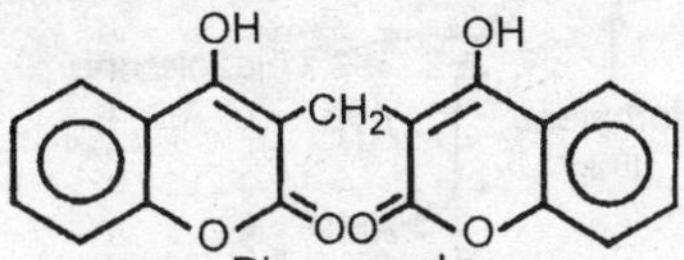

Dicoumarol

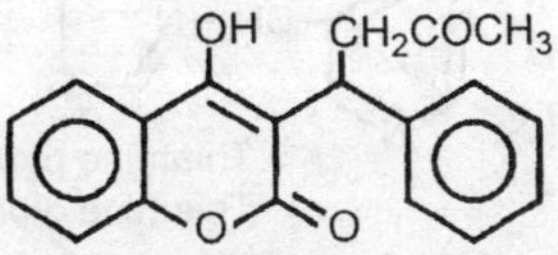

Warfarin

Fig. 23.14 Structures of vit K. antagonists

Dicoumarol and warfarin inhibits epoxide reductase that converts vitamin K epoxide to reduced vitamin K. As a result γ-carboxylation of blood clotting factors is blocked.

3. Salicylates also antagonize vitamin K action.

Toxicity

Is rare in adults. However excessive administration of vitamin K to premature infants produces hemolysis.

WATER SOLUBLE VITAMINS

VITAMIN B COMPLEX

Members of vitamin B complex are (1) Thiamin (Vitamin B_1) (2) Riboflavin (Vitamin B_2) (3) Niacin (4) Pyridoxine (Vitamin B_6) (5) Biotin (6) Folic acid (7) Cyanocobalamin (Vitamin B_{12}) and (8) Pantothenic acid.

THIAMIN

Chemistry

It is a heat labile sulfur containing vitamin. It contains pyrimidine ring and thiazole ring which are joined by methylene bridge (Figure 23.15). It is highly alkaline sensitive.

Absorption and Transport

It is absorbed in small intestine by active transport mechanism and simple diffusion. Then it reaches liver through circulation.

Function

Thiamin pyrophosphate (TPP or TDP) is the active form of thiamin. It is formed from thiamin in presence of ATP in a reaction catalyzed by thiamin kinase present in liver (Figure 23.15).

1. TPP is the prosthetic group of enzymes involved in oxidative decarboxylation of ketoacids like pyruvate dehydrogenase, α-keto glutarate dehydrogenase etc. The role of TPP in pyruvate dehydrogenase reaction is detailed in chapter-9.
2. TPP is also prosthetic group of transketolase reaction of HMP shunt. In this reaction TPP act as carrier of ketol group. Ketol bound TPP is shown in Figure 23.15.

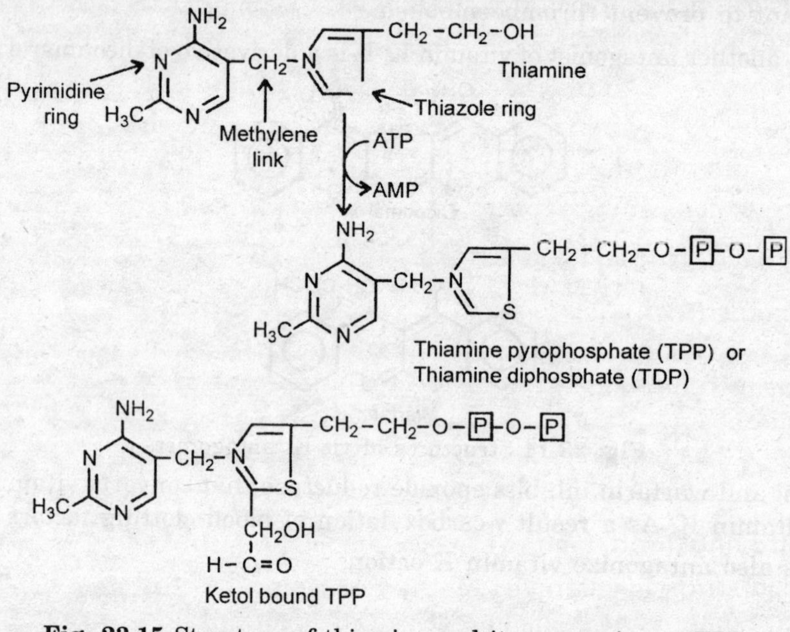

Fig. 23.15 Structure of thiamine and its conversion to TPP
Ketol bound TPP an intermediate in transketolase reaction is also shown

Thiamine Deficiency

Thiamine deficiency is reported from South East Asian countries where consumption of polished rice is common.

1. **Adult beriberi.** In adults thiamine deficiency causes beri beri (I can't, I can't). Early signs of beri beri are insomnia, headache, dizziness, loss of appetite, muscle weakness, numbness and pricking sensation in lower limbs and fatigue. If not treated it leads to
   (*a*) **Wet beri beri.** In which cardiovascular system is affected and it is characterized by edema. Edema appears in lower limbs, trunk, face and serous cavities. Blood pressure becomes abnormal. Heart becomes weak and death occurs due to heart failure.

(b) **Dry beri beri.** In which central nervous system is affected. In addition to early signs severe muscle wasting occurs. As a result individual is unable to walk and becomes bed ridden. Death may occur if not treated.

2. **Infantile beri beri.** In infants thiamine deficiency causes infantile beri beri. It occurs in infants between 2-10 months of age. Wet and dry infantile beri beri are known.
3. **Wernicke-Kor Sakoff syndrome.** Thiamine deficiency in chronic alcoholics gives rise to this syndrome. Symptoms are irregular eye and leg movement, polyneuritis and memory disturbances.
4. In birds and experimental animals thiamine deficiency causes polyneuritis. Birds are unable to fly.

Biochemical Symptoms

Transketolase is less active. Blood pyruvic acid level is high. Lactic acidosis after muscular exercise is common. Blood pyruvate and lactate levels are elevated after ingestion of glucose.

Sources

Rich Sources. Outer coatings of food grains like rice, wheat and yeast.

Good sources. Whole cereals, pulses, oilseeds and nuts.

Fair sources. Meat, liver and egg and fish.

Daily Requirement (RDA)

Since thiamine is essential for carbohydrate metabolism, daily requirement of thiamine depends on carbohydrate content of food. In South East Asian countries where most of the population obtain about 70% of their energy from carbohydrate an intake of about 0.4 mg of thiamine/1000 C has been recommended. So a sedentary worker requires approximately 1-1.2 mg of thiamine per day. It is a round 2 mg for heavy worker.

Thiamine destroying food factors

Thiamine of food stuffs is destroyed by thiaminase present in some fish and Japanese intestinal flora. Some plant foods and sea foods also contain thiamine destroying factors.

Antagonists

Oxythiamine and pyrithiamine are antagonist of thiamine. They are used to produce thiamine deficiency in experimental animals.

RIBOFLAVIN

Chemistry

It contains heterocyclic isoalloxazine ring and ribitol a sugar alcohol (Figure 23.16). It is sensitive to light and alkali but stable to heat and acidic medium.

Absorption and Transport

Absorbed in small intestine and distributed to all tissues by circulation.

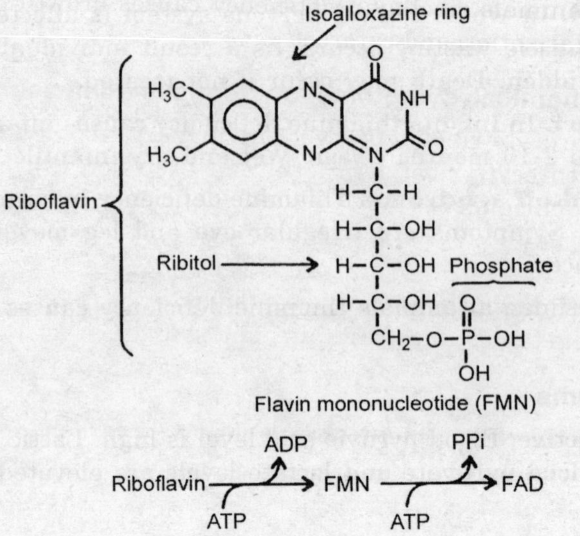

Fig. 23.16 Structure of riboflavin, FMN and formation of FAD

Functions

Active forms of riboflavin are FMN and FAD. They act as prosthetic groups of several enzymes. FMN is flavin mononucleotide (Figure 23.16) and FAD is flavin adenine dinucleotide.

Synthesis of FMN and FAD

In small intestinal cells a flavokinase catalyzes the formation of FMN from riboflavin by using ATP as phosphate donor. This is followed by transfer of AMP from another ATP to FMN to form FAD (Figure 23.16).

Enzymes containing FMN or FAD as prosthetic group are called as flavoenzymes (flavoproteins). As mentioned in Chapter -11 the flavoenzymes catalyzes oxidation-reduction reactions. FMN or FAD act as carriers of hydrogen atoms in such reactions. Isoalloxazine ring participates in oxidation reduction of substrates.

Some FMN requiring enzymes are a L-amino acid oxidase (b) NADH-CoQ reductase. FAD requiring enzymes are a D-amino acid oxidase (b) Succinate dehydrogenase (c) Acyl-CoA dehydrogenase.

Riboflavin Deficiency

1. In humans riboflavin deficiency causes oral, facial, occular lesions and scrotal and vulval lesions.

   Oral, facial and occular lesions are

   (*a*) **Angular Stomatitis.** Lesions of mouth particularly at corners of mouth.

   (*b*) **Cheliosis.** Red swollen and cracked lips.

   (*c*) Dermatitis of nasolabial region.

   (*d*) Vascularization of cornea and conjuctiva and blood shot eyes.

   (*e*) **Glossitis.** Inflammated magenta coloured tongue.

(*f*) Scrotal and vulval lesions are scrotal dermatitis and urogenital lesions.

2. In experimental animals riboflavin deficiency causes growth retardation, corneal and conjuctival vascularization and cataract.

Diagnosis and biochemical symptoms of riboflavin deficiency

Measurement of erythrocyte riboflavin level and urinary riboflavin are used to detect riboflavin deficiency. Erythrocyte riboflavin level and excretion of riboflavin in urine are decreased in riboflavin deficiency.

Sources

Whole grains, legumes, dhals, green leafy vegetables, yeast, eggs, milk and organ meats are good sources. Root vegetables and fruits are fair sources.

Daily Requirement

Like thiamine riboflavin requirement also depends on carbohydrate intake or calorie requirement. A sedentary adult worker needs 1.3 mg/ day. It is about 1.8 mg/day for heavy worker.

NIACIN

Chemistry

The word niacin refers to two pyridine derivatives. They are nicotinic acid and nicotinamide (Figure 23.17). Both are highly stable to heat and stable to alkali and acid.

Absorption and transport

Nicotinic acid and nicotinamide are absorbed in small intestine and reach various tissues through circulation where they are converted to NAD and NADP.

Functions

1. Nicotinamide is component of two coenzymes NAD and NADP. NAD is nicotinamide adenine dinucleotide and NADP is nicotinamide adenine dinucleotide phosphate (Figure 23.17).

Synthesis of NAD and NADP

Dietary nicotinic acid is first converted to nicotinic acid ribose phosphate by phosphoribosyl transferase using ATP which is then converted to NAD by the pathway described for the synthesis of niacin from tryptophan (Chapter 12). A cytoplasmic kinase converts NAD to NADP using ATP as phosphate donor (Figure 23.17).

Both NAD and NADP are co-enzymes of several dehydrogenases which catalyzes oxidation reduction reactions. NAD and NADP act as carriers of hydrogen groups in such reactions. The pyridine ring participates in oxidation reduction of substrates (Chapter 11).

Some NAD requiring enzymes are (*a*) Glyceraldehyde-3-phosphate dehydrogenase (*b*) Malate dehydrogenase (*c*) β-hydroxy acyl-CoA dehydrogenase.

Some NADP requiring enzymes are (*a*) glucose-6-phosphate dehydrogenase (*b*) Glutathione reductase (*c*) Malic enzyme.

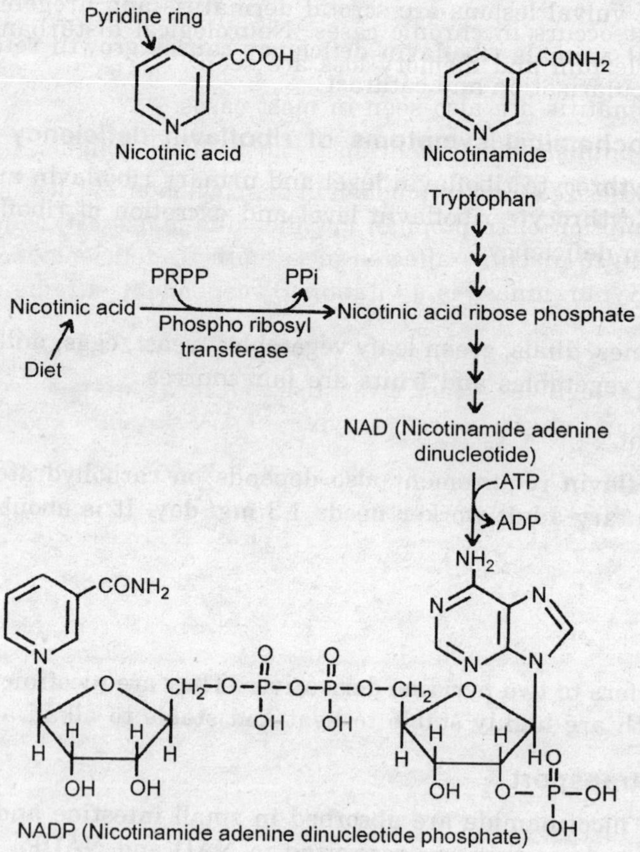

Fig. 23.17 Structures of nicotinic acid and niacinamide. Formation of NAD (P) from dietary nicotinic acid and tryptophan is also shown

Niacin Deficiency

1. It is common in countries where diet of low income group consist of maize only. It is classical nutritional deficiency disease with worldwide distribution. Niacin deficiency in man causes pellagra in which skin, gastrointestinal tract and nervous system are affected. Hence dermatitis, diarrhoea and dementia are characteristic symptoms of pellagra. It is prevalent once in Andhra Pradesh particularly in rocky Deccan plateau. Usually pellagra occurred in maize consuming population of India. But in Deccan plateau it occurred in populations consuming Sorghum (Jower). This conditional niacin deficiency is due to high leucine content in Jower. The excess leucine alters activities of enzymes of tryptophan-niacin pathway. As a result formation of nicotinamide nucleotide from tryptophan is inhibited. This pellagra is not confined to maize eaters but occurs even in sorghum eaters.

   (*a*) **Dermatitis.** It occurs in light exposed areas of skin due to photosensitivity. Initially exposed areas of skin develops sunburn which then progress to pigmentation and ulceration. The most affected areas are neck, forearms and fingers.

   (*b*) **Diarrhoea.** It occurs due to inflammation of mucous membranes of gastrointestinal tract. If it prolongs death may occur.

(c) **Dementia.** It occurs in chronic cases. Neurological disturbances like depression, headache, delerium and memory loss are seen.

2. Glossitis and stomatitis are also seen in most cases.
3. In experimental animals niacin deficiency causes black tongue.

Since niacin is synthesized from tryptophan in man (Chapter 12) disturbances in tryptophan metabolism or consumption of tryptophan low diet like maize can cause niacin deficiency. Tryptophan conversion to niacin is affected in vitamin B_6 deficiency because kynureninase reaction is blocked. Kynureninase is a vitamin B_6 dependent enzyme.

Sources

Whole grains, peanuts, legumes, yeast, liver, fish and meat are good sources. Milk and egg are poor source of niacin but rich source of tryptophan. Vegetables and fruits are poor source of niacin.

Daily Requirement (RDA)

Adults. 15-20 mg/day.

Antagonists

Acetyl pyridine, pyridine sulfonamide and Aminonicotinamide are some of niacin antagonists.

PYRIDOXINE

Chemistry

Three compounds derived from pyridine show vitamin B_6 activity. They are pyridoxine, pyridoxal and pyridoxamine (Figure 23.18). Pyridoxine is stable to heat and sensitive to light and alkali.

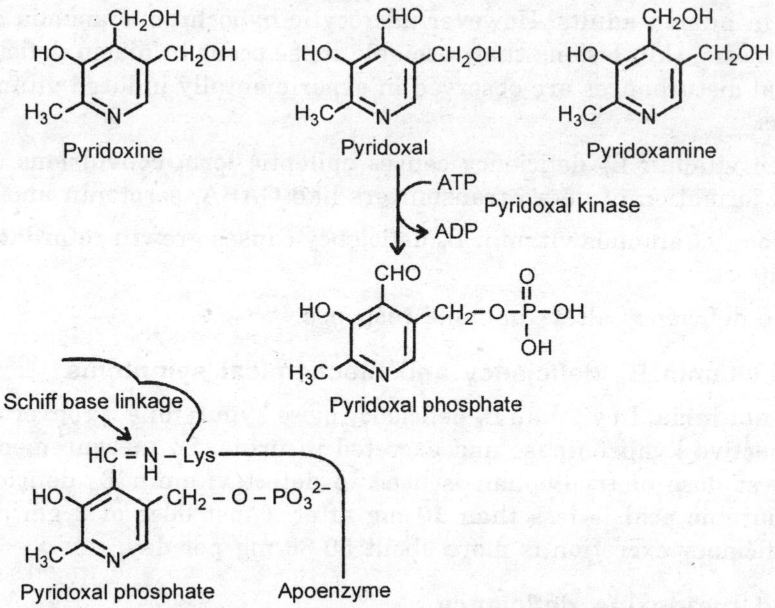

Fig. 23.18 Structures of vit. B_6. Formation of pyridoxal phosphate and its attachement to apo enzyme through schiff base linkage are also shown

Absorption and Transport

Pyridoxine is easily absorbed and reaches various tissues through circulation. In the tissues pyridoxine is converted to pyridoxal and pyridoxamine.

Functions

Pyridoxal phosphate is active form. It is formed from pyridoxal by phosphorylation catalyzed by pyridoxal kinase (Figure 23.18). Tissues also contain pyridoxamine phosphate in small amounts.

Pyridoxal phosphate act as prosthetic group or co enzyme of enzymes which are involved in transamination, decarboxylation, transsulfuration, desulfuration and non-oxidative deamination reactions. Pyriodoxal phosphate is coenzyme for enzymes that are involved in the synthesis of heme, serotonin, catecholamines and coenzyme A synthesis.

1. Pyridoxal phosphate is the prosthetic group of transminases. It is attached to lysyl residue of apoprotein through a Schiff base linkage (Figure 23.18).
2. Pyridoxal phosphate is co-enzyme of glutamate decarboxylase (Chapter - 12) which converts glutamate to γ-aminobutyrate (GABA). Other decarboxylases are dopa decarboxylase and hydroxy tryptophan decarboxylase.
3. Pyridoxal phosphate is a co-enzyme of cystathionine synthase, cystathionine lyase, serine trans hydroxy methylase, serine dehydratase, cysteine desulfhydrase, kynureninase, ALA synthase etc.
4. Phosphorylase of glycogenolysis also contain pyridoxal phosphate.
5. Pyridoxine lowers plasma homocysteine concentration in patients with coronary artery disease.

Pyridoxine Deficiency

1. It is rare in human adults. However microcytic hypochromic anemia due to decreased heme synthesis, skin lesions that resemble those occur in niacin deficiency, depression and mental disturbances are observed in experimentally induced vitamin B_6 deficiency in humans.
2. In children vitamin B_6 deficiency causes epileptic form convulsions (seizures) due to decreased formation of neuro transmitters like GABA, serotonin and catecholamines.
3. In experimental animals vitamin B_6 deficiency causes growth retardation, skin lesions, convulsions etc.
4. Pyridoxine deficiency alters immune response.

Diagnosis of vitamin B_6 deficiency and biochemical symptoms

Xanthurenic aciduria. In vitamin B_6 deficiency more kynurenine is converted to xanthurenic acid due to inactive kynureninase and excreted in urine. So measurement of xanthurenic acid after a test dose of tryptophan is used to detect vitamin B_6 deficiency. In normals urinary xanthurenic acid is less than 10 mg after a test dose of 2 gm of tryptophan. In pyridoxine deficiency excretion is more about 50-60 mg per day.

Drug induced pyridoxine deficiency

Several drugs when used for prolonged periods induce vitamin B_6 deficiency in humans. Most of them act as antagonists of vitamin B_6.

(*a*) **Isoniazid or isonicotinic acid hydrazine (INH) :** It is an anti tuberculosis drug. It forms a hydrazone complex with pyridoxal phosphate which is an inhibitor of pyridoxal kinase. This results in decreased level of pyridoxal phosphate thus leading to convulsions. Cycloserine another anti tuberculosis drug also produces neurological symptoms.

(*b*) **Pencillamine :** It is used in treatment of arthritis and Wilsons disease. It forms complex with pyridoxal phosphate thus leading to deficiency.

(*c*) Oral contraceptives and excessive alcohol consumption also cause pyridoxine deficiency.

Sources

Whole grains, legumes, liver and yeast are good sources. Leafy vegetables, milk, meat and eggs are fair sources.

Daily requirement (RDA)

Adults. 2-2.5 mg/day

BIOTIN

Chemistry

It is a sulfur containing vitamin. It consist of imidozole ring fused to tetrahydro thiophene with valeric acid side chain (Figure 23.19). It is stable to heat but alkaline sensitive.

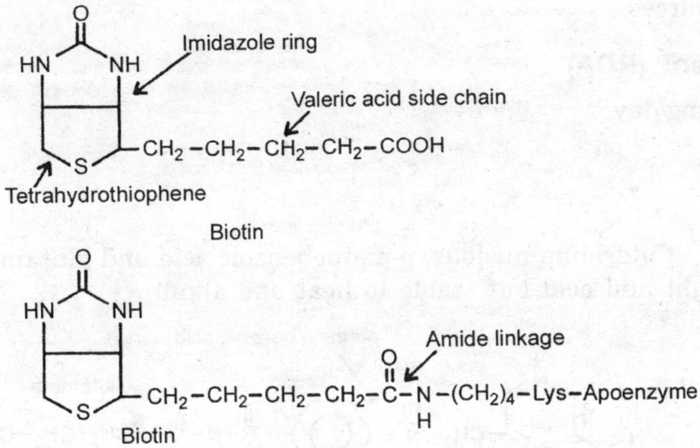

Fig. 23.19 Structure of biotin and its attachment to apoenzyme through ε-amino group of lysyl residue

Absorption and transport

It is absorbed in the small intestine and reaches liver and other tissues through circulation.

Function

Biotin is prosthetic groups of several carboxylases like pyruvate carboxylase, acetyl-CoA carboxylase, propionyl-CoA carboxylase etc. Biotin is attached to ε-aminogroups of lysyl residue of apoenzyme through, amide linkage (Figure 23.19). In carboxylation reaction it acts as a carrier of co_2 (see chapter 12).

Biotin deficiency

1. Biotin deficiency is rare in humans because it is present in most of the common foods.
2. However experimentally induced biotin deficiency, symptoms in man are dermatitis, alopecia, depression, muscular pain and anemia.
3. In experimental animals biotin deficiency produces extensive dermatitis and neurological problems.
4. Biotin deficiency in breast fed infants causes exofoliative dermatitis. It is due to low biotin content of breast milk.

Biochemical symptom

Propionic acidemia occurs in biotin deficiency.

Antagonist of biotin

Avidin a glycoprotein present in egg white combines with biotin to form a complex. One molecule of avidin combines with 3 molecules of biotin. The avidin-biotin complex is not absorbed by intestine. This leads to biotin deficiency. Adults who consumes 4-10 raw eggs are prone to biotin deficieny.

Dietary sources

Whole cereals, legumes, groundnuts, milk, meat and fish are good sources. Vegetables and fruits are fair sources.

Daily requirement (RDA)

Adults. 0.1-0.2 mg/day.

FOLIC ACID

Chemistry

Folic acid consist of pteridine nucleus, p-aminobenzoic acid and glutamate (Figure 23.20). It is sensitive to light and acid but stable to heat and alkali.

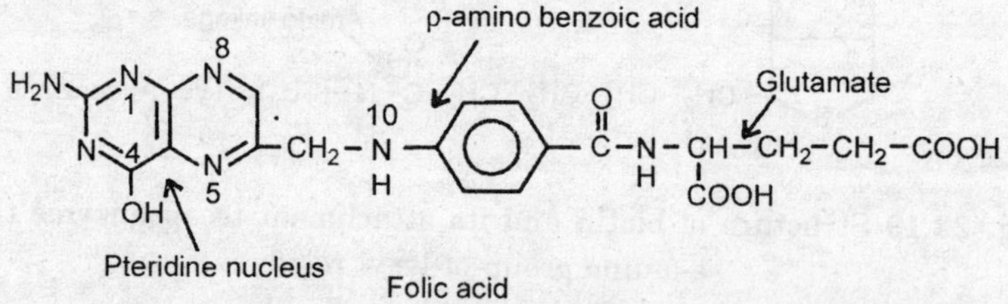

Fig. 23.20 Structure of folic acid

Absorption and transport

Folic acid present in natural foods contain more glutamate (up to 7) residues and it is called as folyl polyglutamate. In the intestinal mucosal cells a lysosomal folyl polyglutamate hydrolase removes excess glutamate residues to form folic acid which is reduced to tetrahydrofolate and methylated to N^5 - methyl tetrahydrofolate. Methyl tetrahydrofolate is the major circulating form probably bound to protein. Liver and other tissues take up circulating methyl tetrahydrofolate and converts to polyglutamate form after the transfer of methyl group (Figure 23.21).

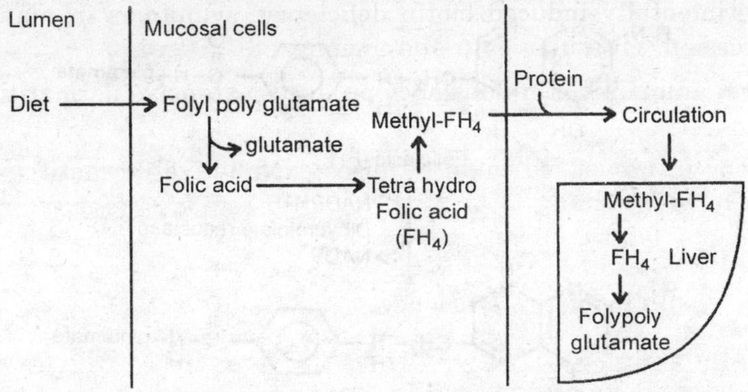

Fig. 23.21 Absorption, transport and fate of folic acid

Function

Tetrahydrofolate or FH_4 which is reduced form of folic acid is carrier of one carbon units.

1. Folic acid prevents neural tube defects (NTD) that occur during fetal development.
2. Defective folate metabolism impairs neural tube closure during development.
3. Folic acid is effective in lowering plasma homocysteine concentration in patients with coronary artery disease.

Synthesis of FH_4

An enzyme dihydrofolate reductase reduces folic acid to FH_4 in two steps using NADPH as hydrogen donor (Figure 23.22). In the first step folic acid is reduced to dihydrofolic acid which is then reduced to FH_4 in second step.

One carbon units carried by FH_4 are methyl (—CH_3), methylene (—CH_2—) methenyl (=CH—), formyl (—CHO), formimino (—CHNH) and formate (—COOH) groups. Formation, inter conversions and utilization of various one carbon derivative of FH_4 is described in chapter-12 under one carbon metabolism subhead. Usually in catabolic pathway one carbon derivative of FH_4 is generated which donates its one carbon unit in a anabolic pathway later.

Folic Acid Deficiency

1. In man megaloblastic anaemia is the main symptom of folic acid deficiency. It is most common in pregnant women and in unweaned children. Since folic acid is required for the synthesis of DNA through nucleotides particularly TMP formation, rapidly dividing cells like bone marrow or erythropoietic cells or intestinal cells are most affected in folic acid deficiency. Hence megaloblastic anaemia is the main symptom of folic acid deficiency. Other symptoms are

   (*a*) Leucopenia and macrocytic hyperchromic anaemia.

   (*b*) Thrombocytopenia.

   (*c*) Diarrhoea and weakness.

2. In experimental monkeys folic acid deficiency produces growth retardation, ulceration of colon and anaemia.

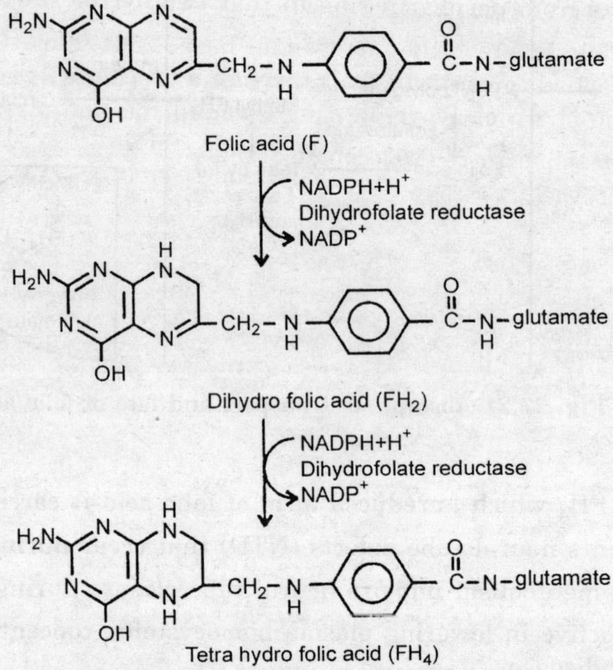

Fig. 23.22 Formation of FH_4 from folic acid (F)

Diagnosis of folic acid deficiency and biochemical symptom

Excretion of FIGLU a metabolite of histidine in urine is more in folic acid deficiency. Hence FIGLU excretion in urine after a test dose of histidine (histidine load test in Chapter - 12) is used to diagnose folic acid deficiency.

Sources

Green leafy vegetables like spinach, cabbage, ladiesfinger, curry and mint leaves, pulses like bengal gram, black gram, green gram, eggs and liver are good sources. Coconuts, whole cereals and milk are fair sources.

Daily Requirement (RDA)

Adults. 0.1 mg/day. Pregnant and lactating women needs 0.15 mg/day.

Antagonists

Use of folic acid analogs like aminopterin, amethopterin etc. is detailed in Chapter 15.

CYANOCOBALAMIN (VITAMIN B_{12})

Chemistry

It has complex chemical structure as shown in Figure 23.23. It is made up of (*a*) Tetrapyrrole ring system called as corrin ring with a central cobalt (Co) atom. Metal is held in centre by four coordinate bonds from N atoms of four pyrroles. Further the corrin ring differs from porphyrin ring in that two pyrroles are linked directly.

(*b*) Unusual nucleotiole in which the nitrogenous base is 5, 6–dimethyl benzimidazole. This nucleotide is attached to central cobalt through a coordinate bond from N of imidazole as well as to side chain of a pyrrole ring through the phosphate.

(*c*) A 'R' group is attached to central cobalt atom.

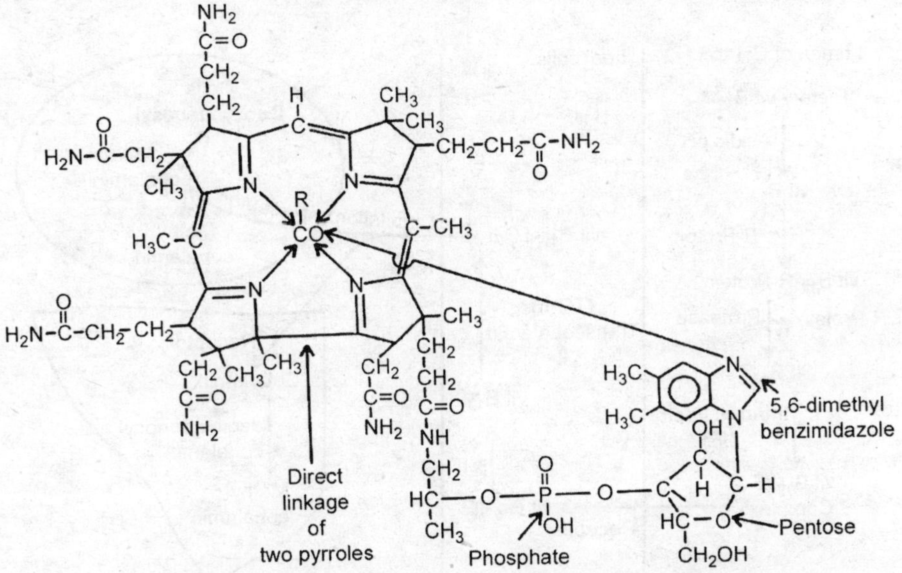

Fig. 23.23 Structure of vit B_{12} (C_{63} H_{88} N_{14} O_{14} PCO)

Various forms of vitamin B_{12} are named according to 'R' group attached to central cobalt atom.

(*a*) If 'R' group is cyanide (CN) then that form of vitamin B_{12} is called as cyanocobalamin.

(*b*) If 'R' group is hydroxyl (–OH) then that form of vitamin B_{12} is called as hydroxy cobalamin.

(*c*) If the 'R' group is methyl ($-CH_3$) then that form of Vitamin B_{12} is called as methyl cobalamin.

(*d*) If the 'R' group is deoxyadenosine then that form of vitamin B_{12} is called as deoxyadenosyl cobalamin.

All the above forms exhibit vitamin B_{12} activity. However most of the therapeutic preparations contain cyanocobalamin. Vitamin B_{12} is sensitive to light. Cyanocobalamin is heat labile.

Absorption and Transport

The absorption of vitamin B_{12} takes place in ileum. The dietary vitamin B_{12} which is bound to some substances dissociates at acidic P^H of stomach. Some kind of R-proteins present in stomach combines with the free vitamin B_{12} to form vitamin B_{12} – R protein complexes. In the duodenum pancreatic protease hydrolyzes vitamin B_{12} – R protein and vitamin B_{12} is released. This vitamin B_{12} combines with intrinsic factor a glycoprotein secreted by parietal cells of the stomach to form vitamin B_{12} intrinsic factor complex. One mg of intrinsic factor binds 3 mg of vitamin B_{12}. Through a receptor mediated mechanism vitamin B_{12} intrinsic factor complex is absorbed in the ileum. In the ileal cells the intrinsic factor is released and the vitamin B_{12} is transferred to a plasma transport protein transcobalamin II.

The transcobalamin II delivers vitamin B_{12} to tissues. The transcobalamin II vitamin B_{12} complex enters the cells through a specific cell surface receptor. In the cytosol of the cell cobalamin is released from transcobalamin II as hydroxycobalamin. In the cells hydroxy cobalamin is converted to methylcobalamin or deoxyadenosylcobalamin (Figure 23.24).

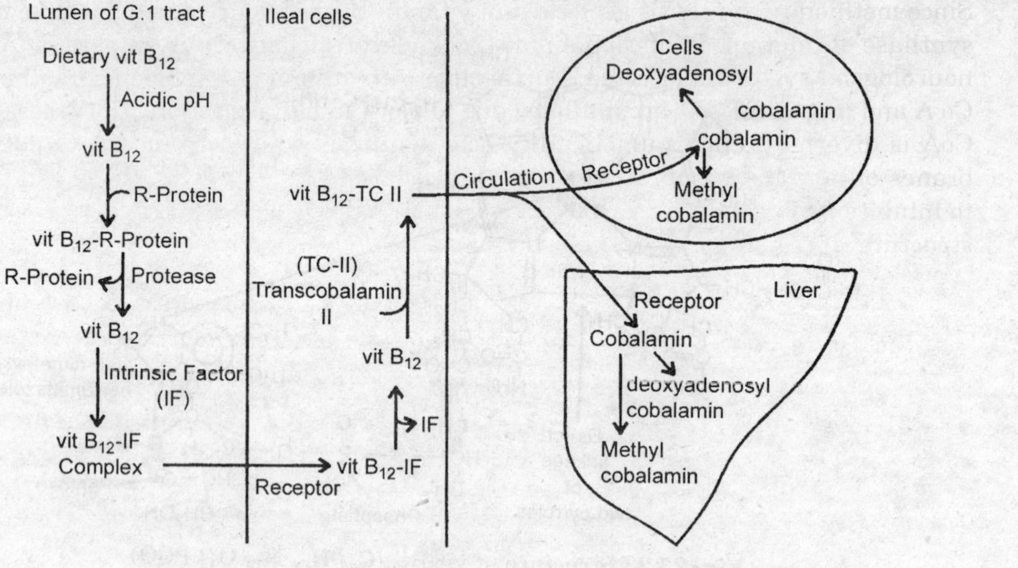

Fig. 23.24 Absorption, transport and fate of vit. B_{12}.

Transcobalamin I is another vitamin B_{12} transport protein present in plasma.

Storage

Unlike other water soluble vitamins vitamin B_{12} is stored in the liver and other tissues which is unique to vitamin B_{12}. The total body content of vitamin B_{12} is 3-4 mg. In the liver it is stored as deoxyadenosylcobalamin. Further liver cobalamins are secreted in the bile and undergo enterohepatic circulation.

Functions

(A) Vitamin B_{12} act as prosthetic group or coenzyme. Vitamin B_{12} coenzymes are called as cobamide coenzymes. Two forms of vitamin B_{12} that are required for activity of enzymes are A) Methylcobalamin or methylcobamide (MC). (B) Deoxyadenosylcobalamin or deoxyadenosylcobamide (DCA).

1. Methyl cobalamin is the coenzyme of methionine synthase (Chapter 12).
2. Deoxy adenosylcobalamin is the prosthetic group of methyl malonyl-COA mutase (Chapter 10).

(B) Vitamin B_{12} is effective in lowering concentration of plasma homocysteine of coronary artery disease patients.

Vitamin B_{12} Deficiency

1. Vitamin B_{12} deficiency affects bone marrow, intestinal tract and neurological system. In vitamin B_{12} deficiency these systems are affected because DNA synthesis, methionine synthesis and fatty acid synthesis are altered. Due to inactive methionine synthase formation FH_4 from methyl FH_4 is blocked in vitamin B_{12} deficiency. So all the FH_4 is trapped as methyl-FH_4 (folate trap). Since FH_4 is required for DNA synthesis erythropoiesis and gastrointestinal cells are affected in vitamin B_{12} deficiency. Bone marrow contains more megaloblasts. This megaloblastosis leads to anaemias (Figure 23.25).

   Since methionine synthesis is blocked in vitamin B_{12} deficiency due to inactive methionine synthase formation of phospholipids and neurotransmitters is impaired. As a result neurological system is affected. Furthermore in vitamin B_{12} deficiency methyl malonyl-Co A and propionyl-CoA accumulates due to block in mutase action. The excess propionyl-CoA is diverted to odd number fatty acid synthesis which are incorporated into membranes of nervous tissue. At the same time normal fatty acid synthesis is affected due to inhibition of acetyl-CoA carboxylase by methyl malonyl CoA. This disturbs the normal structure and function of nerves (Figure 23.25).

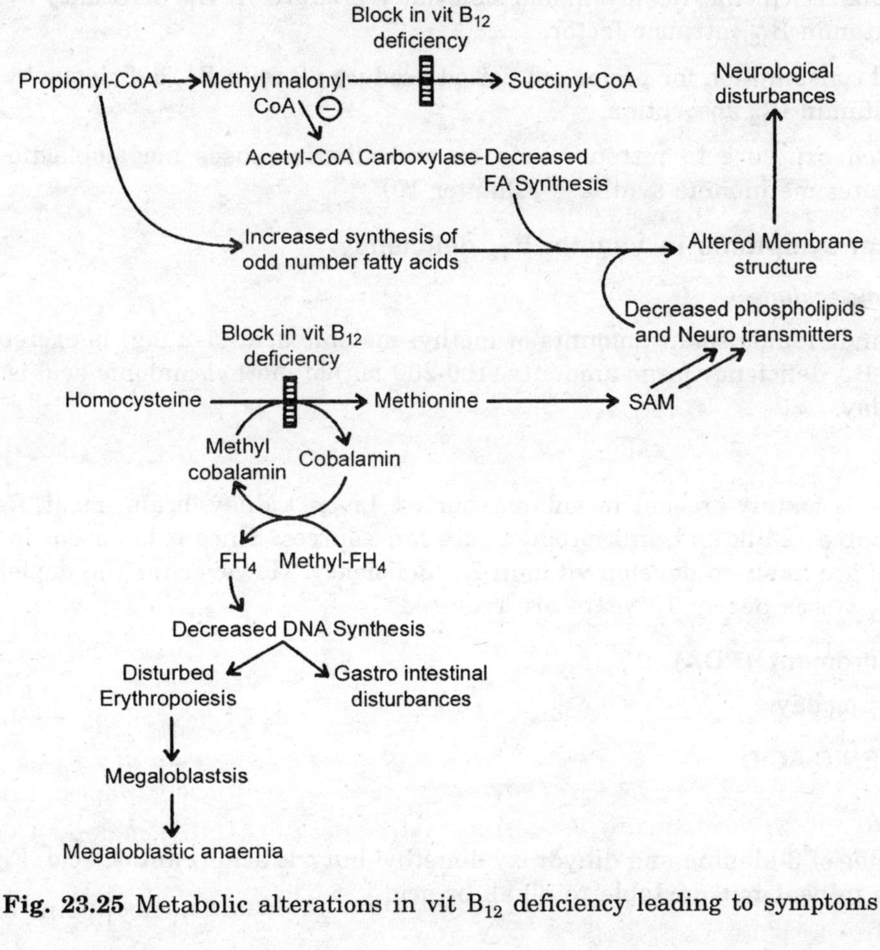

Fig. 23.25 Metabolic alterations in vit B_{12} deficiency leading to symptoms

Therefore the symptoms of vitamin B_{12} deficiency are

(*a*) Megaloblastic anaemia.

(*b*) Neurological disturbances or lesions mainly parasthesia (numbness and tingling sensation in hand and feet) and degeneration of spinal cord.

(*c*) Gastric atrophy and malabsorption.

(*d*) Glossitis (sore tongue).

2. Vitamin B_{12} deficiency due to lack of intrinsic factor gives rise to pernicious anaemia. In this condition also haematopoietic system, gastrointestinal system and nervous system are affected.

Folic acid and megaloblastic anemia

Since megaloblastic anemia that occurs in vitamin B_{12} deficiency is due to non availability of FH_4, folic acid administration cures megaloblastic anemia. However, neurological disturbances are not cured.

Drug induced vitamin B_{12} deficiency

1. Drugs like colchicine, neomycin and salicylates produce vit B_{12} deficiency by interacting with vitamin B_{12} intrinsic factor.
2. Alcohol consumption for prolonged period produce vitamin B_{12} deficiency by interfering with vitamin B_{12} absorption.
3. Repeated exposure to nitrous oxide an anaesthetic causes megaloblastic anemia. It inactivates methionine synthase (Chapter 10).

Biochemical symptoms in vitamin B_{12} deficiency

Methylmalonic aciduria

In normal individuals small amounts of methyl malonic acid (1-2 mg) is excreted per day. In vitamin B_{12} deficiency large amounts (100-200 mg) of methyl malonic acid is excreted in urine per day.

Sources

Vitamin B_{12} is mainly present in animal sources. Liver, kidney, brain, meat, fish and eggs are good sources. Milk and milk products are fair sources. Since it is absent in plant foods vegetarians are likely to develop vitamin B_{12} deficiency. However for the depletion of body vitamin B_{12} stores nearly 10 years are required.

Daily requirement (RDA)

Adults : 3-4 μg/day.

PANTOTHENIC ACID

Chemistry

It is an amide of β-alanine and dihydroxy dimethyl butyric acid (Pantoic acid, Figure 23.26). It is stable to heat but unstable to alkali or acid.

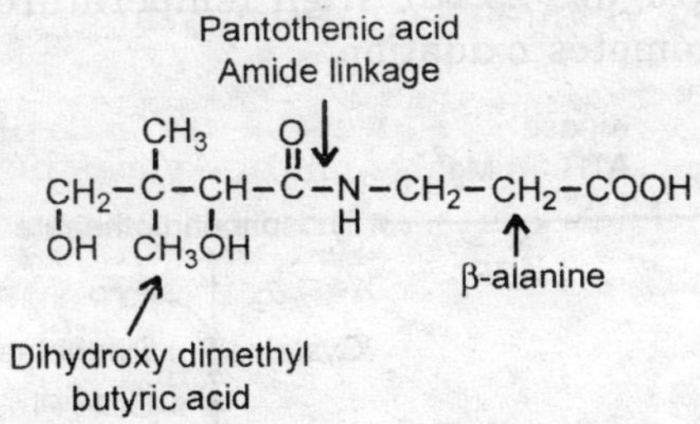

Fig. 23.26 Structure of Pantothenic acid

Absorption and transport

Intestinal phosphatases release pantothenic acid from dietary sources. Free pantothenate or its salts are freely absorbed in the intestine and reach various tissues through circulation.

Functions

1. Pantothenic acid is a component of coenzyme A. Coenzyme (CoA) participates in several enzymatic reactions of carbohydrate, lipid and amino acid metabolism.
2. Pantothenic acid is required for the synthesis of phosphopantotheine of fatty acid synthases complex. Phosphopantotheine of fatty acid synthase complex serve as carrier of acyl groups during fatty acid biosynthesis.

Synthesis of coenzyme A and phosphopantotheine

Synthesis of coenzyme A from pantothenic acid occurs in two stages. In the first stage phosphopantotheine is synthesized from pantothenicacid. This involves phosphorylation, cysteinylation and decarboxylation reactions (Figure 23.27). In the second stage coenzyme A is synthesized from phosphopantotheine by adenosylation and phosphorylation reactions (Figure 23.27).

Pantothenic acid deficiency

1. It is rare in humans. However, experimentally induced pantothenic acid deficiency produce parasthesia of extremities (burning feet), abdominal cramps, restlessness and fatigue in humans.
2. In experimental animals pantothenate deficiency produce dermatitis, graying of hair, fatty liver, growth failure and neurological lesions.

Sources

Organ meat, liver, milk, whole cereals, legumes and eggs are good sources. Vegetables and fruits are poor sources.

Daily requirement (RDA)

Adults : 4-6 mg/day.

VITAMIN C (ASCORBIC ACID)

Chemistry

It is a sugar acid known as hexuronic acid. Ascorbic acid is easily oxidized by atomospheric

O_2 to dehydroascarobic acid (Figure 23.28). High temperature (cooking) accelerates oxidation. Light and alkali also promotes oxidation.

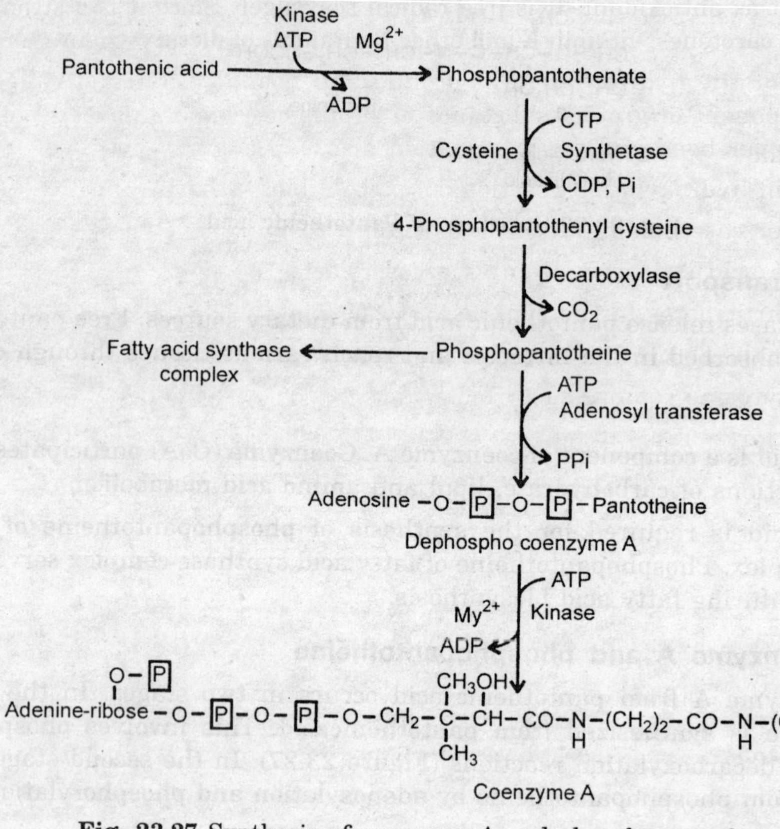

Fig. 23.27 Synthesis of coenzyme A and phosphopantotheine

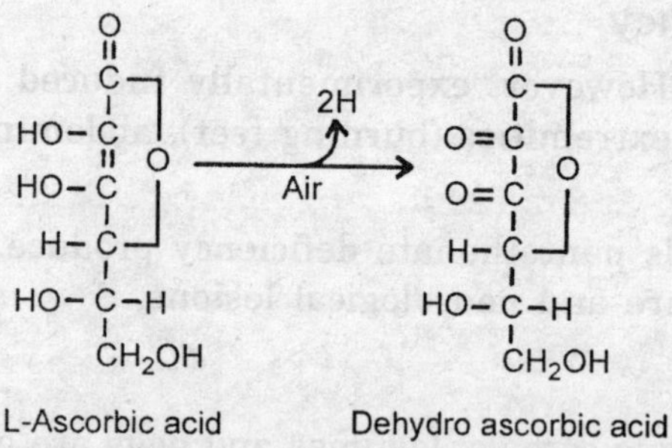

Fig. 23.28 Oxidation of ascorbic acid

Absorption and transport

Vitamin C is readily absorbed in the intestine by sodium dependent active transport mechanism and reaches various body tissues through circulation. Ascorbic acid enters various cells like erythrocytes, leucocytes etc. freely.

Functions

1. Ascorbic acid act as antioxidant. It is free radical scavenger. Since it is a strong reducing agent it protects carotenes, vitamin E and other B vitamins of dietary origin from oxidation.
2. It is required for the hydroxylation of proline and lysine residues of collagen. Since collagen is component of ground substance of capillaries, bone and teeth vitamin C is required for proper bone and teeth formation also.
3. It participates in hydroxylation reactions of steroid biosynthesis.
4. It is required for catecholamine synthesis from tyrosine.
5. In the liver bile acid synthesis requires ascorbic acid.
6. Ascorbic acid participates in the synthesis of carnitine.
7. It is required for the absorption of iron in the intestine. It maintains iron in ferrous form.
8. Catabolism of tyrosine requires ascorbic acid.
9. When given in large doses it reduces severity of cold. However evidence is lacking.
10. Vitamin C is effective in controlling bacterial invasion by inhibiting activity of bacterial hyaluronidase enzyme. It acts as inhibitor of this enzyme due to structural similarity to glucuronate of hyaluronin, the substrate of hyaluronidase.

Vitamin C deficiency

1. In adults deficiency of vitamin C causes scurvy. But it rarely occurs in normal people. The symptoms of scurvy are
   (*a*) Haemorrhages in various tissues particularly in inside of thigh, calf and forearm muscles. It may be due to capillary fragility.
   (*b*) General weakness and anaemia.
   (*c*) Swollen joints, swollen gums and loose tooth.
   (*d*) Susceptible for infections.
   (*e*) Delayed wound healing.
   (*f*) Bone fragility and osteoporosis.
2. Vitamin C deficiency in infants gives rise to infanitle scurvy. It occurs in weaned infants who are fed on diets low in vitamin C.

Diagnosis of vitamin C deficiency

Measurement of plasma ascorbic acid is used to assess ascorbic acid deficiency. In normal individuals plasma ascorbic acid ranges from 0.8-1.4 mg%. In vitamin C deficient individuals its level is below 0.7 mg%.

Sources

Amla (indian gooseberry), guava, coriander and amarnath leaves, and cabbage are rich sources. Fruits like lemon, orange, pineapple, papaya, mango and tomato are good sources. Apples, bananas and grapes are fair sources.

Daily requirement (RDA)

Adults : 60-80 mg/day.

Therapeutic uses

Large doses of Vit C are used to treat common cold, soft tissue infections. Since it is an antioxidant it reduces incidence of cancer, cardiovascular diseases and act as anti aging agent also.

REFERENCES

1. Wald, G. The molecular basis of visual excitation. Nature. **219**, 800-807, 1968.
2. Strader, C.D. Structure and function of G-protein coupled receptors. Ann. Rev. Biochem., **63**. 101-132, 1994.
3. Hargreave, P.A. and Mcdowell, H.M. Rhodopsin and phototransduction a model system for G-protein linked receptors. FASEB. J. **6**, 2322-2331, 1992.
4. Stryer, L. Cyclic GMP cascade of vision. Ann. Rev. Neuro Sci., **9**, 87-119, 1986.
5. Rando, R. R. Polyenes and Vision. Chemistry and Biology **3**, 255-262, 1996.
6. Deluca, H.F. and Schnoes, H.K. Vit. D recent advances. Ann. Rev. Biochem. **52,** 411, 1983.
7. Horwit, M.K. Therapeutic uses of vit E in medicine. Nutr. Rev. **38**, 105, 1980.
8. Benkovic, S.J. and Blakely, R.L. Folates and pterins. Vol. 1, Academic Press, New York, 1984.
9. Halpern, J. Mechanism of vit B_{12}–dependent rearrangements. Science. **227**, 869-875, 1985.
10. Kern *et al*. How thiamin diphosphate is activated in enzymes? Science. **275**, 67-70, 1997.
11. Ruma Benerjee. (Ed.). Chemistry and Biochemistry of B_{12}. J. Wiley, NewYork, 1999.
12. Zhang, K. and Rathod, R.K. Divergent regulation of Dihydrofolate reductase between malaria parasite and human host. Science. **296**, 545-547, 2002.
13. Berkovitch *et al*. Crystal structure of biotin synthase an S-adenosyl methionine dependent radical enzyme. Science. **303**, 76-79, 2004.
14. Gerald Combs. Jr. The vitamins : Fundamental aspects in nutrition and health. Academic Press, 1998.
15. Bouillion. Vitamin proceedings of the Twelfth work shop on vitamin-D. Elsevier, 2004.
16. Bohlke, K. *et al.* Vitamins-A, C and E and risk of breast cancer. Brit. J. Can. **79**, 23-29, 1999.
17. Birringer, M. *et al.* Vitamin E analogues as inducers of apoptosis structure function relationship. Brit. J. Can. **88**, 1948-1953, 2003.
18. Malila N. *et al.* Dietary and serum α-tocopherol, β-carotene and retinol and risk factor for colorectal cancer in male smokers. Eur. J. Clin. Nutr. **56**, 615-621, 2002.
19. Tovar, A.R. *et al.* Biochemical deficiency of pyridoxine does not affect interleukin production of lymphocytes. Eur J. Clin. Nutr. **56**, 1087-1093, 2002.
20. Weil, M. *et al.* Folic acid rescues nitric oxide induced neural tube closure defects. Cell death and Differ. **11**, 361-363, 2004.

21. John, M. Scott. How does folic acid prevent neural tube defects. Nature. Med. **4**, 895-896, 1998.

22. Lee, B.J. *et al.* Folic acid vitamin – B_{12} are more effective than vitamin B_6 in lowering fasting plasma homocysteine concentration in patients with coronary artery disease. Eur. J. Clin. Nutr. **58**, 481-487, 2004.

23. Flemming, A. and Coop, A.J. Embryonic folate metabolism and mouse neural tube defects. Science. **280**, 2107-2108, 1998.

24. Lewerin, C. *et al.* Reduction of plasma homocysteine and serum methyl malonate concentrations in healthy subjects after treatment with folic acid, vitamin B_{12} and vitamin B_6 Eur. J. Clin. Nutr. **57**, 1426-1436, 2003.

25. Liu, M. *et al.* Mixed tocopherols inhibit platelet aggregation in humans. Am. J. Clin. Nutr., **77**, 700-706, 2003.

26. Schuelke, M. *et al.* Urinary α-tocopherol metabolites in α-tocopherol transfer protein deficient patients. J. Lipid. Res. **41**, 1543-1551, 2000.

27. Li, S. *et al.* Vit. C inhibits the enzymatic activity of *S. pneumoniae* hyaluronate lyase. J. Biol. Chem. **276**, 15125-15130, 2001.

28. Tao, Li. *et al.* Identification of gene for vitamin-K epoxide reductase. Nature, **427,** 541-544, 2004.

29. Verboven, C. *et al.* A structural basis for the unique binding features of human vitamin D binding protein. Nat. Stru. Biol. **9,** 131-136, 2002.

30. Van Amerongen, B.M. *et al.* Multiple sclerosis and vitamin D and update. Eur. J. Clin. Nutr., **58**, 1095-1109, 2004.

31. Barker, M.E. *et al.* Serum retionoids and beta carotenes as predictors of hip and other fractures in eldlely women. J. Bone Minerals Res. **20**, 913-920, 2005.

EXERCISES

ESSAY QUESTIONS

1. Describe chemistry, functions, deficiency symptoms, sources and daily requirements of vit. A.
2. Describe chemistry, functions, deficiency symptoms, sources and daily requirements of vit. D.
3. Give an account of vit. K. Add a note on its antagonists.
4. Describe chemistry, functions, deficiency symptoms, sources and daily requirements of vit. C.
5. Describe chemistry, functions, deficiency symptoms, sources and daily requirements of sulfur containing vitamins.
6. Describe functions and deficiency symptoms of vitamin E and vitamin K.
7. Describe sulfur containing vitamins functions and deficiency symptoms.
8. Write coenzyme forms of riboflavin and niacin. Write four reactions showing coenzyme function. Name deficiency symptoms of these vitamins.
9. Write functions and sources of vitamin B_{12}, vitamin C and folic acid.
10. How folic acid coenzymes are formed and utilized? Add a note on clinical uses of folic acid analogs.

SHORT QUESTIONS

1. Define provitamins. Give examples. Write their conversion to vitamins.
2. Write riboflavin coenzyme form. Write two reactions along with cofactors in which it acts as coenzyme.
3. Write functions and deficiency symptoms of vit. E.
4. Explain role of vit. A in visual process.
5. Write mechanistics of vit. E antioxidant action.
6. Write pyridoxine and niacin coenzyme forms. Write a reaction for each with cofactors.
7. Name coenzyme forms of vit. B_{12}. Write deficiency symptoms of this vitamin.
8. How FH_4 is synthesized? Name one carbon units it carries.
9. Write biochemical symptoms in the deficiencies of the following vitamins : a. Pyridoxine b. Vitamin B_{12} c. Folic acid d. biotin.
10. Write briefly on anti-vitamins.
11. Write functions of ascorbic acid.
12. Write deficiency symptoms, daily requirements and sources of vitamin E.
13. Write a note on therapeutic uses of vitamins.
14. Explain symptoms of night blindness and rickets.
15. Write about vitamin binding proteins.
16. Name toxic effects of vitamins.
17. How calcitriol is formed? Write its importance and fate.
18. How FAD is synthesized? Write its coenzyme functions.
19. How NAD and FH_4 are synthesized? Write reactions in which they participate.
20. Name visual pigments. Write their biological roles.

MULTIPLE CHOICE QUESTIONS

1. All the following statements are true for fat soluble vitamins. Except.
   (*a*) They require bile salts for absorption.
   (*b*) They exist in provitamin form.
   (*c*) Liver is their storage site.
   (*d*) Soluble in organic solvents.
2. An example for vit A antagonist is
   (*a*) Citral. (*b*) Benzene.
   (*c*) Dehydroretinol. (*d*) Citric acid.
3. Which of the following is rich vit. E source
   (*a*) Vegetable oils. (*b*) Fruits.
   (*c*) Vegetables. (*d*) Meat.

4. A water soluble vitamin which is a component of coenzyme A is
   (*a*) Biotin.
   (*b*) Pantothenic acid.
   (*c*) Ascorbic acid.
   (*d*) Retinoic acid.
5. FIGLU excretion test is used to detect
   (*a*) Folic acid deficiency.
   (*b*) Biotin deficiency.
   (*c*) Pantothenic acid deficiency.
   (*d*) Vit B_{12} deficiency.

FILL IN THE BLANKS

1. Fat soluble vitamins which act as steroid hormone are.........and ....
2. Excess intake of vitamins leads to............... .
3. Cyanosin is................ containing pigment involved in.............. vision.
4. Daily requirement of vit E depends on.............. and .... content of diet.
5. Biotin is prosthetic group of............... enzymes.

24
CHAPTER

MINERALS

Minerals are inorganic substances. They are not synthesized in the body. Minerals required by the body are obtained through the food. Unlike carbohydrates, fats and proteins minerals do not produce energy. Since most of the minerals are water soluble they are easily absorbed and are excreted in urine and to a lesser extent in feces. About 20-30 g of minerals are excreted per day.

Based on the requirement minerals are divided into :

1. Bulk minerals (macro nutrients)
2. Trace minerals (micro nutrients).

1. **Bulk minerals.** Which are required in the diet in large amounts i.e. greater than 100 mg per day. They are sodium, potassium, chloride, calcium, phosphorous and magnesium. They represents 80% of body inorganic matter.
2. **Trace (minerals) elements.** Which are required in the diet in the small amounts i.e. less than 100 mg/day. They are iron, zinc, copper, iodine, fluorine, selenium, manganese, molybdenum, cobalt and chromium.

MEDICAL AND BIOLOGICAL IMPORTANCE

1. Minerals are present in body tissues and body fluids.
2. Minerals are necessary for the maintenance of physiochemical conditions like secretion of HCl in stomach, blood coagulation, bone matrix, membrane potential, bioluminescence and blood pressure which are essential for life.
3. Minerals are structural components of body soft tissues like liver, muscle etc. For example phospholipids are components of membrane structure.
4. Minerals participate in acid-base balance. Several minerals are components of blood buffers.
5. Minerals are integral parts of several physiologically important compounds like haemoglobin, hormones, cytochromes, iron sulfur proteins, vitamins, enzymes, bile salts, zinc finger proteins, phosphocreatine, nucleic acids and several metabolites.
6. Minerals participates in transport of gases in the body.
7. Minerals are required for several enzymatic reactions.

8. Deficient intake of minerals leads to diseases. In certain populations deficiency of calcium and iron are common. Goitre due to iodine deficiency is common in people living in hill regions in India and other parts of world.
9. In tropical countries iron deficiency occurs due to hookworm, roundworm infestations.
10. Conditions like malabsorption, gastroenteritis, cholera, vomiting and diarrhoea produce mineral deficiency.
11. Environment influences body mineral requirement. Hot climate in tropics like India increases mineral requirement due to loss of minerals in sweat.
12. Excess intake of some minerals leads to diseases. Fluorosis, hemosiderosis and hypertension are associated with excess intake of fluorine, iron and sodium chloride respectively.
13. Mineral metabolism is defective in some inherited diseases. For example Wilson's disease is due to defective copper metabolism.
14. Minerals mediates hormone action.
15. Calcium, phosphorus and magnesium are components of kidney stones, gall stones and pancreatic stones.
16. Minerals are involved in apoptosis.
17. Mineral deficiency is associated with diabetes and apoptosis.
18. Mineral act as chemo preventive agents of cancer.
19. Some minerals act as antioxidants.

Sodium

Human body contain about 150-200 gm of sodium. Soft tissues and bone contains half of it. Extracellular fluid contains rest of sodium.

Functions

1. It is the major cation of extracellular fluid.
2. It is involved in the maintenance of plasma volume and acid-base balance.
3. It is essential for nerve and muscle function.
4. It is required for the absorption of glucose and amino acids in the intestine and kidney.
5. It is required for the formation of bile salts.
6. It is required for the activity of Na^+ K^+-ATPase.

Deficiency and toxicity

Nutritional deficiency is rare. However several other conditions cause low serum sodium levels and excess sodium in body as well as in serum occurs in several diseases as mentioned below.

Normal serum sodium level is 140meq/L.

Hyponatremia

Sodium level in plasma and in other tissues decreases in this condition. It occurs in (*a*) Vomiting, diarrhoea (*b*) Chronic renal failure (*c*) Addison's disease.

Symptoms are low blood pressure and low plasma volume and circulatory failure.

Hypernatremia (toxicity)

Sodium level in plasma and in other tissue is increased in this condition. It occurs in

(*a*) Cushing syndrome (Hyper aldosteronism).

(*b*) Prolonged treatment with ACTH, cortisone and sex hormones.

(*c*) Water retention in body.

Symptoms are high blood pressure (hypertension) and increased plasma volume.

Sources

Pulses, meat, milk, eggs and salt (salted foods) are excellent sources. Vegetables and fruits are poor sources.

Daily requirement (RDA)

Adults. 1.5-3 gm/day.

Potassium

Human body contains about 250 gm of potassium. Most of it (90%) is present in various cells of body. Remaining is present in extracellular fluids.

Functions

1. It is the major cation of intracellular fluid.
2. It plays an important role in nerve-muscle function.
3. It is required for maintenance of plasma volume.
4. It is required for bile salt formation and for the activity of Na^+/K^+-ATPase.
5. It is required to store glycogen in liver and muscle. About 14 mg of potassium is required to store 1 gm of glycogen.
6. It is also required for growth of tissues.

Deficiency and toxicity

Normal serum potassium level is 3-5 meq/L. Nutritional deficiency of potassium is rare. However serum potassium level is decreased (hypokalemia) in many conditions and excess potassium in plasma (hyperkalemia) and in other tissues occurs in several diseases as mentioned below.

Hypokalemia

It occurs in (*a*) Vomiting, diarrhoea (*b*) Cushing syndrome (*c*) prolonged use of diuretics (*d*) During treatment with insulin and digitalis.

Symptoms are muscular weakness, tachycardia, heart enlargement, irritability and paralysis.

Hyperkalemia

It occurs in (*a*) Renal failure (*b*) Addison's disease (*c*) Severe dehydration. (*d*) Excess consumption of potassium salts.

Symptoms are weakness, numbness, paralysis of extremities, low heart sounds and cardiac arrest due to collapse of peripheral vasculature.

Sources

Pulses, oil seeds, eggs, milk, meat, vegetables and fruits are good sources.

Daily requirement (RDA)

Adult. 2-3 gm/day.

Chloride

Human body contains about 120-150 gm of chloride. It is present in major body fluids, soft tissues and erythrocytes. Its distribution among soft tissues varies. For example erythrocytes and nerves contain more than muscle. Bone also contains chloride.

Functions

1. It is the major extracellular anion.
2. It is required for the secretion of HCl, by parietal cells.
3. It is involved in maintenance of electrical neutrality of erythrocytes (chloride shift) and other cells.
4. It is required for maintenance of plasma volume.

Deficiency and toxicity

Nutritional deficiency is rare. Normal serum chloride level is 95-105 meq/L. Serum chloride level is found decreased (hypochloremia) and increased (hyperchloremia) in some diseases.

Hypochloremia

It occurs in (*a*) Prolonged vomiting, diarrhoea (*b*) Pyloric obstruction (*c*) Cholera or ulcerative colitis (*d*) AIDS (*e*) Sun stroke (*f*) Meningitis. Symptoms are muscular spasams (Miners cramps).

Hyper chloremia

It occurs in (*a*) Nephritis (*b*) Prostate enlargement (*c*) Cushing syndrome.

Sources

Pulses, milk, meat and eggs are good sources. Vegetables and fruits are poor sources. Salted foods are excellent sources.

Daily requirement

Adults. 1.5-3.5 gm/day.

Role of sodium, potassium and chloride in membrane potential, action potential and nerve impulse.

Membrane potential

Due to the unequal distribution of sodium, potassium and chloride ions between inside and outside of cell a difference in electrical potential exist between inside and outside of all types of animal cells. This is called as resting membrane potential which is around –70 to –90 mv. The resting potential is negative due to excess cations in outside of the cell. However the movement of these ions across membrane is mediated through special proteins known as ion channels. These ion channels are sensitive to voltage and some are sensitive to certain compounds known as ligands. Hence they are often called as voltage gated channels and ligand gated channels respectively.

Action potential

In nerve cells the resting membrane potential is disturbed when its plasma membrane is stimulated by a neurotransmitter. This leads to production of action potential. When axon membrane of nerve cell is excited by stimulus sodium channels present in membrane are opened and sodium enters into cell. As a result inside of axon becomes more positive and potential difference increases from -70 mv to +30 mv. This leads to generation of action potential due to depolarization of membrane (Figure 24.1) All this occurs within millisecond. During this time potassium channels which are also present in axon are opened and potassium moves out of axon. This leads to restoration of membrane potential within next 2-3 milli seconds and membrane hyper polarization takes place. At the end of the process potassium channels are closed.

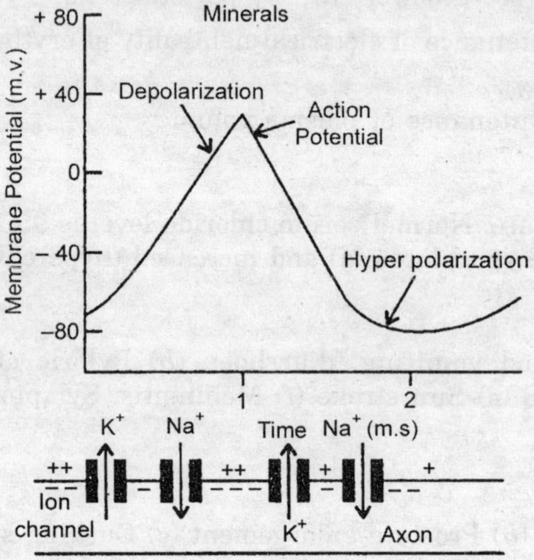

Fig. 24.1 Molecular events associated with action potential

Nerve impulse

Action potential generated is propagated all along axon due to opening of adjacent voltage sensitive sodium channels by depolarisation wave. This propagation is called as nerve impulse.

Patch clamp technique

This technique is used for electrophysiological studies of ion channels. By using this technique it is possible to know number of ions passing through a single ion channel in an action potential. A micro pipette (electrode) containing electrolyte solution and having a narrow opening which can hold one single ion channel is used to study ionic movements. Two principal steps of this technique are given below :

1. A small patch of membrane containing single ion channel is separated by applying suction. The patch sticks to micropipette tip (patch clamping, Figure 24.2).
2. The ionic movements through the ion channel are studied by changing potential across the patch and ionic composition (Figure 24.2).

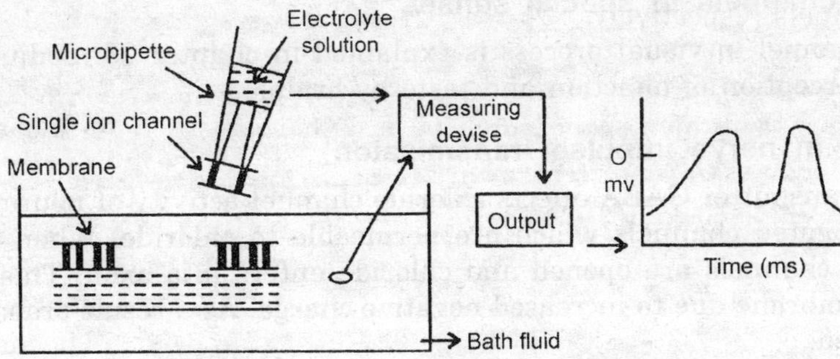

Fig. 24.2 Patch clamp technique

Using this devise it has been calculated that about 7000 sodium ions pass through a single ion channel in a millisecond.

Molecular mechanism of action of voltage gated potassium channel

The potassium channels are transmembrane proteins with central aqueous pore through which ions can flow selectively down electrochemical gradients. The fluxes through these channels are up to 100 millions ions per second.

Now we shall examine how these channels work? How they are able to sense voltage? How they maintain high selectivity? The molecular basis of ion channel function is hot field of research today.

Extensive work carried out in the field of electro physiology, biophysics, molecular and structural biology for the last few decades provided somewhat clear molecular basis of potassium ion channel function.

1. This ion channel or pore is a tetrameric assembly of subunits. Each subunit contains six trans membrane helices and a reentrant pore lining p-loop. The helical segments are designated as S1, S2, S3, S4, S5 and S6. The p-loop of each subunit lines aqueous pore and carries selective ions. (Fig. 24.3A, 3B).
2. The fourth trans membrane segment acts as voltage sensor. It is positively charged due to the presence of arginine or lysine residues at every third position. It is able to move in response to transmembrane potential. This voltage sensing domain is highly conserved.
3. The cytoplasmic part of the channel consists of T1 domain. It is involved in the specificity of channel assembly.
4. The cytoplasmic side of the channel contain pore-occluding ball domain near N-terminus. It is involved in the closure of channel.
5. In response to trans membrane potential the voltage sensor moves. This movement causes rotation of S5 and S6 helices which opens channel pore. As a result of rotation the minimal internal diameter increases sufficiently to allow potassium ions to pass through.
6. An open channel can go back to closed state by reversing rotation of helices.
7. Alternatively an open channel undergo auto inhibitory channel blockade by inactivation of ball domain.
8. The potassium channels are extremely selective in which ions they allow to pass.
9. Potassium channels generate high selectivity by employing filter type architecture. Subunits back bone residues carbonyl oxygen form selectivity filter. This type of oxygen geometry matches precisely with potassium ion only. Hence potassium channel allows only potassium ion in preference to any other ion.

Role of sodium channels in special senses

Role of sodium channel in visual process is explained in chapter 23. Sodium channels are involved in the perception of olfaction and taste by brain.

Role of chloride in nerve impulse transmission

Inhibitory neurotransmitter GABA affects chloride channel activity of neurons. Receptors of GABA are ligand gated channels which are permeable to chloride. When GABA binds to receptors chloride channels are opened and chloride enters into axon. This leads to hyper polarization of membrane due to increased negative charge. As a result propagation of nerve impulse is inhibited.

Medical Importance

1. Several neurotoxins like tetrodotoxin of Japanese puffer fish, saxitoxin of marine plant origin and scorpion venom works by affecting sodium channel activity.
2. Alcohol works by influencing chloride channel.
3. Cystic fibrosis is due to altered activity of cAMP sensitive chloride channel (cystic fibrosis trans membrane conductance regulator, CFTR).

CALCIUM

Human body contain about 1-1.2 kg of calcium. Most of it is present in bone and teeth.

Absorption

Dietary calcium is absorbed in duodenum and in the first part of jejunum by active transport mechanism against concentration gradient in presence of calcitriol.

Factors affecting calcium absorption

1. **Calcitriol :** It increases intestinal calcium absorption by promoting synthesis of calcium binding protein (chapter 23).
2. High protein diet increases calcium absorption.
3. Calcium, phosphorous ratio in the diet. Excess phosphate lowers calcium absorption.
4. Phytic acid present in cereals and oxalates present in certain foods inhibit calcium absorption by forming insoluble calcium salts.
5. Faulty digestion and absorption of fats decreases calcium absorption.
6. Neutral and acidic P^H favours calcium absorption where as alkaline P^H decreases calcium absorption.
7. Dietary fibre if present in excess interferes with calcium absorption.

Functions

1. Calcium is essential for bone and teeth formation.
2. It is essential for blood clotting. It is required for the conversion of prothrombin to thrombin.
3. It is essential for nerve impulse transmission and muscle contraction.
4. Many hormones mediate their action through calcium. Hence it is called as Secondary messenger.
5. It is required for the activity of several intracellular calpains.

6. It is required for the activity of several enzymes like glucose-6 phosphate dehydrogenase, lactonase, phosphogluconate dehydrogenase and trypsin.
7. It is involved in the release of hormones (secretion) and neurotransmitters.
8. It is required for cell motility, mitosis and other micro filament mediated processes.
9. It is involved in membrane transport and for maintenance of membrane integrity.
10. Calcium triggers bioluminescence in marine organisms like jelly fish.
11. **Calcium-apoptosis link.** Calcium has central role in apoptosis. Calcium mediates release of cytochrome C from mitochondria. Calcium mediated processes are also involved in clearance of apoptic cells and cell debris by phagocytosis. So the termination of apoptic death process is also a part of calcium apoptosis link.
12. **Calcium and cancer.** Calcium act as chemopreventive agent of colon cancer. It activates calcium sensing receptor. This results in increased level of intracellular calcium inducing wide range of biological effects. Some of which restrain growth and promote differentiation of transformed colon cells.

Mechanism of calcium mediated actions or calcium signalling systems

Calcium is a versatile intracellular signal molecule that operates over wide cellular or biological processes. Calcium signalling system uses on reactions that introduces calcium into cell. Channels in plasma membrane and endoplasmic/sarcoplasmic reticulum are responsible for on reactions. Calcium signalling system uses off reactions which removes calcium from cell. Pumps and exchangers carry out off reactions.

Most of the calcium signalling components are organized into macro molecular complexes in which calcium signalling functions are carried out within highly localized environment.

Mechanism of Calcium mediated hormone action

Hormones like Catecholamines (α-adrenergic receptors), angiotensin-II, vasopressin, TRH and substance P mediate their action through intracellular calcium. These hormones increases intracellular calcium through G-proteins and inositol triphosphate (IP_3).

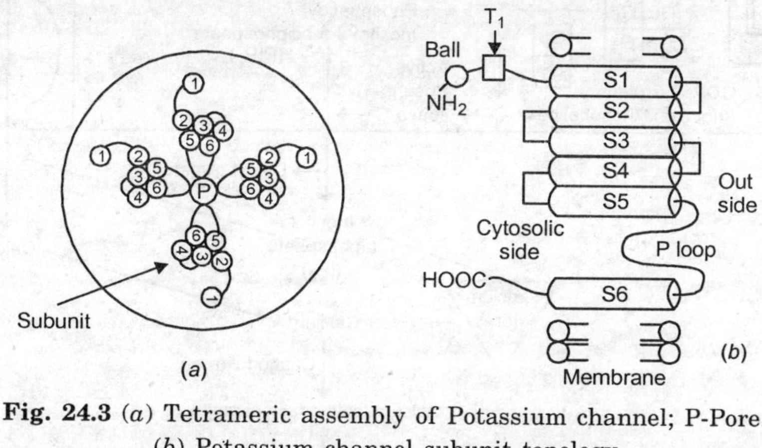

Fig. 24.3 (*a*) Tetrameric assembly of Potassium channel; P-Pore.
(*b*) Potassium channel subunit topology

In the resting cell GDP is bound to nucleotide binding site of G_α-subunit of G-protein which also contain G_β and G_γ subunits (see chapter-23). When hormone combines with receptor of target cell it causes conformational change in receptor which enables it to interact with GDP-

G protein. This leads to exchange of GDP for GTP and formations of G_α-GTP due to dissociation of G_β and G_γ subunits. The GTP-G_α complex activates phospholipase C which in turn acts on membrane phosphotidyl inositol –4.5 bisphosphate (PIP_2) to produce inositol-1, 4, 5-triphosphate (IP_3) and diacylglycerol (Figure 24.3). IP_3 increases intracellular calcium by liberating calcium from calcium stores and by opening calcium channels (Figure 24.4).

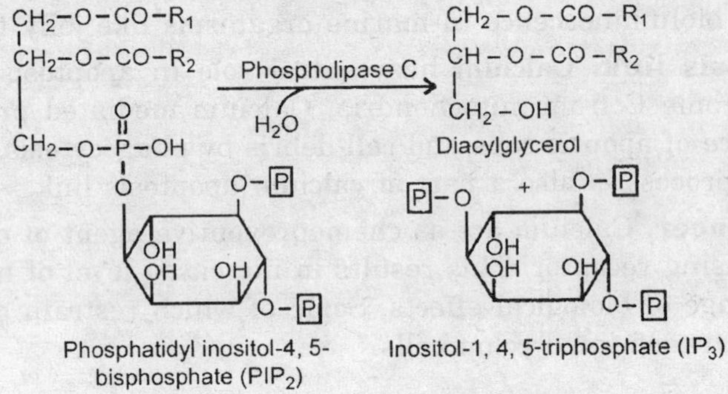

Fig. 24.3 Action of phospholipase C

Then calcium binds to a cytosolic calcium binding protein calmodulin. It is 17 kda protein having four binding sites for calcium. Many effects of calcium are mediated by calmodulin. Binding of calcium to calmodulin causes conformational change in calmodulin-calcium complex which enables it to bind and activate target proteins to produce biological response (Figure 24.4). Some of the enzymes which are activated either directly by calcium or through calcium-calmodulin complex are phosphorylase kinase, glycogen synthase, glyceraldehyde-3 phosphate dehydrogenase, pyruvate kinase, pyruvate dehydrogenase, isocitrate dehydrogenase, α-ketoglutarate dehydrogenase, pyruvate carboxylase, adenyl cyclase, guanylate cyclase and NO synthase. Calmodulin seems to be a subunit of enzyme like glycogen phosphorylase kinase.

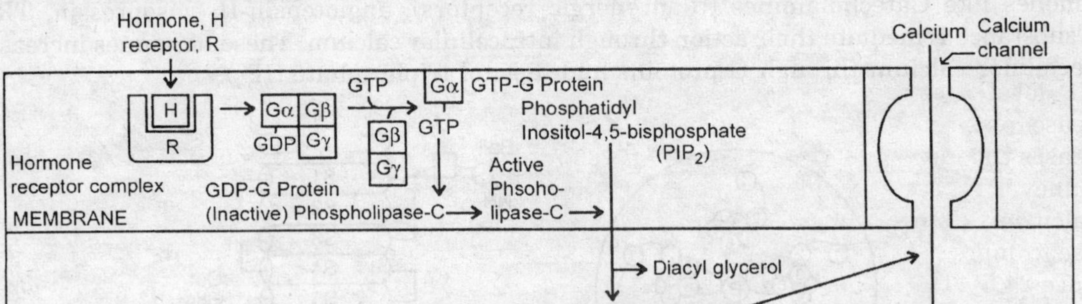

Fig. 24.4 Mechanism of calcium mediated hormone action

Calmodulin-calcium complex also regulates activity of structural elements associated with smooth muscle contraction and microfilament mediated process like endocytosis, cell motility, mitosis, release of secretory granules etc.

Blood Calcium homeostasis

Normal plasma calcium level is 9-11 mg%. In the plasma calcium is present in three forms.

(*a*) **Ionized form.** About 50-60% of total calcium is present in this form. It is physiologically active because it can pass through membranes and capillaries.

(*b*) **Protein-bound.** About 35-40% of the total calcium is present in this form. It is combined with plasma proteins like albumin and hence it is not diffusible through membrane and physiologically inactive.

(*c*) About 6% of total calcium is complexed with organic molecules like citrate and other molecules like phosphate and bicarbonate.

Since calcium plays vital role in several important cellular functions the maintenance of its normal level in plasma is essential. Daily variation of normal plasma calcium level is rarely more than ±3%. These narrow limits are maintained by complex regulatory action of parathyroid hormone (PTH), calcitonin and calcitriol. These hormones keep the calcium level within normal limits by acting on intestine, bone and kidney.

Secretion of PTH

When the plasma calcium level falls below the normal lower limit calcium receptors present in parathyroid cells interact with G-proteins. This leads to increased intracellular calcium due to formation of IP_3 by the action of phospholipase-C which in turn causes release of PTH by increasing intracellular cAMP. Calcium-calmodulin complex increases cAMP probably by inhibiting phosphodiesterase.

Actions of PTH

Parathyroid hormone enters target cells through specific receptor present on membrane surface. The action of PTH on target tissues is mediated by cAMP. PTH increases intracellular cAMP level in target tissues by activating adenyl cyclase. PTH acts on three organs to increase plasma calcium level. Its main action is on bone. Dissolution of bone by PTH increases the movement of calcium from bone to plasma. PTH increases calcium reabsorption in kidney. PTH increases absorption of calcium in the intestine indirectly through the formation of calcitriol. As mentioned in chapter-23 calcitriol increases calcium absorption in kidney. These combined actions of PTH and calcitriol raises plasma calcium level to normal (Figure 24.5). This is followed by inhibition of PTH secretion and production of calcitriol (see chapter-23). Thus all the calcium raising factors are inhibited when plasma calcium level attains normal value.

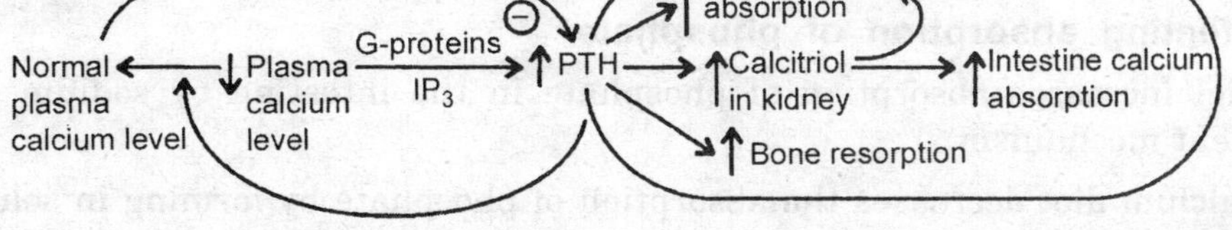

Fig. 24.5 Regulation of plasma calcium by PTH mediated processes

Secretion and action of calcitonin

When plasma calcium level is more than the upper value of normal range calcitonin is produced by the C cells of thyroid gland. Calcitonin lowers plasma calcium level by acting on bone. It enters osteoclasts of bone through receptor mediated process. Its action is also mediated by cAMP. It increases intracellular cAMP level. It decreases release of calcium from bone by preventing bone resorption by osteoclasts.

Deficiency of calcium

Nutritional deficiency of calcium causes growth failure, hyperplasia of parathyroid glands, osteoporosis, hyper irritability and tetany. Howevery it is rare.

Hypocalcemia

The decrease in calcium level leads to tetany and related muscle and neurological disorders (convulsions). It occurs in vitamin D deficiency, hypoparathyroidism, pseudohypoparathyroidism, renal in sufficiency, rickets and osteomalacia. Symptoms of tetany are muscle spasms and hyper excitability of nerves of face and extremities.

Hypercalcemia

It occurs in hyper parathyroidism and hyper vitaminosis of vitamin D. Small increase in plasma calcium is observed in sarcoidosis, milk alkali syndrome, respiratory acidosis and bone cancer. Idiopathic hypercalcemia has been reported in some infants. It occurs within 10 months after birth. Symptoms are depression, mental confusion, anorexia, cardiac arrhythimias, coma and cardiac arrest.

Sources

Milk, sea same seeds, green leafy vegetables, fish are good sources. Egg, nuts, fruits and vegetables are fair sources. Rice is a poor source.

Daily requirement (RDA)

Adults. 800 mg/day (0.8 gm/day).

Children. 0.8-1.2 gm/day.

Phosphorus

Human body contain about 500-700 gm of phosphorus. In the body phosphorus is present as inorganic phosphate complexed with calcium and magnesium in bone and teeth and as organic phosphate associated with phospholipids of membranes, nucleic acids and metabolites.

Absorption

Phosphatases present in the lumen hydrolyzes phosphates from organic substances. Free phosphate is absorbed in jejunum and enters blood by way of portal circulation.

Factors affecting absorption of phosphate

1. Calcitriol increases absorption of phosphate in the intestine by sodium and glucose dependent mechanism.
2. High calcium diet decreases the absorption of phosphate by forming in soluble calcium phosphate.

3. Phosphorus of animal foods is absorbed easily than plant food phosphorus.
4. Anatacids if taken excess interferes with phosphate absorption.

Functions

1. It is present in bone and teeth as hydroxyapatite.
2. It is required for the formation of nucleic acids.
3. It is constituent of blood buffers.
4. It is required for the synthesis of phospholipids.
5. It is constituent of high energy compounds like at ATP, GTP etc.
6. It is involved in modification of several enzymes and cellular proteins.
7. It is required for the formation coenzymes of water soluble vitamins like pyridoxine, thiamine etc.
8. It is constituent of metabolic intermediates like glucose-6 phosphate etc.
9. It is required for the synthesis of milk protein casein which is a phosphoprotein.
10. It is constituent of secondary messengers like cAMP, cGMP etc.

Blood phosphate homeostasis

The normal plasma inorganic phosphorus level is 2.5–4.5 mg%. In children it is slightly higher and ranges from 4-6 mg. Since phosphorus is a constituent of several macromolecules maintenance of its normal level in plasma is essential. Plasma phosphorus level is balanced by several factors under normal conditions (Figure 24.6). However PTH, calcitonin and calcitriol mainly influences plasma phosphorus level. They maintain phosphorus level by acting on kidney. PTH and calcitonin diminishes phosphorus reabsorption where as calcitriol increases reabsorption of phosphorus in the renal tubules.

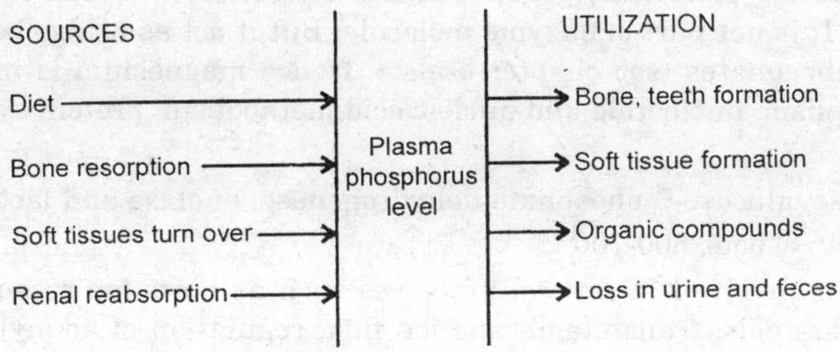

Fig. 24.6 Factors that regulate plasma phosphorus level

Deficiency

The deficiency of phosphate occurs due to impaired absorption or excessive loss through kidney.

Hypophosphatemia

The plasma phosphorus level is decreased in hyper parathyroidism, Fanconi syndrome and vitamin D deficiency. Insulin overdose may cause low plasma phosphorus level.

Hyper phosphatemia

It occurs when kidney fails to remove phosphorus. Therefore hyper phosphatemia is seen in chronic nephritis which progress to renal failure. Hypo parathyroidism and hyper vitaminosis of vitamin D are other diseases in which hyperphosphatemia occurs.

Sources

Pulses, cereals, coconut, groundnut and eggs are good sources. Milk and green leafy vegetables are fair sources.

Daily requirement (RDA)

Adults. 200-300 mg/day.

MAGNESIUM

Human body contains about 25 g of magnesium. Of this 50% is present in bone in combination with phosphate and carbonate. Soft tissues contain about one fifth of total body magnesium. Remaining is present in body fluids.

Absorption

About 40% of ingested magnesium is absorbed in jejunum and ileum. High magnesium content of diet decreases magnesium absorption. Alcohol also interferes with absorption of magnesium. Inverse relationship exists between in take of magnesium and absorption. It suggests that magnesium deficiency treatment requires an extended period.

Functions

1. Magnesium is major intracellular cation like potassium.
2. It is constituent of bone and teeth.
3. It is essential for phosphate group transfer reactions catalyzed by kinases and RNA polymerase. It is not part of enzyme molecule. But it act as bridge between enzyme and nucleoside phosphates (see chapter-4 also). Hence magnesium is involved in carbohydrate metabolism, nucleotide and nucleic acid metabolism, protein synthesis and muscle contraction.
4. Transketolase, glucose-6-phosphate dehydrogenase, enolase and lactonase also requires this metal for activity.
5. Magnesium is involved in several processes such as hormone receptor binding, gating of calcium channels, trans membrane ion flux, regulation of adenylate cyclase, muscle contraction and neuronal activity, control of vascular tone, cardiac excitability and neurotransmitter release.
6. Magnesium increases body's ability to utilize other minerals like calcium, phosphorus, sodium and potassium and vitamins like vitamin C, vitamin E and vitamin B-complex.
7. Magnesium is involved in insulin secretion, binding to receptors and activity.

Regulation of plasma magnesium

Plasma magnesium is carefully regulated within normal range. Kidney is primary regulator of body magnesium balance. Renal magnesium regulation is essentially a filtration and reabsorption process. Normal intake of magnesium is about 300-350 mg per day and about one third is absorbed by gastrointestinal tract. Over a 24 hour period 3500 mg of magnesium is filtered by kidneys. However only 3 to 4% of this amount or about 100 to 150 mg per day is excreted in urine. It is equal to the amount of absorbed magnesium per day. Thus body magnesium balance is determined by renal excretion of magnesium.

Most remarkable change in renal magnesium handling occurs in response to alterations in plasma magnesium concentration. Renal cells are capable of adopting to magnesium availability through receptors which senses the concentration of this cation. Thus when body magnesium status is below normal these receptors senses the need for magnesium retention and cause more reabsorption of magnesium.

Deficiency of magnesium leads to hypomagnesemia. Several other dieseases also cause hypomagnesaemia.

Hypomagnesaemia

The normal serum magnesium level is 1.7-2.4 mg%. Hypomagnesaemia occurs in hyper parathyroidism, chronic alcoholism, kwashiorkor, malabsorption syndromes, vomiting, diarrhoea and pancreatitis. Symptoms are weakness, lethargy, parasthesias, muscle cramps and confusion.

Magnesium deficiency, hypomagnesemia and diabetes

Magnesium deficiency and hypomagnesemia are involved in development of insulin resistance, carbohydrate intolerance, accelerated atherosclerosis, hypertension, diabetic neuropathy and cardiovascular complications.

Deficient intake of magnesium is a risk factor for development of type-II diabetes mellitus independent of age, body mass index, alcohol intake and family history of diabetes.

Close relationship between insulin, glucose homeostasis and intracellular magnesium is recognized. Insulin induces opposite changes in plasma and erythrocyte magnesium concentrations. Intracellular magnesium deficiency impairs action of many magnesium dependent glycolytic enzymes like hexokinase and phosphofructokinase. Magnesium supplementation improves insulin response and action in type-II diabetic patients.

Diabetic patients have low magnesium levels. The mechanism responsible for magnesium deficiency in diabetic patients is not known clearly. It is believed that glycosuria that occurs in diabetic patients impairs renal reabsorption of magnesium from filtrate.

Toxicity

Magnesium overdose leads to hyper magnesaemia which can also occur in other diseases.

Hypermagnesaemia

It occurs in renal failure, diabetic coma and due to excessive intake of anatacids. Symptoms are muscle weakness, nausae, decreased neuromuscular transmission and depression. Death may occur due to respiratory paralysis.

Sources

Nuts, legumes, peas and whole grains are good sources. Fish, meat and green leafy vegetables are fair sources.

Daily requirement (RDA)

Adults. 300-350 mg/day. More during pregnancy and lactation.

IRON

Human body contains about 4-5 gm of iron. A major part of this (65%) is present in hemoglobin. Remaining is present in myoglobin and other iron containing compounds.

Absorption of Iron

In the plant foods iron is present in Fe^{3+} (ferric) state and it is tightly bound to organic molecules. In the stomach where P^H is low Fe^{3+} dissociates and it is reduced to Fe^{2+} (ferrous) by small compounds like ascorbic acid and amino acids like cysteine. Stomach also produces gastroferrin a glycoprotein which combines with small amount of ferric iron (Fe^{3+}). The ferrous iron and gastroferrin are easily absorbed into mucosal cells of duodenum and jejunum by an unknown mechanism. Apart from this, in the mucosal cells ferrous (Fe^{2+}) iron is also formed from dietary heme which is absorbed as such (Figure 24.7).

In the mucosal cells (Fe^{2+}) is oxidized to (Fe^{3+}) by ceruloplasmin a copper containing protein. Ferroxidase is another copper containing protein involved in this oxidation. In the mucosal cells (Fe^{3+}) combines with intracellular carrier molecule (ICM) which is probably responsible for regulation of iron metabolism in the body. Depending on the state of body iron metabolism intracellular carrier (ICM) delivers iron to iron storage protein and plasma iron transport protein in proper proportions (Figure 24.7).

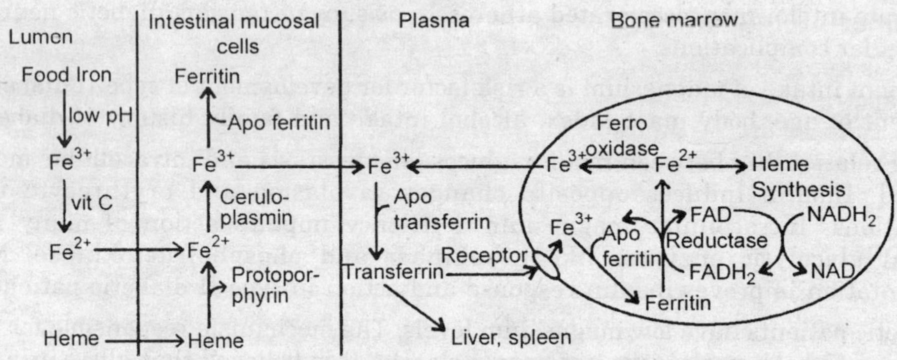

Fig. 24.7 Iron metabolism

Regulation of iron absorption

Under normal conditions iron absorption depends on body iron requirement. ICM plays vital role in absorption of iron. Under normal conditions only 10% of dietary iron is absorbed because ICM is nearly saturated. It transfers absorbed iron in proper proportions to iron storage protein and iron transport protein present in plasma.

In iron deficiency state the ICM is not saturated. So more iron if available in the diet is absorbed. Under these conditions most of iron absorbed is transferred to iron transport protein only.

In iron excess state the ICM is saturated. So minimum iron is transferred to storage protein and transport protein.

Other factors which affect non-heme iron absorption

1. Low phosphate diet increases iron absorption whereas high phosphate diet decreases iron absorption by forming insoluble iron phosphates.

2. Phytates and oxalates decrease iron absorption by forming iron phytate and iron oxalate.
3. High or very low P^H decreases iron absorption.
4. Iron absorption decreases in partial or total gastroctomy.
5. Iron absorption decreases in achlorohydria.
6. Citrate promotes iron absorption.

Transport of Iron

From the mucosal cells ICM releases Fe^{3+} into plasma. Through an unknown mechanism Fe^{3+} enters plasma from intestinal mucosal cells. Since free iron can generate free radicals (chapter 10) in plasma it combines with iron transport protein apotransferrin to form transferrin which transports iron to storage sites. Apotransferrin combines with two molecules of Fe^{3+} to form transferrin (Figure 24.7).

Storage of Iron

Iron is mainly stored in liver, spleen, bonemarrow and intestine. In the intestine apoferritin combines with Fe^{3+} to form ferritin which is iron storage protein. In other tissues transferrin is internalized by receptor mediated process and iron is released. Then apoferritin combines with Fe^{3+} to form ferritin and stored (Figure 24.7).

Transfer of stored iron to transferrin

Ferritin is continuously synthesized and degraded. The transfer of iron from ferritin to plasma apotransferrin involves reduction of Fe^{3+} to Fe^{2+} which causes the release of iron from ferritin. To facilitate its binding to apotransferrin Fe^{2+} is oxidized rapidly. The reduction of Fe^{3+} to Fe^{2+} is catalyzed by ferritin reductase which requires two co-enzymes NAD and FAD where as oxidation is catalyzed by ceruloplasmin (Figure 24.7).

Functions

1. Iron of hemoglobin and myoglobin is involved in transport of oxygen.
2. Iron of cytochromes participates in electron transfer reactions.
3. Iron is constituent of heme enzymes like tryptophan pyrrolase, catalase, peroxidase, xanthine oxidase and cytochrome P_{450}-hydroxylase.
4. It is constituent of iron-sulfur proteins (Non-heme Iron, NHI) like aconitase, succinate-CoQ reductase, NADH-CoQ reductase, CoQ-cytochrome C reductase, adrenodoxin and ferrodoxins.
5. It is a constituent of lactoferrin present in milk and other secretions.

Iron deficiency

Deficiency of iron in blood gives rise to anaemia and condition is called Iron-deficiency anaemia. It is a major nutritional problem in developing countries. Children, adolescent girls, pregnant and lactating women are susceptible to iron deficiency. Microcytic hypochromic erythrocytes are present in blood. The hemoglobin content is less than 9 gm%.

Clinical symptoms are fatique, breathlessness on exertion, giddiness and skin acquires pale colour. In severe cases finger nails become soft and spoon shaped and affected children tend to eat mud.

Other conditions that cause iron deficiency anaemia are excessive menstrual flow, multiple births, gastrointestinal bleeding due to ulcers, hook worm and round worm infestations and pancreatic tumor or infection.

Old people are prone to iron deficiency due to increased frequency of achlorohydria.

Toxicity

If mega doses of iron is taken excess iron is deposited in liver as hemosiderin. Iron stored in this form is not available for use in the body. Hemosiderin deposits are found in pancreas, skin and joints also. The accumulation of hemosiderin in the tissues results in hemosiderosis. It is found in Bentus in South Africa who cook their food in large iron vessels. When the condition is accompanied by bronze pigmentation of skin the condition is called as hemochromatosis.

Other hemosiderosis causing conditions are repeated blood transfusions, idiopathic hemochromatosis in which iron is absorbed in excess due to inherited defect in regulation of iron absorption and alcoholic cirrhosis.

Treatment

Iron chelators like desferyioxamine is useful in removing excess iron from the body. It removes iron from the body by forming water soluble complex which is excreted in urine.

Sources

Cereals, legumes, green leafy vegetables like mint leaves, coriander leaves, spinach and jaggery are good sources. Organ meats like liver, kidney, spleen and farm products like eggs and fish are fair sources.

Daily requirement (RDA)

Adult Male. 10mg/day, female : 18mg/day. During pregnancy and lactation : 30 mg/day.

ZINC

Human body contains about 2-3 gm of zinc. Of this 60% is present in skeletal muscle and 30% is present in bone. Remaining is present in body fluids. Among different organs of the body prostate (86 mg/100 gm) and choroid of eye are rich in this metal.

Absorption and transport

Zinc is absorbed by carrier mediated process in duodenum and jejunum. Phytates affects absorption of plant food zinc. In the plasma albumin transports zinc to various organs.

Functions

1. It is required for the activity of enzymes involved in carbohydrate metabolism, protein and amino acid metabolism, nucleic acid metabolism, bone metabolism, blood pressure, gas transport and removal of superoxides. In most of the enzymes zinc is an integral part and it is attached to protein through coordinate covalent bonds. Over 200 zinc metalloenzymes have been isolated. They are lactate dehydrogenase, malate dehydrogenase, carboxy peptidase, DNA and RNA polymerases, thymidine kinase, alkaline phosphatase, angiotensin converting enzyme, carbonic anhydrase and super oxide dismutase.
2. Zinc is involved in stabilization of hormone insulin.

3. It is involved in vitamin A mobilization from liver (dark adaptation).
4. It maintains structure of chromatin and ribosomes.
5. It is required for tissue growth, development and regeneration.
6. It is a constituent of zinc finger proteins which are involved in regulation of gene expression.
7. Zinc is essential for immune system.
8. It is required for the synthesis of gustin a salivary protein involved in development of taste buds.
9. Zinc is required for normal reproduction.
10. Zinc is required for muscle and bone formation.
11. Zinc function as antioxidant.
12. Zinc act as stabilizer of membranes.
13. Association of tRNA synthatase and tRNA is zinc dependent.
14. Zinc is required for basic cellular functions like DNA replication, transcription, cell division and cell activation.

Zinc deficiency

1. It is uncommon in man. However a deficiency disease due to inborn error has been reported.

   Acrodermatitis enteropathy (AE). It is a rare genetic disease. It causes zinc deficiency due to genetic defect in zinc absorption. Symptoms are diarrhoea, acral dermatitis and alopecia.
2. Zinc deficiency in man has been reported in middle east countries particularly in Egyptian and Iranian dwarfs. Clinical symptoms are hypogonadism and growth retardation.
3. Hypogeusia (loss of taste) is another zinc deficiency symptom observed in man.
4. Patients receiving incomplete parenteral solutions develop zinc dificiency.
5. In experimental subjects zinc deficiency causes dermatitis, sore throat, immune defects.
6. Zinc deficiency potentiates apoptosis.

Toxicity

Though it is less common intake of foods, beverages and milk prepared in galvanized vessels leads to zinc poisoning. Symptoms are nausea, vomiting, diarrhoea and fever. Zinc is an inhibitor of electron transport chain at high concentration.

Sources

Sea foods like oysters and herrings are excellent sources. Meat, liver and eggs are good sources. Cereals, pulses, nuts, vegetables and milk are fair sources.

Daily requirement (RDA)

Adults : 15 mg/day. During pregnancy and lactation, 25 mg/day.

COPPER

Human body contains about 100-150 mg of copper. Of this 40% is in muscle. 15% in liver and 10% in brain. Remaining is present in body fluids.

Absorption

Copper absorption in small intestine probably involves two transport processes. High copper in diet induces metallothionin production by mucosal cells which binds copper and inhibits its absorption.

Functions

1. Copper is required for the activity of enzymes involved in respiratory chain, cross linking of collagen and elastin, blood cell formation, melanin formation, superoxides removal, neurotransmitter formation and neuropeptides. In most of the cases copper is part of enzyme molecule. Some cuproenzymes are cytochrome oxidase, lysyloxidase, superoxide dismutase, ceruloplasmin, tyrosinase, dopamine β-oxidase, amine oxidase and uricase.

Deficiency

1. It is rare in adults. Preterm infants are prone to copper deficiency. Symptoms are hypochromic anaemia, leukopenia, central nervous system lesions, bone demineralization, demyelination of nerves, fragility of large blood vessels, depigmentation of skin and steely hair.
2. **Menkes syndrome.** It is rare inherited deficiency disease in which intracellular copper metabolism is defective. It is due to defective copper binding p-type ATPase of intestinal origin. Symptoms are abnormal kinky hair, growth failure and hypothermia. Hypothermia develops soon after birth and death occurs with in 3 years of age.

Toxicity

1. Copper excess results from ingestion of copper salts or contaminated water. Symptoms are vomiting, diarrhoea and hemolysis.
2. **Wilson's disease.** It is rare inherited disease in which excess copper is present in tissues due to abnormal metabolism of copper in liver. It is due to defective copper binding p-type hepatic ATPase which facilitates removal of copper in bile. Liver, kidney, brain and eye are organs in which copper deposits are found.

Clinical symptoms are acute or chronic liver failure, emotional disturbances and dementia. In the eye copper deposit produce golden brown green ring (Kayser-Fleisher ring) in the cornea. It is a fatal diesase and death occurs within few years after the appearance of clinical signs.

Treatment

Copper chelator like pencilamine is effective in removing excess copper.

Sources

Cereals, pulses, nuts, milk, eggs, and meat are good sources. Vegetables and fruits are fair sources.

Daily requirement

Adults. 2.0 mg/day.

IODINE

Human body contains about 15-20 mg of iodine. Of this 70-80% is in thyroid gland. Remaining is present in muscle, skin, bone, nervous system and other endocrine glands.

Absorption

Under normal conditions iodine is rapidly absorbed in small intestine.

Functions

1. Iodine is required for the formation of thyroid hormones (see chapter-12), thyroxine (T_4) and tri iodotyronine (T_3).
2. Thyroid hormones are essential for growth and development.

Iodine deficiency

1. Most common iodine deficiency disorder (IDD) is goitre, swollen thyroid gland on the neck. Goitre is prevalent in several developing countries. In India occurrence of goitre has been reported in sub Himalayan regions. It is also prevalent in vast mountains of China. IDD are major public health problem in India. About 167 million people of India are at risk for IDD. Among the 457 districts of the country 235 have been found to be endemic to IDD. About 58 millions have goitre and over 8 millions have neurological handicaps. Goitre is reported from hilly areas of Thailand, Myanmar and Indonesia. Iodine content of water from goitrous areas is lower than non-goitrous areas.
2. Decreased I.Q in school children living in iodine deficient areas has been observed.
3. In northern India apathy has been observed in people living in iodine deficient areas.
4. Other iodine deficiency disorders are hypothyroidism, mental disturbances and iodine induced hyperthyroidism.
5. Iodine deficient people are more susceptible to radiation effects.

Goitrogenic factors

Iodine deficiency occurs when foods containing goitrogenic substances are consumed. Goitrogenic factors are present in cabbage, cauliflower and radish. They interfere with iodine uptake by thyroid gland which causes a situation identical to iodine deficiency.

Therapeutic use of iodine

Iodide salts are consumed to prevent accumulation of radio active iodine in thyroid gland in cases of nuclear blasts and accidents.

Sources

Sea foods like sea fish and shell fish are excellent sources. Cereals, milk, meat and eggs are good sources. Green leafy vegetables, root vegetables and fruits are fair sources.

Daily requirement (RDA)

Adults. 150 μg/day or 0.15 mg/day.

FLUORINE

Functions

1. It is essential for development of bone and teeth. It enhances formation of calcium and phosphorus hydroxy apatite crystals. It is present in bone and dentin in the form of fluoroapatite.
2. It prevents the occurrence of dental caries.
3. It may prevent progressive loss of hearing and osteoporosis in adults.

Fluorine deficiency

It causes dental caries. Due to lack of fluorine fluoroapatite of enamel is not formed and tooth substance is susceptible to action of oral acids produced from food residues by oral bacteria. More over fluorine probably prevents acid production by bactria by inhibiting glycolysis. Thus the lack of fluorine produces cavities due to solubilization of enamel by acids produced in oral cavitiy.

Toxicity

High fluoride content in ground water is reported from India, China, Srilanka, West Indies, Spain, Holland, Italy, Mexico, South American and North American countries. In India the extent of fluoride contamination of water varies from 1 to 48 mg per litre. Usually fluoride content of water upto 1 mg per litre is considered safe beyond that limit is considered as unsafe for all practical purposes. Due to high fluoride content in ground water the occurrence of fluorosis which is due to intake of excess fluorine is endemic in several states of India.

Early symptoms of fluorosis

(*a*) Discoloration of enamel surface in front row of the teeth particularly central and lateral incisors of upper and lower jaw.

(*b*) Aches and pain in the joints which may be due to the fluoride toxicity.

(*c*) Non-ulcer dyspepsia, polyuria and polydipsia.

(*d*) Muscle weakness, fatigue, anemia with very low hemoglobin level.

(*e*) Frequent abortions/still births. Fluoride calcify blood vessels and reduces blood flow to growing foetus.

(*f*) Male in fertility with oligospermia, azoospermia and low testosterone levels.

Genu valgum or Knock knees

It is the name given to skeletal abnormality developed in young and adults affected with fluorosis.

There are two types of fluorosis (*a*) Dental fluorosis and (*b*) Skeletal fluorosis.

(*a*) **Dental fluorosis.** It is characterized by mottled teeth. Enamel becomes rough and loses characteristic lustre. Stained, chalky white patches are seen on surface of teeth. Pitting occurs due to loss of enamel and tooth surface appear corroded.

(*b*) **Skeletal fluorosis.** Excess accumulation of fluorine causes skeletal deformities. Deformities of spine and legs are seen in affected people. Stiff and painful joints are other symptoms. Neurological disturbances secondary to spinal deformity are also observed in affected people.

Kidney and thyroid damages have been observed in fluorosis affected people.

In India about 62 million people in 17 out of 32 states are affected with dental or skeletal fluorosis. The number of districts affected differs from state to state. In Andhra Pradesh all districts except Adilabad, Nizmabad, West and East Godavari, Visakhapatnam, Vijayanagarm, Srikakulam are affected with fluorosis. In Karnataka fluorosis is seen in Gulbarga, Raichur, Bellary, Tumkur, Chitradurga and Kolar districts. Districts of other states affected with fluorosis are given in Table 24.1. The first case of endemic fluorosis in humans from India was reported from Prakasam district of Andhra Pradesh in 1937.

Table 24.1 Fluorosis endemic districts in various states of India.

State	District
Tamilnadu	Coimbatore, Dharmapuri, Erode, Madurai, Salem, Tiruchirapalli, Vellore
Kerala	Alleppy, Palghat, Vamanapuram
Orissa	Dhenkanal, Koreput, Pulbeni
Maharashtra	Akola, Amravathi, Bhandara, Bulduna, Chandrapur, Jalagaon, Nagpur, Naded, Sholapur
Madhya Pradesh	Chhindwara, Dindhori, Dhar, Jabua, Mandla, Seoni, Sehore, Shivpuri, Raisen, Vidhisha
Bihar	Daltonganj, Gaya, Gopalganj, Gridh, Palamu, Pashchim, Chemparen, Rohatas
West Bengal	Bankura, Bhardeman, Birbhum, Puruliya
Uttar Pradesh	Aligarh, Allahabad, Agra, Mathura, Meerut, Raibareli, Unnao
Gujarat	All districts except Dang
Delhi	Alipur, Delhi city, Kanjhawala, Najafgarh
Rajasthan	All the 32 districts
Haryana	Bhiwani, Faridabad, Gurgaon, Jhind, Kaithal, Karnal, Kurukshetra, Mohidragarah, Rewari, Rohtak, Sirsa, Sonipat.
Punjab	Amritsar, Bhatinda, Faridkot, Fategarhsahib, Ferozpur, Jalandhar, Mansa, Moga, Muktsar, Ludhiana, Patiala, Ropur, Sangrur
Jammu and Kashmir	Doda
Assam	Karbi Anglong, Nagaon.

Defluoridation

Removal of excess fluorine in drinking water is called as defluoridation. Activated charcol and other absorbents are used in defluoridation.

Sources

Drinking water is the main source of fluorine.

Fluoridation

If drinking water contains inadequate amount of fluorine fluoride salts are added to the water. This process is called as fluoridation.

Daily requirement

Adults. 1.5-4mg/ day or 1-2 ppm (parts per million).

SELENIUM

Human body contains 5-25 mg of selenium. However, it varies according geochemical environment. Liver, kidney, lungs, erythrocytes and heart are rich in this metal.

Absorption and transport

In the foods selenium is present as selenoamino acids like selenomethionine and seleno cysteine. They are absorbed in the small intestine by sodium dependent active transport process. In the plasma selenium is transported by selenoprotein P.

Functions

1. Selenocysteine is constituent of glutathione peroxidase which reduces hydroperoxides like hydrogen peroxide and hydroperoxides of fatty acids to corresponding alcohols in presence of glutathione. This enzyme is present in cytosol of several organs. Since glutathione peroxidase is associated with antioxidant system selenium is essential for effective antioxidant action of vitamin E (chapter 23).
2. Hepatic iodothyronine –5′-deiodinase is another selenoenzyme.
3. A selenoprotein is essential for normal spermatogenesis.
4. In bacteria a seleno protein is involved in the glycine reduction.

Selenium deficiency

1. It causes Keshan disease in China. It is due to low selenium in soil. It commonly affects children and young people. Cardiomyopathy is characteristic symptom.
2. In Russia and China selenium deficiency causes Keshin-Beck disease. Growing children between age of 5-13 years are affected. Osteoarthritis associated with severe joint deformity is characteristic symptom.
3. In experimental animals selenium deficiency disturbs immune function and metabolism of xenobiotics.
4. Since selenium is associated with antioxidant system its deficiency may cause cardiovascular disease, aging, diabetic nephropathy, cataract and cancer (see chapter -10).

Toxicity

Excessive intake of selenium causes selinosis or selenium poisoning. It was reported in China from areas where soil selenium content is high. Symptoms are itchy dermatitis, mottled enamel, brittle hair and nails and peripheral neuropathy with paralysis. Selinosis due to consumption of coco de mono nuts containing high level of selenium has been reported from South America.

Sources

Cereals, meat and fish are good sources. Vegetables and fruits are fair sources.

Daily requirement (RDA)

Adults. 55-75 μg / day or 0.05 – 0.07 mg/ day. PUFA in diet influence selenium requirement.

MANGANESE

Human body contains about 12-20 mg of manganese. Of this 25% is present in bone. It is present in high concentration in liver, kidney, pancreas and pituitary. Body fluids also contain manganese.

Absorption

About 10% of dietary manganese is absorbed in small intestine. Phytates, calcium and phosphate interfers with manganese absorption.

Functions

1. It is a constituent of metalloenzymes like mitochondrial superoxide dismutase, pyruvate carboxylase and arginase.
2. It is required for the activity of glycosyl transferases responsible for the synthesis of proteoglycans and glycoproteins.
3. It is required for the activity of alkaline phosphatase, prolidase, glutamine synthetase, isocitrate dehydrogenase, lactonase and phosphogluconate dehydrogenase.
4. It is required for skeletal growth and development.

Deficiency

1. It is rare in humans. However induced mangnese deficiency causes skin rash and hypo cholesterolemia in man.
2. In animals manganese deficiency causes sterility, skeletal abnormalities, growth failure and fatigue.

Toxicity

Manganese toxicity of dietary origin is rare. However manganese toxicity has been reported in miners exposed to manganese dust due to inhalation. Symptoms are pyschosis and those of Parkinsons disease.

Sources

Whole cereals, vegetables, spinach and meat are good sources.

Daily requirement

Adults. 2.5-5.0 mg/day.

MOLYBDENUM

Small amounts of molybdenum are present in all human tissues. However liver, kidney and milk are rich in this metal. Tissue concentration depends on geographical area.

Absorption

About 80% of dietary molybdenum is rapidly absorbed in the intestine.

Function

1. It is required for the activity of enzymes involved in purine and amino acid metabolism.
2. Molybdenum containing metallo enzymes are xanthine oxidase, sulfite oxidase and aldehyde oxidase.
3. It reduces incidence and severity of dental caries by augmenting effect of fluorine.

Deficiency

Molybdenum deficiency in man is unknown. However inborn error of molybdenum metabolism has been reported.

1. In affected individual metabolism of sulfur containing amino acids and nucleotide is impaired due to genetic defect in the hepatic synthesis of molybdenum containing cofactor. Clinical symptoms are growth retardation, ectopic eye lens and neurological abnormalities.
2. An analogous disease has been reported in patients receiving incomplete parenteral solutions for long time.

Toxicity

Toxicity of molybdenum in man is unknown. However in cattle excess molybdenum causes severe diarrhoea and ill health. It is due to consumption of foliage rich in molybdenum by cattle.

Sources

Cereals, pulses, green leafy vegetables, liver and kidney are good sources. Fruits and other root vegetables are poor sources.

Daily requirement (RDA)

Adults. 150–500 μg/day or 0.15 – 0.50 mg/day.

COBALT

All tissues of human body contain small amounts of cobalt. However liver and kidney are rich in this element.

Absorption

About 70-80% of dietary Cobalt is absorbed in small intestine.

Function

1. It is a constituent of vitamin B_{12}. Hence it is involved in erythropoiesis.
2. It may stimulate erythropoietin production in children and pregnant women.
3. In rats it is required for thyroid hormone production.

Deficiency

It is unknown in man. However in cattle and sheep cobalt deficiency cause anaemia.

Toxicity

It can occur when large amounts of Cobalt salts are used in the treatment of anaemia. Symptoms are polycythemia, thyroid hyperplasia and congestive heart failure.

Sources and daily requirement

Since its only known function in man is as constituent of vitamin B_{12} sources and requirements of this metal are those of vitamin B_{12}. However if body has additional requirement it is met by cobalt found in foods.

CHROMIUM

Human body contains about 6 mg of chromium. It is present in tissues and blood.

Absorption

About 1-2% of dietary chromium is absorbed in the intestine. Organic chromium is rapidly absorbed than inorganic chromium.

Functions

1. It facilitates insulin action by increasing insulin receptors and insulin receptor interaction.
2. It facilitates protein synthesis by increasing transcription.
3. It can influence lipid metabolism via insulin.

Deficiency

1. In man chromium deficiency causes decreased glucose tolerance. Other symptoms are elevated serum lipids, growth retardation, weight loss and peripheral neuropathy.
2. In rats chromium deficiency causes corneal opacity.

Toxicity

Chromium toxicity in man is unknown. In experimental animals oral administration of large dose of chromium causes growth retardation, renal and hepatic necrosis.

Sources

Whole grains, legumes, nuts, yeast, liver, kidney and meat are good sources.

Daily requirement (RDA)

Adults. 50 μg – 200 μg /day or 0.05 – 0.2 mg / day.

OTHER TRACE ELEMENTS

Some other trace elements present in human body whose essentiality in human health is yet to be established are cadmium, vandium, nickel, lithium, bromine and silicon and strontium.

CADMIUM

Human body contains about 30 mg of cadmium. Of this 10 mg is present in kidney and 4 mg in liver. Blood and other tissues also contain this metal.

Absorption

About 20-30% of dietary cadmium is absorbed in the intestine.

Function

1. It is constituent of renal metallothionin.
2. For unknown reasons cadmium is absent in new born kidney but it accumulates in this organ as age advances.

Toxicity

1. Excess cadmium causes hypertension in rats and probably in man.
2. In male and female rats cadmium excess produce reproductive disturbances.

VANADIUM

Human body contain about 10-25 mg of vanadium. Most of it is present in bones, teeth and adipose tissue.

Absorption

Less than 1% of dietary Vanadium is absorbed.

Functions

1. It regulates activity of Na^+/K^+-pump.
2. It regulates phosphorylation of proteins.

Deficiency

Vanadium deficiency causes thyroid, skeletal and neurological defects.

Toxicity

In experimental animals vanadium excess causes diarrhoea and growth failure.

SILICON

Blood and body tissues contain small amounts of silicon. Bone, skin, teeth, muscle, kidney and heart are some organs rich is silicon. Blood silicon concentration is about 200-500 µg%.

Functions

1. It is involved in cross linking of collagen.
2. It is constituent of ground substance where it is complexed with mucopolysaccharides.
3. It is involved in bone calcification.
4. As the age advances silicon content of some organs like skin, heart and thymus decreases.
5. Silicon concentration in several tissues of new born is low compared to adult tissue concentration.

Deficiency

In experimental animals silicon deficiency causes growth retardation and defective bone formation.

Toxicity

Excess silicon causes silicosis. It occurs due to inhalation of silicon dust.

Metallothionins (MTs)

1. Are family of cysteine rich polypeptides. MTs are low molecular weight only 6-7 Kda compounds. They contain about 20 cysteine residues out of total 60-70 amino acids.
2. MTs contain two cysteine rich metal binding domains that give these metalloproteins a dumb bell conformation.
3. MTs are found in vertebrates, mammals, plants and invertebrates.
4. MTs bind metals through mercarpto bonds. MTs are originally thought to be cadmium proteins but are known to bind Zinc, Copper, Mercury and Silver in increasing affinity.

5. MTs donate metal ions in the bio-synthesis of metal containing proteins.
6. MTs are stress inducible proteins with anti-oxidant properties that may act in combination with or independently of glutathione to protect cell from injurious agents.
7. MTs are involved in development of heavy metal tolerance.

REFERENCES

1. Catterwall, W.A. Molecular properties of voltage sensitive sodium channels. Ann. Rev. Biochem. **55**, 953-985, 1986.
2. Farbman, A.I. The cellular basis of olfaction. Endeavour **18,** 2-8, 1994.
3. Dionne, V.E. Emerging complexity of odor transduction, Proc. Natl. Acad. Sci. (USA) **91**, 6253-6254, 1994.
4. Neher, E. and Sakman, E. The patch clamp technique. Sci. Am **266(3)**, 28-35, 1992.
5. Berridge, M. Inositol triphosphate and calcium signalling. Nature **361**, 315-325, 1993.
6. Berridge, M. Inositol triphosphate and diacylglycerol. Ann. Rev. Biochem. **56,** 159-194, 1987.
7. Ohmiya, Y. and Horano, J. Shining the light : The mechanism of bioluminescence reaction of calcium binding photoproteins. Chemistry and Biology **3,** 337-347, 1996.
8. Finch, C.A. and Huebers, H. Perspectives in iron metabolism N. Engl. J. Med. **306,** 1520, 1982.
9. Stadtman, T.C. Selenium dependent enzymes. Ann. Rev. Biochem. **49,** 99, 1980.
10. Messerschmidt. A Ed. Handbook of Metalloproteins. 3 Vols. J. Wiley, New York, 2004.
11. Gerald, Z. (Ed.) Calcium channels in the heart. Landis Bioscience, Texas, 2003.
12. Sigel, Helmut (Ed.) and Sigel, Astrid. Metal ions in biological systems. Dekker/CRC Press, 1996.
13. David, J.A. and Peter, R.S. Ion Channels : Molecules in action. Cambridge University Press, NY, 1996.
14. Celio, Marco, (Ed.) Guide book to calcium binding proteins. Oxford University Press, 1996.
15. Liu, X. and Theil, E.C. Ferritin reactions. Proc. Natl. Acad. Sci. (USA) **101**, 8557-8562, 2004.
16. Berridge, M.J. *et al.* Calcium signalling: dynamics, homeostasis and remodeling. Nat. Rev. Mol. Cell. Biol. **4,** 517-529, 2003.
17. Orrenius, S. *et al.* Regulation of cell death: The calcium apoptosis link. Nat. Rev. Mol. Cell. Biol. **4,** 552-565, 2003.
18. Sigworth, F.J. Structural biology of life's transistors. Nature. **423,** 21-22, 2003.
19. Kuo, A. *et al.* Crystal structure of potassium channel in the closed state. Science. **300,** 1922-1926, 2003.
20. WHO. Elimination of iodine deficiency disorders in South East Asia, 1997.
21. A Treatise on Fluorosis : Fluorosis Research and Rural Development Foundation, Delhi, 2001.

22. Mark P. Mattson and SicL. Chan. Calcium orchestrates apoptosis. Nat. Cell. Biol. **5,** 1041-1043, 2003.

23. Beck, M.A., *et al.* Selenium deficiency and viral infections. J. Nutr. (Suppl.). **133,** 14635-14675, 2003.

24. Calderone, V. *et al.* The crystal structures of yeast copper thione in (CU-MJ): The solution of long lasting enigma, Pro. Natl. Acad. Sci. USA. **102**, 51-56, 2005.

EXERCISES

ESSAY QUESTIONS

1 Describe functions, deficiency symptoms, sources and daily requirements of sodium, potassium and chloride.

2. Describe absorption, transport, functions, deficiency symptoms and sources of iron.
3. Write normal serum calcium level. How it is regulated? Explain role of calcium in hormone action.
4. Describe functions, deficiency symptoms and sources of zinc, iodide and fluorine.
5. Write normal plasma magnesium level. How it is regulated? Name diseases in which it is altered.
6. Write about factors affecting absorption of calcium, phosphorus and Iron.
7. Write deficiency symptoms of Zinc, Iron, Iodine, Fluorine and Selenium.
8. Define minerals. Classify. Give examples for each class. Write about functions, deficiency symptoms, sources and daily requirements of any one example.

SHORT QUESTIONS

1. Explain role of minerals in membrane potential and action potential.
2. Write a note on patch clamp technique.
3. Write functions and sources of phosphate.
4. Explain fluorosis.
5. Write occurrence, functions and toxicity of silicon.
6. Write normal serum phosphorus level. How it is regulated? In what diseases it is increased.
7. Give an account of Zinc functions.
8. What is ceruloplasmin? Write its importance.
9. Write bio-chemical defects in following diseases.

   (*a*) Menke's syndrome. (*b*) Wilson's disease.
10. Write a note on iodine deficiency disorders (IDD).

MULTIPLE CHOICE QUESTIONS

1. Which of the following statement is correct regarding trace minerals

   (*a*) They are required in large amounts.

   (*b*) They are required in less than 100 mg/day.

   (*c*) They account for 80% inorganic matter present in body.

   (*d*) They are required for nerve impulse transmission.

2. Chloride channel of neurons.
   (*a*) Open during propagation of nerve impulse.
   (*b*) Are influenced by hormones.
   (*c*) Are influenced by fluorine.
   (*d*) Are decreased in alcoholism.
3. Calcium is referred as second messenger.
   (*a*) Because many hormones mediate their action through calcium.
   (*b*) Because it carries message from outside to inside of cell.
   (*c*) Because it is related to mRNA.
   (*d*) Because it is involved in nerve impulse transmission.
4. Which of the following is correct regarding serum phosphate level.
   (*a*) In adults its level is 9-11 mg%.
   (*b*) In children its level is 4-6 mg%.
   (*c*) It is increased in Fanconi syndrome.
   (*d*) It is decreased in hypoparathyroidism.
5. Excess cadmimum causes
   (*a*) Hypertension in man.
   (*b*) Hypertension in rabbits.
   (*c*) Dermatitis in man.
   (*d*) Hypopigmentation of skin in rats.

FILL IN THE BLANKS

1. Normal daily excretion of minerals............ .
2. Minerals are present in body..............and body................ .
3. In iron toxicity iron is removed by administering................ .
4. Menke's syndrome is a................ deficiency disease.
5. In cases of nuclear blasts..............are used to prevent radioactive iodine accumulation in thyroid gland.

25

CHAPTER

ENERGY, NUTRIENTS, MEDICINES AND TOXINS OF FOOD

MEDICAL AND BIOLOGICAL IMPORTANCE

1. Food is the source of energy for humans, animals and other living organisms.
2. Carbohydrates, fats and to some extent proteins present in the food provides energy on oxidation.
3. Body uses energy derived from them for
   (*a*) Maintenance of several basic processes like respiration, blood circulation, contraction of cardiac and skeletal muscle, excitability of central nervous system, secretory functions of various glands, membrane potential, excretory function of kidney and other cellular activities. The energy spent for this purpose constitutes basal metabolic rate (BMR).
   (*b*) Various physical activities.
   (*c*) Digestion and metabolizing food.
4. Physiological conditions like pregnancy, lactation and pathological conditions like fever, hyperthyroidism and cancer increases BMR.
5. A sedentary worker requires 2500C of energy whereas heavy worker requires 4500C of energy per day. However, body energy requirement is influenced by environment.
6. Proteins, fats and carbohydrates of food are required for growth and maintenance of body tissues also. For this reason they are called as nutrients. Vitamins, minerals and water are other nutrients required by body.
7. For optimal health a balanced food (diet) that meets energy requirement as well as nutritional requirement is essential.
8. However consumption of excess food or calories causes obesity which in turn progress to several health problems (Chapter–13).
9. Kwashiorkor and Marasmus seen in pre school children of several developing countries are due to consumption of food deficient in nutrients, energy or both.
10. Parenteral feeding meets energy and nutritional requirements of people who are unable to use gastrointestinal tract due to several diseases.

11. Some foods contain medicines (nutraceuticals) in addition to usual nutrients. Such foods have preventive, protective and curative effects on diseases like hypertension, cardiovascular diseases, atherosclerosis, obesity, auto immune diseases and cancers of breast, prostate, lung etc.
12. Fibre present in plant foods reduces incidence of colonic diseases like colon cancer, piles, ulcerative colitis as well as cardiovascular diseases and metabolic diseases.
13. Foods acting as vaccines like banana vaccines (edible vaccines) are being produced by using recombinant DNA technology and soon they may be available in market.
14. Using recombinant DNA technology genetically modified foods (GMF) are being produced in advanced countries. These foods have more shelf life, nutrient quality and good texture etc. Some of them particularly animal derived foods contain medicines also like transgenic milk (Chapter 20).
15. Toxins present in foods are causating agents of diseases like lathyrism, epidemic dropsy, liver damage, botulism and cancer.
16. In South Asian countries maternal malnutrition is due to poverty, inadequate intake of food, false beliefs and taboos.
17. Arsenism (Arsenic poisoning) due to exposure to high arsenic levels in environment is seen in several countries. Arsenic causes cancers in humans.
18. Tobacco smoke an environmental pollutant affects health of non-smokers, children and pregnant women.
19. Mosquito repellants and therapeutic agents also cause environmental pollution and health and ecological hazards.

Energy

We shall now learn about energy requirement of body under various conditions and fuel or energy values of foods which supply this energy under this head. As mentioned earlier food energy is derived from carbohydrates, lipids and proteins present in food. These food components are digested, resulting molecules like glucose, fatty acids and amino acids are absorbed and converted to chemical energy and heat. Carbohydrates, fats and proteins contributes to 50-55%, 30-40% and 10-15% of food energy respectively.

Physical methods used for determination of food energy

Energy or fuel value of food depends on amounts of carbohydrates, fats and proteins present in them. Bomb calorimeter is used to determine energy values of carbohydrates, fats and proteins. The amount of energy they release or their calorific value is determined by oxidizing known amount of food in bomb calorimeter and measuring the heat generated.

Energy Units

Kilocalorie, Kcal (nutritional Calorie, C) or kilo joules (KJ) are the units used to express energy value of foods.

Kilocalorie (Kcal or C) is defined as amount of energy required in the form of heat to raise temperature of 1 Kg water by 1°C. It is thousand times of calorie used in physics. One Kcal or C is equal to 4.186 kilo joules (KJ).

Determination of food energy values using Bomb calorimeter

Bomb calorimeter consist of steel chamber fitted with O_2 under high pressure. A fixed amount of food sample is placed in the chamber. An electrical discharge is used to initiate combustion of food sample. Energy (heat) is released into surrounding which is carried away by water flowing outside the chamber. Energy output of food sample is calculated from difference between the temperature of out going and incoming water.

Energy values obtained with bomb calorimeter for carbohydrates, fats and proteins are given below.

1 gm of carbohydrate	4.1 C or 4.1 Kcal
1 gm of fat	9.45 C or 9.45 Kcal
1 gm of protein	5.65 C or 5.65 Kcal

Energy values for other food stuffs like bread, milk, vegetables etc., may be obtained similarly.

Physiological calorific values of foods (Animal calorimetry)

Calorific values obtained with bomb calorimeter do not reflect *in vivo* values because in bomb calorimeter food is completely oxidized to CO_2 and H_2O where as in body a fraction of food is lost in digestion and nitrogen of protein is eliminated as urea. Furthermore bomb calorimeter is nonliving object. Hence to get clear picture of energy output of food in the body methods involving humans are needed. Direct and indirect calorimetric methods are used to determine energy production (expenditure) in humans when a particular food is oxidized in the body.

Direct Calorimetry

In the direct calorimetry energy production of an individual is measured by estimating his body's heat production. The individual is placed in an insulated chamber then his heat production when a particular food is oxidized in the body is measured directly by recording amount of heat transferred to water circulating through the chamber. The O_2 in take, CO_2 output and nitrogen in urine and feces are also measured.

The calorific values obtained for different foods are given below.

Food stuff	Energy value
Carbohydrates (1 g)	4 C
Fats (1 gm)	9 C
Proteins (1 gm)	4 C
Cooked rice (1 Kg)	290 C
Milk (1 L)	700 C
Bread (1 Kg)	2630 C
Sugar (1 Kg)	4100 C
Cake (1 Kg)	4000 C

The figures obtained for carbohydrates, fats and proteins are slightly less than those obtained with bomb calorimeter due to loss of food (little) in digestion and protein nitrogen as urea.

Indirect Calorimetry

Since oxidation of food in the body is associated with O_2 consumption and CO_2 release in indirect Calorimetry energy production of an individual when a particular food is oxidized in the body is measured by estimating O_2 consumed and CO_2 released.

Respiratory quotient

It is the ratio of the volume of CO_2 produced to the volume of O_2 consumed when particular food is oxidized in the body.

$$\text{Respiratory quotient (R.Q.)} = \frac{\text{Volume of } CO_2 \text{ produced}}{\text{Volume of } O_2 \text{ consumed}}$$

R.Q. for carbohydrate, fat and protein are 1, 0.7 and 0.8 respectively on mixed diet R.Q. is 0.85.

Medical Importance

1. It indicates type of food being oxidized in the body.
2. In diabetes mellitus and starvation R.Q. decreases.

Energy Requirements of an individual

Energy requirement of an individual is made up of several components. They are

(1) Basal metabolic rate

(2) Specific dynamic action of food

(3) Various activities. However, for women pregnancy and lactation are additional components of energy requirement.

Basal metabolic rate

It is the energy expenditure (heat output) of an individual in post absorptive state for the last 12 hours lying at complete physical and mental or emotional rest and having normal temperature.

Measurements of BMR have been made on humans using indirect calorimeter. BMR of an individual can be calculated from a formula given below.

BMR = Weight (Kg) × 24C/day

(24C/day/kg approximately)

Normal BMR : Male = 37.5C/sqm/hour

Female = 35 C/sqm/hour

FACTORS AFFECTING BMR

Many factors influence BMR

1. **Age.** BMR decreases with age. Children have high BMR than adults, old people has low BMR than adults.
2. **Surface area.** BMR is directly proportional to body surface area. Larger the surface area higher the BMR.
3. **Sex.** BMR is high in males than females.
4. **Environment.** In cold BMR is high whereas in warm climate BMR is low.
5. Physiological conditions like pregnancy and lactation increases BMR whereas sleep decreases BMR.
6. **Exercise.** Muscular exercise increases BMR.

Medical Importance

1. In fever BMR increases. For every 1°C rise in body temperature BMR increases by 10%.
2. In hyper thyroidism BMR increases upto 80-90%.
3. BMR increases in conditions like Cushings syndrome, cancer, emphysema and hyper activity of pituitary. Drugs like salicylates and amphetamines increase BMR.
4. BMR decreases in starvation, hypothyroidism, Addisons disease and nephrotic syndrome.

Specific dynamic action (SDA) of food

It has been observed that heat output (energy expenditure) and oxygen consumption of an individual increases upon eating food even when the individual is at rest. It is called as post prandial thermogenesis (PPT) or specific dynamic action of food. It is the extra amount of energy (heat) produced over the normal calorific value of the food stuff when oxidized in the body or used up in the body.

For example when protein having energy value of 100 C is eaten it produces 130 C. This extra 30 C is due to SDA of protein. Therefore SDA of protein is expressed as 30% similarly SDA of carbohydrate, fat and mixed diet are 6%, 4% and 6-10% respectively. The exact source for SDA is unknown. However, probably it may be a result of energy expended in digestion, absorption and transport of ingested food. So while calculating energy requirement for daily activities of an individual 10% of the total calories are added to compensate for expenditure on SDA. However several nutritionists feel it as not necessary.

Energy requirements for various physical activities

Energy required for different daily activities have been determined. For light work (sedentary work) like sitting, standing, dressing and reading 1.5 C/kg body weight/hour is required. About 2.5 C/Kg/hour is required for moderate work like cycling, gardening and walking.

For heavy work like swimming, running and wood cutting about 5.0 C/Kg/hr is required. These values are only approximate because digestion of food varies from person to person.

A sedentary individuals daily energy requirement

Daily energy requirement of 70 Kg adult male engaged in sedentary work has been determined. For this purpose an individuals day has been divided into three phases. Each phase has a duration of 8 hours. They are 1. Sleep 2. Personal activities 3. Office (sedentary) work. Energy requirement for each phase is given below.

	Phase	Energy requirement (C)
1.	8 hours sleep (BMR × body surface area × 8 = 37.5 × 1.7 × 8)	510
2.	Personal activities for 8 hours (off work) it involves both light work for 4 hours and moderate work for 4 hours (1.5 C × 70 × 4 + 2.5 C × 70 × 4)	1120
3.	8 hours office work at rate of 1.5 C/kg/hr (1.5 × 70 × 8)	840
	Total (1 + 2 + 3)	= 2470 C

Thus 70 Kg adult male engaged in sedentary work needs approximately 2500C per day. A college student of 18 years age requires about 2600C per day (assuming his weight as 70 Kg and BMR as 44C/hr/sqm).

In the case of women the daily requirement values are slightly less because of difference in weight. More over in pregnancy and lactation their caloric requirement increases. Energy needed by men and women for various activities is given in Table 25.1.

Table 25.1 Energy needed by men and women for various activities.

Activity	Men (70 kg) C/day	Women (55 kg) C/day
Sedentary work like sitting, standing, reading, typing, teaching	2500	2000
Moderate work like cycling, gardening, walking, digging	3000	2500
Heavy work like wood cutting, running fast, swimming, playing football and basket ball, cricket	4500	3000
Pregnancy	—	2300
Lactation	—	2700

Nutrients

Food we eat contains several substances both organic as well as inorganic substances. Some of them are essential to body and some of them are not essential. For optimal health food must contain essential substances which are not produced in the body. They are often referred as nutrients. Thus nutrients are the chemical substances which are essential for growth and maintenance of body (cells). Some 40-50 chemical substances are essential for human body and they must present in the diet either as such or in preformed form. They are divided into six major groups. 1. Carbohydrates 2. Lipids 3. Proteins 4. Vitamins 5. Minerals 6. Water. The biochemical role of first three group is discussed in previous chapters. They are proximate principles in food. They yield energy and required for growth and maintenance. Their nutritional importance is detailed below. The role of vitamins and minerals in health and disease is also detailed earlier. They are not energy yielding but required for growth and maintenance. Importance of water is discussed in next chapter.

Recommended Dietary Allowance (RDA)

For maintaining good health and for functional efficiency of the body the diet must provide all nutrients in adequate amounts. However daily requirements of different nutrients by an individual are influenced by several factors. They are weight, hight, sex, developmental stage, climate, physical activities and geographical location.

Nutritional expert committee of ICMR have been determined daily allowances for different nutrients. Food and nutrition board of USA and various international societies also recommended daily allowances for different nutrients. They are called as recommended dietary allowances (RDA). In establishing dietary allowances all the above mentioned factors that affect nutrient requirement of an individual are taken into account.

Usually dietary allowances increases gradually from infancy to adulthood. To meet extra requirements of pregnant, lactating and menstruating women increases in nutrients intake have been recommended.

Medical Importance

1. Recommended dietary allowances (RDA) exist for proteins, fats, carbohydrates, vitamins and minerals.
2. Based on daily requirements for different nutrients hospital dietetician designs balanced diet for an individual.

Carbohydrates

Carbohydrate is the major food stuff consumed by humans in most of the countries. As stated earlier carbohydrates contributes to 50-60% of body energy requirement. Principle carbohydrates present in diet are polysaccharides like starch, dextrins, glycogen and trace of inulin. Cereals, legumes, potatoes, sweet potato, bananas, meat and garlic present in food are sources for polysaccharides.

Starch is the dominant carbohydrate in the diet and it is cheapest source of energy. In low income groups it contributes to 75-80% calories. However in high income group it may contributes to 40% calories. Starches of different origin are not digested equally. The digestibility of starch depends on amylopectin content. Starches of cereals are digested rapidly due to high amylopectin where as starches of legumes are digested slowly due to low amylopectin content. The rate of digestibility of different starches is of importance to diabetic patients. Amylase inhibitors present in some foods also affect starch digestibility.

Usually glycogen is absent in plant foods. Even in animal foods also glycogen content is less. Only oysters contain about 6% of its weight as glycogen.

Disaccharides lactose, sucrose and maltose are also present in food. Milk and other dairy products are lactose source in the food. Lactose is the major carbohydrate for infants. It contributes to 35-45% of infants energy requirement. Sucrose is present in candies, sweets, honey, syrups, jams, jellies and jaggery. Some fruits also contain sucrose. Sucrose supplies empty calories. In developing countries sucrose consumption is low where as it is high in developed countries. Excess sucrose is found to raise plasma cholesterol and triglyceride level. Hence sucrose content in the diet should be below 50-70 gm per day. Carbohydrate contents of some common food stuffs are given in Table 25.2.

Table 25.2 Carbohydrate, fat and protein contents of some common food stuffs.

Name	Carbo-hydrate gm/ 100 gm	Fat gm/ 100 gm	Protein gm/ 100 gm	Name	Carbo-hydrate gm/ 100 gm	Fat gm/ 100 gm	Protein gm/ 100 gm
Cereals				**Milk**			
l.Rice	75	1	7	1. Human	7	1.5	4.5
2. Wheat	70	2	12	2. Buffalo	5	7.5	4.0
3. Bread	50	2	8	3. Cow	1.5	3.5	3.0
Pulses				**Cheese**	2.7	0.5	17
I. Black gram	58	6	22	**Cream**	2-0	38	8
2. Red gram	60	5	18	**Eggs**			
Nuts				1. Hen	1	11	13
1. Coconut	8	38	4	2. Turkey	2	11	13
2. Peanut	20	40	27	3, Duck	0.5	15	13

(Contd.)

Vegetables				Meat			
1. Green (cabbage)	5	0.10	0.80	1. Chicken	1.5	8	30
2. Other (cuccumber)	2.0	0.10	0.50	2. Mutton	0.5	14	18
Tubers and roots				Fish	3	10	16
1. Potato	22	0.10	1.50	**Beverages**			
2. carrot	11	0.30	1.00	**Values are in gm/cup**			
Fruits				1. Coffee	18	2	2
1, Banana	25	0.50	1.00	2. Tea	16	1	1
2. Mango	17	0.50	0.80	3. Cocoa	26	8	8
3. Coconut water	5	Traces	Traces				
Mushrooms	5.0	0.70	3.70				

Recommended dietary allowance

Since carbohydrate is synthesized in the body no recommended dietary allowance for carbohydrate. But absence of carbohydrate in the diet for few days leads to keto acidosis and loss of muscle protein. So minimum 100 gm of carbohydrate must present in diet to avoid keto acidosis and wasting of muscle protein.

Lipids

Dietary fat furnishes about 30-40% of body energy requirement. Apart from energy dietary fat provides essential fatty acids, vitamins and cholesterol. In advanced countries dietary fat furnish 40-50% of body energy. However in poor countries it may contribute to 15% of energy requirement. For quick energy high fat intake is essential for dynamic people.

Dietary fat reduces bulkyness of diet. It improves palatability of food and give satiety. Sources of fat in the diet are vegetable oils like peanut oil, safflower oil, cotton seed oil, coconut oil, soybean oil, palm oil, corn oil and sunflower oil. Other sources for fat in diet are butter, cheese, ghee, eggs and chicken fat, beef, cereals, pulses, nuts and other vegetables also contain fats. Cholesterol is present in most of animal fats. Cholesterol rich diet is not good for health as explained in chapter-10. Fat contents of some common food stuffs are given in Table 25.2.

Recommended dietary allowance

Minimum requirement for fat is very low and not yet clearly known. However an ideal diet must contain about 30-50 gm of fat and 5 gm of essential fatty acids. In pregnancy and lactation diet should contain more essential fatty acids.

Proteins

Main function of dietary protein is to provide essential amino acids required for the synthesis of body proteins and other nitrogenous substances. Therefore diet must contain adequate amount of protein to replace essential amino acids and nitrogen lost through normal protein turnover and maintain nitrogen balance. Dietary protein contributes to 10-15% of body energy requirement. In low income groups it may be less. If the diet contains more protein it is used for energy production because it can not be stored. Hence in developing countries where protein in diet is more significant energy is obtained from protein. In Eskimos and traditional hunters of Africa protein furnishes 2/3 of energy requirement. Meat, eggs and milk are main sources. However cereals, pulses, legumes, vegetables and fruits also contain small amount of protein (Table 25.2). Consumption of lean meat leads to digestive problems. So it must be avoided.

Nitrogen Balance

Since protein is the main source of nitrogen in body the dietary protein must make up nitrogen lost from body to maintain nitrogen balance. If an individuals total nitrogen content of the urine and feces equals the amount of dietary nitrogen then the individual is said to be in nitrogen balance or equilibrium

$$\text{Fecal nitrogen (N)} + \text{Urinary nitrogen (N)} = \text{Dietary nitrogen (N)}$$

$$\text{N output} = \text{N intake}$$

i.e.,

$$\frac{\text{N intake}}{\text{N output}} = 1$$

In other words if the ratio of nitrogen intake to nitrogen output is one then the individual is in nitrogen balance or equilibrium. Intestinal flora influences nitrogen balance of an individual.

Positive nitrogen balance

If the ratio of N intake to N output is greater than one then it is called as positive nitrogen balance or if the N output is less than N intake then the individual is in positive nitrogen balance. In the positive nitrogen balance most of dietary nitrogen is retained in the body and less is eliminated from body. More over in positive nitrogen balance the tissue protein content increases due to increased protein synthesis. Usually it occurs during growth, pregnancy, lactation and post operative recovery.

Negative nitrogen balance

If the nitrogen output is more than the N intake then the individual is in negative nitrogen balance or if the ratio of N intake to N output is less than one then the individual is in negative nitrogen balance. In the negative nitrogen balance nitrogen lost is not replaced by dietary nitrogen. It occurs in malnutrition and other wasting diseases where there is tissue breakdown like starvation, uncontrolled diabetes mellitus and cancer. Menstruating women may have transient negative nitrogen balance if proper replacement for nitrogen lost is not possible. Physical exercise trainee may also have transient negative nitrogen balance because of atrophy of muscle.

Protein minimum

It is the minimum amount of dietary protein required to maintain nitrogen balance. It is 1 gm/kg body weight per day.

However protein requirement also depends on the (*a*) Protein quality (*b*) Carbohydrate and fat contents (*c*) Physical activity.

Protein quality

Essential amino acid content determines quality of a protein. An ideal or a good quality protein is the one which has amino acid composition of body protein synthesized at any given time. Further an ideal protein must meet essential amino acid requirement. Unfortunately ideal proteins or good quality proteins are limited.

Limiting amino acid

Proteins of different foods have different proportions of essential amino acids. Some of them may contain required amounts of essential amino acid and few of them may not have adequate amounts of one or more of essential amino acids. An essential amino acid of a protein which is present much below requirement is called as limiting amino acid. Except rice most of the plant proteins contain limiting amino acid.

Examples.

(*a*) Tryptophan is the limiting amino acid in maize, bengal gram and red gram proteins.

(*b*) Lysine is the limiting amino acid in wheat protein.

(*c*) Methionine is the limiting amino acid in peanut protein.

Due to limiting amino acid quality of protein decreases.

Effect of limiting amino acid on protein utilization

When tissue proteins are synthesized all the essential amino acids must be present in proper proportions in tissues. If one essential amino acid is absent in tissues due to lack of dietary supply protein synthesis decreases and nitrogen balance is not maintained. More over biological value of a protein with limiting amino acid is low as we shall see it later.

Protein Supplementation

One way of improving quality of dietary protein with limiting amino acid is by adding another protein containing the missing amino acid. This is termed as protein supplementation. For example cereal proteins are limiting in lysine where as milk proteins are good source of this amino acid. Thus milk protein effectively supplement cereal proteins. Protein supplementation has important role in preparation of vegetarian balanced diet. Supplementation of wheat bread with lysine is commonly done.

Complementary proteins and mutual supplementation of proteins

Complementary proteins are poor quality proteins as such due to limiting amino acids. But they are complementary in limiting essential amino acid composition i.e., a limiting essential amino acid in one protein is present in excess amounts in another protein and *vice versa*. So they supplement each other and make good quality protein in diet. This is known as mutual supplementation of proteins. For example wheat proteins and red gram proteins are complementary proteins and as such both are low quality proteins due to limiting amino acid. Wheat protein is limiting in lysine but good source of tryptophan whereas red gram is limiting in tryptophan but a good source of lysine. When they are mixed they make up good quality protein in diet by supplementing one another i.e., wheat protein effectively supplement pulse protein and *vice versa*. Therefore chapati and dal combination improves quality of protein in diet.

Complementary vegetable proteins form the basis of vegetarian balanced diet. Because of mutual supplementation the net quality of mixture of proteins is higher than the quality of single protein.

Carbohydrate and fat content

If diet contains sufficient amounts of carbohydrate and fat then use of protein for energy production is reduced. Hence protein requirement in diet is minimum. In contrast if the diet contains inadequate amounts of carbohydrates and fats then use of protein for energy production is more. This increases protein requirement in diet.

Physical activity

Protein requirement increases with increases in physical activity due to retention of nitrogen or increased muscle protein in the body.

Recommended dietary allowance for protein and amino acids

For adults daily intake of 55-80 gm (1 gm/kg body weight) of protein has been recommended. Extra amounts are required by pregnant and lactating women.

Minimal daily amino acid requirement of adult male are methionine (16.3 mg/kg), threonine (7 mg/kg), tryptophan (4 mg/kg), valine (11 mg/kg), isoleucine (10 mg/kg), leucine (16 mg/kg), lysine (11 mg/kg) and phenyl alanine (16.4 mg/kg).

Methods to assess protein quality

Few biological methods are available to assess protein quality.

1. Nitrogen balance

If a protein is unable to maintain nitrogen balance then it is a poor quality protein. However nitrogen balance does not indicate anything about digestibility, essential amino acid content and assimilation of products of digestion. Usually good quality protein maintain nitrogen balance if taken in adequate amounts.

2. Biological value (BV)

The biological value of a protein measures the quantity of dietary protein used by animal for growth and maintenance of body function. It is defined as percentage of absorbed nitrogen that is retained by the body.

$$\text{Biological value (BV)} = \frac{\text{N retained}}{\text{N absorbed}} \times 100$$

Biological value of protein may also indicates essential amino acid content, digestibility of protein and availability of digested products for absorption. Biological values for some proteins are given in Table 25.3.

3. Net protein utilization (NPU)

Biological value of protein does not cover nitrogen lost in digestion. In net protein utilization, it is included. It is defined as percentage of dietary nitrogen that is retained in the body.

$$\text{Net protein utilization} = \frac{\text{N retained}}{\text{N intake}} \times 100$$

NPU value of some proteins are given in Table 25.3.

Table 25.3 BV, NPU and PER of some food proteins.

	BV	NPU	PER
Eggs	96	91	4.5
Milk	84	75	3.0
Meat	80	74	2.8
Rice	64	47	2.0
Wheat	58	46	1.7
Bengal gram	57	45	1.6
Ground nut	54	45	1.6

4. Protein efficiency ratio (PER)

It is a better index of protein quality than biological value. It is defined as weight gain per weight of protein eaten. PER value of some proteins are given in Table 25.3.

$$\text{PER} = \frac{\text{Weight gain (gm)}}{\text{Weight of dietary protein (gm)}}$$

Depending on BV, NPV and PER values proteins can be divided into

(*a*) Good quality proteins

(*b*) Low quality proteins

(*a*) **Good quality proteins.** Animal proteins are good quality proteins because they have high BV, NPU and PER values. They are egg, milk and meat proteins.

(*b*) **Low quality proteins.** Plant proteins are low quality proteins because they have low BV, NPU and PER values. They are rice, wheat, bengal gram and groundnut proteins. The plant proteins have low values because they are not digested (absorbed) completely due to several factors.

Diet

Usually diet taken by most of the population contains nutrients of various classes and water. Occasionally diet plays wider role in society than merely providing nutrients and physiological needs of life. Hence composition of diet depends on race, religious restriction, culture, social fads (taboos), income, geographical location and environment. One may feel about diet served at famous restaurant or marriage party as excellent but it can be considered as excellent if it provides all essential nutrients in proper amounts. Thus it is not the palatibility or physical composition of diet that decides what is good for the body or quality of the food.

Balanced diet

A balanced diet contains carbohydrates, fats and proteins in proper proportions and required amounts of vitamins and minerals to meet the energy requirement as well as nutritional requirement of individual. The proportions of carbohydrate, fat and protein in an average Indian balanced diet are approximately 70%, 20% and 10% respectively. Balanced diets for a adult male and adult female who requires 2500C and 2000C per day respectively should contain below shown amounts of carbohydrate, fat, protein and required (recommended) amounts of vitamins, minerals and water.

Male Nutrient	Quantity	Calories (C)	Female Nutrient	Quantity	Calories (C)
Carbohydrate	440 gm	1760	Carbohydrate	350 gm	1420
Fat	50 gm	450	Fat	40 gm	360
Protein	70 gm	280	Protein	55 gm	220
	Total:	2490C		Total:	2000C

Since it is not possible to separate and consume carbohydrates, fats and proteins from common food stuffs the balanced diet described above is of little practical value. The diet we take usually consist of cereals, vegetables, milk, meat etc. Hence balanced diet must be designed using these food stuffs. Vegetarian balanced diet consisting of cereals, pulses, vegetables and milk for adult male and non vegetarian diet consisting of cereals, vegetables and meat for adult male are given below.

Balanced Diet (gm)

	Cereals	Pulses	Greens	Others	Milk	Meat	Fruit	Fat	Sugar
Vegetarian	450	70	100	175	250	—	30	45	40
Non-vegetarian	450	50	100	175	150	30	30	45	40

Malnutrition

Since consumption of adequate amounts of nutrients is essential for growth and maintenance of body function, intake of low quantities of nutrients affects growth and individual. However pregnant and lactating women and growing children are more affected. Consumption of inadequate amounts of protein or calories or both is called as malnutrition. It is common in children of one to five years age. It occurs in starvation and during famine or civil war.

Mild to moderate malnutrition among the children is endemic globally. About 195 million children under age of 5 years are under nourished. Even developed countries are not spared of this curse. In 1992 about 12 million American Children consumed diets that are low in recommended food allowances. The global population of malnourished children below 5 years of age is expected to increase from 193 million to 200 million by 2020 with most of deterioration in Africa.

South Asia has the dubivous distinction of having the highest prevalence of malnutrition in children. About 50% of pre-school children are malnourished in South Asia. Nearly half of all the malnourished children in the world and less proportion of malnourished adult women reside in few South Asian countries India being the largest.

With in the four major countries of South Asia India, Pakistan, Bangladesh and Srilanka the prevalence of under five malnutrition is higher in India and Bangladesh than in Pakistan and Srilanka.

Protein energy malnutrition (PEM)

It is due to consumption of inadequate protein or calories or both in the diet. It is seen all over the world in children of economically weaker sections of the population. It is rarely seen in adults of surgical wards. It is responsible for high rate of mortality and morbidity among pre school children in all states in India. Other name given to this condition is protein calorie malnutrition (PCM). Two forms of protein energy malnutrition are well known in developing countries.

They are marasmus and kwashiorkor.

Marasmus

It is due to inadequate intake of proteins and calories. It is most common protein energy malnutrition disorder in pre school children of below 2 years age of this country and sets in at about one year age. It is a serious condition. A child is said to be marasmic if the weight is 60% below expected weight for his age. It is also seen in South and other South East Asian countries.

Marasmus occurs when infants are withdrawn from breast milk or weaned and given inadequate bottle feedings which are deficient in protein and calories. Marasmus also likely occur when breast feeding was withdrawn for other reason (body line) and processed foods low in protein and calories are given.

Clinical features

1. Growth retardation
2. Severe wasting of muscles and loss of body fat. Legs and arms are skin covered and ribs are visible. Even peristalysis is visible due to thin abdominal wall.
3. Head is big and unproportionate to body size
4. Mental retardation
5. Dry skin and dehydration
6. Eye lesion due to vitamin A deficiency.

Biochemical Symptoms

1. Serum albumin is low
2. Vitamin A content of plasma is also low

Treatment

Intake of adequate amounts of protein and carbohydrate in the diet

Kwashiorkor

It is due to intake of inadequate protein only. Starchy foods consumed by the affected children provide enough calories. Children below 1½years age are commonly affected. It is prevalent in Africa, Central and South America and war infested countries like Somalia. It is less common in India. A child is said to be affected with kwashiorkor when his weight is below 80% of expected weight for age. The mortality rate is about 50%. The affected child may survive into adulthood but he may suffer from irreversible damage due to impaired cellular development.

Generally kwashiorkor occurs when a child is weaned from breast feeding and traditional family foods are given. These foods mainly consist of gruel of colocasia, taro, tapioca, millet or corn and plantain etc. They contain less protein but provide enough calories. This practice is mainly seen in economically weaker population.

Clinical features

1. ***Edema.*** It is seen allover the body including face. But it is more marked in lower limbs.
2. Distanded abdomen or pot belly and poor appetite.

3. **Dematitis.** The skin is hyper or hypo pigmented and becomes thickened. In some areas the thickened skin peels off as flaky paint. As a result cracks or ulceration develops on the skin.
4. Abnormal hair.
5. Apathy and anaemia.
6. Diarrhoea.
7. Prone to infection due to defective immune system.

Biochemical Symptoms

1. Hypo proteinemia.
2. Fatty liver.

Treatment

Intake of good quality protein along with adequate calories in the diet. Both marasmus and kwashiorkor may result from poverty and ignorance. The children are denied food even though it is available because of customs and taboos.

Maternal malnutrition

Maternal malnutrition is one of the major cause of low birth weight new borns. The incidence of malnutrition among girls or adult women is higher in South Asia than any other region. Apart from poverty and in adequate food several false beliefs and food taboos work against nutrition of pregnant and lactating women as well as children.

Food Taboos

1. In India pregnant women often eat less for the fear of baby becoming too big and causing problems during labour.
2. Pregnant women are denied good food due to false beliefs. Papaya a rich source of Vit. A is considered as Abortificient and is banned.
3. Banana eating is believed to produce single child infertility since the banana tree fruits only once in life span.
4. Further malnutrition occurs in new born due to discarding of colostrums which is rich in immunoglobulins, proteins and vitamins.
5. Milk is given to new born only after three days due to false beliefs.

Parenteral feeding

It involves feeding of an individual through parenteral (intravenous) route. It is also called as intravenous hyper alimination. It is given to patients who are unable to take food by mouth or who are unable to use gastrointestinal tract due to various conditions such as surgery, pyloric or intestinal obstruction, pancreatitis, uncontrolled vomiting, cirrhosis, unconscious and cancer.

For maintaining good health parenteral feeding must provide balanced food that meets energy and nutritional requirements of the individual. Using a catheter parental feed containing nutrients is infused into a large blood vessel like superior vena cava or sub clavian vein. Generally parenteral feed contains glucose, amino acids, lipids, electrolytes, essential minerals and vitamins. Composition of a typical parenteral feed is given below.

Glucose = 10-30%

Fat as emulsion = 1 – 4 gm /Kg body weight

Protein hydrolysate = 1 – 1.5gm/Kg body weight

Specified or recommended amounts of vitamins and minerals.

However maintenance of good health in an individual for longer period by parenteral feeding is not possible because individual may develop complications like pneumothorax, septicemia etc. Even maintenance of catheter in proper position is difficult.

Nutraceuticals or food medicines

They are components of foods which have protective, preventive and curative effects on several diseases. They are also called as physiological foods or functional foods or pharma foods or designer foods and new age foods. Several of them have been identified in food stuffs and some are given below together with their beneficial effects.

Dietary fibre

Dietary fibre is defined as part of plant food which is resistant to human digestive enzymes. Plant carbohydrates mostly polysaccharides like cellulose, hemi cellulose, pectin, gums, pentosans and lignin are fibres present in diet. Since dietary fibre is of plant origin, non vegetarien diets are low in (devoid of) dietary fibre. This may be the reason for prevalence of certain cardiovascular and intestinal disease in developed countries where diet mostly consist of foods of animal origin. Cellulose and hemicellulose are water in soluble fibres present in cereals and vegetables. Where as pectins and gums are water soluble fibres present in legumes and fruits. Water in soluble fibres are good for bulking where as water soluble fibres interferes with absorption. Fibre content of some common foods are as follows: cereals (15%) and vegetables(2-8%).

Protective, preventive and curative effects of dietary fibre

1. For optimal health diet must contain fibre.
2. Dietary fibre reduces incidence of colonic diseases like ulcerative colitis, constipation, piles, diverticular disease, cancer of colon etc., probably by promoting movement of bowel contents along the gut, size and consistency of feces, water retention, elimination of toxins etc.
3. Short chain fatty acids produced in the intestine from dietary fibre by the action of flora are involved in the maintenance of structure of intestinal wall.
4. Dietary fibre reduces incidence of metabolic diseases like diabetes mellitus, obesity, ischemic heart disease, hypertension, rheumatoid arthritis, gall stones, varicose veins etc., by interfering with absorption of glucose, cholesterol and bile salts.
5. Fibre rich diet has been found to lower blood glucose, cholesterol and triglyceride levels in humans.
6. Fermentation products of fibre by intestinal flora may meet energy requirement also.

Though the dietary fibre has several beneficial effects it is not without adverse effects. They are

(*a*) In susceptible people high fibre diet produces flatus, abdominal cramps and diarrhoea.

(*b*) Dietary fibre interferes with absorption of vitamins like cobalamin and minerals like calcium and iron in the intestine.

Several designer foods containing varying amounts of fibre are now available in market in advanced countries. While designing these foods advantages and disadvantages of fibre have been considered.

ω-3 poly unsaturated Fatty acids (ω-3 PUFA)

Eicosapentaenoic acid (EPA, 20:5, $\Delta^{5,8,11,14,17}$) and Docosa Hexaenoic Acid (DHA,20:6, $\Delta^{4,7,10,13,16,19}$) are two ω-3 poly unsaturated fatty acids present in fish oils. They are also present in eggs, milk and other fats but at low concentration. However because of their beneficial effects designer eggs containing adequate quantities of these ω-3 PUFA are being produced in several advanced countries by feeding chicks diet (fish oils) rich in ω-3 fatty acids. They are not essential fatty acids. However DHA and EPA are required for photo receptors present in retina and development of brain. In the body DHA is synthesized from linolenic acid an essential ω-3 PUFA.

Beneficial effects of ω-3 PUFA

1. They reduce incidence of cardiovascular diseases and atherosclerosis. Hence they are often referred as cardiovascular nutraceuticals.
2. They reduce incidence of inflammatory and autoimmune diseases.
3. They protect the body from developing cancer of lung, colon, pancreas and prostate.

Antioxidants of fruits, vegetables and spices

1. Beta carotenes, tocopherols and ascorbic acids are antioxidants present in fruits, vegetables etc. reduce incidence of several diseases by eliminating free redicals (see chapter-10).
2. Curcumin of turmeric, caffeine of tea and coffee, capsaicin of chillies, piperine of pepper and euegenol of cloves are other antioxidants present in diet. They also act as scavengers of free radicals and hence they have also beneficial effects on health.

Curcumin, Cancer and AIDS

1. Curcumin (diferuloyl methane) the main yellow bioactive compound of turmeric has anti carcinogenic action as well as antiviral action.
2. Turmaric is considered as traditional Indian medicine.
3. The average intake of turmeric by Asians varies from 0.5 to 1.5 g/day/person which produce no toxic symptoms.

Anticarcinogenic action of curcumin

1. Curcumin act as potential anti-carcinogenic compound.
2. It induces apoptosis and inhibits cell cycle progression both of these prevents cancerous cell growth.
3. It induces apoptic cell death by DNA damage and fragmentation.
4. It causes rapid decrease in mitochondrial membrane potential and release of cytochrome-C to activate caspase 9 and caspase 3 for apoptic cell death.
5. It suppress tumor growth through other ways. Nitric Oxide and its derivatives play major role in tumor promotion. Curcumin inhibits iNOS and COX2 production.

Anti-Viral effect of Curcumin

1. Curcumin shows anti HIV activity. It inhibits activity of HIV-I integrase needed for viral replication. It also causes HIV protease inhibition.
2. It inhibits ultraviolet light induced HIV gene expression.
3. Thus Curcumin has potential for novel drug development against HIV.

Ripened and unripened bananas

Ripened and unripened bananas are found to be useful in cardiovascular and digestive disorders.

1. Ripe and unripe bananas have anti hypertensive action. They contain inhibitors of angiotensin converting enzyme (ACE) which plays key role in blood pressure regulation. Hence they lower blood pressure by inhibiting action of ACE.
2. Unripe bananas cure stomach ulcers by promoting growth of mucosal cells of stomach and inhibiting growth of bacteria. Cysteine protease inhibitors present in these bananas may be responsible for this due to their antibacterial action.
3. Ripened banana is reported to be useful as laxative. Trypsin inhibitors present in ripened bananas may be responsible for this beneficial effect of bananas.
4. Bananas also promote healing of lesions of ulcerative colitis.
5. Banana fruit is effective in treatment of celiac disease and sprue.

Allylsulfides

They are present in garlic and onion. They reduce incidence of Cardiovascular diseases by lowering blood cholesterol and blood pressure.

Lycopene of tomatoes

Red color of tomatoes is due to lycopene. It acts as antioxidant. It prevents cancers of lung, prostate, breast and colon. It even slow down progression of prostate cancer.

Hydroxy citrate

It is present in malabar tamarind. It reduces body fat. Hence it is useful in treatment of obesity.

Epigallo catechin-3-gallate (EGCG)

It is present in green tea. It inhibits growth of lung and esophagus cancers by blocking angiogenesis.

Resveratrol

It is present in grapes. It reduces incidence of skin cancer in experimental animals. Grapes also contain compounds which prevent growth of new blood vessels that are needed for growth of tumors.

Phenyliso-thiocyanate

It is present in cabbage. It prevents lung cancer.

In addition to above mentioned nutraceuticals, attempts towards production of genetically modified foods containing medicines like vaccines (edible vaccines), antibodies and hormones like insulin by using recombinant DNA technology (transgenic plants and transgenic animals) are in progress in several developed as well as developing countries.

Glucosinolates

1. Glucosinolates (GLS) are group of thio glucosides present in vegetables like cabbage, cauliflower, broccoli, turnip, radish, horse radish, white mustard, brown mustard and rape seeds.
2. These compounds and their products formed in the body act as chemoprotective agents against chemically induced carcinogenesis.
3. They block initiation of tumors in several organs. They induce cytochrome P_{450} enzyme systems and thus help in excretion of carcinogen.

Food toxins

Food we eat contains toxins some times in addition to nutrients. These toxins enter into human body when foods containing them are eaten. Body may remove some of them by detoxification but few of them are harmful to health because body is unable to neutralize their toxicity. Several types of toxins of different sources have been identified in foods.

Natural toxins

They are naturally present in foods and most of the cases they are part of food. Some toxins are added by humans (food adulteration). Some toxins becomes part of food when used by humans to control pest during cultivation.

1. β-N- oxalyldiaminopropionate (BODA)

It is a neurotoxin and present in lathyrus seeds (masoor dal) which are used as cattle and other animal feed. It is harmless when consumed in small quantities. However consumption of these seeds in large amounts cause lathyrism. It also occurs when dals adulterated with these seeds are consumed. In India lathyrism was reported in Andhra Pradesh and Madhya Pradesh. Lathyrism is a disease of spinal cord and initially it starts with heavyness in lower limbs and restricted movements. In later stage permanent paralysis of lower limbs occurs due to atrophy of muscles. B-oxalyl aminoalanine (BOAA) is another related substance which cause lathyrism.

2. Sanguinarine

It is an alkaloid present in seeds of poppy weed *argemone maxicana*. It also grows as weed in mustard crop. Consumption of mustard oil adulterated with argemone oil produces epidemic dropsy which is endemic in parts of India (Bihar and West Bengal) where mustard oil is main cooking medium. Sanguinarine inhibit pyruvate oxidation. Symptoms of epidemic dropsy are cardiomyopathy, edema, skin rash, vomiting and diarrhoea.

3. Goitrogens

Thiocyanates and isothiocyanates present in edible oils like rape seed and mustard oils are known as goitrogens. They prevent utilization and uptake of iodine by thyroid gland and this leads to goitre. Cabbage contain another goitrogen a thioglycoside.

4. Hypoglycin A

It is toxic amino acid present in uripe fruits of akee plant. It inhibits fatty acid oxidation and causes Jamaican vomiting sickness.

5. Cyanogenic compounds

They are cyanide producing compounds present in cereals, tubers and legumes. Cooking destroys their toxicity. Lima bean contains 10-20mg of cyanide/100gm. The cyanogenic compounds containing foods cause toxicity when taken raw. So animals eating raw tapioca develops fatty degenaration of liver and kidney.

6. Anti vitamins

These food components interfere with absorption or utilization of vitamins. For example orange peel used in some foods contains citral an anti vitamin of vitamin A. So consumption of such foods cause vitamin A deficiency. Linseed contain linetin which interfers with pyridoxine. Like wise thiaminase of fish, red cabbage and black berry may reduce availability of thiamine. Other anti vitamins present in food are avidin of egg and dicoumarol of sweat cloves.

7. Pressor amines

Amines like tyramine is present in cheese and beer. It is removed by monoamine oxidase (MAO). Hence persons taking drug that inhibit MAO get hypertension due to accumulation of tyramine. Since bananas contain serotonin and catecholamines excess consumption of bananas must be avoided.

8. Solanine

It is an alkolid present in skin of potato. Green potatoes may contain this in excess. When excess is taken it causes potato poisoning. Symptoms are head ache, vomiting and diarrhoea.

9. Protease inhibitors

Several legumes, cereals and bananas contain inhibitors of trypsin, chymotrypsin and elastase. However most of them are inactivated during cooking. In experimental animals they cause digestive problems.

10. Gossipol

It is present in cotton seeds. It prevents absorption of lysine by forming complex.

11. Favism

People with less active glucose-6-phosphate dehydrogenase develops hemolytic anaemia when they consume fava beans. It is called favism.

12. Shell fish poisoning

Consumption of shell fish containing saxitoxin and okadaic acid produces gastrointestinal problems and cancer respectively. Actually the toxins are present in marine plankton. Consumption of this plankton by shell fish leads to their accumulation in shell fish. For this reason shell fishing has been banned in areas where the above plankton is present.

13. Mushroom poisoning

Mushroom poisoning occurs due to consumption of two types of mushrooms. They are amanita phalloides and amanita serna. They contain phallotoxins and anatoxins. The former causes abdominal pain, vomiting, diarrhoea and later causes liver damage and renal failure.

14. Insecticides

Extensive use of insecticides like DDT and chlordane to increase crop yields and eliminate mosquitoes led to their accumulation in water and soil. Since they are not biodegradable they enter human body through natural food chain. DDT is extremely toxic to all forms of life. Most of the vegetables and milk we consume contain DDT. Even it is found in milk of lactating women.

Panmasala

1. It is consumed by people of several Asian countries including India. It consists of arecanut, catechu, lime, cardamom and unspecified flavouring agents with or without tobacco. It is gaining tremendous popularity among school children also. Both boys and girls are attracted equally to panmasala consumption.
2. Arecanut and catechu are also part of pan commonly consumed in several Asian countries.
3. Epidemiological studies shows association between chewing pan and risk of oral cancer in Indian population.
4. In experimental animals panmasala with or without tobacco produces cancer of lungs, testis, liver etc. Hence habitual pan masala used in humans may promote carcinogenesis.

Microbial, fungul toxins and helminths

When food is contaminated with pathogenic bacteria or fungus or helminths consumption of such food causes health problems (food poisoning) and parasitic infections. Pathogenic bacteria present in food releases toxins into the food making food unsuitable for consumption. Food poisoning due to microbial toxins is common in developing countries due to lack of regulatory acts.

1. Botulism

It is due to consumption of food containing toxin producing pathogenic bacteria *clostridium botulinus*. Characteristic symptoms are muscle paralysis and death due to respiratory failure. It may occur due to consumption of defectively processed fish and meat.

2. Aflatoxins

Fungus *aspergillus flavus* which grows on moist food grains and nuts like maize and ground nut produces aflatoxins (mycotoxins). Aflatoxins cause liver damage and cancer in animals. Aflatoxin B_1 is most potent hepato carcinogen. Usually food grains stored in moist condition or without proper drying are likely to get contaminated with this fungus. Aflatoxin epidemics due to consumption of aflatoxin contaminated maize and ground nut have been reported from Gujarat, Rajesthan and Andhra Pradesh respectively. Clinical symptoms are jaundice, ascites and portal hypertension.

3. Helminth infections

Consumption of under cooked pork and beef infected with tape worms causes tape worm infection. Like wise consumption of salads consisting of raw vegetables and uncooked fish contaminated with eggs of parasites can cause parasite infections.

Food preservatives and additives

Food preservatives are the chemical substances used to preserve foods. Food additives are chemical substances used to improve physical appearance like color, texture etc., of foods. However some of food additives and preservatives act as toxins.

1. Nitrates

They are used to preserve foods particularly meat products. However in the body they are converted to carcinogenic nitrosamines,

2. Monosodium glutamate (MSG)

Most of Chinese restaurants add MSG to food to increase flavour. Most of the people tolerate well but some people are allergic to MSG. Clinical features include numbness, palpitation and weakness. Most of these symptoms are transient and disappear within 2 hours. MSG may be converted to GABA in the body.

3. Cyclamate and saccharine

They are artificial sweeteners. Since saccharine is carcinogenic its use is banned and even cyclamate is permitted as food additive only upto specified amount.

Toxins of food processing

Some toxins are incorporated into food during processing of food.

Mutagens and carcinogens

High temperature cooking of meat and fish like roasting, frying and grilling produces potent mutagens and carcinogens like amino imidazo-aza-arenenes (AIAs) or benzpyrenes. However their exact role as causating agents of cancer in man is not known with certainity.

Environmental or Industrial pollution

Industrial waste containing heavy metals is usually discharged into near by rivers and lakes by Industries. The heavy metals which are toxic enters into human body through food chain and cause health problems. Like wise automobile exhaust contributes to excess levels of lead and carbon monoxide and other suspended solid matters in the environment. When air polluted with such toxic chemicals is inhaled they enter human lungs and exerts toxic effects. They enter human body through food chain also. Even nuclear blasts which were carried out in the environment and present day nuclear power reactors also create radioactive elements in environment. These radio active elements enter human body through food chain and emit harmful radiation in the body.

1. Mercury poisoning (Minamata disease)

An out break of mercury poisoning due to consumption of sea fish contaminated with mercury has been reported from Japan. Dumping of Industrial waste containing mercury into Minamata bay led to this tragedy. Initially mercury was absorbed by the algae present in the bay which is later concentrated in fish. Initial symptoms of Minamata disease are numbness of extremities, unable to use hands for holding things and writing etc; abnormal gait, weakness and sensory disturbances. These symptoms progress to paralysis, difficulty in swallowing and death can occur.

2. Lead poisoning

Excessive lead present in atmosphere enters human body through natural food chain. Symptoms of lead poisoning are decreased liver and kidney function, sperm count and mental performance. Lead concentration in the air of most of cities is beyond normal permissible limit.

3. Strontium-90(^{90}Sr) and iodine-131 (^{131}I)

Nuclear explosions, nuclear accidents (Chernobyl disaster) and radiation from nuclear power reactors produce radionuclides ^{90}Sr and ^{131} I in the atmosphere. These radionuclides gradually enter human body through natural food chain. ^{131} I get concentrated in thyroid gland and may cause thyroid cancer. ^{90}Sr get concentrated in bone and teeth. Radiation from ^{90}Sr stored in bone may damage adjacent bone marrow. In addition ^{90}Sr is also get concentrated in milk. Consumption of such milk by infants and children may pose threat to their normal health.

Arsenic poisoning

Arsenic poisoning occurs in humans when they are exposed to high arsenic levels in the environment. Exposure to high levels of arsenic in the air, diet, soil and drinking water causes arsenism disease in humans. Pollution of air, water, soil and food with this metal is threat to plant, animals including human race. It is not only an environmental pollutant but also potential human carcinogen. It is associated with skin, liver and lung cancers.

Exposure to high levels of arsenic have been found in India, Bangladesh, China, Thaiwan, Japan, Thailand, Chile, Argentina, Hungary, Canada, Combodia, Vietnam, U.K. and U.S.A.

Arsenic poisoning causes skin lesions dermatoses, melanosis, keratosis, rhagades (skin cleft on palm and feet), liver damage, mucous membranes and digestive, respiratory, circulatory and nervous system damages. Lesion of skin progress to cancer. Exposure to high arsenic levels also leads to development of diabetes mellitus.

Two kinds of endemic arsenism are known. One is drinking water type which is based on the consumption of arsenic contaminated food and water. WHO maximum permissible level of arsenic in drinking water is 50 µg/L. Arsenic contamination of drinking water is global problem. How ever it is more severe in West Bengal, India and Bangladesh. Here over twelve million people reside where ground water arsenic concentration is 2 to 40 times higher than recommended permissible level.

Another type is coal smoke pollution. Inhalation of smoke from combustion of high arsenic coal causes arsenism. Arsenic pollution in the air occurs in mining areas, coal based thermal power plants, arsenic based industrial units. The arsenic present in the air around such places enters water through down winds and causes drinking water pollution. In Thailand arsenic poisoning around mining areas is reported. In Kolkata arsenic based pesticide paris green manufacturing factory contaminated drinking water with arsenic affecting several thousand people of the region with arsenism.

Molecular mechanism of arsenic induced carcinogenesis

Arsenic is able to induce cancer in skin and lung. Arsenicosis is the name given to cancer induced by arsenic. Arsenic induce cancer by affecting DNA methylation. Both hypo and hyper methylation of DNA causes aberrant expression of oncogenes, tumor suppressor genes which in turn cause abnormal proliferation leading to carcinogenesis.

Tobacco

Environmental tobacco smoke from smokers and tobacco based agricultural activities, industrial activities like bidi and cigarette making companies causes pollution of environment with tobacco. Tobacco smoke contains thousands of toxic chemicals implicated in many diseases including Benzene, cyanide, lead, cadmium, radio active polonium, benza(O) pyrenes, carbon monoxide, nicotine etc. Breathing of this smoke by non-smokers, children and women which is known as passive smoking (second hand smoke) can affect their health several ways.

Second hand smoke causes about 3000 lung cancer deaths a year compared to less than 100 lung cancer deaths per year from normal outdoor air pollution. Cardiovascular diseases also occur in passive smokers. In pregnant women second hand smoke affects baby health before and after birth. Exposure of children to environmental tobacco smoke contributes to neurological impairment, allergic diseases like asthma, ear diseases, respiratory infections and cardiovascular diseases.

Working with tobacco has adverse health effects. Nicotine is rapidly absorbed through skin and causes green tobacco sickness (GTS) in agricultural workers of tobacco. Bidi rollers are exposed to tobacco also contain high levels of nicotine in blood. High rate of tuberculosis and asthma are reported from bidi workers of Bihar and Tamilnadu. Young girls engaged in bidi making suffers from growth impairment, menstrual disorders and body pains etc.

Mosquito repellents

Due to environmental degradation mosquito breeding reached all time high level. Most of the rural and urban areas of South Asia are invaded by mosquitoes through out the year except for a brief period during summer and winter. Mosquitos transmit diseases such as malaria, filariasis, dengue haemorrhagic fever, yellow fever and Japanese encephalitis.

Several types of mosquito repellents are widely used in South Asian countries including India to combat mosquito menace. Repellents are available in the form of lotions, vapourizers, creams, mats, coils etc. Marketing of repellents in India is highly organized and many brands can be found throughout the country.

Now researchers are finding harmful effects of repellents used against mosquitos. These repellents used allethrin group of compounds. The main site of action of these compounds is sodium channel. They keep sodium channel open for prolonged period which causes sodium current to flow for longer time. It leads to hyper excitation of nervous system. A recent study shows that these repellents are harmful to human health. So their use should be limited and avoided. Acute toxic symptoms are breathing problems, allergy, asthma etc. These symptoms disappear on withdrawl of repellent use. Prolonged exposure to these repellents may be neurotoxic and immunotoxic hazard.

Bhopal gas tragedy

Bhopal gas leak is worst environmental disaster that occurred on the night of 3rd December, 1984. It took heavy toll of human lives. More than 2000 dead in first few days. Gas that leaked contained methyl isocyanate (MIC) and possibly hydrogencyanide (HCN).

Initial clinical symptoms are irritation of eye, throat, cough and drowsiness. These are followed by severe pulmonary edema leading to cardiovascular distress. Finally convulsions and death due to cardiovascular arrest. Intense fatigue and muscular weakness are other common symptoms. Cherry red discoloration of lungs is another characteristic observed in autopsy specimens.

Symptoms and signs seen in victims and autopsy specimens are due to actions of MIC and its products. MIC binds free amino group of valine residue of hemoglobin and other tissue proteins. It leads to N-carbamoylation of these proteins which thought to be responsible for cherry red discoloration of lungs. HCN caused some degree of acute cyanide toxicity in victims.

Biocides

These are therapeutic compounds which are lethal to non target species. Until recently the impact of therapeutic compounds and personal health care products on environment are ignored. Since each species has role in maintenance of ecosystem balance elimination or reduction in population of particular species by biocides leads to ecological disturbances.

Recent dramatic decrease in vulture population in some Asian countries India and Pakistan is result of poisoning by residue of diclofenac sodium a therapeutic substance. Diclofenac is widely used antipyretic as well as analgesic. Diclofenac poisoning causes renal complications, gout and consequent mortality. Since vultures are efficient scavengers decline in their population leads to environmental degradation. Other biocides are analgesic acetaminophen kills Indonasian snakes, anticoagulant war farin kills rodents. Therefore therapeutic compounds must be evaluated for their environmental hazards prior to their approval.

REFERENCES

1. James, W.P.T and Schofield, C. Human energy requirement. Oxford University Press, Oxford, 1990.
2. Neuberger, A. and Jukes, T.H. Eds. Biochemistry of nutrition. Vol. Ia-Ib, Baltimore, 1979.
3. Kritchevsky, D. Dietary fibre. Ann. Rev. Nutr. **8**, 301, 1988.
4. Kinsella, J.E. Dietary fish oils. Nutrition Today, 7-14, Nov. Dec. 1986.
5. Rao, N.M. Banana and hypertension. Curr. Sci. 76, 1064, 1999.
6. McMillan, M. and Thomason, J.C. An out break of suspected solanine poisoning in school boys. Quart J. Med. 227-244, 1979.
7. Sarkar, S.N. Isolation from argemone oil of disanguinarine and sanguinarine. Toxicity of Sanguinarine. Nature **162**, 265-266, 1948.
8. Krishnamachari, K.A.V.R. Bhat R.V. Nagarajan, V. and Tilak, T.B. G. Hepatitis due to aflatoxins; An out break in western India. Lancet **1**, 1061, 1975.
9. Eyan. *et al*. Curcumin a major constituent of turmeric corrects cystic fibrosis defects. Science. **304**, 600-602, 2004
10. Brody, Tom. Nutritional Biochemistry, Academic Press, 1998
11. Martha, H.S. Biochemical and physiological aspects of human Nutrition, W.B. Saunders & Co, 1999.
12. Casimir, C. Akoh. Food lipids: Chemistry, Nutrition and biotechnology. Dekker/CRC,2002
13. Marlin Kohlmeier. Nutrient Metabolism, Elsevier, 2003.
14. Ann Coulston, Cherryl Rock and Elaine Monsen. Eds. Nutrition in the prevention and treatment of diseases, Academic Press, 2001
15. Dean Oliver and Hans Reimann, Steve Taylor. Food Born diseases, Academic Press, 2002.
16. Angelika, I. New balanced diet: Enhance your well being with delicious pH Balanced Food, Silver Back Books, 2000.

17. Radomir. L.(Ed.). Amino acid composition and biological values of cereal proteins. Kluwer Academic Publisher, 2002.

18. Jana, N.R. *et al.* Inhibition of proteosomal function by curcumin induces apoptosis through mitochondrial pathway. J. Biol. Chem. **279**, 11680-11685,2004.

19. Khar, A. *et al.* Anti tumor activity of curcumin is mediated through the induction of apoptosis in tumor cells. FEBS Lett. **445**, 165-168, 1999.

20. Breslin, K. Arsenic in Asia: Water at its worst. Environ. Health Perspect. **108**, 393-397, 2000.

21. Taher, M.M. *et al.* Curcumin inhibits UV-light induced HIV virus gene expression. Mol. Cell. Biochem. **254**, 289-297, 2003.

22. Tseng, C.H. *et al.* Long term arsenic exposure and incidence of non-insulin dependent diabetes mellitus in Taiwan. Environ. Health Persopect. **108**, 847-851, 2000.

23. Tobacco or Health. WHO, Geneva, 1997.

24. Gana, K. *et al.* Immunomodulation of isolated human neutrophils by green tea extract J.Nutraceuticals, Functional and Medical Foods.**4(1)**, 15-26, 2003.

25. Carol, T.C. Functional Foods-New Perspectives: A Functional Food Symposium. J.Nutraceuticals, Functional and Medical Foods.**4(1)**, 67-77, 2003.

26. Dulak, J. Nutraceuticals as antiangiogenic agents. J. Physiol. Pharmacol. **56**, 51-692, 2005.

EXERCISES

ESSAY QUESTIONS

1. Name components of an individuals daily energy needs. Describe each one. Determine daily energy requirement of a sedentary worker.
2. Name proximate principles in food. Explain nutritional importance of each one. Give their RDA values.
3. Define limiting amino acid. How it effects protein quality? Suggest ways to improve quality of protein of vegetarian diet.
4. Define malnutrition. Describe its disorders.
5. Define new age foods. Describe various new age foods present in diet.
6. Give an account of food toxins.

SHORT QUESTIONS

1. Define calorie. How you determine food energy values? Give energy values of common food stuffs.
2. Define BMR. Write normal BMR values for male and female. Name diseases in which BMR is altered.
3. Define SDA. Write SDA values of protein, carbohydrate, fat and mixed diet. Write its significance in energy requirement.
4. Define complementary proteins. Write their importance in vegetarian diet.

5. Define balanced diet. Write composition and components of a vegetarian balanced diet.

MULTIPLE CHOICE QUESTIONS

1. Which of the following is correct regarding respiratory quotient.
   (*a*) It provides energy values of common food stuffs.
   (*b*) It decreases in diabetes.
   (*c*) It decreases in starvation.
   (*d*) It decreases in diabetes and starvation.
2. Normal woman energy requirement per day
   (*a*) Is higher than normal man energy requirement.
   (*b*) Is equal to normal man daily energy requirement.
   (*c*) It lower than normal man daily energy requirement.
   (*d*) Increases with age.
3. All of the following statements are correct for nitrogen balance. Except
   (*a*) It is influenced by nitrogen intake.
   (*b*) It is influenced by nitrogen output.
   (*c*) It is influenced by dietary protein.
   (*d*) It is influenced by dietary carbohydrate.
4. Which of the following has high biological value
   (*a*) Vegetable proteins. (*b*) Animal proteins.
   (*c*) Derived proteins (*d*) Denatured vegetable proteins.
5. Parenteral feed contains nutrients like
   (*a*) Glucose. (*b*) Denatured proteins.
   (*c*) Amylose. (*d*) Starch.

FILL IN THE BLANKS

1. ______________ is used to determine energy values of food stuffs.
2. Respiratory quotient of mixed diet is______________.
3. Dietary allowances increases from ________ to ________.
4. Dietary fat ________ bulkyness of food.
5. Minamata disease is due to __________ poisoning.

CASE

1. To a rural primary heath centre physician a one year boy was brought by his parents. The boy had distanded abdomen, edema of lower limbs and hyper pigmented skin over buttocks and on one side of head. His plasma protein and immunoglobulins levels were low and prothrombin time increased. Write your diagnosis.

26
CHAPTER

WATER, ELECTROLYTES AND ACID BASE BALANCE

WATER

Water occupies 75% space of this plant. Likewise water occupies about 70-75% of human body mass.

MEDICAL AND BIOLOGICAL IMPORTANCE

1. Water is essential constituent of all forms of life.
2. Water is present in every cell. It is the medium in which all cellular events occurs.
3. It is required for enzyme action and for the transport of solutes in the body.
4. Water aids the folding of biomolecules like proteins, nucleic acids etc.
5. Semi-fluid nature of body is due to water.
6. Water regulates body temperature.
7. Water accelerates biochemical reactions by providing ions.
8. Water content in the body alters in dehydration and edema.

Water dynamics, Protein structure and function

Thorough knowledge of dynamics of water at the surface of protein in solution is required to understand function of protein molecules. In addition to stabilizing native state of protein water molecules in the hydration shell around a protein play an important role in its biological activity. Role of water in mediating protein receptor interaction is well documented.

The water molecules present in active centre of protein molecule are more mobile and participates in ligand binding process. Removal of these water molecules results in loss of biological activity. On the other hand water molecules in the hydration shell stabilizes three dimensional structure of protein by forming water protein hydrogen bond which are not easily removed by dehydration. Thus these water molecules are dynamically slow while the ones that are biologically active are relatively fast ones.

Distribution of water in the body

Nearly 45 litres of water is present in 70 Kg adult male. Of this 30 litres is found in intra cellular fluids including bone and rest (15 litres) is present in extracellular fluids. Water distribution among various extracellular fluids is 8.5 litres in interstitial fluid, 3.0 litres in plasma and 4.5 litres in trans cellular fluids like secretions of respiratory, gastrointestinal tract, skin, ear, nose, vitreous humor of the eye and cerebrospinal fluid.

Since fat is water insoluble, water content of body alters according to fat present in the body. In obese people water constitutes low percentage (55-65%) of body weight. In lean people water constitutes high percentage (70-75%) of body weight. Females have low water percentage (65%) because of relatively high percentage of fat compared to males. The daily water intake and water output of an adult leading sedentary life is given below.

Water intake	mL/day	Water output	mL/day
Drinking water	1200	Urine	1200
Food water	1000	Skin	900
Metabolic water	300	Lungs	300
		Fecal water	100

Factors affecting water intake and water output

1. Environment influences water intake and water output of an individual. In hot weather water output decreases (urine) and water intake increases. Water intake is less in cold climate and water output (urine) is more.
2. In disease like diabetes and renal diabetes, output of urine is more.

Maintenance of water balance

Fluid intake (thirst) and urine volume are involved in water balance maintenance. They play crucial role in body water homeostasis. When the water is deficit, it stimulates thirst centre in hypothalamus to cause thirst and at the same time another centre in hypothalamus is stimulated to release antidiuretic hormone (ADH). More fluid is taken because thirst centre is activated. ADH increases reabsorption of water in kidney. Thus water deficit is compensated. When the body contains excess water the reverse process occurs i.e. the thirst centre is inhibited drinking ceases and in the absence of ADH reabsorption of water in kidney decreases. These mechanisms come into action with deficit or excess of 200-300 ml in body water. Therefore total body water in a healthy 70 Kg man varies by no more than 500 ml under normal physiological conditions.

Disorders of water balance

1. **Dehydration (water depletion).** It is due to deficiency of water. It occurs in vomitting, diarrhoea, diabetes incipidus and in lesions of hypothalamus.
2. **Over hydration (Edema).** It is due to excess water in body. It may leads to edema. It occurs in water intoxication, excessive administration of intravenous fluids, increased secretion of ADH, protein deficiency, cancer and drugs.

Electrolytes

Charged solutes or electrolytes are present in body fluids like intracellular fluid (ICF), extra cellular fluid (ECF), various secretions, blood plasma and in bone. The two types of solutes present in body are inorganic and organic. The inorganic solutes or electrolytes consist of cations and anions. The organic electrolytes are mainly anions. The inorganic cations are sodium (Na^+), potassium (K^+), calcium (Ca^{2+}) and magnesium (Mg^{2+}). The inorganic anions are chloride (Cl^-), bicarbonate (HCO_3^-), phosphate (PO_4^{3-}) and sulphate (SO_4^{2-}). The organic anions are contributed by proteins, organic acids and organic phosphates.

Medical and biological importance

1. Physiological processes like membrane potential, neuromuscular excitability, nerve impulse transmission, HCl secretion and gas transport are dependent on ICF and ECF electrolyte composition.
2. Blood clotting, enzyme catalysis, bone formation and muscle contraction are dependent on electrolytes.

Distribution of electrolytes

Sharp differences in the distribution of anions and cations in the ICF and ECF exist. Na^+ is the major cation of extracellular fluid whereas K^+ predominates in ICF. Similarly Cl is the major anion in ECF whereas organic anions predominates in ICF. Concentrations of electrolytes in ICF and ECF are given below :

Fluid	Cations	Total (Meq/L)	Anions	Total (Meq/L)
ICF	Na^+, K^+, Ca^{2+}, Mg^{2+}	203	Cl^-, HCO^{3-}, PO_4^{3-}, SO_4^{2-}	203
ECF	Na^+, K^+, Ca^{2+}, Mg^{2+}	151	Cl^-, HCO^{3-}, PO_4^{3-}, SO_4^{2-},	151

Electrolytes of blood plasma : The important anions in blood plasma are bicarbonate, chloride, phosphate, sulfate, iodide and fluoride.

Bicarbonate : Normal plasma bicarbonate level is 24-30 meq/L. It is responsible for the maintenance of blood pH. It is component of carbonic acid bicarbonate buffer system. Plasma bicarbonate level undergo changes in acid base and electrolyte disturbances.

Chloride : It is the major anion in plasma. The normal range is 100-110 meq/L. It is required for maintenance of water distribution between plasma and cells. Chloride level decreases in vomiting and diarrhoea.

Phosphate : Normal phosphate level in plasma ranges from 2-4 mg/dl. It is involved in maintenance of plasma pH. It is component of phosphate buffer system.

Cations in plasma are sodium, potassium, calcium, magnesium, iron and copper.

Sodium : It is the major cation in plasma. Its normal range is 133-146 meq/L. Its level decreases in vomiting and diarrhoea.

Potassium : Its level ranges from 3.8-5.4 meq/L. Its level also decreases in vomiting and diarrhoea.

Calcium : Normal plasma range is 9-11 mg/dl. Its level decreases in rickets.

Maintenance of electrolyte balance

1. For normal function of body electrolytes concentrations of body fluids must be controlled. Many mechanisms operate to control body electrolyte balance. One such mechanism is sodium pump. It maintains low intracellular level of Na^+ and high extracellular level. Hormone aldosterone maintains electrolyte balance by acting on kidney. It increases Na^+ absorption and K^+ excretion by kidney.
2. Diet, water and salt intake influences the concentration of electrolytes in body fluids.

3. Kidney maintains plasma bicarbonate concentration. Further, kidney maintain electrolyte balance by excreting salts or by retaining salts depending on diet and environmental condition.

Renin-Angiotensin System (RAS)

It is involved in the maintenance of electrolyte balance. It is also involved in blood pressure regulation. It regulates electrolyte balance by affecting aldosterone level. Angiotensin-II is the main player of the system.

Liver produces angiotensinogen which is an α_2-globulin. It is substrate for renin an enzyme produced by juxtaglomeruler cells of kidney. These kidney cells are sensitive to changes of Na^+ and Cl^- concentrations in tubular fluids as well as to blood pressure changes. Any factor that decreases NaCl or blood pressure stimulates renin release by juxtaglomeruler cells.

When released renin acts on angiotensinogen and produce angiotensin-I which is a decapeptide. Angiotensin converting enzyme (ACE) present in endothelial cells of lung, blood vessels and plasma acts on angiotensin-I and produce angiotensin-II an octapeptide by removing a dipeptide from carboxy terminus.

Angiotensin-II acts on glomeruler cells and promotes aldosterone synthesis from chloesterol. Aldosterone acts on renal tubuler cells and causes Na^+ retention. It also promotes secretion of K^+, H^+ and NH_4^+ by kidney.

Angiotensin-II increases blood pressure by causing vaso constriction and hydrolyzing bradykinin a powerful vasodilator. Thus angiotensin-II affects blood pressure as well as electrolyte balance.

Inhibitors of angiotensin converting enzyme or ACE inhibitors are powerful antihypertensive agents. They act as antihypertensive agents by decreasing production of angiotensin-II and blocking hydrolysis of bradykinin.

Renin-angiotensin system is shown in Fig. 26.1A. Captopril, lisinopril and enelapril are some of the commonly used ACE inhibitors in the treatment of hypertension.

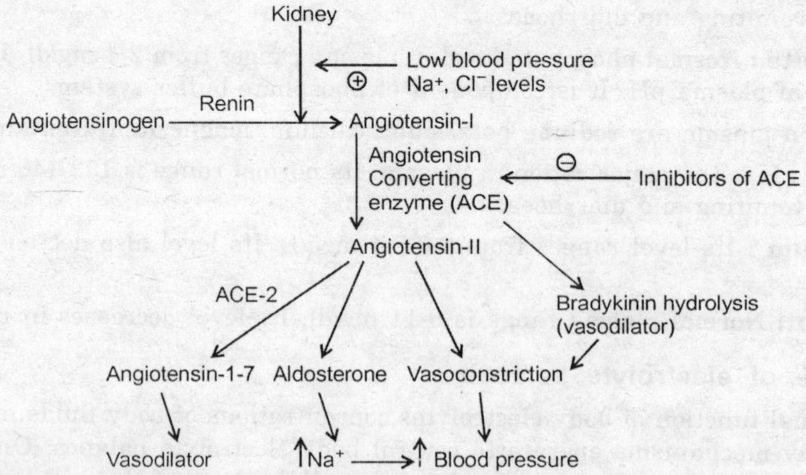

Fig 26.1. (*a*) Renin-Angiotensin system (RAS), ⊕ activation, ⊖ inhibition.

Recently an isoform of ACE is discovered in endothelial cells of heart, kidney, testis. It is designated as ACE-2. It is also a zinc metalloprotease. It converts angiotensin-II to angiotensin

1-7 by removing a single amino acid residue from carboxy terminus. Angiotensin 1-7 is a vasodilator. Unlike ACE, ACE2 is not inhibited by ACE inhibitors like captopril, lisinopril and enalopril. It is believed to be a part of second arm of RAS which is involved in normotension.

Electrolyte disturbances

Loss of body fluids due to vomiting, diarrhoea, haemorrhage, burns and sunstroke results in electrolyte disturbances.

Acid base balance or Hydrogen (H^+) Homeostasis

The word acid base balance refers to maintenance of stable level of pH of body fluids. During metabolic processes both acids or bases are formed. Under normal conditions they are neutralized by specific systems involved in maintenance of pH level. Under pathological conditions excessive amounts of acids or bases may accumulate in body fluids and tissues leading to disturbances in acid base balance. In a normal healthy person the blood pH ranges from 7.35-7.45. Throughout ones life this blood pH remains constant.

Medical and biological Importance

1. Proper pH is required for the optimal action of enzymes and for the transport of molecules within the body and between cells and its surroundings.
2. Proper pH is required for the maintenance of structure of nucleic acids, proteins, coenzymes and various metabolites.
3. Acidosis and alkalosis are two important disorders of acid base balance.

Hydrogen (H^+) Homeostasis

Three different systems are involved in the maintenance of stable blood pH level. They are :

I. Buffer systems of blood plasma, tissue fluids and cells like erythrocytes.

II. Lungs.

III. Kidneys.

By the combined action of these systems constant H^+ concentration is maintained in the body.

Buffer systems

They are responsible for the maintenance of pH of plasma, ICF, ECF and tissues of the body. For the good understanding of role of buffer in the regulation of body pH, some physical chemistry of buffer is required.

The pH of a buffer system is related to concentration of its weak acid as well as salt or conjugate base of weak acid and pK of weak acid. In logarithmic form the relationship is expressed as Henderson-Hassel balch equation

$$pH = pK + \log \frac{\text{Salt (conjugate base)}}{\text{Acid (weak)}}$$

This equation can be used

1. To know pH of a buffer solution if pK of weak acid and ratio of acid and its base are known.
2. To determine the concentration of weak acid and its base if the pH of buffer system and pK of weak acids are known.

Further, when the concentrations of weak acid and its conjugate base are equal the above equation becomes

$$pH = pK$$

Thus pK value can be defined as pH at which the concentration of acid and its conjugate base (salt) are equal. In simple words pK is the pH at which acid is half dissociated or neutralized. Based on titration of weak acid against base it was found that each buffer has maximum buffering action at its pK value. The effective buffering range of a given buffer system is about one pH unit on either side of pK value. For example acetate buffer consist of acetic acid as weak acid and sodium acetate as its salt (conjugate base). The pK of acetic acid is 4.75. So acetate buffer has maximum buffering action in pH region of 3.75-5.75.

Action of buffer

By taking acetate buffer as example action of a buffer is given below.

The two components of acetate buffer are acetic acid (CH_3COOH) and sodium acetate (CH_3COONa). When acid like HCl is added the base component of buffer reacts as shown below.

$$CH_3COONa + HCl \rightarrow NaCl + CH_3COOH$$

Since acetic acid is weak acid compared to HCl, the pH change is little on addition of HCl to acetate buffer.

When alkali like NaOH is added acetic acid of buffer reacts and neutralizes change in pH caused by addition of alkali.

$$NaOH + CH_3COOH \rightarrow CH_3\ COONa + H_2O$$

Thus buffer resist change in pH when acid or alkali is added.

Buffers of blood plasma

1. **Bicarbonate and Carbonic acid (HCO_3^-/H_2CO_3) buffer.** It is present in greater concentration and plays major role in regulating pH of blood with in normal limits. Even though the pK of H_2CO_3 is 6.1, the HCO_3^-/H_2CO_3 function as major buffer at pH 7.4 by maintaining ratio of 20 : 1 for conjugate base ($H\ CO_3^-$) to weak acid (H_2CO_3).

The ratio of conjugate base to weak acid required to keep the blood pH 7.4 is obtained by substituting pH and pK values in Henderson - Hasselbalch equation as shown below :

$$7.4 = 6.1 + \log \frac{HCO^-_3}{H_2CO_3}$$

$$\text{Log} \frac{HCO^-_3}{H_2CO_3} = 7.4 - 6.1$$

$$\text{Log} \frac{HCO^-_3}{H_2CO_3} = 1.3$$

Since the antilog of 1.3 is 20, $\frac{HCO^-_3}{H_2CO_3} = \frac{20}{1}$

The pH of blood remain 7.4 as long as this ratio is maintained. Increase or decrease in pH due to entry of acids or bases into blood is met by adjustment in this ratio. Any alteration in the ratio for prolonged time leads to disturbances in acid base balance.

Mechanism of action of bicarbonate buffer in controlling blood pH

Bicarbonate buffer acts against metabolic acids or nonvolatile acids produced. Metabolic acids are aceto acetic acid, β-hydroxy butyric acid, lactic acid, pyruvic acid and small amounts of phosphoric and sulphuric acids. The bicarbonate neutralizes more than 50% of all the acids stronger than carbonic acid. The bicarbonate that remain in plasma after neutralization of all acids is referred as alkali reserve. In blood HCO^-_3 is in association with Na^+. When acid enter blood Na^+ HCO^-_3 is used to convert strong acid to weak acid as shown below :

$$Na^+ \ HCO^-_3 + NaH_2PO_4 \rightarrow Na_2HPO_4 + H_2CO_3$$

$$2Na^+HCO^-_3 + H_2SO_4 \rightarrow Na_2SO_4 + 2H_2CO_3$$

$$Na^+HCO^-_3 + \text{Acetoacetate} \rightarrow \text{Sodium acetoacetate} + H_2CO_3$$

$$Na^+HCO^-_3 + \text{Lactate} \rightarrow \text{Sodium lactate} + H_2CO_3$$

Since H_2 CO_3 is a weak acid hydrogen ion (pH) concentration in the blood changes a little. Further, there is slight decrease in the ratio of HCO^-_3 / H_2CO_3 of bicarbonate buffer. This is immediately brought back to normal temporarily by disposal of carbonic acid by lungs. The sodium salts are removed from blood by filtration in kidney. Further, sodium and bicarbonate are recovered in kidney tubule cells and enters plasma. Thus the ratio of HCO^-_3 : H_2CO_3 returns to normal and blood pH remains 7.4. Restoration of HCO^-_3 : H_2CO_3 ratio to normal by kidney requires many hours or few days but it is complete and permanent.

2. **Phosphate ($H_2PO^-_4$/HPO_4^{2-}) buffer and protein (protein ⁻/protein) buffer.** Their concentration is low in blood so they play minor role in regulating blood pH. The phosphate buffer is more effective than bicarbonate buffer because pK of HPO^{2-}_4 (6.8) is close to blood pH 7.4 but its concentration is low.

Buffers of red blood cells

Most important buffer in R.B.C. is haemoglobin (Hb^-/HHb) buffer system. It is the major buffer system of blood as well as erythrocytes. The pK value of imidazole group (6.0) of histidine (part of haemoglobin) is close to body pH and hence Hb buffer system is effective at body pH. Further high Hb concentration (14 gm/dL) makes it major buffer of blood.

Lungs

Respiratory system (Lungs) serve as immediately available temporary mechanism for maintenance of acid base balance. Lungs affect acid-base balance by altering carbonic acid component of bicarbonate buffer. The carbonic acid content of blood depends on partial pressure of CO_2 (PCO_2) in plasma which is in turn controlled by lungs. Further, in lungs carbonic acid formation from CO_2 and H_2O is catalyzed by carbonic anhydrase.

$$H_2CO_3 \leftrightarrow \uparrow CO_2 + H_2O$$

When blood pH falls, the plasma HCO^-_3 concentration decreases and the ratio of HCO^-_3: H_2 CO_3 is decreased. In this acidotic state respiratory centre is stimulated and respiratory rate (Hyper ventilation) is increased. So, more of CO_2 is blown off. This results in decreased PCO_2 and less carbonic acid formation. Now the ratio of HCO^-_3 : H_2CO_3 increases and blood pH returns to normal. When the blood pH increases exactly reverse occurs. Due to decreased H^+ concentration in blood, the H_2 CO_3 is less and the ratio of HCO^-_3 : H_2 CO_3 is increased. This acid base disturbance is compensated by decreasing respiratory rate (Hypoventilation). Hypoventilation raises the plasma PCO_2 and hence H_2 CO_3 is increased. As a result of this the ratio of HCO^-_3 : H_2CO_3 come back to normal and blood pH is restored to pH 7.4.

Role of kidneys in acid base balance

Kidney regulates acid base balance by several mechanisms

1. Kidney removes sodium salts of acids formed by the action of bicarbonate on acids from circulation by glomerular filtration. In the lumen Na^+ is exchanged for the H^+ ions formed in tubular cells. This exchange is facilitated by Na^+ / H^+ antiporter system. H^+ enters lumen whereas Na^+ enters tubule cell by this process.
2. **Kidney absorbs bicarbonate from filtrate in the form of CO_2.** In the lumen of the kidney the $HCO^-{}_3$ combines with H^+ to form $H_2CO^+{}_3$ which is dehydrated to CO_2 and H_2O. The luminal membrane is impermeable to $H\ CO^-{}_3$ but permeable to CO_2. So, CO_2 diffuses into renal proximal tubule cells where it is rehydrated by carbonic anhydrase to carbonic acid. The bicarbonate ion formed from the dissociation of H_2CO_3 in the tubule cell diffuses into the blood plasma along with Na^+ by symport mechanism. Thus the kidney restores alkali reserve or bicarbonate level of plasma. Both the events are shown in Figure 26.1.

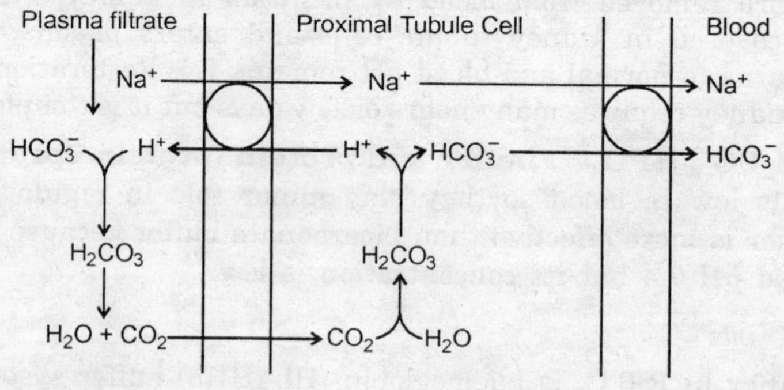

Fig. 26.1 Reabsorption of sodium and bicarbonate in proximal tubule

3. **Hydrogen ion excretion.** In the distal tubule cell of kidney, H^+ is formed by the dissociation of $H_2\ CO_3$. These H^+ ions are exchanged for Na^+ by antiport system. In the lumen H^+ combines with $Na\ HPO^-{}_4$ to form NaH_2PO_4 and excreted as such in urine. Na^+ enters blood along with $HCO^-{}_3$ by symport. The hydrogen ion excretion conserves Na^+ in tubule cells. The pH of the urine becomes acidic at this stage. This process is shown in Figure 26.2.

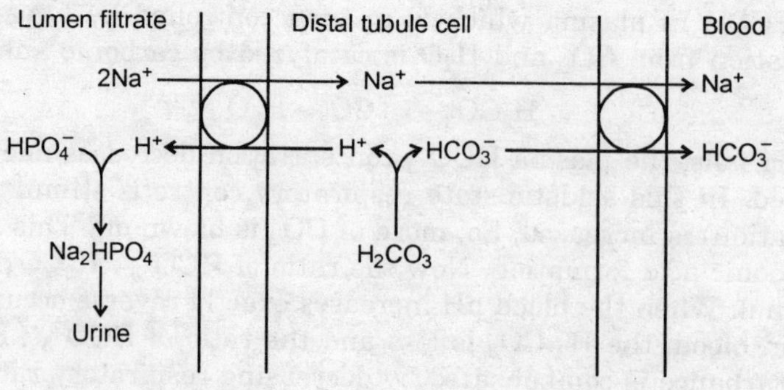

Fig. 26.2 Hydrogen ion excretion in distal tubule

4. **Formation and excretion of ammonia.** Ammonia is formed in the kidney from glutamine extracted from blood. Plasma enzyme glutaminase hydrolyses glutamine to ammonia and glutamate. H^+ ions are translocated from renal cells into lumen by energy dependent proton pump. Ammonia formed in renal cells diffuses into lumen. In the lumen ammonia binds to H^+ ions to form NH^+_4. The NH^+_4 present in the urine contributes to acidity of urine. It is shown in Figure 26.3.

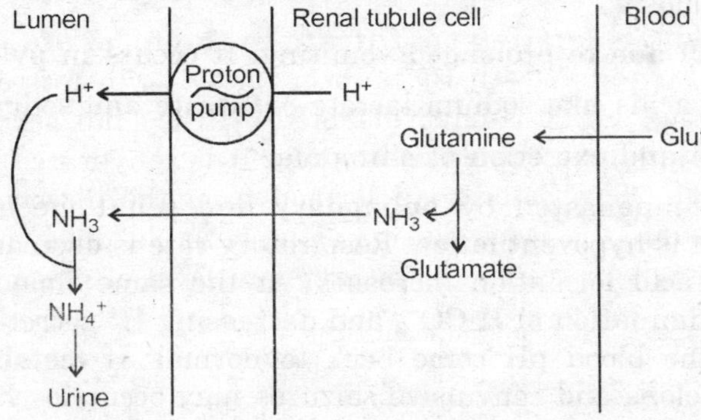

Fig. 26.3 Formation and excretion of ammonia in kidney

Thus kidney plays major role in H^+ homeostasis by regulating HCO^-_3 concentration in plasma and by removing H^+ ions produced in the body. Kidney also recovers Na^+. Since HCO^-_3 and Na^+ are electrolytes kidney regulates electrolyte composition of the body also.

Disturbances in Acid base balance

They are grouped into acidosis and alkalosis.

Acidosis. It is due to accumulation of acids and blood pH is below 7.4.

Alkalosis. It is due to accumulation of alkali and blood pH is above 7.4.

Acidosis or alkalosis due to less or more of bicarbonate are called as metabolic acidosis or metabolic alkalosis respectively. Like wise acidosis or alkalosis due to more or less of carbonic acid are called as respiratory acidosis and respiratory alkalosis respectively. These disturbances can be acute or chronic and always body attempts to restore normal acid base balance or HCO^-_3 / H_2CO_3 ratio by changing the removal of CO_2 by lungs or by altering the reabsorption of HCO^-_3 and H^+ removal in kidney. If the normal ratio of HCO^-_3, H_2CO_3 is restored then the acidosis or alkalosis is compensated. If body fails in its attempt then the acidosis or alkalosis is uncompensated.

Metabolic acidosis. It is the most common acid base disturbance. In this condition the plasma bicarbonate level is low. Metabolic acidosis may result from

(*a*) Excess production of acids which occurs in diabetes mellitus, starvation, phenyl ketonuria and maple syrup urine disease. Intense muscular exercise may lead to accumulation of lactic acid then the condition is called lactic acidosis.

(*b*) Ingestion of mineral acids. Excessive administration of certain drugs.

(*c*) Loss of HCO^-_3. It occurs in vomitting, diarrhoea, loss of pancreatic fluids or upper intestinal contents due to intestinal obstruction.

(*d*) Decreased H^+ secretion in kidney. It occurs in nephritis.

(*e*) Increased elimination of HCO^-_3 by kidney. It occurs in renal failure.

Metabolic acidosis is compensated by lungs and kidney. Increased respiration elminates CO_2 faster and carbonic acid content diminishes. The renal compensatory mechanism involves excretion of more ammonia and acid phosphates. These compensatory mechanisms may restore pH of blood. If acidosis is not compensated the pH falls and patient may go into coma. Chronic metabolic acidosis cases are treated by administration of sodium lactate or citrate.

Metabolic alkalosis. It is rare. It is due to more bicarbonate in plasma.

Causes for metabolic alkalosis

(*a*) Excessive loss of HCl due to prolonged vomiting. It occurs in pyloric obstruction.

(*b*) Ingestion of salts of acids like sodium lactate or citrate and sodium bicarbonate.

(*c*) Excessive production and excretion of ammonia.

This condition is compensated by pulmonary and renal mechanisms. Pulmonary compensatory mechanism is hypoventilation. Respiratory rate is decreased CO_2 accumulates in plasma and carbonic acid formation increases. At the same time kidney compensates alkalosis by increasing elimination of $H\ CO^-_3$ and decreasing H^+ secretion. By the combined action of these organs the blood pH come back to normal. If metabolic alkalosis is not compensated, tetany develops and convulsive seizures may occur in children.

Respiratory acidosis. It is due to more plasma PCO_2 level.

Causes for respiratory acidosis

(*a*) **Depression of respiration (Hypoventilation).** Hypoventilation occurs due to excessive dosage of morphine, barbiturates and other respiratory depressents.

(*b*) **Obstruction to air passage.** It occurs in pneumonia, emphysema, asthma and tracheal obstruction.

Mainly renal mechanism compensate this condition by absorbing more HCO^-_3 and eliminating more H^+ and ammonia in urine.

Respiratory alkalosis. Plasma PCO_2 level is low in this acid base imbalance. Respiratory alkalosis may result from.

Hyperventilation. Stimulation of respiratory centre in the brain leads to hyperventilation. It occurs in fever, head injury, anxiety, hysteria, salicylate poisoning, hot climate and high altitude.

Kidney compensates this imbalance by elimination of more HCO^-_3 and decreasing H^+ secretion.

Laboratory diagnosis of acid base disturbances. Determination of the type of acidosis or alkalosis can be made by measuring plasma pH, PCO_2 and HCO^-_3. Various blood parameters in acid base disturbances are given bleow :

Blood Parameters in acid-base disturbances

Condition	Plasma pH	Plasma $H\ CO^-_3$ Meq/L	Plasma PCo_2 mm Hg
Normal	7.4	25	40
Metabolic acidosis	7.25	18	40
Metabolic alkalosis	7.50	35	40
Respiratory acidosis	7.15	24.50	75
Respiratory alkalosis	7.50	25.50	20

REFERENCES

1. Daven Port, H.W. The ABC of acid base chemistry. 6th ed. University of Chicago Press, Chicago, 1974.
2. Christensen, H.N. Body fluids and acid-base balance. W.B. Saunders Co., Philadelphia, 1964.
3. Muntwyler, E. Water and electrolyte metabolism and acid-base balance. The C.V. Mosby Co., St. Louis, 1968.
4. Masoro, E.J. and Siegel, P.D. Acid-base regulation. W.B. Saunders Co., Philadelphia, 1978.
5. Gold berger, E.E. Water, electrolytes and acid-base syndromes. 4th ed. Lea and Fabigger, Philadelphia, 1975.
6. Pitts, R.F. The role of ammonia production and excretion in regulation of acid-base balance. N. Engl. J. Med., **184**, 32, 1971.
7. Juha, K. Kidney Kinetics and Chloride ion pumps. Nature Genetics. **21**, 67-68, 1999.
8. Shapiro, B.A. *et al.* Clinical application of blood gases. Mosby, 1993.
9. Weldy, Norma, J. Body fluids and electrolytes. A programmed presentation. 7th ed. Mosby, MO, USA, 1995.
10. Adam, T.S. William, T.S. and James, F.A. Editors. Clinical acid base balance. Oxford University Press, 1997.
11. Hogan, M.A. Fluids, Electrolytes and acid-base balance : Reviews and Rational. Prentice Hall, 2001.
12. Burton David Rose. Clinical physiology of acid-base and electrolyte disorders. MC Graw-Hill, 2000.
13. Jeffrey M. Brensilver. Primer of water, electrolyte and acid-base syndromes. Oxford University Press, 1996.
14. Joyce Lefeuerkee. Handbook of fluid, electrolyte and acid-base imbalances. Delmar Learning, 2003.
15. Mattos, C. Protein-water interactions in a dynamical world. Trends Biochem. Sci. **27,** 203-208, 2002.
16. Pal. S.K. *et al.* Biological water at the protein surface. Dynamical solvation probed directly with femto second resolution. Proc. Natl. Acad. Sci. USA, **99,** 1763-1768, 2002.
17. Yagil, Y. and Yagil, C. ACE2 modulates blood pressure in the mammalian organism. Hypertension, **41**, 871-875, 2003.
18. deGroot, B.L. *et al.* The dynamics and energetics of water permeation and proton exclusion in aquaporins. Curr. Opin. Structu. Biol. **15**, 176-180, 2005.

EXERCISES

EASSAY QUESTION

1. Describe the role of body buffers and lungs in maintenance of body fluids pH or acid base balance or H^+ homeostasis.

SHORT QUESTIONS

1. Write distribution of water in body. How water balance is maintained?
2. Write electrolyte distribution in ICF and ECF. How electrolyte balance is maintained?
3. Define buffer. Explain its action with example.
4. Write Henderson-Hasselbalch equation. Write its importance.
5. Explain role of kidney in acid-base balance.
6. Name different types of acid-base balance disturbances.
7. Define metabolic acidosis. How it is compensated?
8. Write conditions that cause respiratory acidosis and alkalosis.
9. Write role of renin-angiotensin system in electrolyte balance.
10. Write components of renin-angiotensin system. Write importance of this system in the body.
11. Explain mechanism of action of buffer in pH maintenance.
12. Write normal plasma sodium and potassium levels. How sodium level is maintained? In what disease it is altered?

FILL IN THE BLANKS

1. ....regulates body temperature.
2. Increased secretion of ADH causes................ .
3. Normal plasma bicarbonate level is.............. .
4. Plasma potassium level decreases in .... and.............. .
5. A buffer has maximum buffering action at...........value of its acid component.

27
CHAPTER

DETOXIFICATION OF XENOBIOTICS

A variety of toxic substances or potentially toxic substances may enter human body. They are food additives, poisons, toxins, certain drugs, chemicals, environmental pollutants, pesticides and other foreign substances. They are called as Xenobiotics (Xenos (Greek) - Strange). When they are ingested either accidently or some other way they may be absorbed from the gastrointestinal tract and gain access to the organs and tissues of the body. In the body xenobiotics undergo changes. These changes reduce the toxicity of xenobiotics. The conversion of highly toxic xenobiotics to less toxic substances is called detoxification or detoxication or biotransformation.

MEDICAL IMPORTANCE

1. Detoxification protects body and its organs from deleterious effects of toxins.
2. Detoxification removes most of drugs consumed from the body. Because of this drugs must be taken frequently during recovery from illness or disease.
3. Occasionally detoxification may generate toxic substance from relatively non-toxic substance.
4. Many anticancer agents work by inducing enzymes of detoxification.
5. Polymorphisms of enzymes of detoxification is associated susceptibility to diseases like myocardial infarction, cancer, inflammatory disease, alcoholic cirrhosis etc.

Generally detoxification converts less soluble toxic substance to more polar water soluble and hence the compound is easily excreted in urine. Some detoxified compounds may be excreted in feces through the bile. Liver is the organ involved in detoxification reactions. Detoxification of xenobiotics occur mainly in two stages (phases). In the first phase (stage) xenobiotics undergo three types of chemical reactions. They are oxidation, reduction (hydroxylation) and hydrolysis. The second phase involves conjugation of xenobiotics with variety of substances. Occasionally the detoxified products are sometimes more toxic than the original substance. Biotoxification is the word used to indicate such process.

I(*a*) Oxidation. Indole and Skatole are produced from tryptophan by the action of microbes. They are responsible for the disagreeble odour of the feces. They undergo oxidation.

Skatole → Skatoxyl, indole → Indoxyl

Benzene → Phenol, Benzaldehyde → Benzoic acid

Chloral → Trichloro acetic acid, Toluene → Benzoic acid

Ethylalcohol may be oxidized completely to CO_2 and water. Similarly methanol may be oxidized to formaldehyde and formate.

Methanol → Formaldehyde → Formate

(*b*) **Reduction.** It is less common and less important than oxidation.

$$\text{Picric acid} \xrightarrow{\text{Reduction}} \text{Picramic acid}$$

$$\text{Chloral hydrate (Sedative)} \xrightarrow[\text{Reduction}]{} \text{Trichloro ethyl alcohol}$$

(*c*) **Hydroxylation.** Detoxification of number of drugs and steroids occur by hydroxylation. These reactions are catalyzed by cytochrome P_{450} dependent monooxygenases.

$$\text{Phenobarbitol} \xrightarrow{\text{CytP}_{450}} \text{Hydroxy phenobarbitol}$$

$$\text{Meprobamate (Tranquilizer)} \longrightarrow \text{Hydroxy meprobamate}$$

Felbamate is structurally related to meprobamate. It is used in the treatment of epilepsy. It is eliminated by hydroxylation.

$$\text{Felbamate} \xrightarrow{\text{Hydroxylation}} \text{Hydroxyfelbamate}$$

Cytochrome P_{450} (CYP) Enzymes

They are most important phase-I enzymes. They are involved in the detoxification and bio activation of xenobiotics present in food, organic solvents, tobacco smoke, drugs, pesticides, environmental pollutants and alcoholic drinks. They are products of CYP super family of genes. Over 100 mammalian CYP genes and their products are studied extensively. Some members of CYP super family with their function are given below :

CYP Form	Function
CYP1A1	Inducible member of CYP super family helps in detoxification of carcinogens, toxins.
CYP1A2	Catalyzes activation of carcinogenic aryl amines and aflatoxin B.
CYP3A4	Involved in biotransformation of many drugs.
CYP2E1	Involved in oxidation of volatile environmental chemicals and anesthetics.

Medical Importance

1. CYP enzymes are involved in biotransformation of several endogenous compounds and activation of certain carcinogens. Certain compounds of dietary origin inhibit activities of these enzymes thus acting as selective inhibitors of carcinogens or toxicity of chemicals.
2. Polymorphisms in the genes coding for CYP enzymes is associated with susceptibility to different diseases including alcohol related diseases like alcoholic cirrhosis and alcoholic pancreatitis.

(*d*) **Hydrolysis.** Many drugs are detoxified by hydrolysis.

$$\text{Aspirin (Acetyl salicylic acid)} \xrightarrow[\nwarrow H_2O]{\text{Esterase}} \text{Salicylic acid + Acetic acid}$$

Atropine (Psychoactive) $\xrightarrow{H_2O}$ Tropic acid + Tropine

II. Conjugation. Conjugation means the chemical combination of one compound with another compound. Many toxic substances are detoxified after combining with compounds like glucuronic acid, glutathione, sulfate, cysteine, acetate, glycine and glutamine.

(*a*) **Conjugation reaction using glucuronic acid.** Glucuronic acid participates in detoxification reactions as its UDP derivative.

Phenol is detoxified by conjugation with glucuronic acid.

UDP-Glucuronic acid

Phenol ⟶ Phenyl glucuronide

UDP Glucuronyl transferase

UDP-Glucuronic acid

Paraacetamol (Analgesic and Antipyretic) ⟶ Conjugated product

UDP

UDP-Glucuronic acid

Benzoic acid ⟶ Glucuronide monobenzoate

UDP

Antibiotic chloramphenicol undergo conjugation with glucuronate.

UDP-Glucuronic acid

Chloramphenicol ⟶ Complex with glucuronate

UDP

Lamotrigine an antiepileptic drug is conjugated with glucuronic acid and excreted in urine.

UDP-Glucuronic acid

Lamotrigine ⟶ Conjugated product

UDP

Diclofenac sodium an analgesic and antipyretic is eliminated from the body by conjugation with glucuronic acid.

UDP-Glucuronic acid

Diclofenac Sodium ⟶ Conjugated product

UDP

Morphine, menthol, camphor, chloralhydrate, salicylic acid, PABA are excreted in conjugation with glucuronic acid.

(*b*) **Conjugation with glutathione.** Aliphatic or aromatic halogen substituted hydrocarbons are conjugated with glutathione. The conjugation is catalyzed by an inducible enzyme glutathione-S-transferase.

Dichloronitrobenzene is a halogen substituted aromatic hydrocarbon undergo conjugation with glutathione. The conjugated product is further acted upon by other enzymes to produce mercapturic acids which are excreted in urine.

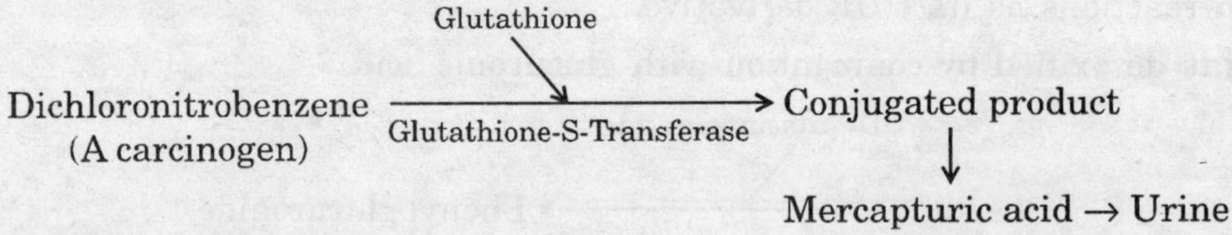

Glutathione transferases (GST)

Glutathione-S-transferases are major enzymes of detoxification. They are involved in bioactivation and detoxification of xenobiotics present in food, tobacco smoke, alcoholic drinks, pesticides, drugs, environmental pollutants, antitumor agents etc. They catalyze binding of large variety of electrophiles to sulfhydryl group of glutathione. Three types of mammalian glutathione-S-transferases are identified. They are cytosolic, mitochondrial and microsomal GST.

Medical importance

1. Glutathione-S-transferases are involved in removal of chemical carcinogens. Since reactive ultimate carcinogenic form of chemical carcinogens are electrophiles GST is considered as important detoxification mechanism of carcinogen.
2. GST are involved in activation of unsaturated aldehydes, quinones, epoxides and hydroperoxides formed during oxidative stress.
3. Mammalian cytosolic GST exhibits polymorphism which increases susceptibility to carcinogenisis and inflammatory diseases.
4. Polymorphism of human microsomal GST is associated with increased risk of myocardial infarction and stroke.

(*c*) **Conjugation reactions using sulfate.** Paraacetamol, phenol, cresol, indoxyl and skatoxyl are compounds conjugated with sulfate. PAPS or active sulfate donates sulfate group.

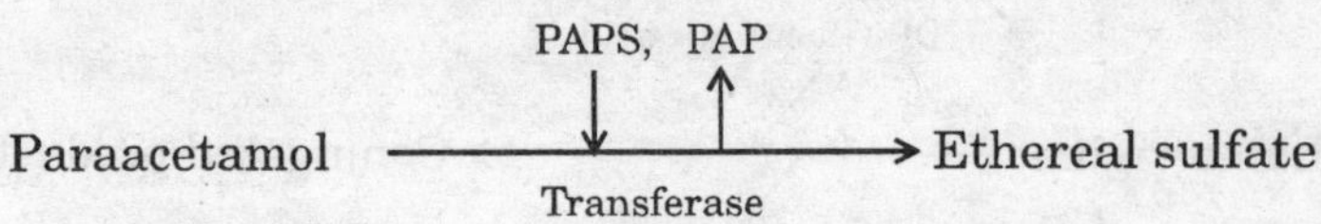

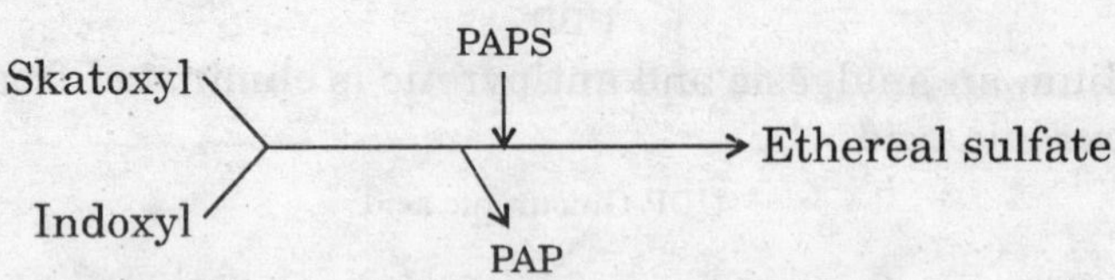

Pain killer diclofenac sodium is conjugated with sulfate.

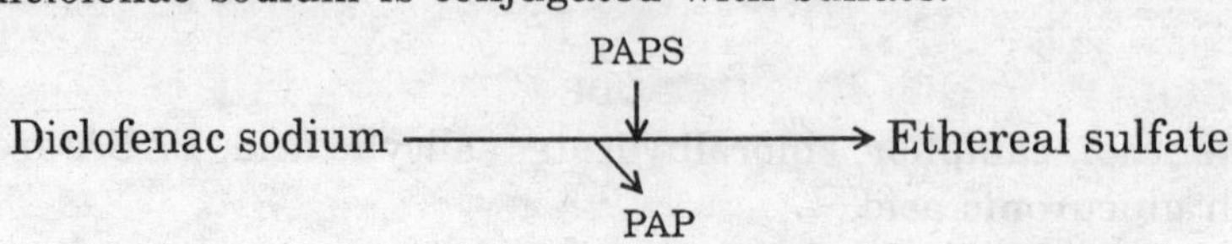

(*d*) **Conjugation reactions using cyteine.** Naphthalene, anthracene, bromobenzene, chlorobenzene, iodobenzene and benzyl chloride are converted to mercapturic acids by conjugation with cysteine and acetylation.

$$\text{Bromobenzene} \xrightarrow[\text{Acetyl-CoA}]{\text{Cysteine}} \text{Bromo phenyl mercapturic acid}$$

(*e*) **Conjugation reactions using acetate.** Sulfa drugs are detoxified by acetylation.

$$\text{Sulfa Drug} \xrightarrow{\text{Acetyl-CoA}} \text{Acetylated sulfa drug}$$

Zonisamide an epilepsy drug is acetylated and excreted in urine.

$$\text{Zonisamide} \xrightarrow[\text{CoA}]{\text{Acetyl-CoA}} \text{Acetylated sulfa drug}$$

Isonicotinic acid hydrazide used in treatment of tuberculosis undergo acetylation.

$$\text{Isonicotinic acid hydrazide} \xrightarrow[\text{Acetyl-CoA}]{} \text{Acetylated product}$$

(*f*) **Conjugation reactions using glycine.** An example of conjugation with glycine is the detoxification of benzoic acid.

$$\text{Benzoic acid} \xrightarrow[\text{CoA}]{\text{Activation}} \text{Benzoyl-CoA} \xrightarrow[\text{Glycine}]{\text{CoA}} \text{Hippuric acid}$$

(*g*) **Conjugation with glutamine.** Phenyl acetate is conjugated with glutamine.

$$\text{Phenyl acetate} \xrightarrow{\text{Glutamine}} \text{Phenylacetyl glutamine}$$

Detoxification of cyanide : Cyanide is converted to thiocyanate. The reaction is catalyzed by Rhodanase.

$$\text{HCN (Cyanide)} + \text{S (Sulfur)} \xrightarrow{\text{Rhodanase}} \text{HSCN (Thiocyanate)}$$

Methylation. Some compounds are detoxified by methylation. S-adenosyl methionine serve as methyl donor.

$$\text{Nicotinamide} \xrightarrow[\text{SAM} \quad \text{SAH}]{\text{Methylation}} \text{Methyl Nicotinamide}$$

BAL (British anti Lewisite) is methylated and excreted. BAL removes toxic metals such as arsenic, mercury and cadmium from body.

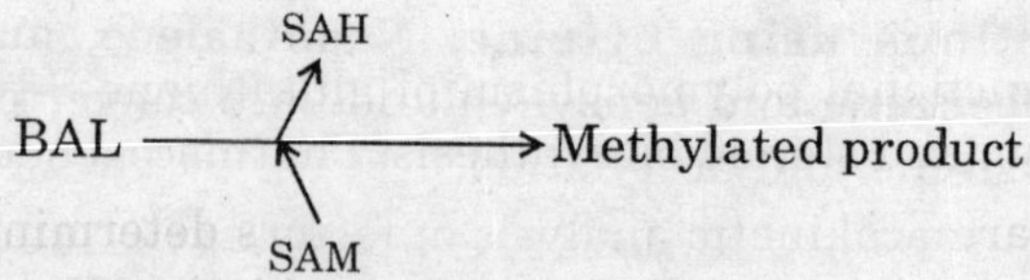

BAL is used as antidote for arsenic poisoning.

Biomethylation

Arsenic ingested is detoxified by methylation and excreted in urine. Biomethylation reduces toxicity of arsenic and facilitates its elimination from the body. Initially inorganic arsenic is methylated to monomethylarsenic acid and finally to dimenthyl arsenic acid.

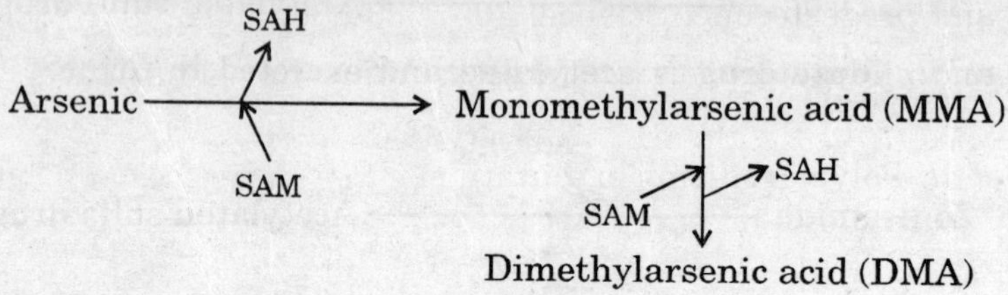

Anti carcinogens and enzymes of detoxification

1. Several anticarcinogens exert their effect by inducing phase-I and phase-II enzymes. Most important phase-I enzymes are CYP enzymes.
2. Phase-II enzyme induction is common feature of many chemoprotectants of cancer. Induction of phase-II enzymes before or during exposure to carcinogen decreases or inhibits carcinogensis.
3. Glucuronyl transferases and GST of phase-II enzymes are induced by some anti-carcinogens.

REFERENCES

1. Mulder. Detoxification or toxification? Modification of toxicity of foreign compounds by conjugation in the liver. Trends Biochem. Sci. **4**, 86-90, 1979.
2. Jakoby, W.B. and Ziegler, D.M. The enzymes of detoxification. J. Biol. Chem. **265,** 20175, 1990.
3. Mannervick, B. *et al*. Glutethione conjugation : reaction mechanism of glutathione s-transferase. In conjugation Reactions in Drug Biotransformation. Alto, A. (Ed.). Elseiver, Amstardam, pp 101-122, 1978.
4. Mannervick, B. and Danielson, U.H. Glutathione-s-transferases. Structure and catalytic activity. CRC Crit. Rev. Biochem. **23**, 283-337, 1988.
5. Gulick, A.M. and Fahl, W.E. Forced evolution of glutathione-s-transferase to create a more efficient drug detoxification enzyme. Proc. Natl. Acad Sci. (USA). **92,** 8140-8144, 1995.
6. Vahter, M. Methylation of inorganic arsenic in different mammalian species population groups. Sci. Prog. **82,** 69-88, 1999.

7. Tetlow, N. *et al.* Functional polymorphism of glutathione-S-transferase A3 : effects on xenobiotic metabolism and steroid biosynthesis. Pharmacogenetics. **14(10),** 657-663, 2004.
8. Nishida, C. *etal.* Pharmacokinetic analysis of factors determining elimination pathways for sulfate and glucuronide metabolities of xenobiotics. Xenobiotica. **34 (5),** 439-448, 2004.
9. Leslie, E.M. Haimeur, A. and Waalkes, M.P. Arsenic transport by the human multidrug resistance protein. Evidence that a triglutahione conjugate is required. J. Biol. Chem **279**, 32700-32708, 2004.
10. Williams, P.A. *et al.* Crystal structure of human cytochrome P_{450} 3A4 bound to metyrapone and progesterone. Science. **305**, 683-686, 2004.
11. Hayes, J.D. *et al.* Glutathione transferases. Annu. Rev. Pharmacol. Toxocol. Aug. 17, 2004.
12. Burim, R.V. *et al.* Polymorphisms in glutathione-S-transferases and cytochrome P_{450} and susceptibility to cirrhosis or pancreatitis in alcoholics. Mutagenesis **19,** 291-298, 2004.
13. Daniel, K.N. *et al.* A brain detoxifying enzyme for oxgano phosphorus nerve poisons. Proc. Natl. Acad. Sci. USA. **102**, 6195-6200, 2005.

EXERCISES

ESSAY QUESTION

1. Define detoxification. Give an account of different phases of detoxification with suitable examples.

SHORT QUESTIONS

1. Define xenobiotics and biotoxification. How they differ?
2. Name toxins that can enter human body. Name toxins that are detoxified by reduction.
3. Write role of glutathione and acetyl-CoA in detoxification.
4. Define conjugation. Write detoxification reactions involving conjugation.
5. Write on glutathione-S-transferases.
6. Write about role of cytochome P_{450} enzymes in cancer.
7. How cyanide, arsenic, phenol are detoxified?

28
CHAPTER

ISOTOPES

Basic chemistry tells us that an element in nature is made up of electrons, protons and neutrons. The protons and neutrons are present in nucleus of the element where as electrons are found around nucleus. Further the number of protons in nucleus equals to the number of electrons. The total number of protons and neutrons determines atomic weight or mass number of the element which is shown in a superscript numeral before the chemical symbol of the element. For example carbon (C) atomic weight is 12 and it is written as ^{12}C.

Isotopes are multiple forms of an element. They occur in nature. They differ in atomic weights due to different number of neutrons in nucleus. Nuclide is the another alternative word for isotopes. For example carbon has four isotopes. They are ^{11}C, ^{12}C, ^{13}C and ^{14}C. They have different atomic weights due to differences in intranuclear neutrons. ^{11}C has five neutrons, ^{12}C has six neutrons, ^{13}C has seven and ^{14}C has eight neutrons. Likewise hydrogen (H) has three isotopes. They are ^{1}H, ^{2}H and ^{3}H and oxygen (O) has three isotopes ^{16}O, ^{17}O and ^{18}O.

MEDICAL AND BIOLOGICAL IMPORTANCE

1. Isotopes revolutionized biochemistry, molecular biology and biotechnology.
2. Biomolecules like enzymes, hormones, genes and cytokines present in picomoles (10^{-12}M) or femalo moles (10^{-15}M) that can not be detected by usual chemical methods can be measured or detected using isotopes.
3. Isotopes are widely used in treatment and diagnosis of various types of cancers.
4. Isotops greatly expanded our knowledge of cell biology and are found to be useful in agriculture and food industry also.
5. Human body composition and body pools have been determined using isotopes.
6. Life span, turn over (rate of synthesis) or biosynthetic pathway of a compound of interest can be determined by labelling (tagging) the compound or its precursor with an isotope.
7. Isotopes are used to establish absorption site, inactivation or various ways of utilization of given vitamin.
8. Isotopes are found to be useful in assessing functions of body organs (organ function studies).

9. Isotopes are used to know way in which a compound of interest is degraded inside the body.
10. Isotopes are found to be useful in positron emission tomography (PET) studies involving *in vivo* measurements of enzyme kinetics, metabolism of compound, receptors, blood flow, blood volume, uptake of a metabolite etc.
11. Isotopes are used in nuclear magnetic resonance (NMR) studies of protein structure and dynamics.
12. *In vivo* NMR can be used to know changes in metabolites in an organ under different conditions.
13. Isotopes are used to measure rate of absorption of minerals in the body.
14. Isotopes are useful in establishing enzyme reaction mechanisms.
15. Way of entry of environmental pollutants into body, their distribution and biotransformation are studied using radio isotopes.
16. Isotopes are widely used in genetic engineering and molecular biology.
17. Radioactive high performance liquid chromatography (RHPLC) is used to separate and quantitate radio metabolites produced in experimental subjects.
18. Radio isotopically labelled compounds are used as a markers of apoptosis.
19. Fate of hormones inside the body, presence of hormone receptors in cell membrane or cells are established by using radio isotopes.
20. Post translation modification, protein phosphorylation etc. are studied with the help of radio isotopes.
21. *In vivo* NMR is used in exploring biochemistry and physiology of humans and other living things. It is used in distinguishing disorders of glycogenolysis and glycolysis. It is used in evaluation of brain pathologies. Energy metabolism in human skeletal muscle is studied using *in vivo* NMR techniques.
22. *In vivo* NMR spectroscopy is useful in studying metabolism of anti neoplastic agents as well as efficacy of treatment.
23. Cardiac MRI is used in cardiac morphology, cardiac ischemia and functioning of cardiac walls.
24. MRI angiography is used to know vascular abnormalities like flow, occlusions, thrombosis etc.
25. fMRI is used to explore functional areas of brain involved in various tasks.
26. FDG-PET is used to study pathophysiology of epilepsy and actions of antiepileptic drugs.

Classification of Isotopes

Isotopes can be grouped into two types. (1) Radio isotopes and (2) Stable isotopes.

Radio isotopes

They are unstable isotopes and undergoes conversion to another element with emission of radiation. The conversion may take place in hours to years. Some commonly used radio isotopes are ^{3}H, ^{11}C, ^{14}C, ^{24}Na, ^{32}P, ^{35}S, ^{45}Ca, ^{59}Fe, ^{59}Co and ^{131}I.

Radioactivity

Emission of radiation by a radio isotope is called as radioactivity. Radio isotopes emit three different types of radiations. They are alpha (α)-rays, beta (β) -rays, and gamma (γ)-rays. The three emissions α, β and γ have mass, charge and energy. Some radio isotopes that give these emissions are given below.

α-rays

Radio isotope of element uranium ^{235}U emits α-rays and undergoes conversion to another element thorium as shown below:

$$^{235}U \rightarrow {}^{231}Th + \alpha \text{ rays}$$

β-rays

Radio isotope of element carbon ^{14}C emit β-ray and undergoes conversion as shown below.

$$^{14}C \rightarrow {}^{14}N + \beta \text{ ray}$$

γ-rays

Radio isotope of element cobalt ^{59}Co emit γ-rays as shown below.

$$^{59}Co \rightarrow {}^{59}Co + \gamma \text{ rays}$$

Properties of radio isotopes

The characteristic properties of radio isotopes due to α, β and γ emissions are 1. Ionization 2. Penetrating solid matter 3. Production of luminosity. Usually one or more of these properties are used for detection and quantitation of radio isotopes.

Production of radio isotopes

1. Since isotopic form of an element exist in nature they can be isolated and purified from enriched natural sources. However it is rare practice. Most of the radio isotopes used in biochemistry are produced in nuclear reactors. Neutrons (n) generated in nuclear reactors combines with an isotope of an element to produce radio isotope. For example ^{14}C is produced from ^{14}N when it combines with neutron as shown below.

$$^{14}N + {}^{1}n \rightarrow {}^{14}C + \beta \text{ rays}$$

Likewise ^{24}Na is produced from ^{23}Na when it captures a neutron as shown below.

$$^{23}Na + {}^{1}n \rightarrow {}^{24}Na + \gamma \text{ rays}$$

2. Isotopes also can be produced in a cyclotron by bombardment of nucleus of an element with proton.

Production of radio labelled compounds

The radio isotopes produced from either of above mentioned ways are converted to labelled (tagged) biochemical compounds like ^{14}C-glucose, ^{14}C-acetate, ^{14}C-cholesterol, ^{32}P-ATP, ^{32}P-DNA etc. by chemical and enzymatic synthesis.

Stable isotopes

Isotopes which do not undergo further change due to internal stability are called as stable isotopes. They do not emit radiation. Some stable isotopes are ^{1}H, ^{2}H, ^{12}C, ^{13}C, ^{15}N and ^{18}O.

Radioactive decay

The unstable nucleus of radio isotope undergoes conversion to another element with emission of radiation. The radioactive decay of any radio isotope shows first order reaction kinetics. Hence the number of decay events in a fixed time interval is entirely dependent on the number of radio active atoms present and decay is not affected by other atoms present, temperature and decay events occurred earlier. This is the law of radioactive decay which is expressed mathematically as

$$N = N_O e^{-kt}$$

where N = The number of atoms, N_O = Number of atoms at Zero time
T = time, k = decay constant of radio isotope.

Since this equation simply states that part of nuclei that decays in a given time interval is constant for a radio isotope, it has little practical value. Even decay constants for various radio isotopes can not be calculated by this equation. Half life of a radio isotope is more convenient parameter than decay constant. It is defined as time required for half the amount of given radio isotope to disintegrate and it is written as t½. The half life is also intrinsic property of isotope like K. Half life of several commonly used isotopes in biochemical research are given below :

Isotope	Half life (t½)	Emission
^{14}C	5568 years	β-rays
^{3}H	12 years	β-rays
^{45}Ca	165 days	β-rays
^{35}S	87 days	β rays
^{59}Fe	45 days	β and γ-rays
^{32}P	14.2 days	β-rays
^{131}I	8 days	β and γ-rays
^{24}Na	15 hours	β and γ-rays

Half life and decay constant of isotope are related as shown below.

$$t½ = \frac{0.693}{K}$$

So by using above equation decay constant for an isotope can be calculated when its t½ is known.

Radioactive decay units

Curie (Ci) is the basic unit of radio active decay. It is defined as the amount of isotope that undergoes 3.7×10^{10} distintegrations per second (dps). It is equivalent to approximately 16.66 mg of radium. More commonly used decay units are millicurie (mCi) and microcurie (μCi) which corresponds to 3.7×10^{7} dps and 3.7×10^{4} dps respectively.

Roentgen

It is unit of radiation exposure and is based on ionization produced by radiation. It is defined as amount of radiation that produces ions carrying one electrostatic unit of electricity of either sign per 1CC of air at normal temperature and pressure.

Measurement of radioactivity

Devices used for measurement of radioactivity are called as counters. Two types of counters are used for radioactivity measurement. They are commonly used for measurement of radio isotopes that emit β-rays.

Geiger counter or Geiger Mueller Counter

Since interaction of radiation with matter produce ions measurement of radioactivity in Geiger counter is based on ion collection. The Geiger counter consist of chamber filled with inert gas like helium or argon. When β-rays emitting radio isotope is brought close to the chamber radiation passing through gas ionizes gas and produce electrons and positive ions. Movement of electrons to anode and positive ions to cathode develops potential difference. This potential difference is proportional to radiation which is detected as count.

Scintillation counter

Scintillation counters are more efficient than Geiger counters. Measurement of radioactivity in scintillation counter is based on transfer of energy of electrons released from matter when it is hit by radiation to a fluorescent substance (fluors). For this reason in scintillation counting radioisotope is dissolved in appropriate solvent. When β-ray is emitted by radio isotope it interact with solvent molecule and electrons are produced. The energy of these electrons is transferred to outer orbital of fluor which in turn get excited. The excited fluor returns to ground state with the emission of light or photon. A photo-multiplier tube amplifies this light signal and converts it to an electrical signal which is detected as count.

Uses or applications of radio isotopes

Much of our current biochemical knowledge is the result of applications of isotopes. Radioisotopes are also widely used in immunodiagnostics, cancer therapy, organ scaning, agriculture and food industry.

1. Radioisotopes as tracers

Normally in vivo changes of given metabolite is impossible to follow because they are invisible. But if that metabolite is labelled or tagged with radio isotope we can follow or trace its biochemical transformations in presence of other non-labelled compounds by detecting radiation from radio labelled compounds. For this reason isotopes are called as tracers.

Some of compounds labelled with radio isotopes are ^{14}C glucose and ^{14}C acetate in which one of the carbon is replaced by ^{14}C radio isotope. Likewise ^{15}N-glutamate, ^{14}C-aspartate and $^{18}O_2$ are other labelled compounds. Usually labelling of compound with radio isotope does not affect its chemical properties and it undergoes same transformations as that of unlabelled compound in vivo. The choice of which isotopic label to use depends on type of experiment that is planned.

The isotope tracer methods are used to determine various metabolic processes in intact body. Several of known metabolic pathways have been elucidated by using isotopes as tracers. Some examples are given below.

(*a*) An isotopic tracer is used to establish whether a metabolite is a precursor of particular compound.

(*i*) Acetyl-CoA as precursor of cholesterol has been established by using ^{14}C-acetate as tracer.

(*ii*) Sources of various atoms of purine ring have been established by isotopic tracer methods.

(*iii*) Co_2 as precursor of glucose in plants has been established by using $^{14}Co_2$ as tracer.

(*b*) Information on the action of branching enzyme of glycogenesis has been obtained by ^{14}C labelled glucose tracer.

(*c*) An isotopic tracer can be used to know degradative product of given compound. For example uric acid as end product of purine degradation has been established by using ^{14}C-labelled guanine as tracer.

(*d*) Rate of synthesis of a given compound can be established by using isotopic tracers. For example rate of synthesis of DNA or replication has been determined using ^{3}H labelled thymidine tracer.

(*e*) Isotopic tracer may be used to establish whether a metabolite is predominant precursor of a given compound.

(*f*) Information on site of destruction, metabolic abnormalities and reuses of a given compound may be obtained by following movements of its isotopic tracer through different parts of the body.

(*g*) Information on rate of absorption and defects in absorption of a given mineral can be obtained by using labelled mineral as tracer. For example radio iron tracer (^{59}Fe) is used to know factors affecting iron absorption in the intestine.

2. Radio isotopes in absorption of minerals

1. Beans labelled with ^{55}Fe and ^{70}Zn are used to study absorption of iron and zinc in human subjects. Iron and zinc absorption levels are calculated from radioactivity of iron in RBC and from urinary excretion of zinc isotopes after feeding bean meal containing labelled iron and zinc.
2. Calcium absorption in humans is studied by administering test meal containing ^{47}Ca. Then calcium absorption is determined from excretion of ^{47}Ca in 2 hour urine sample collected after meal.

3. Isotopes in space, volume and pool measurements

Isotopes are found to be useful in measurement of body mass, body water, extracellular fluid and body pools of various substances.

a. Using ^{3}H labelled tritium oxide body mass, water and extracellular fluid have been established as 41%, 62% and 17% respectively.

b. Using ^{14}C labelled uric acid body uric acid pool has been established as 1.1 gm.

c. Using ^{24}Na and ^{42}K body pools of sodium and potassium have been established.

d. Using ^{51}Cr erythrocyte volume has been established.

Radio isotopes in volume measurements

Radio iodinated serum albumin is used to measure lung liquid volume and secretion which is important in understanding respiratory distress syndrome of infants.

4. Isotopes in life span measurements

Isotopes have been used to establish life span of proteins and cells.

(a) Using ^{15}N labelled glycine erythrocyte life span has been determined as 120 days.

(b) Half lifes of several plasma proteins have been established by using ^{131}I labelled plasma proteins.

(c) Using ^{15}N labelled glycine half lifes of several tissue proteins have been established.

5. Isotopes in measurement of hormones and other molecules

Radioimmuno Assay (RIA): Since hormones are present in nano or picomole concentration in blood they can not be measured by most of standard methods. But by using radioimmuno assay (RIA) technique they can be measured. RIA is based on antigen-antibody reaction. Moreover it is highly sensitive due to involvement of isotopes. It can detect pico mole or femtomole amounts of hormones or other similar compounds. Different steps of RIA are given below :

(a) Since RIA is based on antigen-antibody reaction first antibodies to hormone to be measured are produced by injecting hormone into animal. This hormone act as antigen and antibodies are produced.

(b) After isolating antibody (Ab) from the serum of animal it is incubated with radiolabelled hormone (antigen, An^+). This results in formation of labelled antigen-antibody complex (An^+-Ab).

(c) Sample containing unlabelled antigen (hormone) is allowed to react with labelled antigen-antibody complex. Unlaballed antigen (hormone) of sample displaces labelled antigen from antigen-antibody (An^+-Ab) complex. Higher the amount of antigen (hormone) in sample then higher the amount of displaced radio labelled antigen at equilibrium.

(d) Using a calibration curve the amount of hormone in the sample is calculated by measuring the amount of labelled antigen displaced.

Different steps of RIA are shown in Figure 28.1.

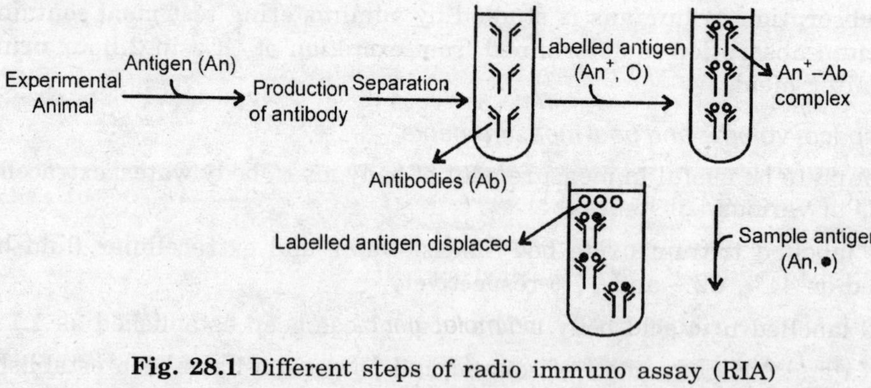

Fig. 28.1 Different steps of radio immuno assay (RIA)

(e) Calibration curve is prepared by using known amounts of unlabelled antigen equilibrated with definite amount of labelled antigen antibody complex (Figure 28.2).

RIA is also used to measure cyclic nucleotides, drugs, steroids, cancer antigens, antibiotics, peptide, prostaglandins etc.

6. Radio Isotopes in Hormone function

1. ^{125}I labelled insulin is used to study insulin metabolism in the body.

2. Presence of specific receptors for progesterone in uterine endometrial cell membrane and receptors for estradiol in the membrane of intestine, uterus, breast etc. are established by using ^{3}H progesterone and ^{3}H estradiol respectively.

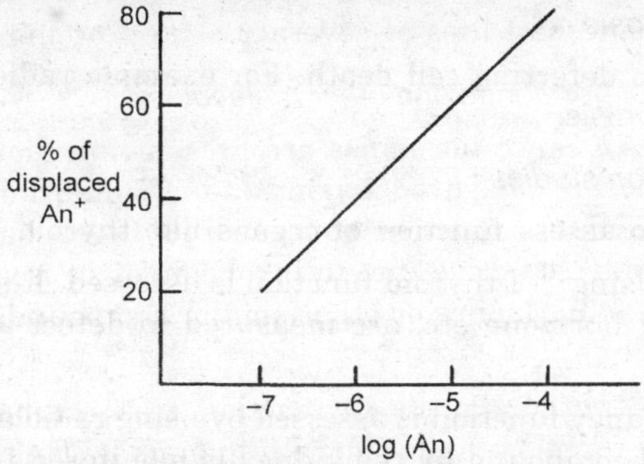

Fig. 28.2 A calibration curve for radio immuno assay (RIA)

7. Radio isotopes and transport across membrane

In porphyrias ALA accumulation is commonly observed in cells. ^{14}C labelled ALA is used to establish transport system for the uptake of ALA by various cells.

8. Post translational modifications of proteins

Radio isotopes are used to study post translation modification of proteins.

(*a*) For example acylation of proteins i.e. protein palmitoylation and protein myristoylation are studied by using ^{3}H palmitate and ^{3}H myristate.

(*b*) ^{32}P labelled orthophosphate and nucleotides are used in protein phosporylation studies by kinase etc.

9. Radio isotopes and effects of environmental pollutants

Some environmental pollutants are absorbed through skin and later distributed to various organs of the body. Radio nuclides are used to study absorption and distribution of environmental pollutants. DDT is still one of the major environmental pollutant that creates health risks for humans and other mammals. DDT absorption through the skin and its distribution in body organs is determined by using ^{14}C labeled DDT.

Mercury is another environmental pollutants highly toxic to humans. Biotransformation of mercury is studied by using ^{203}Hg labelled mercury chloride.

10. Radio isotopes in genetic engineering and molecular biology

1. ^{32}P labeled DNA probes are used in recombinant DNA technology, DNA chip technology, blotting or hybridization techniques, DNA finger printing, RFLP etc.
2. ^{32}P labeled nucleotides are used in DNA sequencing, DNA polymerase action etc.
3. ^{3}H thymidine is used to follow DNA replication.

11. Radio active high performance liquid chromatography (RHPLC)

1. It is another form of HPLC with radio analyzer. Radioactive compounds are separated and detected by using RHPLC.

2. ^{14}C labeled malonyl-CoA and Stearyl-CoA are used to study the fatty acid chain elongation in microsomes of blood vessels, brain, liver etc. RHPLC is used to identify metabolites formed in this study.

12. Radio isotopes in apoptosis

Radio isotopes are used in detecting cell death. For example radio labeled annexin is used as *in vivo* marker of apoptosis.

13. Isotopes in organ function studies

Radio isotopes are used to assess function of organs like thyroid, kidney etc.

(*a*) **Thyroid function.** Using ^{131}I thyroid function is assessed. Rate of hormone production, rate of elimination of hormone etc. are measured to detect abnormal function of thyroid.

(*b*) **Kidney function.** Kidney function is assessed by using radiolabelled hippuric acid. Rate of removal of labelled compound by the kidney is monitored to detect abnormal kidney function.

14. Isotopes in organ imaging

Radio isotopes are used to obtain diagnostic radiological images of organs. When a isotope is injected intravenously or given orally it is taken by organ of interest. Then images of organ are obtained by using scanner. These images provide information on shape, size, location of abnormal lesion if any. ^{131}I is used to obtain images of lung and thyroid. Indium isotope ^{133}In is used to obtain brain scan images.

15. Radio autography

It is widely used technique in biochemistry, cell biology and molecular biology. It is based on interaction of radiation from radio isotope with photographic emulsion. Different steps of radio autography are given below.

1. First radio labelled precursor (molecule) is incorporated into biomolecule (sample) or cell of interest using appropriate method.
2. Later sample or cell containing radio labelled compound is brought close to photographic film. Ionizing radiation from sample falls on photographic film and interacts with photographic emulsion.
3. After a given period of exposure the film is developed and radioautogram is obtained.
4. Dark areas on the film indicates localization of biomolecule in the cell or localization of radio isotope in the sample.

A radio autogram of intestinal villi of an experimental animal injected with ^{3}H uridine is shown in Figure 28.3.

Usefulness of radioautography in situ hybridization techniques is explained in chapter 20.

16. Isotopes in cancer radio therapy

Radio isotopes are found to be useful in treatment of cancer. Tumor cells are sensitive to radiation exposure compared to normal cells.

(*a*) ^{131}I is used in the treatment of thyroid cancer and hyperthyroidism.

(*b*) ^{60}Co is used in the treatment of tumors situated deep in the body because of its γ-ray emission.

(*c*) ^{32}P is used in the treatment of leukemia and lesions of skin.

(*d*) Radio nuclide bearing monoclonal antibodies are used in cancer therapy. It is a major development in monoclonal antibody therapeutics.

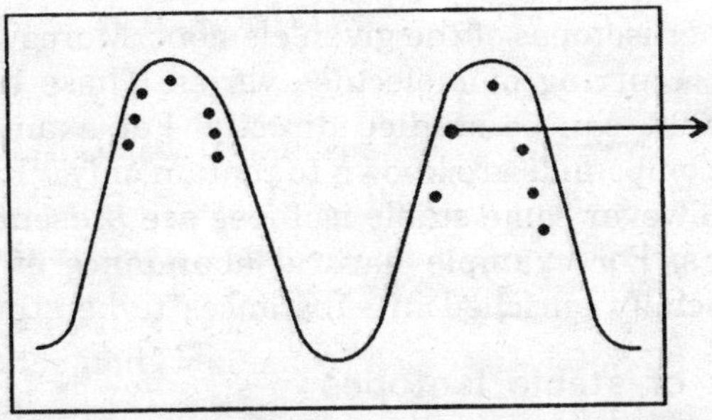

Fig. 28.3 Radio autogram of intestinal villi showing incorporation of ^{3}H-Uridine into RNA

17. Isotopes in enzyme measurement

Some enzyme levels in plasma and tissues are measured using radio labelled substrates. Isotopes are also used to identify active site of enzyme or to elucidate mechanism of enzyme action.

Radio isotopic enzyme assays

1. ^{3}H labeled glycerol-3-phosphate is used to measure the activity of glycerol phosphate dehydrogenase.
2. ^{14}C labelled α-ketoglutarate is used to measure glutamate dehydrogenase activity.
3. Glutamate decarboxylase activity is measured by using ^{14}C labelled glutamate.
4. ^{3}H labelled hippuryl-glycyl-glycine and ^{14}C, ^{3}H labelled angiotensin-1 are used to measure angiotensin converting enzyme activity.

Radio isotopes in enzyme catalysis

Bacterial resistance to most of the antibiotics is well documented. However molecular mechanisms by which antibiotics are inactivated by bacteria are not clear. β-lactamases are enzymes involved in bacterial resistance of β-lactam antibiotics. They catalyzes hydrolysis of β-lactam antibiotics. Involvement of carbamylated lysine residue in catalytic function of D class of β-lactamases is established by using $NaH^{14}CO_3$ which is an expansion of catalytic capabilities of amino acids in nature beyond 20 common amino acids in the development of biological catalysts.

18. Isotopes in agriculture

Radio isotopes are widely used in agriculture. Plant biochemistry and molecular biology are two areas of agriculture where isotopes are used. For example uptake of nutrients by root system from the soil has been established using radio isotopes.

19. Isotopes in food industry

In food industry isotopes are used to increase shelf life of foods and dairy products.

(*a*) For example milk pasteurized by exposing to radiation (radio pasteurization) has more shelf life.

(*b*) For example foods sterilized by exposing to radiation (Radio sterilization) have increased shelf life.

Sources for stable isotopes

Usually they occur alongwith other isotopes of the given element. Moreover natural abundance of a given isotope in naturally occurring biomolecules varies. Those biomolecules in which isotope of interest is close to 100% can be studied directly. For example biomolecules like nucleic acid and phosphorylated compounds are known to contain only ^{31}P isotope of phosphorus (natural abundance is 100%). However some stable isotopes are present in small amounts in naturally occurring biomolecules. For example natural abundance of ^{13}C is only 1% such stable isotopes have to be artificially enriched in substances to be studied.

Detection and measurement of stable isotopes

Mass spectrometer is used for detection and measurement of stable isotopes. Detection and measurement of stable isotopes by mass spectrometer is laborious and expensive compared to detection and measurement of radio isotopes.

Application of stable isotopes

1. Stable isotopes like ^{1}H, ^{2}H, ^{7}N, ^{13}C, ^{14}N, ^{15}N, ^{19}F, ^{23}Na, ^{35}P, ^{35}Cl and ^{39}K are used in NMR based techniques like NMR spectroscopy and magnetic resonance imaging (MRI).
2. Occasionally some stable isotopes are used as tracers.
3. Stable isotopes are found to be useful in gradient centrifugation.

Nuclear Magnetic resonance (NMR)

The nuclei of above mentioned stable isotopes behave like small magnets and have spin or orientation of two types. The two types of spin have different energy levels an high energy spin level and low energy spin level (Figure 28.4). When a magnetic field and electromagnetic radiation is applied to such nuclei they absorb electro magnetic radiation of specific frequency and resonate or assume other high energy spin state. For example in a magnetic field of 84000 gauss strength ^{1}H resonates at frequency of about 360 megahertz (360 MHZ, 360 million cycle per second). Likewise ^{31}P resonates at 146 MHZ and ^{13}C resonates at 90 MHZ. The frequency at which an isotope resonate is called as resonance frequency and the phenomenon is called as nuclear magnetic resonance (NMR). Conversely resonance can be achieved by fixing electromagnetic radiation and varying magnetic field strength.

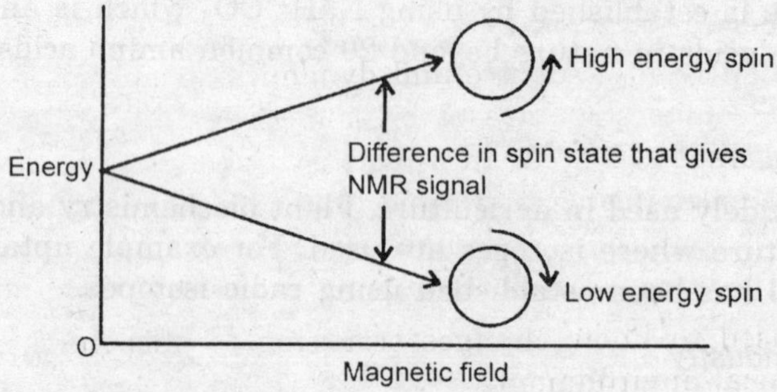

Fig. 28.4 Principle of nuclear magnetic resonance (NMR)

The energy level of spinning nucleus in a magnetic field is sensitive to its surrounding chemical environment. Hence nuclei in different chemical environment resonate at different frequency. The differences in resonance frequency are expressed as chemical shifts (symbol δ) with respect to reference material added in the sample. The resonance of a inorganic phosphate (Pi) is shown as absorption band or peak in Figure 28.5. It is designated as ^{31}P NMR spectrum of inorganic phosphate. In the NMR spectrum chemical shift (δ) is expressed as ppm (part per million) relative to reference material. Instruments used to measure resonances are called as NMR spectrometers.

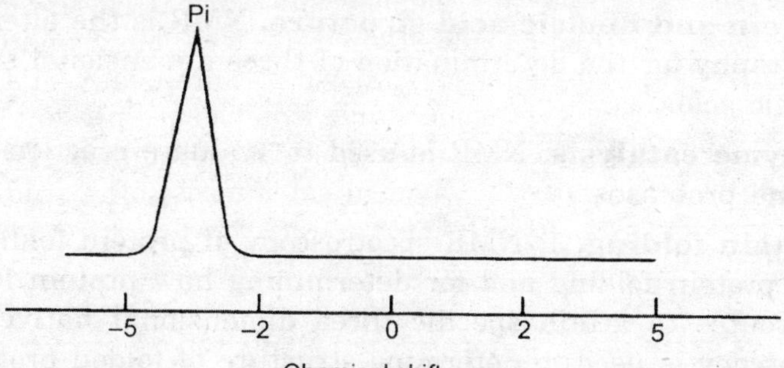

Fig. 28.5 ^{31}P NMR spectrum of inorganic phosphate.

With large NMR spectrometers it is possible to resolve resonances of most of the parts of large molecule like protein. An NMR spectrum showing resonances of different groups of a part of bovine pancreatic trypsin inhibitor in the form of absorption bands or peaks is shown in Figure 28.6. The peak indicates intensity of particular group in sample.

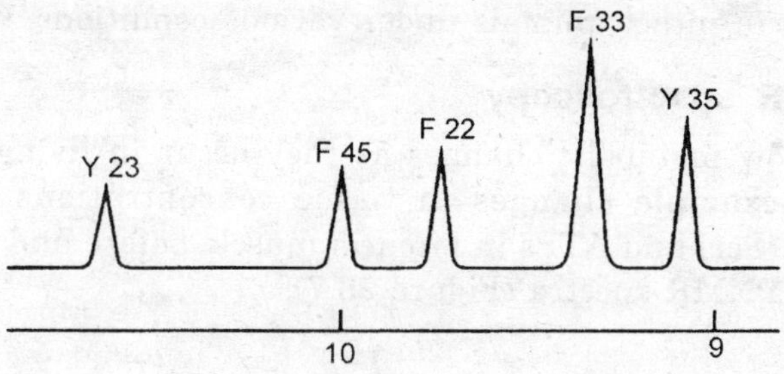

Fig. 28.6 ^{1}HNMR spectrum of a part of bovine pancreatic trypsin inhibitor. Resonances of specific groups are shown with letters.

Applications of NMR

1. Since NMR is sensitive to structure and dynamics at molecular level, NMR is widely used to study molecular structure of big molecules like proteins, nucleic acids etc., molecular changes that can occur in a molecule when its surrounding environment is changed, reaction mechanisms and molecular changes which occurs when a protein molecule undergoes conformational change. All these applications of NMR are usually considered under *in vitro* NMR spectroscopy. Some typical examples are given below.

   (*a*) ^{31}P NMR is used to know changes occurring to phosphate of nucleic acid under different chemical environment.

(*b*) ^{13}C NMR has been used to establish predominant form of D-glucose in solution.

(*c*) ^{13}C NMR is used to know changes which occurs when a protein molecule undergoes conformational change like from α-helix to random coil conformation.

2. NMR is used to study protein folding and dynamics.
3. NMR is widely used non invasive technique for studying metabolic changes in intact organism or organs or cells (*in vivo* NMR Spectroscopy) and for obtaining diagnostic radiological images (Magnetic resonance imaging, MRI).
4. **NMR and protein and nucleic acid structure.** NMR is the alternative to the older X-ray crystallography for the determination of three dimensional structure of proteins as well as nucleic acids.
5. **NMR and Enzyme catalysis.** NMR is used to evaluate reaction mechanisms of enzymes like serine proteases.
6. **NMR and Protein folding.** 1. NMR spectroscopy of protein folding is used to know early events of protein folding and for determining how protein folding is channeled along specific routes to attain specific three dimensional native protein structure. 2. NMR spectroscopy is used to determine structure of folded proteins.
7. **NMR and Diagnosis.** ^{1}HNMR techniques are used as an adjunct to histological identification of types of different grades of tumours non-invasively in soft tissue sarcomas like fibrosarcoma.

In vivo NMR spectroscopy

It is a non-invasive technique based on NMR principle that is used for detection of metabolites in living cells, organs in intact animals under various conditions.

Applications of NMR spectroscopy

1. It is used to follow metabolic changes as they occur in living animals under various conditions. For example changes in tissue concentrations of metabolites like Pi, Phosphocreatine (Pcr) and ATPs in forearm muscle before and after exercise have been detected using ^{31}PNMR spectra (Figure 28.7).

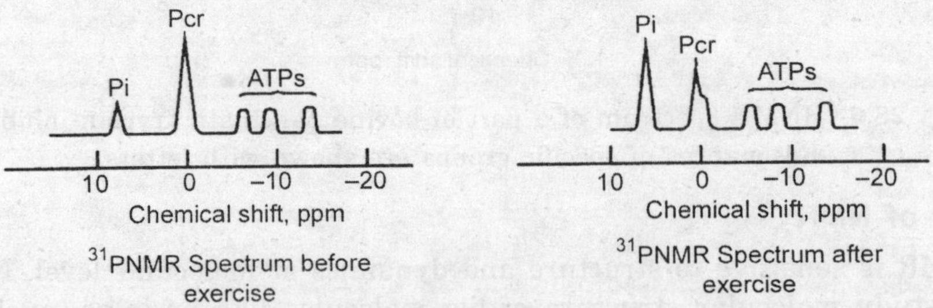

Fig. 28.7 Changes in concentrations of Pi, Pcr and ATPs as shown by ^{31}PNMR spectra in forearm muscle before and after exercise.

2. Using NMR spectroscopy biochemical information on pathological process of tissue of interest can be obtained. ^{31}PNMR spectra are used to study differences in metabolism of cancer tissue from that of normal tissue. Typical ^{31}PNMR spectrum of a normal breast tissue has several peaks which corresponds to phospho creatine (Pcr) and ATPs

(Figure 28.8a). However in breast cancer ^{31}PNMR spectrum in the place of phospho creatine peak three peaks which corresponds to phosphate monoester (PME), Pi and phosphate diester (PDE) are seen (Figure 28.8b).

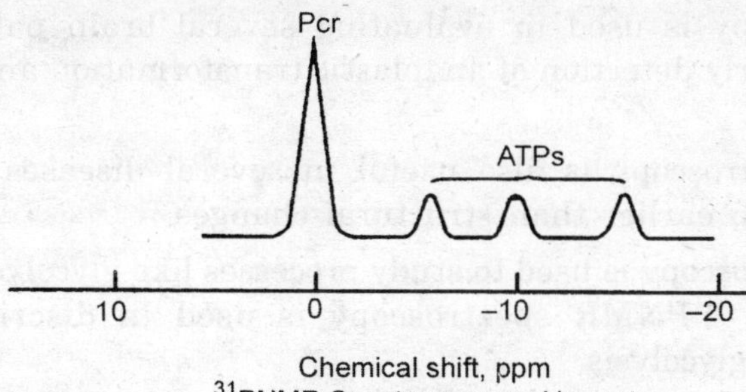

^{31}PNMR Spectrum normal breast

(*a*)

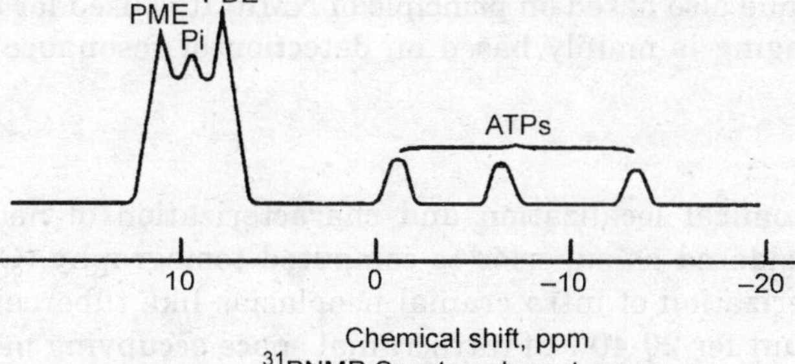

^{31}PNMR Spectrum breast cancer

(*b*)

Fig. 28.8 ^{31}PNMR spectra showing concentrations of various metabolites in (*a*) Normal breast (*b*) Breast cancer.

3. It is used to monitor drugs and their metabolites directly in human body.
   (*a*) Concentrations of psychoactive drugs like trifluoperazine and fluoxetine in brain are measured directly by using ^{19}FNMR spectroscopy.
   (*b*) ^{7}Li NMR spectroscopy (*in vivo* NMR) is used to measure concentration and distribution of lithium (Li) in brain to know therapeutic effects as well as toxic effects of lithium. Usually lithium is used to treat mania and manic depressive disease.
4. ^{31}PNMR spectroscopy of muscle allows indirect study of glycolysis and oxidative phosphorylation. ^{31}PNMR is extensively used to study energy metabolism of human muscle since its discovery. For example, wide variations in Pcr/Pi, Pi/ATP, Pcr/ATP ratio in muscle of normal individuals of world over are found to be due to the differences in lifestyle, nutrition, race, etc.
5. Changes in muscle metabolism of rest, during exercise and recovery are studied using ^{31}PNMR spectroscopy.
6. *In vivo* fluorine-19 nuclear magnetic resonance (^{19}FNMR) spectroscopy is used to study metabolism and kinetics of 5-fluorouracil (5-FU) an anti-neoplastic agent in human liver. ^{19}FNMR spectroscopic study of 5-FU metabolism offer a non-invasive means to assess efficiency of treatment.

7. *In vivo* NMR spectroscopy is used for exploring biochemistry and physiology of humans and other living organisms. ^{1}HNMR spectroscopy is routinely used now to study biochemistry of brain, muscle, breast etc.
8. ^{1}HNMR spectroscopy is used in evaluating several brain pathologies. It is used in tumour grading, early detection of anaplastic transformation and monitoring treatment methods.
9. *In vivo* NMR spectroscopy is also useful in several diseases where molecular level changes occur much earlier than structural changes.
10. *In vivo* NMR spectroscopy is used to study processes like glycolysis and lipid metabolism in human muscle. ^{31}PNMR spectroscopy is used in discriminating disorders of glycogenolysis and glycolysis.

Magnetic resonance imaging (MRI)

This non invasive technique also based on principle of NMR. It is used for obtaining diagnostic radiological images. Imaging is mainly based on detection of resonance signal from proton (^{1}H) of water.

Applications of MRI

1. It is used for anatomical localization and characterization of neoplastic (cancerous) lesions. MRI is considered as superior to computed tomography (CT) for better localization and characterization of intra cranial neoplasias like tuberculoma of cerebellum. Tuberculomas account for 20-40% of intracranial space occupying mass lesions in developing countries.
2. MRI is also used to study neurodegenerative disease like Alzheimers disease (AD). MRI of AD patient shows loss of cortical tissues and reduction in volume of hippo campus.
3. It is used to determine total lesion volume of neural tissue in demyelinating disease like multiple sclerosis (MS). The total lesion volume reflects overall disease burden and thus useful in quantifying the lesion.
4. ^{14}FMRI : In this MRI technique ^{19}F containing perfluorocarbons (^{19}F PFC) are used to obtain images. ^{19}FPFC are organic molecules in which all hydrogens are replaced by ^{19}F stable isotope. Since ^{19}F magnetic resonance (MR) signal is sensitve to tissue O_2 partial pressure, ^{19}F PFCMRI is used to measure oxygenation of tumor tissue. When ^{19}FPFC are injected intravenously they are taken up by tumor cells. Then ^{19}F MRI is carried out. PFC have been used as blood substitutes to supply O_2 directly to lungs in experimental animals.

Cardiac MRI

Cardiac use of MRI include cardiac morphology, myocardial ischemia, infact and imaging of wall motion deficits.

MRI Angiography (MRIA)

MRIA is used to study vascular anatomy in health and disease. In head and neck region, MRIA is useful for evaluating flow in carotid artery, the circle of Willis, cerebral artery and venous sinuses and for determining presence of vascular occlusions, vascular malfunctions, etc.

Functional MRI (FMRI)

1. It is based on paramagnetic nature of deoxyhaemoglobin. Since deoxyhaemoglobin is paramagnetic substance in the presence of external magnetic field it alters magnetic field in its vicinity.
2. This in turn affects magnetic resonance behaviour of water protons within the surrounding blood vessels which manifest as changes in image intensity.
3. An increase in neuronal activation by stimulus or task lead to an increase in arterial blood with proportionate decrease in venous deoxyhaemoglobin in capillaries. This manifest as increase in signal intensity in MRI images.

Applications of fMRI

1. fMRI is powerful non-invasive technique used for mapping brain areas activated during sensory or motor task. fMRI is used to detect increased cerebral blood volume, flow, blood oxygenation that occurring in association with increased neuronal activity during activation.
2. fMRI is used to localize brain areas involved in post ejaculatory refractive period in young healthy males.
3. fMRI is used to map primary motor cortex location for fingers, toes, elbows and tongue.
4. fMRI is used to study brain function in various psychiatric disorders like depression, anxiety, psychosis, schizophrenia etc. Schizophreniac patients show overall diminished response to motor tasks.
5. fMRI is used in unraveling the mystery of the human brain.

Positron Emission Tomography (PET)

It is a computed tomography (CT) based on positron emitting radio isotopes. Some of the radio isotopes emit positrons (anti electrons) which combines with electrons to produce γ-rays. The images of γ-ray emitting regions of organ of interest are obtained by using scanner. The half lifes of these positron emitting radio isotopes ranges from 2-100 minutes. They are ^{11}C, ^{13}N, ^{15}O and ^{18}F. Since carbon, nitrogen and oxygen are constituents of large number of biomolecules and drugs these compounds are labelled with ^{11}C, ^{13}N and ^{15}O and used in positron emission tomography. Some of the compounds labelled with positron emitting radio isotopes are ^{11}C-glucose, ^{11}C-glutamate, ^{13}N-glutamate, ^{18}F-captopril and ^{18}F-Fluorodeoxy glucose (^{18}F-FDG).

Applications of PET

1. PET is used for *in vivo* quantitative measurement of metabolism of particular substance. For example defective dopamine metabolism in brain of Parkinsons disease affected patient has been demonstrated with ^{18}F-Fluro dopa PET.
2. PET is used for *in vivo* measurement of rates of enzyme catalyzed reactions. For example *in vivo* kinetics of pulmonary angiotensin converting enzyme (ACE) has been studied with ^{18}F-captopril PET.
3. PET is also used for *in vivo* measurement of blood flow, blood volume, receptors etc.
4. FDG and receptor PET are used to study pathophysiology of epilepsy and mechanism of action of antiepileptic drugs.

REFERENCES

1. Freifelder. Physical Biochemistry (Chapter 5) 2nd ed. Freeman, Sanfrancisco, 1982.
2. Van Vunakis, H. and Langone, J.J. Eds. Methods of Enzymology, Vol. 70, Academic Press, New York.
3. Bock, K. and Pedersen, C. ^{13}C NMR spectroscopy of monosaccharides. Adv. Carbohydrate chem. Biochem. **41,** 27-66, 1983.
4. Barker, R. and Serianni, A.S. Carbohydrates in solution. Studies with stable isotopes. Acc. Chem. Res. **19,** 307-313, 1986.
5. Shulman, R.G. NMR spectroscopy of living cells. Sci. Am. **248(1),** 86-93, 1983.
6. Radda, G.K. The use of NMR spectroscopy for the understanding of disease. Science. **233**, 640-645, 1986.
7. Higgins, C.B. MRI of heart, Anatomy, physiology and metabolism, Am. J. Roentgenol, **151,** 239, 1988.
8. Phelps, M.E. and Mazziotta, J. Positron Emission Tomography. Human brain function and biochemistry. Science **228,** 799, 1985.
9. Schuster D. P. *et al. In vivo* measurements of pulmonary angiotensin converting enzyme kinetics. J. Appl. Physiol. **78(3),** 1158-1168, 1995.
10. Ishma, R. and Torchia, D.A. Protein dynamics from NMR. Nature Structural Biology, **7**, 740-743, 2000.
11. Slater, R.J. Ed. Radio isotopes in Biology : A practical approach. IRL Press, Oxford, 1990.
12. Gareth, R.E. Wiley, D.C. Oleg, J. Editors. Structure and mechanisms. From ashes to enzymes. American Chemical Society, 2002.
13. Gosling, J.P. Immunoassays : A practical approach. Oxford University Press, 2000.
14. Tim Chard. Introduction to Radio immunoassays and related techniques. Elsevier Science, 1995.
15. John, C. *et al.* Hetero nuclear NMR investigation of dynamic regions of intact *E. Coli* ribosomes, Proc. Natl. Acad. Sci. USA **101,** 10949-10954, 2004.
16. Leclare, X. *et al.* The potential of proton magnetic resonances spectroscopy (^{1}H-mRS) in the diagnosis and management of patients with brain tumours. Curr. Opin. Oncol. **14,** 292-298, 2002.
17. Arjov. Z. *et al.* Insights into muscle diseases gained by phosphorus magnetic resonance spectroscopy. Muscle and Nerve. **23,** 1316-1334, 2000.
18. Gonzalez, R.G. *et al.* Measurement of human brain lithium *in vivo* by MR spectroscopy. Am. J. Neuroradiol. **14,** 1027-1037, 1993.
19. Juneja, J. *et al.* NMR studies of protein folding. Curr. Sci. **84,** 157-172, 2003.
20. Detre, J.A. and Floyd, T.F. Functional MRI and its applications to the clinical Neurosciences. Neuro. Scientist. **7,** 64-79, 2001.
21. Stanly, J.A. *In vivo* magnetic resonance spectroscopy and its application to neuro psychiatric disorder. Can. J. Psychiatry. **47,** 315-326, 2002.

22. Milenic, D.E. and Brechbiel, M.W. Targeting of radio isotopes for cancer therapy. Cancer Biol. Thera. **3**, 361-370, 2004.

23. Robert, H.H. *et al.* Probing site specific conformational distributions protein folding with solid state NMR. Proc. Natl. Acad. Sci. USA. **102**, 3284-3289, 2005.

EXERCISES

ESSAY QUESTIONS

1. Give an account of radio isotopes applications in biochemistry and medicine.
2. Define nuclear magnetic resonance (NMR). Name instruments used to measure NMR. Explain applications of NMR.

SHORT QUESTIONS

1. Define radio isotope and stable isotope. Give two examples for each.
2. Define t½. Write equation used to calculate t^{Y2}. Write half lifes of 14^{C} and 32^{P}.
3. Define curie (C_i), millicurie (mC_i) and roentgen.
4. Name devices used to measure radioactivity. Explain working principle of any one.
5. Write principle and applications of radio immunoassay (RIA).
6. Write a note on autoradiography.
7. Write applications of magnetic resonance imaging (MRI).
8. Write principle and applications of positron emission tomography (PET).

29 CHAPTER

BIOCHEMICAL COMMUNICATIONS

MEDICAL AND BIOLOGICAL IMPORTANCE

1. It deals with mechanism of communication between cells.
2. In the body cells of different organs communicate with each other through specific chemical substances which may be referred as biochemical messengers.
3. Hormones produced in the body by various glands are involved in regulation of blood glucose (Chapter 9), calcium and phosphorus (chapter 23) and water, electrolyte levels (Chapter 26).
4. G-Protein coupled receptors (GPCR) are key player in several physiological process like neurotransmission, cell growth, differentiation, cell metabolism, inflammation, immune response, taste and odor perception.
5. Neurotransmission involves ligand induced dimerization of GPC receptors which is considered as major target for development of drugs.
6. Anti inflammatory, immuno suppressive and anticancer activities of glucocorticoids involves inhibition of target genes.
7. Thyroid function tests are widely used in diagnosis of thyroid diseases which are most prevalent endocrine disorders in India.
8. Depression and Parkinsonism are due to defective processing of catecholamines.
9. Psychosis and schizophrenia are due to increased sensitivity of dopamine receptors (DARs). Some antipsychotic drugs and antagonists of DARs and agonists are drugs for Parkinsonism.
10. Different types of memory formation involves structural and functional changes in synapse.
11. Understanding of cellular and molecular mechanism of memory lead to development of new therapeutic agents for dementia patients and improvement of memory function.
12. Loss of dopamine making cells which occurs in Parkinsonism is treated by administering (a) Dopamine precursor L-dopa (*b*) Dopamine receptor agonist like bromocriptine (*c*) Embryonic stem cells.
13. Alzheimer's disease (AD) which is characterized by severe dementia is treated with acetylcholine esterase inhibitors like tacrine, physostigmine etc.

14. Alteration in taste is common disorder associated with several types of illness and use of drugs. Hence knowledge of molecular mechanisms involved in taste signal transduction is useful in development of drugs for treatment of taste disorders.
15. Olfactory disturbances occurs in cold infection, drug use and diseases. Knowledge of olfactory signalling is useful in treatment of odor disturbances.
16. Hormones arc involved in development and maintenance of secondary sex characteristics, menstrual cycle and pregnancy.
17. Hormones like catecholamine prepare body to fight against stressful situations.
18. Over production and diminished synthesis of hormones leads to pathological conditions. For example over production of thyroxine causes thyrotoxicosis and decreased synthesis leads to goitre.
19. Hormone agonists and antagonists have clinical applications. Progesterone agonists are used as contraceptives and estrogen antagonists are used as anticancer agents.
20. Pregnancy tests are based on identification of hormone human chorionic gonadotrophin (hCG) in urine. Implanted embryo produces this hormone.
21. Several toxins like cholera, pertusis, stimulants like caffeine and theophylline work by affecting second messenger levels by which hormone action is mediated. Lithium used in treatment of manaic depression also work by altering second messenger levels in brain.
22. Botulinus toxin produced by *clostridium botulinum* which causes food poisoning syndrome botulism work by inhibiting release of neurotransmitter at neuromuscular junction.
23. β-blockers like propranolol, metoprolol used in treatment of hypertension and cardiac arthymias etc. work by blocking binding of catecholamines to β-receptors.
24. Glyceryl trinitrate used in angina pectoris work by releasing local mediator NO gas.
25. Nerve gas DFP, Sarin, parathion and physostigmine used in treatment of myasthenia gravis work by altering neurotransmitter levels.
26. Pheromones act as mating signals in lions, tigers etc.
27. Phytohormones regulates growth and reproduction in plants.

Chemical nature of biochemical messengers

Biochemical messengers differ in their chemical nature. They may be proteins (polypeptides), peptides, amino acids, amino acid derivatives, steroids, fattyacid derivatives and gas.

Classification of biochemical messengers

Based on their ability to communicate over a distance they are classified into endocrine hormones, local mediators and neurotransmitters.

1. **Endocrine hormones.** They act on cells which are far away from their site of synthesis. Blood carries these hormones from site of formation to site of action. Usually tissues that produce this type of biochemical messengers are called as endocrine glands.
2. **Local mediators.** They act on cells which are close to their site of formation. Usually they are not carried by blood. The tissues which produce this type of biochemical messengers may be called as paracrine glands.

3. **Neurotransmitters:** They act between nerves (cells) and nerve and muscle at which they are formed. Usually they are not carried by blood.

Some common biochemical messengers, their chemical nature, origin, effects (actions) are given in Table 29.1 and Table 29.2.

Table 29.1 Some biochemical messengers and their properties and action.

Name	Origin	Chemical nature	Major effects (actions)
Hormones			
Insulin	Pancreas	Protein	Promotes glycogenesis and lipid synthesis
Glucagon	Pancreas	Protein	Promotes glycogenolysis and gluconeogenesis
Cholecystokinin	Intestine	Protein	Promotes secretion of enzymes by pancreas
Parathyroid hormone	Parathyroid	Protein	Stimulates Ca^{2+} absorption in intestine and kidney.
Calcitonin	Thyroid	Protein	Inhibits calcium resorption
Thyroxine	Thyroid	Amino acid derivative	Involved in BMR
Catecholamines	Adenal medulla	Amino acid derivatives	Promotes glycogenolysis and lipolysis in liver and adipose tissue
Glucocorticoids	Adrenal cortex	Steriods	Promotes gluconeogenesis
Progesterone	Ovaries and placenta	Steroid	Maintain menstrual cycle and pregnancy

Table 29.2 Biochemical messengers, properties and actions

Name	Origin	Chemical nature	Major effects
Local mediators			
Nitric oxide (NO)	Several cells	Gas	Smooth muscle relaxation, Penile erection
Prostaglandin E_2	Many cells	Fatty acid derivative	Decreases acid secretion in stomach
Neurotransmitters			
Catecholamines	Adrenergic neurons	Amino acid derivatives	Main neurotransmitters of sympathetic nervous system. Raises blood pressure and heart rate etc.
Acetylcholine	Cholinergic neurons	Aminoacid derivative	Neurotransmitter at synapse and neuromuscular junction
γ-aminobutyric acid (GABA)	Many cells	Aminoacid derivative	Inhibitory neurotransmitter
Glutamate and glycine	Neuronal cells	Aminoacids	Inhibitory neurotransmitters
Substance P	Brain	Peptide	Neurotransmitter in brain

Mechanism of action of hormones and local mediators

Now we shall examine molecular mechanisms by which messages present in chemical substances like hormones and local mediators are converted into biochemical effects or biological responses in the target cells or organs. Usually translation of chemical message into biochemical effect involves two or three steps as given below. However number of steps depends on chemical messenger (Fig. 29.1 A).

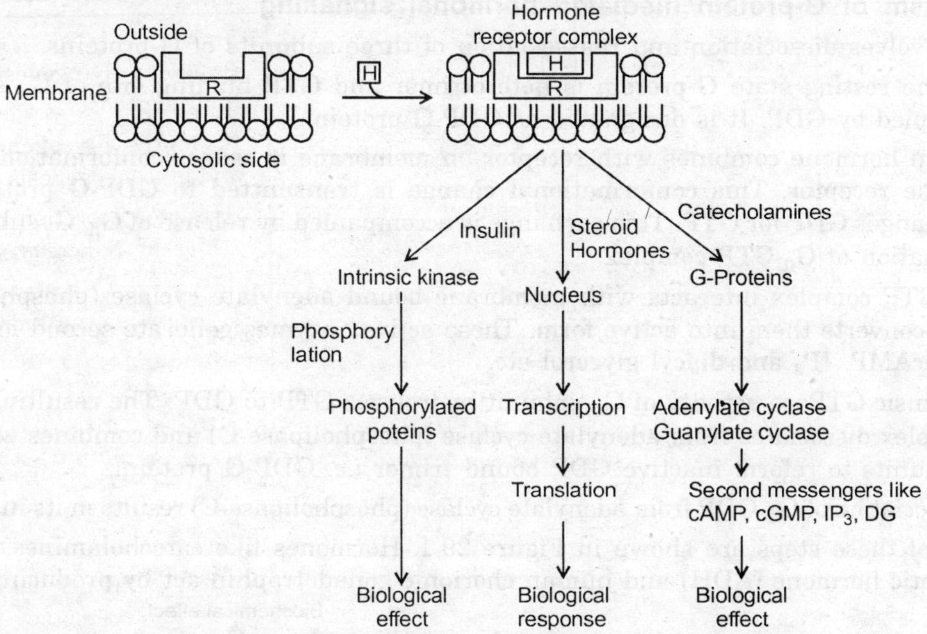

Fig. 29.1 (*a*) General mechanism of hormone action. H-hormone, R-receptor.

1. Binding of hormone to receptor on membrane of target cells or intracellular receptor initiates conversion of signal or message. The remaining steps of conversion process varies from one chemical messenger to other.
2. (*a*) In the case of insulin binding of insulin to receptor activates intrinsic tyrosine kinase activity of receptor which inturn regulates activities of cytoplasmic proteins by phosphorylation and produce biochemical effect.

   (*b*) In the case of catecholamines the hormone-receptor complex activates enzymes like adenylate cyclase and phospholipase C through G-proteins. This generates second messenger molecules like cAMP, IP_3, diacyl glycerol (DG) etc. (Chapters-9 and 23).

   (*c*) In the case of steroid hormones the hormone -receptor complex activates transcription.
3. The second messengers produces final biochemical effect of hormone by inducing changes in enzyme activities etc.

Guanine nucleotide dependent proteins or G-proteins

1. They are peripheral membrane proteins present on cytoplasmic side of various cells. Several types of G-proteins have been identified.
2. They are able to move laterally through membrane.
3. They are heterotrimers *i.e.* consist of three different subunits G_α, G_β and G_γ. The subunits vary among G-proteins.

4. The α-subunit has unique characteristics.
   (a) It has site to interact with hormone-receptor complex.
   (b) A site to combine with β, γ sub units.
   (c) A site to combine with GTP and GDP.
   (d) It possesses intrinsic GTPase activity i.e. ability to hydrolyze GTP to GDP.

Mechanism of G-protein mediated hormonal signalling

1. It involves dissociation and reassociation of three subunits of G-proteins.
2. In the resting state G-protein is heterotrimer and GTP binding site of G_α subunit is occupied by GDP. It is designated as GDP-G protein.
3. When hormone combines with receptor on membrane it causes conformational change in the receptor. This conformational change is transmitted to GDP-G protein which exchanges GDP for GTP. This exchange is accompanied by release of G_β, G_γ subunits and formation of G_α-GTP complex.
4. G_α-GTP complex interacts with membrane bound adenylate cyclase (phospholipase-C) and converts them into active form. These active enzymes generate second messengers like cAMP, IP_3 and diacyl glycerol etc.
5. Intrinsic GTPase activity of G_α subunit hydrolyzes GTP to GDP. The resulting G_α-GDP complex dissociates from adenylate cyclase (phospholipase-C) and combines with G_β, G_γ sub units to reform inactive GDP bound trimer *i.e.* GDP-G protein.
6. Dissociation of G_α-GDP from adenylate cyclase (phospholipase-C) results in its inactivation.

All of these steps are shown in Figure 29.1. Hormones like catecholamines, glucagon, antidiuretic hormone (ADH) and human chorionic gonadotrophin act by producing cAMP.

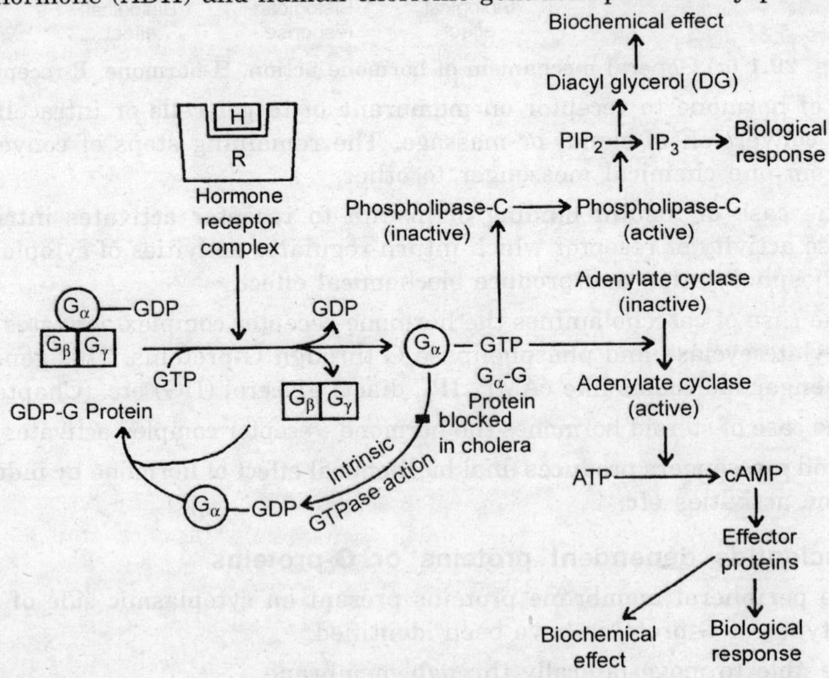

Fig. 29.1 Mechanism of G-protein mediated hormonal signal transmission. H = hormone, R = receptor.

Medical Importance

1. *Vibrio cholerae* microorganism which causes cholera acts by irreversible activation of G-proteins of intestinal mucosal cells. Toxin produced by this organism is called as cholerae toxin. It catalyzes ADP-ribosylation of arginine side chain of G_α subunit. This modification abolishes intrinsic GTPase activity of G_α subunit. Hence modified G_α-GTP cannot dissociate from adenylate cyclase leading to excess production of cAMP. Increased cAMP causes Cl^- flux from intestinal cells and it is accompanied by water. As a result more fluid enters intestinal lumen and patients get diarrhoea (Fig. 29.1 B).

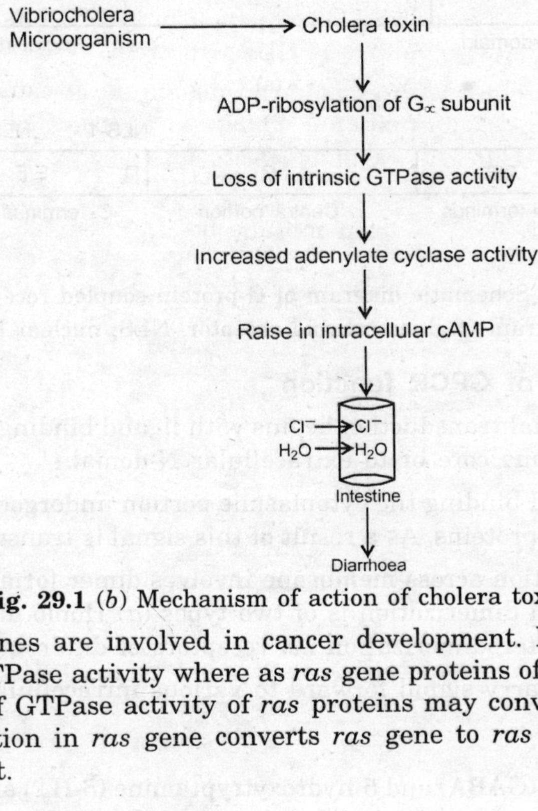

Fig. 29.1 (*b*) Mechanism of action of cholera toxin.

2. Mammalian *ras* genes are involved in cancer development. Ras oncogene proteins of cancer cells lack GTPase activity where as *ras* gene proteins of normal cells has GTPase activity. The loss of GTPase activity of *ras* proteins may convert normal cell to cancer cell. Usually mutation in *ras* gene converts *ras* gene to *ras* oncogene which leads to cancer development.

G-Protein coupled receptors (GPCR)

They are super family of cell surface receptors involved in signal transduction. This largest single super family of receptors include over 2000 receptors which responds to varieties of molecules.

Structure

All GPCR share some common structural features. They have an extracellular N-domain, seven trans membrane domains which form transmembrane core and an intracellular C-domain (Fig. 29.2 A).

Functions

1. GPCR function is to transmit information across cell membrane from extracellular environment to the interior of cell. They provide communication between exterior and interior of cell.

2. They act as key players in several physiological process such as cellular metabolism, cell growth and differentiation, cell secretion, neurotransmission, inflammation, immunity, taste and odor perception.
3. Neurotransmitters, hormones, photons (light), tastants, odorant substances binds to GPCR.

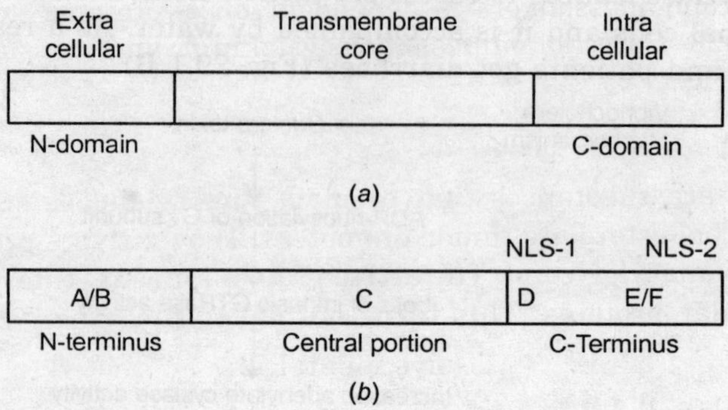

Fig. 29.2 (*a*) Schematic diagram of G-protein coupled receptor (GPCR). (*b*) Schematic diagram of glucocorticoid receptor. NLS, nuclear localization signal.

Molecular mechanism of GPCR function

1. GPCR mediated signal transduction begins with ligand binding. The ligand binds either within transmembrane core or to extracellular N-domain.
2. In response to ligand binding the cytoplasmic portion undergoes conformational change and interact with G-proteins. As a result of this signal is transmitted across membrane.
3. The signal transduction across membrane involves dimer formation of two receptors in the membrane. Such dimerization is of two types (*a*) Homo dimerization *i.e.* receptors of same kind (*b*) Heterodimerization *i.e.* receptors of different kinds.
4. Finally G-proteins carry signal forward to various intracellular messengers.

Medical importance

1. γ-amino butyric acid (GABA) and 5-hydroxytryptamine (5-HT) are two neurotransmitters implicated in epilepsy, anxiety and behaviour. GABA neurotransmission involves heterodimerization of two GABA receptors namely GABAR1 and GABAR 2. Neither of these monomers are functional on their own. Unlike GABA receptors 5-HT receptors 5-HT_{1B} and 5-HT_{1D} receptors form homodimers when expressed alone and heterodimers when coexpressed.
2. The ligand induced dimerization of GPCR is major target currently for development of novel drugs.
3. About 30% of clinically prescribed drugs function as either agonists or antagonists of GPCR.

GPCR interacting proteins (GIP)

GPCR interact not only with G-Proteins but also with accessory proteins called GPCR interacting proteins (GIP). These proteins are transmembrane proteins. Some are ion channels, ionotrophic receptors etc. These proteins have important functions. They are involved in

GPCR targeting to specific cellular compartments, in their assembling into large functional complexes like receptosome, in their trafficking to and fro from plasma membrane and in the fine tunning of signalling properties.

Hormonal signalling through IP_3 and diacylglycerol

Action of many hormones is mediated through IP_3 and diacylglycerol. The production of these intracellular second messengers is dependent on G-proteins and calcium influx as mentioned in chapter 23. Catecholamines, cholecystokinin, angiotensin II and oxytocin act by producing IP_3 and DG.

Medical Importance

1. Tumor promoters are substances that promote tumors and as such they may not be carcinogenic. Phorbol esters are tumor promoters. They activate protein kinase C which is also activated by diacylglycerol. The active protein kinase C catalyzes phosphorylation of some intracellular proteins. This turns normal cell to cancer cell.
2. Lithium used to treat manic depressive mental illness work by blocking production of inositol phospholipids in brain.

Cyclic GMP (cGMP) as second messenger

Effects of hormone like atrial naturetic factor (ANF) produced by heart and NO gas on target tissues involves generation of cGMP as second messenger. ANF and NO causes smooth muscle relaxation. However they generate cGMP from GTP by acting on two different guanylate cyclase enzymes.

Binding of ANF to membrane receptor of target cell leads to activation of membrane bound guanylate cyclase which in turn rises cGMP level. cGMP inturn activates cGMP dependent protein kinases which phosphorylates serine and threonine residues of effector proteins.

NO gas produced in endothelial cells in response to vasodilation signal enters smooth muscle where it binds soluble guanylate cyclase. This leads to its activation and production of cGMP. cGMP causes relaxation of smooth muscle. Mechanism of cGMP mediated signalling is shown in Figure 29.2.

Hormonal signalling through tyrosine phosphorylation

Insulin effects on target cells involves phosophorylation of tyrosine residues of intracellular protein substrates.

Insulin receptors

1. About 20000 insulin receptors are found on most of mammalian cells. Insulin receptor is a glycoprotein and it is a tetramer.
2. It is made up of four subunits of two types and designated as $\alpha_2\beta_2$. Both subunits are glycosylated.
3. The two α-subunits are located on extracellular side and are involved in insulin binding.
4. The two β-subunits spans entire membrane and are involved in signal transduction. The cytoplasmic domain of β-subunit possess intrinsic tyrosine kinase activity and an autophosphorylation site.

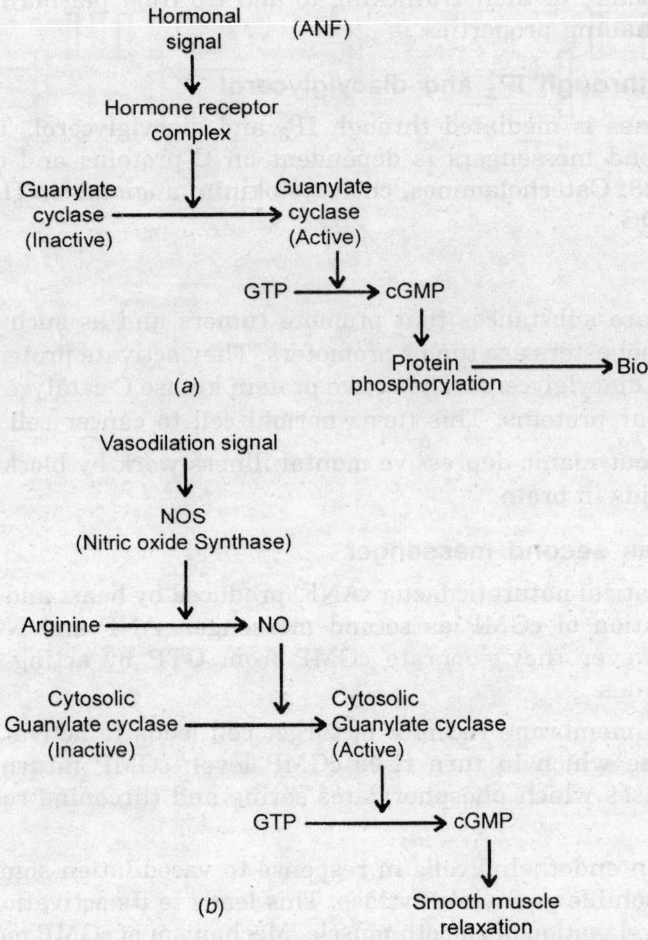

Fig. 29.2 Mechanisms of cGMP mediated signalling of ANF (*a*) and NO (*b*)

Mechanism of insulin action

1. Action of insulin begins with binding of this hormone to its receptors.
2. When insulin binds to receptor, tyrosine kinase activity of β-subunit of receptor is stimulated. As a result β-chain undergoes autophosphorylation.
3. The phosphorylated insulin receptor phosphorylates tyrosine residues of insulin receptor substrate-1 (IRS-1).
4. Now the phosphorylated IRS-1 binds to variety of intracellular proteins like kinases, phosphatases etc. and activates them through some unknown mechanism. These active kinases and phosphatases regulates activities of enzymes of various metabolic pathways by phosphorylation and dephosphorylation (Figure 29.3).

Other hormones that act by tyrosine phosphorylation are insulin like growth factors (IGF), nerve growth factor, prolactin, erythropoietin etc.

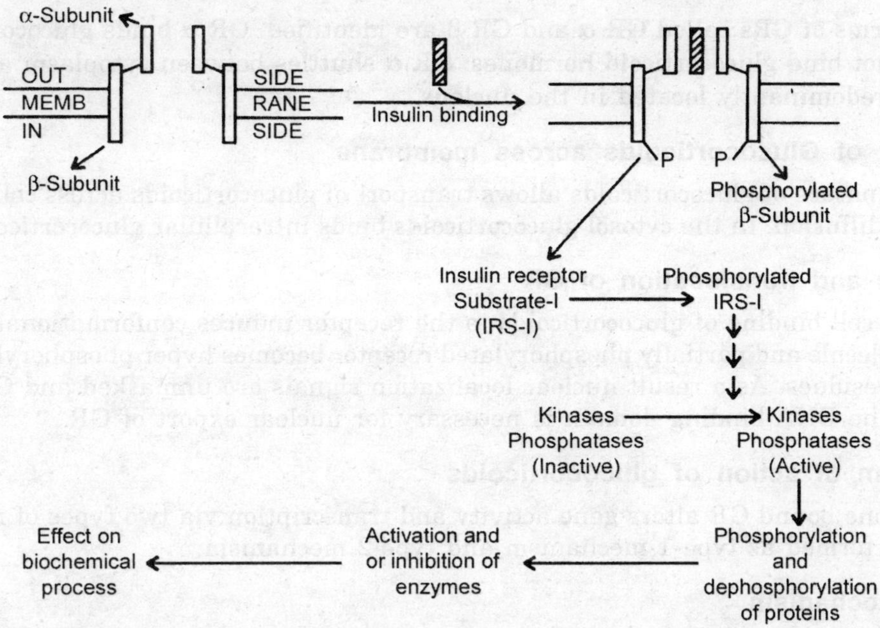

Fig. 29.3 Mechanism of insulin action on biochemical processes

Hormonal signalling through intracellular receptors

Action of steriod hormones, retinoic acid and thyroid hormone is mediated through intracellular receptors. The hormone-receptor complex initiates signal transduction in target tissues. The effect of these hormones on target cells is mainly increased expression of certain genes as mentioned in chapter 19.

Glucocorticoid signalling

Glucocorticoid signalling occurs through their specific intracellular glucocorticoid receptor (GR) and produce stimulatory or inhibitory actions by stimulating or inhibiting gene activity and transcription.

Glucocorticoid Receptors (GR)

They are super family of steroid receptors. All members of super family share three characteristic structural or functional domains. A typical glucocorticoid steroid receptor contain six regions or domains A, B, C, D, E and F. The variable N-terminal domain (A/B region) is involved in activation of genes and interacts with transcription machinery or transcription factors. It is also known as trans activating domain. The central portions of the receptor contains conserved DNA-binding domain (C-region) in which two zinc fingers are also situated. The DNA-binding domain participates in receptor dimerization, nuclear translocation and transactivation. The two zinc fingers has different roles. One of the fingers projects into major groove of the DNA where it recognizes and binds to glucocorticoid responsive element (GRE) sequence. It is also known as recognition helix. Other zinc finger is involved in the formation of GR homodimers. The less conserved C-terminal domain (D/E/F region) is known as hormone binding domain which binds to hormone. It also contains two nuclear localization signals (NLS) (Fig. 29.2.B).

Iso forms of GR

Two iso forms of GRs called GR α and GR β are identified. GR α binds glucocorticoids and GR β cannot bind glucocorticoid hormones. GR α shuttles between cytoplasm and nucleus. GR β is predominantly located in the nucleus.

Transport of Glucocorticoids across membrane

Lipophilic nature of glucocorticoids allows transport of glucocorticoids across cell membrane by simple diffusion. In the cytosol glucocorticoids binds intracellular glucocorticoid receptor.

Activation and translocation of GR

Inside the cell binding of glucocorticoids to the receptor induces conformational changes in the GR molecule and partially phosphorylated receptor becomes hyper phosphorylated mostly at serine residues. As a result nuclear localization signals are unmasked and GR moves to nucleus. The DNA binding domain is necessary for nuclear export of GR.

Mechanism of action of glucocorticoids

The hormone bound GR alters gene activity and transcription via two types of mechanisms which are termed as type-1 mechanism and type-2 mechanism.

Type-1 mechanism

Direct activation or repression of target genes by glucocorticoid bound GR is known as type-1 mechanism.

Type-2 mechanism

In direct inhibition of target genes by hormone activated GR is termed as type-2 mechanism.

Type-1 mechanism of glucocorticoid action

1. In the nucleus hormone bound GRα (HGRα) undergoes homodimarization, hetero dimerization or nodimerization.
2. The homodimerization leads to formation of HGRα-HGRα complex and hetero dimerization involves formation of HGRα-HGRβ complex.
3. Binding of HGRα-HGRα homodimer to glucocorticoid responsive element (GRE) activates the transcription of gene. Binding of HGRα hoodimer induces chromatin remodeling in promoter region which facilitates transcription.

   In contrast binding of HGRα-HGRβ heterodimer to GRE leads to suppression of GR α stimulated gene transcription. GRβ represses stimulatory action of GR α by specifically inhibiting GRE mediated transcription.
4. Binding of HGRα complex without involving dimerization to negative glucocorticoid responsive element (nGRE) inhibits gene transcription. The mechanism of action of GR on nGRE involves displacement of positive regulatory protein from promoter site. In Fig. 29.4. Type-1 mechanism of action of glucocorticoids is shown.

Type-2 mechanism of action of glucocorticoid

1. In this type of hormones action, glucocorticoid bound GR α binds to transcription factor (TF).
2. Then it inhibits transcription of target genes stimulated by transcription factor (Fig. 29.5).

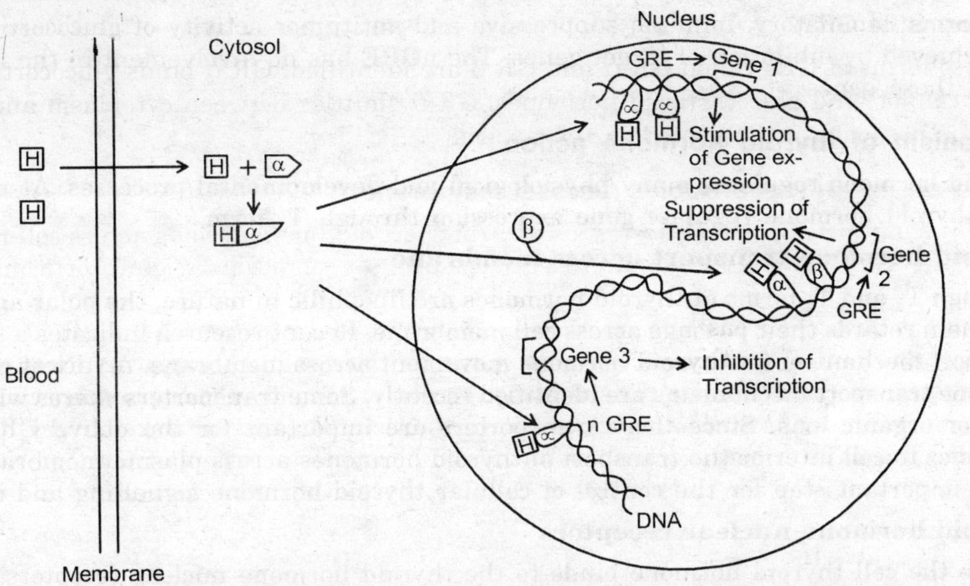

Fig. 29.4 Type-1 mechanism of action of glucocorticoid hormone.
H, hormone, α-α isomer of glucocorticoid receptor; β-β isomer of glucocorticoid receptor, GRE, glucocorticoid responsive element; nGRE, negative glucocorticoid responsive element.

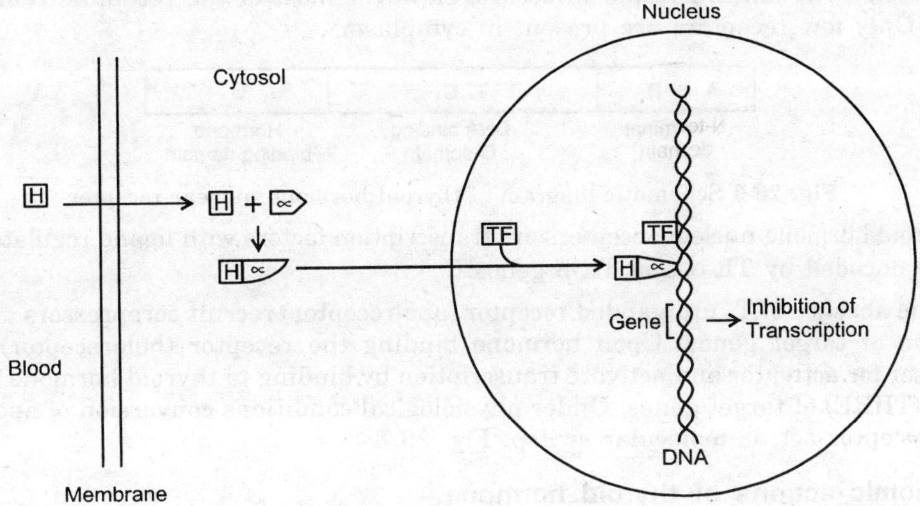

Fig. 29.5 Type-2 Mechanism of action of glucocorticoid hormone. H, hormone; α-α isomer of glucocorticoid receptor; TF, transcription factor

Medical importance

1. Glucocorticoids are essential for normal physiology and survival of mammals including man. Hence it is essential to understand molecular basis of glucocorticoids action.
2. Glucocorticoids arc involved in the regulation of carbohydrate metabolism, lipid metabolism, protein metabolism, oxidative metabolism, electrolyte balance, reproduction, growth, apoptosis, immuno suppression, anti inflammatory action, anti tumor activities etc.

3. Anti inflammatory, immuno suppressive and antitumor activity of glucocorticoids are achieved by inhibition of target genes. The nGRE has no involvement in the inhibition of these genes.

Mechanism of thyroid hormone action

Thyroid hormone regulates many physiological and developmental processes. At molecular level thyroid hormone regulate gene expression through T_3 form.

Thyroid hormone transport across membrane

Although T_3 and T_4 forms of thyroid hormones are lipophilic in nature, the polar amino acid side chain retards their passage across cell membrane. Recent research indicates a saturable transport mechanism for thyroid hormone movement across membrane. A variety of thyroid hormone transport mechanisms are identified recently. Some transporters shares with amino acids or organic ions. Since these transporters are important for the delivery of thyroid hormones to cell interior the transport of thyroid hormones across plasma membrane is one of the important step for the control of cellular thyroid hormone signalling and action.

Thyroid hormone nuclear receptors

In side the cell thyroid hormone binds to the thyroid hormone nuclear receptors. Thyroid hormones nuclear receptors belong to super family of nuclear receptors which consist of several domains. They are N-terminal A/B domain, DNA-binding C domain and hormone binding D-domain (Fig.29.6). Shuttling of these receptors between nucleus and cytoplasm and between DNA and nucleoplasm occurs. However most of the receptors remain in the nucleus. Only few receptors are present in cytoplasm.

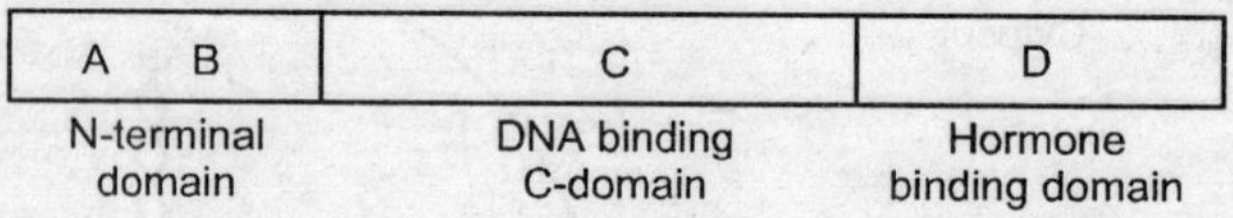

Fig. 29.6 Schematic diagram of thyroid hormone nuclear receptor.

Thyroid hormone nuclear receptors are transcription factors with ligand regulated activity. They are encoded by TR-α and TR-β genes.

In the absence of T_3 unliganded receptor (apo-receptor) recruit corepressors and repress expression of target genes. Upon hormone binding the receptor (holoreceptor) exchange corepressor for activator and activate transcription by binding to thyroid hormone responsive element (THRE) of target genes. Under physiological conditions conversion of apo-receptors to holo receptor act as molecular switch. Fig. 29.7.

Non-genomic actions of thyroid hormone

A number of thyroid hormone effects occur rapidly and unaffected by inhibitors of transcription and translation. They are known as nongenomic actions of thyroid hormone. They are observed in various cell types, brown adipose tissue, heart and pituitary.

The non genomic actions are localized to cytosol, plasma membrane and cell organelles. These non genomic actions include regulation of ion channels, oxidative phosphorylation and mitochondrial gene transcription and involves generation of intracellular secondary messengers and induction of Ca^{2+}, cAMP, proteinkinase signalling cascades.

Thyroid disorders

Thyroid disorders are the most common among all the endocrine diseases in India. The estimated disease burden in the country due to these disorders is approximately 42 million. Endemic goiter and thyrotoxicosis are widely prevalent disorders of thyroid in India. Thyroid goiter is found in the entire country where as thyrotoxicosis is seen in north Indian states.

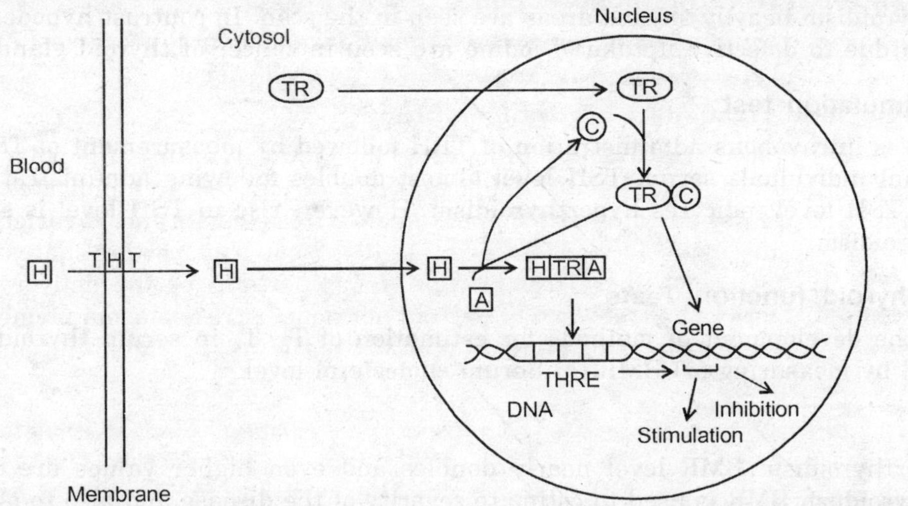

Fig. 29.7 Mechanism of action of thyroid hormone. TR, thyroid hormone receptor; A, activator; THRE, thyroid hormone responsive element; C-corepressor; THT, thyroid hormone transporter.

Thyroid function Tests

Since thyroid disorders are common among endocrine disorders in this country, several tests are used to assess the level of functioning of thyroid gland. They are popularly known as "Thyroid function tests".

Most important thyroid function tests are

1. Estimation of T_3, T_4 and TSH in serum.
2. Radioactive iodine uptake studies.
3. TRH stimulation Tests.

Estimation of thyroid hormone in serum

Measurement of T_3, T_4 and TSH levels in serum is useful in diagnosis of thyroid diseases. Currently RIA and ELISA methods are available for estimation of thyroid hormones in serum. Normal values of these hormones are given below

T_3 : 100-250ng/100 ml, T_4: 4.0-16.0 μg/100ml.

TSH: 1-3μU/ml.

In hypothyroidism T_3 T_4 levels are decreased and TSH level is increased. In hyperthyroidism T_3 and T_4 levels are increased and TSH level is decreased due to feedback inhibition. If hypothyroidism is due to defective hypothalamus or pituitary gland then the level of all three hormones *i.e.* T_3, T_4 and TSH in serum is decreased.

Radioactive iodine uptake test

Since iodine is required for the synthesis of thyroid hormones thyroid gland take up iodine and concentrates it in the cells. Radioactive iodine uptake test is based on this thyroid function.

It involves intravenous administration of fixed dose of radioactive iodine ^{131}I to the patient. After few hours neck region of the patient is scanned for radio active emission. In hyperthyroidism heavily shaded areas are seen in the scan. In contrast hypodense areas in the scan due to defective uptake of iodine are seen in cancer of thyroid gland.

TRH stimulation test

It involves intravenous administration of TRH followed by measurement of TSH in blood. In normal individuals serum TSH level almost doubles following administration of TRH. Normal TSH level indicates hyperthyroidism. However, rise in TSH level is suggestive of hypothyroidism.

Other thyroid function Tests

Before the development of methods for estimation of T_3, T_4 in serum thyroid function is assessed by measuring (*a*) BMR (*b*) Serum cholesterol level.

BMR

In hyperthyroidism BMR level nearly doubles and even higher values are obtained. In hyperthyroidism BMR is used to estimate severity of the disease and also to observe effect of treatment. BMR is reduced in hypothyroidism and in severe cases less than half of the normal values are obtained. Here also BMR estimation is used both in diagnosis and in following treatment.

Regulation of hormone action

So far I explained mechanisms by which hormonal message is translated into biochemical effect or biological response in target cells. Now we shall examine when and how endocrine gland receives signal to secrete or stop production of hormones. Usually release or secretion or inhibition of hormones by endocrine glands is under control of higher centres in brain. Depending on needs of organism or individual a particular hormone is produced or inhibited and this signal is delivered to target gland through chemical substances known as releasing factors or release inhibiting factors and trophic hormones.

Releasing factors or release inhibiting factors are produced by hypothalamus where as trophic hormones are produced by anterior pituitary gland. However hypothalamus being part of brain it is under control of other brain centres. Usually releasing factors or release inhibiting factors of hypothalamus reach anterior pituitary gland through direct circulatory connection where as trophic hormones of pituitary reaches target gland through blood circulation.

Chemical nature of releasing factors and trophic hormones

Most of the releasing factors or release inhibiting factors are proteins. Likewise trophic hormones are also proteins (peptides).

Hypothalamic releasing or release inhibiting factors

The releasing or release inhibiting factors produced by hypothalamus are thyrotrophin releasing factor (TRF), growth hormone release inhibiting factor (GRF) or somatostatin, corticotrophin releasing factor (CRF) and gonadotrophin releasing factor (GRF).

Regulation of hormone action by releasing and trophic hormones

When hypothalamus is activated by higher brain centres releasing or release inhibiting factors are produced. In response to hypothalamic signal through releasing or release inhibiting factor anterior pituitary either generates trophic hormone or stops its release. The trophic hormone if released acts on target endocrine glands to produce hormone.

For example thyrotrophin releasing factor when released by hypothalamus in response to higher centre stimulation acts on anterior pituitary to release thyrotropic or thyroid stimulating hormone (TSH). This in turn acts on thyroid gland to release thyroxine.

Other trophic hormones produced by anterior pituitary, their target glands and hormones secreted by target glands are given in Table 29.3.

Table 29.3 Action of some trophic hormones of anterior pituitary gland.

Name	Target gland	Hormones Secreted
Adreno cortico trophic hormone (ACTH)	Adernal cortex	Gluco corticoids
Follicle stimulating hormone (FSH)	Testes/Ovary	Testosterone, estrogen / progesterone
Lutinizing hormone (LH)	Testes/Ovary	Testosterone, estrogen / progesterone

Regulation of hormone action by feedback inhibition

This is another way of controlling hormone action. Usually hormone action is self limiting. It controls its own production. For example hormones of adrenal cortex inhibit release of CRF and ACTH (Figure 29.8).

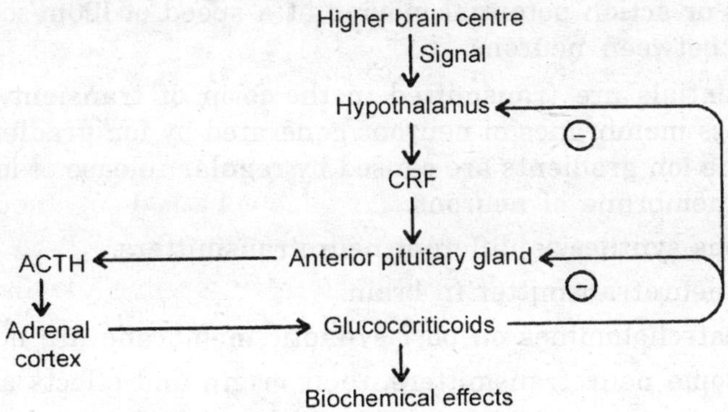

Fig. 29.8 Regulation of hormone action by feedback inhibition. ⊖ indicates inhibition.

Agonists and antagonists of Hormones

Agonists

Agonists are hormone analogs which are structurally not related to hormone. They are like alternative substrates of an enzyme. However they are able to bind to hormone receptor. Sometimes agonists bind to receptor more tightly than hormone. Usually binding of agonist to receptor produces an effect similar to that of hormone. Some agonists are more potent than hormone itself.

Antagonists

Antagonists are also hormone analogs but their binding to receptor does not produce biological effect characteristic of the hormone. Antagonists of hormones are very much like competitive inhibitors of an enzyme. However antagonist abolishes hormone effect.

Medical Importance

1. Hormone agonists and antagonists are used to explore molecular structure of receptors. This information is used to design new potent drugs.
2. Some agonists and antagonists have clinical applications.
3. Isoproterenol which is an agonist of catecholamines is used in treatment of asthma.
4. Diethyl stilbestrol is an estrogen analog used for isolation of estrogen receptor.
5. Progesterone agonists like norethindrone and medroxy progesterone acetate are used as oral contraceptives and to inhibit ovulation for months respectively.
6. Nicotine is agonist of acetyl choline.
7. Clomiphene citrate is an estrogen antagonist used to promote conception.
8. Estrogen antagonist tamoxifen is used in the treatment of breast cancer.
9. Toxins like tubo curarine and cobra toxin are antagonists of acetyl choline.

Neurotransmitters

1. They establish communication between nerve cells, nerve and muscle. The communication is in the form of nerve impulse.
2. They are involved in nerve impulse transmission.
3. Nerve impulses or action potential moving at a speed of 100m/sc provide intercellular communication between neurons.
4. The action potentials are transmitted in the form of transient changes in potential differences across membranes of neurons generated by ion gradients involving Na^+, K^+ and Cl^- ions. The ion gradients are caused by regular release of ions from ion channels located in the membrane of neurons.
5. Different neurons synthesize different neurotransmitters.
6. Dopamine is a neurotransmitter in brain.
7. The effects of catecholamines on post synaptic membrane are not clear.

In Table 29.2 some neurotransmitters, their origin and effects are presented.

Synaptic transmission

A neuron transmit signal to another neuron through synapse or synaptic cleft characterized by space between two adjoining neurons. In the synapses action potential causes secretion of neurotransmitter by pre synaptic cell. The secreted neurotransmitter binds its receptor on postsynaptic membrane to initiate a cascade of events leading to specific response or generates action potential.

Receptors for neurotransmitters

Post synaptic membranes have neurotransmitter receptors associated with ion pumps or channels. A neurotransmitter that is released by synaptic vesicle in the synaptic cleft binds to these receptors and influences membrane potential of post synaptic neuron directly and indirectly by several different mechanisms. The signal to open or close ion pumps is not determined by chemical properties of this neurotransmitter alone but also by the type of neurotransmitter that is released.

1. One type of receptor has ion channels associated with it to which neurotransmitter binds directly and bring about conformational change leading to opening of ion channel immediately.
2. The second type of receptor gates these ion channels indirectly with second messenger system. A neurotransmitter bound to such receptor causes release of regulatory proteins with in cell membrane that act on family of ion channels.

Medical importance

1. The direct stimulation is faster and lasts only few milliseconds and used in the circuitary that produce behaviour.
2. The second messenger system is slower and involves lasting changes in connection strength and alteration in excitability of neurons. This makes it possible to learn new behaviour.
3. Reduction in number of postsynaptic receptors leads to neurological diseases.
4. A neurotransmitter can inhibit or excit neurons depending on receptor.

Mechanism of action of acetylcholine

1. Acetylcholine is involved in transmission of nerve impulse between nerves and between nerve and muscle.
2. In the presynaptic end of neuron acetylcholine is stored as vesicle.
3. The arrival of nerve impulse causes release of vesicle into synaptic cleft where acetylcholine is released.
4. Binding of acetylcholine to specific cholinergic receptors present in postsynaptic membrane causes depolarization of postsynaptic membrane due to influx of Na^+. This leads to generation of nerve impulse in post synaptic neuron.
5. Choline esterase present in synaptic cleft hydrolyzes acetylcholine when it dissociates from receptor.

   Acetyl choline mediated nerve impulse transmission and action of acetylcholine esterase are shown in Figure 29.9A, 29.9B respectively.

Medical Importance

1. Wargases (Nerve gases) insecticides like parathion work by inhibiting acetylcholine esterase.
2. Neostigmine used in the treatment of myasthenia gravis work by increasing level of acetylcholine at neuromuscular junction. It raises acetylcholine level by inhibiting acetylcholine esterase.
3. Cobra toxin work by binding to acetylcholine receptor at neuromuscular junction. The binding of cobra toxin to acetylcholine receptor inhibits postsynaptic nerve impulse transmission.
4. Succinylcholine used as muscle relaxant prior to anaesthesia work by binding to acetylcholine receptor for longer time. This prolonged binding of succinylcholine to acetyl choline receptor leads to permanent depolarization of postsynaptic membrane.

5. **Acetylcholine Estrase Inhibitors (AChEI).** Alzheimer's disease (AD) a neurodegenerative disease is characterized by severe dementia is treated with inhibitors of acetylcholine estrase. Inhibitors of this enzyme increase availability of AChE by reducing its breakdown. Tacrine, Physostigmine and Rivastigmine are inhibitors of AChE used in treatment of AD patients.

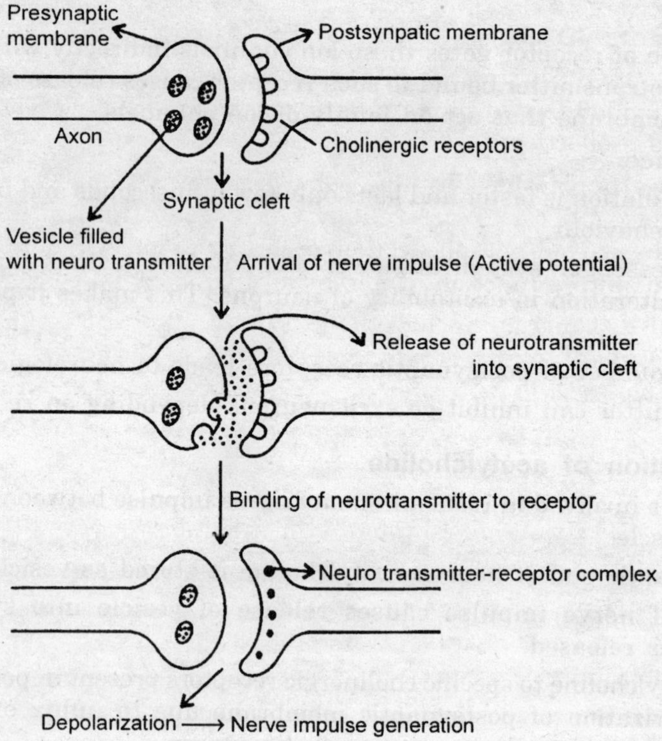

Fig. 29.9 (*a*) Acetylcholine mediated nerve impulse transmission.

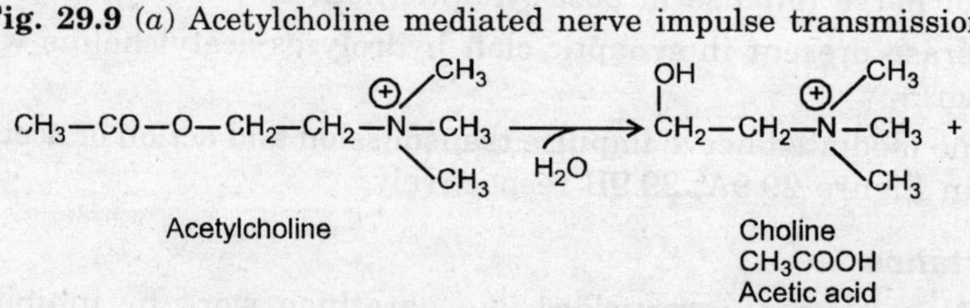

Fig. 29.9 (*b*) Action of acetylcholine esterase.

γ- Amino butyric acid (GABA)

1. It is an inhibitory neurotransmitter. It blocks nerve impulse transmission by hyper polarizing postsynaptic membrane.
2. When it binds to receptor of postsynaptic membrane Cl^- enters from outside to inside of post synaptic neuron through pore like opening present in receptor. The pore present in receptor opens only when GABA binds to it.
3. Entry of Cl^- leads to hyperpolarization of postsynaptic membrane. This makes depolarization of postsynaptic membrane difficult. As a result nerve impulse is not produced and nerve impulse transmission is inhibited.

Catecholamine neurotransmitters

Catecholamines noradrenaline (NE) and dopamine (DA) are used as neurotransmitters in the brain. Dopamine is highly concentrated in basal ganglia. NE and DA are packaged in synaptic vesicle and are released in synaptic cleft where they bind to their receptors in the post synaptic membrane to elicit specific responses.

Dopamine receptors (DARs)

They are members of GPCR super family and consist of five structurally distinct subtypes. These can be subdivided to two sub groups on the basis of their structure, pharmacological and transductional properties.

1. The first sub group termed D_1 like comprises the D_1 and D_5 DARs that stimulates adenylate cyclase and raises intracellular cAMP level. This leads to activation of protein kinase and brings about phosphorylation of certain proteins in nerve cell. Phosphorylation of ion channels alters function of nerve cell like excitability.
2. The second DARs subgroup includes D_2 to D_4 receptors and termed D_2 like. The D_2 like DARs are coupled to inhibitions of adenylate cyclase as well as turnover of phosphatidylinositol and activation of K^+ and Ca^{2+} channels.
3. DARs are subjected to various regulatory mechanisms which can either positively or negatively modulate their expression and functional activity.
4. Dopamine can both excite and inhibit neurons through DARs.
5. D_2 receptors form heterodimmers.
6. Dopamine release excites direct pathway by stimulating D_1 receptor and inhibit indirect pathway by stimulating D_2 receptor.

Fate of catecholamines

After performing their function NE and DA are removed from the synaptic cleft and are taken up by either by presynaptic membrane or by other glial cell membranes with the help of membrane transporters or uptake proteins available in these membranes

In the presynaptic membrane they are packaged again in the synaptic vesicle to start another cycle. The catecholamine neurotransmitters are also metabolised and inactivated by two enzymes catechol-o-methyl transferase in the synaptic cleft and monoamine oxidase -B (MAO-B) in the mitochondria, Fig. 29.10.

Medical importance

1. Hypersensitivity to dopamine receptors cause psychosis and schizophrenia.
2. D_2 like DARs are primary target for all known antipsychotic drugs (Antagonists) and drugs used to treat Parkinsonism (agonists).
3. Defects in catecholamine processing are responsible for many neurological diseases including depression involving NE and Parkinsonism involving dopamine.
4. Anti depressants like desipramine and inhibitors of MAO-B work either by increasing level of catecholamines in the brain or by facilitating prolonged stimulation of postsynaptic receptors.
5. Parkinsonism is characterized by death of dopamine making cells. Dopamine receptors agonist like bromocriptine is used to counter degeneration of dopaminergic neurons in the brain.

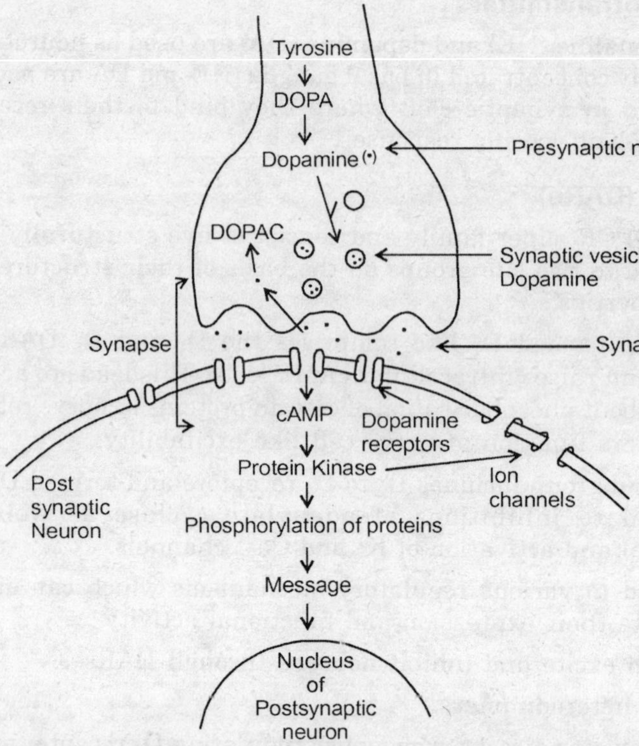

Fig. 29.10 Dopaminergic synapse with synthesis, storage, release and removal of dopamine. DOPAC, dihydroxy phenyl acetate.

L-Dopa a precursor of dopamine is also used to treat Parkinsonism. However it does not stop further deterioration of dopaminergic cells and hence not suitable for long term use.

Transplantation with genetically engineered embryonic stem cells or mouse embryonic stem cells are used to treat Parkinsonism. When they are grafted or injected into the brain of Parkinsonism patients they give rise to dopamine producing cells.

Signal transduction for memory

1. Our memory is located in the synapse. Structural and functional changes takes place in synapse when different types of memories are formed. Synaptic plasticity is word used to describe alterations as well as differences in the strength of synapses. So, memory involves restructuring of synapses.
2. Shortterm memory which lasts for minutes to hours and long term memory which can remain for weeks are governed by synaptic plasticity.
3. Weaker stimuli give rise to short term memory. It involves phosphorylation of ion channel proteins leading entry of more calcium ions. This leads to increased amount of neurotransmitter release at synapse and amplification of the signal, Fig. 29.11.
4. Strong stimuli give rise to long term memory. It involves increased levels of second messenger molecules like cAMP and proteinkinase A. These signals reach cell nucleus and leads to increased synthesis of specific proteins. If the synthesis of new protein is blocked by use of inhibitors only long term memory is affected.

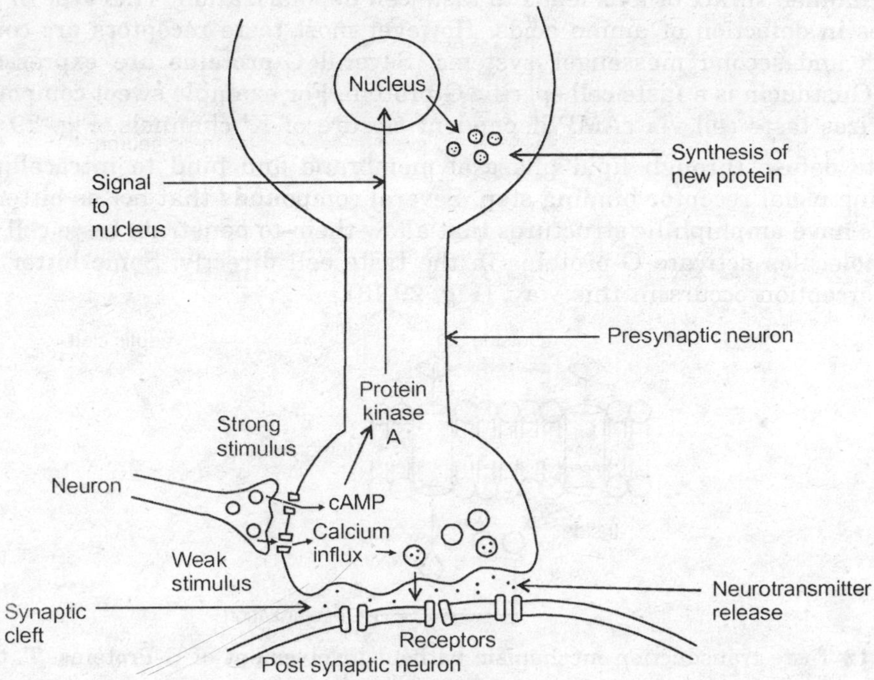

Fig. 29.11 Signal transduction for Memory.

Medical importance

1. Knowledge of cellular and molecular mechanism of memory may be used for development of new drugs to improve memory function of patients with different types of dementia.

Taste signaling

Taste sensation is initiated when tastants interact with taste cells (buds) present on the tongue epithelium. Tastants, taste cells and taste receptors interaction activates cascade of events that lead to release in neurotransmitter at afferent nerve fibres.

The mechanisms of taste transduction are diverse and involve wide array of signaling components.

Mechanism of taste transduction

Taste transduction mechanisms received much attention recently and have been the focus of considerable research. The tastants interact with the taste cells in many ways which depends of the type of tastants or type of taste perception.

1. Tastants directly interact with ion channels and produce taste cell depolarization. It may involve either direct penetration of ion channel by tastants or by blocking an open ion channel. For example mechanism by which we taste saltyness is due to direct permeation of Na^+ ions through sodium channels. This transfer of charge from outside to inside of the cell leads to development of depolarizing potential. In contrast bitter taste transduction involves blocking of an open potassium channels, Fig. 29.12.
2. Tastants bind taste receptors linked to ion channels or to G-proteins involved in generation of second messengers. When tastant binds to receptor it causes conformational change

in ion channel. Influx of ions leads to taste cell depolarization. This type of mechanism operates in detection of amino acids. However most taste receptors arc coupled to G-proteins and second messenger systems. Several G-proteins are expressed in taste bunds. Gustducin is a taste cell specific G-protein. For example sweet compound sucrose depolarizes taste cell via cAMP dependent closure of K^+ channels, Fig. 29.13.

3. Tastants defuse through lipid phase of membrane and bind to intracellular targets bypassing usual receptor binding step. Several compounds that act as bitter and sweet tastants have amphiphilic structures that allow them to penetrate taste cell membrane. Such molecules activate G-proteins in the taste eell directly. Some bitter compounds taste perception occurs in this way. (Fig. 29.13).

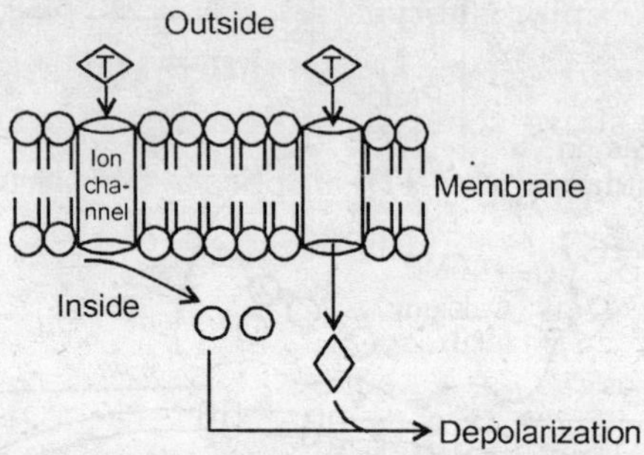

Fig. 29.12 Taste transduction mechanism without involvement of G-Proteins. T, tastants.

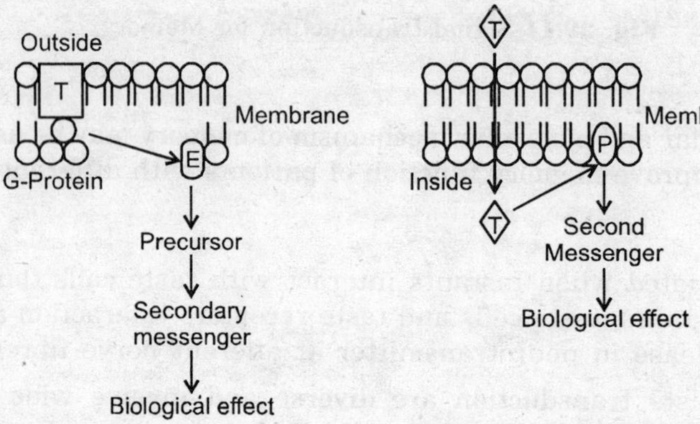

Fig. 29.13 G-Protein involved taste signal transduction. T, tastant, E-enzyme, P-protein.

Medical Importance

1. Alteration in taste is common disorder associated with several types of diseases as well as use of drugs.
2. Knowledge of cellular and molecular mechanism involved in taste transduction is useful, in developing drugs for the treatment of taste disorders.

Odor signalling

Eukoryotic organisms including man evolved complex olfactory system which give ability to identify odors, chemicals or scents in environment. The molecular mechanisms involved in this perception of odor are currently being investigated intensively using molecular biology, electrophysiology, Neurobiology techniques. Odor signalling pathways are elucidated to some extent by using these techniques.

Briefly odor perception involves initial interaction of odorant molecule with receptor proteins of olfactory system which is then transmitted to brain where it is processed and interpreted.

Olfactory Receptors (OR)

In the wall of nasal cavity olfactory epithelial cells contain olfactory neurons. Each olfactory neuron carries on its surface at least ten hair like cilia containing receptor proteins which recognizes and binds odorant molecules. These receptors are members of G-protein coupled receptors (GPCR) super family. Over thousand members of OR super family are identified. They are coded by thousand different genes. From more than thousand genes each olfactory neuron expresses only one receptor subtype.

Each OR specifically recognizes a set of odorants that share common molecular features. However all members of OR share some structural and functional features. They are

1. A seven transmembrane domain (7-TD) implicated in structural integrity.
2. A functional motif involved in ligand binding.

Odor signaling pathway

Odor signaling occurs through receptor mediated second messenger pathway.

1. The first step in odor perception or odor signalling pathway is the activation of one or more of OR.
2. When odorant molecule binds to OR cells containing these receptors are get activated. Each OR first activates G-protein G_{olf} to which it is coupled.
3. The G-protein inturn stimulates formation of olfactory cyclic nucleotide cAMP by activating adenylatecyclase.
4. cAMP binds to ligand gated cation channel leading to channel opening. This in turn leads to activation of olfactory neuron and electrical signals are generated.
5. Through thin nerve processes these signals directly pass through distinct micro domain known as glomeruli in the olfactory bulb of the brain.
6. From the glomeruli in the olfactory bulb information is passed to the other parts of the brain for interpretation. In Fig. 29.14 odor signalling pathway is shown.

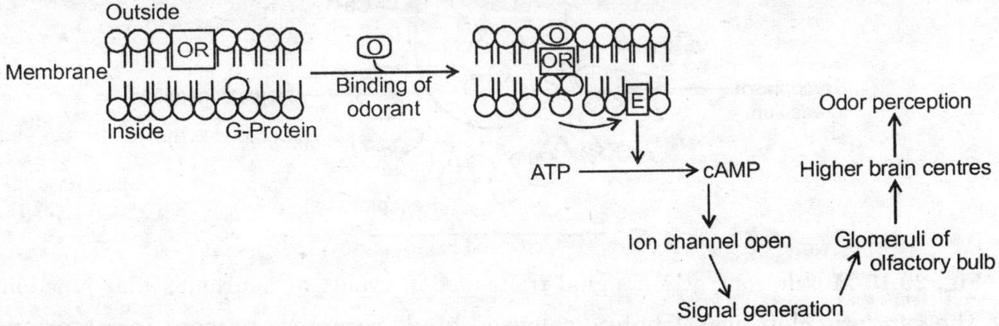

Fig. 29.14 Odor signalling pathway. O, odorant; OR, olfactory receptor; E, enzyme.

Our nose is able to detect and discriminate among thousands of odorants with diverse chemical structures and properties which requires enormous molecular recognition capacity. This is achieved through distinct receptor proteins present in the nasal cavity which are able to bind only specific molecules. A distinct odorant activates only one type of receptor. Further specific odorant detection may involve a signalling pathway that is distinct from those used by other odorants. However receptors appears to be non-specific i.e. specific odorant may activate multiple receptors and *vice versa*.

Medical importance

1. Knowledge of odor signalling may prove useful for treatment of olfactory disturbances or smell disturbances associated with infections like cold, drug use and diseases.
2. Molecular basis of odor recognition is useful in development of electronic nose or sensors for odorants present in environment.

Signal transduction for muscle contraction

Neuromuscular junction is the site of signal transduction for muscle contraction. It is the junction between motor nerve terminal and muscle. Nerve impulse is transmitted to muscle via neuromuscular junction. The part of muscle membrane that is in contact with nerve terminal is known as motor end plate. It is thrown into several folds which increases surface area for neurotransmitter action. The nerve end contains several vesicles filled with neurotransmitter acetylcholine.

The sequence of events that occur at neuromuscular junction during signal transduction for muscle contraction are as follows.

1. Arrival of nerve impulse at motor nerve end open ion channel for Ca^{2+}. This allows entry of Ca^{2+} form outside into inside of nerve terminal.
2. This leads to rupture of vesicle by the calcium ions and release of acetylcholine into synaptic cleft. In Fig. 29.15. Sequence of event involved in muscle contraction signal transduction are shown.

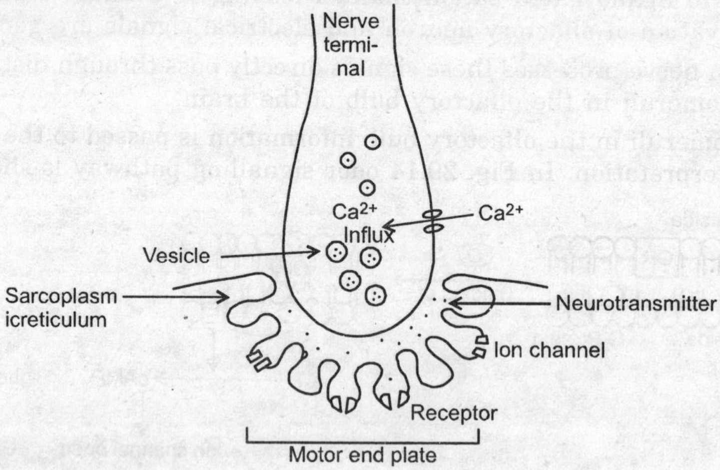

Fig. 29.15 Muscle contraction signal transduction events at neuromuscular junction.

3. In the synaptic cleft acetylcholine released binds receptors present in motor end plate. When two molecules of acetylcholine binds to receptors it undergoes conformational change and opens cation channels present in motor end plate.
4. Rapid influx of cations Na^+/ Ca^{2+} into muscle fibre occurs. It results in depolarization of muscle membrane and production of end plate potential.

5. Transmission of the end plate potential to adjacent muscle membrane leads to generation of action potential which results in muscle contraction.
6. Acetylcholine dissociates from its receptors with in two milliseconds by diffusion and hydrolyzed by acetylcholine esterase.
7. Choline is taken up by nerve terminal through active transport process and used for synthesis of acetylcholine.

Medical importance

1. Botulinum toxin interfere with muscle contraction by inhibiting acetylcholine release into synaptic space at neuromuscular junction and cause muscle paralysis.
2. **Snake venoms and neuromuscular junction.** There are approximately 420 venomous species of snakes living on this planet. Neuromuscular junction is one favorite target of these venoms. Those venoms affecting release of acetylcholine from the presynaptic membrane are called beta neurotoxins. They cause clinical myokymia.
3. Muscular dystrophies are due to defects in neuromuscular junction structure.
4. Mysthania gravis is caused by antibodies against acetylcholine receptor (AchR) which produce compromise in end plate potential reducing effective synaptic transmission. Auto antibody production is T-cell dependent process.
5. **Prion disease (Mad cow disease) and neuromuscular junction.** Prion protein which causes mad cow disease localizes in neuromuscular junction of tongue on exposure to meat products containing prion agent that is possible mechanism for prion agent transmission in animals.

REFERENCES

1. Barritt, G.J. Communication within animal cells. Blackwell, Oxford, 1992.
2. Barridge, M.J. The molecular basis of communication within cells. Sci. Am. **253(4)**, 142-152, 1985.
3. Coleman, D.E. and Sprang, S.R. How G-proteins work : a continuing story. Trends Biochem. Sci. **21**, 41-46, 1996.
4. Berridge, M.J. Inositol triphosphate and calcium signalling. Nature. **361**, 315-325, 1993.
5. Holmgrean, J. Actions of cholera toxin and the prevention and treatment of cholera. Nature. **292**, 413-417, 1981.
6. Kikkaww, U. Kishimoto, A. and Nishizuku, Y. The protein kinase C family : Heterogenity and its implications. Ann. Rev. Biochem. **58**, 31-44, 1989.
7. White, M.F. and Kahn, C.R. The insulin signalling system. J. Biol. Chem. **269**, 1-4, 1994.
8. Schally, A.V. Coy, D.H. and Meyers, C.A. Hypothalamic regulatory hormones. Ann. Rev. Biochem. **47**, 89-128, 1978.
9. Snyder, S.H. Drugs and neurotransmitter receptors in brain. Science **224,** 22-31, 1984.
10. Gomperts, Bastein, D. (Ed.). Signal Transduction. Academic Press, 2002.
11. Haga, T. and Berstein, G. G-protein coupled receptors. CRC Press, Florida, USA, 1999.
12. Reith, M.E.A., (Ed.) Neurotransmitter transporters: structure, function and Regulation. Humana Press; NJ, 1997.

13. Huber, Z. Guide book to small GTPases. Oxford University Press, 2002.
14. Hardie, D.G. Biochemical messengers, hormones, neurotransmitters and growth factors. Chapman & Hall, 1991.
15. Mueller-Schwarze, D. and Silver stain, N., (Eds.). Chemical signals in Vertebrates VI Plenum, NY, 1992.
16. Wilson, R.D. and Hare, J.F. Animal communication: Ground squirrel uses ultrasonic alarms. Nature. **430**, 523, 2004.
17. Shu-oushan and P. Water. Induced nucleotide specificity in GTPase. Proc. Natl. Acad. Sci. USA **100**, 4480-4485, 2003.
18. I. Ruiz-Stewart *et al.,* Guanylyl cyclase is an ATP sensor coupling nitric oxide signalling to cell metabolism. Proc. Natl. Acad. Sci. USA **101,** 37-42, 2004.
19. Damartino, M.V. *et al.* Interaction of glucocorticoid receptor and chicken ovalbumin upstream promoter transcription factor-II: Implications for actions of glucocorticoids on glucose, lipoprotein and xenobiotic metabolism. Ann. N.Y. Acad. Sci. **1024**, 72-84, 2004.
20. Shirasaki, H. *et al.* Expression and localization of steroid receptor in human nasal mucosa. Acta otolaryngol. **124(4),** 958-963, 2004.
21. Schoneveld, O.J. *et al.* Mechanisms of glucocorticoid signalling. Biochim. Biophys. Acta. **1680(2),** 114-128, 2004.
22. Hayashi, R. *et al.* Effects of glucocorticoids on gene transcription. Eur. J. Pharmacol. **500**, 51-62, 2004.
23. Kohrle, J. Guard your master: Thyroid hormone receptors protect their gland of origin from thyroid cancer. Endocrinol. **145(10),** 4427-4429, 2004.
24. Gurnell, M. *et al.* Nuclear receptors in disease: Thyroid receptor beta, PPar gama and orphan receptors. Essays in Biochem. **40**, 168-189, 2004.
25. Mai. W. *et al.* Thyroid hormone receptor alpha is a molecular switch of cardiac function between fetal and postnatal life. Proc. Natl. Aced. Sci. (USA). **101(28)**, 10332-10337, 2004.
26. Bockaert, J. *et al.,* G-Protein coupled receptors (GPCR) interacting proteins (GIP). Pharmacol. Thera. **103(3)**, 203-221, 2004.
27. Foley, P. *et al.,* Dopamine receptor agonists in therapy of Parkinson's disease. J. Neurol. Trans. **111,** 1375-1446, 2004.
28. Namkung, Y., Sibley, D.R. Protein C kinase mediates phosphorylation, desensitization and trafficking of the D_2 dopamine receptor. J. Biol. Chem. Sept.3, 2004.
29. Hashimoto, K. *et al.* An unliganded thyroid hormone receptor causes severe neurological dysfunction. Proc. Natl. Acad. Sci.(USA) **98(7),** 3998-4003, 2001.
30. Paul, M. Yen. Physiological and molecular basis of thyroid hormone action. Physiol. Rev. **81**, 1097-1142, 2001.
31. J.E. Silva. The thermogenic effect of thyroid hormone and its clinical implications. Ann. Inter. Med. **139**, 205-213, 2003.
32. Maruvada, P. *et al.* Dynamic shuttling and intra nuclear mobility of nuclear hormone receptor. J. Biol. Chem. **278**, 12425-12432, 2003.
33. Fujiwara, K. *et al.* Identification of Thyroid hormone transporters in humans: different molecules are involved in a tissue specific manner. Endocrinol. **142**, 2005-2012, 2001.

34. Lindamann, B. Receptors and transduction in taste. Nature. **413**, 219-225, 2001.
35. Andres-Barquin, P.J. Conte, C. Molecular basis of bitter taste. The T2R family of G-protein coupled receptors. Cell Biochem. Biophys. **41(l)**, 99-112, 2004.
36. Bagiani, A. *et al.* Channels as taste receptors in vertebrates. Prog. Biophys. Mol. Biol. **83(3)**, 193-225, 2003.
37. Friedrich, R.W. Neturobiology: Odorant receptors make scents. Nature. **430**, 511-512, 2004.
38. Katada, S. *et al.* Odorant response assays for a heterologously expressed olfactory receptor. Biochem. Biophys. Res. Commun. **305(4)**, 964-969, 2003.
39. Cartaud, A. *et al.* Muscle specific kinase (MSK) is required for anchoring acetylcholine estarase at the neuromuscular junction. J. CelI. Biol. **165**, 505-515, 2004.
40. Trinided, J.C. and Cohen, J.B. Neuregulin inhibits acetylcholine receptor aggregation in myotubes. J. Biol. Chem. **279**, 31622-31628, 2004.
41. Nakata, K. *et al.* Ultrastructural localization of high affinity choline transporter in rat neuromuscular junction. Synapse, **53**, 53-56, 2004.
42. Gales, C. *et al.* Real time monitoring of receptor and G-protein interactions in living cells. Nature Methods. **2**, 177-184, 2005.

EXERCISES

ESSAY QUESTIONS

1. Define biochemical messengers. Classify. Give examples. Write their chemical nature and functions.
2. Describe general mechanism of hormone action.
3. Define G-proteins. Explain their structure. Write mechanism of G-protein mediated hormonal signalling. In what diseases G-protein function is altered.
4. Define synapse. Synaptic cleft. Write mechanism of synaptic transmission of nerve impulse.
5. Write normal plasma thyroid hormone level. How they are translocated across membrane? Write mechanism of thyroid hormone action. Add note on thyroid function tests.
6. Describe mechanism of action of glucocorticoid hormones.
7. Write molecular mechanisms involved in taste and olfactory signal transduction.
8. Write an essay on neurotransmitters and their receptors.

SHORT QUESTIONS

1. Write about G-protein coupled receptors.
2. Explain insulin signalling pathway.
3. Write mechanism of acetylcholine mediated neurotransmission.
4. Write a note on dopamine receptors.
5. How dopamine is formed and utilized? Name clinical conditions associated with this process.
6. How hormone action is regulated?
7. Write mechanism of thyroid hormone action.
8. Write briefly about glucocorticoid receptors.

9. Write biochemical alterations in following diseases.
   (*a*) Psychosis, (*b*) Depression, (*c*) Parkinsonism (*d*) Alzhemeir's disease
10. Explain type-1 mechanism of glucocorticoid action.
11. Write mechanism of short and long term memory formation.
12. Define neuromuscular junction. How signal is mediated through the junction? In what diseases it is affected?
13. How sweet, bitter and salty tastes are generated?
14. Write briefly about taste and olfactory receptors.

30
CHAPTER

BIOCHEMISTRY OF APOPTOSIS

Occurrence

Apoptosis occurs in most of the life forms. So far it is found in plants, bacteria, invertebrates and mammals including humans.

MEDICAL AND BIOLOGICAL IMPORTANCE

1. It deals with molecular mechanisms underlying apoptosis.
2. Apoptosis is a process involved in many physiological and pathological conditions.
3. It is a cellular suicidel mechanism that occurs during development. It is also known as programmed cell death (PCD).
4. It plays major role in controlling cell number of tissues like gastrointestinal tract, reproductive tract, skin etc.
5. It plays crucial role in tissue sculpting, pattern formation and tissue homeostasis.
6. It is involved in immunity and inflammation. It has a role in lymphocytes turnover.
7. Several diseases are due to alterations in the balance between cell death and cell division.
8. Decreased apoptosis is a cause for cancer, autoimmune diseases like rheumatoid arthritis (RA), systemic lupus erythromatosus etc.
9. Increased apoptosis occurs in Alzheimers disease (AD), Parkinsons disease (PD), AIDS etc.
10. Recent evidence indicates involvement of apoptosis in acute renal failure.
11. Genes of apoptosis are evolutionarily conserved. Death genes manipulation may be beneficial to biotechnology industries. Industrially useful cell lines with longer life span may be obtained by death genes genetic engineering. In otherwords immortalization of cell or tissues may be accomplished by manipulating death genes.
12. Substances that can induce apoptosis in cells particularly cancer cells are present in common fruits and vegetables. They are useful in the treatment and prevention of some types of cancer.

Apoptic Pathway

1. Apoptosis involves many biochemical and cytological events.

2. In response to death signal/stimuli cell enters apoptic pathway.
3. Death receptors translate death signal into metabolic reactions by activating prodeath enzymes.
4. Active death enzymes in turn hydrolyze death substrates.
5. As a result cell death occurs and apoptic bodies or cell debris are formed due to fragmentation of cell.
6. Phagocytosis clears cell debris leaving no trace of prior existing cell (Fig. 30.1).

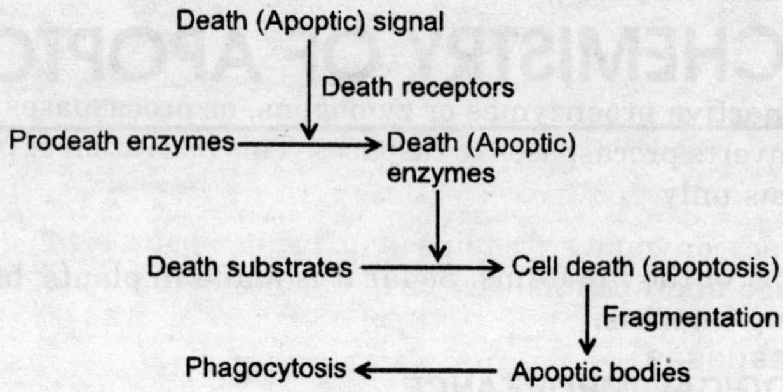

Fig. 30.1 Simplified view of apoptic pathway.

Death Signals

Death signals are not common to all types of cells. They vary according to cell type. Death signals may originate from the cell itself or outside of cell or combination of both. Some of the events that act as signals for apoptosis are

1. An increase in reactive oxygen species (ROS).
2. Collapse of mitochondrial membrane potential that causes release of death substance cytochromes.
3. Increased intracellular calcium level.
4. Loss of essential survival factors.
5. Radiation exposure, hormones, drugs and toxins action on cell.
6. Increased intracellular ceramide level.
7. Increased expression of phosphatidyl serine on outer cell membrane.
8. Environmental and developmental signals.

Signal Transduction

Some apoptic signal conversion to active apoptosis requires death receptors and adaptors. However conversion of death signal into active apoptosis is found to require synthesis of protein in the case of other apoptic signals.

Death Receptors, Death factors and Adaptors

Death receptors are membrane bound proteins. They have three types of domains. Ligand or death factor binding domain located on extracellular side, a transmembrane domain and death domains (DDs) which are located on cytosolic side. Some known death receptors are Fas (Apo-1, or CD 95) the receptor for FasL, Tumor necrosis factor receptor TNFR etc. Some known death factors are Faslignd (FasL or CD95L), TNF- related apoptosis inducing ligand (TRAL) and tumor necrosis factor (TNF).

Adaptors are cytoplasmic proteins. They have two types of domains, its own death domain (ODD) through which its recognizes DD of death receptor and death enzyme domain (DED) through which it binds to death enzymes via their respective death enzyme domains (DEDs). Some known adaptor proteins are FADD (Fas associated death domain. Apaf-1 (apoptosis protease activating factor-1) and factors released by mitochondria.

Death Enzymes

Proteases, granzymes and nucleases are involved in apoptosis. Proteases are cysteine proteases that has specificity towards aspartate - X - bonds. Hence, they are named as cysteine aspartate specific protease or caspases. Granzyme is a serine protease but had specificity towards aspartate - X - bonds like caspases.

Prodeath Enzymes

All caspases exist as inactive proenzymes or zymogens, or procaspases or prodeath enzymes. Limited proteolysis converts procaspases to caspases. This activation of procaspases to caspases occurs during apoptosis only.

Active caspases act on many proteins and bring about cytological changes like cell condensation, shrinkage and apoptic body formation.

Classification of Caspases

More than 15 different caspases are identified in animals. They have high level of substrate specificity. Some caspases are involved in activation of procaspases of apoptic path way and some are involved in the cleaving of death substrates.

Based on their function caspases are divided into

1. Upstream instigators and 2. Downstream terminators.

1. Upstream instigators

Are those caspases that incit proteolytic activation.

Example :

(*a*) DED containing caspase 8 and 10.

(*b*) Caspase recruiting domain (CARD) containing caspase 9.

Upstream active caspases then directly activate down stream caspases.

2. Down stream terminators

Are those caspases which kill cell by cleaving intracellular death substrates.

Examples:

(*a*) Caspase 3

(*b*) Caspase 7

Death Substrates

Terminator caspases cleave many death substrates and structural proteins. Some death substrates are poly ADP ribose polymerase (PARP), inhibitor of caspase activated DNA ase (ICAD), DNA dependent protein kinase (DNA-PK), DNA fragmentation factor etc. Cleavage of death substrates leads to death of cells. Terminator caspases also proteolyze many structural proteins like gel solin, microfilament protein and nuclear lamins.

Mechanism of Apoptosis

Molecular events associated with apoptosis are

(*a*) Initiation

(*b*) Activation of caspases

(*c*) Proteolysis

(*d*) DNA fragmentation.

These events may vary according to cell types.

Cytological events associated with apoptosis are chromatin condensation, disintegration of cell into membrane surrounded apoptic bodies.

Initiation

1. Apoptic process is initiated with binding of death ligand or death factor to death receptor. This is followed by clustering of death domains (DDs) of death receptors.
2. An adaptor protein then binds through its own death domain (ODD) to the clustered receptor death domains and thus form death inducing signalling complex (DISC) Fig. 30.2.
3. This is followed by recruitment of death domain of procaspase to adaptors death enzyme domain (ADED).

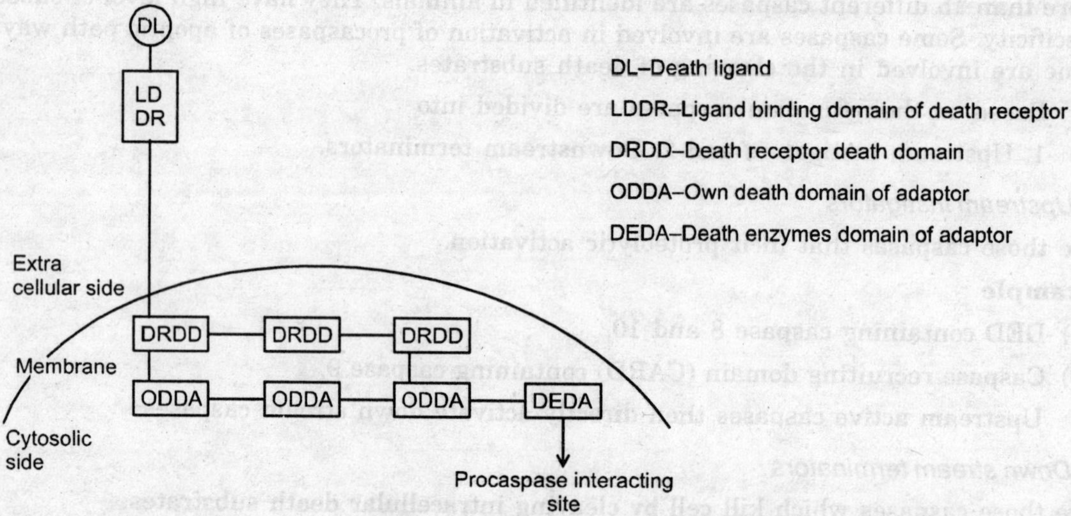

Fig. 30.2 Schematic view of death inducing signalling complex (DISC).

Activation of Caspases

1. Recruitment of DED-bearing procaspase into DISC leads to activation of this upstream procaspase.
2. Procaspase is composed of N-terminal DED, a large domain and a small domain. The three domains are separated by aspartate residues.
3. Activation of procaspase to active caspase involves proteolytic processing at aspartate residue and involves removal of N-terminal domain and formation of a oligomer which is composed of large and small domains.

4. The DED of procaspase plays an important role in the initiation of activation. It mediates interaction of procaspases with respective DED of adaptor molecule.

   Since caspases are specific towards aspartate - X - bonds they may be responsible for their own activation (autocatalysis) and for the activation of other caspases.

5. The active upstream caspase then activates downstream caspases.

Proteolysis

Active down stream caspases act on many death substrates and bring about dissembly of cytoplasm.

DNA Fragmentation

1. Down stream caspase cleaves CAD-ICAD complex thus releases CAD. Activity of CAD results in DNA fragmentation.
2. PARP is also cleaved to apoptic fragments.
3. Fragmentation of DNA takes place at the nucleosome linker sites.
4. The length of oligonucleosomal fragments is found to be of 180 base pairs (bp).
5. Electrophoretic separation of these DNA fragments shows characteristic ladder formation. The rungs of ladder are multiples of 180 basepair fragment.

   Mechanism of apoptosis is summarized in Fig. 30.3.

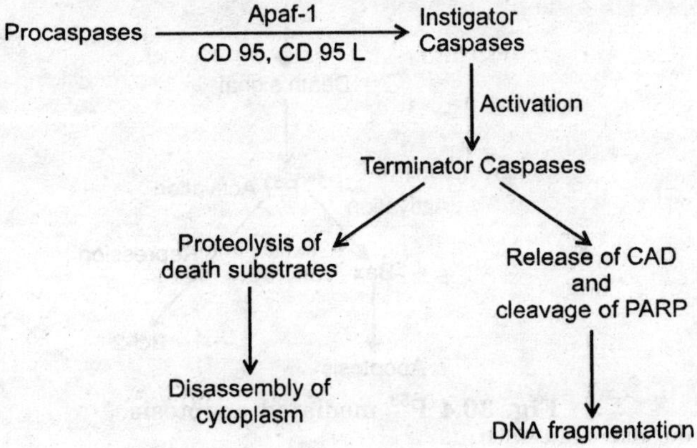

Fig. 30.3 Mechanism of apoptosis.

Apoptic Regulators

1. Many proteins influence apoptosis by interacting with adaptors/cofactors.
2. Some promote apoptosis and hence they are known as death promoters. Some known death promoters are Bax, Bcl-X, Bak, Bok etc.
3. Some inhibit apoptosis and hence they are known as death inhibitors. Some known death inhibitors are Bcl-2 (B-cell lymphoma-2), Bcl-XL, Bcl-W etc.
4. Death promoters mainly releases death promoting substances like cytochrome C from mitochondria by forming pores in mitochondrial membrane.
5. In contrast death inhibitors may prevent release of cytochrome C from mitochondria or inhibit caspase activation.

Apoptic Inducers

1. Some exogenous substances are found to induce apoptosis.
2. Induction of apoptosis in cancer cells is useful in the management, therapy and prevention of cancer.
3. Recent studies indicated presence of tumor inhibitory compounds in some plants.
4. Infact several anticancer agents act by inducing apoptosis in cancer cells. Apoptic induction is now mechanism based drug discovery.
5. Curcumin of turmeric, gingerol of ginger, resveratrol of grapes, epigallocatechin gallate of green tea, limonene of orange peel are found to induce apoptosis in several types of cancer cells.

Role of P^{53} in Apoptosis

Apoptosis under certain conditions like radiation, hypoxia, cell cycle disturbances is P^{53} dependent. Even cytotoxic effects of some anticancer drugs are mediated through p^{53} dependent pathway.

P^{53} controls apoptosis by transcriptionally dependent and independent mechanism. It shifts cell balance towards cell death by Bax activation and Bcl-2 repression. It strongly transactivates Bax promoter and thus induces marked elevation in Bax protein level (Fig. 30.4). However presence of P^{53} independent negative regulatory element (NRE) in Bcl-2 gene suggests P^{53} independent control of apoptosis.

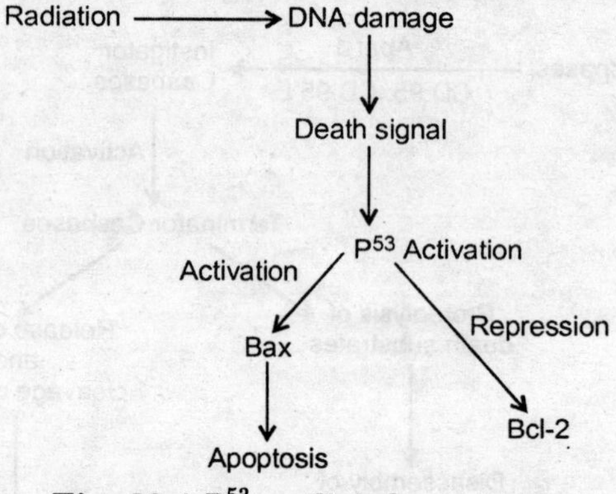

Fig. 30.4 P^{53} mediated apoptosis.

Death Genes

1. Genes responsible for cell death are evolutionarily conserved. They are known as cell death defective genes (*ced* genes).
2. Some of the genes promote apoptosis and some inhibit cell death.
3. In nematode C. *elegens* two genes *Ced* 3 and *Ced* 4 promote apoptosis and ced 9 inhibits apoptosis.
4. Some genes involved in dispersal and degradation of dead cells are also identified.
5. *Ced* 3 codes caspase. *Ced* 4 codes a cofactor that binds caspase and causes its activation. *Ced* 9 codes a protein that prevents apoptosis.
6. A gene called reaper (rpr) controls apoptic death in fruit fly Drosophile. The rpr gene product is similar to mammalian CD95, TNFR.
7. Bcl-2 was first gene identified in human chromosome. It is similar to *Ced* 9 of *C. elegens*.

REFERENCES

1. Winkler, J.E. (Ed.). Apoptosis and inflammation, Bir khauser Verlag, Basel, 1999.
2. Xiang, J, Chao, D.T and Korsmeyer, S.J. Proc. Natl. Acad. Sci, USA. **93**, 14559-14563, 1996.
3. McCarthy, N.J. Whyte, M.K., Gilbert, C.S. and Evan, G.I.J. Cell Biol. **136**, 21 5-227, 1997.
4. Inohara, N. Kosiki, J.C., Benedict, M.A. and Nunez, G.J. Biol. Chem. **274**, 270-274, 1999.
5. Gress, A. *et al*. J. Biol. Chem. **274**, 1156-1163, 1999.
6. Kroener, G. Cell death Differ. **5**, 547-552, 1998.
7. Lockshin, R. Zakari. Z and Tilly, J. (Eds.). When cells die; A comprehensive evaluation of apoptosis and programmed cell death. Wiley-Liss, New York, 1998.
8. Maureen E. Murphy *et al*. P^{53} moves to mitochondria: A turn on the path to apoptosis. Cell Cycle. July, 2004.
9. Grabbarek, K. J. *et al*. Sequential activations of caspases and serine proteases (serpases) during apoptosis. Cell Cycle. **1**, 124-131, 2002.
10. New Comb, W.E. *et al*. Flavopiridol induces mitochondrial mediated apoptosis in Murine Glioma cells via release of cytochrome C and apoptosis inducing factor (AIF). Cell Cycle. **2**, 243-250, 2003.
11. Halen, A. Papadaki and George D.E. The role of apoptosis in pathophlsiology of chronic neutropenaias associated with Bone marrow failure. Cell Cycle. **2**, 447-451, 2003.
12. Leslie D. Burntnick. *et al*. Structure of the N-terminal half of the gelsolin bound to actin: Roles in severing, apoptosis and FAF. The EMBO Journal. **23**, 2713-2722, 2004.
13. N.R. Jana, *et al*. Inhibition of proteosomal function by curcumin induces apoptosis through mitochondrial pathway. J. Biol. Chem. **279**, 11680-11685, 2004.

EXERCISES

ESSAY QUESTIONS

1. Write an essay on death signals, death receptors, death factors, death enzymes, death substrates and death adaptors.
2. Define apoptosis. Write mechanism of apoptosis. Add a note on apoptic regulators.

SHORT QUESTIONS

1. Write medical and biological importance of apoptosis.
2. Outline apoptic pathway.
3. Give an account of death signals.
4. Classify caspases. Give examples for each class.
5. Write a note on death and prodeath enzymes.
6. Write role of P^{53} in apoptosis.
7. Define apoptic inducers. Give examples. Write their importance.
8. Define death genes. Give examples. Mention role of each on apoptosis.
9. Name prodeath enzymes. How they are activated?

31
CHAPTER

BIOCHEMISTRY OF CELL CYCLE

MEDICAL IMPORTANCE

1. It deals with molecular events associated with cell division cycle (CDC) or cell cycle.
2. Some cancers are due to disturbances in cell cycle. For example breast cancer, retinoblastoma etc.
3. An understanding of cell division at molecular level may lead to development of new therapies and diagnostics for cancer.
4. Reversible phosphorylation of proteins is involved in regulation of cell cycle.
5. Blocks in proteolysis of cell cycle proteins leads to uncontrolled cell division and cancer. This information may be exploited for development of new cancer therapies.
6. Tumor suppressor protein p^{53} blocks progression of cell cycle with damaged DNA. Loss of p53 gene promotes cancer development in some cases.

Cyclins

They are proteins involved in cell cycle regulation. Several cyclins have been identified in animals and bacteria.

Classifications of cyclins

Cyclins are classified based on their occurrence during various phases of cell division cycle.

1. **S-phase cyclins**. They occur during S-phase of cell.

   Example : cyclins of A type.
2. **G-phase cyclins**. They occur during G-phase of cell cycle.

   Example : cyclins C, cyclins-D, E, F types.
3. **M-phase cyclins :** They occur during M-phase of cell cycle. They are also known as mitotic cyclins.

   Example : Different B-type cyclins.

Cyclin dependent kinases (CDKs)

1. They are another type of proteins involved in the regulation of cell division cycle. Several of them have been identified in mammals and bacteria.

2. They are cdk_1, cdk_2, cdk_3, cdk_4, cdk_5 etc.
3. They undergo reversible phosphorylation. Tyrosine and threonine residues are site of phosphorylation.

Classification of cdks

1. They may be classified according to their abundance during various phases of cell cycle.
2. So like cyclins we have S-phase cdks, G-phase cdks, M-phase cdks.

Cyclin dependent kinase-cyclin complex (CDK) Or Cell cycle's engine

1. It consists of two subunits namely cdks and cyclins.
2. In the absence of cyclins, cdks are inactive and lacks kinas activity. cdks combine with cyclins to form cyclin dependent kinase-cyclin complex (CDK), cdk of CDK complex is active.
3. cdk-cyclin complex (CDK) is known as cell cycle's engine due to its role in regulation of cell cycle.

Role of CDK In Cell Cycle

1. During cell cycle different cdks combines with cyclins to form CDKs which facilitates passage of cell through various phases and check points of the cell cycle.
2. cdk_2 complexed with S-phase cyclins induces S-phase. G1/S check point of cell cycle is crossed.
3. cdk_1 complexed with M-phase cyclins induces M-phase.
4. This allows crossing of G2/M check point of cell cycle by dividing cell (Fig. 31.1).

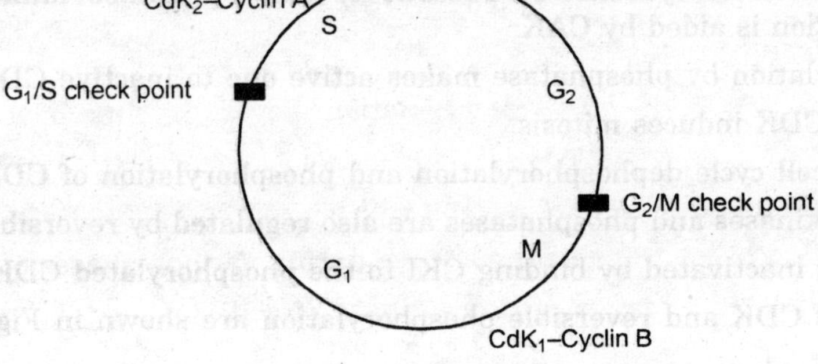

Fig. 31.1 Role of CDKs in cell cycle.

5. Other cdks are required for the transition from G_0 to G_1 in mammals.
6. During cell cycle cdks undergoes activation by phosphorylation and dephosphorylation.
7. A phosphatase dephosphorylates cdk_1 of cdk_1 - cyclin B complex. This leads to activation of cdk_1.
8. In contrast cdk_2- cyclin A complex is phosphorylated by a kinase. This leads to activation of cdk_2.
9. Active forms may stimulate their own activation and inactivation. Phosphorylation and dephosphorylation of cdks are shown in Fig. 31.2.

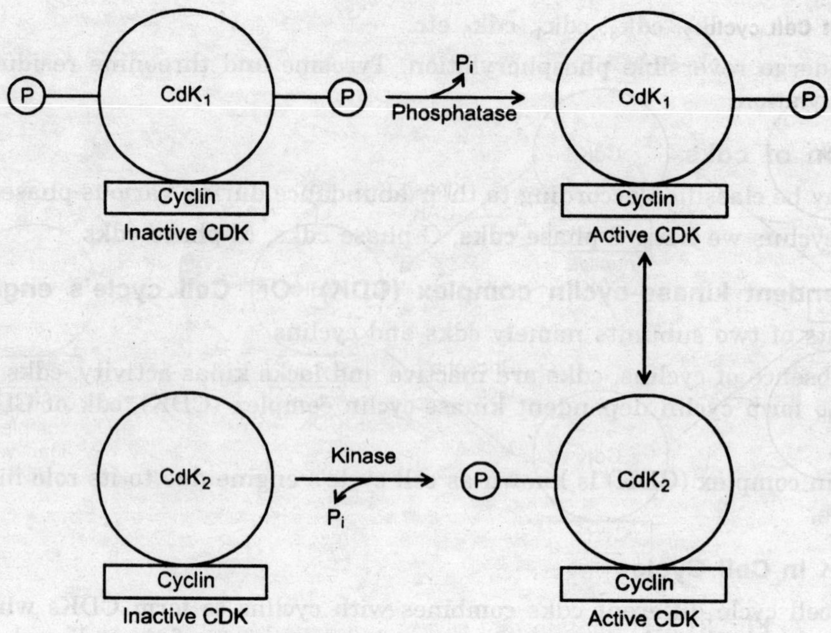

Fig. 31.2 Activation of CDK.

Reversible phosphorylation of CDKs

1. During cell cycle CDKs activity is regulated by this process.
2. Kinases and phosphatases activities of some proteins are responsible for reversible phosphorylation of CDKs.
3. Phosphorylation of tyrosine-15 residue of cdk by kinase makes it active. This phosphorylation is aided by CAK.
4. Dephosphorylation by phosphatase makes active one to inactive CDK.
5. Only active CDK induces mitosis.
6. In the next cell cycle dephosphorylation and phosphorylation of CDK occurs.
7. Activities of kinases and phosphatases are also regulated by reversible phosphorylation.
8. CDK may be inactivated by binding CKI to the phosphorylated CDK.

Formation of CDK and reversible phosphorylation are shown in Fig. 31.3.

Activators and inhibitors of CDKs

CDKs activity during cell cycle is also regulated by specific activators and inhibitors present in cell.

CDK activators (CAKs)

1. CDK activators are known as CAKs.
2. The activators of CDKs themselves can be cdks.
3. Some CAKs are transcription factors so that activates transcription together with progression of cell division.
4. They activates kinases that phosphorylates cdks of CDK.

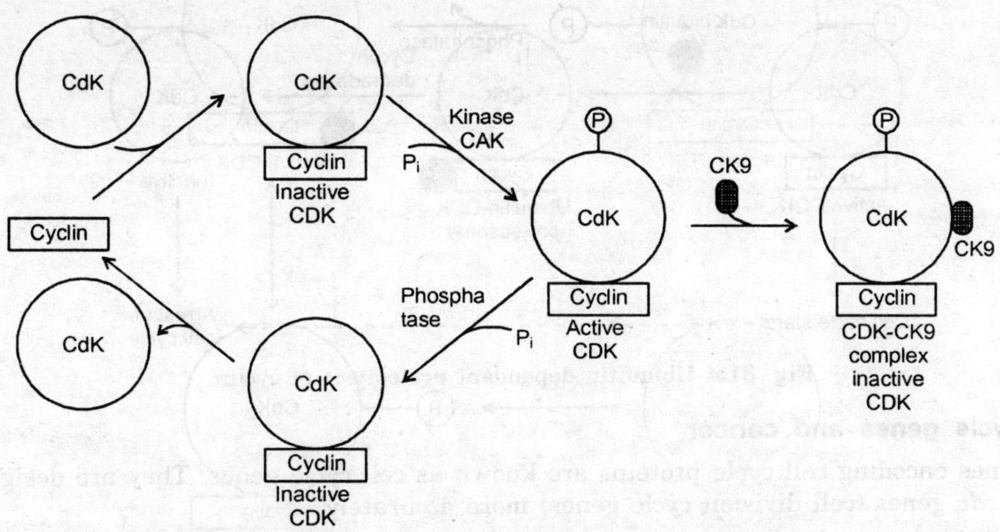

Fig. 31.3 Formation and reversible phosphorylation of CDK.

CDK inhibitors (CKIs)

1. A number of CDK inhibitors have been identified.
2. These CKIs respond to signals of growth inhibitors.
3. CKI binds cdk of CDK. This leads to inhibition of cell cycle progression due to inactivation of active CDK.

Non-cyclin proteins of cell cycle

1. Many non-cyclin proteins are involved in cell cycle regulation.
2. p^{53}, product of tumor suppressor gene (TSG) is one such non cyclin protein.
3. It act as transcription promoter. It activates a gene coding CDK inhibitor.
4. Production of CDK (cdk–cyclin) inhibitor results in the arrest of cell cycle.

Proteolysis of cell cycle proteins

1. Like many proteins cell cycle proteins also undergo degradation.
2. So proteolysis of cell cycle proteins plays an important role in the regulation of cell cycle.
3. Cell cycle proteins that undergo proteolysis are M-cyclins, G_1-cyclins and CKIs.
4. M-cyclins are degraded to control mitosis.
5. G_1-cyclins are degraded after G_1 phase.
6. CKIs are degraded for initiation of S -phase.

Cell cycle proteins degradation pathway

1. An ubiquitin dependent pathway is responsible for degradation of cell cycle proteins.
2. Ubiquitin forms a proteosome with cell cycle protein to be degraded.
3. Degradation of cyclin of a CDK leads to inactivation of a CDK.
4. This results in arrest of cell cycle progression. (Fig. 31.4).

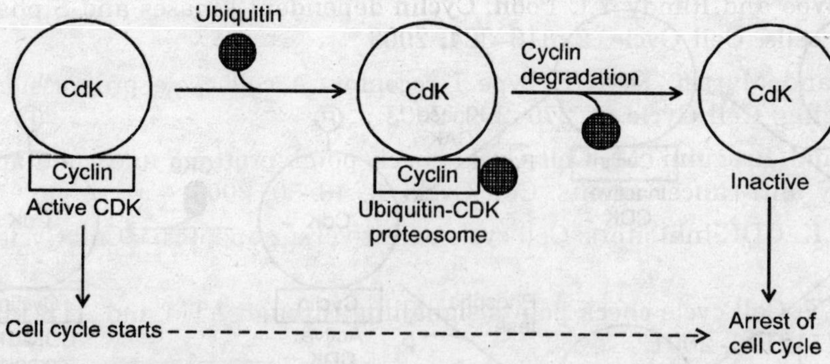

Fig. 31.4 Ubiquitin dependent proteolysis of cyclin.

Cell cycle genes and cancer

1. Genes encoding cell cycle proteins are known as cell cycle genes. They are designated as *cdc* genes (cell division cycle genes) more accurately.
2. Some of *cdc* genes are found to be oncogenes.
3. Defects or mutations in *cdc* genes may lead to certain cancers.
4. Defective *cdc* genes produce defective cell cycle proteins which may cause cancer.
5. Sometimes products of *cdc* genes interact with P^{53} protein which accounts for many human cancers.
6. Some genes of cell cycle are known as check point genes, because they prevent cell with damaged DNA undergoing cell division particularly at G2/M checkpoint.
7. Mutations in the check point genes leads to development of cancer.

Polo like kinases (plk) in cell cycle

1. The polo like kinase family plays a vital role in many cell cycle related events.
2. Members of the family are polo like kinase 1 (plk1), polo like kinase 2 (plk2), polo like kinase 3 (plK3) etc.
3. These enzymes are so named because they contain polo box(s) in the c-domain. These box (s) are highly conserved among kinases. However kinase activity is shown by N - terminal domain.
4. These enzymes are involved in activities of cdc 2, maturation and assembly of centrosome, cytokinesis, promotion of metaphase transition etc.

REFERENCES

1. Hutchinson, C. and Glover, D.M. (Eds.). Cell cycle control, Oxford University Press, New York, 1995.
2. Murray, A.W. and Hunt, T. The cell cycle. Freeman, New York, 1993.
3. Brown, N.R. *et al.* Structure, **3**, 1235–1247, 1995.
4. Nguyen, V.Q. Co., C. and Li, J.J. Nature, **411**, 1068–1073, 2001.
5. Simon, J.A. *et al.* Cancer Res. **60**, 328–333. 2001.

6. Richard A. Woo and Randy Y.C Poon. Cyclin dependent kinases and S phase control in mammalian cells. Cell Cycle. **2**, 316–324, 2003.
7. Dupont, J. and Martin, H. IGF Type I receptor. A cell cycle progression factor that regulates Aging, Cell Cycle. **2**, 270–272, 2003.
8. Damia, G. and Broggini. M. Cell Cycle check point proteins and cellular response to treatment by anti cancer agents. Cell Cycle, **3**, 46–50, 2004.
9. Schwartz, G.K. CDK inhibitors: Cell cycle arrest versus apoptosis. Cell Cycle. **1**, 122–123, 2002.
10. Abraham, R.T. Cell cycle check points signalling through ATM and ATR kinases. Genes Dev. **15**, 2177–2196, 2001.
11. Brown, E.J. and Baltimore, D. Essential and dispensable roles of ATR in cell cycle. Genes Dev. **17**, 615–628, 2003.
12. Van Btahant, A.J. *et al*. An origin deficient yeast artificial chromosome triggers a Cell cycle checkpoint. Mol. Cell. **7**, 705–713, 2001.
13. Mart Roo, G. *et al*. Cyclin specificity in the phosphorylation of cyclin dependent kinases substrates. Nature **434**, 104–108, 2005

EXERCISES

ESSAY QUESTIONS

1. Describe cyclins and cyclin dependent kinases of cell cycle.

SHORT QUESTIONS

1. What is known as cell cycle engine? How it is formed? Write its role in cell cycle.
2. Explain non-cyclin proteins of cell cycle.
3. How cell cycle proteins are degraded?
4. Write a note on activators and inhibitors of CDKs.
5. Explain role of reversible phosphorylation in cell cycle.
6. Write briefly on cell cycle genes and polo like kinases.

32

CHAPTER

BIOCHEMISTRY OF BLOOD

MEDICAL AND BIOLOGICAL IMPORTANCE

1. Blood is a fluid present in multicellular and multi organ organisms like mammals, humans etc. About 5 litres of blood is present in a 70 kg human adult.
2. It is the connecting fluid among organs of humans. It act as a link between organism and environment and cell and its surrounding.
3. Absorded food materials are transported to various locations in the body by the blood.
4. It carries waste products from tissues to kidneys for elimination from the body.
5. It regulates body temperature by distributing body heat.
6. Plasma proteins are involved in several physiological processes like blood pressure, transport of organic, in organic elements, water and acid base balance etc.
7. Plasma protein levels are altered in many diseases. Plasma protein levels are increased in dehydration, burns etc. and decreased in edema.
8. Acute phase reactants are increased in inflammatory conditions and injuries or surgeries.
9. Allergic reactions, auto immune diseases are due to alterations in immune systems.
10. Amyloidosis occurs by deposition of fragment derived from immunoglobulins. Amyloid deposits are found in several neuro degenerative diseases in brain and blood vessels. Further immunoglobulins are increased in multiple myeloma.
11. Plasma protein electrophoresis is part of day today's modern medical diagnosis.
12. Haptoglobin one of the plasma protein is involved in the transport of hemoglobin within the body.
13. Hemoglobin, red pigment of blood is involved in O_2 transport. Decrease in hemoglobin level causes anaemia.
14. Blood clotting a process that prevents bleeding is due to several proteins present in blood. They are known as blood clotting factors. Several clinically used anticoagulantes work by blocking blood clotting. Hemophilia, a bleeding disorder is due to deficiency of blood clotting factors.

15. Complement system that act as mediator of inflammation is present in blood. It consist of several proteins. Deficiencies of complement components are associated with diseases like systemic lupus erythromatosus, glomerulonephritis, recurrent infections etc.
16. Several enzymes are present in normal blood. Their level raises in many pathological conditions.
17. Many organic substances like carbohydrates, lipids, vitamins, polypeptide hormones, steroid hormones, cytokines and acids like acetoacetic acid, pyruvic acid, lactic acid etc. are found in blood. Estimation of these organic constituents of blood is useful in diagnosis and prognosis of diseases.
18. Non protein nitrogenous substances like urea, uric acid, creatinine, bilirubin, aminoacids and bile acids are present in blood. Their levels are altered in several diseases.
19. Several inorganic molecules are also present in blood. They exist as anions and cations. In several diseases their levels are altered.
20. Blood group ABO and Rh are due to presence of blood group substances on membranes of erythrocytes. Knowledge of blood group system is required for safe blood transfusion and organ transplantation.
21. Leukemias are malignant neoplasma of white blood cells.
22. In seveal cancers, tumor markers are present in blood. Their detection and quantitation is useful in the diagnosis and prognosis and management of cancer patients.
23. Poisons, drugs, alcohol are found in blood when they are consumed during course of treatment of diseases or in suicide or murder.
24. Foreign organisms or their products are found in blood during infections. Further blood contain substances produced by body in response to these infections. Several such diseases are diagonized by detecting these compounds in blood.
25. Saliva of several blood feeding insects like ticks, mosquitoes etc. contain wide array of bioactive compounds which facilitates continuous flow of blood during feeding by affecting various steps of host coagulation (hemostesis) process.

Blood, Plasma, Serum

The total volume of blood present in a human adult is about 8% of his body weight. It has pH of 7.35-7.45 and specific gravity of 1.05-1.06. It consist of red blood cells (RBC), white blood cells (WBC), platelets, proteins, organic and inorganic substances.

The cells free portion of blood is known as plasma. About 3 litres of plasma is present in 70kg human adult. Plasma consist of water and variety of solute molecules. Water makes up about 90% of plasma and remainder consist of solutes. Solutes of plasma are proteins, organic and inorganic substances. Proteins constitutes 7% of plasma whereas organic substances constitutes 2% and remainder consist of inorganic substances.

When the blood`is allowed to clot then a clear fluid separates which is known as serum. Usually the clot consist of blood cells and fibrin. Centrifugation is used to separate plasma or serum from remaining constituents of blood. Plasma is obtained after adding the anti coagulant to blood.

Plasma Proteins

Structure, functions, diseases associated with changes in levels of plasma proteins are detailed in chapter 4.

Electrophoresis of plasma proteins

Different plasma proteins are easily separated by electrophoresis. In addition electrophoresis is used to show differences in plasma proteins. In several diseases plasma proteins are changed. These changes in amount of plasma proteins in diseases are visualized by electrophoresis.

Several types of electrophoresis are used to know changes in plasma proteins in diseases. They are paper electrophoresis, cellulose acetate electrophoresis and agar gel electrophoresis. Among these agar gel elecrophoresis is commonly used.

Some examples of electrophoretic patterns and densitometre scans are given in Fig. 32.1. In nephorsis albumin and γ-globulin are decreased but α-globulins increased and β-globulins remained normal. In cirrhosis albumin is less but γ-globulin is more and other globulins are normal. In multiple myeloma an extra (M) band appears between β-and γ-globulins. In rheumatoid arthritis γ and β-globulins are increased and other fractions are normal. In Hodgkins disease albumin and γ-globulin are decreased but α-globulins are increased significantly.

Polyacrylamide gel electrophoresis (PAGE)

It is another type of electrophoresis that is useful for the separation of plasma proteins. In this technique separation is based on size as well as charge. Polyacrylamide gel is used as supporting material for separation which also act as molecular seive. It separates plasma protcins into 30 components.

Red Blood Cells (RBC)

An adult male has about 4.5 to 6.0 million RBC per microlitre of blood. In adult females RBC count is 4.0–5.5 million per microlitre of blood. The packed RBC volume (hematocrit) is 40–50% and 35–45% for men and woman respectively.

Synthesis

Bonemarrow is the site of RBC formation. Production of RBC is mainly regulated by erythropoietin, a glycoprotein that is produced by kidney. Hypoxia stimulates release of erythropoietin from kidney into circulation. After reaching bone marrow through circulation it acts on bone marrow (stem) cells which differentiate and proliferate to mature erythrocytes. Apart from erythropoietin other proteins insulin like growth factor, interleukins etc. are needed for the synthesis of erythrocytes.

Structure of Erythrocyte Membrane

Erythrocyte membrane is lipid bilayer consisting of lipids, proteins and carbohydrates.

Lipids

Lipids constitutes of 50% membrane. Lipids present in membrane, are phospholipids, glycosphingolipids and cholesterol.

Proteins

They make up about 50% cell membrane. About 10 major proteins and more than 100 minor proteins are identified in erythrocyte membrane. The major proteins are mainly integral and peripheral membrane proteins. Glycophorins, glucose transporter and anion exchange canal are integral membrane proteins. Spectrin, ankyrins, actin and tropomyosin are peripheral proteins. The peripheral proteins form cytoskeleton network on cytosolic side of erythrocyte membrane. They interact with integral proteins to regulate shape and flexibility of erythrocyte.

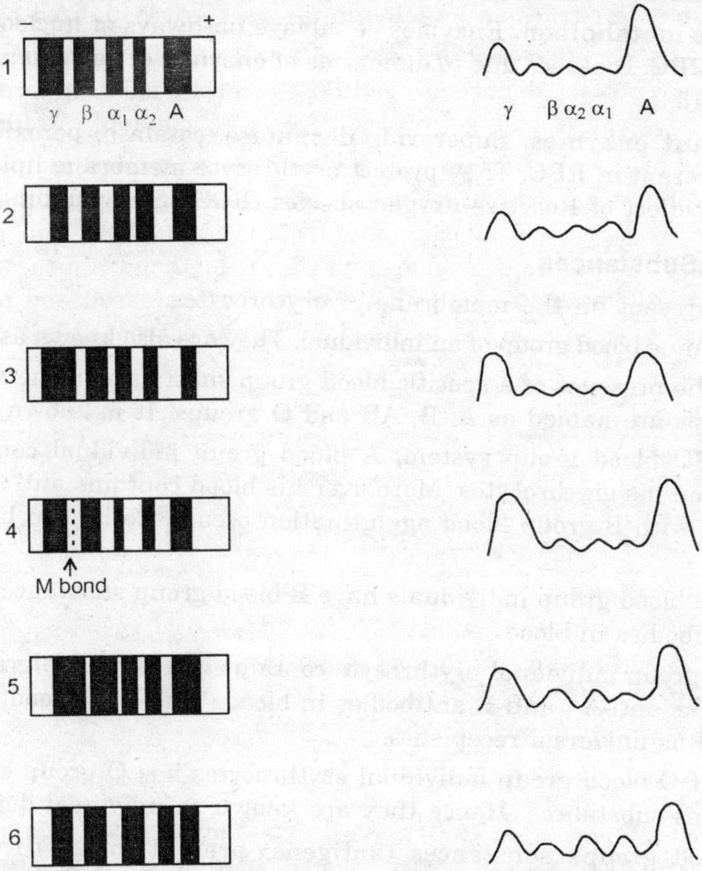

Fig. 32.1 Electrophoretic patterns and densitometer scans of serum proteins in health and diseases. A, Albumin; α_1, α_2, β, γ-globulin fractions. 1. Normal 2. Nephrosis 3. Cirrhosis 4. Multiple Myeloma 5. Rheumatoid arthritis 6. Hodgkin's disease.

Medical importance

Hereditary spherocytosis and elliptocytosis are inherited diseases characterized by presence of sphere shaped and ellipsoid shaped RBC in blood of affected individuals respectively. They are due to abnormal spectrin and ankyrin production.

Metabolic Pathways of RBC

(*a*) **Hemoglobin metabolism.** Major red pigment of erythrocyte is hemoglobin. Synthesis, degradation, structure, functions and diseases associated with these aspects of hemoglobin are described in chapter-22.

(*b*) **Carbohydrate Metabolism.** Glycolysis, HMPshunt, 2-3 bis phosphoglycerate cycle are involved in function of erythrocyte. Diseases due to deficiencies of enzymes of these pathways are explained in chapter–9.

(*c*) **Metabolism of glutathione.** RBC takes up glutathione from circulation. Liver produces glutathione and releases into circulation. Glutathione keeps -SH groups of membrane lipids and proteins in reduced form. RBC may produce some amount of glutathione.

(*d*) **Nucleotide metabolism.** Enzymes of salvage pathways of nucleotide biosynthesis are present in RBC. Diseases due to defiencies of enzymes of salvage pathways are detailed in chapter-15.

(*e*) **Anti oxidant enzymes.** Superoxide dismutase, catalase, peroxidase are antioxidant enzymes present in RBC. They protect erythrocyte membrane lipids and proteins from deleterious effect of Reactive oxygen species (ROS). See chapter-10 for more details.

Blood Group Substances

1. They are present on the membrane of erythrocytes.
2. They determine blood group of an individual. They are also known as blood group antigens.
3. Based on the presence of a specific blood group substance on the surface of erythrocyte blood groups are named as A, B, AB and O groups. It is known as ABO system.
4. In this ABO blood group system, A blood group individual contains A blood group substance on his erythrocytes. More over his blood contains anti -B antibodies. If he is transfused with B group blood agglutination occurs. So he can be given only A group blood.
5. Likewise B blood group individuals have B blood group substances on erythrocytes and anti A-antibodies in blood.
6. A B blood group individual erythrocyte contains both A and B groups blood substances and he lacks anti-A , anti-B antibodies in blood. Thus A B blood group individuals are considered as universal recepients.
7. In contract O blood group individual erythrocytes has O group substancses, and lacks A, B groups substances. Hence they are known as universal donors.

The ABO blood groups substances (antigens) present on erythrocyte membrane are glycosphingolipids with oligosaccharide chain. They are shown below.

```
                                     Fucose
                                       |
Ceramide - oligosaccharide - Galactose -N-Acetylgalactose
        A group substance.
```

```
                                     Fucose
                                       |
Ceramide - oligosaccharide - Galactose - Galactose
        B group substance.
```

```
                                     Fucose
                                       |
Ceramide - oligosaccharide - Galactose
        O group substance.
```

They consists of ceramide, oligosaccharide, fucose and terminal galactose. The oligosaccharide is a trisaccharide and composed of glucose, galactose and N-acetylgalactose. In A group substance N-acetyl galactose and in B group substance galactose are attached to terminals galactose respectively.

Other minor blood groups are Rh and M, N. The Rh blood group is due to substance known as Rh factor which is an integral membrane protein of erythrocytes. Individuals having Rh factor are known are Rh positive individuals. The Rh factor passes from father to child. Some individuals (about 9% of whites) lacks this proteins and they are known as Rh negative individuals. They may produce anti Rh antibodies if they are exposed to Rh positive blood. So they must be transfused with Rh negative blood. Determination of Rh blood groups is important in the case of woman who may become pregnant. If infant is Rh positive and mother is Rh negative abortion due to production of antibodies may occurs. The MN blood groups are due to glycophorin A polymorphism. However MN blood groups system is not important for blood transfusions.

White blood cells (WBC)

Normal adult has 5,000-8,000 WBC per microlitre of blood. The WBC are divided into granulocytes or polymorphonuclear leukocytes (PMN), monocytes and lymphocytes. The granulocytes are further divided into subgroups like neutrophils, basophils and eosinophils. Each group, subgroup have unique functions.

Neutrophils

They are part of body's immune system. They are also involved in inflammation.

Metabolism

Some pathways of carbohydrate metabolism are active in neutrophils. They are glycolysis and HMPshunt. Several proteases and anti proteinases are present in neutrophils. They are involved in hydrolysis of proteins. Neutrophils also contain enzymes involved in phagocytosis like myeloper oxidase, NADPH-oxidase, lysozyme etc.

Basophils, Eosinophils and monocytes

Basophils are involved in hypersensitivity reactions. Anticoagulant heparin, histamine etc. are products of basophils. Eosinophils are involved in allergic reactions. Parasitic infections are also associated with increased eosinophils in blood. Monocytes are precursors of macrophages. Macrophages are involved in immune response. They are involved in phagocytosis.

Lymphocytes

They are classified into B-lymphocytes and T-lymphocytes. B-lymphocytes are derived from bone marrow. T-lymphocytes are derived from thymus.

T-lymphocytes are further sub divided into T-helper cells and T-cytotoxic cells.

T-lymphocytes produce cytokines like interleukins and interferons. T-helper cells contain CD-4 (cluster differentiation -CD) receptor on its surface where as cytotoxic T-cells contain CD-8 receptor. All types of lymphocytes are part of immune system. Th1-helper cells type I, Th2-helper cells type II, Ts-suppressor T cells are also exist.

Immune System

It is a network of organs, cells and their products that protects individual from pathogens or disease causing agents like bacteria, virus etc. Spleen, thymus, bone marrow, tonsils, lymph nodes are organs and neutrophils (granulocytes), monocytes, and lymphocytes are cells which forms immune system.

Immune response

When an immunogen (antigen) or pathogen enters into body it elicits an immune response. The ability of an antigen to elicit immune response depends on complexity of antigen. The immune response consists of several sequences of events. Many components of immune system and their products are involved in immune response. Elimination of antigen that elicited immune response is final outcome. Two types of immune responses are known. They are

1. Innate immune response and
2. Adaptive immune response.

1. Innate immune response

It is first line defence. It is a quick and non-specific response. No memory cell are produced. Hence it is unable to fight future infections. Neutrophils and monocytes (macrophages) are involved in this types of immune response. Natural killer cells also has role in innate immune response.

When bacteria enters into body, neutrophils present in blood comes out of capillaries to fight infections or invading bacteria. Then they reach site of infections. Chemotactic substances like leukotriens, chemotacticpeptide etc. aids migration of neutrophil towards bacteria. Neutrophils pass through blood capillares endotheliel cells by receptor mediated process. Intergrins, integral membrane proteins of neutrophils plays very important role in this process.

Binding of neutrophils to bacteria leads to their activation and elimination of bacteria after phagocytosis. Reactive oxygen species (ROS) are produced by activated neutrophils which kill bacteria (See chapter-11). Role of neutrophils in immune response is shown in Fig. 32.2.

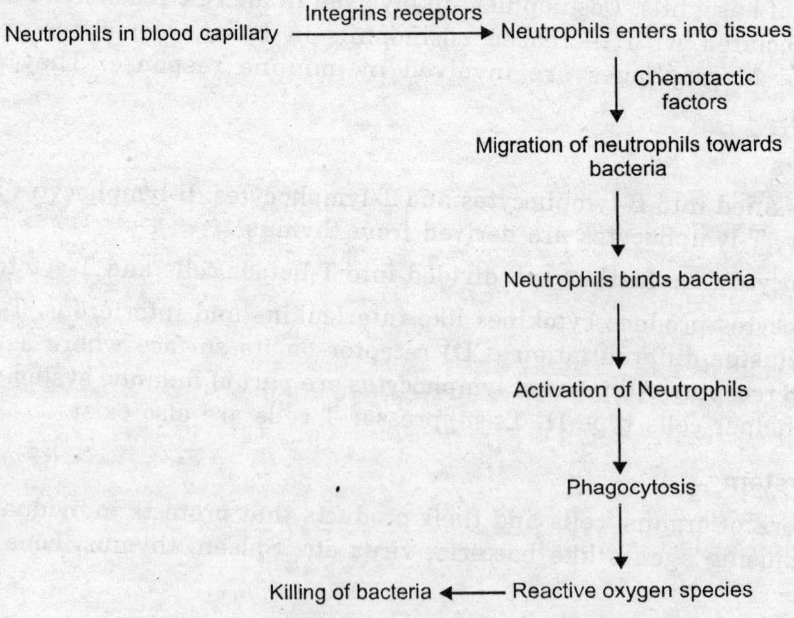

Fig. 32.2 Role of Neutrophils in Innate Immune response.

2. Adaptive immune response

It is second line of defence. It is slow and highly specific response. It displays memory, i.e. it is capable of fighting future infections. It is sub divided into

(*a*) Humoral immune response.

(*b*) T-cell mediated immune response.

Humoral immune response

1. It is mediated by B-lymophocytes or B-cells.
2. On binding antigen naive B-cell get activated and differentiated into plasma cells or clones.
3. The plasma cells secretes immunoglobulins and later undergoes apoptosis.
4. Some B cells remain as memory cells to fight furture infections.
5. The immunoglobulins forms complex with circulating antigen.
6. Antigen-antibody complex is cleared from circulation (Fig. 32.3). Immunoglobulins classifications, structure and functions of various classes of immunoglobulins are detailed in chapter-4.

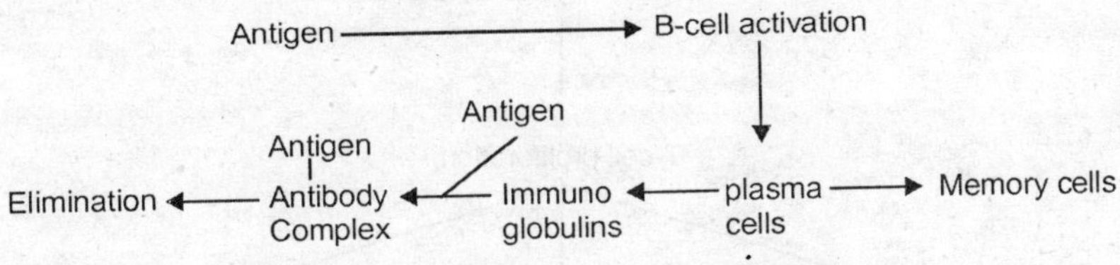

Fig. 32.3 Humoral Immune response

7. Cytokines like interleukins produced by T-helper cells modulate B-cell mediated humoral immune response.

T-cell mediated immune response

Unlike B-cell which recognizes antigen, T-cell recognizes cell surface major histocompatibility complex (MHC) molecules containing pathogen derived peptides present in the membrane of antigen presenting cells (APC). MHC molecules are proteins present on surface of all types of cells. MHC cell surface proteins are of two types, class I and II. These cell surface molecules are also known as human leucocyte antigen (HLA). MHC proteins has another important function. MHC class proteins presents on cell surfaces makes it to be recognized by immune systems as self.

Natural killer (NK) cells a sub group of cells belonging to innate immune response survey body cells for MHC class proteins, cells which lack MHC class proteins are killed. Only MHC class, proteins containing peptides derived from antigen (pathogen) are recognized by T-cells as foreign. Thus immune system is capable of differentiating self from non-self based on expression of MHC class proteins. Knowledge of MHC classification is also required for successful organ transplantation. Sequence of events of T-cell mediated immune response are out lined (Fig. 32.4) below.

1. Naive T-cells are released into circulation by thymus. They enter T-cells zones (TCZ) of lymph nodes as well as spleen.

2. Immunogen or pathogen that enters during infections is degraded by macrophages. Macrophages containing pathogen derived products migrate to lymph node. A small proportion of peptides derived from pathogen bind to MHC class molecules and are expressed on cell surface of antigen presenting cell (APCs).

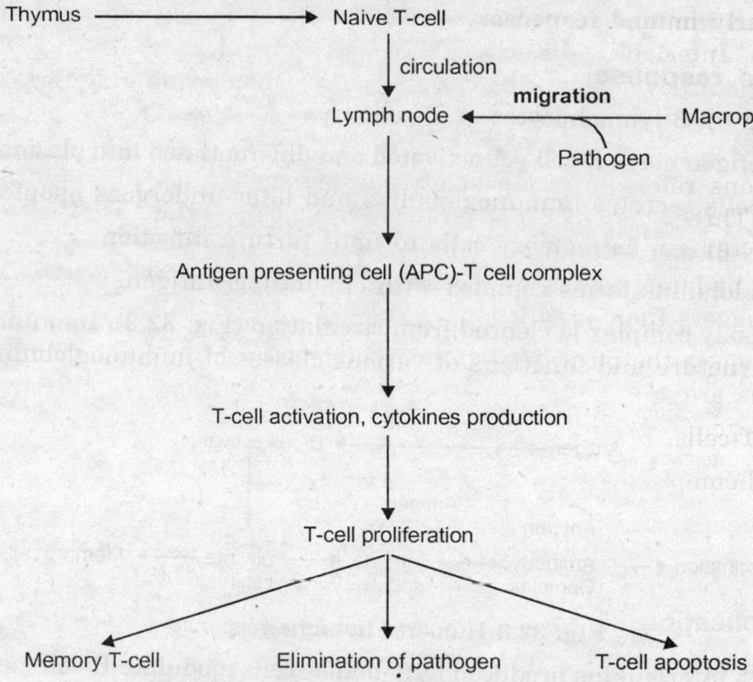

Fig. 32.4. T-cell mediated immune response

3. Specific T-cells recognizes MHC/peptide complex on APC via T-cell receptor (TCR).
4. T-cells are activated. High level of interleukins, interferons, etc. are produced. T-cells undergoes differentiation and proliferation. Depending on types or nature of pathogen various sub classes of T-cells are produced.
5. Pathogens as well as infected cells are cleared by T-cells.
6. As levels of interleukins drops activated T-cells undergo apoptosis. A few memory T-cells remains to fight future infections.

Cytokines

The term cytokines refers to group of non antibody proteinaceous molecules produced by chiefly T-lymphocytes on contact with antigen. Usually they are small molecular weight compounds. Now it is known that cytokines are produced by other cell. They mainly act as intercellular mediators of immune response. They are also involved in inflammation, tissue repair, hemopoiesis, cancer etc. Some important cytokines, their origin and functions are detailed below.

Interleukins (ILs)

About 20 interleukins are identified. Each one has unique origin and functions. They are interleukin-1 (IL-1), interleukin -2 (IL-2), interleukin-3(IL-3), interleukin-4 (IL-4), interleukin-5 (IL-5), to interleukin-20 (IL-20).

They are produced by T-lymphocytes, antigen presenting cells (APCs), macrophages, natural killer (NK) cells, monocytes, mast cells, basophils, eosinophils, epithelial cells and other types of cells.

They support growth and proliferation of T-cells, B-cells. IL-4 act as regulator of allergic reactions particularly immediate hyper sensitivity. Some interleukins are involved in release of hormones. Interleukin-16 act as chemoattractant. They also act on hemopoietic system. They promote development of various cells of hemopoietic system.

Interferons (IFNs)

The term interferons refers to group of glycoprotein molecules that interfere with viral infections of cells. Three classes of interferons are identified. They are interferon-α (IFNα), interferons -β (IFN-β) and interferon-γ (IFN-γ). Several subclasses in each class also exist. They are produced by lymphocytes, macrophages, monocytes, fibroblasts and epitheliel cells. Viral infections triggers their production.

Anti viral action is the most important property of interferons. Other important functions of interferons are

(*a*) Inhibition of T-cells, B-cells proliferation.

(*b*) Inhibition of hemopoiesis.

(*c*) Anti tumor agents.

(*d*) Increased expression of MHC class proteins.

Therapeutic application

IFNs have clinical application in the treatment of viral infections. They are used in the treatment of HIV infection as adjuvants. They are also useful in the treatment of several types of cancers like leukemia, lymphoma, renal cell cancer, multiple myloma, melonoma etc.

Tumor necrosis factors (TNFs)

Two Tumor necrosis factors (TNFs) are identified. They are Tumor necrosis factor-α and Tumor necrosis factor-β. They are produced by activated macrophages, monocytes, antigen presenting cells, T-cells, B-cells, natural killer cells and endothelial cells. They are released in repsonse to pathogens.

Tumor necrosis is the most important property of tumor necrosis factors. They are also involved in immune response. They act as modulators of immune response. They induce apoptosis in certain types of cells. They are associated with septic shock and inflammation.

Chemokines (CKs)

They are family of low molecular weight proteins. Some 30-50 cytokines are identified. They are classified into three classes according to their amino acid sequences around conserved motif that is made up of four cysteine residues.

They are produced by T-cell, B-cells, macrophages, polymorpho nuclear leukocytes, antigen presenting cells, monocytes, NK cells, endothelial cells and epithelial cells. Some chemokines are monocyte chemotactic proteins (MCPs), lymphotactin (LTN), granulocyte chemotactic proteins (GCP), eotaxin etc.

Chemotaxis is the principal function of cytokines. They cause migration and orientation of leucocytes. They act as modulators of immune response. They are involved in activation of T-lymphocytes. They have role in development of diseases like asthma, allergy, rheumatoid arthritis, sarcoidosis, pulmonary fibrosis, atherosclerosis and cancer.

Complement system

1. Immune system alone is unable to eliminate pathogens. Hence, for protection of body against infections, immune system requires complement system.
2. The complement system consists of 20 different proteins.
3. They are complement-1 (Cl), Complement-2 (C2), Complement-3 (C3) and from complement-4 (C4) to Complement-20 (C20). The components of complement system are mainly produced by liver. Monocytes and other cells synthesize only small amounts.

When activated complement system generates biological effector molecules. Antigen antibody complex, C-reactive proteins (CRP), neutrophils and plasma proteases activates complement system. During activation many components of complement system are cleaved into two fragments one large fragment and a small fragment. These fragments are responsible for many biological actions of complement system.

Effector molecules of complement systems are involved in

(*a*) Elimination of antigens or pathogen by lysis or phagocytosis. They solubilizes immune complexes for uptake by reticulo endothetial cells.

(*b*) Anaphylaxis, chemotaxis

(*c*) Initiation of inflammation

(*d*) Increasing production of phagocytes

(*e*) Regulation of anti body response.

Platelets(Thrombocytes)

About 1.5-4 lacs of platelets are present per microlitre of blood. They are produced by bone marrow. Thombopoietin controls synthesis of platelets.

Cell membrane

Platelet cell membrane is similar to structure of other types of cell membranes. However it invaginates extensively to form canalicular system which is in contact with extra cellular fluids. It contains several receptors for binding of collagen, fibrinogen and platelet adhesion promoting factor known as von-Willebrand's factor (VMF) which is a glycoprotein released at the site of injury.

Subcellular organelles

Platelets contain several subcellular organelles like mitochondria, golgi apparatus, lysosomes, endoplasmic reticulum and granules. Granules present in platelets contain adenine nucleotides, ADP, ATP, serotonin, clotting factors V and XIII, platelet derived growth factor (PDGF), protein C inhibitor, platelet factor IV and thromboxane A_2.

Functions

Platelets are involved in hemostasis, i.e. arrest of bleeding, blood clotting, chemotaxis, vasoconstriction and tissue repair.

(*a*) **Formation of platelet plug (platelet aggregation).** When blood vessel is injured clumping of platelets occurs at injured site. It is mediated by thrombin. On endothelial cells thrombin receptors are present. These receptors are exposed upon injury. Binding of thrombin to this receptor leads to activation of the receptor. Platelets binds to activated receptor through von-willebrand's factor that is released at the site of injury. Von-willebrand factor serve as link between platelets and thrombin activated receptor. Binding of platelets to activated receptor leads to initiation of platelets activation. Activated platelets release, ADP, serotonin, platelet activating factor and thromboxane A_2 which further activates platelets. This results in the formation of platelet aggregation which inturn causes stoppage of bleeding from ruptured blood vessel.

Intact normal endothelium of blood vessel does not promote platelet aggregation due to lack of activators and secretion of prostacyclin (PGI) a potent inhibitor of platelet aggregation.

(*b*) **Blood clotting.** Platelets are involved in blood clotting. Fibrin cross links formation requires platelets derived transglutaminase.

(*c*) **Chemotaxis.** Platelet factor IV act as chemotactic agent for neutrophils and monocytes.

(*d*) **Vasoconstriction.** Serotonin released by activated platelets causes vasoconstriction. Hence blood supply to injury site is decreased.

(*e*) **Tissue repair.** Platelet derived growth factor stimulates repair of damaged tissue.

Blood Clotting

It is the one of the essential biological process divised by nature to prevent bleeding or leakage of blood from injured (damaged) blood vessels. Damage to blood vessel may occur due to infections, diseases, ageing, cuts, surgery etc. It involves initial formation of platelet plug to arrest bleeding and fibrin clot formation later which covers injured area and stop any further leakage of blood.

Platelet plug formation is detailed earlier. Clot formation is brought about by several clotting factors present in blood (Table 32.1). Most of these blood clotting factors are proteins and possess catalytic activity. They exist in two forms an inactive zymogen form and active form. Roman numbers are used to indicate blood clotting factors. For example V indicates factor five. Further 'a' letter after Roman number of factor indicates an activated factor. For example 'Va' indicates activated factor five.

Table 32.1 Blood clotting factors

Factor	Name	Factor	Name
I	Fibrinogen	VIII	Antihemophlic factor
II	Prothrombin	IX	Christamus factor
III	Tissue factor	X	Stuert factor
IV	Calcium	XI	Thromboplastin antecedent
V	Proaccelerin	XII	Hageman factor
VII	Proconvertin	XIII	Proglutamidase

Two separate pathways: 1. Extrinsic pathway and 2. Intrinsic pathway are involved in blood clotting. These pathways bring about activation of factor X. Clot formation from activated factor X occurs in one final common pathway.

Extrinsic Pathway Factors

Tissue factor or factor III and factor VII are two factors unique to extrinsic pathway.

1. **Tissue factor:** It is also known as factor III of blood clotting. It is an integral membrane protein containing 263 amino acid residues. Extracellular side of this integral membrane protein act as receptor for factor VII.
2. **Factor VII:** It is gla (γ-carboxglutamyl residues) containing protein. Gla residues are calcium binding sites. It exist in two forms an inactive zymogen and an active form. Zymogen is converted to active form by two ways.

   (*a*) Protein-protein interaction between zymogen and tissue factor.

   (*b*) Proteolytic cleavage of zymogen by thrombin.

Extrinsic Pathway

1. It is also known as tissue factor pathway.
2. Blood clotting or blood coagulation is initiated by extrinsic pathway. It is so named because a factor which is not present in circulating blood is required for blood clotting. This factor is identified as tissue factor (TF) or factor III.
3. When blood vessel rupturs extracellular domain of tissue factor is exposed. In presence of Ca^{2+}, factor VII binds to exposed part of tissue factor to form initial enzyme complex TF-VII-Ca^{2+} that initiates blood clotting. Factor VII of TF-VII-Ca^{2+} complex is activated to VIIa through protein-protein inter action. Now TF-VIIa-Ca^{2+} complex combines with factor X to form TF-VIIa-Ca^{2+}-X complex. Factor VIIa is a serine proteinase that activates factor X to factor X a by cleaving six amino acid peptide. TF-VIIa-Ca^{2+}-Xa complex also exist in circulating blood. Free VIIa is catalytically inactive. Various steps of extrinsic pathway are shown in Fig. 32.5.

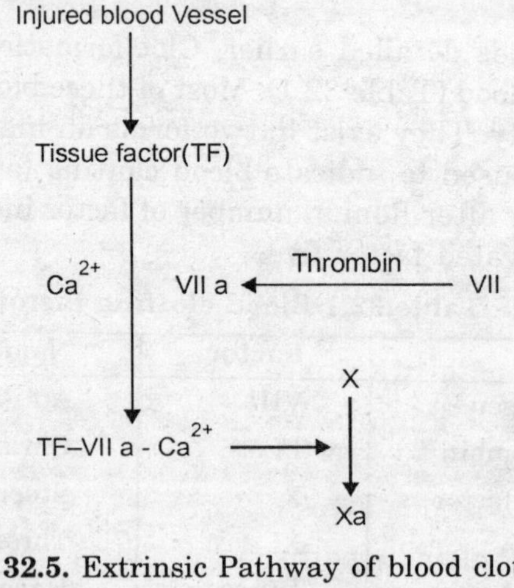

Fig. 32.5. Extrinsic Pathway of blood clotting.

Intrinsic Pathway Factors

Factor VIII, IX, XI and XII are unique to intrinsic pathway. High molecular weight kininogen (HMWK), prekallikrein and kallikrein are non factor components of intrinsic pathway.

1. **Factor VIII.** It exist in two forms an inactive zymogen and an active form. In circulating blood it is complexed with von-wille brand's factor (VMF). Activated factor VIII is released from the complex by thrombin involving cleavage of Arg-X bonds. Factor VIIIa is a heterotrimer which also contains Ca^{2+}.
2. **Factor IX.** It is another gla containing protein of blood clotting. It also exist an inactive and an active form. Proteolytic cleavage of arg-X bonds of factor IX leads to its activation with release of peptide. Factor XIa activates factor IX to factor IXa which is an endopeptidase.
3. **Factor XI.** In circulating blood it is complexed with high molecular weight kininogen (HMWK). It exist in two forms zymogen form and active form. Inactive zymogen is converted to active form by proteolytic cleavage catalyzed by factor XIIa. The active factor XI is an endopeptidase which activates factor IX to factor IXa.
4. **Factor XII.** It exist in two forms an inactive zymogen form and an active form. A conformational change that occurs due to binding of factor XII to exposed anionic membrane surface of endotheliel cells of blood vessel leads to activation of zymogen. Factor XIIa is an endopeptidase which converts factor XI to factor XI a and prekallikrein to kallikrein. Kallikrein further activates factor XII to factor XIIa. Factor XIIa releases bradykinin from HMWK.
5. **High Molecular Weight Kininogen (HMWK).** It is a high molecular weight protein present in circulating blood. It has binding site for two proteins of intrinsic pathway, prekallikrein and factor XI.
6. **Pre kallikrein (PK) and Kallikrein.** They are non factor proteins of intrinsic pathways present in blood. In plasma PK combines with HMWK to form PK-HMWK complex. Factor XIIa converts PK of PK-HMWK complex to kallikrein by cleavage of peptide bond. Kallikrein is catalytically active it activates factor XII to factor XIIa.

Intrinsic Pathway

1. It is also known as contact factor pathway.
2. When blood vassel in injured anionic sites of membrane phospholipids are exposed. Factor XII binds to these sites and undergoes conformation change to factor XIIa. The exposed anionic sites are also binding sites for two circulating complexes, XI-HMWK and PK-HMWK. Hence, these complexes binds to anionic surfaces. Now the membrane bound factor XIIa activates PK of PK-HMWK complex to kallikrein and factor XI to factor XIa in presence of Ca^{2+}. Kallikrein releases bradykinin from HMWK.
3. Factor XIa activates factor IX to factor IXa in presence of calcium.
4. Factor IX a inturn activates factor X to factor Xa in presence of factor VIIIa by cleaving six amino acid peptide. Various steps of intrinsic pathway are shown in Fig. 32.6.

Thus both extrinsic and intrinsic pathways converts factor X to factor Xa.

Final common Pathway Factors

Prothombin (factor II), fibrinogen (factor I), factor V and factor XIII are unique to final common pathway.

1. **Prothrombin.** It has molecular weight of 750 kilodaltons and contains gla residues which acts as calcium binding sites. It is a circulating plasma protein. Prothrombin is

activated to thrombin by factor Va-Factor Xa (prothrombinase) complex by proteolytic cleavage with elimination of gla residues. Thrombin is a serine protease. Fibrinogen is its substrate. Anticoagulants like anti thrombin heparin and hirudin inhibits action of thrombin. Thrombin mediates clumping of platelets at site of injury.

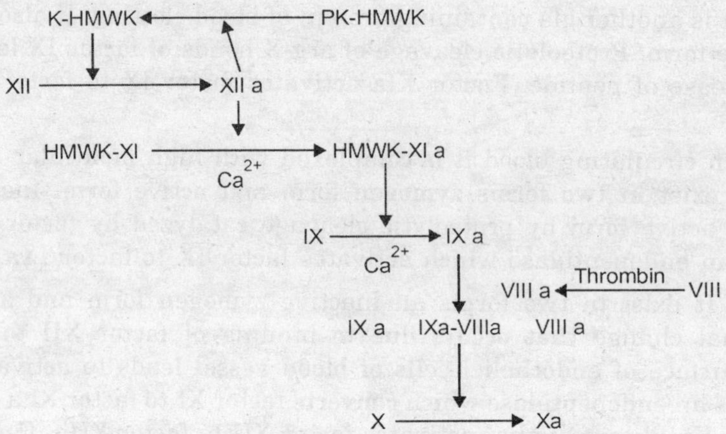

Fig. 32.6 Intrinsic pathway of blood clotting.

2. **Fibrinogen.** It is another globular protein with molecular weight of 340 kilodaltons that is present in circulating plasma. It consists of six subunits. They are αα′, ββ′ and γγ′. Like subunits are joined at their N-terminal regions by disulfide bonds. Short segments of free N-terminal regions projects outwards where subunits are joined. These segments are highly negatively charged due to presence of large number of aspartate and glutamate residues. The highly negatively charged fibrinogen molecules repel each other. Thus charge to charge repulsion of fibrinogen molecules prevents their aggregation.

3. **Factor V.** It is a 330 kilodalton protein. Thrombin activates factor V to factor Va by proteolytic cleavage. Factor Va is a heterodimer which consists of large subunit and a small subunit. These subunits are held together by Ca^{2+}.

4. **Factor XIII.** It is transglutaminase (glutamidase or transpeptidase). Protrans glutaminase is its corresponding inactive zymogen. Thrombin activates factor XIII to factor XIIIa by cleavage of a peptide bond.

Final common pathway of Blood Clotting

1. At site of blood vessel injury anionic sites of membrane phospholipids are exposed. Positively charged calcium, Ca^{2+}, binds to these sites. Prothrombin also binds to exposed anionic sites which is facilitated by gla residues through their interaction with Ca^{2+}. At the same time factor Va binds to factor to Xa to form Va-Xa complex. This inturn binds prothrombin and converts prothrombin to thrombin.

2. Thrombin removes negatively charged N-terminal regions of fibrinogen molecules. The resulting fibrin molecules aggregates to form soft clot.

3. Factor XIIIa (transglutaminase) strengthens and stabilizes soft clot by forming crosslinks between fibrin molecules. This enzyme catalyzes formation of iso peptide bond between amide group of glutamine of one fibrin molecule and ∈-amino group of lysine of another

fibrin molecule. These cross linkages converts soft clot to hard clot. Various steps of final common pathways are shown in Fig. 32.7.

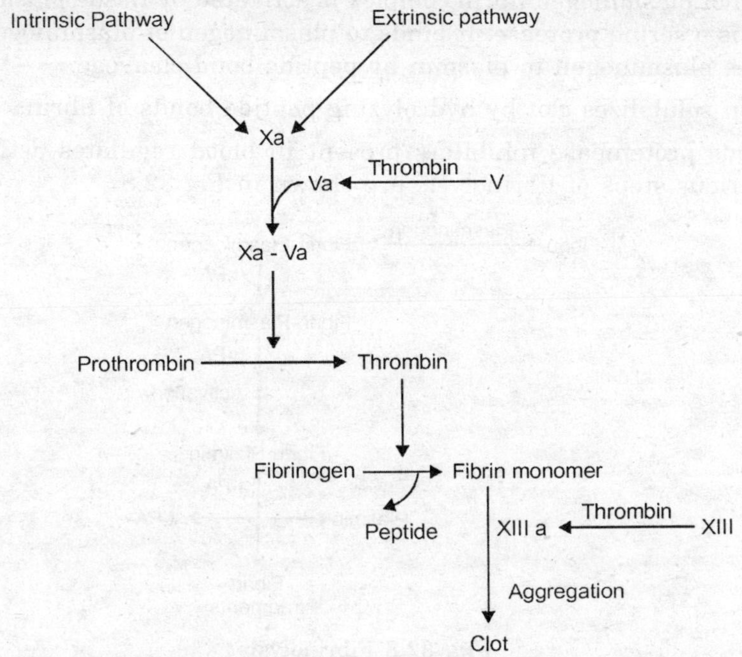

Fig. 32.7 Final Common pathway of Blood clotting.

Blood clotting regulation

Activities of blood clotting factors are carefully controlled to prevent unwanted clot formation as well as to stop blood clotting that has been initiated. Proteinacious Proteinase inhibitors present in blood inactivates active proteinases of blood clotting to control clot formation. Inhibition of proteinase involves formation of proteinase inhibitor complex.

(*a*) **Anti thrombin III (AT III).** It is a major proteinacious serine proteinase inhibitor (serpin) that inhibits several proteinases of blood clotting. It specifically inhibits thrombin and factor Xa.

(*b*) **Anti convertin.** It is also known as tissue factor pathway inhibitor (TFPI). It is an inhibitor of extrinsic pathway. It is a protein with molecular weight of 32 kilodaltons. It contains three domains which are functionally homologous to pancratic trypsin inhibitor (PTI). Hence, it is considered as multienzyme inhibitor. It combines with TF-VIIa-Ca^{2+} Xa complex of extrinsic pathway. Each of its domain inhibit action of one of the enzymes of TF-VIIa- Ca^{2+}-Xa complex.

Fibrinolysis

1. It clears clot form site of injury. Unwanted clot formed in circulatory system are also cleared by this process.
2. Plasmin a serine protease formed from plasminogen dissolves fibrin clots.

3. Plasminogen has high affinity towards fibrin clots and forms a complex with fibrin molecules of clot.
4. Plasminogen of plasminogen fibrin complex is activated by tissue plasminogen activator (*t*-PA). *t*-PA is a serine protease. It binds to plasminogen of plasminogen fibrin complex and activates plasminogen to plasmin by peptide bond cleavege.
5. Plasmin then solubilizes clot by hydrolyzing peptide bonds of fibrin.
6. Proteineacious proteinease inhibitors present in blood regulates activity of *t*-PA and plasmin. Various steps of fibrinolysis are shown in Fig 32.8.

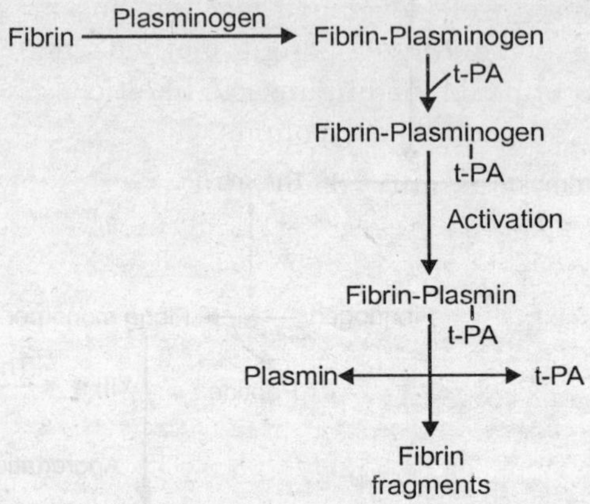

Fig. 32.8 Fibrinolysis

Medical importance

Some diseases are due to defective blood clotting. Some drugs work by affecting blood clotting and fibrinolysis.

1. **Hemophilia.** It is an X-chromosome linked inherited diseases of blood clotting. It is characterized by spontaneous bleeding. It is due to defficiency factor VIII. The blood level of this factor is less than 5% of normals in hemophiliacs. Due to deficiency of this factor blood clotting is impaired in hemophiliacs. Treatment involves frequent blood transfusion or factor VIII administration which is obtained by using recombinant DNA technology.
2. **Anticoagulants.** Several agents that block or prevent blood clotting are used as anti coagulants.

   (*a*) **Heparin.** It acts as anticoagulant by combining with antithrombin. This inturn inhibits thrombin actions.

   (*b*) **Hirudin.** It is an anticoagulant isolated from saliva of leech. It combines with thrombin and blocks its action.

   (*c*) **Chelating agents.** They act as anticoagulants by forming complexes with Ca^{2+}. They are fluoride, citrate, oxalate, EDTA etc.

   (*d*) **Warfarin and di coumarol.** They inhibit formation of gla residues of blood clotting factors. How ever in test tube they are ineffective as anti coagulants.

3. **Urokinase, streptokinase and recombinant t-PA.** They are enzymes which facilitate dissolution of fibrin clot. They promote plasminogen conversion to plasmin. They are used as thrombolytic agents or clot busters in the treatment of myocardial infarction. They restore blood flow to affected cardiac tissue by dissolving clot formed in coronary artery.
4. **Aspirin.** It is an anti platelet drug. It prevents platelet aggregation by blocking production of thromboxane A_2 and prostacyclin. It is used as adjuvant in thrombolytic treatment.
5. **Anti hemostatic (coagulation) compounds of insect saliva.** Even though humans and other vertebrates have well developed mechanisms for prevention of blood loss the blood feeding insects evolved highly potent methods to bypass the host coagulation (hemostasis). The saliva of blood feeding insects like ticks, mosquitos etc. contain several bioactive (pharmacologically active) compounds which affects various steps of coagulation.

Saliva of these insects contains anti coagulants like thrombin inhibitors and factor Xa inhibitors which target blood clotting factors thrombin and factor Xa or both. Apyrase is an enzymes present in tick saliva prevents platelet aggregation by breaking down ADP to AMP and Pi. Vasodilators presents in insect saliva like PGI_2, PGE_2, and tachykinin counter balance vasoconstriction, which is also a part of blood coagulation (hemostasis).

The blood feeding insects are responsible for the transmission of several diseases like malaria, Kyasanur forest disease in India, some forms of encephalitis in Afro-Asian countries and Lyme disease in U.S.A, Europe and Asia.

Enzymes of Plasma

Plasma contains many enzymes. Further details are given in chapter –4 under heading clinical enzymology.

Other organic compounds or constituents of Blood

They are non protein nitrogenous compounds, carbohydrates, lipids, amino acids, porphyrins, bilirubin, organic acids, vitamins and hormones.

Non protein nitrogenous Substances

Urea, uric acid and creatinine are non protein nitrogenous substances present in blood. Importance of urea, and creatinine is detailed in Chapter-12. Uric acid importance is detailed in chapter -15. Likewise plasma amino acids, porphyrins and bilirubin details are given in chatper - 12 and chapter - 22 respectively.

Carbohydrates

Monosaccharides like glucose, fructose and sugar acids are present in blood. Most important carbohydrate is glucose whose importance is given in chapter-9.

Lipids

Triglycerides, cholesterol and free fatty acids are most important.

Triglycerides

Normal triglyceride level is 75-240 mg%. They are used by peripheral tissues for energy production. In diabetes, starvation and on high fat diet triglyceride level is more.

Cholesterol

Its normal level is detailed in chapter-10.

Free fatty acids

Normal free fatty acids level in plasma is 10-25 mg%. Plasma free fatty acids level is more in diabetes, starvation, von Gierkes disease and on high fat diet.

Organic acids

Pyruvate, lactate, acetoacetate, succinate, citrate, malate etc. are some of the organic acids present in blood.

Vitamins

Normal blood contains fat soluble as well as water soluble vitamins in very small quantities. For example, about 30-80 μg of Vit A is present per 100 ml of blood. About 0.5-1.8 mg of vit. E is present per 100ml of blood. Some water soluble vitamins presents in blood along with their levels are vit. C 0.4-1.5 mg per 100 ml blood and folicacid 0.3-2 μg per 100 ml of blood.

Hormones

Hormones of adrenal medulla, adrenal cortex, testes, ovaries and thyroid hormones are non protein hormones present in blood. They are epinephrine, norepinephrine, glucocorticoids, mineralocorticoids, estradiol, progesterone and thyroxine. The level of these hormones are increased or decreased due to hyper or hypoactivity of glands that are involved in their production.

Polypeptide hormones are also present in blood. Some of them are insulin, glucagon, growth hormone, ADH and trophic hormones, like ACTH, FSH, LH, TSH etc.

Inorganic constituents of blood plasma

They exist as anions and cations. Further details are given in chapter-26 under electrolytes heading.

REFERENCES

1. Shriver, Z. Sundaram, M. Venkataraman, G. Freed. J. Linhardt, R. Biemann, K. and Sasi Sekharan, R. Cleavage of antithrombin III binding site in heparin by heparinases and its implication in the generation of low molecular weight heparin. Proc. Natl. Acad. Sci. USA. **97,** 10365, 2000.
2. Brummel, K.E. Butenes, S. and Mann, K.G. An integrated study of fibrinogen during blood coagulation. J. Biol. Chem. **274,** 22862, 1999.
3. The MHC consortium, Nature. **401,** 921-923, 1999.
4. Nobel, A. Immunology. 101, 289-299, 2000.
5. Hemmi, H. *et al.* Nature. **408,** 740-745, 2000.
6. Roth, G.J. and Calverely, D.C. Aspirin, Platelets and thrombosis. Blood **83,** 885, 1994.
7. Dickason, R.R. and Huston, D.P. Creation of a biologically active interleukin-5 monomer. Nature. **379,** 652-655, 1996.
8. Beldwin, W.M. *et al.* Complement in organ transplantation. **59,** 793-808, 1995.

9. Ibrahim, M.A. Gnazy, A.H. Mahrem, T.M. and Khalil, M.I. Factor Xa (Fxa) inhibitor from camel tick. Comp. Biochem. Physiol. B. Biochem. Mol. Biol. 130, 501-512, 2001.

10. Balkwill Fran. Ed. The cytokine network. Oxford University Press, 2000.

11. Morgan, B. Paul and Harris, C.L. Eds. Complement regulatory proteins. Academic Press, 1999.

12. Marion, E. Reid and Christine Lomas Francis. The Blood group antigen Facts Book, 2nd Ed; Academic Press, 2003.

13. Paola, L. *et al.* Crystal structures of human urokinase plasminogen activator receptor bound to an antagonist peptide. The EMBO Journal. **24**. 1663-1665, 2005.

EXERCISE

ESSAY QUESTIONS

1. Write components of immune system. Define immune response. Classify. Write about any one type.
2. Explain erythrocyte structure. Mention important metabolic pathways of erythrocyte. Add a note on blood group substances of erythrocytes.
3. Define adaptive immune response. Describe its various types.
4. Describe structure and function sources of cytokines and chemokines.
5. Describe structure and functions of platelets.
6. Name blood clotting factors. Describe intrinsic pathway of blood clotting.
7. Describe final common pathway of blood clotting. Add a note on inhibitors of blood clotting.

SHORT QUESTIONS

1. Define plasma, serum. How they differ? Write method for obtaining them from blood.
2. Write briefly about plasma protein electrophoresis in health and disease.
3. Briefly describe blood group substances.
4. Write role of neutrophils in innate immune response.
5. Explain T-Cell mediated immune response.
6. Write a note on interferons.
7. How platelet plug is formed?
8. Outline extrinsic pathway of blood clotting.
9. Define fibrinolysis. Write various steps of fibrinolysis.
10. Define clot busters. Give examples. Write their importance.
11. What are anticoagulants? Give example. Mention their clinical importance.

33

CHAPTER

ORGAN FUNCTION TESTS

MEDICAL IMPORTANCE

1. These are laboratory tests done to assess function of specific organ of human body.
2. If these tests are performed to assess function of liver then they are named as liver function tests. Likewise other functional tests are named.
3. Function of an organ is altered due to infections, toxins, genetic factors, altered immunity, cancer or neoplasms etc.
4. Number of tests to be performed to assess function of an organ depends on the functional roles of that organ and pathological conditions.
5. In the case of organs having multiple functions a single test may not be adequate to assess functional integrity. Further more a change that occurs in one functional test may not be observed in another functional test. Hence organs which have multifunctions are assessed by an array of tests.
6. Apart from providing an insight into dysfunction of an organ these tests are useful in detection, diagnosis and prognosis of diseases affecting specific organ.
7. Blood and urine of subject under investigation are generally used for these tests. If the function of an organ is normal, values within normal range are obtained. Any increase or decrease in value suggests dysfunction.
8. Some of these tests are even part of routinely done investigations of a clinical biochemistry laboratory.
9. These tests are more useful in differential diagnosis.
10. These tests are useful in evaluating degree of dysfunction (severity), classification of diseases and directing further management of illness.

LIVER FUNCTION TESTS

We shall first learn about functions of liver. Then proceed to tests done to assess liver function.

Functions of liver

1. Liver is an essential organ. It has diverse functions.

2. Liver is involved in secretion or excretion of several components like bilirubin and bile acids.
3. It is involved in the synthesis of plasma proteins and blood clotting factors.
4. It is involved in metabolism of carbohydrates, lipids and proteins.
5. It is sensitive to actions of several hormones.
6. It is involved in xenobiotics metabolism.

Liver function tests based on each of above functions are done routinely in laboratory. In addition measurement of serum enzymes specific to liver is helpful in assessing liver damage (Chapter 4).

Tests based on Secretory or Excretory function

1. Liver is involved in secretion of bilirubin and bile acids.
2. So measurement of bilirubin in serum and urine and serum bile acids is helpful in assessing liver damge.
3. Measurement of urine urobilinogen is also useful test of liver function.

Serum bilirubin

1. Serum bilirubin is elevated in jaundice.
2. Elevated levels of unconjugated bilirubin occurs in prehepatic jaundice because liver cells are unable to process excess bilirubin formed.
3. Conjugated bilirubin level raises in post hepatic jaundice because of obstruction to flow of secreted bilirubin.
4. Both conjugated and unconjugated bilirubin levels are elevated in hepato cellular damage that occurs in hepatitis or hepatic jaundice.

Urine bilirubin

1. Bilirubin is absent in normal urine.
2. It is found in the urine of post hepatic jaundice cases.
3. In prehepatic cases bilirubin is absent in urine.

Urine Urobilinogen

1. Excretion of urobilinogen is increased in prehepatic (hemolytic) jaundice.
2. Decreased excretion of urobilinogen occurs in post hepatic jaundice.

By combining these tests different types of jaundice can be easily differentiated (Fig. 33.1).

Serum bile acids

1. Serum bile acid level ranges from 0.3-1.3 mg/dl.
2. Elevated serum bile acid level suggests hepato cellular diseases like hepatitis, cirrhosis and obstruction of portal system.
3. Serum bile acid concentration is more due to impaired uptake or secretion by hepatocytes.
4. Increase in serum bile acid level is more marked in cholestasis.

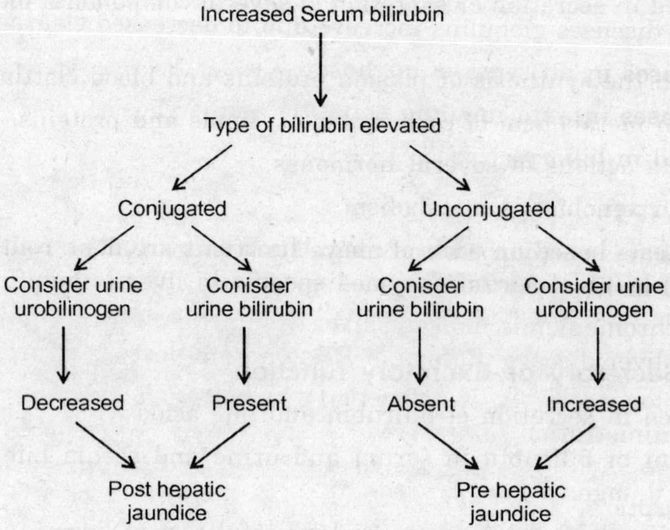

Fig. 33.1 Scheme showing utilization of serum, urine bilirubin and urine urobilinogen tests in differential diagnosis of liver diseases.

Tests based on excretion of xenobiotics or Clearance Tests

Liver clears several xenobiotics rapidly from blood stream. Very little of them is cleared by other organs. Therefore elimination of these xenobiotics from the blood stream depends on functions of liver. Liver takes up these molecules by active transport mechanism involving a carrier molecule and excretes later in bile.

Liver clears xenobiotics either as such or its conjugates or both and hence they are used to study liver function. Usually these tests are performed on non-jaundiced patients. Some of the xenobiotics used in clearance tests are bromosulfophthalein, aminopyrine, indocyanin green, caffeine, rose bengal and sodium benzoate. Any retention of these substances in blood after administration indicates liver cell dysfunction. However with the development of more specific tests and due to side effects associated with the use of these compounds clearance tests are performed only rarely.

Tests based on Synthetic function

1. Liver synthesizes many plasma proteins, blood clotting factors lipoproteins and urea.
2. Synthesis of these compounds may be affected in pathological conditions. Hence their concentration in plasma may decrease. However due to their long half life and regenerating capacity of the liver the decrease may be apparent only on long standing liver diseases.
3. In addition liver clears immunoglobulins like IgA, IgG and IgM. In chronic liver diseases plasma concentration of these immunoglobulins is affected.

Serum albumin

1. In several liver diseases hypoalbuminemia occurs. Since half life of albumin is 20 days decrease in albumin level occurs in chronic liver diseases.

Serum globulins

1. In chronic liver diseases globulins increase due to decreased clearance by hepatocytes.
2. IgA level increases in all types of cirrhosis.
3. IgG level increases in auto immune hepatitis and cirrhosis.
4. IgM is increased in biliary cirrhosis.

Prothrombin Time (PT)

1. Since prothrombin is one of the blood coagulation factor synthesized by liver its synthesis is decreased in liver disease.
2. Hence hypoprothrombinemia indicates liver dysfunction. Further prothrombin time (PT) is prolonged in liver disease. Return of PT to normal level is of prognostic importance.
3. Since PT is prolonged in vit. K deficiency it is ruled out by estimating PT before and after vit. K administration.
4. PT may be prolonged in chronic obstructive jaundice due to resultant vit. K deficiency due to malabsorption.
5. Thus PT is useful in differential diagnosis of jaundice.

In addition, measurement of other plasma proteins like ceruloplasmin, antitrypsin, haptoglobulin and transferrin is also used in liver functional studies.

Blood Urea

1. Since liver is the only organ involved in the production of urea its level decreases in liver failure cases.

Tests based on metabolic function

Liver is involved in the conversion of galactose to glucose and distribution of ammonia.

Galactose tolerance test

1. Liver is the only organ involved in disposal of galactose. So, measurement of galactose clearance by liver is useful in assessing hepatic function.
2. After an intravenous galactose injection blood samples are collected for every 10 minutes until one hour. Galactose in measured in blood samples.
3. Normally liver clears galactose within 10-15 minutes. Delay of clearance indicates cirrhosis and hepatitis.
4. In galactosemics also galactose clearance is less.

Blood Ammonia

1. Since liver converts ammonia to urea through urea cycle reactions ammonia level is elevated in liver diseases.
2. When ammonia accumulation reaches toxic level hepatic coma develops.

Enzyme Tests

1. Several enzymes are released from diseased hepatocytes.
2. They may be of cytosolic, mitochondrial and membrane associated enzymes.

3. Type of enzyme released depends on severity and specific diseases of liver.
4. The amount of enzyme in plasma is thus altered in liver diseases.
5. Such enzyme tests are useful in evaluation of liver functions as well as diseases affecting liver.
6. Transaminases, alkaline phosphatase, γ-glutamyl transpeptidases and 5′-nucleotidase are the enzymes tests that are usually done to assess liver function.

Transaminases

1. Alanine aminotransferase (ALT), aspartate aminotransferase (AST) are two enzymes present in liver. They have different half lifes. The half life of ALT is 47 hours and AST is 17 hours. Further liver contains more of ALT and AST is present in other organs like heart and skeletal muscle.
2. So, AST test is useful only in the absence of secondary disease and ALT test is a specific indication of liver dysfunction.
3. However, due to their presence in liver cells both the enzymes are elevated in liver disease. The degree of elevation indicates quantum of hepatic cellular damage and return to normal level is suggestive of recovery.
4. Due to higher half life ALT returns to normal slowly in acute hepatitis and its level is higher than AST.
5. In alcoholic liver disease AST level in higher than ALT level.

Alkaline Phosphatase (ALP)

1. It is a membrane bound enzyme concentrated in sinusoids and endothelium of portal venous system. Only small amounts are present in bile canaliculi.
2. Any types of biliary tree obstruction increases synthesis of ALP by hepatocytes which then leaks into plasma. As a result plasma ALP level raises.
3. In extra hepatic obstruction elevation is more marked about three fold and in intra hepatic obstruction elevation is about 2.5 fold.
4. However, in infective hepatitis its level may remain normal or moderately elevated.
5. Thus ALP test is useful in differential diagnosis.

γ-Glutamyl transpeptidase (GGT)

1. It is membrane bound enzyme. GGT activity is elevated in all forms of liver disease.
2. About 10 to 30 times it is elevated in biliary obstruction.
3. It is more sensitive than ALP and transaminase in the detection of obstruction.
4. It is only moderately elevated in infective hepatitis.
5. Alcoholic cirrhosis is another liver disease in which GGT is elevated.
6. In fatty livers also GGT level is elevated.

5′-Nucleotidase (5′-NT)

1. It is another membrane bound enzyme.
2. Several fold increase in 5′-NT activity is found in conditions where there is obstruction to flow of bile which may be either intrahepatic or extrahepatic.

3. Normal or moderately elevated 5′-NT activity is found in infective hepatitis.
4. In biliary cirrhosis also 5′-NT activity is elevated.

Changes in enzyme tests in various liver diseases are presented in Table 33.1.

Table 33.1 Enzyme tests in various liver diseases.

	ALT	AST	ALP	GGT	5′-NT
Hepatitis (Acute or chronic)	↑↑↑	↑↑	↑	↑	↑N
Cholestasis (Intra or extra hepatic)	↑	↑	↑↑↑	↑↑	↑↑↑
Cirrhosis	N↑	N↑↑	—	↑	↑

KIDNEY FUNCTION TESTS

Functions of Kidney

1. Kidney is an essential organ. It has several diverse functions.
2. Nephron is functional unit of kidney. It consists of glomerulus and renal tubules
3. Kidney maintains water, electrolyte and acid base balance of the body through filtration and reabsorption process. Glomerulus is responsible for filtration and renal tubules are involved in reabsorption. In addition renal tubules secretes some solute molecules.
4. Kidney clears several non-protein metabolic waste products like urea, uric acid, creatinine etc., from circulation.
5. Kidney produces erythropoietin, calcitriol, renin and prostaglandins.

Since glomerulus and renal tubules are major functional units of kidney most of the kidney function tests done to assess renal damage are based on either function of glomerulus or renal tubules.

Tests of glomerular function

1. The glomerulus is involved in filtration of blood.
2. It is a sieve and act as selective permeability barrier.
3. The rate at which filtrate is formed in glomerulus is known as glomerular filtration rate (GFR). It largely depends on number of functioning nephrons. Hence it is a sensitive index of renal function.
4. Clearence tests are used to assess glomerular filtration rate.

Clearance Tests

1. These tests measures clearance of a substance by kidney from blood which may be of endogenous or exogenous origin.
2. Clearance is a theoretical concept. It is defined as volume of plasma which is completely cleared of a substance by kidneys per minute. It is expressed as *ml* of plasma cleared per minute (ml/min).
3. A substance that meets following criteria is used for clearance studies.

(*a*) The substance must be freely filterable.

(*b*) The substance does not undergo reabsorption.

(*c*) The substance is not secreted by renal tubules.

4. Formula for calculation of clearance is given below:

$$\text{Clearance of substance (ml/min)} = \frac{UV}{P}$$

U = Concentration of the substance in urine.

V = Volume of urine in ml per minute

P = Concentration of the substance in plasma

Creatinine Clearance Test

Since creatinine is neither secreted nor reabsorbed creatinine is used as endogenous marker of renal GFR. Production of creatinine is also not influenced by diet, age etc. Creatinine clearance test is used to assess renal GFR world wide.

In this test first patient is given 500 ml water. So that his body is hydrated properly. After an hour his bladder is emptied and urine is discarded. Then the urine passed for a 4 hour period is collected and volume is measured. Blood samples are also collected during collection of urine. Creatinine concentration in blood and urine samples is determined and by substituting thc values in the above mentioned formula creatinine clearance is obtained.

Normal creatinine clearance values are 90-110 ml/min/1.73 square meter body surface area. Low GFR indicates renal dysfunction. It occurs in various kidney diseases and several pre renal conditions.

Urea clearance Test

Like creatinine urea is another endogenous substance used as marker for the measurement of GFR. Like creatinine, measurement of urea in urine and plasma can be easily done in clinical laboratory. However, diet influences urea production and it undergoes reabsorption to some extent. So urea clearance test may not reflect the true GFR values.

In this test about 200 ml of water is given to the subject after a normal breakfast. His bladder is emptied immediately and urine is discarded. After an hour his bladder is completely emptied and urine is collected and its volume is measured. A blood sample is also taken at the same time. Then urea concentration in blood and urine is measured. Formula given below is used to get urea clearance values.

$$\text{Urea clearance (ml/min} = \frac{UV}{P}$$

U = Urea concentration in urine.

V = Volume of urine excreted per minute.

P = Urea concentration in blood.

Normal urea clearance is 75 ml/minute. However, normal urea clearance value is influenced by urine output per minute. Maximum clearance occurs when urine output is 2 ml per minute. Then the urea clearance value is referred as maximum. If the urine output is less than 2 ml per minute then it is known as standard urea clearance which is usually 54 ml per minute. The clearance values decreases with progressing renal diseases.

Inulin Clearance Test

Several exogenous substances are also used as markers of GFR. Exogenous substances as markers of GFR are used in assessment of slowly progressing renal diseases such as that of diabetic nephropathy. Inulin is a poly fructosan i.e. fructose is building block of polymer. It is neither secreted nor reabsorbed and does not undergo changes. Hence it measures GFR.

In the inulin clearance test 500 ml water is given to the fasting patient one hour before begining of the test. Then for every 30 minutes 100 ml is given until the end of test. Usually the test ends in about 4 hours. The patient is given single dose of insulin 70 mg/kg body weight is infused within 5 minutes. Then urine and blood samples are collected at 2 hours, 3 hours and 4 hours after the infusion. Concentration of inulin in urine and blood samples is determined.

Normal inulin clearance values are 100-120 ml/min/1.73 sq. m. body surface area. Less values indicates renal dysfunction.

Tests of tubular function

1. In renal tubules glomerular filtrate is converted to urine due to absorption of solutes like glucose, amino acids, bicarbonate, water, sodium, chloride etc., from filtrate and secretion of hydrogen, ammonia, uric acid etc., into filtrate.
2. Further water absorption in the tubules in influenced by antidiuretic hormone (ADH).
3. So, in diseases affecting tubular function specific gravity, osmolality and volume of urine are altered.

Specific gravity measurement

Specific gravity of urine depends on concentration of solutes. Normal specific gravity is 1.03. It increases due to presence of glucose or protein in urine. Specific gravity decreases when water reabsorption is affected due to lack of ADH. Specific gravity measurement is part of concentration and dilution test.

Urine osmolality measurement

Normal individuals urine osmolality ranges from 300 to 900 mosm/kg. It is influenced by water in take. In renal failure osmolality is high. Measurement of urine osmolality is part of concentration dilution tests.

Urine volume measurement

In normal individuals volume of urine passed during night is half of volume of urine output of the day time. High urine output during night time indicates tubular dysfunction. Further urine out put is more in diabetics and ADH deficient people.

Concentration-Dilution tests

These tests assess renal tubular function.

(A) Concentration test

ADH injection is given in this test to assess concentrating ability of kidney. Specific gravity and osmolality of the urine are measured. In normals the specific gravity and osmolality must be within normal limits. Decreased specific gravity indicates loss of concentrating ability of kidney due to disease.

(B) Dilution Test

In this test a test load of water is given to assess capacity of kidney to excrete water. Urine samples are collected. Volume, specific gravity and osmolality of urine are measured. Normal individual excretes almost all of water load and specific gravity and osmolality of at least one of the urine sample are very much low.

Tests to assess renal tubular Secretory activity

Some of the foreign substances are completely removed by kidneys when they are introduced into blood. Phenolsulfonphthalein (PSPL) is one such compound frequently used to test renal efficiency.

Phenolsulfonphthalein test (PSPL)

In this test initially 200 ml of water is given to the patient and bladder is emptied after 15 minutes. Then PSPL dissolved in water is given by intramuscular route. Bladder is emptied after 2 hours. PSPL is measured in the urine sample.

Normal kidney removes most of the PSPL from circulation in two hours. The rate of elimination decreases with progressive renal impairment.

In addition to the tests described so far urine analysis that is routinely carried out in clinical bio-chemistry laboratories for blood, albumin, bile may be helpful in assessing renal dysfunction. However these analysis are of little value when renal dysfunction is minimal due to regenerating capacity of kidney.

Levels of blood urea, uric acid, creatinine, calcium, phosphorus, electrolytes also may indicate renal dysfunction because kidney is involved in handling of these compounds. Usually their levels in blood are elevated in renal diseases.

REFERENCES

1. Adacti, Y. Horii, K. and Takahashi, Y. Serum glutathione-s-transferase activity in liver disease. Clin. Chem. Acta. **106,** 243-255, 1980.
2. Black, E.R. Diagnostic strategies and test algorithms in liver disease. Clin. Chem. **43,** 1555-1560, 1997.
3. Murray, M.P$_{450}$ Enzymes: inhibition mechanism genetic regulation and effects of liver disease. Clin. Pharmacokinet. **23,** 132-146, 1992.
4. Women, H.J. Molecular biological methods in diagnosis and treatment of liver diseases Clin. Chem. **43,** 1476-1486, 1997.
5. Fossati, P. Ponti, M. and Passoni, G. A step forward in enzymatic measurement of creatinine. Clin. Chem. **40,** 130-137, 1994.
6. Newman, D.J. Thakkar, H. and Dwards, R.G. Serum cystatin c measured by automated immunoassay. A more sensitive marker of changes in GFR than serum creatinine. Kidney. Int. **47,** 1312-1318, 1995.

7. Perrone, R.D. Medias, N.E. and Levey, A.S. Serum creatinine as an idex of renal function. New insights into old concepts. Clin. Chem. **38,** 1933-1953, 1992.

8. Sokoll, L.J. Russell, R.M. Sadonski, J.A. *et al*. Establishment of creatinine clearance. Reference values in older women. Clin. Chem. **40,** 2276-2281, 1994.

9. Hikaru Koide. Ed. Cellular and Molecular biology of kidney, Karger, S. 1992.

10. Paoliccni, A. *et al*. Gamma Ilutamyl Transpeptidase in fine needle liver biopsies of subjects with chronic hepatitis. C.J. Virol. Hepat. **12**, 269-273, 2005.

EXERCISE

ESSAY QUESTIONS

1. Write functions of liver. Describe various liver function tests.
2. Mention kidney functions. Give an account of tests performed to assess kidney function.
3. Write an essay on clearance tests used to study kidney and liver function.

SHORT QUESTIONS

1. Explain importance of bilirubin and urobilinogen in differential diagnosis of liver disease.
2. Write liver functions based on xenobiotics elimination.
3. Define prothrombin time. Explain its role in diagnosis of liver disease.
4. Give an account of enzyme tests in liver disease.
5. Define clearance, clearance tests. How clearance is calculated? Write criteria for chosing a substance for clearance test.
6. Write normal creatinine clearance. Write procedure of this test. Mention its clinical importance.
7. Write about phenolsulfonphthalein test.
8. Explain concentration dilution test.
9. Write changes in the levels of the following in liver disease.
   (*a*) Serum bilirubin (*b*) Serum AST (*c*) γ-GGT (*d*) Alkaline phosphatase.

34

CHAPTER

BIOCHEMICAL TECHNOLOGY

MEDICAL AND BIOLOGICAL IMPORTANCE

1. This chapter deals with techniques used to study various aspects of biochemistry as well as techniques useful in diagnosis, treatment and management of diseases.
2. Differential centrifugation is used for isolation of cell organelles. Isolated cell organelles are used to study structure, function, metabolic pathways etc.
3. Electrophoresis is used for the separation of plasma proteins and to study changes in plasma proteins in diseases.
4. Paper chromatography is used for the separation and identification of amino acids, sugars etc. in biological samples.
5. Spectrophotometric methods are employed for measurement of enzyme activity in the biological fluids.
6. Enzymes are isolated from organs or cells by using an array of separation techniques in sequence which usually begins with homogenization and may terminates with affinity chromatography or high performance liquid chromatography (HPLC).
7. In hospital biochemistry laboratory many biomedical equipments like colorimeter, spectrophotometer, flame photometer, spectrofluorimeter and auto analyzers are used to estimate blood constituents in health and diseases.
8. A wide range of methods are used for estimation of various blood constituents. Estimation of blood constituents is useful in diagnosis, prognosis and management of diseases.
9. Urine composition is altered in several diseases. Qualitative tests are used for identification of normal as well as abnormal constituents of urine. Further urine constituents are estimated by several quantitative methods.
10. Qualitative as well as quantitative analysis of urine is useful in diagnosis, treatment and management of diseases.

Isolation of cell organelles or subcellular Fractionation

1. Detailed study of structure and function of each cell organelle requires isolation of the organelle in pure form without any contamination with other cell organelles.
2. This is accomplished by a process known as subcellular fractionation traditionally.

3. It involves. (*a*) Homogenization and extraction

   (*b*) Centrifugation.

4. However isolation of cell organelles of all types of cells may not be possible with these processes alone.
5. They may be modified accordingly to the type of cell or additional steps may be required.

Homogenization and extraction

1. Separation or isolation of an organelle from cell requires breaking of cell under suitable conditions.
2. Cells of organs like liver, kidney etc. are broken by a process known as homogenization.
3. In this process motor driven teflon pestle is rotated within a glass tube containing organ slices in a suitable medium.
4. Rotation of pestle exerts mechanical shearing forces on cells and breakes cells releasing their contents into medium. Thus homogenization results in extraction of organelles into medium.
5. The solution (medium) containing intact organ is known as 'Homogenate'.
6. Since cell organelles are labile and subject to loss of biological function they must be homogenized and extracted under mild conditions. Use of extreme pH and temperature is not desirable.
7. Hence most of the isolation of cell organelles is carried out in cold room.
8. Due to action of enzymes like proteinases, nucleases that are released when cell is broken significant loss of biological function of organelles may occur at room temperature.
9. Commonly used medium for homogenization and extraction of cell orgeanelles is 0.25M sucrose pH 7.4 containing ions Na^+, K^+, Mg^+ at physiological concentration.

Centrifugation

1. In this technique separation of orgeanelles is acheived using instrument known as centrifuge.

Principles of Centrifugation

1. If a solution containing large particles is left to stand at room temperature for a period of time then the particles sediments under the influence of gravitational force.
2. In centrifugation force which is greater than gravitational force is used so that the particles sediment faster in a short time period.
3. Force required for separation of organelles in centrifuge is relative certrifugal force (RCF). It is calculated using below mentioned formula.

   $$\text{RCF} = 1.118 \times 10^{-5} \times n^2 \times r.$$

   Where r = Distance from the centre of rotation to the bottom of tube in rotor cavity or bucket.

   n = Speed of rotor in revolutions per minutes (r.p.m.).

4. Generally RCF is expressed as number of times greater than gravity *i.e.* 800 × g or 800g.

Components of a Centrifuge

1. Centrifuges contains rotor or centrifuge head, driveshaft and a motor. Homogenate is taken in centrifuge tubes and placed in rotor.
2. Additional components like timer, refrigeration unit etc. may be present in some centrifuges.

Types of centrifuges

Various types of centrifuges currently in use are

1. **Table top ordinary nonrefrigerated centrifuge.** It gives RCF up to 5000g and without timer or refrigerating unit.
2. **Table top high speed refrigerated centrifuge.** It gives RCF up to 25000g and with timer and refrigerating unit that gives 4°C temperature.
3. **Ultra centrifuge.** It is a very high speed centrifuge. It contain refrigerating unit, timer etc. It gives RCF of above 100000g.

Differential Centrifugation

1. Centrifugal separation depends on size, molecular mass and density of cell organelles. Each subcellular organelle sediments when specific centrifugal force is applied for a period of time. Hence homogenate prepared is subjected to centrifugation at different centrifugal forces for different time periods etc. and fractions of nucleus, mitochondria, ribosomes etc. are obtained.
2. In each centrifugation step particular cell organelle sediments through solution to give pellet and supernatant containing unsedimented particles.
3. At the end of each centrifugation the pellet and supernatant are separated and pellet is washed with homogenization medium then it is recentrifuged.
4. This process is repeated several times using different centrifugal forces (RCFs) till all cell organelles are isolated.
5. Various steps involved in isolation of cell organelles of liver cell are given below (Table 34.1). The centrifugation is carried out using refrigerated ultracentrifuge.
   (*a*) Liver homogenate prepared using teflon/glass homogenizer in 0.25 M sucrose pH 7.4 is subjected to centrifugation at 800g for 10 minutes. The pellet obtained is washed in 0.25 M sucrose and recentrifuged. The pellet obtained now is resuspended in 0.25 M sucrose and named as nuclear fraction.

   (*b*) This supernatants obtained in the above steps are pooled in a separate tube and subjected to centrifugation at 4000g for 10 minutes. The pellet obtained is washed and recentrifuged, pellet and supernatant are obtained. This pellet is named as mitochondrial fraction after resuspending it in 0.25 M sucrose.

   (*c*) The supernatants obtained in above steps are pooled and centrifuged at 18000g for 20 minutes. The pellet obtained in this step is resuspended in sucrose and designated as lysosomal fraction.

   (*d*) The supernatant obtained in the above step is transferred to another tube and centrifuged at 40000 g for 30 minutes. A pellet containing golgi complex is obtained and resuspended in sucrose.

(*e*) The supernatant of the above step is centrifuged at 100000g for 30 minutes and microsomal fraction is obtained as pellet.

(*f*) The above step supernatant is centrifuged at 105000 g for 20 minutes and ribosomes are obtained as pellet.

(g) The supernatant obtained in the final centrifugation is named as cytosolic fraction.

Table 34.1. Isolation of cell organelles by differential centrifugation.

Centrifugal force applied	Time in minutes	Cell organelle isolated
800g	10	Nucleus
4000g	10	Mitochondria
18000g	20	Lysosomes
40000g	30	Golgi complex
100000g	30	Microsomes
105000g	20	Ribosomes
Supernatant of final step	—	Cytosol

ELECTROPHORESIS

It is a commonly used separation technique. The term electrophoresis refers to movement of charged molecules under influence of an applied current. It is used to separate variety of compounds like proteins, lipoproteins, hemoglobins, oligonucleotides, amino acids etc. It is also used to know purity of isolated enzymes or proteins. In this technique separation is based on migration of charged molecules under influence of electrical field. The rate of migration of charged molecules also depends on the size, pH, temperature, strength of current etc.

Usually positively charged molecules moves towards cathode and negatively charged molecules moves towards anode under influence of applied current. Using a buffer of appropriate pH all compounds in mixture to be separated are converted to either positively charged molecules or negatively charged molecules. For example all fractions of plasma proteins carry negative charge at alkaline pH. Therefore all of them move towards anode. The distance each fraction can travel depends on their net charge, size etc. Proteins that are highly negatively charged moves ahead of fractions that are less negatively charged molecules. Thus they get separated.

Depending on supporting material used for separation electrophoresis is named as paper electrophoresis, cellulose acetate electrophoresis, agar gel electrophoresis, polyacrylamide gel electrophoresis etc. Any type of electrophoresis requires electrophoretic tank and power pack.

Paper electrophoresis

In this technique plasma proteins are subjected to electrophoresis on paper. The paper commonly used is what man No.1. The paper is kept horizontally in horizontal type of electrophoresis. In the case of vertical electrophoresis the paper is kept vertically. The horizontal type of electrophoretic tank consist of two buffer compartments that are separated by bridge. Further, an electrode is present in each compartment. From power supply unit current enters buffer compartment through electrodes. The two compartments of electrophoretic tank are filled to a uniform level with a buffer. Usually barbitone buffer pH 8.6 is used for the separation of plasma proteins.

The paper is soaked with buffer and placed on the bridge of electrophoretic tank. Then with micropipette sample is applied at one end of paper that is close to the cathode. This provides sufficient distance on paper for fast moving proteins so that they can migrate to maximum extent. The movement of proteins is followed by adding bromophenol dye to sample (serum). The paper is connected to buffer compartment through paper wicks. After closing electrophoretic tank with lid direct current (D.C.) of about 1mA per cm width of paper is applied for about 12-16 hours. At the end of run the current is switched off and the paper is removed, dried in an oven and stained with bromophenol blue.

The separated proteins appear as bands on paper. Paper electrophoresis of normal plasma proteins yields 5 bands. They are albumin, α_1-globulin, α_2-globulin, β-globulin, and γ–globulins. Albumin shows maximum mobility where as γ-globulin, has minimum mobility towards anode α and β globulin show intermediate mobility. A typical horizantal paper electrophoretic set up is shown in Fig. 34.1.

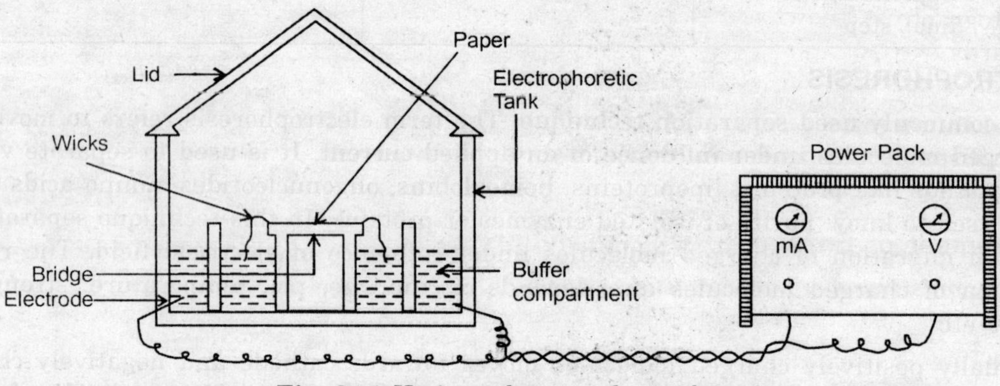

Fig. 34.1 Horizontal paper electrophoresis.

Separation and identification of amino acids

Separation and identification of aminoacids of body fluids or biological samples of other origin is a part of diagnosis of disease and research. Several methods are available for the separation and identification of amino acids of body fluids. Paper chromatography is one such method.

PAPER CHROMATOGRAPHY

It is one of the several chromatographic methods. It requires few micrograms of samples and hence highly sensitive. It separates closely related compounds like amino acids, sugars, peptides, nuclotides etc. based on their partition between two solvent phases. The two solvent phases are stationary phase and mobile phase. During separation of mixture stationary phase remains static where as mobile phase moves over stationary phase. The paper serve as support to hold stationary phase.

The partition of compounds to be separated between two phases depends on partition coefficients of each compound of mixture. Hence closely related compounds having different partition coefficients move differently when mobile phase is allowed to move over stationary phase. After separation compounds are identified as colored spots over the paper by using coloring reagent.

In this technique sample containing mixture of amino acids (sugars) is applied in microgram quantities as small spot with help of micropipette at one end of paper. Then the solvent system is allowed to pass over the spot for about 12-16 hours. The water of the solvent is held back by paper and act as stationary phase where as organic solvent moves over the paper and act as mobile phase. The solvent system used for separation depends on type or nature of compounds to be separated. Generally for separation of aminoacids solvent system consisting of butanol, aceticacid and water in the ratio of 4 : 1 : 5 is used. When mobile phase moves over stationary phase, compounds of the mixture move different distances on the paper according to their partition coefficient. Nonpolar aminoacids like phenylalanine moves fastest of all the aminoacids. Highly polar aminoacids like aspartic and glutamic acids moves faster than amino acids like arginine, histidine. Thus mixture get separated in this way. The separated compounds are identified by spraying proper coloring reagents or R_f values. R_f values is defined as ratio of distance moved by compounds to the distance moved by solvent or mobile phase. After separation aminoacids are identified by using ninhydrin reagent. The paper with color spots is known as chromatogram. Carbohydrates are identified by using dinitro salicylicacid as coloring agent. Usually this type of chromatography is known as descending paper chromatography because mobile phase moves downwards over sample. If the mobile phases moves upwards over the sample then it is known as 'ascending paper chromatography'.

Medical importance. Using this paper chromatography amino acids or sugars excreted in urine in diseases are identified by comparing their R_f values with the R_f values of the known amino acids or sugars.

Measurement of Enzyme activity and study of Enzyme Kinetics

1. Enzyme activity is measured in several ways. Likewise enzyme kinetics are studied by many methods. The term kinetics refers to study of changes in reaction rate when a reactant is converted to a product.
2. Majority of methods are based on study state conditions. If enzymes kinetics are studied under steady state conditions then they are called as steady state kinetics.
3. Under steady state conditions concentration of enzymes substrate complex [ES] in an enzymatic reaction is constant.
4. Some methods of enzyme estimation are based on presteady state conditions.

Spectrophotometric Methods

1. They are a kind of methods used to measure enzyme activity as well as kinetics like K_m, V_o, V_{max} etc.
2. They are simple and accurate but requires expensive spectrophotometer.
3. They are based on absorption of light by either a substrate or product of the enzymatic reaction at a particular wave length. None of the other reactants or products of that reaction absorb light at that particular wavelength.
4. Enzymatic reactions that produce or consume NADH are commonly measured by these methods. NADH absorbs light at 340 nm but NAD^+, oxidized form of NADH does not absorb at 340nm. Hence absorption at 340 nm increases in NADH generating reactions and decreases in NADH consuming reactions.

5. Lactate dehydrogenase (LDH) produces lactate from pyruvate by consuming NADH. Hence absorption at 340 nm decreases due to activity of LDH. Therefore by measuring this change in absorption LDH level is determined. Likewise alcohol dehydrogenase (ADH) activity is determined by following formation (increases in absorption) of NADH. Generally change in absorption is measured for few minutes. Then enzyme activity is calculated by using below given formula. It is known as kinetic method of enzyme estimation.

   Enzyme activity

   Units per milli litre = change in absorption per minute × Volume of enzyme used.

6. Even if substrate or product of enzyme of interest does not absorb light it may be measured by coupling the reaction to the another reaction that absorb light. For example none of the compounds of aspartate transaminase (AT) catalyzed reaction (see below) absorb light but it is estimated by coupling this reaction to malate dehydrogenase (MDH) catalyzed reaction. MDH converts oxaloacetate of AT reaction to malate by consuming NADH (see below). Decrease in absorption due to use of NADH corresponds to transaminase activity. Thus by measuring decrease in absorption at 340 nm AT level is determined.

   Aspartate transaminase catalyzes reaction given below.

   $$\text{Asparatate} + \alpha - \text{ketoglutarate} \xrightleftharpoons{\text{AT}} \text{Glutamate} + \text{Oxaloacetate}$$

   Malate dehydrogenase catalyzes following reaction.

   $$\text{Oxaloacetate} + \text{NADH} + \text{H}^+ \longrightarrow \text{Malate} + \text{NAD}^+$$

7. Study of enzyme kinetics like K_m, V_o, V_{max} etc. by using spectrophotometric methods is explained later in substrate concentration of study of properties of enzymes.

ISOLATION (PURIFICATION) OF ENZYMES

Medical Importance

1. To study structure and properties, enzymes has to be separated from the cell or tissues because enzyme is present in thousands of different types of molecules or compounds of cell.
2. Isolated enzymes are useful in fermentation industry, detergent making, medical instruments or electronics like biosensors.
3. Immobilized enzymes are used in clinical chemistry, food industry, pharmaceutical industry, immunodiagnostics etc.

To separate enzyme of interest from other compounds differences in properties like size, mass, electrical charge, solubility and affinity for other compounds are exploited. Enzyme isolation begins with selection of tissues rich in that enzyme and suitable method for its measurement. Generally isolation of enzymes involves use of variety of techniques in a sequence beginning from homogenization (Table 34.2). Some are given below.

1. **Homogenization.** A tissue rich in enzyme of interest is homogenized in mixer or blender and homogenate is obtained.
2. **Dialysis.** In this technique a semipermeable membrane like cellulose membrane with pores is used to separate high molecular mass enzymes from low molecular mass compounds. Sample (homogenate) is placed in dialysis bag and equilibrated with suitable

medium for 6-12 hours. Molecules of smaller size comes out through pores where as molecules of larger size remain in the dialysis bag. Thus low molecular mass compounds are separated from high molecular mass enzyme of interest.

3. **Centrifugation.** It separates enzymes of interest from nucleus, mitochondria, lysosomes and other cell or tissue debris.
4. **Fractional precipitation by salts.** This separation technique is based on solubility of proteins in salt solutions. Some proteins are more soluble in salt solutions like ammonium sulfate or potassium sulfate where as some are less soluble. So when salt is added proteins that are soluble remain in solution and less soluble proteins are precipitated. This way separation of desired enzyme is achieved from other unwanted proteins.

Column Chromatography

(*a*) It is a most commonly used technique for isolation of enzymes.

(*b*) In this technique a column packed with a material that adsorbs (interact) molecules based on differences in their structure or other properties is used for separation of desired enzyme from others.

(*c*) When mixture or sample to be separated is allowed to pass through the column some compounds of the mixture interact weakly with column material and lightly absorbed and others are strongly adsorbed due to their strong interaction with column material. Some molecules does not interact with column material and come out of column.

(*d*) The lightly adsorbed compounds comes out of the column first when the column is washed and strongly adsorbed molecules comes out later.

(*e*) Thus mixture is separated with this technique.

(*f*) Several column chromatographic techniques are available for isolation of enzymes.

(*g*) They are named according to basis of separation. Some are given below.

5. **Ion-Exchange chromatography.** In this method separation is based on charge of molecules. The column material used for separation is called as ion-exchange resin. Usually ion-exchange resins are either polycationic i.e. containing positive charges or polyanionic. i.e. containing negative charges. Negatively charged resin binds to cations strongly and called as cation exchange resin. Positively charged resin binds anions tightly and called as anion exchange resin. For example a cationic resin is used for separation of mixture containing highly negatively charged molecules, weakly negatively charged molecules and positively charged molecules. When this mixture is allowed to pass through the column positively charged molecules comes out of the column due to lack of interaction. The remaining two types of molecules are adsorbed or retained. However weakly negatively charged molecule bind less strongly. When the column is eluted with NaCl less tightly bound molecules comes out at low NaCl concentration where as tightly bound molecules comes out later at high NaCl concentration. NaCl causes release of adsorbed molecules by breaking electrostatic interaction between resin and bound molecules. So by using ion exchange chromatography mixture is separated in this way.
6. **Gel Chromatography:** In this method separation is based on molecular size or weight. The column material is gel beads. Gel beads are porous i.e. contain pores of specific size. Large molecules cannot penetrate pores but small molecules entrers pores easily. So when mixture or sample containing molecules of various sizes is allowed to pass

through the column, large molecules comes out first. Small molecules remain in the column because they enters pores of gel beads. They comes out of the column on elution. Thus separation of mixture is acheived.

7. **Affinity Chromatography:** It is highly specific chromatography method. In this technique separation is based on natural tendency of coming together of two molecules like enzyme or substrate or inhibitor. Using this technique enzyme may be purified from homogenate. Substrate or inhibitor of desired enzyme is covalently attached to column material through a spacer. It is loosely called as ligand. So when mixture containing enzyme is allowed to pass through column except enzyme all other molecules comes out and enzyme is bound to ligand or substrate or cofactor or inhibitor. Later enzymes is collected by breaking interaction between enzyme and substrate.

   Most of these chromatographic methods are slow because elution is carried out at low pressure. Hence separation requires many hours. This may cause loss of activity of sensitive enzymes.

8. **High performance liquid chromato graphy (HPLC):** It is an advanced separation technique. It is very rapid i.e. takes less time. It is most commonly used for the separation of highly sensitive enzymes. In HPLC separation is carried out at very high pressure. Since columns used for other chromatographic methods cannot with stand this pressure steel columns are used in HPLC. Material used for separation in the columns may be ion-exchange resins, gel beds etc. HPLC requires sample injector, monitor, detectors etc. unlike other chromatographic methods.

Table 34.2. Isolation of an enzyme

Steps	Enzyme activity Units/ml	Fold purification
1. Homogenate	0.5	1.00
2. Dialysis	0.75	1.25
3. Centrifugation	1.00	2.00
4. Precipitation by salt	2.00	4.00
5. Ion exchange chromatography	8.00	16.00
6. Gel chromatography	10.00	20.00
7. Affinity chromatography	25.00	50.00
8. High performance liquid chromatography(HPLC)	75.00	150.00

Study of properties of enzymes

Highly purified enzymes are used to study properties. Spectrophotometric methods or colorimetric methods are used to study enzyme properties.

1. **Substrate concentration.** Effect of substrate concentration on rate or velocity of enzymatic reaction is studied measuring enzyme activity at different concentration of the substrate. Then graph is obtained by plotting substrate concentration against velocity. Kinetic parameters like K_m, V_o, V_{max} are calculated from the graph.
2. **Cofactors or inhibitors.** Effect of cofactors or inhibitor is studied by measuring enzyme activity in presence of cofactor. If enzyme activity increases then the cofactor is activator and if enzymes activity decreases then the cofactor is inhibitor.

3. **Temperature.** Effect of temperature is studied by measuring enzyme activity at different temperatures. Then a graph is obtained by plotting temperature against enzyme activity. From the plot optimum pH is obtained.
4. **Hydrogen ion concentration (pH).** Effect of pH on enzyme activity is studied by measuring enzyme activity at different pH. Then enzyme activity is plotted against temperature. From the plot optimum pH of enzymes is obtained.

Methods for estimation of blood constituents

The levels of organic constituents of blood like glucose, urea, uric acid, proteins, bilirubin, hormones, enzymes and vitamins as well as levels of inorganic constituents of blood like sodium, potassium, chloride, bicarbonate and phosphate are altered in many pathological conditions. So their estimation in blood is useful in diagnosis, prognosis and management of diseases. Many biomedical equipments are used for their estimation. They are colorimeters, spectrophotometers, flame photometers, spectrofluorimeters and more recently blood gas analyzers and autoanalyzers. Even in autoanalyzer estimation of constituents of blood involves colorimeter, spectrophotometer etc. which are photometric instruments.

Blood glucose, urea, uricacid, cholesterol, phosphate and proteins are estimated by colormetric methods. Enzymes, proteins, amino acids, nucleic acids and vitamins are estimated by spectrophotometric methods. Water soluble vitamins thiamine and riboflavin are estimated by spectrofluorimetric methods. Flame photometer is used for the estimation of sodium, potassim, calcium, lithium etc.

Apart from photometric methods estimation blood constituents is carried out by other methods also. For example calcium is estimated by titrametric methods. Hormones are estimated by radio immunoassay (RIA) and non-isotopic immunoassays. Blood pH, Pco_2, and bicarbonate are estimated by blood gas analyzer. Some blood constituents are estimated by several methods. For example blood glucose is estimated by several colorimetric methods.

Photometry

It is a most widely used technique is biochemistry laboratory. Unlike electrophoresis and chromatography it is not a separation technique. It is used for quantitative estimation of substances or compounds present in biological sample or fluid i.e. it enables to know amount of substance. Very small amount of substance is needed for estimation. It is also used to detect compounds in biological samples. Now a days it is used to study protein folding and dynamics.

It is based on light absorption property of compounds. Certain compounds containing double bonds absorb light to attain stable configuration. The light absorption by these compounds must obey Beer-Lambert's law.

According to Beer's law light absorption by light absorbing compounds is proportional to concentration of that substance. It is expressed as equation below.

$$A = K_1C$$

Where A = absorption, K_1 = Constant, C = Concentation

Lambert's law states that light absorption by light absorbing substance is proportional to the depth of light absorbing material. This relationship is expressed as equation below.

$$A = K_2b$$

Where K_2 = Constant, b = depth of light absorbing substance

By combining the above two laws we get below given equation.

$$A = abc$$

Where A = absorption or extinction coefficient of light absorbing substance and A is called as optical density (O.D).

Thus in all photometric measurements light absorption by light absorbing substance is proportional to concentration and depth of light absorbing substance.

COLORIMETRY

If light absorbing substance in photometry is colored then photometry becomes colorimetry. The instruments used for photometric measurments are called as photoelectric colorimeter or colorimeter or spectrocolorimeter. Most of the colored substances absorb light in visible range i.e. 400-700 nm. Usually a colored substance absorbs light of a particular wavelength that is determined by its molecular structure as well as its own color.

In hospital laboratory or any biochemistry laboratory concentration of glucose, uric acid, urea, cholesterol and transaminases etc. in blood are estimated by using colormetric methods. In most of these colorimetric methods concentration of substance in unknown samples (test, T) is calculated from optical density values of unknown and a standard (s) which contain known amount of substance to be estimated by applying Beer-Lambert's law.

So according to Beer - Lambert's law.

$$O.D_T = A\,bc_T \quad ...(1)$$

$$O.D_s = A\,bc_s \quad ...(2)$$

By dividing 1 with 2 we get

$$\frac{A\,bc_T}{A\,bc_S} = \frac{O.D_T}{O.D_S}$$

By cross multiplying we get

$$C_T = O.D_T / O.D_S \times C_S \quad ...(3)$$

By substituting $O.D_T$ $O.D_S$ and C_S values in equation 3 concentration of test is calculated.

In equation 1 and 2 A remains same because light absorbing substance is same in both test and standard. Likewise b remains same because optical density values of test and standard are measured by using same cuvette.

Instead of single standard, number of standards are used to eliminate error that may arise from using single standard. Then optical density (O.D) values are plotted against concentration of standards. A straight line indicates that the light absorption by light absorbing color solution obeys Beer-Lambert's law. From the straight line graph concentration of unknown is obtained by drawing perpendicular from the point where a line drawn from O.D values of unknown intersected the straight line (Fig. 34.2).

Components of Colorimeter

A light source, slits, filter, cuvette, detector and meter are components of a colorimeter (Fig. 34.3). The light source is a tungsten lamp that provides light ranging from 400-700nm. Only a narrow beam of light that comes out of the slit falls on filter. The filter provides light of only specific wavelength required for measurement by eliminating unwanted light. The light of specific wavelength passes through cuvette in which absorbing material is present. The light which is not absorbed by substance comes out and fells on detector. This light is converted to electrical energy by the detector and shows on meter or read out device.

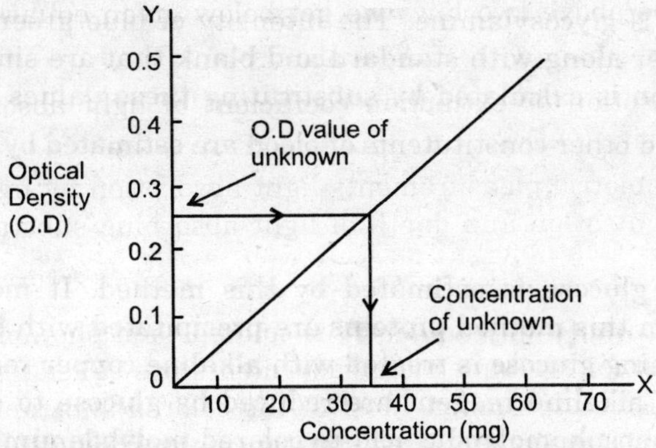

Fig. 34.2 Standard graph of colored compound.

Estimation of blood constituents by colorimetric methods

As mentioned earlier several blood constituents are estimated by using colorimetric methods. However as such these substances are colorless. Hence they are converted to colored substance by using appropriate chemical reagents. However, these reagents may absorb light and contributes to optical density values of standard and test. Therefore a blank which contains all reagents used for color development is always run alongwith standard and test and optical density value is obtained.

This optical density value is subtracted from optical density values of test and standard to eliminate absorption of reagents. Accordingly, equation 3 used for calculation of concentration of test is modified.

$$C_T = \frac{O.D_T - O.D_B}{O.D_S - O.D_B} \times C_S \qquad ...(4)$$

Where $O.\,D_B$ = Optical density of blank

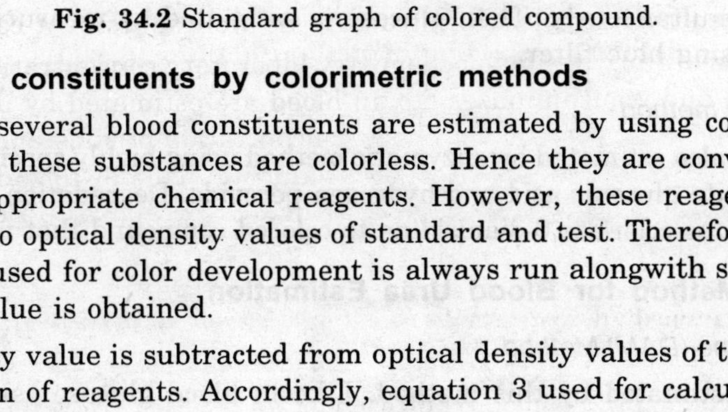

Fig. 34.3 Components of photoelectric colorimeter.

Colorimetric Methods for blood glucose estimation

O-Toluidine Method

It is based on the reaction of glucose with O-toluidine. In this method initially proteins in blood are removed by precipitating with trichloroacetic acid. Then protein free filtrate containing glucose is treated with O-toluidine at 100°C in presence of glacial acetic acid to produce blue green N-glycosylamine. The intensity of blue green color is measured at 630 nm or using red filter along with standard and blank that are similarly treated. Then blood glucose concentration is calculated by substituting these values in equation 4.

Blood glucose and other constitutents of blood are estimated by more than one colorimetric method.

Folin-wu method

Traditionally blood glucose is estimated by this method. It measures other sugars also alongwith glucose. In this method proteins are precipitated with tungstic acid. Then protein free filterate containing glucose is treated with alkaline copper reagent at elevated temperature. Cupric ions of alkaline reagent are reduced by glucose to cuprous ions which inturn reduces colourless phosphomolybdic acid to colored molybdenum blue. Standard and blank are also run simultaneously. Then glucose is estimated by measuring intensity of color at 490nm or by using blue filter.

Glucose oxidase method

Blood glucose is also estimated by enzymatic method using highly specific glucose oxidase which converts glucose to gluconic acid and hydrogen peroxide. Degradation of hydrogen peroxide by peroxidase oxidizes colorless 0-dianisidine to colored compound that is measured.

Colorimetric Method for Blood Urea Estimation

Diacetyl monoxime (DAM) Method

Blood urea is estimated by this method. Like in blood glucose estimation in this method initially proteins in blood are precipitated with trichloroacetic acid. Then urea present in protein free filtate is made to react with diacetyl monoxime under strong acidic conditions at high temperature in presence of catalyst like iron and thiosemicarbazide to give pink color. Standard containing known amount of urea and blank are also treated similarly. Then urea is estimated by measuring optical density values at 540nm or by using green filter.

Colorimetric method for estimation of serum total protein

Total protein in the serum is estimated by biuret method. It is based on the formation of violet colored complex when peptide bonds in the proteins react with cupric ion in alkaline medium. Total protein in serum is estimated by treating serum with biuret reagent. Standard containing known amount of protein and blank are also treated with biuret reagent. Intensity of violet color is measured at 540nm or using green filter in terms of optical density values. Then total protein in serum is calculated from. O.D values.

Colorimetric estimation of serum uric acid

It is based on reducing property of uric acid. In alkaline medium uric acid reduces phosphotungstic acid to blue tungsten which is measured at 710 nm or using red filter. Proteins in the blood are precipitated by treating with tungstic acid.

Serum bilirubin estimation by colorimetric method

It is based on principle of Vanden Bergh reaction. Bilirubin reacts with diazotized sulphanilic acid to produce purple pink color azobilirubin which is measured at 540nm or using green filter. Total bilirubin level is obtained by allowing diazotization in presence of methanol.

Conjugated bilirubin is determined by treating serum directly with azoreagent. Unconjugated bilirubin is obtained by subtracting conjugated bilirubin from total bilirubin.

Colorimetric estimation of blood cholesterol

Zak's method is used for estimation of blood cholesterol. Initially proteins are precipitated with ferrichloride and acetic acid reagent. Then protein free filtrate containing cholesterol is treated with ferrichloride Sulphuric acid mixture in acetic acid solution to give red color which is measured at 540 nm or using green filter.

Estimation of phosphate in serum by colorimetric method

Fiske-Subbarow method is used for estimation of phosphate in serum. In this method initially proteins are precipitated with trichloroaceticacid (TCA). Then protein free filtrate containing phosphate is treated with molybdic acid to produce phosphomolybdic acid. This is reduced to blue molybdenum by using reducing 1-amino-2-naphthol-4-sulfonic acid (ANSA). The blue color is read at 660 nm or using red filter.

Spectrophotometry

Spectrophotometry involves use of an instrument called Spectrophotometer. Spectrophotometer is superior to colorimeter in several aspects. Spectrophotometers are used for measurement in ultraviolet and infrared regions in addition to visible region. Prisms or gratings are used to get light of specific wave length. Hence spectrophotometric estimations are more accurate. A deuterium lamp provides ultraviolet light in an UV-Spectrophotometer. Sample volume required for measurement is very less compared to colorimetric measurement. Further very small amount can be detected or measured. Quartz cuvettes are used in spectrophotometry in place of glass cuvettes that are used in colorimetry.

Spectrophotometers are used to study role of coenzymes or metals in enzyme catalysis and enzyme kinetics. Protein folding and dynamics are studied by using spectrophotometer. Further spectrophotometers are also used to detect and quantify compounds like proteins, vitamins, amino acids and nucleic acids etc.

1. **Enzyme activity measurement.** There are two types of spectrophotometric methods for measurment of enzyme activity. They are
   (*a*) Kinetic method
   (*b*) End point method
   (*a*) **Enzyme estimation by kinetic method.** In this method enzyme activity is calculated by measuring changes in absorption for ten minutes. Enzyme is not inactivated or enzymatic reaction is not terminated in this type of method.
   (*b*) **Enzyme estimation by end point method.** In this method enzyme activity is calculated by measuring absorbtion of product formed in a specific period of time after inactivating enzyme or terminating enzymatic reaction.
2. **Estimation of proteins and amino acids.** UV light absorption by tryptophan at 280 nm allows direct estimation of proteins by spectrophotometry. Ordinary colorimetric methods are not useful when protein concentration is very less and takes more time because color development is involved. So estimation of protein by measuring absorption

at 280 nm is frequently used in purification of enzymes or proteins where several samples are to be measured at a time.

Aromatic aminoacids like phenylalanine and tyrosine that absorb light in UV region are also identified and quantified by using spectrophotometer.

3. **Estimation of Vit. A.** Vit. A absorbs light at 325nm. So it is estimated by using spectrophotometry.
4. **Estimation of nucleic acids, purines, pyrimidines and nucleotides.** UV light absorption by adenine, guanine, thymine, cytosine and uracil allows their detection and quantification as well as nucleic acids and nucleotides which contains these compounds.

Flame photometry

In this type of photometry light emission by excited atoms is measured rather than light absorption. Atoms of metalic elements get excited when energy is supplied. Electrons of certain orbitals of these elements absorb energy and attains high energy (excited) state. Since electrons are unstable in the excited state they return to ground state by emitting light of certain wavelength which may be colored also. The light emitted or color produced when excited atoms return to ground state is characteristic of that element. For example metalic element sodium produces yellow, potassium violet and lithium red when excited in flame. Further the intensity of the color is proportional to number of atoms present in flame which inturn proportional to the concentration of that element.

Flame photometer

They are the instruments used for flame photometric measurement. The components of a flame photometer is similar to photoelectric colorimeter except an atomizer and flame. Flame is used to excite atoms of elements. The atomizer draws sample through aspirator and converts it to fine mist which then enters flame. The detector measures light emitted and converts light energy to electrical energy.

Sodium, potassium, calcium and lithium are measured in various biological samples like blood, urine, C.S.F etc. by using flame photometer.

Spectrofluorimetry

It is also based on emission of light by excited atoms. The emission of light by excited atoms is often known as fluorescence and hence the name spectrofluorimetry. Spectorflurometers are instruments used for estimation of substances by spectrofluorimetric methods. In this technique instead of flame, light of particular wave length is used to excite atoms of the sample. Either filter or gratings are used to get a light of specific wavelength. Another difference is detector is placed perpendicularly to light path because the excited atoms emit light in all directions while returning to ground state.

Substances present in very very less concentrations that is in nanogram quantities in biological samples are measured using spectrofluorimetry. Water soluble Vitamins like thiamine and riboflavin in blood and urine are estimated by spectrofluorimetric methods.

Autoanalyzers

Due to advances in frontier areas of biochemistry number of constituents to be analyzed as well as number of blood samples to be analyzed increased to several folds in hospital biochemistry laboratories worldwide. This led to introduction of automation in clinical chemistry labs. The automated instruments are able to perform tests repetitively in short span of time with only minimal human involvement. Since these automated instruments analyses variety of constituents of biological samples like blood, urine, C.S.F. etc. they are known as autoanalyzers . Further, use of automation minimizes error that occurs due to boredom when repetitive type of work is done by humans. Moreover, use of autoanalyzer improves reproducibility of results. Another advantages is reduction in overall cost of medical care. However autoanalyzers are very costly equipments which can be afforded by only very large hospitals with sufficient financial backup.

A sampler, proportionate pump, dialyzer, waterbath, colorimeter, spectrophotometer or spectrofluorimeter and recorder are main components of an autoanalyzer. Usually number of components and type of components of an autoanalyzer may vary according to the type of autoanalyzer. Further, method employed for estimation of an analyte in an autoanalyzer is largely choice of its maker or manufacturer. Various components of autoanalyzer are connected by plastic tubes which allows flow of solutions from one component to another.

Operation of an autoanalyzer begins with loading of sampler with samples. The proportionate pump aspirates small volume of sample from each of samples that are loaded. Then the aspirated samples are channeled to dialyzer where dialyzable and non dialyzable constituents of samples get separated. Appropriate reagents in specified amount are added by proportionate pump to these constituents for the color development. The water bath provides proper temperature required for color development. Now the intensity of color developed is read by colorimeter or any other measuring device and recorder does calculation and gives a printout containing values obtained for each analyte.

Many types of autoanalyzers are currently available. They differ in manner in which they analyze various constituents of a sample or number of samples.

1. **Continous flow autoanalyzer.** This type of autoanalyzer is able to analyze samples in a sequence for more than one analyte. Further reagents and diluents are pumped continuously through tubings along with samples and every sample is subjected to same type of methods. For examples if blood glucose of one sample is analyzed with glucose oxidase method remaining samples glucose is also estimated by using same method.
2. **Multichannel autoanalyzer.** This type of autoanalyzer subjects samples to a set of tests (many tests) and results are given as printout. Using multichannel autoanalyzer more than 18 tests can be done on single sample simultaneously and 60-100 samples can be processed per hour.
3. **Single channel autoanalyzer.** This type of autoanalyzer subjects each sample to only one test (single analyte) and results of many samples are given as printout.
4. **Discrete autoanalyzer.** This type of autoanalyzer analyzes sample for an analyte by using more than one methods. It is capable of analyzing each sample in a specific manner. In other words, in this type of autoanalyzer all samples are not processed in the same manner.
5. **Semi autoanalyzer.** This type of autoanalyzers are able to do only some steps of analysis and remaining steps are manually done. Introduction of desired volume of sample, mixing with reagents, color development etc. involved in estimation are done

by operator or technician. Channelling of colored solution to photometer, measurement of absorption, calculation and printout of results are done by auto analyzer.

Some semi autoanalyzers are able to analyze only one analyte at a time (single channel analyzer) but continously it can analyze many samples in a sequence. Some semi auto analyzer are able to analyze more than one analyte (multichannel analyzer).

Blood constituents are estimated by other methods also. For example serum calcium is estimated by titrametric method.

Serum calcium estimation by titrametric method

After 12hours fasting blood is collected. Then serum is separated within one hour after centrifugation. Ammonium oxalate is added to serum to precipitate calcium in serum as calcium oxalate. The excess ammonium oxalate is removed by washing precipitate with dilute ammonium hydroxide. Now calcium oxalate is dissolved in sulphuric acid. Released oxalicacid is titrated with potassium permanganate solution. Pink color development indicates end point of titration. Titre value (A) is obtained. A balnk containing only sulphuricacid is also titrated and titre value (B) is obtained. One ml of potassium permanganate is equal to 0.2 mg of calcium . The amount of calcium in serum is obtained by multiplying the A-B with 0.2 mg.

Urine

1. Urine is fluid excreted by human body.
2. Kidneys of the body are responsible for the production of urine.
3. They produce urine from the blood to maintain water, electrolyte, acid-base balance of the body and normal composition of extracellular, intracellular fluids.
4. Acids, bases formed, various metabolic end or waste products, detoxified substances, compounds that are produced in excess and present in blood in excess are eliminated from blood by kidneys.

Physical characteristics of normal urine

Urine produced by normal healthy individual is known as normal urine. The physical characteristics of normal urine are (*a*) Volume (*b*) Color (*c*) pH (*d*) Specific gravity (*e*) Odor (*f*) Turbidity.

(*a*) **Volume.** The volume of urine excreted per day ranges from 1-1.5 litres. However several factors influences volume of urine excreted. Environment, food, exercise, temperature, fluid intake and physiological conditions affects volume of urine output. In cold and emotional conditions urine volume increases. In contrast urine volume decreases in hot climate and on exercise. Further urine output is more during day time and less during night. However in night shift workers it is reversed.

(*b*) **Color.** Fresh urine has an amber yellow color. The color of the normal urine is due to a pigment. Urochrome is the yellow pigment present in urine. It consist of urobilinogen (urobilin) and peptide fragment. The color of the urine intensifies on standing due to conversion of colorless compounds to color compounds by atmospheric O_2.

(*c*) **pH.** Normal urine pH ranges from 5.0-7.5. Usually normal urine is considered as acidic and has pH of 6.0. The pH of urine is influenced by acid, basic, organic as well as inorganic ions present in urine. The organic and mineral (inorganic) acids present in urine contributes to titrable acidity of urine. Another factor that influences pH of urine is diet. On protein diet urine pH decreases where as urine pH increases on fruit and vegetable diets. The urine excreated following meal is alkaline. Due to secretion of H^+ ions into gastric juice urine passed soon after a meal is alkaline. It is reffered as 'alkaline tide.'

(*d*) **Specific gravity.** Normal urine has a specific gravity of about 1.015 to 1.025. It is due to solids present in urine. Urinometer is instruments used to determine specific gravity of urine. The specific gravity of urine depends on urine output (volume). Specific gravity is inversely proportional to volume. Hence specific gravity of urine passed during night is more than specific gravity of the urine passed during day time.

(*e*) **Odor.** Normal urine has some aromatic odor. Odor of urine depends on diet. Urine passed in disease conditions lacks its characteristic odor.

(*f*) **Turbidity.** Fresh urine is a clear transparent liquid. However on standing urine may appear slightly cloudy (turbid) due to mucoproteins and epithelial cells that may enter into urine from linings of urinary tract.

Chemical composition of Normal urine

Normal urine contains mostly water, nitrogenous organic compounds, non-nitrogenous organic compounds and inorganic salts.

Nitrogenous organic compounds

Metabolic waste products like urea, uric acid, creatinine and ammonium are non protein nitrogenous (NPN) compounds excreted in urine. Detoxified products like indican, hippuric acid are also excreted in urine. Urine also contains very small amounts of amino acids, urobilinogen, vitamins, hormones, enzymes, porphyrins and low molecular weight peptides.

1. **Urea.** It is the only nonprotein nitrogenous substance that is excreted in large amounts in the urine of humans. It is the waste product of protein catabolism. About 20-35 gm of urea is excreted per day. However excretion of urea in urine is influenced by diet particularly protein diet. Further excretion of urea increases in wasting diseases due to increased protein catabolism. Urea clearence test is used to assess kidney function.

2. **Creatinine and creatine.** Creatinine present in urine is derived from skeletal muscle. About 1-2 gms of creatinine is excreted per day in the urine. Since urine creatinine is derived from muscle creatinine excretion is more in men and less in women. However diet has no effect on urine creatinine excretion. Creatinine clearence is used to assess renal function.

   About 60-150 mg of creatine is excreted in the urine per day. However it is not constant. Creatine which is not taken up by muscle escapes into urine. So if muscle mass is affected in any disease condition then creatine excretion in urine increases. Myasthenia gravis and muscular dystrophy are two diseases where skeletal muscle is badly affected. Therefore creatine excretion in urine increases in these diseases. In wasting diseases also creatine excretion in the urine is more.

3. **Uric acid.** About 0.6-0.7 gm of uricacid is excreted per day in urine. It is a metabolic waste product. Purine nucleotide catabolism or nucleic acid catabolism yields uric acid. Hence uric acid excretion in urine depends on nucleic acid intake. Also rate of degradation of endogenous nucleic acids affects uric acid excretion. Meat, meat products and leukemia causes increased excretion of uric acid in urine.
4. **Ammonia.** It is mainly a product of amino acid catabolism. Other amino group containing compounds like purines and pyrimidine breakdown also yield ammonia. About 1 gm of ammonia is excreted in urine per day. In the urine it exist as ammonium salts. Diet especially protein diet increases ammonium excretion in urine. In acid base disturbances also ammonia excretion changes.
5. **Amino acids.** About 150-250 mg of amino acids are excreted in urine per day. Amino acids excretion is more in urine in inherited diseases of amino acid metabolism. They are known as amino acid urias. Amino acid excretion is more in other diseases also like Fanconi syndrome, muscular dystrophy etc.
6. **Indican.** About 10-20 mg of indican is excreted in urine per day. It is detoxified form of indole which is produced in colon by bacteria from tryptophan. Indole is eliminated as indoxylsulfate which is also known as indican in urine. It is also known as ethereal sulfate or organic sulfate of urine. Amount of indican in urine is proportional to formation of indole from tryptophan. Putrifaction of intestinal contents by bacteria increases excretion of indoxylsulfate in urine.
7. **Hippuric acid.** About 0.5-0.7 gm of hippuric acid is excreted in urine per day. Vegetable food stuffs are main source of hippuric acid in urine. Benzoates present in plant foods are detoxified as hippuric acid and excreted in urine.
8. **Urobilinogen.** About 4 mg of urobilinogen is excreted in urine per day. On standing urine urobilinogen is converted to urobilin. It is derived from bilirubin and contributes to color of urine. Urobilinogen excretion in urine is altered in diseases associated with bilirubin metabolism. Urobilinogen excretion is more in urine in hemolytic jaundice. Urobilinogen is absent in urine in obstructive jaundice.
9. **Vitamins.** Ascorbic acid, riboflavin and FI GLU are excreted in urine. However if these and other water soluble vitamins are taken in excess their excretion in urine becomes more.
10. **Hormones.** Steroid hormones like male sex hormones, female sex hormones and aldosterone are excreted in urine. Small amounts of catecholamines and their metabolites are also excreted in urine.
11. **Enzymes.** Urine contains enzymes like urokinase, pepsin, trypsin, amylase, γ-glutamyltranspeptidase, angiotensin converting enzymes etc. in very small, amounts. When concentration of these enzymes in blood is elevated their excretion in urine is more.
12. **Porphyrins.** Very small amounts of porphyrins and its precursors are excreted in urine. In porphyrias their excretion in urine is more.

Non-Nitrogenous organic constituents of normal urine

Very small amounts of non nitrogenous organic compounds are found in urine of normal individuals. Usual laboratory tests are unable to detect these small amounts that are present in urine. Some of them are glucose, glucuronides, organic acids like citric acid, oxalic acid, acetoacetic acid, pyruvic acid, lactic acid etc.

Inorganic constituents of normal urine

Anions and cations are the inorganic constituents of normal urine.

Anions of normal urine

1. **Chloride.** About 10-15 gm of chloride is excreted in urine per day. It is the major inorganic constituent of urine. Chloride excretion in urine is influenced by diet, fluid intake and acid-base status of the individual. Chloride excretion is altered in disease conditions. In Addisons disease chloride excretion is more but it is less in vomiting and diarrhoea.
2. **Phosphates.** About 0.5-1.5 gm of phosphate is excreted per day in urine. In urine phosphate exists as salts of phosphoric acid. Phosphate content of diet influences urinary phosphate level. Further urinary phosphate levels alters in several diseases. In rickets, Vit-D deficiency, hypoparathyroidism, pregnancy, kidney disease less phosphate is eliminated in urine but in hyperparathyroidism excretion of phosphate in urine is increased.
3. **Sulfate.** About 0.5-1.8 gm of sulfate is excreted in urine per day. Both organic and inorganic sulfates are present in urine. However sulfur containing amino acids are the only source for urine sulfate. Inorganic sulfate is about 80% and remainder is organic sulfate. Ethereal sulfate is the name given to organic sulfate of urinary sulfate. Sulfate excretion increases in fever due to in increased breakdown of proteins. Anesthetics, cyanides and nitrites also increases urinary sulfate because they are detoxified to sulphur compounds and eliminated through urine.

Cations of normal urine

Sodium and potassium are the major cations present in urine. About 80-180 meq of sodium and 40-80 meq of potassium are excreted in urine. Some cations are excreted in trace amounts in urine. They are calcium, magnesium, iron, zinc and copper.

Abnormal constituents of urine

In pathological conditions physical characteristics of urine like color, volume, pH etc. are altered. Likewise excretion of certain compounds which are usually excreted in very small amounts is increased markedly in diseases conditions. Further some compounds which are usually absent in normal urine are excreted in urine in some diseases. Excretion of organic as well as inorganic constituents is altered in diseases. Some of the diseases in which excretion of organic and inorganic constituents of urine is altered are mentioned earlier.

Physical characteristics of abnormal urine

Urine, volume, color, pH, specific gravity, odor and turbidity are altered in several diseases.

1. **Volume.** Urine volume increases in pathological conditions. It is known as polyuria. In some diseases urine volume decreases and it is known as oligouria. Sometimes urine formation is completely blocked. It is known as anuria. Diabetes mellitus, diabetes insipidus, renal diseases, drugs and endocrine dysfunctions causes polyuria. Vomitting, diarrhoea, fevers, excessive sweating and nephritis cause oligouria. Anuria occurs in shock, poisoning, bilateral urolithiasis, incompatible blood transfusion and in renal failure.
2. **Color.** Due to presence of blood, bile, drugs, certain metabolites color of urine is altered. Urine appears brown when blood is present. Urine appears darkbrown when

urobilinogen is excreted in more amount. Bilirubin excretion makes urine yellowish. Melanin makes urine black. Sometimes urine color changes on standing or exposure to atmospheric o_2. Due to excretion of homogentisic acid urine becomes dark on standing. Urine color turns from pink to brown due to excretion of porphyrins on exposure to light. Urine color turns dark yellow when vitamin supplements are taken.

pH. Acidic urine is passed in uncontrolled diabetes, starvation and fevers. In alkalosis and alkali therapy urine becomes alkaline.

Specific gravity. Specifc gravity of urine decreases in diseases associated with increased urine volume like diabetes insipidus. Specific gravity of urine increases in diabetes due to more glucose in urine. In fever and acute nephritis also specific gravity of urine increases.

Odor. In uncontrolled diabetes urine of fruity aromatic odor is passed. It is due to excretion of more of acetone in urine. When urine is retained in bladder a putrid or strongly ammonical odor develops due to decomposition of urine by bacteria.

Turbidity. Due to excretion of lipids urine appears cloudy or turbid. Presence of pus and bacteria also makes urine turbid.

Organic constituents of abnormal urine

Sugars, protein, ketone bodies, bilirubin (bile pigment), bile salts, blood, lipids, porphyrins and its precussors are abnormal constituents of urine.

1. **Sugars.** Sugars excreted in urine are mostly monosaccharides and disaccharides. Monosaccharides are glucose, fructose, galactose and pentose. Lactose is disaccharide usually excreted in urine.
   (*a*) **Glucosuria.** It occurs in diabetes mellitus and renal diabetes. It also occurs in hyperactivity of pituitary, adrenals and thyroid glands. Asphyxia and ether anaesthesia also causes glucosuria.
   (*b*) **Lactosuria.** It occurs in pregnant and lactating woman.
   (*c*) **Fructosuria.** It occurs in essential fructosuria and hereditary fructose intolerance.
   (*d*) **Galactosuria.** It occurs in galactosemia.
   (*e*) **Pentosuria.** Pentoses are excreted in essential pentosuria.
2. **Proteins.** Excretion of protein in urine is known as proteinuria. Detectable amount of proteinuria occurs in several physiological and pathological conditions. Albuminuria is other name given to this condition. Albuminurias or proteinurias are divided into functional and pathological proteinuria.
   (*a*) **Functional or benign proteinuria.** It occurs on severe excercise, exposure to cold and standing for long time(orthostatic proteinuria). A transient albuminuria also occurs in pregnant women.
   (*b*) **Pathological proteinuria.** It occurs mainly in renal diseases. However several prerenal and postrenal conditions also causes proteinuria.
      (*i*) Prerenal diseases that cause albuminuria are cardiac disease, liver disease, convulsions, fevers, tumor in abdomen, hypertension etc.
      (*ii*) Renal diseases associated with proteinuria are glomerulonephritis and nephrosis.

(iii) Postrenal conditions that causes proteinuria are lesions of ureters, urethra, bladder and prostate.

(*c*) **Microalbuminuria.** It occur in long standing diabetic people who are prone to develop diabetic nephropathy. Usually, if daily urinary albumin excretion (UAE) exceeds 30 mg then the condition is known as microalbuminuria. The routine tests employed in laboratory to detect proteinuria are unable to detect albumin excreted in this condition.

3. **Blood (Haematuria).** Blood or hemoglobin are excreted in urine in urinary tract infections, stone in kidney, in compatible blood transfusion, metal poisoning, cancer of kidney, introduction of catheter etc.
4. **Ketone bodies.** Ketone bodies are excreted in urine in diabetes, starvation, ether anaesthesia, toxic pregnancy, von Geirke's disease etc.
5. **Bilirubin (Bile pigment).** It is found in urine of jaundice patients. However, it is excreted more in obstructive jaundice.
6. **Bile salts:** In obstructive jaundice bile salts are excreted in urine.
7. **Lipids (Lipuria).** Excretion of lipids in urine makes appearance of urine as that of milk. It occurs in chyluria. High fat diet may also produce lipuria.
8. **Porphyrins and its precursors.** In porphyrias porphyrins and its precursors are excreted in urine in large quantities. δ-ALA excretion is more in lead poisoning.

Urine analysis

Urine is analysed for its physical characteristics as well as chemical constituents in hospital biochemistry laboratory. The physical characteristics as well as chemical constituents of urine are altered in several diseases as mentioned earlier. So detection as well as quantitative measurement of the constituents of urine is useful in diagnosis, prognosis as well as management of diseases. Usually urine is subjected to qualitative analysis and quantitative analysis. Qualitative analysis is used to identify various constituents of urine in normal and disease conditions. Quantitative analysis involves estimation of various constituents of urine in normal and disease conditions.

Generally urine collected for 24 hours period is used for analysis. Organic constituents like urea, uricacid, creatinine, urobilinogen and ammonia in urine are detected by performing qualitative test. Likewise by using qualitative tests inorganic constituents of urine like chloride, phosphate, sulfate etc. are detected in urine. Even abnormal constituents of urine like glucose, protein, ketone bodies, bilirubin, blood etc. are detected by performing qualitative tests.

Tests for abnormal constituents of urine

1. **Benedict's test.** It is used for detection of sugar in urine. The reducing sugar tautomerizes to enediol under alkaline conditions. These enediols are unstable and gives rise to powerful reducing agents. They reduce cupric ion to cuprous ion. Under hot conditions red cuprous oxide is formed.
2. **Heat and acetic acid test.** It is used for detection of protein in urine. Protein present in urine denatures on exposure to heat. Due to decreased solubility denatured protein forms coagulum or precipitate.

3. **Rothera's test for ketone bodies.** Ketone bodies forms a purple colored complex with sodium nitroprusside in presence of ammonia.
4. **Hay's test.** It is used for detection of bile salts in urine. Bile salts reduces surface tension of water hence sulfur powder sinks to bottom.
5. **Petenkofer's test.** It is another test for bile salts identification. Sucrose undergoes dehydration to furfural derivatives which condenses with bile salts to give violet ring.
6. **Fouchet's test.** It is test for bilirubin. Wet barium sulphate adsorbs bilirubin which is oxidized to green biliverdin by fouchet's reagent.
7. **Benzidine test.** Blood is detected by this method. Heme oxidizes hydrogen peroxide to O_2 which in turn oxidizes benzidine to green or blue colored products.

Methods for estimation of urine constituents

1. Photometeric method, titrometric method etc. are used for estimation of urine constituents.
2. Urine creatinine is estimated by colorimetric method.
3. Sodium and potassium in urine are estimated by flame photometric method.
4. Urinary riboflavin is estimated by spectrofluorimetric method.
5. Urinary enzymes are estimated by spectrophotometric methods.
6. Urine chloride, sugar, titrable acidity and ammonia etc. are estimated by titrametric method.
7. Urine urea is estimated by using Doremus ureometer.
8. Protein in urine is estimated by using Esbach's albuminometer.
9. Hormones in urine are estimated by radioimmunoassay and non-isotopic immunoassays.

Urine creatinine estimation

It is based on Jaffe's reaction. Creatinine in urine reacts with picric acid under alkaline conditions to produce creatinine picrate which is orange color. Standard and blank are also treated similarly. Then creatinine in urine is calculated from optical density values which are obtained by using green filter or at 540 nm.

Reducing sugars in urine

Reducing sugar in urine is estimated in cases of severe diabetes which are usually associated with excretion of large quantities of glucose in urine. It is based on the principle of Benedict's qualitative test. It is titrametric method in which urine is titrated against blue colored Benedict's quantitative reagent. The Benedict's quantitative reagent contains potassium thiocyanate and potassium ferrocyanids along with copper in alkaline medium. Potassium ferrocyanide keeps cuprous oxide formed during titration in solution. At elevated temperature glucose present in urine reduces copper of Benedict's reagent to cuprous oxide which inturn get converted to cuprous thiocyanate by reacting with potassium thiocyanate. The appearance of white color due to consumption of all of blue colored copper gives end point of titration. Then glucose in urine is calculated from volume of Benedict's reagent used for titration. Generally Benedict's quantitative reagent is made in such way that 20 mg of glucose of urine reduces 10 ml of Benedict's reagent.

Estimation of Chloride in urine

Chloride present in urine is precipitated as silver chloride by treating with an excess of silver nitrate and concentrated nitric acid. The precipitate is removed by filtration. The unreacted silver nitrate in filterate is titrated with ammonium thiocyanate using ferric alum as indicator. During titration silver nitrate reacts with ammonium thiocyanate to form silver thiocyanate which get precipitated. When silver nitrate is completely converted to silver thiocyanate, ammonium thiocyanate react with ferric alum to form dark brown color ferric thiocyanate which is end of titration. The titre value is the measure of unreacted silver nitrate. Then silver nitrate reacted with urine is obtained from the titre value. One ml of silver nitrate is equal to 10mg of sodium chloride. Finally amount of chloride in urine is obtained by multiplying volume of silver nitrate reacted with 10.

Estimation of titrable acidity and ammonia in urine

The titrable acidity of urine is due to acids present in urine. The titrable acidity of urine is measured by titrating with sodium hydroxide using phenophthalein as indicator. When all the acid is neutralized further addition of sodium hydroxide produces pink color. The titre values corresponds to titrable acidity of urine.

Ammonia in urine is estimated by formal titration method. When formaldehyde is added to urine containing ammonia H^+ ions are released which are titrated with sodium hydroxide as described above. One ml of sodium hydroxide is equal to 1.7 mg of ammonia. So amount of ammonia in urine is calculated by multiplying volume of sodium hydroxide used with 1.7 mg.

Titrable acidity and ammonia of urine are 200-300 ml and 0.5-0.8 gm per day respectively. In starvation, diabetes, acidosis, on high protein diet titrable acidly and ammonia are increased. In alkalosis both titrable acidity and ammonia of urine decreases.

Estimation of urine urea

Since amount of urea excreted in urine is high a less sensitive method based on principle of alkaline hypobromite is used for estimation of urine urea. A special instrument known as Doremus ureometer is used for estimation of urine urea. Using this apparatus volume of nitrogen released on addition of alkaline hypobromite to urine sample is measured.

Doremus ureometer contains an open broader limb and a narrow closed limb that is graduated. Each sub division is equal to 0.01 gm of urea. A stopcock connects two limbs. When urine reacts with alkaline hypobromites in open limb N_2 is released. From the amount of nitrogen released quantity of urea is calculated.

Estimation of albumin in urine

In diseases large quantities of albumin is excreted in urine. It is estimated by using Esbach's albuminometer. It is based on protein precipitation by picric acid. In this method urine albumin is precipitated by using picric acid.

Esbach's albuminometer is a test tube like apparatus with mark U near middle and mark R near the top. The portion below U is graduated from 0-12 that gives albumin in gm/liter. In this technique urine is taken upto U mark and Esbach's reagent containing picric acid is added up to R mark. Protein is precipitated by inversion mixing. Then after one hour urine albumini in gm/liter is obtained from the reading corresponding to meniscus of the precipitate.

REFERENCES

1. Dudley, A.W. Lin, J.J. and Ley, N.C. Automatic balancing centrifuge. Am. J. clin. Pathol. **101**, 399, 1994.
2. Gersten, D. Gel electrophoresis of proteins. John Wiley & Sons, New York, 1996.
3. Cushman, D.W. and Cheung. U.S. Spectrophotometric assay and properties of angiotensin converting enzymes of rabbit lung. Biochem. Pharmacol. **20,** 1637-1648, 1971.
4. Meng, Q.C., King, S.J. Branham, K.E. Deluces, J.L. Lorber, B. and Oparil, S. Preparative isolation of angiotensin converting enzymes from human lung. J. Chromatography. **579,** 63-71, 1992.
5. Warner, L.M. Soper, S.A. and Mogrown, I.B. Molecular fluorescence phosphorescence and chemiluminescence spectrometry, Anal. Chem. **68,** 73R-91R, 1996.
6. Boyd, J.C., Felder, R.A. and Savory, J. Robotics and changing face of clinical laboratory, J. Auto. Chem. **16,** 35, 1994.
7. Wilson, G.S. Zhang, Y. and Reach, G. Progress towards development of implantable sensor for glucose. Clin. Chem. **38,** 1613-1617, 1992.
8. Hans Bisswanger. Practical Enzymology. Wiley, New York, 2004.
9. Bisswanger, H. Enzyme kinetics: Principles and Methods. Wiley, New York, 2002.
10. Farrell, S. and Ryan, T.R. Experiments in Biochemistry: A Hands on approach. Brooks/ Cole, 1999.
11. Wilson K. and Walker, J.M. Principles and Techniques of Practical Biochemistry. Cambridge University Press, 2000.
12. Alexander, J.N. *et al.* Fundamental laboratory approaches for Biochemistry and Biotechnology; John Wiley, New York, 2003.
13. Brunzel, N.A. Fundamentals of Urine and body fluid analysis. W.B. Saunders, PA, 1994.
14. Oliver, R.W. Ed. HPLC of macromolecules. Oxford University Press, England 1998.
15. Matejtschuk, P.Ed. Affinity separations: A practical approach. IRL Press, Oxford, 1997.
16. Hames, B. David. Gel electrophoresis of proteins: A practical approach, Oxford University Press, 2002.
17. Hargis, L.G. Howell, J.A. and Sutton, R.E. Ultraviolet and light absorption spectrometry. Anal. Chem. **68,** 169R-183R, 1996.
18. Morimobu. T. *et al.* Measurement of Vit.E metabolites by high performance liquid chromatography during administration of high dose of Vit. E. Eur. J. Clin. Nutr. **57,** 410-414, 2003.

EXERCISES

ESSAY QUESTIONS

1. Describe differential centrifugation method for isolation of cell organelles.
2. Write principles and applications of the following.

   (*a*) Paper chromatography

   (*b*) Electrophoresis

3. Discuss importance of spectrophotometric methods in enzyme studies with examples.
4. How enzymes are isolated? Write importance of isolated enzymes.
5. Give an account of methods of blood constituents estimation.
6. Write about colorimetric methods used for estimation of blood constituents with examples.
7. Describe photometry.
8. Write principles and applications of spectrophotometry. Write components of spectrophotometer.
9. Describe flame photometry and spectrofluorimetry.
10. Define autoanalyzer. Write its components and operation. Explain various types of auto analyzers currently available.
11. Give an account of organic constituents of normal urine.
12. Describe physical characteristics of normal and abnormal urine.
13. Give an account of abnormal constituents of urine. How they are identified?
14. Describe column chromatography.
15. Write about methods of urine analysis.

SHORT QUESTIONS

1. Write principles and applications of centrifugation.
2. Write components of a centrifuge. Classify centrifuges. Give examples.
3. Write a note on principles and applications of electrophoresis.
4. Draw horizontal electrophoresis. Label parts.
5. Explain principles of paper chromatography. Write its importance in biochemistry.
6. Write briefly about dialysis and fractional precipitation.
7. Define homogenization. Write on homogenizers.
8. Write note on affinity chromatography.
9. Define HPLC. Write its components. How it is superior to other forms of chromatography? Write its applications.
10. Write laws of absorption. Name instrument works on absorption. Draw its components. Label.
11. Define spectrophotometry. Write components and applications of spectrophotometer.
12. Write briefly about photometry.
13. Explain principles and applications of flame photometry.
14. What is spectrofluorimetry? Write components of spectrofluorimeter. Write its applications.
15. What are autoanalyzers? Write components of autoanalyzers. Briefly explain each one.
16. How an autoanalyzers work? Write about types of autoanalyzers used in clinical labs.
17. Write a note on semi autoanalyzers.
18. Write a note on automation of clinical chemistry lab.
19. Explain advantages and disadvantages on use of autoanalyzer in hospital lab.
20. Write note on NPN substances of urine.
21. Write on tests of glucose, proteins, blood, ketone bodies of urine.
22. Explain proteinurias.
23. Write importance of urine analysis in diagnosis with examples.
24. Write clinical importance of urine urea. Name the instrument used for estimation of urine urea.
25. Write about ions of normal urine.

GLOSSARY

A

Adipose tissue : A specialized tissue found under skin which is involved in triglyceride storage.

Aerobic : In presence of oxygen.

Algorithm : Process used in problem solving.

Allergy : An exaggerated susceptibility of an individual to foreign substances. From Greek, Allos-other, ergon-activity.

Analogs : A substance which is similar in many respects to a given substance. From Greek, Ana-according to, logos-similar.

Anaerobic : In absence of oxygen.

Angstrom (A^o) : A unit of length equal to 10^{-8} cm.

Antiparallel : Opposite in direction.

Array : Sequential arrangement.

B

Bilayer : A double layer.

Biopsy : Observation of living tissue which is excised from living body under a microscope to establish diagnosis. From Greek, bios-life, opsis-vision.

C

cDNA : Complementary DNA synthesized from mRNA using reverse transcriptase. Usually radio labelled nucleoside triphosphates are used for polymerization by reverse transcriptase.

Chondrocyte : Cartilage forming cell.

Chemi informatics : It involves development and use of computer technologies to process chemical data.

Chemotactic : Molecules which attracts cells towards it.

Chip : Small piece cut from hard material on which electrical circuits are printed.

Cholestasis : Obstruction to flow of bile. From Greek, chole-bile, statis-standing still.

Clone : A genetically identical individual (organism) derived from single cell.

Configuration : Spatial arrangements of constituent groups of a asymmetric carbon.

Computational Biology : It involves development and use of computer based programmes to process life sciences data.

Covalent bond : A chemical bond formed between elements due to sharing of electrons.

Co-ordinate bond : A linkage between two elements involving one sided sharing of electrons.

Cytoskeleton : A fibrous net work found in cytosol.

D

Dalton : It is single hydrogen atom weight (1.66×10^{-27} mg).

De novo : Total synthesis from new organic compound.

E

E. Coli (*Escherichia coli*) : A bacteria found in human intestine.

Edema : Swelling due to water retention.

Electrophile : Positively charged or electron deficient groups.

Electro motive force : Electrical energy generated due to unequal distribution of charged species.

Endo peptidase : An enzyme that cleaves internal peptide bonds of a protein. From Greek, Endo-within.

Excited state : High energy state of substance or molecule which occurs when energy is absorbed.

Exopeptidase : An enzyme that cleaves peptide bonds from either N or C terminus of protein or polypeptide. From Greek, Exo-outside.

F

Familial : Related members of a family. From Latin, Famila-house hold.

Filariasis : Infestation with filaria organisms having thread like shape found commonly in tropics.

Fistula : An abnormal connection between two systems (organs) of body.

Fluoroscence : Light (energy) emission by excited molecule when it returns to ground state.

Functional genomics : It involves study of functions of genes and their products.

G

Genesis : Production.

Genomics : It involves study of structure and genes of DNA.

Ground state : Normal stable form of molecule.

H

He La cells : A human cell line derived from a cervical cancer patient named Henrietta Lach.

Hereditary : Inherited. From Latin Hereditas – Heirship.

Hibernation : Polar animals winter sleep.

Homoserine : Higher analog of serine.

Host : The organism upon which parasite lives.

Hybridoma : A new cell line arising from fusion of two different cells.

Hydrophobic : Uncharged water insoluble molecules.

Hydrophilic : Charged water soluble molecules.

Hydrolysis : Cleaving of big molecule into two molecules in water dependent reaction.

Hypoxia : Decreased O_2 in tissues. From Greek, Hypo-under, oxys-sharp.

I

Immortalization : conversion of an organism or cell having finite life span to one with infinite life span.

Infant : A child whose age is less than a year. From Latin, Infans without speech.

Infestation : Presence of parasites in the body. From Latin, Infestare to infest.

Infarction : Death of a part of tissue due to blocked blood supply. From Latin, Infarcire–to stuff into.

Infusion : Flow of fluid into body by gravity. From Latin, infundareto pour into.

Insomania : sleeplessness.

Insitu : In undisturbed state.

Inversion : Upside down.

In vitro **:** In the test tube or laboratory.

In vivo **:** In the body or living cells.

L

Lesion : Injury.

Ligand : A molecule bound to another molecule like protein.

Lysis : Dissolution or breaking open.

M

Multienzyme complex : Group of enzymes present as single polypeptide.

N

nm (nanometer) : It is used to indicate wave length of light and equals to 10^{-9}m.

Nonheme iron (NHI) : Iron present in none hemoproteins.

Nucleophile : Negatively charged or electron excess groups.

O

Oxidation : Loss of electrons.

Organelle : Membrane covered structures in cell.

Olfaction : Smell

P

Pharmacogenomics : It is study of impact of an individuals genes on body response to drugs.

Pleated sheet : Side by side arrangement of polypeptide chain.

Pi : Inorganic phosphate.

PPi : Inorganic pyrophosphate

Prion : Proteinacious infective agent.

Proteomics : It is study of protein-protein interactions, prediction and modeling of proteins (proteome).

Polymorphism : Many forms.

Photon : Smallest unit of light energy.

R

Reduction : Gain of electrons.

Reducing equivalents : It is used to indicate electron or hydrogen or hydride.

Residue : Monomer of a polymer.

Reverse genetics : It starts with DNA sequence and concludes with analysis of pheno type.

S

Sarco : Flesh. From Greek, Sarkos.

T

Transducer : A device which converts energy from one form to other form.

Transduction : Transfer of a signal from one system to another. It may involve conversion of one form of signal to other form.

Transgenic animal : An animal with foreign DNA.

Transformation : Genetic modification of a bacterial cell due to incorporation of foreign DNA into that cell.

U

UV light : Ultraviolet light in the region of 200-400 nm

V

Vaccines : Extract of dead disease causing organisms used to produce active antibodies.

Vesicle : A hallow structure. From Latin, vescula-small bladder.

Virus : An ultra microscopic organism. From Latin.

Z

Zwitter ion : A dipolar molecule with equal numbers of positive and negative charges.

ANSWERS TO EXERCISES

CHAPTER 1

Multiple Choice Questions

1. (*a*) 2. (*a*)
3. (*a*) 4. (*c*)

Fill in the blanks

1. Nucleus.
2. Cell membrane
3. Cardiolipin
4. Lysosomes.
5. Microtubule.

CHAPTER 2

Multiple Choice Questions

1. (*a*) 2. (*c*)
3. (*a*) 4. (*b*)
5. (*d*)

Fill in the blanks

1. Aromatic amino acids.
2. Aspartame.
3. Peptide.
4. γ-Aminobutyric acid.

CHAPTER 3

Multiple Choice Questions

1. (*d*) 2. (*a*)
3. (*a*) 4. (*b*)
5. (*c*) 6. (*a*)

Fill in the blanks

1. Collagen, elastin.
2. 4, 6.
3. Prolamines.
4. Interchain.
5. 4.
6. α_i antitrypsin.
7. Bence-Jones proteins.
8. Abzymes or catalytic anti bodies.

CHAPTER 4

Multiple Choice Questions

1. (*d*) 2. (*a*)
3. (*a*) 4. (*c*)
5. (*c*) 6. (*a*)
7. (*a*) 8. (*a*)

Fill in the blanks

1. Cleansing agents.
2. Non-enzyme.
3. Optical specificity.
4. Drugs.
5. Decreases.
6. Poisons.
7. Metallo, activated.
8. Tense, relaxed.

CHAPTER 5

Multiple Choice Questions

1. (*a*) 2. (*a*)
3. (*a*) 4. (*b*)
5. (*c*) 6. (*c*)

Fill in the blanks

1. Glycogen.
2. Ascorbic acid.
3. Blood groups.
4. Sucrose
5. Sialic acid.

CHAPTER 6

Multiple Choice Questions

1. (*d*) 2. (*a*)
3. (*a*) 4. (*b*)
5. (*c*) 6. (*c*)
7. (*b*)

Fill in the blanks

1. Thermal insulator.
2. Dipalmitoyl lecithin.
3. Tripalmitin.
4. Gangliosides.
5. Sulfate.
6. Cis-trans.
7. Polar, non-polar.
8. Lipid bilayer.

CHAPTER 7

Multiple Choice Questions

1. (*c*) 2. (*b*)
3. (*b*) 4. (*a*)

Fill in the blanks

1. Receptors.
2. Iodide transporter.
3. Changes.
4. Non-covalent bonds.
5. Difference.
6. H^+/K^+-ATPase.

CHAPTER 8

Multiple Choice Questions

1. (*a*) 2. (*c*)
3. (*c*) 4. (*b*)
5. (*c*)

Fill in the blanks

1. Allergic.
2. Filariasis.
3. Pyranose.
4. Chole cystokinin.
5. Pancreatitis and Cystic fibrosis.

CHAPTER 9

Multiple Choice Questions

1. (*c*) 2. (*c*)
3. (*c*) 4. (*a*)
5. (*a*)

Fill in the blanks

1. Metabolism.
2. Glucose.
3. Enolase.
4. Pompe's.
5. Galactose-1-phosphate Uridyl transferase.

CASES

1. Hereditary fructose intolerance.
2. Von Gierke's disease.

CHAPTER 10

Multiple Choice Questions

1. (*c*) 2. (*d*)
3. (*c*) 4. (*d*)
5. (*c*) 6. (*b*)

Fill in the blanks

1. 15 Kg.
2. Energy, water.
3. Carbon-carbon bond.
4. Malonyl-CoA.
5. Fatty liver.
6. Cyclooxygenase.
7. Good cholesterol.
8. LDL variant.

CASES

1. Carnitine deficiency.
2. Atherosclerosis due to hypercholesterolemia.

CHAPTER 11

Multiple Choice Questions

1. (*a*) 2. (*c*)
3. (*c*) 4. (*c*)
5. (*c*)

Fill in the blanks

1. Cancer.
2. Currency.
3. Gain.
4. 3.
5. Dissociates, phosphorylation.

CHAPTER 12

Multiple Choice Questions

1. (*d*) 2. (*d*)
3. (*a*) 4. (*c*)
5. (*c*) 6. (*a*)

Fill in the blanks

1. Aspargine.
2. Liver.
3. Leucine.
4. No, nitropusside.
5. Anticancer.
6. H-2 receptors.

CASES

1. Primary hyperoxaluria.
2. Phenylketonuria.
3. Alkaptonuria.

CHAPTER 13

CASES

1. Diabetes.
2. Ketoacidosis due to starvation.

CHAPTER 14

Multiple Choice Questions

1. (*c*) 2. (*c*)
3. (*d*) 4. (*a*)

Fill in the blanks

1. Stimulants.
2. Nucleic acids
3. Unusual.
4. Vitamin.
5. Orotidylic.

CHAPTER 15

Multiple Choice Questions

1. (*c*) 2. (*c*)
3. (*b*) 4. (*d*)
5. (*a*)

Fill in the blanks

1. HMP shunt.
2. Erythrocytes, leucocytes, brain.
3. Endo.
4. Suicide.
5. Leukemia, radiotherapy.

CASES

1. Lesch-Nyhan syndrome.
2. Severe combined immuno deficiency disease (SCIDD).

CHAPTER 16

Multiple Choice Questions

1. (*c*) 2. (*c*)
3. (*c*) 4. (*c*)
5. (*c*)

Fill in the blanks

1. Two separate.
2. TGCGTAT.
3. Same.
4. A-DNA.
5. Tψ C, Anticodon.

CHAPTER 17

Multiple Choice Questions

1. (*d*) 2. (*b*)
3. (*b*) 4. (*a*)
5. (*a*)

Fill in the blanks

1. Multiplication.
2. Transfer, nucleus, cytosol.
3. ATP.
4. GMP.
5. RNA.

CHAPTER 18

Multiple Choice Questions

1. (*a*) 2. (*c*)
3. (*b*) 4. (*c*)
5. (*c*)

Fill in the blanks

1. Energy.
2. Adaptor.
3. Releasing factor and GTP.
4. Purine.
5. Removed.

CHAPTER 20

Fill in the blanks

1. Non-existant.
2. Single stranded.
3. Asexual.
4. Hybridoma.
5. Satellite DNA.

CHAPTER 22

Multiple Choice Questions

1. (*d*) 2. (*b*)
3. (*a*) 4. (*c*)
5. (*b*)

Fill in the blanks

1. Metalloporphyrino.
2. Photosensitive.
3. Oxidation.
4. Active transport.
5. Reduction.

CASES

1. Carbon monoxide poisoning.
2. Obstructive Jaundice.

CHAPTER 23

Multiple Choice Questions

1. (*b*) 2. (*a*)
3. (*a*) 4. (*b*)
5. (*a*)

Fill in the blanks

1. Vit. A, Vit. D.
2. Hyper vitaminosis.
3. Vit. A, color.
4. Selenium, PUFA.
5. Carboxylase.

CHAPTER 24

Multiple Choice Questions

1. (*b*) 2. (*a*)
3. (*a*) 4. (*b*)
5. (*a*)

Fill in the blanks

1. 20-30 gm.
2. Tissues, Fluids.
3. Desferrioxamine.
4. Copper.
5. Iodide salts.

CHAPTER 25

Multiple Choice Questions

1. (*d*) 2. (*c*)
3. (*d*) 4. (*b*)
5. (*a*)

Fill in the blanks

1. Bomb calorimeter.
2. 0.85
3. Infancy, adult hood.
4. Reduced.
5. Mercury.

CASE

1. Kwashiorkor.

CHAPTER 26

Fill in the blanks

1. Water.
2. Over hydration.
3. 24-30 meq/L.
4. Vomiting, diarrhoea.
5. p^K.

INDEX

Symbols

Numbers

B

C

F

G

I

J

M

O

P

Q

R

U

V

Y

Z